Foundations of Nursing Practice

For Elsevier:
Senior Commissioning Editor: Ninette Premdas
Development Editor: Mairi McCubbin
Project Manager: Morven Dean
Senior Designer: Sarah Russell
Illustration Manager: Bruce Hogarth
Illustrator: Antbits, Graeme Chambers

Foundations of Nursing Practice

Fundamentals of Holistic Care

Edited by

Chris Brooker
BSc MSc RGN SCM RNT
Author and Lecturer,
Norfolk, UK

Anne Waugh
BSc(Hons) MSc CertEd SRN RNT ILTM
Senior Lecturer, School of Acute and
Continuing Care Nursing,
Napier University, Edinburgh, UK

Foreword by

Roger Watson
PhD RN FIBiol FRSA
Professor of Nursing, School of Nursing and
Midwifery, The University of Sheffield,
Sheffield, UK

MOSBY

ELSEVIER

EDINBURGH • LONDON • NEW YORK • OXFORD • PHILADELPHIA • ST LOUIS • SYDNEY • TORONTO 2007

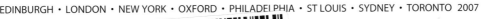

MOSBY
ELSEVIER

First published 2007

ISBN-13: 9780723433569
ISBN-10: 0 7234 3356 9

British Library Cataloguing in Publication Data
A catalogue record for this book is available from the British Library

Library of Congress Cataloging in Publication Data
A catalog record for this book is available from the Library of Congress

Notice
Knowledge and best practice in this field are constantly changing. As new research and experience broaden our knowledge, changes in practice, treatment and drug therapy may become necessary or appropriate. Readers are advised to check the most current information provided (i) on procedures featured or (ii) by the manufacturer of each product to be administered, to verify the recommended dose or formula, the method and duration of administration, and contraindications. It is the responsibility of the practitioner, relying on their own experience and knowledge of the patient, to make diagnoses, to determine dosages and the best treatment for each individual patient, and to take all appropriate safety precautions. To the fullest extent of the law, neither the Publisher nor the Editors assume any liability for any injury and/or damage to persons or property arising out or related to any use of the material contained in this book.

The Publisher

The Publisher's policy is to use **paper manufactured from sustainable forests**

Printed in China

Contents

Contributors

Branch experts

Carol Chamley BA MA CertEd DipN MSSM RCNT RSCN RNT RGN ONC
Senior Lecturer, Coventry University, Faculty of Health and Life Sciences, Coventry, UK
Child branch

Jayne Donaldson BN MN PhD PGCE RN
Senior Lecturer, Clinical Skill Development, School of Acute and Continuing Care Nursing, Napier University, Edinburgh, UK
Clinical skills

Susanne Forrest MPhil DipCNE PGCertEd RGN RMN
Senior Lecturer in Mental Health, Faculty of Health Studies, School of Community Health, Napier University, Edinburgh, UK
Mental health

Elaine Kwiatek MSc CertEd RCT RGN RNMH
Senior Lecturer and Teaching Fellow in Learning Disability, School of Community Health, Napier University, Edinburgh, UK
Learning disabilities

Contributors

Aurea Amos BSc PGCert DipCNE CertEd RGN RCNT RNT
Formerly Lecturer, School of Acute and Continuing Care Nursing, Napier University, Edinburgh, UK
24 Caring for the person having surgery

Irene Anderson BSc(Hons) PGCE DPSN RGN
Senior Lecturer, Tissue Viability, School of Nursing and Midwifery, University of Hertfordshire, Hatfield, UK
25 Wound management

Emma Briggs BSc(Hons) PhD PGCert(Research) PGCert(Academic Practice) RN
Lecturer in Nursing, Florence Nightingale School of Nursing and Midwifery, King's College London, London, UK
13 Safety in nursing practice

Chris Brooker BSc MSc RGN SCM RNT
Author and Lecturer, Norfolk, UK
19 Promoting hydration and nutrition

Norrie Brown MEd PhD DipCNE CertEd RMN RGN ILTM
Senior Lecturer and Senior Teaching Fellow, School of Acute and Continuing Care Nursing, Napier University, Edinburgh, UK
3 Health and social care delivery systems

Christine Burton BSc MN RGN RCNT RNT ILTM
Lecturer, School of Acute and Continuing Care Nursing, Napier University, Edinburgh, UK
22 Promoting the safe administration of medicines

Carol Chamley BA MA CertEd DipN MSSM RCNT RSCN RNT RGN ONC
Senior Lecturer, Coventry University, Faculty of Health and Life Sciences, Coventry, UK
23 Pain management – minimizing the pain experience

Jane Christie MSc PGDE RN
Lecturer, School of Acute and Continuing Care Nursing, Napier University, Edinburgh, UK
2 Evolution of contemporary nursing

Christine Donnelly BA PhD DipHV RGN RNT ONC
Lecturer/Programme Leader, Complementary Therapies, School of Community Health, Napier University, Edinburgh, UK
18 Mobility and immobility

Jayne Donaldson BN MN PhD PGCE RN
Senior Lecturer, Clinical Skill Development, School of Acute and Continuing Care Nursing, Napier University, Edinburgh, UK
22 Promoting the safe administration of medicines

Jacqui Fletcher BSc(Hons) MSc PGCert RGN
Senior Lecturer, School of Nursing and Midwifery, University of Hertfordshire, Hatfield, UK
25 Wound management

Maria J. Grant BA(Hons) MSc PGCE
Research Fellow (Information), Salford Centre for Nursing, Midwifery and Collaborative Research (SCNMCR), University of Salford, Manchester, UK
5 Evidence-based practice and research

Morag Gray MN PhD DipCNE CertEd ILTM RGN RCNT RNT
Head of Curriculum Development, Faculty of Health and Life Sciences, Napier University, Edinburgh, UK
4 Learning and teaching

Janis Greig BSc MSc DipLSN RMN RGN RNT MIHPE
Lecturer, School of Community Health, Napier University, Edinburgh, UK
1 Understanding health and health promotion

Pauline Hamilton MN DipAsthma RNT RCNT RGN RMN
Lecturer, Adult Nursing, School of Nursing, Midwifery and Community Health, Glasgow Caledonian University, Glasgow, UK
14 The nursing process, holistic assessment and baseline observations

George Hoggarth BSc(Hons) MA RGN RMN RNT ENB655, 769, A74
Lecturer, Mental Health, School of Nursing, Salford University, Manchester, UK
11 Stress, anxiety and coping

Dorothy Horsburgh BA(Hons) MEd PhD DipCNE RGN RNT RCNT
Lecturer, School of Acute and Continuing Care Nursing, Napier University, Edinburgh, UK
7 The NMC Code of conduct *and applied ethical principles*

Michelle Howarth MSc PGCE RGN
Lecturer, Salford Centre for Nursing, Midwifery and Collaborative Research, University of Salford, Manchester, UK
5 Evidence-based practice and research

Gay James BSc MSc DipN RGN RCNT RNT
Senior Lecturer, Adult Nursing, School of Health and Social Sciences, Coventry University, Coventry, UK
23 Pain management – minimizing the pain experience

Catriona Kennedy BA(Hons) PhD DipNurs RN DN RNT DNT PWT
Senior Lecturer, School of Acute and Continuing Care Nursing, Napier University, Edinburgh, UK
12 Loss and bereavement

Rosie Kneafsey BSc MRes PGCE RGN
Lecturer, Salford Centre for Nursing, Midwifery and Collaborative Research, University of Salford, Manchester, UK
5 Evidence-based practice and research

Karen Lockhart BSc MSc PGCE RGN
Lecturer, School of Acute and Continuing Care Nursing, Napier University, Edinburgh, UK
12 Loss and bereavement

Maureen S. MacMillan BSc(Hons) PhD RGN SCM(pt1)
Senior Lecturer, School of Acute and Continuing Care Nursing, Napier University, Edinburgh, UK
3 Health and social care delivery systems

Neil Murphy BSc(Hons) MSc DipHE RMN ENB812, 655, 870
Lecturer/Practitioner, School of Nursing, Mental Health branch, Salford University, Manchester, and Moorside Unit, Bolton, Salford and Trafford Mental Health Trust, Trafford, General Hospital, Manchester, UK
11 Stress, anxiety and coping

Sherri Ogston-Tuck BSc MA PGDipHE RN
Nursing Lecturer, Acute Adult Nursing and Pain Management, Florence Nightingale School of Nursing, King's College University, London, UK
6 Legal issues that impact on nursing practice

Ah Nya Plant BSc(Hons) MSc DipAA RGN RM RCNT RNT MNIMH
Lecturer/Programme Leader, School of Community Health, Napier University, Edinburgh, UK
10 Sleep, rest, relaxation, complementary therapies and alternative therapies

Theresa Price BSc(Hons) MSc CertEd FE RN RNT ILTM
Lecturer, School of Nursing, Midwifery and Community Health, Glasgow Caledonian University, Glasgow, UK
14 The nursing process, holistic assessment and baseline observations

Kate Rennie-Meyer BSc RGN RCT RNT
Lecturer, School of Acute and Continuing Care Nursing, Napier University, Edinburgh, UK
15 Preventing the spread of infection

Jillian Riley BA(Hons) MSc RGN RM

Head of Post-Graduate Education for Nurses and Allied Health Professionals, Department of Education, Royal Brompton Hospital, London, UK

17 Breathing and circulation

Naomi Sharples BA(Hons) MBA PGCE RNLD RMN Master Practitioner NLP

Senior Lecturer, School of Nursing, Faculty of Health and Social Care, University of Salford, Manchester, UK

9 Relationship, helping and communication skills

Martin Steggall BSc(Hons) MSc DipN RN

Senior Lecturer, Applied Biological Science and Urology; Honorary Urology Nurse Specialist, St Bartholomew School of Nursing and Midwifery, City University, London, UK

20 Elimination – urine

David Tait BSc(Hons) MSc RMN RGN RNT

Lecturer, School of Acute and Continuing Care Nursing, Napier University, Edinburgh, UK

8 The human lifespan and its effect on selecting nursing interventions

Linda Veitch BSc(Hons) MSc RGN RNT

Lecturer, School of Acute and Continuing Care Nursing, Napier University, Edinburgh, UK

2 Evolution of contemporary nursing

Susan Walker BSc(Hons) MA PGCE RGN

Lecturer, Nursing/Clinical Skills, School of Nursing, University of Salford, Manchester, UK

21 Elimination: faeces

Anne Waugh BSc(Hons) MSc CertEd SRN RNT ILTM

Acting Head, School of Acute and Continuing Care Nursing, Napier University, Edinburgh, UK

16 Caring for the person with physical needs, sensory impairment and unconsciousness

24 Caring for the person having surgery

Foreword

Good text books have a habit of coming out just after you really needed them, and this book is no exception. My daughter recently qualified as a nurse and, while I recommended many good books to her – and usually had to buy them for her – including several of the mighty tomes on nursing to which I have contributed, I usually gave them with a health warning. Either they were just under the mark or provided too much information that would not be needed at her stage in her university programme. However, the present book edited by Chris Brooker and Anne Waugh could have been recommended without reservation – as I now recommend it to readers of this Foreword.

There is a prevailing opinion, held mostly by people whose opinions are more significant than the evidence on which they base those opinions, that current nursing education is simply stuffing the heads of future nurses full of nonsense; material which they will never need and which leads them astray from the core function of nursing: to care for people. I simply do not accept this argument; my own background is in biological sciences and, along the road to graduating, I studied chemistry (in all its forms), physics, mathematics and statistics. I don't recall more than an ounce of all that now and have probably never used much of it since but I have never heard a criticism of any programme of study in another discipline expressed in this way. My point is that the contents of the present book – which is foundational – should dispel any doubts about the content and purpose of modern nursing. The 'nay sayers' regarding current nursing education will probably be most comfortable starting at the back of the book where absolutely fundamental aspects of nursing practice: safety, infection control, nutrition and elimination (two chapters on this!) are each headlined.

However, what is important for me – if the book is approached the right way round – is that it begins by putting nursing in context, its recent history and professional development. This is surely the right way round: develop the professional and then give them the skills. However, so much of what has happened lately in nursing education in the UK has been an emphasis on a return to skills – albeit their fundamental importance – and a downplaying of the professional and educational aspects. Doing it the other way round, starting with skills in the hope that professional attributes will develop later leads to the 'why do we/do we really need to know this?' mentality with which many in nursing education are familiar. *Foundations of Nursing Practice* approaches its subject matter in the appropriate direction and at the appropriate level. It may have been published just in time for my next daughter to study nursing.

Sheffield, 2006 — Roger Watson

Preface

This book has been written specifically to meet the needs of nursing students undertaking the common foundation programme and is reflected in the title *Foundations of nursing practice: the fundamentals of holistic care*. It aims to explain how and why sensitive and holistic nursing care which is evidence-based is carried out. It is therefore relevant to students who will enter all branches of nursing and includes material that is both common to all and specific to each branch. There is an emphasis not only on the theory that underpins nursing practice in the common foundation programme but also on nursing skills which form an increasingly emphasized part of the programme. The authors come from diverse nursing backgrounds and represent many different universities. An expert in clinical skills has reviewed each chapter together with experts from each branch to ensure the content reflects each branch accurately and appropriately.

The curriculum and outcomes for entry to the branch programmes laid down by the Nursing & Midwifery Council which are largely focused on health, health promotion, social and life sciences as they apply to nursing has been used as the basis for the book.

The book is organized in four sections:

1. Health, nursing and health care in the 21st century – the chapters in this section explore theories of health and health promotion (Ch 1), the emergence of contemporary nursing (Ch 2) and the systems within which contemporary healthcare is delivered (Ch 3).
2. Professional practice – this requires knowledge from several fields that are integrated into contemporary nursing practice and those explored are learning and teaching (Ch 4), evidence-based practice (Ch 5) and legal (Ch 6), moral and ethical (Ch 7) frameworks.
3. Nursing and lifespan implications – many nursing interventions are specific to patients'/clients' stage of development and/or stage on the lifespan (Ch 8) – Chapter 12 considers loss and bereavement. All nursing interventions rely on effective communication, which is discussed in Chapter 9. Rest and sleep are considered in Chapter 10 and stress, anxiety and coping are examined in Chapter 11.
4. Developing nursing skills – this section explains nursing skills which must always be underpinned by safe practice (Ch 13) and begin with assessment (Ch 14). Preventing the spread of infection is explained in Chapter 15. A wide range of fundamental nursing interventions is explored in the remaining chapters within the final section.

Each chapter contains a range of activities to assist your learning – these are explained on page xvii. Many informative 2-colour illustrations, photographs and tables explain or expand the material in each chapter.

This textbook therefore provides a comprehensive introduction to nursing which will meet the needs of students, nurses returning to practice, mentors and other registered nurses.

Norfolk and Edinburgh, 2007

Chris Brooker
Anne Waugh

Acknowledgments

We would like to thank the experts for their constructive comments and helpful advice:

Susanne Forrest – Mental health
Carol Chamley – Child health
Elaine Kwiatek – Learning disabilities
Jayne Donaldson – Clinical skills
John Tingle – Chapter 6: Legal issues that impact on nursing practice.
Dave Holman – Safeguarding children

Several people at Elsevier have kept us on track in order to ensure the book reached publication especially Sarena Wolfaard, Mairi McCubbin, Ninette Premdas and Morven Dean. Graeme Chambers has skillfully interpreted our ideas into clear and attractive illustrations that complement the text. In addition we are grateful to the authors, experts and their families and not least our families, David and Andy for their patience and support throughout the project.

How to use this book

This book will help you develop the knowledge base and nursing skills needed to provide holistic patient/client care. Each chapter has the same format and many features to assist your learning. These are outlined below to help you get the best from this book.

Glossary terms – a selection of terms is included at the beginning of the chapter. They are defined and used in the chapter, and the definitions have been collated into a glossary at the end of the book (p. 731) for easy reference.

Learning outcomes – these provide guidance about what you can expect to learn after reading the chapter and carrying out the activities within it.

Boxes with information – different types of boxes have been used to assist learning, break up the text and to highlight information in a concise manner.

Box X.XX

Plain/text: these are generally a concise list of relevant information that relates to a topic within the text, e.g. Box 1.16 UK groups most susceptible to poverty (p. 16), Box 13.21 When handwashing is carried out (p. 337).

Nursing skills boxes: these provide the principles of nursing skills that are included within the common foundation programme, e.g. Box 15.8 Handwashing (p. 401), Box 22.7 Principles of drug administration (p. 640).

First aid: these contain a summary of the principles of first aid for common conditions, which is a Nursing and Midwifery Council requirement of the common foundation programme, e.g. Box 15.16 Management of needlestick injuries (p. 408), Box 18.2 Sprains and strains (p. 504).

Activity boxes – these contain scenarios and related activities that will help you explore particular topics in more depth. Many are referenced and/or include further resources to help you extend your knowledge. The activities are intended to help you consider the following aspects of nursing practice in more detail:

Reflective practice, e.g. Box 14.3 Sharing personal information (p. 356), Box 19.17 Using benchmarks of best practice (p. 550).

Evidence-based practice, e.g. Box 1.18 Effects of poverty (p. 17), Box 15.21 Good cleaning practices (p. 413).

Health promotion, e.g. Box 13.9 Falls prevention (p. 326), Box 19.22 Safe alcohol limits (p. 555).

Ethical issues, e.g. Box 7.2 Maintaining confidentiality? (p. 167), Box 18.12 Condoning unsafe practice (p. 517).

Critical thinking, e.g. Box 1.7 Lay and professional conflict (p. 7), Box 13.8 Promoting independent living and social activities (p. 325).

Cross referencing – there are extensive cross references within the text that signpost links to material and topics from:

- other parts of a chapter – denoted (see p. XXX)
- other chapters – denoted (see Ch. XX).

Summary – this is a list of bullet points summarizing key areas explored within the chapter.

Self test – a variety of activities can be found at the end of each chapter for you to test your learning. The answers are provided on pages 727–730.

Key words and phrases for literature searching – suggestions are included to help you begin to find out more about key topics within the chapter (see also Ch. 5 – Literature searching).

Useful websites – these direct you to simple but reliable sources of Internet information about relevant topics. They are wide-ranging and include charities and organizations; many provide general information about the topic although some provide more detailed information about common conditions and illnesses for both lay people and health professionals.

References – extensive use is made of in-text references. The list of references to material used within the text is included at the end of the chapter. These aim to be straightforward and many are easily accessible using the Internet. Learning how these have been incorporated into the text and also how they are listed at the end are essential skills for nursing students. Although the method used varies between universities, the principles are similar.

Further reading – a selection of further reading suggestions is provided at the end of the chapter. These give you the opportunity to access a wider range of related information in order to expand your knowledge base.

Glossary – this is a collated list of the glossary terms identified at the beginning of each chapter that can be used for easy reference (see p. 731).

Index – an extensive index has been compiled to enable you to locate information quickly and easily.

SECTION 1

Health, nursing and health care in the 21st century

Understanding health and health promotion

1

Janis Greig

Glossary terms

Demography

Epidemiology

Health determinant

Health education

Health promotion

Morbidity

Mortality

Public health

Statutory bodies

Learning outcomes

This chapter will help you:

- Reflect on personal and official definitions of health
- Discuss common lay health beliefs and their effects on behaviour
- Explain the relationship between attitudes, values and behaviours
- Review the factors that influence health
- Show awareness of the effects of poverty as the key determinant of health
- Understand the place of health promotion in modern nursing
- Describe common methods and approaches to the measurement of health
- Appreciate individual responses to illness.

Introduction

The health White Paper, *Saving Lives: Our Healthier Nation* (DH 1999a, Section 11.14) states that nurses, midwives and health visitors play a crucial role in promoting health and preventing illness. People have close contact with health professionals at key points in their lives – in infancy, during adolescence, pregnancy and childbirth, and in sickness and older age – creating significant opportunities for health promoting interventions.

The *Code of professional conduct: standards for conduct, performance and ethics* (NMC 2004) states that nurses must protect and support the health of individual patients, clients and the wider community (see Ch. 7). To achieve this, it is important for nurses to have an understanding of their own and others' health definitions and beliefs. Apart from increased self-awareness, nurses can better understand and relate to their patients and their health and illness behaviour.

Nurses also need to know the factors that affect health and health beliefs in our increasingly multicultural society. This allows accurate assessment of care needs, the planning of sensitive care and the targeting of relevant information. The ultimate aim may be to help people change their health-related behaviour. Furthermore, the increasing focus on evidence-based healthcare means that nurses need to have an understanding of how and why health and illness are measured.

This chapter lays the foundation for the rest of the book by discussing definitions of health, models of health and illness, health beliefs, attitudes and values, factors influencing health, health promotion and health education, measuring health and illness and illness behaviour. It is important to consider the different terms used to describe people in a variety of health and social care settings. Adult, mental health, children's and learning disability nurses use language that gives clues to their underlying values and assumptions of power and passivity about the person in receipt of care (Ch. 7):

- *Patient*: A traditional word to describe the recipient of care. Commonly used by nurses, doctors and other healthcare workers, it may imply a relative passivity or inequality in the relationship with professionals – 'experts know best'. It is widely used in adult nursing, child health nursing and other clinical settings within the NHS.
- *Client*: May imply a more active recipient of care and is sometimes used in situations where a fee is charged, e.g. complementary therapies. The perception is one of greater equality in relationships with professionals rather than a medical or clinical

focus. The term is widely used in social work, mental health, learning disability and other community-based settings.

- *Service user or user of services*: This terminology is commonly used in mental health and learning disability work but is becoming widespread in other settings. It may at first seem to be a more neutral phrase than 'patient' or 'client', more accurately describing a person in relation to the services received rather than reflecting issues of passivity or power. However, it is also a political statement. For example, people with mental health problems may define themselves this way and, by so doing, reject the medicalization of their experience and situation, including the mental illness diagnosis. They may prefer to use the word 'distress', rather than the diagnostic label given. Even more radical is the use of the term 'survivor' to describe a person's experience of mental health services.
- *Resident or tenant*: A term which may be used in care of older people. Workers in care homes in the community often use this word to describe recipients of their care, whether it is health or social care.

Definitions of health

Before reading this section you should undertake the activity in Box 1.1.

The word 'health' is derived from the old English word *hael* meaning whole and, despite being the subject of much research, it cannot be neatly defined. There is no universal definition of health as everyone has their own idea of what it means. When asked to define 'health' in class or during research, people may highlight the physical functioning of their body, their ability to carry out tasks, feeling content and happy or even respond in terms of relationships with family and friends. In other words, health is multidimensional, composed of different but interrelated dimensions.

Dimensions of health

Six dimensions of health are usually described, five at an individual level surrounded by a further one at the level of society:

- *Physical* – body shape, size, function
- *Mental* – or intellectual health; means the ability to think clearly and coherently, making rational judgements
- *Emotional* – or affective health; means the ability to recognize emotions, adapt to and cope with stress and anxiety
- *Social* – the ability to make and sustain relationships with people
- *Spiritual* – relates to personal beliefs and behaviour, being content or at peace and may include religious beliefs and practices
- *Societal* – relates to everything surrounding a person in their immediate or wider environment, including working and living conditions, employment, income, social norms and the political context.

The dimensions of health are interrelated and problems in one area may well affect another. A social dimension issue, e.g. a relationship problem, may cause mental health problems. A person with a chronic physical illness may develop an accompanying mood or emotional problem. Societal issues such as poverty and low income determine people's diet and lifestyle, affecting their physical health. It is important to recognize that the relatedness of the dimensions is so strong that it is artificial to try discussing them as separate issues (Box 1.2).

Holistic health

Nurses applying this multidimensional approach to healthcare need to assess all aspects of health and consider each patient/client as a whole person (see Ch. 2). This is called a holistic approach and derives from the Greek word *holos* meaning whole. Kerr (2000) reminds us that a holistic approach to nursing care is based on ancient beliefs that the spirit is a legitimate focus for nursing care as much as the body.

REFLECTIVE PRACTICE Box 1.1

Your view of health

Student activities

1. Think about your own view of health and write down your own personal definition, or even just some key words.
2. Compare your ideas with those of a friend or co-worker and discuss any similarities or differences.
3. Ask yourself:
   - What attributes might a healthy person have?
   - What would a healthy person look like?
   - Have you always defined health in this way or has it changed since you were a child?
   - Do you think this might change in the future?

REFLECTIVE PRACTICE Box 1.2

Dimensions of health

Student activities

Look back at the six dimensions of health:

1. From your own life, identify examples of how problems in one dimension may impact on another.
2. Do the same again, but this time thinking about patients/clients you have met in placements.
3. Consider the following situations and suggest the dimensions in which the individual may have problems:
   - A 35-year-old married woman with postnatal depression
   - A 54-year-old man who has been made redundant
   - A 14-year-old boy undergoing treatment for cancer
   - A 78-year-old widow living on minimum benefits.

The body as a machine

During assessment interviews or other interactions with people, it is common for nurses to hear descriptions related to the physical dimension of health, where anatomy and physiology are described in an oversimplified way, comparing the body to the workings of a machine. This is called mechanistic functioning and descriptive words commonly used include pipes, blockages, tubes, plumbing, waterworks, ticker and pump. This type of comparison is also used by people to describe the workings of the mind or brain, using words such as wheels or cogs turning, whirring, ticking or breakdown. You should now try the activity in Box 1.3.

The continuum of health

Figure 1.1 shows how health can be viewed positively or negatively with extremes of positive and negative health states at opposite ends of a health continuum. This reflects the reality that health is much more complex than merely 'I'm ill' or 'I'm not ill'. The continuum allows for movement along the line, reflecting the dynamic nature of health, which varies over time, with age and stage of development and changing circumstances.

Mental health as a continuum

The idea of a single continuum may be seen as unhelpful in mental health. Some people experience high levels of well-being as a symptom of mental illness. For example, a person may experience elation arising from a bipolar mood disorder and would report feeling 'great'. Tudor (2004) describes the use of the two continua concept where one axis represents mental health and well-being and the other mental ill-health.

REFLECTIVE PRACTICE Box 1.3

The body as a machine

Lay people sometimes describe anatomy and physiology of the mind or body as if it is a machine.

Student activities

- Do you use this terminology yourself?
- If so, think of examples of the words or phrases used.
- Next time you are interacting with people in a practice placement, listen for examples of mechanistic functioning.

Positive and negative health

Words indicating positive health imply the presence of positive and additional qualities such as fitness, wellness or well-being. The positive aspect of health tends to be less dominant, with a tendency to describe health states in a negative way, not focusing on positive health but instead on the absence of disease. For example, describing health as being free from the symptoms of illness or not having a medically defined condition – 'I don't have any major illness so that means I'm healthy'. Words indicating negative health states include disease, illness, deformity, abnormality, ill-health, injury, disability, handicap, mental distress or disorder.

It is interesting to note the large number of words used to indicate negative health compared to the few describing positive health states – wellness, well-being, fitness. The word 'disease' tends to be used in an official way by doctors, nurses and others for physical conditions with observable physical changes. However, like health, illness cannot be easily defined and is often described as a subjective experience, personally defined by each individual.

WHO definitions of health

The most well-known definition of health is that of the World Health Organization (WHO 1946): 'Health is a state of complete physical, mental and social well-being and not merely the absence of disease or infirmity.'

This definition has many strengths and it:

- Is historically important
- Was written in the post-World War 2 optimism of 1946
- Was one of the first authoritative attempts to define health and was proposed by a prestigious international agency
- Promotes a positive view of health by mentioning well-being
- Is a holistic definition, including different dimensions of health
- Can be seen as an idealistic target to aspire for – health as an ideal state.

However, it has been widely criticized. Some of the criticisms centre on the word 'state' which implies a lack of change and does not fit with modern views that health is dynamic, changing with life circumstances. The word 'complete' seems to make this an absolute statement and one which, although idealistic, is unrealistic and unattainable. Lastly, the authority of the WHO to define health has been questioned, as it is acknowledged that everyone has their own definition.

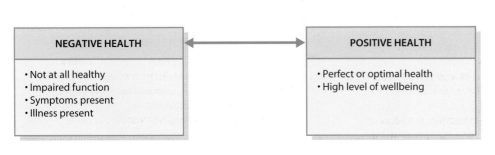

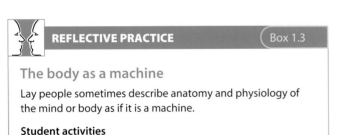

Fig. 1.1 Health as a continuum

Box 1.4 Theories of health

1. Health as an ideal state – the most well-known example is the WHO (1946) definition of health.
2. Health related to physical/mental fitness and role/function – health allows people to carry out normal daily tasks.
3. Health as a commodity – underlying medical practice, health is seen as an external entity which can be given or even bought.
4. Health as a personal strength or ability – health is seen as related to innate or developed strengths, which can be physical or intellectual. It is possible, in this theory, to be 'healthy' even if disabled or suffering from a disease, illness or social problem.

[Adapted from Seedhouse 2001]

Although the original 1946 definition is still commonly quoted, the World Health Organization amended their definition of health in the Ottawa Charter (WHO 1986) to:

> Health is the extent to which an individual or group is able to realize aspirations, to satisfy needs, and to change or cope with the environment. Health is, therefore, seen as a resource for everyday life, not the objective of living. Health is a positive concept emphasizing social and personal resources, as well as physical capacities.

The 1986 definition remains valid today and is considered to be realistic in comparison to the unattainable 'ideal state' of the earlier definition. This definition focuses on health as enabling adaptation to change and emphasizes the dynamic nature of health, the importance of social aspects of health and the link between health and economic productivity. The WHO definitions of health (1946, 1986) are only two of many, and Seedhouse (2001) summarizes the vast range of health definitions into four major groups (Box 1.4).

Defining mental health

Mental health problems are widespread in society (see Box 1.5). Despite these problems being so common, there is a lack of awareness about mental health among the general public and perhaps even among health professionals. Check your awareness of mental health by carrying out the quiz in Box 1.6.

Mental health problems may be the most common reason for people visiting their GP yet mental health remains difficult to define. It is common to define mental health subjectively, i.e. as something each person defines individually. Barker (2003, p. 7) says that 'mental illness and mental health . . . possess no clear, accepted definition. However, they are used in everyday conversation as if their meaning is unambiguous'. Mental health can be taken to mean the opposite of mental illness or even a state of well-being.

It is interesting to note that there is no WHO definition of mental health or mental illness. Instead they use the term mental disorder, which implies a clinically

Box 1.5 UK mental health – what are the issues?

The *Choosing Health* consultation (DH 2004) showed that:

- 1 in 6 adults at any one time has a mental disorder – as many as 9 million people in the UK
- 1 in 10 children under the age of 15 years has a mental health disorder, as do 45% of children and young people looked after by local authorities
- Up to 1 in 4 consultations with a GP are concerned with mental health
- Up to 670 000 people in the UK have some form of dementia
- 500 000 people in the UK consider they are experiencing serious work-related stress
- Suicide has strong links with mental health and is increasing in young people aged 15–19 years, especially males
- Adult male suicides hit a 30-year low in 2003, having reduced steadily since 1998 while adult female suicides have remained steady. Males account for 75% of all suicides
- Mental health problems are strongly linked to social inequality, e.g. urban deprivation, low household income and unemployment.

? CRITICAL THINKING Box 1.6

Mental health awareness quiz

Student activities

The quiz is designed to test your knowledge of mental health and to help you think about your attitudes to people with mental health problems. Circle your response to each question.

1. People with schizophrenia have a split personality. TRUE/FALSE
2. You cannot recover from a mental illness. TRUE/FALSE
3. Most people who have a mental illness end up in hospital. TRUE/FALSE
4. One-third of all absences from work are due to emotional distress. TRUE/FALSE
5. You can always tell if a person has had a mental illness. TRUE/FALSE
6. People are born with a mental illness. TRUE/FALSE
7. There is no point speaking to someone with a mental illness about their problems. TRUE/FALSE

[Resource: Alexander A 2001 Mental health awareness quiz. Napier University, Edinburgh (unpublished)]

- Go to the MIND (National Association for Mental Health) website (www.mind.org.uk) and find out more about the mental health issues raised above.
- Answers: 1. F; 2. F; 3. F; 4. T; 5. F; 6. F; 7. F.

recognizable set of symptoms or behaviour associated in most cases with considerable distress and substantial interference with personal functions.

Many authors have tried describing mental health as one or more of the following:

- Living happily
- Having good self-esteem
- Being able to relate well to other people
- Having a sense of self and identity
- Living productively
- Autonomy
- Maturity
- Coping effectively with stress
- Problem-solving
- Adapting to change (Seedhouse 2002).

The Department of Health (2001a) describes the importance of mental health and well-being to overall health and productivity and defines mental health as:

> Essentially about how we think and feel about ourselves and others and how we interpret the world around us. It affects our capacity to communicate and to form and sustain relationships.

Lay and professional definitions of health

Lay definitions of health refer to the ideas, beliefs and opinions of ordinary members of the public. Studies into lay people's definitions of health show that people perceive that health can coexist with even serious disease. It is only the last group of theories in Box 1.4 that allows for this, the first three groups must have absence of illness and disease. Professional definitions of health arise from people 'educated in health' such as nurses, doctors, allied health professionals (AHPs) or from official sources, e.g. government experts and agencies. Lay and professional definitions of health vary considerably and may result in differing expectations, lack of understanding or even conflict in issues of relationship, diagnosis, treatment and care. Box 1.7 shows an example of lay and professional conflict.

CRITICAL THINKING Box 1.7

Lay and professional conflict

Jim is 28 years old and has a history of mild asthma going back to childhood. He has had several episodes of bronchitis in the past which have always responded well to treatment with antibiotics. He smokes 30 cigarettes a day.

Jim visits his practice nurse with a heavy cold and a sore throat and requests a prescription for antibiotics. The practice nurse explains that since his cold is caused by a virus, she will not advise antibiotics. Instead she starts asking about his smoking habits.

Student activity

After reading the scenario above, identify:

- How Jim might feel about his request being denied and how he may react to this
- What the practice nurse may be thinking
- The differing expectations within the consultation
- The possible effects of any conflict on the future relationship.

Models of health and illness

The word 'model' has many meanings but in the study of health and illness refers to a conceptual framework or a perspective, a way of viewing or thinking about health and illness which informs research or practice (Seedhouse 2001). The implication is, therefore, that there may be as many different models in this area as there are different ways of thinking about health and illness. The most common models of health and illness are medical, social and patient-centred.

The medical model

Many health professionals ascribe to the medical model, also known as the biomedical model, which tends to focus on illness rather than health. It has tended to be dominant, although this is now changing. The medical model is underpinned by the growth of scientific thinking, technological progress and research that has developed from the 18th century to the present day. The focus is on being objective when identifying physical problems.

Observed symptom clusters lead to diagnosis, which in turn determines treatment options. Cure and repair are emphasized, with treatment often involving drugs or surgery. The intention is usually to remove the identifiable cause of the problem, returning the patient to a 'normal state'. The medical model assumes that a diagnosis is not valid unless made by expert practitioners. A further assumption is that patients are relatively passive during the process.

Mental health language and the medical model

Foucault (1973) believed that use of language is crucial in determining the way people think and therefore that there could be problems in the use of medical model terminology in the areas of mental distress or mental health problems. The phrase 'mental illness' tends to reflect the medical model, which is neither accurate nor helpful when applied to problems that are often largely social or behavioural. Even use of the adjective 'mental' has been criticized as it relates to the mind rather than to the brain or even to abnormal behaviour where many problems might manifest. It is more accurate to use the term 'mental distress' which fits with modern thinking and is usually preferred by clients.

The social model

Whereas the medical model tends to focus on causes of illness within the individual, the social model considers the society in which the individual lives. This approach arose in the 19th century from the idea that improved health comes from improved environmental and living conditions, e.g. better housing, public health programmes and improved sanitation. The language of the social model is not of symptoms but instead uses terms including barriers, exclusion, distress and disability.

The patient-centred model

Yet another view of health and illness is the patient-centred or client-centred model. It derives from Carl Roger's (1951) work on person-centred therapy and is a dominant model in modern healthcare, especially in mental health, learning disability and complementary therapies. Of key importance in this approach is the patient's own perception of their physical or psychological health. This forms the starting point for a more equal, negotiating type of relationship, with the potential for more holistic assessment. This approach is based on the premise that people have significant and unique knowledge of their own symptoms or problems from which healthcare professionals can learn.

Expert patients

The belief that patients can develop successful strategies for coping with symptoms forms the basis of the Expert Patient Programme, a training scheme delivered by the NHS in England since 2004.

The aim is to provide opportunities for some of the 17.5 million adults living with a long-term health condition to take more control over their health. In effect, to become expert patients by understanding and managing their condition better and thereby improve their quality of life (DH 2001b). The programmes involve attending a series of classes based in primary care settings to learn about issues such as symptom management, medication, relating to health professionals, community resources and stress management. You can find out more about expert patients by carrying out the activities in Box 1.8.

REFLECTIVE PRACTICE Box 1.8

'Expert patient' – dream or nightmare?

Student activities

1. Locate the article below and, from your reading, answer the following questions:
   - Why do some health professionals criticize the idea of expert patients?
   - Why would some health professionals prefer the use of other names such as autonomous patient, resourceful patient or involved patient?
2. Ask a patient/client to tell you about their health problem and how it affects them.
3. Consider how you would feel about providing care for people that know more about their condition or treatment than you do?

[Resource: Shaw J, Baker M 2004 'Expert patient' – dream or nightmare? The concept of a well-informed patient is welcome, but a new name is needed [editorial]. British Medical Journal 328:723–724]

Health beliefs

Interpersonal relationships are often seen as the central role of nurses (see Ch. 9). It is therefore essential that nurses are aware of, and understand, the beliefs and perceptions of their patients/clients to facilitate relationship forming. Nurses need to have an informed understanding of the diversity of health beliefs because of their significant position as 'intermediaries' between medical and lay belief systems, acting as translators of patient/client experience to doctors and vice versa. To accomplish this, nurses need sensitivity to people's subjective experience of illness and an open-mindedness regarding the limitations of the medical approach (Jones 1994). Contemporary health beliefs are better understood by briefly considering how they have developed over time.

Early health beliefs

Early health belief systems date from 3000 BC. The orthodox Chinese system, Ayurvedic medicine and ancient Greek/Roman civilizations were among the first to have a written, systematic categorization of illness for the purposes of diagnosis and treatment. All had ideas of systems in balance or harmony, were person-centred, holistic and made links between health, illness and the individual's personality, the climate, stage of lifespan and the environment.

Although these belief systems seem like 'ancient history', it is important to note that orthodox Chinese and Ayurvedic medicine are still practised by millions of people throughout the world. In general, non-Western ideas of health are becoming increasingly common in UK society. Chapter 10 provides more information about the emergence of complementary therapies.

Religion and health

There has been a long and enduring link between religion, moral behaviour and health. The central idea is that illness may be caused by moral failure or some lapse in good behaviour. There is also the notion that the person may 'deserve to become ill because they have brought it on themselves through their own actions' (see Box 7.5, p. 171, for a contemporary example that explores withholding treatment for smokers).

The Latin word for pain, *poena*, comes from the same root as the word for punishment and the Bible describes pain in childbirth as punishment for Eve's sin in the Garden of Eden. The idea of illness as punishment for moral failure may seem very old-fashioned yet it is still a commonly held belief in current society (Jones 1994). This kind of thinking about 'deserving' illness or being punished for bad behaviour by becoming ill is the norm for children of primary school age. Children's views of health and illness are considered later (p. 10).

From research into lay people's health beliefs, it is common to hear phrases like 'You get what you deserve, people bring things on themselves' or 'It's in God's hands, everything is for a reason'. Helman (2000) also notes that one common image often used in the press is of acquired immune deficiency syndrome (AIDS) as moral punishment, with sufferers divided into two groups: the 'innocent' (children and people with haemophilia) and the 'guilty' (everyone else).

Supernatural ideas and health

Centuries ago, when illness arose for no apparent reason, people sometimes believed that someone had wished them harm by thought, the casting of spells or giving of the evil eye (Helman 2000). Belief in special powers and witchcraft were very common in ancient times but are still held by many people in the UK today, especially as its population becomes more culturally diverse. Large numbers of British people, e.g. those of Afro-Caribbean descent, still hold these beliefs. It is therefore important for student nurses and other healthcare professionals to be sensitive to cultural aspects of health belief and related behaviour (Box 1.9).

Strong supernatural beliefs may result in people having feelings of not being fully in control of their own destiny. In some circumstances, this can lead to a type of fatalism, especially if the person believes in an afterlife or in reincarnation. This is a major issue for health promoters as some people may not value the need to change their health behaviours or lifestyle.

Scientific developments and health

From the 18th century onwards, there was rapid development in scientific knowledge accompanied by technological advance. The emphasis was on research, evidence and objectivity and the beginnings of the medical model are based here. The medical model remains the most common professional view, with its current focus on evidence-based practice (see Ch. 5).

REFLECTIVE PRACTICE Box 1.9

Culture and nursing practice

Cultural background has an important influence on many aspects of people's lives, including their beliefs, behaviour, perceptions, emotion, language, religion, rituals, family structure, diet, dress, body image, concepts of space and time, and attitudes to illness, pain and other forms of misfortune – all of which may have important implications for health and healthcare.

(Helman 2000, p. 3)

Student activities

1. Read the quote above and reflect on your personal or clinical experience.
2. Try to think of examples of diversity in clients'/patients' beliefs and behaviours which you have encountered in practice, e.g. in relation to:
   - Family roles and involvement
   - Gender roles, clothing and privacy
   - Personal hygiene practices
   - Dietary habits.

By the 19th century, there were two main models of health and illness: contagion and miasma. The contagion model stressed that the causes of illness were through contact or touch, magic, diabolism, lack of discipline and moral control. This was the dominant model until the 'germ theory' emerged. Again, although historical, some people still hold notions of contagion in today's society, e.g. people of strong religious faith, minority ethnic groups.

The miasma model, as espoused by Florence Nightingale in her *Notes on Nursing* of 1859, centred on belief systems which considered that illness was caused by bad air or smells, poor atmospheric conditions, rotting food and sewage. It followed then that the treatment of illness involved personal and environmental cleanliness, usually involving fresh air, scrubbing, boiling and bleaching. It is still common these days to hear people voice miasma concerns which tend to be about dampness in the air or cleanliness.

Throughout the 20th century and up to the present day, the medical model has grown and remains dominant. Secularization of beliefs has increased so that, for most people, illness tends not to be linked with either moral failure or religious belief. Non-Western notions of health are common, with an increasing interest in, and rise in the use of, complementary therapies (see Ch. 10). All of these advocate holism by stressing that illness is of the whole self, not merely a problem in an aspect of body function. Complementary therapies are now embedded in many mainstream NHS settings.

Current lay health beliefs

The trend is towards a huge diversity of health beliefs in the UK, which is increasingly multicultural. It is therefore inevitable that nurses will care for people with beliefs that are different from their own. The concept of balance or moderation remains common in modern health beliefs and is often expressed as the idea of trade-off, where individuals regulate their behaviour, e.g. 'I walked to work today so I can have pudding for lunch.'

Categories of lay health beliefs

There is a multitude of common health beliefs noted in this intensively studied area. Blaxter (1990) studied the health beliefs of lay people and observed that these changed according to age, gender, family responsibilities and cultural background. She found young men tended to emphasize physical fitness and function whereas older adults described health as linked to social and emotional relationships. Blaxter (1990) summarized lay health beliefs into 10 categories:

1. Health as never thinking about being healthy or ill
2. Health as behaviour, the healthy lifestyle
3. Health as not ill, not going to the doctor
4. Health as social relationships
5. Health as absence of illness
6. Health as ability to function, to carry out tasks
7. Health despite disease
8. Health as energy or vitality

9. Health as a reserve of strength
10. Health as psychosocial well-being.

Box 1.10 provides an activity to help you recognize common, contemporary health beliefs.

Lay beliefs about the causes of illness

The study of lay theories of illness causation, also known as lay aetiology, refers to people's attempts to make sense of their own or family experience of illness or disease. They try to describe what has happened to someone and why. Jones (1994) described humans as natural scientists, with an innate drive to understand and ascribe meaning to the world around them. However, lay people usually have limited scientific understanding of the structure and functioning of the body, the causes of disease and the reasons for body malfunction. They may hold logical but incorrect assumptions about the cause of illness (Helman 2000), e.g. cold (temperature or weather) causes a cold (viral infection).

Like the medical model, lay theories of illness are multifactorial, placing the causes in one of the following four sites: within the individual, in the natural world, in the social world or in the supernatural world (Box 1.11).

CRITICAL THINKING Box 1.10

Recognizing health beliefs – quotes about health and illness

- 'I think that babies should get aired every day – fresh air in all weathers.'
- 'I smoke, have asthma and bronchitis for which I need inhalers, I'm overweight and am partially deaf in one ear but overall I would say that I am healthy.'
- 'I am healthy, I can always manage to get to work.'
- 'I really think if you've got to go, you've got to go. It's all mapped out you know.'
- 'I can do everything I need to do, earn money, look after my family – to me that's real health.'
- 'I'm very healthy, I've got great family and faithful friends.'
- 'He lived until he was 89, mind you he was from sturdy stock, they were all long-lived in that family.'
- 'Her son was disabled and her husband left her but she just got on with it, she never made any fuss and coped with everything.'

[Adapted from Greig J 1995 Men talking about health: a qualitative study. Unpublished MSc thesis, Edinburgh University]

Student activities

- Read the quotes above from lay people expressing their own ideas about health and illness and try to identify what type of belief is being expressed. It may help to look back at Blaxter's 10 categories of health beliefs, the Seedhouse groups of health definitions and the section on history of health beliefs.
- Next time you are on placement, listen for lay health beliefs expressed by patients/clients.

The first two explanations relate to the Western industrialized world while the last two usually arise from non-industrialized or rural communities (Helman 2000).

Children's health and illness beliefs

There is distinctive progression in children's understanding of health and illness-related concepts with age. Children's understanding corresponds to their stage of cognitive development, using Piaget's theoretical framework as comparison (see Ch. 8). 'Draw and write' techniques are commonly used to explore children's health perceptions and, by the age of 6, children may have already developed distinct ideas about the causes of health and illness.

Preschool children see illness occurring as if by magic and sometimes perceive it as punishment for past misconduct and may even believe that healthcare professionals intentionally set out to hurt them (Hart & Chesson 1998). They know the names of some external body parts but internal bodily functions remain largely unknown.

Children aged 6–7 years tend to have a view of health which describes healthy people as being young, sporty, happy, smiling and actively involved in outside activities (Kerr 2000). In this age group, children may believe that illness is caused by a single factor, often a germ (Hart & Chesson 1998). They are familiar with the names for external body parts and some internal organs and bodily functions. Little is known about children's concepts of mental health, other than feelings related to being happy or sad.

Children aged 9–10 years understand the principles of germ transmission but many believe that all illness is caused this way, even cancer and eczema (Hart & Chesson 1998). Given this, it follows that they sometimes have difficulty in understanding prescribed treatment. Perrin and Gerrity (1981) noted that medical terms were

Box 1.11 **Lay beliefs about the causes of illness**

- *Individual level theories*: Emphasize malfunction within the body. Causes of illness tend to centre on notions of vulnerability, resistance, wear and tear, hereditary predisposition, imbalance and mechanical damage or blockage
- *Natural world theories*: Seek explanation in climatic conditions. Causes of illness typically centre on air quality and seasons, microorganisms which are commonly described as insects (e.g. tummy bug), astrology, accidental injuries, parasites and environmental irritants
- *Social world theories*: Tend to blame other people, emphasizing interpersonal conflict, witchcraft, sorcery, 'evil eye', spells, potions, rituals
- *Supernatural world theories*: Seek explanation in gods, ancestors or spirits. Illness is seen as a reminder for a lapse in behaviour. In industrialized settings, individuals are more likely to blame fate, luck or Acts of God.

[Adapted from Helman (2000)]

frequently misinterpreted by children, giving examples of oedema perceived as 'demon in my belly' and diabetes perceived as 'die of betes'.

Children aged 11 years have begun to develop a more detailed understanding of health and illness and by 13 years grasp the complexity of illness with its multiple possible causes. They are able to discuss the complex interplay between biological, lifestyle and environmental factors that influence health and illness (Helman 2000). They can readily identify health determinants (see p. 14) and understand health-damaging behaviours such as passive smoking (Kerr 2000). They have studied at school and can relate, for example, aspects of body functioning to the components of a healthy diet. They are also more likely to appreciate the impact of psychological factors, grasp the notion of drug-related side-effects and the time delay often experienced in response to treatment (Hart & Chesson 1998), e.g. it may take several days before antibiotic medicine is seen to 'work'.

In all age groups, the most common symptoms described as ill-health by children were fever, headache, dizziness or rash (Helman 2000). Thermometers feature strongly in children's 'draw and write' descriptions. Children perceive fever to be the key symptom used by their parents to determine whether or not they are ill. This reflects their own experience, which is usually limited to common illnesses of childhood such as viral infections.

It is also noteworthy that, unlike adults, positive aspects of illness feature strongly in children's drawings and descriptions of being ill. These include staying off school, being the centre of attention, having visitors, treats and special foods.

Becker's health belief model

There are many health belief models that provide an overview of the factors influencing health beliefs. One is the health belief model (HBM) devised by Becker (1974) to explain how people behave in relation to their health. A person's beliefs about whether they are likely to contract an illness and the degree to which they see an illness as being severe can be considered as a perceived threat and is the basis by which their behaviour is influenced. The HBM (Fig. 1.2) has been shown to be highly predictive of health behaviour.

According to the HBM, participation in preventative health behaviour, i.e. behaviour which should decrease the risk of illness, is predicted on the basis of the following:

- How an individual perceives their susceptibility to a given disorder – what is the likelihood of being affected?
- How an individual perceives the seriousness or severity of the disorder – how bad would it be?
- How an individual perceives the benefits of taking action – what will be gained?
- How an individual perceives the barriers to action – how hard is it to change, what will be lost?
- The individual's experience of cues to action – what has been seen or heard which triggers health behaviour action, e.g. GP advice, a health scare or major life event
- Health motivation – how highly a person values health.

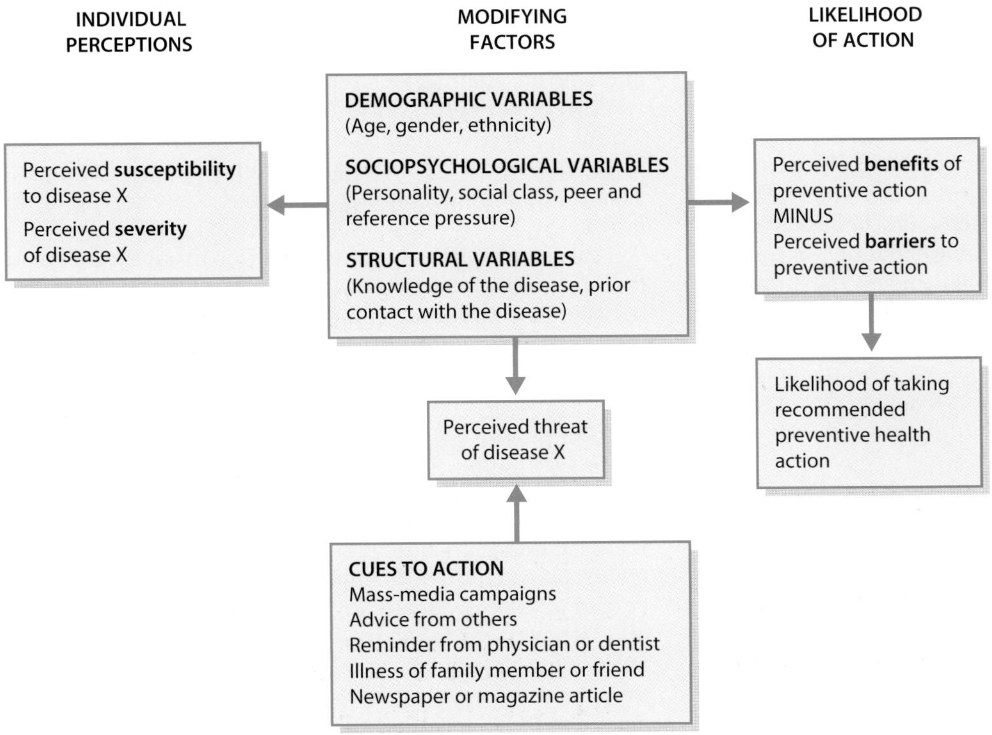

Fig. 1.2 Becker's health belief model (reproduced with permission from Naidoo and Wills 2000)

Values in health are discussed below and Chapter 7 considers values and ethics in nursing practice. Originally, the HBM had four key beliefs affecting the central concept of health motivation. Later, the HBM was extended to include the fifth key belief: perceived self-efficacy, which refers to a person's confidence in their ability to make/maintain a change in health behaviour. Modifying factors may include sociocultural factors, age and gender. It suggests that people will consider the advantages and disadvantages of engaging in positive health behaviour, even if the existing behaviour is not changed, and relies on a particular cue for action to be taken.

The nurse's role and application of the HBM

Nurses can help people to change their health behaviour in many ways. It is important to realize that any contact with health professionals, however brief, is often a 'cue to action' in itself. It is important to use this contact to discuss health behaviours – people expect it and may be surprised if the subject is not broached. Nurses and other health professionals have high credibility with patients/clients and a brief discussion may be all that someone, who has been considering positive health-related change, needs to move forward and actually make a change.

There is a need for nurses to offer factual, balanced health information that clearly indicates individual susceptibility or risk. The language and images used are important considerations, especially in children and people with learning disability. Shock tactics, moral judgements or emotive language are unhelpful and may alienate patients/clients. Interaction between nurses and patients/clients should stress not only the benefits of preventative health behaviour but also offer encouragement and strategies for dealing with barriers to change.

Attitudes, values and behaviours

This is a complex area of social psychology important in nursing and health promotion since attitudes combine aspects of people's values, feelings and beliefs. An attitude is defined as a relatively stable tendency to respond consistently to particular people, objects or situations. The use of the word 'stable' rather than 'fixed' implies an ability of the attitude to change or be changed. An attitude represents a person's general feelings towards someone or something. It can be negative or positive, strongly held or weak. Attitudes have three components, summarized as ABC:

- A – affective component or 'feeling' aspects
- B – behavioural aspects
- C – cognitive component or knowledge and belief aspects.

Nurses are often involved in assisting patients/clients to change their health-related attitudes with the aim of causing a positive behaviour change. For example, to explore dietary issues with a person newly diagnosed with diabetes, the nurse needs to:

- Allow time for them to express their feelings about the diagnosis before assessing their understanding of the symptoms and dietary changes needed
- Answer any questions and explore the person's usual eating habits at their own pace
- Provide reinforcement and supplementary reading
- Assess where any practical changes can be made.

To ensure success, all of this must be done sensitively and with the person as participant as possible in the interaction. Care with use of language, visual aids and the opportunity for rehearsal would be of particular benefit to people with a learning disability (Box 1.35, p. 27).

Public and private attitudes

An attitude openly expressed by a person in public is usually called an opinion. Attitudes may or may not be predictive of people's behaviour. Publicly stated opinions may, or may not, reflect a person's true, privately-held attitude that tends to be divulged only to trusted and close family members and friends. People may express different attitudes to researchers in an attempt to help the interaction, give a more 'textbook' answer or appear more acceptable. An example of this in nursing might be when carrying out an admission assessment, a person who drinks heavily may purposely underestimate their alcohol units consumed per week and describe themselves as a social drinker.

Cognitive dissonance

Festinger's (1964) idea of cognitive dissonance is based on the three components of attitudes mentioned above. It is common for a person who knows and understands the adverse effects of smoking (cognitive component) and who has poor self-esteem because they smoke (affective component) to continue to smoke (the behaviour). This is known as smoking dissonance and is experienced as psychological discomfort or guilt because of the inconsistency that exists among the three components of an attitude.

Festinger (1964) suggested that it is usual for a person feeling this discomfort to have a drive to resolve the conflict between the different components of their attitude and therefore reduce the dissonance experienced. Cognitive dissonance therefore can be viewed as a possible precursor of a positive health-related behaviour change. If nurses or other healthcare professionals perceive a person's cognitive dissonance, then this may be a first step along the road to attitude change and, possibly, behaviour change. Mass media campaigns may purposely seek to induce or increase dissonance for this very reason, e.g. the British Heart Foundation anti-smoking advertisements which verged on the physically revolting, using emotive images of a fatty substance oozing out of cigarettes. It is important to note that this type of mass media campaign is not understood by a large proportion of people with a learning disability (NHS Health Scotland 2004).

Values

Attitudes are underpinned by values, which are broad and less specific than attitudes. Values underpin an individual's 'philosophy of life' which are then applied to everyday life. They may relate to moral, ethical or religious issues as well as health, gender roles, family life and the environment. How much a person values their health is a key part of the health motivation section of Becker's health belief model (see Fig. 1.2).

A person's value system is composed of broad beliefs developed through early learning, upbringing and socialization within the family and later at school, with peers and through life experiences and work. The cultural context in which this develops is also very important.

Each value may have multiple attitudes associated with it. Although it may be possible to cause attitude change, it is more difficult to change a person's value system as it is an integral part of their early upbringing and life experience. For example, values relating to moral conduct in life may have associated attitudes about crime and punishment, sexual behaviour, marriage and the rearing of children.

Stereotyping

Although the term 'stereotype' originally referred to a printing stamp used to make multiple copies, it began to be used in the early 20th century to describe the way society categorizes people by 'stamping' them with a set of characteristics. Stereotypes are underpinned by direct expressions of beliefs and values and may offer a shorthand way to generalize about a person or a group of people (Box 1.12).

It may seem natural to try to classify people in society but stereotypes are to be avoided in nursing because they do not acknowledge individual differences and are usually oversimplified and negative. Stereotypes form the basis of prejudice, or unfavourable opinion, formed against a person or group of people, usually based on the following characteristics:

- Age
- Gender
- Mental or physical disability
- Occupation
- Race
- Religion
- Nationality.

Fear of the unknown, e.g. of minority groups, may fuel stereotypes. When people are judged on stereotypes and there is resulting prejudice, this is known as discrimination.

People with mental health problems have historically suffered serious discrimination and can be considered one of the most socially excluded groups in British society. Public fear of mental illness has been fuelled by well-publicized cases in the media where a mentally distressed person has behaved violently. However, two-thirds of all media reports on mental health issues portray a direct association between mental distress and violence. This shows how stereotypes are often untrue because, statistically, people with mental health problems are no more likely than anyone else to engage in violent behaviour. In addition, data show that people with mental distress are much more likely to harm themselves than other people. Discriminatory behaviour includes:

- Ignoring or avoiding people
- Abusive language, especially 'jokes'
- Dehumanizing slang
- Name-calling
- Excluding behaviour such as restricted membership of clubs and societies
- Lack of equal access to jobs or promotion.

The result can be segregation and isolation for individuals and, in extreme cases, discrimination is expressed as physical violence.

Discriminatory behaviour which targets children is referred to as bullying and, increasingly, this term is also used by adults in the workplace. Bullying is a common form of discrimination with 51% of primary school children and 28% of secondary school children reporting some experience of being bullied (DfES 2003). Bullying refers to deliberately hurtful actions, encompassing a broad spectrum of behaviours. In the case of children, name-calling is the most common type of bullying but other behaviours include teasing, rumour-spreading, theft of possessions or money, abusive text messages or emails, coercion,

REFLECTIVE PRACTICE Box 1.12

Stereotyping

Discriminatory behaviour can result from negative stereotypes and should be avoided by nurses. It is important to be non-judgemental and form effective relationships with all patients/clients. Nurses must be self-aware and recognize stereotyping both within themselves and in everyday life. Carry out the short quiz below to find out if you hold negative stereotypes.

Student activities

1. Brainstorm words or phrases which briefly describe and summarize your mental image of the following:
   - Male nurses
   - Blondes
   - Cowboys
   - Social workers.
2. Complete the sentences below and then ask yourself where you 'learned' this:
   - Everyone over 65 is . . .
   - Women drivers should . . .
   - People with red hair are . . .
3. Now look back at your answers and consider what forms of discriminatory behaviour could result from these stereotypes.
4. Next time you watch TV or read a newspaper, look out for perpetuated stereotypes. Is this different in different types of newspaper?

Box 1.13 **Bullying and children**

- Vulnerability to bullying often relates to physical and individual characteristics such as body shape, size, physical disability or learning difficulty such as dyslexia
- More than 20 000 children in the UK call the telephone helpline 'Childline' each year about bullying; 20% say that the current 'tormentor' is a former friend
- Bullying causes shame, humiliation and fear. It can also cause feelings of powerlessness and low-self-esteem which can last into adulthood
- Concentration problems and increased school avoidance can lead to behavioural problems and deterioration in academic performance
- In some cases, children may attempt self-harm.

[Adapted from Department for Education and Skills (2003) and Childline (2004)]

being excluded or ignored in play, class, sports and other activities or physical threats and abuse (Childline 2004) (see Box 1.13).

Lifestyle, health behaviours and locus of control

In relation to health, lifestyle means health-related behaviours over which a person has some choice. These include:

- Sexual health practices
- Tobacco use
- Alcohol use
- Diet
- Exercise
- Non-prescribed or recreational drug use
- Stress management
- Use of preventive health services.

Becker (1974) described adaptive health behaviour as being either preventative health behaviour or sick role behaviour. Examples of preventative health behaviours include exercising, not smoking and eating a healthy diet; sick role behaviours include seeking medical help, using services and complying with treatment (p. 33).

The term 'internal locus of control' is used to describe the beliefs held by some people that they have the power to make health-related choices, and to influence and control their health behaviour. In short, the individual feels and believes that they are ultimately responsible for their own health. Other people demonstrate an external locus of control where they see outside factors controlling their health and health behaviour, with the tendency to blame luck, fate, God, the climate or the environment. You may hear people say things like 'If the bullet's got your name on it . . .' or 'If you've got to go, you've got to go'. These are examples of fatalism and evident in some of the quotes in Box 1.10 (p. 10).

It is arguable whether everyone is equally free to make meaningful health-related choices. Some people are severely constrained by issues such as income, education, knowledge and peer group pressure. For example, on a very low income it is hard to afford a healthy wholemeal loaf rather than the cheaper, and less healthy, white alternative.

Factors influencing health

Factors that influence or determine health are called health determinants. The same factors that determine health also determine ill-health, and each determinant may have either positive or negative effects on health, e.g. housing. Positive health effects related to housing as a health determinant include warmth, space, comfort, well-being and psychological security. Negative aspects of housing as a health determinant are well documented and include overcrowding, noise and safety concerns leading to stress and depression, and dampness and mould resulting in physical illness, e.g. asthma.

Determinants are many, varied yet interrelated and are described by Dahlgren and Whitehead (1991) as being on five levels. The multifactorial view shown in Figure 1.3 illustrates health determinants as layers surrounding a core and allows differentiation between individual and sociopolitical factors. The core factors – gender, ethnicity, age and heredity – are inherited characteristics and largely fixed, while the surrounding layers of influence may be open to some modification. The next layer is individual lifestyle where personal behaviours may not be rationally or voluntarily chosen, but are heavily influenced by family, friends and peer group, and by social and community networks. Wider influences on health include:

- Living and working conditions
- Issues related to housing
- Access to health services
- Clean drinking water and sanitation
- Work environment or unemployment
- Access to education
- Agriculture and food supply.

It is important to note that these wider determinants are not open to action by individuals but need collective action at the level of government. For example, although individuals can play their part in environmental issues in a small way – by choosing environmentally friendly cleaning products and adopting recycling behaviours – it requires policy, legislation and action at national and international levels to achieve positive changes in some health determinants, e.g. water and air quality.

The outermost layer contains the socioeconomic, cultural and environmental conditions prevalent in society including interest rates, unemployment rates and political stability. Access to health and social services is a major determinant of health and one attempt to address this is the Children's National Service Framework (DH 2004). This is a 10-year programme intended to promote fair, high-quality, integrated health and social care from pregnancy to adulthood. There are three parts: Part 1

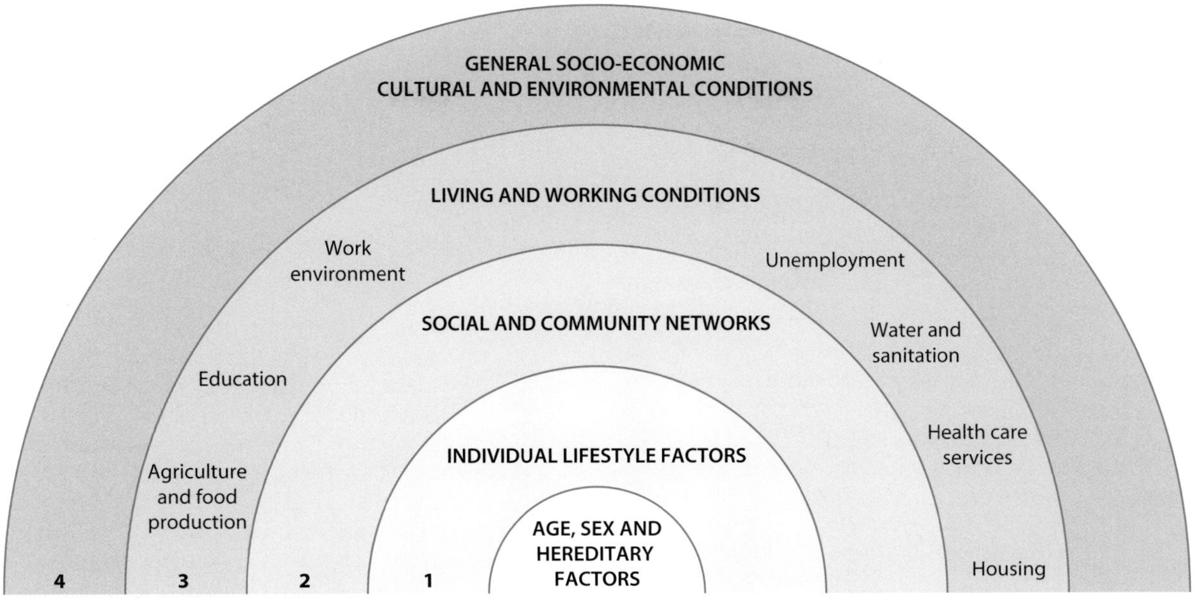

Fig. 1.3 The main determinants of health (reproduced with permission from Naidoo and Wills 2000)

provides core standards for all children and young people (Box 1.14); Part 2 contains standards relating to those with illness, complex needs or mental health and well-being needs and those in hospital; Part 3 covers maternity services.

Determinants of mental health and well-being

Determinants of mental health and well-being are shown in Figure 1.4. Factors influencing mental health are grouped into four spheres:

- Individual
- Family and community
- Societal
- Spiritual.

Each sphere relates to dimensions of self-esteem which together influence mental health and well-being (Box 1.15).

Poverty as the key determinant of health

The most important health determinant is poverty but there is no clear consensus on how it is best defined or measured. Poverty can be defined as absolute or relative.

- *Absolute poverty* is the inability to meet basic biological needs such as food, warmth and shelter. This relates to the first level of Maslow's hierarchy of needs (see Ch. 8). Box 1.16 shows the UK groups most susceptible to poverty.
- *Relative poverty* is usually defined by a comparison to a country's average living standards, as measured by income level or ownership of certain goods, e.g. a car, or access to services, e.g. child care (Box 1.17).

Box 1.14 **Children's National Service Framework (DH 2004) Part 1: Five core standards**

Standard 1. Promoting health and well-being, identifying needs and interventions
The health and well-being of all children and young people is promoted and delivered through a coordinated programme of action, including prevention and early intervention wherever possible, to ensure long-term gain, led by the NHS in partnership with local authorities.

Standard 2. Supporting parents
Parents or carers are enabled to receive the information, services and support that will help them to care for their children and equip them with the skills they need to ensure that their children have optimum life chances and are healthy and safe.

Standard 3. Child, young person and family-centred services
Children and young people and families should receive high-quality services which are coordinated around their individual and family needs and take account of their views.

Standard 4. Growing up into adulthood
All young people have access to age-appropriate services which are responsive to their specific needs as they grow into adulthood.

Standard 5. Safeguarding and promoting welfare
All agencies work to prevent children suffering harm and to promote their welfare, provide them with the services they require to address their identified needs and safeguard children who are being or who are likely to be harmed.

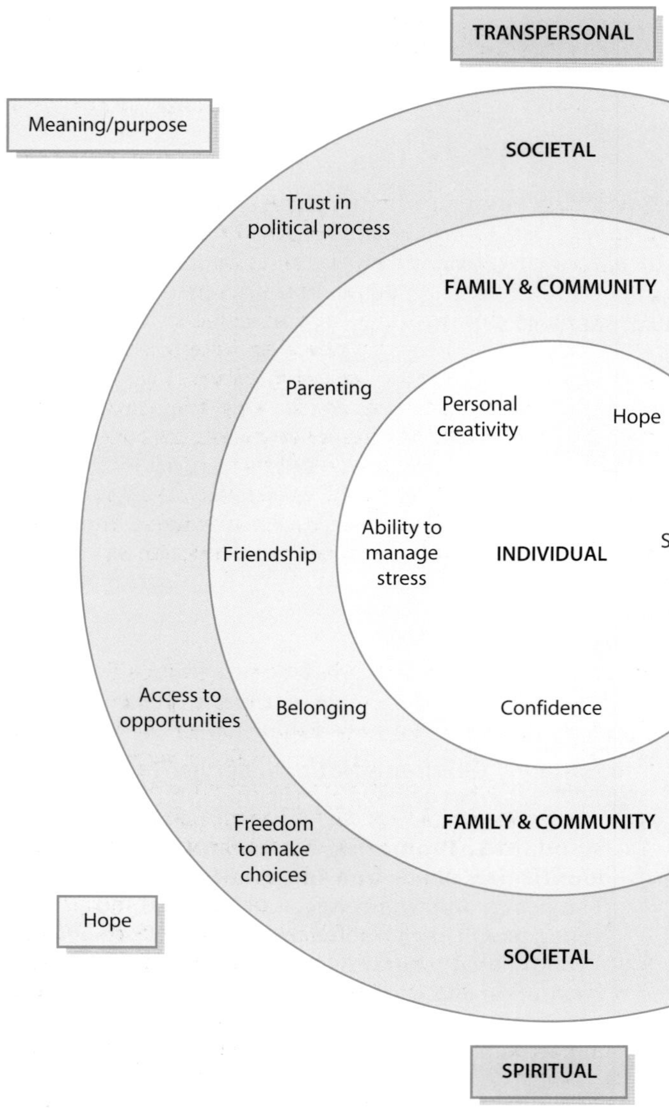

Fig. 1.4 The confidence spiral: determinants/components of mental health and well-being (reproduced with permission from Kennedy 2002)

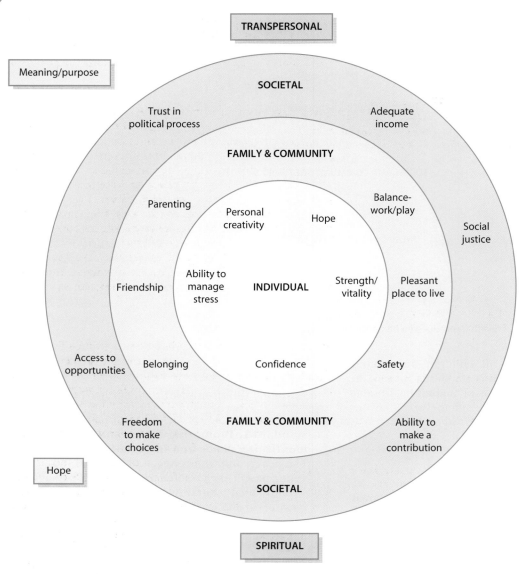

CRITICAL THINKING Box 1.15

Mental health and well-being

Student activities

- From your own experience, reflect on what factors influence your self-esteem and mental well-being positively or negatively.
- Think about patients/clients you have cared for and consider the factors that are likely to influence their self-esteem and well-being.

The European Anti-Poverty Network (EAPN 2003) urge that people's own perceptions of poverty are acknowledged. However, the most commonly used official definition of poverty is living in a household with an income under 60% of the average for the country in which

Box 1.16 **UK groups most susceptible to poverty**

- People in social housing
- Households dependent on state benefits
- Young people aged 16–22 years
- Large families, e.g. four or more dependent children
- Families with children under 11 years of age
- Households with no paid workers
- Separated or divorced households
- Women and children
- Lone parent households
- Adults in one-person households, including single pensioners.

[Adapted from Gordon D 2000 Poverty and social exclusion in Britain. Joseph Rowntree Foundation, York]

CRITICAL THINKING Box 1.17

A satisfactory standard of living?

Student activities

- Reflect on the household items or daily activities you consider essential for a 'normal' standard of modern living.
- Lack of car ownership is one key measure of deprivation and relative poverty. Consider how lack of car ownership might impact on day-to-day life and on health in general today.

EVIDENCE-BASED PRACTICE Box 1.18

Effects of poverty

Poverty and disadvantage in childhood are key determinants of future mental health for children and young people. A tendency toward adult depression and also physical problems is strongly associated with social deprivation.

Children of low-income families:

- Are three times more likely to have mental health problems than those from professional families (15% compared with 5%)
- Are more likely to have low birth weights and associated developmental problems
- Have higher teenage conception rates.

[Resource: Office for National Statistics 2004 The health of children and young people. Online. Available: www.statistics.gov.uk/children]

Student activity

Make an online search of the Office for National Statistics website (above) and find out more about low-income families and any of the following:

- Low birth weight babies
- Teenage pregnancy
- Mental health in children
- Accidental deaths in children.

they live. Sometimes, this definition of poverty is further refined by deducting housing costs. This relative measure changes over time and in 2000–2001, 12.9 million people in the UK were living below this threshold (after deducting housing costs), 4 million of whom were children (JRF 2003). Box 1.18 shows the disproportionate effect of poverty on children.

Relative poverty and participation in society

Relative poverty involves more than merely income; it also includes the idea that someone with a low income is unlikely to be able to participate in mainstream society. The European Anti-Poverty Network (EAPN 2003) describe the effects of relative poverty as being unable to or precluded from meeting one or more needs without outside help. These needs relate to aspects of life which enable self-determination, i.e. assuming one's responsibilities and exercising one's rights, or fundamental services such as education, housing and health.

Components of poverty

Poverty is complex and multidimensional, linking to fundamental issues including housing, healthcare and also to factors such as social exclusion. A combination of low pay, inadequate benefits or unemployment can lead to poverty. Low income gives rise to separate components of poverty including poverty of food, fuel, housing, transport, access to recreation/social facilities and, over time, leads to relative powerlessness. Ongoing poverty can negatively influence an individual's physical and psychological health, with associated behavioural changes including increased use of alcohol or nicotine, sometimes called 'drugs of comfort'. Box 1.18 highlights the links between childhood poverty and mental health.

Social class and health inequalities

Poverty has been linked to health inequalities for many years. Chadwick's 1842 *General Report on the Sanitary Conditions of the Labouring Population of Great Britain* showed that richer people had a life expectancy more than double that of the poorest in society. Although life expectancy has improved steadily since then, there has not been an even improvement across social classes; inequalities still remain and may be growing.

Social class was previously categorized according to the Registrar General's Classification of Social Class which was largely unchanged between 1921 and 2000 (see Box 1.19). People were allocated to one of five classes on the basis of the occupation of the head of the household. Although suited to men of working age, criticism of this classification centred on the exclusion of people lacking occupation, e.g. students, retired or unemployed people. Women were not included in their own right, their class being derived from that of their husband or father. Publications before 2001 use this classification.

For the 2001 census, classification of social class was revised and now the National Statistics Socioeconomic Classification (NS-SEC) is used. Eight categories were introduced to take account of changes in the labour market and the role of women. It included categories for the self-employed and those who have never worked or who are long-term unemployed. More information is available from the Office for National Statistics website.

Research into health inequalities

In 1977, the Labour government appointed Sir Douglas Black to chair a working group to review the information on health inequalities and then identify policy and research that should follow. In 1980, by the time the Black Report was due to be published, there had been an election and a change of government from Labour to Conservative. At first, the Black Report was circulated to academics in a very low-key way. It clearly showed that during the first 35 years of the NHS there had been an

Box 1.19 **Classification of social class**

Registrar General's Classification of Social Class (used in publications prior to 2001)

Class
1 Professional
2 Semi-professional
3a Skilled non-manual
3b Skilled manual
4 Partially skilled
5 Unskilled

National Statistics Socioeconomic Classification (NS-SEC) (used in publications since 2001)

Class
1. Higher managerial and professional
   1.1 Company directors, bank managers, senior civil servants
   1.2 Doctors, barristers, teachers, social workers
2. Lower managerial and professional, e.g. nurses, actors, police, soldiers
3. Intermediate, e.g. secretaries, clerks
4. Small employers and own account workers, e.g. publicans, farmers, taxi drivers
5. Lower supervisory, craft and related occupations, e.g. printers, plumbers, butchers
6. Semi-routine occupations, e.g. shop assistants, traffic wardens, hairdressers
7. Routine occupations, e.g. waiters, road sweepers, cleaners, couriers
8. Never worked and long-term unemployed

Box 1.20 **Summary of the Acheson report recommendations**

Acheson (1998) made 39 recommendations that were wide-ranging and included the following:

- Raising of state benefits, especially for women and children
- Additional resources for schools in deprived areas
- Increased employment and training opportunities
- More social housing
- Access to healthcare for homeless people
- Free school fruit for primary 1 and 2 pupils
- Affordable, high-quality day care for preschool children
- A focus on the health and nutrition of women
- A focus on breastfeeding
- Better housing and job opportunities for minority ethnic groups.

CRITICAL THINKING Box 1.21

Comparing the Black Report and the Acheson Report

Student activities
- Locate and read the following article which compares the Black Report to the Acheson Report.
- Note the similarities or differences between these two milestone reports.

[Resource: Davey Smith G, Morris J, Shaw M 1998 The independent inquiry into inequalities in health (editorial). British Medical Journal 317:1465–1466]

improvement in health across all social classes. However, there was still a strong relationship between social class and life expectancy, infant mortality and inequalities in the use of health services (Townsend et al 1992).

The Black Committee recommended a comprehensive anti-poverty programme with detailed and costed targets. The two main elements were:

- Fairer distribution of resources
- Provision of the necessary educational and employment opportunities for active social participation.

The Black Report advocated that the key approach to tackling health inequalities was preventative work in childhood and in particular the 'first years of life'. This has been borne out by subsequent research and remains the main emphasis in current health promotion targets. The Black Report's recommendations were not implemented but, nevertheless, stimulated extensive research and raised the issue of inequalities around the world.

Some 20 years after the Black Report, the Acheson Report was commissioned by the newly elected Labour government in 1997 to review inequalities in health in England. It was published in 1998 and the main findings were that poor neighbourhoods are characterized by poor health. Also noted was that health inequalities still affect society and that they are cumulative from before birth to old age and that poverty has a disproportionate effect on children. The incidence of premature death was noted to be highest amongst the poor, directly linked to inequalities in income. The Acheson Report made recommendations in three main areas:

- All policies likely to have an impact on health should be evaluated
- High priority should be given to the health of families with children
- Further improvements should be made to reduce income inequalities and raise the living standards of poor households.

Box 1.20 gives an overview of the Acheson Report recommendations.

The Acheson Report stated that individual lifestyle and personal choice were not responsible for the 'health gap', arguing instead that income levels, changes in society and constraints prevent individuals from choice. For example, changes in transport and shopping contributed to the creation of 'food deserts' – areas of social housing with no shops or services, or only one small and expensive corner shop. This makes the purchase of fresh food at reasonable prices almost impossible for some families.

Unlike the Black Report which largely led to further research, the Acheson Report prompted actual policy change and engendered a climate focusing on health inequalities. Undertaking the activities in Box 1.21 will help you compare the findings of the Black Report and the Acheson Report.

Changing trends in health and illness

Health and illness issues change over time. During the last century, there was a shift in the pattern of disease from infectious diseases prevalent in the 19th and early 20th centuries to chronic physical conditions and mental health issues for the 21st century (see Box 1.5, p. 6). Diabetes is one example of a chronic physical disease causing premature death and disability. In the UK, it affects 1.3 million of the population and is increasing so rapidly that by 2010 it is estimated that 3 million people will be affected (BMA 2004). Diabetes rates in children are increasing and are linked to obesity. Suicide is increasing in children and young people. The UK also has some of the worst death rates in the world for coronary heart disease (CHD), strokes (British Heart Foundation 2003), cancer and respiratory diseases. These chronic diseases are strongly linked to lifestyle factors such as cigarette smoking, poor diet, physical inactivity and excessive alcohol consumption. Strong links exist between social class and the prevalence of these risk factors, which predominate in the poorest sections of society.

Other health trends related to lifestyle include sexual health and sexually transmitted infections (STIs). The sexual health of young people in the UK is poor and linked to unsafe sexual behaviours such as unprotected sex, which has contributed to high rates of STIs and unwanted pregnancies (Box 1.22).

Apart from the increase in chronic illness and lifestyle-related diseases, another important issue is the development of new communicable diseases such as Ebola virus, human immunodeficiency virus (HIV) and AIDS, variant Creutzfeldt–Jakob disease (vCJD), severe acute respiratory syndrome (SARS) and bird flu. Longstanding infectious conditions previously thought to be curable are now re-emerging and are resistant to conventional treatments, e.g. tuberculosis (TB) and methicillin-resistant *Staphylococcus aureus* (MRSA).

Changing issues in health and illness have focused interest in health promotion and increased government funding of initiatives. The rationale is based on the large preventable component of many illnesses, e.g. smoking and lung cancer. There is a huge potential for health gains if morbidity and mortality are reduced, e.g. publicizing the effects of passive smoking on children's health (Box 1.23).

The 'greying' of the population refers to a growing elderly population with an associated shift from acute to chronic illness. Older adults often have several, concurrent illnesses, known as 'multiple pathology'. This situation has been described as living longer, but not healthier. Chronic illness and multiple illnesses mean a changing emphasis on 'care' rather than 'cure'.

The health needs of people with a learning disability are also changing because of increasing life expectancy and the increasing trend for more people with very complex health needs (NHS Health Scotland 2004).

The huge and growing financial cost of inpatient care, compared to health promotion funding, makes prevention of ill-health and health improvement an attractive

Box 1.22 UK trends in sexual health and STIs

- The conception rate in all females has decreased slowly over the last 10 years except for young women aged 13–15 which has remained constant
- Over half of all conceptions in women under 16 years end in a termination and this has increased slightly
- During the 1980s and early 1990s, many STI rates were falling or stable, possibly reflecting changes in sexual behaviour in response to the emergence of HIV
- Chlamydia is the most common STI and the number of new cases has risen steadily since the mid 1990s, doubling since 1996. There was a 14% rise in the number of cases between 2001 and 2002. The highest rates of chlamydia are in young women aged 16–19
- The second most common STI is gonorrhoea with a 9% increase between 2001 and 2002.

[Resource: Office for National Statistics 2004 Sexual health: chlamydia rates continue to rise. Online. Available: www.statistics.gov.uk 14 July 2006]

Box 1.23 The effects of passive smoking on children's health

Exposure to smoking during infancy and childhood increases the risk of the following and accounts for:

- 10% of middle ear infections in children
- 15% of lower respiratory tract infections
- 25% of wheezing
- 20–50% of sudden infant death syndrome.

In addition, exposed children may also experience reduced lung function and impaired physical growth and academic attainment compared to children of non-smoking mothers.

[Adapted from NHS Health Scotland/ASH Scotland 2003 Reducing smoking and tobacco-related harm – a key to transforming Scotland's health. NHS Health Scotland/ASH Scotland, Edinburgh]

Box 1.24 Key changes driving UK health and social care

The economic and political context

- Information and service sector growth replacing manufacturing
- Extreme poverty will be eliminated but there will be a persisting gap between rich and poor
- Long-term unemployment will increase
- Increasing migration and number of refugees.

Demographic changes

- Increasing elderly population, both in absolute terms and as a percentage of the total population
- Fastest growing age segment is older adults over 80 years
- Declining birth rate, deferred child rearing.

Epidemiological trends

- Increase in non-communicable diseases
- Growth in mental ill-health
- Overeating and obesity
- Emerging and resurgent infectious diseases.

Consumer wants

- Choice as a fundamental of political ideology
- Increase in well-informed, demanding consumers
- Empowerment of older people – gerontocracy
- Access to IT-based information.

[Resource: Warner M, Longley M, Gould E et al 1998 Healthcare futures 2010. Welsh Institute Health and Social Care, University of Glamorgan, Pontypridd]

strategy for governments. The key changes driving health and social care until 2010 are varied and are summarized in Box 1.24. They provide the current context for health promotion, which is explored below.

Health promotion

Health promotion encompasses all the activities below:

- Monitoring children's height, weight and developmental progress
- Encouraging 'flu jab' uptake by TV campaigns
- Organizing access to clean needles for intravenous drug users
- Assessing a surgical patient's smoking status
- Encouraging tooth brushing with learning disability residents
- Explaining to parents how their child should use an inhaler
- Teaching stress reduction to people with mental distress
- Helping people access their full benefit entitlements
- Supporting the rights of non-smokers to have a smoke-free workplace
- Immunizing children
- Supporting people with weight loss programmes

HEALTH PROMOTION Box 1.25

Exploring health promotion initiatives

Student activities

1. From the list below, choose a health promotion initiative that interests you:
   - Free fruit schemes in school
   - Paths to Health – walking activity for over 50s
   - SureStart – positive parenting
   - Don't suffer in silence – anti-bullying
   - Baby Friendly Initiative – breastfeeding
   - See Me – reducing stigma for those with mental distress
   - NHS mammography.
2. Using an online search engine, find out more about the specific initiative, noting:
   - Its aim, methods and focus
   - Its target group
   - Whether it is delivered nationally or locally.

- Undertaking blood pressure checks in workplaces
- Developing an anti-bullying programme in primary schools
- Working with community groups about local traffic issues, e.g. calming measures.

These different activities have a common aim in that they are all positive actions to improve health which, in summary, is what health promotion is all about. It is of note that only some of the activities above relate to physical health and it is important to recognize that health promotion encompasses all dimensions of health (p. 4). Contemporary health promotion often focuses on social and economic issues such as poverty and inequalities in access to healthcare and services.

The focus of health promotion activity could be the whole population but often activities are targeted to meet particular needs, focusing on one or more of the following:

- Key stages of the lifespan – pregnancy and breastfeeding, child development, parenting, retirement
- Certain age groups – preschool or secondary school children or people over 50 years
- High risk groups – homeless people, children and young people looked after by local authorities
- Excluded groups – inequalities of access for minority ethnic groups, travelling people, people with mental distress or learning disability
- Specific physical illnesses – CHD, diabetes, high blood pressure
- Gender-specific issues – testicular cancer, breast or cervical cancer, menopause
- Lifestyle-related issues – smoking, drugs and alcohol, diet, activity levels, sexual health
- Mental and emotional health – awareness raising, suicide prevention, anti-stigma, anti-bullying
- Settings and situation related – schools, prisons, workplaces, community (Box 1.25).

HEALTH PROMOTION Box 1.26

Mental health promotion

Mental health promotion operates at three levels within the population:

1. *Strengthening individuals*, e.g. promoting life skills, parenting skills, improving self-esteem at any stage of the lifespan
2. *Strengthening communities*, e.g. social support, social inclusion, improving neighbourhoods, anti-bullying, workplace health, safety and accident prevention, childcare and self-help networks
3. *Reducing structural barriers to mental health*, e.g. reducing discrimination and inequalities, combating stigma, promoting equal access to education, housing, services and support.

[Adapted from NeLH/Mentality 2002 What is mental health promotion? Online. Available: www.nelh.nhs.uk 14 July 2006]

Student activity

Thinking back to your recent practice experience, consider which levels of mental health promotion you have been involved with.

Health promotion is a useful summary phrase that covers a broad range of activities aimed at improving positive health and preventing ill-health. The most well-known definition is that of the WHO (1984) who define health promotion as 'the process of enabling people to increase control over, and to improve, their health'.

The National Service Framework for Mental Health (DH 1999b) defines mental health promotion as any action to enhance the mental health and well-being of individuals, families, organizations and communities (Box 1.26). Standard 1 aims to ensure that health and social services working with individuals and communities reduce discrimination and promote social inclusion. In the policy document *Making it Happen: A Guide to Delivering Mental Health Promotion* (DH 2001a) there is a focus on preventing mental health problems by tackling issues related to wider health determinants which contribute to mental distress, e.g. bullying at school or in the workplace, reducing fear of crime and improving access to environmental or recreational services.

Emergence of health promotion

Health promotion grew from the WHO Health for All (HFA) movement, the original title being HFA by the Year 2000 (WHO 1977). The Declaration of Alma-Ata (WHO 1978) was the birth of the HFA movement and its values underpin contemporary health promotion, with its aims and principles cascading from international level to inform national legislation. The Alma-Ata declaration states that health for all:

- Involves the population as a whole in the context of their everyday life, rather than focusing on people at risk of specific diseases
- Is directed towards action on the causes or determinants of health to ensure that the total environment which is beyond the control of individuals is conducive to health
- Combines diverse, but complementary, methods or approaches
- Aims particularly at effective public participation, supporting the principle of self-help movements
- Is an activity in the health and social fields but is not a medical service, yet health professionals in primary care have an important role.

Box 1.27 **The Declaration of Alma-Ata**

This declaration was made in the context of:

- 800 million of the world's population being in absolute poverty
- A third of all deaths being in the under-5 age group
- Up to 95% of people in developing countries having no access to health services.

It expressed the need for urgent action by all governments, health and development workers and the world community to protect and promote the health of all of the people of the world.

The main foci of the Alma-Ata declaration were:

- State responsibility for health
- Action in social/economic sectors
- Recognizing health inequalities in and between countries
- Sustainable economic and social development leading to increased quality of life
- Participation by individuals and communities to increase their health.

[Based on WHO 1978]

The centrality of primary care (or primary healthcare) to health promotion was first acknowledged here and it remains a key feature of all HFA declarations. Primary care is the first tier of health provision, provided by generalists in the local community 'as close as possible to where people live and work' (WHO 1978). Members of the primary healthcare team include general practitioners (GPs), practice nurses, health visitors, dentists, opticians and pharmacists. Other key aspects of the Alma-Ata declaration are summarized in Box 1.27.

The Ottawa Charter (WHO 1986) is arguably the most important health promotion document, providing the underpinning philosophy and setting the scene for all later developments. It described prerequisites of health as peace, education, shelter, food, income, social justice, a stable economy and sustainable resources. Five major types of health action were to:

- Build healthy public policy
- Create supportive environments
- Strengthen community action

Box 1.28 **Principles of health promotion**

Health promotion programmes, policies and other organized activities should be planned and implemented so that health promotion can be:

- *Empowering*: Enabling individuals and communities to assume more power over the personal, socioeconomic and environmental factors that affect their health
- *Participatory*: Involving those concerned (the stakeholders) in all stages of planning, implementation and evaluation
- *Holistic*: Fostering physical, mental, social and spiritual dimensions of health
- *Intersectoral*: Involving the collaboration of agencies from relevant sectors
- *Equitable*: Guided by a concern for equity and social justice
- *Sustainable*: Bringing about changes that individuals and communities can maintain once initial funding has ended
- *Multistrategy*: Using a variety of approaches including policy development, organizational change, community development, legislation, advocacy, education and communication, in combination with one another.

[From WHO 1984]

- Develop personal skills
- Reorient health services towards primary care.

The Ottawa Charter also highlighted a future commitment to health promotion with emphasis on developing health-promoting policies and environments and working with communities, not just focusing on individual lifestyle behaviours.

Principles of health promotion

The WHO used the HFA principles to devise the principles of health promotion (WHO 1984), the key principles of which are shown in Box 1.28.

Health promotion and public health

It may be a source of confusion for students, and indeed health professionals, that there are two similar sounding phrases describing similar types of work – health promotion and public health. Health promotion means different things to different people and there are difficulties in distinguishing between this and public health. The Acheson Report (Acheson 1998) described public health as the science and art of preventing disease, prolonging life and promoting health through the organized efforts of society.

When comparing health promotion and public health, there are three main views expressed:

- Health promotion and public health are different
- Health promotion and public health are the same
- Health promotion overlaps with, or is part of, a broader concept called public health (Box 1.29).

Box 1.29 **Health promotion and public health**

1. Health promotion and public health are different

Health promotion can be seen as deriving from a more social model of health with a focus on healthy public policy, addressing determinants such as inequalities, using community approaches and advocacy. Public health can be described as an elaboration of the medical model, traditionally involving a focus on communicable disease, environmental health, screening and immunization.

2. Health promotion and public health are the same

Increasingly the two terms are used synonymously in the literature. Many universities have changed their postgraduate programme titles from Health Promotion to Public Health and in primary care the term public health is more commonly used than health promotion. Other phrases including health improvement and health gain also appear frequently in modern health policies.

3. Health promotion overlaps with, or is part of, a broader concept called public health

This may be the most common prevailing view. It is seen as unhelpful to describe health promotion as a separate entity and it should be seen as an integral part of public health. The Acheson Report (1998) clearly defines health promotion as part of the broader concept of public health. Health promotion has been described as the implementation arm of public health. The two entities can also be seen as having overlapping spheres of activity such as health education, strategic planning and legislation. Sometimes the phrase 'new public health' is used to include health promotion.

Box 1.30 shows the current focus in UK public health practice.

National health promotion organizations

Each UK country has its own agency or authority for health promotion. Students should explore the relevant links to their own country (see 'Useful websites', p. 35). Covering the whole of the UK, the Health Development Agency emerged in 2000 from the Health Education Authority (HEA), which it replaced.

England no longer has a national health education body and its core functions are undertaken by the Department of Health whose website covers specific topics including alcohol, children and families, drugs, immunization and sexual health.

Box 1.30 Current focus in public health practice

- Surveillance and assessment of the population's health and well-being
- Promoting and protecting the population's health and well-being
- Developing quality and risk management within an evaluative culture
- Collaborative working for health and well-being
- Developing health programmes and services and reducing inequalities
- Policy and strategy development, and implementation to improve health and well-being
- Working with and for communities to improve health and well-being
- Strategic leadership for health and well-being
- Research and development to improve health and well-being
- Ethically managing self, people and resources to improve health and well-being.

[Resource: Skills for Health 2004 Public health practice national competence framework. Online. Available: www.skillsforhealth.org.uk]

The Health Promotion Agency for Northern Ireland supports those working in the areas of health promotion and public health, as well as members of the public.

Health Promotion Wales arises from the Welsh National Assembly. Their website has links to the Chief Medical Officer website and supports the promotion of health and well-being in Wales. The National Public Health Service for Wales (NPHS) coordinates the activities of the public health resources of all health authorities in Wales, including laboratory services and communicable disease surveillance.

Scotland's agency is NHS Health Scotland which provides a national focus for collaborative work to improve health and reduce inequalities.

Values in current health promotion practice

The values that nurses and health promoters need for effective practice that underpins health promotion skills in the 21st century (Health Education Board for Scotland 2000) are:

- Being aware of and understanding health-related beliefs, attitudes and skills
- Creating opportunities to enable individuals to make choices and decisions for themselves
- Encouraging individuals, families, groups and communities to identify their health-related needs and to work in partnership together
- Developing and supporting health promoting environments and encouraging different sectors to work together
- Considering health as an integral aspect of life
- Promoting the view that social and emotional security, and mental and spiritual well-being, are as important to overall well-being as physical health
- Recognizing influences working against health, e.g. marketing of cigarettes or advertising of junk food, unemployment, pollution and homelessness
- Recognizing the impact that life circumstances have on health
- Working towards reducing life and health inequalities.

Settings and skills for health promotion

Health promotion covers a wide range of activities which take place in many settings. NHS settings include hospitals and primary care. It also takes place in communities, voluntary organizations, workplaces, schools, in self-help groups and through the media. The skills used in health promotion also vary depending on the:

- Type of activity undertaken
- Client group
- Setting (see Chs 3, 9 and 14).

Health promotion skills are very similar to those of modern nurses and include needs assessment, planning and research, evaluation, communication, a counselling approach, management, networking, teaching, marketing, influencing policy and practice change, writing and publication.

Approaches to health promotion

Bottom-up and top-down approaches are the two main views of health promotion. They represent issues of power, control and relationships differently and this underpins their use in health promotion settings.

'Bottom-up' refers to the generation of issues, concerns and expressed needs from clients themselves rather than the experts being in charge. In this approach, clients are encouraged to be participative, taking an active part, or even the lead role, in identifying what they need in terms of information or assistance.

'Top-down' is the opposite approach and describes situations where the nurse or health promoter takes the lead and identifies concerns for, or on behalf of, clients. This approach is also described as expert led. Here, there is less client participation and less equality in the relationship. Sometimes, there is no contact with the client at all as in the case of TV health campaigns. Health advertisements try to market health in the same way as other products and often use celebrity endorsement. Health promotion through the media is also top-down as it has been planned and designed by experts and is one-way and impersonal. It is increasingly common for health and illness-related themes to be addressed through TV dramas and soap operas.

There are five ways of thinking about or viewing health promotion: medical, behavioural change, educational, client-centred and societal approaches.

The medical approach

This approach to health promotion is about encouraging people to seek medical help and to comply with prescribed treatment. It employs top-down methods to ensure that patients to cooperate and comply. The aim is to reduce risk factors and prevent ill-health. Methods include preventative procedures such as immunization and screening, in addition to information-giving and persuasive advice about lifestyle changes, e.g. giving up smoking. The latter can be carried out in person, by leaflets or through the mass media, e.g. television advertisements.

The behavioural change approach

Using this approach encourages individuals to make positive health-related changes, however small, e.g. encouraging people in the workplace to increase their exercise levels by using the stairs instead of taking the lift. Other commonly targeted lifestyle behaviours include smoking, alcohol use, diet and nutrition. The aim of this approach remains the prevention of disease by reduction of associated risk factors. It remains a top-down, expert-led approach, although participation may be encouraged.

The educational approach

This approach can be undertaken with individuals but more often involves group work. Group work is considered to be essential to explore and challenge people's attitudes, clarify misconceptions and ensure that the knowledge which people need to make informed decisions is available. Communication skills are key to this approach (see Ch. 9).

This approach may also focus on skills development as well as knowledge and attitudes. For example, within the subject of healthy eating, budgeting or cooking skills may be practised.

This approach can either use bottom-up strategies or be directive and expert-led, depending on the design of the session.

The client-centred approach

This is a wholly bottom-up strategy where clients, either individuals or groups, identify their own concerns or areas where they need more information or assistance. Clients are seen as full equals in the process and the aim of this approach is empowerment, i.e. clients are enabled to maintain or increase control over their own lives. This means that the health promoter does not take charge of the situation but acts only as a facilitator. Often this approach is carried out in community groups where, for example, a local mother and toddler group may raise concerns about safety and local road crossings.

The societal approach

This approach is large scale and often seen as political. It frequently involves a focus on broader social and environmental determinants of health. It can be bottom-up in approach, e.g. where night-duty nurses organized a petition, lobbied managers and caterers and then successfully negotiated healthier food choices at night in their hospital canteen. It can also be top-down, e.g. when central government made seat belt wearing compulsory by law or local rules enforced no-smoking areas at work.

Societal change usually requires fundamental and far-reaching political action which is beyond the scope of individuals. This is especially true when trying to reduce inequalities in health by, for example, addressing minimum wage legislation and levels of state benefits.

Models of health promotion

Models of health promotion are theoretical frameworks giving examples of health promotion activities such as preventative health services, health education, community-based work, public policies and organizational development, and economic and regulatory activities. These activities can be at international, national, regional or local levels.

Tannahill's model of health promotion

The Tannahill model (Fig. 1.5) defines health promotion as comprising efforts to enhance positive health and prevent ill-health, though the three overlapping spheres of:

- Health education
- Prevention (of ill-health)
- Health protection.

Health education is defined in Tannahill's model as communication activity aimed at enhancing positive health and preventing or diminishing ill-health. This can be carried out with individuals or groups, through influencing the beliefs, attitudes and behaviour of those with power and of the community at large. This is considered further in the next section.

Prevention of ill-health is described by Tannahill as activities concerned with reducing the risk of occurrence of ill-health, or an unwanted event. Different levels of

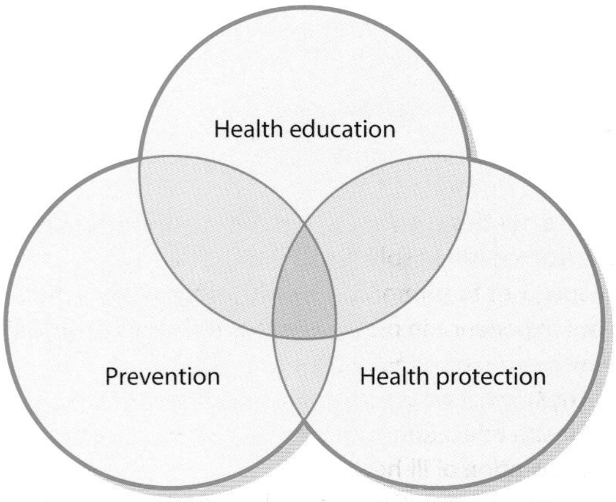

Fig. 1.5 The Tannahill model (reproduced with permission from Naidoo and Wills 2000)

prevention exist and activities from adult nursing are used as examples:

- Primary prevention of the first occurrence of a given illness or other unwanted phenomena, e.g. immunization
- Secondary prevention of the avoidable consequences of an illness through early detection and treatment, e.g. screening
- Tertiary prevention of the avoidable complications of an established irreversible disease, e.g. rehabilitation.

Box 1.31 shows levels of prevention applied to other nursing settings.

The third sphere of activity in the Tannahill model is health protection which includes the public policy framework for prevention of ill-health and positive enhancement of well-being. It includes legal, fiscal and political measures, e.g. tobacco tax, or policies, laws and codes of practice, e.g. seat belt legislation. Another example of legislation for health is the policy document *Valuing People: A New Strategy for Learning Disability for the 21st Century* (DH 2001c) which was the first government White Paper about people with learning disabilities for 30 years and seeks to legislate to address the inequalities of access to services (see also Valuing people website in 'Useful websites', p. 35).

The Tannahill model is straightforward and easy to use, fitting well with nursing and other healthcare practice in primary care and NHS settings. However, it has been criticized for its medical model approach, its largely individual focus and the lack of emphasis on social determinants of health and illness. It may be less helpful in community settings and when working with disadvantaged or excluded groups. The activities in Box 1.32 will help you apply the Tannahill model of health promotion to nursing practice.

HEALTH PROMOTION Box 1.31

Levels of Prevention

Learning disability nursing
- Primary prevention – self-care education, e.g. dental hygiene
- Secondary prevention – screening for sensory deficits
- Tertiary prevention – management of epilepsy.

Mental health nursing
- Primary prevention – self-care education, e.g. safe use of prescribed medicines, stress management
- Secondary prevention – screening, using a mental health assessment tool
- Tertiary prevention – rehabilitation techniques for schizophrenia.

Child health nursing
- Primary prevention – positive parenting strategies, accident prevention for toddlers
- Secondary prevention – preschool child development checks
- Tertiary prevention – nebulizer training for parents of children with asthma.

REFLECTIVE PRACTICE Box 1.32

The Tannahill model in practice

Student activities
1. Look at the 'three spheres of activity' that the Tannahill model uses to summarize health promotion. Think about your experience in practice and identify nursing activities which could be defined as:
   - Health protection
   - Health education
   - Prevention of ill-health.
2. Identify opportunities for health promotion in your placement.

The Tones model

An empowerment model of health promotion was devised by Tones in 1993. It aims to enable people to gain control over their own health and in this way it sounds very similar to the important WHO (1986) definition of health promotion. A summary of the model (Tones & Tilford 2001) reads like a formula:

Health promotion = health education × healthy public policy.

The full model is more complex than the Tannahill model. Starting at the bottom of Figure 1.6, education is seen as critical to the process of raising awareness so that people can make informed health choices, participate in and influence health policy. This applies to both lay people and health professionals. In this model, healthy social and environmental factors are emphasized and this view fits better with bottom-up, community-based approaches as in mental health, learning disability and voluntary organizations. It may be harder to envisage this model in relation to working within a traditional NHS setting.

Health education

Although people may use the terms health promotion and health education interchangeably, they are not the same. As seen above, health education is just one part of health promotion and is only one of many methods available to the nurse or health promoter. It has been mentioned above as one of the five approaches to health promotion (see p. 24) and forms one-third of health promotion according to the Tannahill model (see Fig. 1.5). Health education was also described as one half of the summarized Tones Model (see Fig. 1.6).

There are many diverse definitions of health education, some of which are listed below. Health education (as adapted from Kiger 1995) can be described as:

- A communication activity, e.g. the Tannahill model
- Persuading people to adopt and sustain healthful life practices

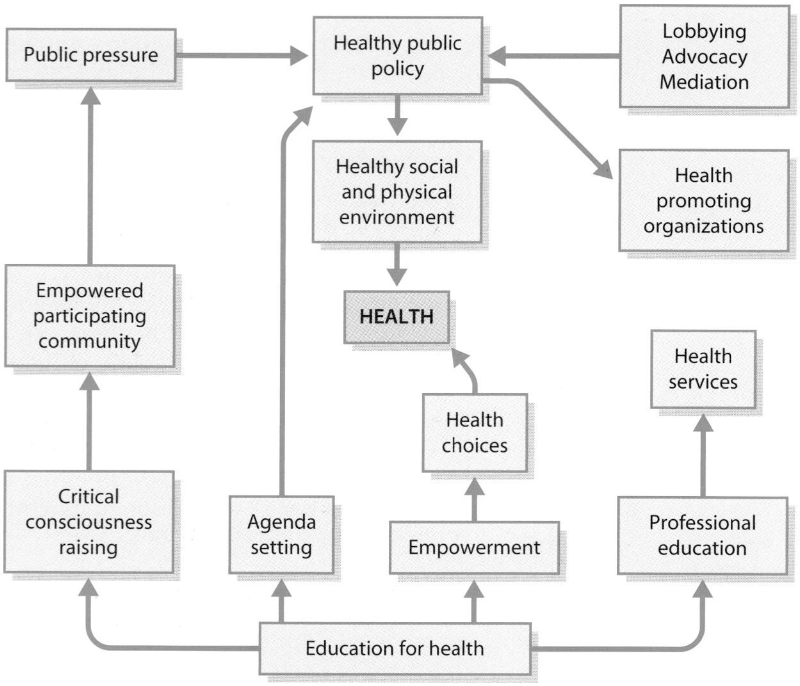

Fig. 1.6 The Tones model of health promotion (reproduced with permission from Naidoo and Wills 2000)

- Developing people's skills in decision-making and clarifying beliefs and values about health
- Changing the knowledge, feelings and behaviour of people
- An information-giving activity
- Persuading people to use available health services wisely
- Enabling people to improve their own health
- Enabling people to control their own health, e.g. the Tones model
- Assisting communities to engage in conflict with powerful authorities
- Seeking to modify behaviours responsible for disease
- Seeking the roots of health problems and finding them in social, economic and political factors.

HEALTH PROMOTION Box 1.33

Health education approaches

Student activities

- Look at the list of health education definitions (pp. 25–26) and identify similarities and differences in their approaches.
- Consider the five approaches to health education and the examples of related health education activities and compare them with the health promotion approaches described on p. 24. Note the similarities.
- Identify which of the approaches to health education are used in health education activities in your placement.

Approaches to health education

Kiger (1995) described five approaches to health education: medical, educational, media/propaganda, community development and political action. These can be compared to the five approaches to health promotion explained earlier (p. 24). The approaches to health education are outlined below with examples of the likely methods used:

- The medical approach to health education assumes that rational facts will persuade people to change their health-related behaviour. Methods include expert advice, talks, lectures, booklets and leaflets, alone or in combination.
- The educational approach to health education does not mean instruction in the same way as the medical model but rather 'leading to learning'. It uses people-centred methods such as discussion groups, problem-solving, values clarification, skills teaching, role play and peer work.
- The media/propaganda approach to health education has been described as manipulation for health. Like the medical model it uses the mass media, TV and radio advertisements and markets health as if it were a product.
- The community development approach centres on enabling and empowering people. It uses bottom-up methods that include assisting people to organize, change, raise awareness or gain consensus.
- The political action approach seeks to promote societal or political change. It uses methods such as providing evidence, lobbying, mobilizing local support and exploring anti-health agencies.

The activities in Box 1.33 will help you think about health education approaches used in your placement.

EVIDENCE-BASED PRACTICE Box 1.34

The positive effects of health information

Hayward (1975) found that the positive effects of preoperative health information and education for patients included:

- Improved informed consent
- Greater patient satisfaction
- Increased compliance with treatment programmes
- Better progress and outcomes
- Reduced levels of distress during invasive procedures
- Reduced anxiety levels
- Reduced pain and need for analgesic drugs (see Ch. 23)
- Faster recovery times
- Shorter hospital stays.

Student activities

- Reflect on the possible benefits of patient education listed above and identify examples from your personal experience when having information helped you or a family member.
- Identify examples from your placement experience when having information helped a patient/client or their family.

Health education in the NHS

A medical approach to health education is sometimes known as patient education in NHS settings. Methods such as 1:1 talks/interactions, group work and written information, alone or in combination, have been shown to increase patients' knowledge and understanding of their symptoms, illness, surgery, drugs or other treatments. Effective communication skills are vital to people's understanding of information provided (Ch. 9).

As long ago as 1975, Hayward's research demonstrated that there are positive effects when patients know what to expect and are prepared by being provided with suitable information prior to clinical procedures (Box 1.34).

Levels of health education

As well as having different approaches, health education is also described as having different levels: primary, secondary and tertiary.

Primary health education

Primary health education involves a focus on the structure and function of the body or mind, how bodies or relationships work and how to promote and maintain them. Nurses carry out much primary health education in their everyday practice, e.g. each time information is given before informed consent is sought, lifestyle advice is offered or a procedure or treatment is explained to patients. It is usually undertaken with individuals but can be carried out in groups.

Undertaking health education with learning disability clients can be challenging because they have more complex health needs than the general population but tend not to have equity of access to health services (Gates 2003). This is also true for people from black or ethnic minority communities (NHS Health Scotland 2004). The Scottish Executive (2000) identifies seven fundamental principles, which state that people with learning disability should be:

- Valued
- Treated as individuals
- Asked about what they need and be involved in choices
- Given the help and support to do what they want to do
- Able to get local services like everyone else
- Able to get specialist services when they need them
- Able to have services which take account of age, abilities and needs.

Some people with learning disabilities learn at a slower pace and key considerations for health education are summarized in Box 1.35.

HEALTH PROMOTION Box 1.35

Health education for people with learning disabilities

Gates (2003) identifies key considerations when planning health education for clients with learning disabilities. Activities should be:

- Interactive and designed to meet the needs of particular clients
- Conducted in an unhurried fashion, in a supportive and non-judgemental environment
- Systematic in planning and delivery so that material is presented in small chunks lasting no more than 30–40 minutes
- Based on everyday life, e.g. healthy eating education being reinforced during shopping trips
- Planned so that repetition and opportunities to practise are provided
- Provided using the appropriate level of language for each client, with suitable visual aids and other learning materials.

Student activity

Review the principles above and reflect on your placement experience with a client who had learning disabilities.

Secondary health education

This takes the form of information and advice about services to improve and maintain health, how to get the best out of healthcare and other systems, what is available and how to complain if necessary. Nurses may also carry out secondary health education in their everyday practice, but perhaps less often than primary level health education. In all settings, but especially in community nursing, nurses have to help people to:

- Understand their rights
- Obtain contact details for community-based services
- Be referred to agencies, e.g. housing associations
- Gain access to complaints/suggestions forms.

HEALTH PROMOTION Box 1.36

Examples of health education

Student activity

Reflect on which level(s) of health education you have seen used in nursing practice and identify examples of:

- Primary health education
- Secondary health education
- Tertiary health education.

Another empowering resource for people is the Patient Advocacy Liaison Service (PALS). This government initiative ensures that each Trust has PALS officers to provide help, information, advice and support locally and to help address any concerns or problems experienced by patients and their families.

Tertiary health education

The highest level is tertiary health education which focuses on raising awareness of the sociopolitical health determinants such as unemployment, education, pollution, water and food quality, and traffic levels. Another focus is the activities of the anti-health sector of the economy such as advertising and sponsorship by tobacco companies. This is sometimes called consciousness raising and is common in bottom-up work with community-based groups. In general, it is less common for nurses to carry out this level of health education compared to the other two. Although not often part of mainstream NHS work, tertiary health education features in the education of health professionals and may include study of poverty, inequalities and other health determinants. Box 1.36 will help you consider levels of health education in nursing practice.

UK health policy context

By 1986, the WHO's main target for the following decades was that all citizens of the world should attain a level of health that would permit them to lead socially and economically productive lives by the year 2000. The European region of the WHO later introduced Health21, namely 21 targets for the 21st century, to achieve this goal (WHO 1998).

The first UK national targets for health were set in 1992 and each UK country devised its own targets and strategy documents. A further round of revised White Papers on health and healthcare appeared in 1999 following political devolution. *The Jakarta Declaration on Health Promotion into the 21st Century* (WHO 1997) was incorporated into all four national documents with collaborative working as the dominant theme.

While the aims described in the policy documents of all four UK countries are similar in their focus on tackling health inequalities and social exclusion, they are quite different in the use of language, approach and in their organizational development. Despite emphasis on integrated policies and collaborative services, the UK has been described as developing four distinct health services (Muir & Sidey 2000). This is complex for health professionals so it is recommended that emphasis be placed on the policies relating to the reader's own UK country. These policies can be accessed on links from the homepages of each country's national agency for health. Box 1.37 gives examples of some key health policy documents.

Box 1.37 **Key health policy documents**

England
- *The New NHS* (DH 1997)
- *Saving Lives: Our Healthier Nation* (DH 1999)
- *NHS Plan* (DH 2000)
- *Wanless Reports* (HM Treasury 2002/2004)
- *Choosing Health* (DH 2004)

Scotland
- *Designed to Care* (DH 1997)
- *Towards A Healthier Scotland* (Scottish Executive 1999)
- *Improving Health in Scotland – The Challenge* (Scottish Executive 2003)
- *Partnerships in Care* (Scottish Executive 2003)

Wales
- *Putting Patients First* (DH 1997)

Northern Ireland
- *Fit for the Future* (DH 1999)

The health White Paper, *Saving Lives: Our Healthier Nation* (DH 1999a) was heavily influenced by the Jakarta Declaration, the Health21 targets, and the political and ideological changes of the Labour government that came to power in 1997. It was described as 'the first comprehensive Government plan' (DH 1999b). This public health strategy for England was published with twin goals: to improve health of everyone, and to reduce the health of the worst off in particular.

It was the first time that a government had formally acknowledged that poverty equated directly with poorer health. The strategy aimed to prevent up to 300000 untimely and unnecessary deaths by the year 2010. 'Tougher but attainable targets' sought to reduce the:

- cancer death rate in people under 75 by at least 20%
- CHD and stroke death rates in people under 75 by at least 40%
- accident death rate by at least 20% and the serious injury rate by at least 10%
- death rate from suicide by at least 20%.

The NHS Plan (DH 2000) recognizes that, despite its many achievements, the NHS has failed to keep pace with changes in society. It states that there is no greater injustice than inequalities in health, and outlines options for funding healthcare and for investments in NHS facilities and NHS staff in England. The plan outlines a new delivery system for the NHS as well as changes between health and social services, and changes for NHS doctors, nurses, midwives, therapists and other NHS staff. The plan also outlines changes for patients and in the relationship between the NHS and the private sector. In addition, the plan sets out strategies for cutting waiting times for treatment, improving health and reducing inequality. Actions for tackling clinical priorities and for services to older people are discussed and the reform programme outlined.

Derek Wanless, the former chief of the NatWest Bank, was commissioned by the UK government to review the future of healthcare with emphasis on preventative health measures and health inequalities. In 2002, Wanless published his first report *Securing Our Future Health: Taking a Long-term View* and later updated this. His final report *Securing Good Health for the Whole Population* was published in 2004.

The reports assessed the resources required to provide high quality health services in England, how public health spending decisions are taken and how to ensure cost effectiveness. The report included information on the main causes of mortality, morbidity and key risk factors in England, including trends over time. Wanless avoided making specific recommendations but broadly stated that more research should be carried out before embarking on expensive public health initiatives. Furthermore, he stated that the government should assemble stronger evidence on cost effectiveness, before setting priorities.

The White Paper *Choosing Health: Making Healthier Choices Easier* (DH 2004) sets out key principles for supporting the public to make healthier and more informed choices regarding their health. It seeks to provide information and practical support to motivate people, and improve their emotional well-being and access to services so that healthy choices are easier to make. The key areas of action include inequalities, children and young people, the health-promoting NHS, work and health, and national and local delivery.

CRITICAL THINKING Box 1.38

Demographic trends in the UK

The data below come from the 2001 Census and are available from National Statistics online:

- The live birth rate has risen slightly and, combined with falling death rates, has contributed to the population of the UK slowly increasing. 2003 figures put the total UK population at just over 59 million
- In 2002, 19.8 million of the population were 50 years or over. By 2031 this is projected to rise to 27 million
- Older women outnumber older men and by age 85 years there are 2.6 women for every man
- The average age for women giving birth is 29.4 years.

Student activity

Go to National Statistics online at www.statistics.gov.uk and search the database for information on other health-related topics, e.g. life expectancy, ethnicity, lone-parent families, disability or age on marriage.

Measuring health and illness

Demography refers to the study of populations, with data gathered on the age, gender and size of groups within the population and the geographical spread or migration of those groups. It also covers what are known as vital statistics: births, marriages, divorces, separations and deaths. Box 1.38 shows some examples of UK demographic trends.

Epidemiology is the study of the occurrence, patterns and spread of disease in a population. The data can demonstrate the scale of a health problem and its trends, showing changes in mortality and morbidity over time. Epidemiological data can highlight the natural history and progression of a disease, e.g. Snow's 19th century work demonstrated that cholera spread from infected water pumps and was important in proving the existence of germ theory. Causation can be established when there is evidence that exposure to a particular environmental, lifestyle or socioeconomic factor contributes to ill-health and it was using these methods that the causal link between smoking and lung cancer was proven. Epidemiology can also show the severity of a problem and predict the ways in which individuals or communities may be affected. It can assess the likelihood, or probability, of a disease or condition occurring as well as suggesting how it can be tackled or prevented. Later, follow-up evaluation studies may show whether changes can be attributed to particular interventions.

Purposes of measuring health and illness

Health and illness can be measured in many ways and for many reasons. Measuring health and illness in communities provides the opportunity for:

- Assessing a population's health status
- Describing the patterns of disease in populations, in either small groups or whole countries
- Analysing differences between one population and another and, over time, identifying trends
- Directing interventions appropriately, therefore increasing the population's health and maximizing health potential
- Identifying and responding to specific needs of minority groups or sections of the population whose health needs have not been fully met
- Targeting at-risk groups to reduce inequalities in health
- Making resource allocation more equitable
- Influencing policy, research or development of priorities (Pencheon et al 2001).

In addition to measuring ill-health or death, information on the health status of people is also collected, e.g. height, weight and dental health. Such data act as a baseline, allowing comparisons over time and identification of trends. Another area of study is health behaviour

Box 1.39 **Examples of demographic and epidemiological data**

- Mortality and morbidity rates
- Reasons for primary healthcare consultations
- Immunization rates
- Screening rates
- Accident rates
- HIV, AIDS notifications
- NHS waiting lists
- Children at risk register
- Child developmental health records
- Poverty/inequality measures, e.g. Jarman index of disadvantage
- Sociodemographic statistics.

[From Naidoo and Wills 2000]

indicators related to individual lifestyle, e.g. smoking status. Environmental indicators are also measured, e.g. air and water quality, housing type and density. Social environment indicators include wealth, income and social class, with one particular focus being the measurement of deprivation. There are many measurements used to identify underprivileged areas with a view to improving or targeting services. Two of the most well-known deprivation measurement tools are the Jarman index and the Townsend index, both of which take into account indicators such as social housing and lack of car ownership.

The advantage of epidemiological and demographic studies is that information is collected regularly, it is relatively consistent and readily available. It is sometimes known as routinely available data and examples are shown in Box 1.39. Both of these quantitative sciences are largely concerned with numerical descriptions relating to groups of people. They do not focus on individuals but instead study the vital statistics or the ill-health of populations within society.

Common methods of health and illness measurement

The common methods of measurement are counts and rates:

- Counts are the simplest numerical description, e.g. 14 people in a nursing home have diarrhoea.
- Rates are the number of affected people expressed as a proportion of a total population. Following the example above, if 14 people are affected out of a total nursing home population of 56, then the rate is 14/56 or 25%.

Percentages are the commonest way to express proportions. Sometimes, the numbers per 1000, per 10 000 or per 1 000 000 are used instead of per 100 (percentage).

Incidence

Incidence, or incidence rate, refers to the rate of development, i.e. the new cases, of a disease or problem rather than the total number of people affected in a given period, usually 1 year. The number of people developing a disease in a group of known size over a specific period of time can be expressed in this way. For example, the incidence of depression in men aged 55–59 years in a particular country was 252 per 100 000 for the year 2002–2003. This means that there were 252 new cases of depression for every 100 000 of the population in this age group during the given year.

A mortality rate is similar to incidence except it refers to the number of deaths from a condition in a particular group during a period of time. SMR refers to standardized mortality ratio and uses the formula below:

$$\text{SMR} = \frac{\text{observed deaths in study population}}{\text{expected deaths in study population}} \times 100$$

The observed death rate in a defined population is compared to the rate expected in a standard population, e.g. the ratio of the rate of lung cancer deaths in smokers compared to that of non-smokers. Therefore, if the SMR is less than 100, the mortality experience of the study population is less than that of the reference population.

Prevalence

Prevalence, or prevalence rate, refers to the total number of people with a disease or condition in a group at a specific time. For example, the prevalence of chickenpox in a preschool nursery on a given day was 10%.

Distribution

Another key term used in epidemiology and demography is distribution. This refers to the spread of a problem or disease by age, gender, race, ethnicity, socioeconomic class, geography or other variable.

Other approaches to measurement of health and illness

Other than epidemiological study, there are three other main approaches commonly used in health and illness measurement: needs assessment, social audit and community profiling. The agency undertaking the measurement exercise and the purpose of the study determine the approach taken. The focus of study may be:

- Using routinely available data or gathering primary data (new research)
- At the individual level or whole populations
- Exploring illness and disease or broader health determinants
- Top-down or bottom-up (see p. 23)
- Primarily using epidemiological data or community participation.

Needs assessment

This is commonly used in health and social care settings, especially in community-based work. It is described as the first phase in health promotion planning, namely identifying what a client or population group needs to enable them to be more healthy (Naidoo & Wills 2000).

An individual approach to needs assessment focuses on a person's lifestyle and behaviours, such as smoking status. The purpose of this is to gather data directly from the individuals in the community under study to inform health promotion planning for behaviour change and risk factor modification. No account is taken of the socioeconomic context or the social and environmental health determinants affecting individuals' lives, leading to criticism that this is measurement of 'behaviour in a vacuum' (Perkins et al 1999).

Population-based needs assessment, or health needs assessment, is used by statutory bodies to measure health needs in defined populations. In the health arena, statutory bodies are centrally funded agencies, e.g. health authorities, local authorities and health promoting organizations, which undertake health-related work on behalf of the government.

One example of a population-based needs assessment is the Learning Disability Needs Assessment (NHS Health Scotland 2004), which highlighted changes in demographical trends, such as the:

- Increasing number of people with learning disability
- Increasing number of people with complex and multiple needs related to physical and learning disability
- Increasing number of older adults with learning disability
- High prevalence of health need, especially unmet health needs
- Different mortality causes, e.g. high rates of oesophageal cancer.

Needs assessment uses an epidemiological approach and tends to be top-down, with limited community involvement. Quantifiable, secondary information is used with heavy reliance on available data such as Census and electoral ward information. Electoral wards are the key building blocks of UK administrative geography and data are held by the Office for National Statistics (see 'Useful websites', p. 35).

Needs assessment focuses on ill-health and the determinants of disease by measuring the incidence, prevalence and degree of severity of various health problems in a population, although causal links are not always obvious (Perkins et al 1999). For example, an increase in the level of youth suicide may be identified in a town but not the reasons behind it.

Social audit

Social audit is a broader approach to health and illness measurement than needs assessment. This is used by a wide variety of voluntary, statutory or community organizations to assess need at local, city or district levels and is wider in scope than lifestyle factors or ill-health rates. Social audit is underpinned by a broad and more social definition of health and health determinants. The interplay of resources, e.g. environment, housing, transport and employment, is a major focus.

Social audit often involves the collection of new primary data and is increasingly called health impact assessment. It tends to be top-down but includes a variable amount of community participation. It has been described as a socioeconomic approach to needs assessment which uses a wide range of quantitative, secondary data to give a view 'of' a community, rather than 'from' a community (Perkins et al 1999). This approach is professionally led and encourages multiagency working because different disciplines need to be involved, e.g. health promoters may be working with local councillors, transport consultants and environmental health specialists to consider the impact of traffic in a community.

Community profiling

Community profiling is the approach commonly used by local health boards, local authorities and councils to measure and evaluate the health and social needs of their populations. Its focus is how local people view their health and social needs in their community. The aim of community profiles is to obtain accurate and appropriate information from local people which is then used to support epidemiological and population data. This is often considered to be the most balanced and helpful approach to measurement of health and illness, as it uses both top-down and bottom-up strategies in the assessment. Community nurses, health visitors and those working in health promotion and public health are often involved in compiling these profiles. Many student nurses undertake a small community profile as part of their coursework.

Community profiling is sometimes known as the community participation approach to needs assessment. It uses client-centred methods and is underpinned by the concept of empowerment. It is described as 'done with' not 'done to' the community (Perkins et al 1999). The degree of community involvement is highly variable in this approach but it tends not to be dominated by professionals.

One potential problem in community profiling is trying to encourage meaningful community participation. Any assessment of community needs seeking public involvement needs to use creative methods of data collection to prevent 'tokenism'. In addition to questionnaires and local surveys, more creative methods of community participation in data collection or evaluation include focus groups, 1:1 interviews, photographs, collage, examples of work from community groups, audiotapes, video work and drama.

Another potential problem is that community involvement can raise unrealistic expectations. Community profiling tends to identify large numbers of needs that cannot all be tackled due to staff, time and financial constraints. Delays or perceived inaction can dishearten participants in the data collection who may have high expectations of change and improvements in their community health and social services.

Priorities

Of the many identified health needs arising from the assessment process, some needs take precedence because

HEALTH PROMOTION Box 1.40

Health Improvement Programmes

Health Improvement Programmes (HImPs) are a cornerstone of current health promotion strategy.

Student activity
Find the HImP for your local area using an online search engine and identify:

- Local priorities for funding and programme development
- National and local targets within the HImP.

they are considered more important than others. They are therefore tackled first and this is called prioritizing, or priority setting. Health economists refer to this as rationing, describing finite resources but infinite needs.

The reasons why one particular issue becomes a priority are many and varied. It may be simply that the local health professional's personal interest area or expertise is the deciding factor in which need is tackled first or in what order needs are addressed. Usually, however, priorities are set in line with a central or local policy either alone or in combination, for example:

- National or central government agenda and targets
- Local authority agenda and targets
- Resources and funding availability
- Local people's identified priority.

Health Improvement Programmes (HImPs)

Needs assessment and priority setting at a local level are requirements of each primary care trust in England in collaboration with key stakeholders, e.g. local authorities, voluntary organizations, health professionals and community representatives. This collaborative activity forms the basis of HImPs which are strategic plans to address health, healthcare and services needs in a local area. A key aim of HImPs is to encourage different agencies to work together in a more integrated manner. Programmes can then be developed to tackle inequalities and promote social inclusion.

Priorities for HImPs can be nationally set targets arising from *Saving Lives: Our Healthier Nation* (DH 1999a) such as the delivery of SureStart, services for preschool children and their parents. Local targets for health improvement can also be listed as priorities when they are issues of particular relevance to an area, e.g. under-age drinking in a town centre. Find out about the HImP for your local area by undertaking the activities in Box 1.40.

Illness behaviour

When people are ill their reactions to it are described as illness behaviour, i.e. what they do and how they respond to their changing health state. Illness behaviour is complex and occurs in the context of the family or support system and it is sometimes said that it is not individuals who become ill, but the whole family. The study of illness behaviour focuses on people's experience of illness, their interpretation of, and reactions to, symptoms which may limit their normal function or activities, and how chronically ill individuals cope with the practical and emotional demands of their illness.

Increasingly, instead of illness behaviour, it is called 'illness action' to emphasize the fact that people are active participants in dealing with their own (and others') illness. Each person reacts differently to illness, or the threat of it, in terms of both their behaviour and emotions. Different illness reactions make it crucial that nurses understand and empathize with the experiences of their patients and clients in order to plan suitable, individualized care interventions. The components of Becker's health belief model (p. 11) – including culture, gender, the person's attitude to the illness and their family's reaction to it – are variables which may affect illness behaviour. Another major influence is the nature of the illness itself as patient/client reactions may depend on whether the problem is:

- Short or long term
- Life threatening or not serious
- Sudden or acute in onset
- Chronic, recurring or progressive in pattern (see Ch. 11)
- Disfiguring or not.

Self-help

Most symptoms are dealt with by people themselves without seeking formal medical help. Self-treatment with over-the-counter (OTC) medicines bought from supermarkets, corner shops or pharmacies is increasingly common as is the use of homeopathic and other complementary treatments.

It is common for people to use a lay referral system where they ask trusted friends, colleagues or family members for advice about symptoms or treatment. Sometimes it is the lay 'referees' who diagnose and recommend an OTC medicine from the pharmacy. They may also strongly suggest that the person seeks medical help and exert pressure until they comply. This is known as 'sanctioning by significant others'.

The effects of illness

Illness, especially when serious, chronic or life threatening, can have far-reaching effects on a wide range of issues such as the ability to function physically or mentally, coping with increased stress, family roles and dynamics, caring roles, work roles, finances, body image, self-concept and self-esteem. Reactions to serious illness sometimes resemble loss and bereavement responses such as shock, denial and disbelief (see Chs 11, 12).

Help-seeking behaviour

In the sociology of health and illness, help-seeking behaviour is a major theme for study which seeks to answer questions such as:

- Why do some people seek medical help for particular symptoms while others do not?
- What factors increase the likelihood of people seeking medical help?

The more visible, frequent and disruptive in day-to-day life a symptom is, the more likely a person is to seek medical help (Box 1.41). This, however, must be set in the context of the person's knowledge, their estimate of the seriousness of the symptoms and the family's tolerance of any restriction of role function caused by it.

There is sometimes a problem with the view that interruption to normal activity is seen as the main trigger for seeking help. For conditions with a slow, insidious onset, e.g. cancer, HIV or Alzheimer's disease, the person can carry on with normal activities for a lengthy period and there may be a considerable delay in seeking help, allowing symptoms to become more advanced before help is sought.

Box 1.41 **Determinants of help-seeking behaviour**

Mechanic (1978) described 10 determinants of help-seeking behaviour, i.e. factors that influence a person's decision to seek medical help:

- How visible a symptom is, e.g. obvious skin rash or limp
- The person's estimate of the seriousness of the symptom, e.g. sleep disturbance
- The person's knowledge and understanding about the symptom
- How much the symptom disrupts usual roles and function, e.g. family, work, social activities
- Frequency or persistence of symptoms, e.g. headache daily for more than 1 week
- How much the symptom is tolerated by family and friends, e.g. smoker's cough
- How much basic needs are affected by the symptom, e.g. dental pain restricting eating
- How much other needs compete with illness responses, e.g. too busy with child care to rest swollen feet
- How much the person has other reasons for the symptoms, e.g. low mood and tearfulness described as tiredness in the mother of a newborn infant
- How available medical help or treatment is in terms of access, cost and time as well as emotional costs like stigma, e.g. a person with possible symptoms of a sexually transmitted infection delays seeking help because of embarrassment.

[Resource: Mechanic D 1978 Medical sociology. Free Press, New York]

The sick role

Triggers that strongly influence a person's decision to see medical help frequently relate to the wider context of their life rather than the symptoms of ill-health directly. For example, someone experiencing interpersonal problems in their wider life is much more likely to notice physical symptoms and then seek help.

In 1952, Talcott Parsons proposed the concept of the sick role where illness is seen as abnormal and/or disrupting an individual's usual activities. Parsons believed that people learn the sick role through socialization starting in childhood and change their behaviour when trying to cope with illness. The sick role was described as temporary and conditional on the sick person cooperating to get well again as soon as possible. Parsons (1991) described three main tenets of the sick role:

- The sick person is not held personally responsible for their illness, meaning that they cannot be blamed for their situation as the cause of the illness is beyond their control. Illness is therefore seen as not resulting from personal behaviour or actions. Critique of this first tenet may involve its lack of application to some illnesses or conditions where blame is attributed, e.g. self-harm, STIs or substance misuse which all have moral overtones.
- The sick person has certain special rights including the privilege of withdrawing from normal tasks or responsibilities. The sick person may be expected not to attend work or school and is allowed to withdraw from household tasks. It might be permissible for the sick person to stay in bed and require to be looked after, but this is strictly temporary. Impolite behaviour may well be tolerated or excused because of the illness. Critique of this tenet is that it does not extend to people with disability. Restriction of activity and staying in bed is neither suitable nor required for people with chronic mental or physical illness. Withdrawal from activities, except in the short term, does not fit with modern concepts of rehabilitation (see Ch. 11).
- The sick person must actively try to get well by seeking expert help and following instructions in the 'patient role'. Parsons believed that the true sick role can only be conferred by a medical expert whose job it is to legitimize the illness. This removes any doubt that the sick person is malingering and makes the illness official. The patient is expected to cooperate and try to recover as soon as possible by obeying instructions such as adhering to prescribed treatments. Sick role status will not be granted, and sympathy and special rights quickly evaporate, if the sick person will not seek medical help or cooperate. There has been widespread criticism of the inappropriateness of the sick role concept in relation to people with incurable or terminal illness.

CRITICAL THINKING Box 1.42

The sick role

Student activities

Consider Parson's sick role and think about your experiences, both personal and from your clinical practice.

1. How well does the sick role explain your own experiences of ill-health?
2. Review the following situations and consider how appropriate the sick role is for:
   - A child with chickenpox
   - A teenager with appendicitis
   - A man with longstanding depressive illness
   - A woman with chronic fatigue syndrome/ME
   - A child with a learning disability and cerebral palsy
   - A woman who has recurrent migraine headaches.

The activities in Box 1.42 will help you think further about the sick role. It is interesting to note how congruent Parson's sick role concept is with the bio-medical view, reinforcing ideas that patients are passive. However, since the sick role was first described in the 1950s, nurses and healthcare workers are much more likely to expect patients to be actively involved in all aspects of their care.

Summary

- Personal definitions of health may vary widely from official definitions.
- Health is multidimensional in nature, encompassing physical, mental, emotional, social, spiritual and societal dimensions.
- The medical model is less dominant in contemporary approaches to health promotion.
- Health beliefs vary widely and understanding them is an essential part of nurses' involvement in health promotion activities.
- Changes in health behaviour often need to be preceded by change in people's attitudes and values but this is often difficult to achieve.
- Many factors influence health, the key determinant being poverty which is linked to inequalities in health.
- The Health for All movement and subsequent legislation underpin health promotion activities, which may take place at global, national and local levels.
- Health promotion includes a wide range of activities that are often targeted to particular groups. It takes place in many different settings and forms part of the role of all nurses. The overall aim determines the approach taken and methods used.
- Health education is part of health promotion – it also takes many forms and is carried out in a range of settings.
- Measuring health and illness can involve nurses and provides valuable information for healthcare planning.
- Illness behaviour includes self-help, lay referral systems, help-seeking behaviour and the sick role.
- People today have high expectations of health and healthcare.

Self test

1. State the WHO (1946) definition of health, explaining the phrase 'health is multidimensional'.
2. Outline some key determinants of health.
3. Differentiate between relative and absolute poverty.
4. Name some ancient health beliefs which are still prevalent today.
5. Compare and contrast approaches to health promotion and health education.

Key words and phrases for literature searching

Determinants of health
Dimensions of health
Health beliefs
Health definitions
Inequalities
Poverty

Useful websites

National agencies

Health Promotion Agency of Northern Ireland	www.healthpromotionagency.org.uk Available July 2006
Health Promotion Wales	www.hpw.wales.gov.uk Available July 2006
Health Protection Agency	www.hpa.org.uk Available July 2006
National Institute for Health and Clinical Excellence (*incorporates the former Health Development Agency*)	www.publichealth.nice.org.uk/ Available July 2006
National Public Health Service for Wales	www.wales.nhs.uk/sites/home.cfm?ORGID=368 Available July 2006
NHS Health Scotland	www.hebs.scot.nhs.uk Available July 2006
Patient Advice and Liaison Services (PALS)	www.dh.gov.uk/PolicyAndGuidance/OrganisationPolicy PatientAndPublicInvolvement/PatientAdviceAndLiaison Services/fs/en Available July 2006

Health topics

Alcohol	www.wrecked.co.uk Available July 2006
Drugs	http://talktofrank.com Available July 2006
Immunization	www.immunisation.nhs.uk *or* www.mmrthefacts.nhs.uk Available July 2006
Sexual health	www.playingsafely.co.uk Available July 2006

Health information and advice

Department of Health	www.dh.gov.uk Available July 2006
Learning disability policy	www.valuingpeople.gov.uk Available July 2006
Office for National Statistics	www.statistics.gov.uk Available July 2006

NHS Direct (Tel: 0845 4647) is a national helpline staffed 24 hours a day by qualified nursing staff. It offers information on the NHS and current health and illness issues.

NHS Direct Online (www.nhsdirect.nhs.uk) is the internet arm of NHS Direct and has links with NHS Direct Wales and NHS 24.

NHS Direct Wales (Tel: 0845 4647) offers the same service in Wales.

NHS 24 (Tel: 0845 24 24) provides a similar service in Scotland.

References

Acheson D 1998 Independent enquiry into inequalities in health. TSO, London
Barker P (ed) 2003 Psychiatric and mental health nursing. Arnold, London
Becker MH (ed) 1974 The health belief model and personal health behaviours. Slack, Thorofare, NJ
Blaxter M 1990 Health and lifestyles. Tavistock Routledge, London
British Heart Foundation 2003 CHD statistics database. BHF, London
British Medical Association 2004 Diabetes mellitus: an update for health professionals. BMA, London
Childline 2004 Bullying: information for teachers and professionals working with young people. Childline, London
Dahlgren G, Whitehead M 1991 Policies and strategies to promote social equity in health. WHO, Copenhagen
Department for Education and Skills 2003 Tackling bullying: listening to the views of children and young people. DfES, London
Department of Health 1999a Saving lives: our healthier nation. TSO, London
Department of Health 1999b National Service Framework for mental health. Online: www.dh.gov.uk Available July 2006
Department of Health 2000 The NHS plan. TSO, London
Department of Health 2001a Making it happen: a guide to delivering mental health promotion. Online: www.dh.gov.uk Available July 2006
Department of Health 2001b The expert patient: a new approach to chronic disease management in the 21st century. TSO, London
Department of Health 2001c Valuing people: a new strategy for learning disability for the 21st century. Online: www.dh.gov.uk Available July 2006
Department of Health 2004 Choosing health: making healthier choices easier. Online: www.dh.gov.uk/PublicationsAndStatistics/Publications/fs/en Available July 2006
EAPN 2003 European project on poverty indicators. Final report. Online: www.eapn.org Available July 2006
Festinger L 1964 Conflict, decision and dissonance. Tavistock, London

Foucault M 1973 The birth of the clinic. Tavistock, London
Gates R (ed) 2003 Learning disabilities: towards inclusion. 4th edn. Churchill Livingstone, Edinburgh
Hart C, Chesson R 1998 Children as consumers. British Medical Journal 316:1600–1603
Hayward J 1975 Information, a prescription against pain. RCN, London
Health Education Board for Scotland 2000 Team working. HEBS, Edinburgh
Helman C 2000 Culture, health and illness. 4th edn. Butterworth-Heinemann, Oxford
Jones L 1994 The social context of health and health care. Macmillan Publishing, Basingstoke
JRF 2003 Progress on poverty 1997–2003/4. JRF Findings Ref. 043. Online: www.jrf.org.uk Available July 2006
Kennedy A 2002 Sorted not screwed up. Report for the Aberdeen Foyer. Online: www.aberdeenfoyer.com/foyer_report.pdf Available July 2006
Kerr J (ed) 2000 Community health promotion: challenges for action. Baillière Tindall/RCN, London
Kiger AM 1995 Teaching for health. Churchill Livingstone, Edinburgh
Muir J, Sidey A (eds) 2000 Textbook of community children's nursing. Baillière Tindall/RCN, Edinburgh
Naidoo J, Wills J 2000 Health promotion: foundations for practice. 2nd edn. Baillière Tindall, Edinburgh
NHS Health Scotland 2004 People with learning disability in Scotland. Health needs assessment report. Online: www.phis.org.uk Available September 2006
Nursing and Midwifery Council 2004 *Code of professional conduct: standards for conduct, performance and ethics*. NMC, London. Online: www.nmc-uk.org/aFramedisplay.aspx?documentID=201 Available July 2006
Parsons T 1991 The social system. Routledge, London
Pencheon D, Guest C, Melzer D et al (eds) 2001 Oxford handbook of public health practice. Oxford University Press, Oxford
Perkins E, Simnett I, Wright L 1999 Evidence-based health promotion. Wiley, Chichester
Perrin EC, Gerrity PS 1981 There's a demon in your belly: children's understanding of illness. Pediatrics 67(6):841–849
Rogers CR 1951 On becoming a person. Constable, London
Scottish Executive 2000 The same as you? A review of services for people with learning disabilities. TSO, Edinburgh
Seedhouse D 2001 Health: the foundations for achievement of potential. 2nd edn. Wiley, Chichester
Seedhouse D 2002 Total health promotion: mental health, rational fields and the quest for autonomy. Wiley, Chichester
Tones K, Tilford S 2001 Health promotion: effectiveness, efficiency and equity. Nelson Thornes, Cheltenham
Townsend P, Davidson N, Whitehead M 1992 Inequalities in health: the Black Report and the health divide. Penguin, London
Tudor T 2004 Mental health promotion. In: Norman I, Ryrie I (eds) The art and science of mental health nursing. Open University Press, Milton Keynes, Chapter 2
WHO 1946 Preamble to the constitution. WHO, Geneva
WHO 1977 Health for all by the year 2000. WHO, Geneva
WHO 1978 Alma-Ata 1978: primary health care. WHO, Geneva
WHO 1984 Health promotion: a discussion on the concept and principles. WHO, Copenhagen
WHO 1986 Ottawa charter for health promotion. WHO, Ottawa
WHO 1997 The Jakarta declaration on health promotion into the 21st century. Online: www.who.dk Available July 2006
WHO 1998 Regional health for all targets: Health21 health for all. WHO, Copenhagen

Further reading

Helman C 2000 Culture, health and illness. 4th edn. Butterworth-Heinemann, Oxford
Naidoo J, Wills J 2000 Health promotion: foundations for practice. 2nd edn. Baillière Tindall, Edinburgh
Perkins E, Simnett I, Wright L 1999 Evidence-based health promotion. Wiley, Chichester
Seedhouse D 2001 Health: the foundations for achievement of potential. 2nd edn. Wiley, Chichester

2 Evolution of contemporary nursing

Linda Veitch and Jane Christie

Glossary terms

Accountability
Autonomy
Clinical nurse specialist (CNS)
Humanism
Nurse consultant
Patient allocation
Person-centredness
Primary nursing
Professionalism
Proficient
Task allocation
Team nursing

Learning outcomes

This chapter will help you:

- Understand how nursing has evolved since the 1700s
- Explore contemporary nursing and how it is influenced by society
- Discuss how nurses influence policy and practice in health and social care by responding positively to the needs of society and the requirements of health policy
- Outline the different approaches to organizing nursing care
- Describe how to become a nurse in the 21st century
- To be aware of the diverse roles undertaken by nurses in different settings.

Introduction

Since early times nursing has developed in response to the changing needs of society. As the structure of society alters, new nursing habits, customs, values and knowledge emerge in response to the composition and health of the population. This chapter outlines the evolution of nursing from the 1700s to the present day and will demonstrate how nursing, which does not exist in isolation, has been influenced by society and the sociopolitical agenda of the day. It explores how contemporary nursing roles have developed in response to the challenges facing healthcare delivery – for example, increased workload, reduction in junior doctors' working hours, nurses wishing to advance their practice, the focus on person-centred care, increasing the accessibility of healthcare for all and the shift of responsibility for those with chronic illness from the acute sector to the community. In addition, detail is provided about how to become a nurse in the 21st century. By outlining the key roles of the nurse and service users in different settings we hope that this will provide a useful introduction on which to build for those undertaking a common foundation programme.

Evolution of nursing

This section outlines the different values and beliefs about nursing and nurses at different periods since the 1700s, together with the events and context that influenced the changes in thinking. The roles of influential nurses including Florence Nightingale and Mary Seacole, and that of Mrs Ethel Fenwick – a force in the campaign to introduce the nurse registration – are explored. Also considered are major events in nursing such as professional registration and statutory regulation, and the influence of both World Wars (1914–1918, 1939–1945), the inception and development of the NHS and the more recent developments in professional regulation and education. The development of specialist nursing such as the care of children and people with mental health problems is also explored.

Nursing in the 18th and 19th centuries

In the 1700s, in times of accident or sickness, being in the comfort of one's own home was normal and lay people largely carried out the nursing role in the community.

Catholic nuns who had taken vows of poverty first staffed hospitals and many nurses were expected to work not for monetary gain but from religious inspiration or a 'calling'. 'Nursing' was also associated with maternity care, where women were expected to show the same love and devotion when caring for complete strangers that they naturally showed to their children. The underlying values of the time have been described as asceticism (Pearson et al 1996), which were:

- Dedicated individuals who committed their lives to the care of others
- Carers who denied their own needs in order to serve others
- Provision of the basic needs of food, shelter and comfort.

Carers often lived within the institution where care was provided and consequently their employers commonly exploited their 24-hour presence.

During the 1800s, the foundation of the Royal College of Surgeons led to a closer relationship between medical education and hospitals. The governors appointed matrons who were responsible for household affairs, supervision of nurses and other hospital servants. The best matrons tried to select women of good character to be head nurses and staff nurses. However, the majority of nurses were for the most part rough, dull and poorly educated women. Sairy Gamp, described by Charles Dickens in *Martin Chuzzlewit*, epitomized the nurses of the day. Many nurses worked in appalling surroundings with little or no education. Their work was considered to be a particularly repugnant form of domestic service. Motivated by the desire to earn money rather than by self-sacrifice or devotion to their job, they drank large amounts of alcohol, took snuff, were generally unkempt and lacked delicacy, discretion, tact and concern for their patients.

The influence of Florence Nightingale

Florence Nightingale was born in Florence, Italy, in 1820 of wealthy, middle-class parents. After several attempts to receive formalized training in 1850 and 1851, she spent brief periods in Germany at a Protestant institution that trained deaconesses in childcare and nursing. Soon afterwards Florence Nightingale became Superintendent of Nurses at the Institution for the Care of Sick Gentlewomen in Distressed Circumstances in London. For this she received no pay but was able to display her skills in nursing and nursing administration, which included greatly improved standards of nurses and nursing care and also the expectation that care should be based on compassion, observation and knowledge.

In 1854 the Secretary for War appointed Florence Nightingale to travel with a group of 38 women to Crimea to provide nursing services. Later, other nurses joined them so that by the end of the war Florence had 125 nurses under her supervision. Despite resistance from the medical establishment, Florence and her team worked long hours to establish hygienic standards of care. She was obsessed with discipline and through determination and persistence improved ventilation and reduced overcrowding, thereby reducing the mortality rate of wounded soldiers. One of her legacies was the 'Nightingale ward', a ward layout where long rooms have beds spaced out on each side, which are still found in some areas today. Florence recognized the soldier's human dignity and in return they held her in high esteem. She became known as the 'Lady with the Lamp' and was glorified by the public and press back home and her reputation grew.

On her return to England, Florence had developed revolutionary ways of collecting statistics known as 'model forms' and consequently many now regard her as the first research nurse. Although Florence found she was a heroine, she never enjoyed her fame and disliked the sentimental reference that her name inspired. The only testimonial she would accept was a fund, heavily subscribed by the public and named in her honour, which she used to found training schools for nurses.

The success of the Nightingale reforms led to the rapid expansion of nurse training schools, initially in London voluntary hospitals, then to larger provincial voluntary hospitals and finally to new hospitals being built by local government and poor law authorities (Baly 1995). Despite this there was still a need for nursing at home and Florence worked closely with William Rathbone to establish training for district nurses. District nursing started as a voluntary service, run by voluntary committees, until the value of the service was recognized and local authorities gradually began to accept more responsibility for sick people in the community. It was also recognized that certain occupations carried a particular risk to health and some firms employed a nurse to look after the health of their employees.

As a result of her work, Florence was able to define the nature of nursing clearly and how nursing was distinct from and not subservient to medicine (Box 2.1). This paved the way for the establishment of nursing as a profession with a sound and specific educational base.

Mary Seacole

Mary Seacole was another nurse and healer who contributed to the welfare of allied soldiers in the Crimean War. She was of mixed Scottish and Jamaican descent. Although experienced in the treatment of fevers and wound care, the authorities in England rejected her, so she visited battlefields, dispensing comfort and provisions to the wounded. In 1856, she returned bankrupt to England and published a book about her travels, which was one of the few published writings of any black woman before the 20th century. She was helped financially through funds raised by the soldiers she had nursed and finally received a pension from Queen Victoria. Until the centenary of her death in 1981 Mary had been forgotten but renewed interest in her achievements resulted in a nursing award being named after her. In 2003 a campaign was launched for a permanent memorial of her in London and in February 2004 in an online poll she was voted the greatest black Briton.

Health visiting

The first home health visiting began in the mid-1850s as a public health service which focused on problems

REFLECTIVE PRACTICE Box 2.1

Florence Nightingale's values

Nursing is a calling

- Religious beliefs in the existence of 'natural laws' could be discovered and used to help people improve their health and existence
- Nursing was all-consuming in terms of time commitment, i.e. more than an occupation
- Nursing work was so important that it should be thought of as a religious vow.

Nursing is an art and a science

- The science of nursing needs formal education
- The art of nursing gave freedom to act, to be creative, proactive and function as an advocate for the patient.

Mankind can achieve perfection

- People can control the outcomes of their lives
- People can pursue perfection by understanding 'nature's laws'. This understanding would enable people to readily use these laws to benefit their existence, so pursuing perfect health
- The role of the nurse was to provide the optimum environment in which perfect health could be achieved.

Nursing requires a specific education

- Education for nurses was revolutionary in the 19th century
- The Nightingale approach required a blend of theoretical and clinical experience.

Nursing is distinct and separate from medicine

- Although, physician and nurse deal with the same client population, nursing is aimed at discovering the 'natural laws' that will assist in putting the patient in the best possible condition so that nature can affect a cure.

(Adapted from Selanders 1993)

Student activity

Reflect on the values above and consider the extent to which they influence nursing today.

of sanitation and epidemics; nurses, sanitary engineers or lay visitors were sent into the homes of families with young children to offer advice about health and hygiene (Kamerman & Kahn 1993). At the same time a 'Sanitary Association' was formed to teach the 'laws of health', followed 10 years later by the 'Ladies Sanitary Association' enabling respectable women, known as 'Health Missioners', to teach health to mothers. From the voluntary work of these health missioners, health visitors (HVs) emerged and the importance of lowering the infant mortality rate ensured that their work became recognized and brought under the direction of the Medical Officer of Health. The work of early HVs was mainly educative and persuasive; they visited as counsellors to the whole family rather than either inspectors or nurses. The first training-specific health visiting course was established in 1892, around the same time as the first social work courses in the United States.

Development of nursing specialties

Specialist nursing services such as children's nursing and mental health nursing have their origins in the 1800s.

Children's nursing

Early accounts of paediatric home visiting started during the mid 1800s (Royal College of Nursing 1984). Charitable dispensaries were established as the most appropriate means of treating sick children (Carter & Dearmun 1995) and there was strong opposition to admission of children to hospital (Lansdown 1996). Other fears arose because children were often malnourished and susceptible to infection and hospitals were widely viewed as a major source of infection (Watt & Mitchell 1995). However, in recognition of need for specialist services for sick children, Dr Charles West founded The Hospital for Sick Children in Great Ormond Street, London, in 1852. This was followed by the Edinburgh Sick Children's Hospital in 1860. The aims of Great Ormond Street Hospital were to teach women the specialist skill of children's nursing and to provide advice for mothers. By 1888 it was recognized that sick children required specialized nursing and sick children's nurses required specialist training. A 2-year training programme was introduced almost 10 years before the start of training for adult nurses (Carter & Dearmun 1995).

Mental health nursing

During the 1800s there was also a change in attitude towards the mentally ill. At that time, people with mental distress were labelled as 'insane' and commonly marginalized. Those who could afford treatment were cared for in institutions known as asylums, while many of those who could not were sent to prison.

In the early 19th century there was a desire to tackle poverty, sickness and ignorance and general acceptance of a common ethical principle, namely that society had a responsibility for the weak. It was also recognized that mental health nursing (then known as asylum nursing) should be a skilled profession, needing intellectual and personal gifts rather than just strong nerves and powerful muscles.

Browne, Medical Superintendent at the Royal Edinburgh Asylum in 1838, recognized that the people who were closest to the patients, who spent most of their time with them and who managed them when they became distressed were untrained attendants (Nolan 2000). In attempting to improve this he started a course of lectures, which were a landmark in the history of mental health nursing. The first manual for attendants working in Mental Hospitals, *The Handbook for the Instruction of the Attendants of the Insane*, was published in 1885. This 'Red' Handbook became the content of training, run by the Medico-psychological Association in the late 1880s, for attendants working with the mentally ill. It included basic anatomy and physiology, principles of general nursing, the mind and its disorders, care of the insane and general duties of the attendant/nurse.

The beginning of education and regulation

By the 1880s nursing leaders were beginning to question whether nurses should be required to pass a public examination before entry to a register, as medical practitioners had been required to do since 1858. Opposition came from a number of quarters, perhaps most significantly from Florence Nightingale who thought that a central examination might undermine her philosophy of nursing. The matron of the London Hospital was also against registration but the matron at St Bartholomew's Hospital in London, Ethel Gordon Manson, was convinced of the need to raise standards and gain professional status for nursing. In 1887 she married Dr Bedford Fenwick who was active in medical politics and shared his wife's aspirations concerning the registration of nurses. In 1893, Mrs Fenwick took over the publication of the *Nursing Record* and then used this to underpin her campaign for registration. In 1903 the name changed to the *British Journal of Nursing*, with Mrs Fenwick remaining as editor, a position she occupied for nearly 50 years.

In 1887 Mrs Fenwick founded the Royal British Nursing Association (RBNA). Around the same time she refused to include graduates of an examination set by the Medico-psychological Association for asylum attendants. In 1895, Mrs Fenwick explained grounds for this exclusion:

> No person can be considered trained who has only worked in hospitals and asylums for the insane . . . considering the present class of persons known as male attendants, one can hardly believe that their admission will tend to raise the status of the association.
>
> Adams (1969, p. 13)

The fact that asylum attendants had to care not only for people with mental health problems but also their physical needs suggests that they should have been eligible. However, Brooking et al (1992) argue that this snub did not greatly trouble the attendants as their main concerns related to pay and conditions of service.

The success of the nursing reforms led to a rapid increase in the number of training schools. Advances in medical science demanded a more conscientious type of nurse. Middle-class women viewed nursing as a worthy career and at that time only teaching or the newly developing civil service offered an alternative. However, as a result of the rapid change, the tradition of discipline began to disappear. Criticism was stifled and orthodoxy and conformity were the norm and, despite Miss Nightingale's remarks about obedience being 'suitable praise for a horse', obedience was seen as a cardinal virtue.

Nursing in the 20th century

The Society for the State Registration of Nurses was formed in 1902, with Ethel Fenwick as Secretary and Treasurer. The National Council of Trained Nurses of Great Britain and Ireland was established 1904, with Ethel Fenwick as President (Royal British Nurses' Association 2003).

Two other legacies of the Nightingale reforms soon became a travesty – the nurses' home and the method of payment. The nurses' home that was originally supposed to provide a cultural and educational background for young women who had left middle-class homes, and to raise the sights of those who had not, had become a cheap way of housing the labour force who had to work around the clock. The first student nurses, known as probationers, were supernumerary to the workforce but as low pay was introduced under the auspices of 'getting the right type of girl' it became questionable whether probationers were actually pupils or workers.

In trying to change the negative image of nursing and make it more respectable, nurses were torn between delivering care and maintaining their knowledge, independence and status. This was managed by linking nursing firmly to medicine and describing the function of nursing as 'carrying out doctors' orders'.

In 1902 the Midwives Act required that all practising midwives undertook training and registered with the Central Midwives Board. The Central Committee for the State Registration of Nurses was formed 1909 with Ethel Fenwick as joint honorary secretary. Between 1910 and 1914 the Central Committee introduced annual parliamentary bills on nurse registration but these were blocked. The impact of World War 1 (1914–1918) and the unqualified female volunteers, the Voluntary Aid Detachment, sent to assist nurses that threatened to dilute nursing led to the establishment of an organization for trained nurses.

The College of Nursing (that later became the Royal College of Nursing) was established 1916, and in 1917 there were inconclusive discussions about a merger between the RBNA and the College. The principal objectives of the college were to:

> - Promote better education and training of nurses and advancement of nursing as a profession
> - Promote uniformity of the curriculum
> - Recognize approved nursing schools
> - Make and maintain a register of persons to whom certificates of training or proficiency had been granted
> - Promote Bills of Parliament for any object connected with the interests of the nursing profession and, in particular, with their education, organization and protection or for their recognition by the state.
>
> Baly (1995, p. 151)

The College of Nursing refused further pleas by the Medico-psychological Association to allow attendants to join, despite an increasing number taking the Associations course and examination.

In 1919, the Nurses Bill received royal assent and the General Nursing Council (GNC), chaired by Mrs Fenwick, was established 1920, with the duty of setting up a register of qualified nurses and a syllabus for instruction and examination. The GNC register of qualified nurses included:

- A general part containing the names of all nurses who satisfied the conditions of admission
- Supplementary parts for:
  - male nurses

- nurses trained in the care of persons suffering from mental disease
- nurses trained in the nursing of sick children.

Later the register included parts for nurses of infectious disease and nurses trained in the care of 'mental defectives' (people with learning disabilities).

Women were attracted to sick children's nursing because the age of entry into training was 21 years rather than 23–24 years for general nurses (Carter & Dearmun 1995). The new GNC started its own course and examination for asylum attendants but this carried little weight as the qualification was not required to gain a senior position in an asylum (Brooking et al 1992).

In 1921 the GNC set up a Disciplinary and Penal Committee, which had the power to deal with state registered nurses (SRNs) who were not 'fit and proper persons', and was able to prosecute those purporting to be registered nurses (RNs) when they were not. Although standards for competence were tested by examination, the most crucial characteristics of professional status were personal behaviour including obedience, tidiness and unquestioning loyalty. However, the profession had handed over control of entry qualifications and the requirements for basic training to the government who were also responsible for staffing hospitals as cheaply as possible. Although the GNC tried to overcome this disadvantage, statutory control was present and the first hallmark of a profession, that it controls its own standards of entry and training, was lost (Baly 1995).

A review of mental health nursing in 1924 identified the number of mental health nurses in England and Wales and recommended that:

- Consideration be given to the suitability of people for mental health nursing
- Work could be made more attractive if hours were reduced and holiday entitlement and salaries increased to be 10% higher than general nurses and for male nurses to receive 20% more than female nurses
- Nurses' accommodation and recreational facilities be improved
- Mental health nurses be trained alongside general nurses
- General nurse tutors be appointed to mental hospitals in order to raise standards of general nursing care.

However, due to the poor prevailing economic conditions at the time, none of these recommendations was seriously addressed (Nolan 2000).

General nursing gradually became acceptable work for middle-class women. The advantages included the ability to lead an independent life in respectable company and an occupation that was no longer menial, but one that involved training and exercise of intelligence. Working class women also flocked into nursing as they could earn more, do less menial work than in domestic service and move up the social ladder.

The British College of Nurses (BCN) was founded by Mrs Fenwick in 1926, with herself as President and Dr Fenwick as Treasurer. In 1927 the College of Nursing applied for its Royal Charter and the application, which was opposed by the RBNA, was granted in 1928 and it was renamed the Royal College of Nursing (RCN) in 1939. The BCN closed in 1956 (Royal British Nurses' Association 2003).

The 1930s

During the 1930s the public image of general nursing continued to be that of 'heroine' but the media was recognizing that nurses required education, which included development of both skills and knowledge, for practice. Nurses were depicted as brave, rational, decisive, humanistic and autonomous. It was an era of fantasy, romance and adventure where the focus of nursing was loyalty to physicians and patients. Gradually the new values of 'romanticism' were taken on board and were likened to hero worship of the leaders and doctors as nurses had a subservient relationship to them. Nursing was dependent on medicine to take the main responsibility for decision-making and nurses became adept at suggesting a course of action to a doctor in a way that allowed the doctor to perceive he had initiated it (Stein 1967). During the 1930s there was a considerable influx of men into mental health nursing, especially from depressed areas.

High unemployment and a lack of alternative careers made it easy to recruit nurses. However, there was widespread dissatisfaction in the profession over recruitment, pay and conditions, which led the government to set up a committee chaired by Lord Athlone to consider issues of shortages, wastage and training of nurses. This committee made a number of recommendations to improve staff conditions that would encourage nurses to stay in the profession. This included:

- Increasing hospital staff numbers to relieve nurses of non-nursing duties
- Organizing part of nurse training under general education
- Recognizing the role of the nurse assistant who was to be on an official GNC 'roll'.

However, the report was low key and by 1939 the country was under the shadow of World War 2.

The impact of World War 2 (1939–1945)

The war changed the situation from an apparently adequate supply of nurses to one of acute shortage. Nurses from all fields were recruited for the armed forces, which resulted in too few nurses to care for civilians. The Ministry of Health set up an Emergency Nursing Committee to organize a Civil Nursing Reserve to assist employing authorities to meet additional staffing needs occasioned by the war. This supplied upwards of 1800 nurses and unwittingly through this the Ministry of Health played an important part in the development of nursing by:

- Becoming the direct employer of nurses
- Introducing a second grade of assistant nurse, for whom there was no definition or standard of training
- Introducing a third grade called auxiliaries, who had received no training

- Increasing the burden of supervision for trained nurses
- Introducing part-time working
- Paying higher salaries to nurses in the Reserve than those in civilian posts, leading to a rift between the two.

The consequence of this was that in 1941 the Ministry of Health recommended that all hospitals paid salaries equivalent to those in the reserve. To assist the Ministry of Health in its new role as employer, a Division of Nursing was created and the first Chief Nursing Officer appointed. In 1943 the pay of nurses was put on a level with that of teachers but this made little difference to the recruitment figures so steps were taken to improve conditions of service (see Box 2.2). The Nurses Act 1943 came into force and State Enrolled Assistant Nurses became subject to the discipline of the GNC.

During World War 2 the recruitment and distribution of nurses was subject to specific controls:

- Certain nurses were no longer permitted to join the armed forces
- All nurses had to register and, if not employed, were urged to take a post in an area of shortage
- Employment had to be through the Ministry of Labour and nurses could only give up their posts in order to undertake further training. Without this intention they were regarded as available for work in an area of shortage with the consequence that nurses chose to gain a second qualification in midwifery rather than a spell in a sanatorium
- Nurses could be directed to posts not of their choosing; however, as a consequence of the war, this never really happened.

By the end of World War 2 hospital beds had to be closed due to shortages of nursing staff. Through the necessity to attract sufficient recruits, entry qualifications and the age of entry were lowered. Students and auxiliaries were the main recruits and qualified nurses became frustrated. Training began to suffer as there was insufficient support and supervision for students who began to feel that their preparation was inadequate. Many of those who stayed were rapidly promoted to positions of responsibility for which they were ill prepared. During the war years, some nurses took on increased responsibilities, for example on military ships they were expected to conduct physical and psychiatric assessments and initiate treatments, often without any medical support. Their efficiency, confidence and skills demonstrated what could be achieved outwith institutional bureaucracy. However, their experience was by no means comprehensive and they lacked knowledge and skills in managing the chronic conditions prevalent in civilian life (Nolan 2000).

Post war, nurses continued to administer doctors' orders and to monitor their patients closely. Military nurses maintained their allegiances and the number of male nurses increased as demobbed servicemen with medical experience joined the profession. Many joined the Society of Registered Male Nurses as the RCN remained closed to them until 1960. Through this they sought to improve the status and practice of mental health nursing.

REFLECTIVE PRACTICE Box 2.2

Conditions of service in 1943

Proposal of the Nurses Salaries Committee

- Working fortnight to be reduced to 96 hours
- Continuous night duty should not exceed 3 months for student nurses and 6 months for trained nurses
- All nurses entitled to 28 days' holiday a year, taken as stipulated by the hospital, plus 1 day off per week
- Sick pay according to length of service
- Higher salaries according to number of beds.

Student activities

- Reflect on the changes in conditions of service for nurses since the 1940s.
- Try to talk to someone who qualified as a nurse during the 1940s and find out how they felt about their conditions of service.

[Resource: Oxtoby K 2005 A lifetime in nursing. Nursing Times 101(24):24–25]

The influence of the National Health Service (NHS) on nursing

The NHS was established in 1948 with the aim of healthcare being free at the point of delivery (see Ch. 3). Nurses were in favour of the NHS and felt part of the service. Hart (2004, p. 55) notes that in the *Nursing Times* that year Mary Witting said 'the great principle has been accepted; never again need any of us suffer disease through lack of money'. However, from the outset there was a serious shortage of nurses and many hospitals were critically dependent on students. Significantly, during the planned introduction of the NHS, no provision for the education of nurses had been considered. In 1950 the following recommendations were made:

- Bedside work essential for training
- Hospitals not to exploit student nurses
- Part-time working to be encouraged
- Adequate pay for all nursing posts, equal pay for equal work
- Nurses should help shape NHS policy.

Large mental hospitals were usually located in the countryside and operated as self-sufficient communities, even down to having their own graveyards. There was strict regulation with rather impersonal procedures for patients, and tight discipline and a much-feared hierarchy for nurses. Nevertheless, there was a sense of common purpose in a community that was virtually self-contained and self-maintaining (Brooking et al 1992). Increasingly, mental hospitals developed open-door policies, enabling patients to take weekend leave and enjoy a broader range of activities including art and industrial therapies such as assembling components to provide rehabilitation and occupy their time with meaningful activities. Accommodation and recreational facilities improved for staff and alliances were built between doctors and nurses.

During the 1950s attitudes to children being cared for in hospital began to change. It was suggested that emotional damage might occur if children were separated from their parents for lengthy periods. The Ministry of Health commissioned the Platt Report (Ministry of Health 1959), a report on the welfare of children in hospital. At the same time it was recognized that nurses needed better communication skills and the ability to give patients information prior to admission. There needed to be better signposting within hospitals/care settings, flexible visiting times and easier access for families to speak to a doctor and/or nurse. In addition, attitudes to people with disabilities, older adults and those with rehabilitation needs were also changing, which had implications for hospital nurses, district nurses and HVs who all needed to be aware of increasing resources and appliances available for people with disabilities.

The influence of the medical model

During the late 1950s, with the growth of technology, romanticism began to lose favour and the value system of pragmatism began to evolve. Pragmatism is associated with a practical approach to assessing situations and acting on them in a practical way. Nurses were expected to extend their role to incorporate the impact of new technical knowledge. At this time, the nursing profession had a poor image regarding relationships with other hospital staff and colleagues (see Ch. 9). There were many complaints about 'petty discipline' and authoritarian attitudes existed for the following reasons:

- The influence of the armed forces during the evolution of the NHS
- The ratio of trained staff to untrained was low and simple authoritative rules reduced the need for supervision
- Technical knowledge advanced so rapidly that it created insecurity, which led to defensive behaviour, e.g. not listening to other people and the creation of petty rules. In addition, technology encouraged specialization and the new knowledge conferred both power and status.

The trend towards specialization reflected the reductionist approach where, as a result of the need for knowledge, the body is split into parts or systems and each part is studied independently. Subsequently, innumerable specialties in both nursing and medicine emerged, each concerned with only a small part of the whole person.

Research undertaken at this time recognized nursing as a particularly stressful occupation (see Ch. 11) as nurses were in constant contact with people who were ill or injured and whose recovery was not always certain or complete (Menzies 1961). To avoid intense anxiety, nursing care was based on a patient's medical diagnosis rather than on their individual needs. Nursing actions were based around familiar ward routines and conformity was expected. Along with this went depersonalization and categorization of patients according to bed numbers and disease. This approach to practice reflected the medical model.

Davies (1976) emphasized the importance of the power and control invested in the role of the traditional hospital matron who was perceived to be managing an obedient and highly useful nursing workforce. The matron was seen as the powerful figure and nurses as quiet, obedient followers of routine. Nevertheless, by carrying out all jobs, however humble and routine, that were necessary for patient comfort and recovery, nurses gained public sympathy and state support. Their daily work was usually organized around 'ward routines' that focused on carrying out a series of tasks, e.g. bedpan rounds, dressing rounds, getting everyone who was able out of bed for breakfast. Some of the benefits of this task approach were:

- Reduction of nurses' stress
- Protection of nurses from arbitrary whims of their superiors or doctors
- Easy and safe organization of work, particularly when there is a high turnover of staff, meaning that important actions were not missed.

In the 1960s a formal management structure was introduced as career development for senior nursing staff. This aimed to increase the status of the profession in hospital management and consequently the role of matron was abolished. The Salmon Report based nursing management on three tiers:

- Ward sisters/charge nurses, *accountable to*
- Nursing officers, *accountable to*
- Senior nursing officers and principal nursing officers.

This extended the career prospects for nurses by creating nursing officers who had responsibility for nursing. Many nurses did not take readily to these new roles and there was no career progression for those who wanted to continue having patient contact. Also, at this time, nurse theorists were beginning to challenge the traditional view of nursing characterized by:

- Its dependence on the medical profession
- Hierarchical structures
- Centralized decision-making without the input of clinicians
- Fragmentation of care by using task allocation to deliver care (see p. 48)
- The seeming unimportance of nurse–patient relationships.

The influence of nursing theory

During the 1960s there was a dramatic change in attitudes acknowledging the shift away from nurses as doctors' assistants, which was increasingly encouraging nurses to accept direct responsibility and accountability for their actions and their consequences, and for the decision-making processes that led to those actions. An influential quote from Henderson (1961, p. 42) at that time, stated that:

> The unique function of the nurse is to assist the individual, sick or well, in the performance of those activities contributing to health or its recovery (or to a peaceful death) that he would perform unaided if he had the necessary strength, will or knowledge, and to do this in such a way to help him gain independence as rapidly as possible. This aspect of her work, this part of her function, she initiates and controls; of this she is master.

At the same time other nurse theorists also began to describe what nursing was about and saw the development of the first nursing models, which are descriptions of what nursing is (Pearson et al 1996). Nursing models are based on beliefs about the following factors:

- *The person* – the individual receiving care
- *Health* – where the patient lies on the health and wellness continuum (see Ch. 1)
- *The care environment* – setting for individual/practitioner interaction
- *Nursing* – the roles of nurses and the knowledge and skills they need to carry out their roles.

Nursing models are explored in detail in Chapter 14. There are many models, each reflecting the diverse perspectives of nursing roles and care settings (Box 2.3).

Emergence of nursing models saw the beginning of the move away from the medical model (see p. 43 and Ch. 1) and a move towards the holistic approach (see p. 47) which focuses on the value of the person and the quality of their existence and experience. However, as medicine became more technical and more scientific, nurses increasingly took on more skills and procedures that had previously been carried out by doctors. At that time student nurses were part of the workforce and provided most of the nursing care with minimal supervision.

Box 2.3 **Examples of models used in different care settings**

Adult nursing	
Biomedical	*Medical model*
Goal attainment	King – 1981
Adaptation	Roy and Andrews – 1999
Activities of living	Marriner Tomey et al – 2000
Self-care	Orem – 1991
Systems	Neuman – 1995
Transformative	Dunphy & Winland-Brown – 1998
Mental health/learning disability nursing	
Developmental	Peplau – 1952
Normalization	O'Brien – 1981
Human becoming	Parse – 1987
Human caring	Watson – 1988
Humanistic	Paterson & Zderad – 1988
Children's nursing	
Partnership and negotiation	Casey's partnership model, Casey – 1988
Partnership and negotiation	Nottingham model, Smith – 1995

The early influence of nursing research

In the early 1970s the Briggs Report (Department of Health and Social Security 1972) set the expectation that nursing courses would incorporate research methods and that their findings would be used in nursing practice. The first nursing research was undertaken around that time; however, it had little impact on nursing practice. The Briggs Report also recommended the replacement of the existing regulatory body (the GNC) and the Nurses, Midwives and Health Visitors Act was passed in 1979. Consequently, the United Kingdom Central Council for Nursing, Midwifery and Health Visiting (UKCC) and four National Boards for nursing were established, one for each UK country, with a specific responsibility for education. The core functions of the UKCC were to maintain a register of UK nurses, midwives and health visitors, provide guidance to registrants and handle professional misconduct complaints (see Chs 6, 7). The main functions of the national boards were to monitor the quality of nursing and midwifery education courses and to maintain the training records of students on these courses.

The influence of humanism

Since the 1960s the underlying values and beliefs of nursing have become those of humanism, which explores the value of human beings, their uniqueness as individuals, quality of life and freedom of choice. These beliefs value the ability of others to know and understand people's feelings and their lived experience. The values of humanism include:

- Valuing humanness and the uniqueness of humans as individuals
- Understanding the meaning and purpose of people's lives from their perspective
- Giving freedom to individuals to make decisions for themselves
- Taking physical, psychological, spiritual, emotional and social needs into account.

Many nurses feel strongly that caring lies at the very heart of nursing. Kitson (1996) argues that in addition to the capacity of nurses to care for others, they also have the abilities to develop a nurse–patient helping relationship (see Ch. 9) and to share professional knowledge.

The nursing profession was recognized as being unique because it addresses the responses of individuals and families to actual and potential health problems in a humanistic and holistic manner (Marriner Tomey et al 2000). However, the NHS was originally built around the idea that the 'professional management' function was the same regardless of the organization or person to which it related. This new approach challenged the traditional professional ethos and healthcare professionals were forced to consider care in terms of its cost effectiveness. The new style also focused on quality assurance and the identification of standards of care. This raised a problem with the ethos of 'caring'. Caring was difficult to measure and for influential managers who sought value for money it did not provide the hard evidence needed to measure outcomes (Norman & Cowley 1999). Consequently, the cost-driven management style of the late 1980s continues to influence nursing and to increase the drive for technical competence and scientific nursing skills.

Code of professional conduct

The UKCC developed the first code of conduct for nurses, midwives and HVs in 1984, which set out for the first time key expectations for professional practice and accountability. Its purpose was to protect the public through providing professional standards, to inform the public of the standard of professional conduct they could expect, to ensure accountability and to make it clear that RNs, midwives and HVs have a duty of care to their patients and clients. This has been refined and is currently published by the Nursing and Midwifery Council (NMC) as *The NMC code of professional conduct: standards for conduct, performance and ethics* (NMC 2004a) (see Ch. 7).

Project 2000

In the 1980s it was recognized that, as a result of changing disease patterns and social contexts and the introduction of reforming modes of care delivery, there would be new healthcare needs that required a different kind of nurse. In order to meet this need the UKCC (1985) put forward a different approach to the education of nurses. The main proposals included:

- Links between Colleges of Nursing and Higher Education Institutions
- New parts of the professional register, one for each branch of nursing for those completing the new education programmes
- Supernumerary status for learners made possible, in part, by creating an alternative workforce of healthcare assistants (HCAs) (Box 2.4)
- New professional competencies to be achieved
- A programme at the level of a higher education diploma
- A common foundation programme (CFP) for all types of nursing before pursuing one of four branch programmes.

CRITICAL THINKING Box 2.4

Nursing skill mix before Project 2000

Before Project 2000 a typical ward might have had the following staff to cover the day shifts:

- A senior and a junior sister/charge nurse
- Two or three qualified nurses, including enrolled nurses
- Between six and 10 student nurses, some from each year of training
- Two or three auxiliary nurses.

Student activities

- Consider the practical issues involved in provided nursing care to patients/clients during the transition from 'learner as worker' to supernumerary student.
- Ask people who were qualified nurses at the time and those who were training as nurses in the old and new systems about their experiences.

Moving from rituals to evidence-based practice

The development of education and regulation for nurses and midwives failed to bring nursing the power and prestige that were anticipated by early nursing leaders. Over the last 15–20 years there has been a shift from 'the practitioner knows best' to the belief that one can never take one's own practice for granted. However, nursing had still only developed a limited body of knowledge that could be defined as nursing and which was exclusive of other disciplines. Consequently, the purpose of nursing research is to establish a body of nursing knowledge which in turn increases the professional status of nursing (see Box 2.5 and Ch. 5).

The attributes of a profession include:

- Having its own body of specialist knowledge
- Having a role in society that is valued
- Employing some means of internal regulation (Chinn & Kramer 1995).

The introduction of the nursing process during the 1980s enabled nurses to develop a more systematic approach to care (see Ch. 14). There was the expectation that nurses should carry out best practice that was in the interest of their patients and that they would be accountable for their actions. The systematic nursing process gradually evolved into evidence-based decision-making, a process of turning clinical problems into questions and then systematically locating, appraising and using current research findings as the basis for clinical decisions (see Ch. 5). By using a structured problem-based approach practitioners can logically apply the best available evidence to their care, i.e. evidence-based practice (see Ch. 5). Table 2.1 summarizes the major events influencing the evolution of nursing discussed in this section.

EVIDENCE-BASED PRACTICE Box 2.5

Professional status – body of specialist knowledge

Select an area of care that is relevant to your practice.

Student activities

- Is there a body of specialist nursing knowledge that relates to your chosen area?
- What evidence is available to support the existence of specialist nursing knowledge?
- What is the benefit of specialist nursing knowledge to the patients/clients there?

Table 2.1 Major events in the evolution of nursing

Date	Context	Influences on nursing practice
1700	Care was largely carried out in people's homes by lay people	Catholic nuns staffed hospitals and many nurses were expected to work not for money but from religious inspiration or a 'calling'
1800	Foundation of the Royal College of Surgeons led to a closer relationship between medical education and hospitals	Governors appointed matrons responsible for household affairs, supervision of nurses and other hospital servants Ordinary nurses were of lower status, received some money and a beer allowance, endured appalling working conditions and had little or no education
1834	Poor Law Amendment Act	Workhouses with intolerable conditions for poor, sick and needy people Sick people nursed by elderly pauper women
1854–1856	Crimean War	Florence Nightingale introduced measures such as sanitary principles, which contributed to a reduction in mortality rates of wounded soldiers Mary Seacole visited battlefields, dispensing comfort and provisions to the wounded
1856	Florence Nightingale described as the first research nurse	Using statistics she collected during the Crimean War, she illustrated the need for sanitary reforms in all military hospitals
1858	Improvement of standards	Doctors who passed a public examination entered on a register. By 1880 nurse leaders were suggesting that nurses should be required to do the same
1860	Florence Nightingale founded the first nursing training school Attitudes towards the poor changed, poverty implied sickness	The Nightingale Training School and Home for Nurses based at St Thomas' Hospital in London Poor Law Hospitals and 'probationer' nurses
1914–1918	World War 1	Young women known as Voluntary Aid Detachment (VAD) assisted nurses
1919	Nurses Act	Registration of UK nurses
1920	General Nursing Council was established	The three Councils had clearly prescribed duties and responsibilities for the training, examination and registration of nurses and the approval of training schools for the purpose of maintaining a register of nurses for England and Wales, for Scotland and for Ireland
1939–1945	World War 2	Nurses joining military services led to recruitment problems at home Dissatisfaction over nurses' pay and conditions
1943	Recruitment of nurses remained a problem	Pay parity with teachers Introduction of nursing assistants, later to become enrolled nurses (second level nurses)
1960	More policy decisions for nurses	Salmon Report – formal nursing management structure but no clinical career structure
1979	Nurses, Midwives and Health Visitors Act	Review of registration and education of nurses, midwives and health visitors United Kingdom Central Council for Nursing, Midwifery and Health Visiting (UKCC) and four National Boards were established
1983	Griffiths report	Introduction of general management culture – NHS to be run as a business
1986	Project 2000	Higher education qualification for nurses proposed; supernumerary status for nursing students
1989	Review of pay scales	Clinical grading structure for nurses introduced
1990	Working for patients; purchaser/provider	Financial performance prominent in healthcare
1997–1999	The new NHS: modern, dependable (DH 1997) A first class service: quality in the new NHS (DH 1998a) Making a difference (NHS Executive 1999) Fitness for practice (UKCC 1999)	Expansion of the nursing workforce Strengthening of nursing leadership Clinical governance – corporate accountability for the quality of care Widening access to nursing education, common foundation programme followed by branch programmes
2000	The NHS plan (DH 2000)	Outlined healthcare reforms which would lead to extra beds, more hospitals, modernized GP surgeries, more consultants, more nurses, more IT support, better food and cleaner wards

(*Continued*)

Table 2.1 (*Continued*)

Date	Context	Influences on nursing practice
2002	UKCC becomes Nursing and Midwifery Council (NMC)	The principal functions of the Council shall be to establish from time to time standards of education, training, conduct and performance for nurses and midwives and to ensure the maintenance of those standards
2004	Agenda for change	Modernized NHS pay system with new pay bandings, job evaluation scheme and knowledge and skills framework
2005	Reduction in junior doctors' hours; review of nurses' roles	Nurses increasingly undertaking advanced roles
2006	Reorganization of NHS structures Some NHS trusts report financial overspends	Redundancies amongst NHS staff including nursing posts Nurses speak out against the speed of reorganization and policy implementation, arguing that the change is detrimental to patient care

Approaches to nursing practice

This section outlines holistic care and patient centredness and then explains the four main approaches to organizing nursing care.

Holistic care

Caring that involves looking after the 'whole person' is truly holistic and healing. Holistic care recognizes the uniqueness of each human being, their individuality, personality and human frailty (Makinen et al 2003). It can be argued that every nurse knows that the subtle process of caring has physical, psychological, social and spiritual dimensions but that this is often hard to express in words. It involves the integration and coordination of interpersonal, technical and professional skills that results in a complex network of interactions that contribute to successful nurse–patient relationships (Adams et al 1998). Holistic care (see also Ch. 1) therefore requires nurses to think beyond the concept of cure which is based on scientific facts and technical competence.

Person-centred care

Nursing is moving in this direction with increasing emphasis on therapeutic relationships with patients/clients and making changes in care delivery that give patients/clients more power and choice, and pays more regard to their needs and wishes (Salvage 2002). Recently, holistic care has been developed further to embrace the concept of person-centredness (Box 2.6). This is concerned with the rights of people to have their values and beliefs as individuals respected, i.e. their personhood (McCormack 2003). It is said that it is these values that give people their uniqueness and authenticity. Maintaining person-centredness is now central to decision-making and determining the actions of all healthcare professionals in their practice.

The principles of person-centredness can be applied across health and social care settings and all branches of nursing. Everyone experiencing healthcare is on a journey or pathway of care that involves new situations so uncertainty is to be expected. Uncertainty can be challenging but it also provides opportunities for learning and solutions, resolutions and outcomes that, with the appropriate support, can be uniquely created and tailored to meet individual needs.

> **Box 2.6 Person-centredness**
>
> Person-centredness involves respecting the rights of each person to make rational decisions, to determine their own goals and to enable them to reach their own decisions. This involves:
>
> - Sharing information
> - Recognizing other people's values as being truly important
> - Making explicit the intentions and motivations for nursing actions
> - Involving patients/clients in planning and negotiating their care
> - Responding to cues that maximize coping resources through the recognition of important things in their daily life
> - Offering personal support and practical expertise while enabling the person to follow a path of their own choosing in their own way. This may also require the person to be informed about the harmful consequences of their own choices.
>
> [After McCormack 2003]

Involving users and carers

The patient/client/carer (or consumer) is the most important person in the healthcare system. The nurse has an important role in ensuring continuity and maintaining consumer autonomy (the ethical principle that individuals should make their own decisions about their lives) within the maze of the healthcare system, which can be challenging. This may include helping the consumer to:

- Understand what the treatment options are, the benefits and disadvantages of each

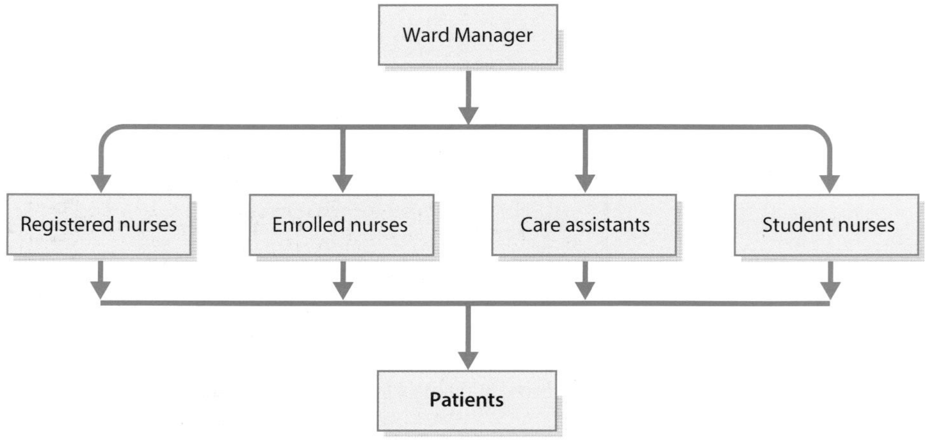

Fig. 2.1 Channels of communication in task allocation or functional nursing

- Know who will carry out treatment
- Ensure their rights regarding choice are upheld.

This helps to reduce feelings of anxiety and isolation. Patient/client/carer involvement has become the norm in contemporary nursing practice as it promotes patient decision-making and partnership working, ensuring that services provided meet the service user's needs (DH 2004). This approach considers service users as experts in their own lives and also often in their disease/condition, i.e. it encourages expert patients to manage their own chronic condition. People's perceptions of what constitutes quality care are formed by their encounters with an existing care structure and by their expectations and experiences (Larsson & Larsson 2003).

Contemporary health and social care provision encourages bridging the hospital/community divide through delivery of more flexible and seamless services, including intermediate care, that are built round the patient care pathway rather than institutions or budget systems.

Approaches to organizing nursing care

There are four approaches that have been used and elements of these underpin nursing practice in most settings today.

Task allocation

Task allocation was the main method of organization when hospitals were established and still persists to some extent in many areas of nursing (Fig. 2.1). Where it continues, this is usually due to autocratic leadership styles (see Ch. 9) and the continuing use of the biomedical model (see p. 43 and Ch. 1). Task allocation is based on a hierarchy of tasks where tasks are carried out according to the status of the caregiver and has much in common with an industrial production line, with each carer carrying out a limited range of care-related tasks for many patients/clients. It also reflects the hierarchical, ecclesiastical and military roots of nursing that value obedience and subservience. For example, in a hierarchy, tasks are allocated by seniority where:

- *Senior nurses* – administer drugs, change dressings, speak to relatives, serve meals
- *Junior nurses* – carry out bed baths, give bedpans, complete fluid balance charts, take observations
- *Untrained nurses/care assistants* – help people to wash, serve drinks, feed patients/clients, undertake general tidying up, arrange flowers
- *Domestic staff* – undertake general cleaning, tidying and washing up.

Patient allocation

This was introduced in the 1970s to enable nurses to focus on caring for individual patients/clients rather than on a range of tasks. Nurses were allocated specific patients to care for. The aim was to provide continuity of care; however, both the nursing hierarchy and relationships between charge nurses and other nurses remained the same and essentially task allocation continued but for smaller groups of patients/clients.

Team nursing

In 1956, the RCN developed a theory of team nursing but a number of issues prevented this approach being developed:

- When a patient's needs were greatest they were nursed by a team in intensive care units
- There was too much hostility between RNs and nursing assistants
- Interprofessional rivalries between nurses and others including doctors
- Financial cuts and shortages meant reverting to task allocation for speed
- Those RNs who aspired to a higher status had no wish to return to nursing tasks they regarded as menial.

However, during the 1980s, team nursing evolved and allowed care to become more individualized. Nurses are allocated to a team who provide care to a specific group of patients/clients (Fig. 2.2). The team leader shares responsibility for patient care, communication and coordination with the ward manager. Ideally, the same team cares for the same group of patients for the duration of their stay. This increased continuity of care provides more meaningful work for nursing teams.

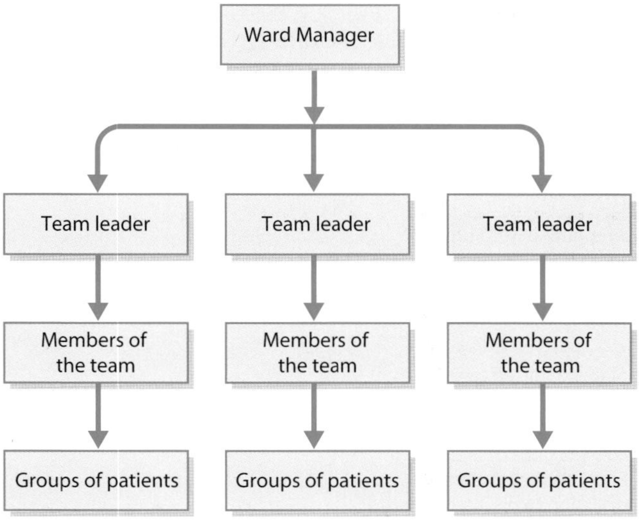

Fig. 2.2 Channels of communication in team nursing

Primary nursing

This involves patients/clients being allocated to an individual RN rather than a team of nurses (Fig. 2.3). The focus is on individual holistic care, where the participation of patients/clients and relatives is encouraged. The primary nurse has 24-hour responsibility for their group of patients, known as a caseload, throughout their stay. Primary nurses have the knowledge and ability to make decisions, and also the authority to carry them out. In the primary nurse's absence, an associate nurse, another RN or primary nurse carries out the planned care with the involvement of students and HCAs. In settings where primary nursing is practised, the sister/charge nurse acts as consultant, role model (managing a small caseload), ward manager and in-service educator. In common with other care delivery systems, primary nursing has advantages and disadvantages (Box 2.7).

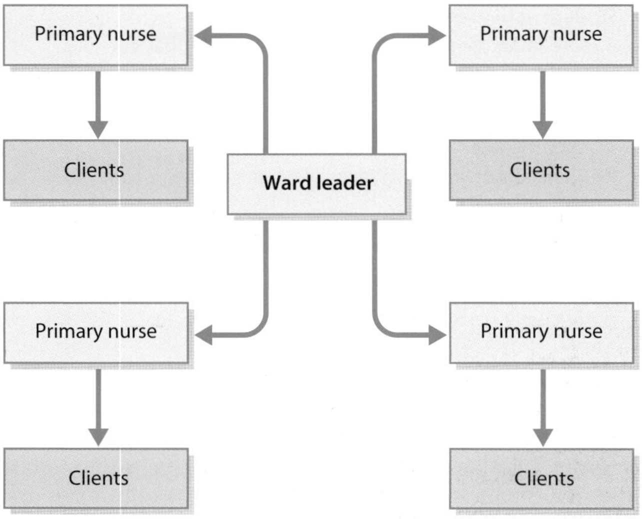

Fig. 2.3 Channels of communication in primary nursing

Box 2.7 Advantages and disadvantages of primary nursing

Advantages

- Patients have the opportunity to develop a therapeutic relationship with one nurse
- Clear documentation by the major care giver should ensure 24-hour continuity of care
- Primary nurses are accountable for their actions and are encouraged to develop clinical skills, leadership skills and interpersonal skills
- Increased job satisfaction for primary nurses
- Improved communication as relatives and members of the multidisciplinary team (MDT, see p. 53) approach the primary nurse to obtain information about patients/clients.

Disadvantages

- Patients may not like the primary nurse
- Nurses may not have the time to develop this relationship
- 24-hour cover is difficult or impossible within many settings
- Requires good education and understanding of the role
- Increased responsibility requires authority and support from the manager
- Can be stressful without adequate support
- Members of the MDT used to a hierarchical system may find it difficult to communicate with primary nurses rather than the sister/charge nurse
- Supervision and normal lines of reporting are different, which – if not agreed – can lead to breakdown in communication.

[After Sparrow 1986]

Care delivery in practice

It has been recognized that when team or primary nursing is used as a method for organizing patient care, less stress is reported by the practitioners involved. Alongside this, there is the belief that patients feel better cared for and their individual needs are met, practice is enhanced, teamwork is more evident and there is greater job satisfaction.

Figure 2.4 summarizes the key characteristics of the four approaches to organizing care. There is growing evidence that nurses do not work in the four ways described above, but that care settings are organized in more complex ways using attributes from more than one of the different approaches to care delivery (Adams et al 1998) (Box 2.8). It is interesting to note that patients' perceptions of the quality of care are often dependent on individual nurses rather than the system of care delivery (Jupp 1994).

Contemporary nursing

This section explores the fundamental role of the nurse, how society influences nursing and contributes to the

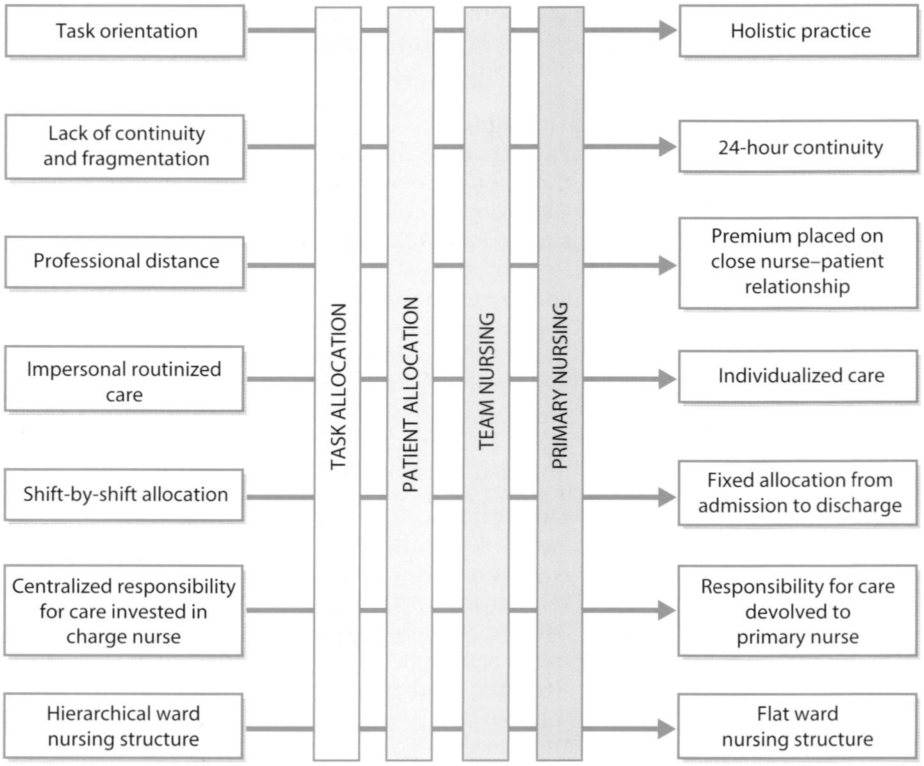

Fig. 2.4 The key characteristics of the four main ways of delivering nursing care (after Adams et al 1998)

REFLECTIVE PRACTICE Box 2.8

Organization of nursing care

Think back to aspects of nursing care in your last placement.

Student activities

- Which practitioners, including members of the MDT, provided care?
- Were patients/clients/parents involved?
- How was care allocated – by tasks or by patients/clients?
- Did patients/clients have the same nurses allocated to them every day?
- Did you feel the nurses had time to get to know the patients?
- Who was the coordinator of care? Who did the ward rounds?
- What was the role of the ward manager?
- What was the main system of care delivery used?

CRITICAL THINKING Box 2.9

ICN definition of nursing

Nursing encompasses autonomous and collaborative care of individuals of all ages, families, groups and communities, sick or well and in all settings. Nursing includes the promotion of health, prevention of illness, and the care of ill, disabled and dying people. Advocacy, promotion of a safe environment, research, participation in shaping health policy and in patient and health systems management, and education are also key nursing roles.

Student activities

After reading the *ICN Definition of Nursing*, look back at Henderson's definition (p. 44) and:

- Compare them and consider how nursing has changed over the last 40 years.
- Think about your own ideas of what 'nursing' is today

[Resource: International Council of Nurses 2004 The ICN definition of nursing. Online: www.icn.ch/definition.htm Available: July 2006]

development of nursing in different settings and the role of the nurse as a member of the MDT. In addition, there is consideration of how nurses and nursing continue to influence policy and practice in health and social care by responding positively to the needs of society and the requirements of health policy.

Nursing today

The fundamental role of the nurse is about 'caring', which involves spending time with the person promoting health or supporting those who are ill, distressed or disturbed by disease or injury (Box 2.9). It involves demonstrating a capacity to observe, listen and think about individual patient's/client's needs, being able to engage them in a way that enables the nurse and the patient/client to work together to reach an understanding of the problems from the patient's/client's own perspective before identifying ways by which these can be addressed. It is important also to recognize that cure is not always an attainable goal.

Nurses remain the core of the NHS workforce and are essential in maintaining services on a 24-hour basis. Role changes are emerging from the demand for high quality care in response to patients'/clients' needs and there are numerous opportunities for motivated RNs to lead innovative services that cross the boundaries of hospital and community settings, following patient journeys, providing continuity and ensuring a seamless service for those in their care. A nurse from any branch can be a practitioner, manager, researcher, educator, coordinator of services and health promoter, all within the same shift. These diverse roles put a nurse in a unique position to influence healthcare that is responsive to individual needs. In order to fulfil such diverse roles, special attributes are needed:

- A coordinating function
- A teaching function, for careers, patient and professional (see Ch. 4)
- Developing and maintaining programmes of care
- Technical expertise, exercised personally or through others
- Concern for the ill but also for those currently well
- Special responsibility for frail and vulnerable groups (see Ch. 7).

Department of Health (2002)

Influences on nursing today

The future of nursing holds a myriad of challenges, which include external forces as well as influences from within the profession as the role of the nurse evolves further. External factors that will continue to influence healthcare and nursing include increasing technology, demographic changes, changing patterns of disease, consumerism and increasing recognition of people's rights, e.g. the Human Rights Act 1998 (see Ch. 6), safety at work, globalization and the impact of increased travel.

Technology

Technological advances, e.g. in telecommunications and imaging techniques, are shaping the ways in which nurses work. To measure up to the future needs of the profession, nurses must be computer literate and able to embrace the new technologies and ways of working. Patients' records are being computerized and patient data are becoming available via information systems, e.g. laboratory results, prescriptions and integrated care pathways (ICPs, see Chs 3 and 14). ICPs enable healthcare professionals in any setting to document care against agreed standards, not only to monitor patients' health but also the performance of individuals and teams.

Demography

In mid-2004 the UK population was 59.8 million people (National Statistics Office 2004) with an average age of 38.4 years; one in five people in the UK was under 16 and one in six was aged 65 or over. As a result of declining fertility rates and increasing life expectancy, the UK has an ageing population. International migration into the UK from abroad has been an increasingly important factor in the population change. In response to this, healthcare has to develop new ways of working; for example, to increase the expertise and partnership working with frail older adults and to promote understanding of other cultures and changing disease patterns. With the breakdown of the extended family and the increased need to demonstrate status through the acquisition of material possessions, people are becoming more isolated and stressed.

Changing disease patterns

Modern healthcare and medical technology have begun to transform the health of the nation and life expectancy for many has increased but not to the same degree in all social groups (see Ch. 1) and geographical areas. The development of vaccines has dramatically improved health by reducing mortality and morbidity from infectious diseases. People are less physically active and are eating more sugar and fat and insufficient fresh fruit and vegetables, which has led to increasing obesity. This is also contributing to the increased incidence of chronic conditions such as diabetes, cardiovascular disease and cancers. Chapter 1 discusses the UK Government health targets that have been devised as a focus for health promotion and aim to reduce the incidence of these common and largely preventable conditions.

Smoking is the greatest preventable cause of illness and premature death and despite an overall fall in prevalence (DH 1998b) there is an increase among younger people (DH 1998c). Adolescent pregnancy is a major cause for concern, as is the increased incidence of drug and alcohol misuse and other mental health problems (The Scottish Office 1999).

Consumerism

The users of health services today are sophisticated and informed, having been educated by the media, advertising campaigns and other spheres of consumer behaviour. There is much more interaction between healthcare consumers (patients/clients/parents) and healthcare providers than in the past. Over time, patients/clients have been transformed into consumers whose perceived needs, wishes and expectations influence the delivery of healthcare. It appears that health is an important concern of all age groups, that many individuals see themselves as responsible for their own health and that people are more actively taking control of their healthcare. Those people with an internal locus of control, who take responsibility for their own health, are usually well informed, educated and articulate, and among the healthiest groups in society, whereas those groups with the poorest health may have an external locus of control where they feel that they have little or no control over health and well-being.

Diversity and equity

Diversity is about recognizing and valuing human differences for the benefit of patients/clients, carers, staff and the public at large. Diversity goes hand in hand with equity and equality, which is about creating a fairer society in which everyone can participate and has the same opportunity to fulfil their potential. In reality, there is no equity or equality of opportunity if differences cannot be recognized and valued (Scottish Executive Health Department 2005).

Human rights

People's rights have become more widely acknowledged, particularly since the passing of the Human Rights Act in 1998 (see Ch. 6) and the European Union Social Charter. These have wide-ranging implications for the profession as they impact on nursing practice and nursing research. Examples include conscientious objection, age and disability, right to life, patient advocacy, role expansion, healthcare resource allocation, emergency contraception, do-not-resuscitate orders, rights to privacy and dignity, confidentiality and anonymity, ethics, genetics and informed consent, advance directives (called advance decision to refuse treatment in the Mental Capacity Act 2005) and patients'/clients' right to choice (see Chs 6, 7).

The healthcare system must challenge discrimination, promote diversity and respect human rights. It is not uncommon for certain groups of people to be discriminated against, including older adults, drug users, homeless and unemployed people, minority ethnic groups and those with mental health problems. In practice, diversity should mean that all people are treated as equal and can access free healthcare at the point of need.

Nursing in different settings

In response to societal influences new nursing roles have developed in different settings. Society has changed and a new approach to healthcare is needed. Health choices will be made easier by providing better information and advice. This means developing the talents, commitments and strength among nurses to ensure they maximize their contacts with patients, clients and local communities to make every contact a health-promoting opportunity wherever they work, be it in the community, at home, GP surgeries or hospitals.

Roles in the community

The National Health Service and Community Care Act (1990) has led to significant changes in the place of care delivery, heralding a move from largely hospital-based provision to care within community settings (see Ch. 3). The emphasis on community services will further increase with the implementation of the English White paper *Our Health, Our Care, Our Say: a New Direction for Community Services*, which provides for a shift of resources from hospital- to community-based services (DH 2006). Nurses are increasingly the first point of contact for patients/clients, whether in NHS walk-in clinics or via NHS direct (England and Wales) or NHS 24 (Scotland). In addition, nurses are increasingly taking a lead in providing services for some people with mental health problems and chronic physical health conditions. These services tend to focus on the health of the patient/client, rather than their illness, and are largely community based. Nursing roles in the community include those of specialist community public health nurses (school nurses with specialist practice qualifications, HVs and occupational health nurses) and community practitioners such as district nurses, community mental health nurses (see Ch. 3) and community learning disability nurses. Some of these roles are discussed below.

School nursing

School nurses provide an essential link between schools, home and the community, which helps to safeguard the health and well-being of children and young people. In order to do this they work with children/young people, parents/carers, teachers and a multidisciplinary team (MDT) of other health and social care professionals. Their responsibilities include supporting children with complex health needs, immunization and drop-in clinics, assessing the health needs of every 5-year-old and providing health promotion programmes for young people, e.g. on health issues such as safe sex, stress management, discrimination and bullying.

Health visiting

HVs focus on health and social needs, working in collaboration with other NHS disciplines and other agencies. Their clients include children and mothers, families, older adults and marginalized groups including asylum seekers and travelling people.

The HV undertakes health promotion activities. This may include assessing the health needs of children in the community to identify vulnerable groups and provide effective programmes of support and care that will protect and promote health and well-being. HVs work with social workers and others to safeguard children by identifying if they are vulnerable, i.e. their safety or welfare is at risk. They also deliver public health programmes that address national and local health priorities such as reducing inequalities, smoking cessation and tackling obesity. They help healthy people to stay well and ill people to come to terms with their illness. They generally have a caseload of clients of one age group, usually children, but some have caseloads of older adults and people with other needs.

Public health nursing

Specialist community public health nurses aim to reduce health inequalities by working with individuals, families and communities to promote health, prevent ill-health and protect health. The emphasis is on partnership working that cuts across disciplinary, professional and organizational boundaries that impact on social and political policy to influence the determinants of health (see Ch. 1) and promote the health of whole populations (NMC 2004b). The HV role may evolve and develop through further education to become this newly defined practitioner.

Family health nursing

The World Health Organization Europe (2000) proposed a new type of nurse that would be based in local communities. The envisaged role of this family health nurse (FHN) was multifaceted and included helping individuals, families and communities to cope with illness and to improve their health. The FHN and the family health physician were presented as the key professionals at the hub of a network of primary care services.

In 2001, the Scottish Executive Health Department saw this as a potential solution to some of the problems of providing healthcare in Scotland's remote and rural regions and undertook a pilot project which was then evaluated (Scottish Executive Health Department 2003). This role is still in its infancy and further development and evaluation are required.

District nursing

District nurses (DNs), also known as community nurses, provide nursing care for people of all ages in a variety of non-hospital settings including patients' homes, GP surgeries and residential nursing homes. Their work involves, for example, health assessments and health promotion, wound management, administering medication, risk assessment and palliative care. It may also involve running clinics for people with chronic conditions such as diabetes. DNs often manage a caseload of patients and they work with other healthcare professionals in supporting patients' families and carers.

Hospital nursing

In hospitals many nurses are expanding their roles to meet demands for increasingly complex care needs based on innovative technologies and to compensate for a shortage of medical staff. Many RNs, along with midwives and therapists, undertake a wide range of clinical activities including the right to make and receive referrals, admit and discharge patients, order investigations and diagnostic tests, run clinics and prescribe drugs.

Intermediate care

Intermediate care is sometimes required on discharge from an acute hospital for patients who cannot return home immediately and require some form of rehabilitation. These are often GP beds in a community hospital. Increasingly, nurses work across hospital and community settings, an example of which is the clinical nurse specialist role (see p. 66).

Nurses as members of a multidisciplinary team

The multidisciplinary approach is increasingly recognized in healthcare as a valuable way of working. Nurses are often part of a MDT that may include doctors, physiotherapists, pharmacists, dietitians and many other health and social care professionals (see Ch. 3). It is important to understand the roles of all the members and how they interlink to provide 'seamless' healthcare.

The key to multidisciplinary care is collaboration, the coming together of different health and social care professionals as partners to develop a collective understanding, which requires effective coordination, a flattened hierarchy and transformational leadership style (West 1994). The following characteristics are outcomes by which success can be measured:

- Members should feel that they are important to the group
- Individual tasks should be meaningful and rewarding
- Individual contributions should be identifiable and subject to evaluation and comparison
- Teams should have interesting tasks to perform
- Clear group goals with inbuilt performance feedback.

Effective teamwork within the MDT

Teamwork is about working together and requires cooperation and understanding (see Ch. 9). The readiness to develop a collaborative approach is recognized by a group's capacity to experience and manage competition, conflict, risk and stress, and their willingness to communicate (Rowe 1996). Team members must be aware that their behaviour not only affects others but also the overall performance of the team. The aim should be to adopt the helpful roles outlined in Table 2.2. Moving towards the helpful behaviours involves self-awareness and a team with members who are ready to change and learn from others (see Ch. 9).

However, effectiveness is not down to individuals alone. An effective team requires skilful coordination which West and Field (1995) argue involves:

- A key professional acting as team coordinator or key worker
- Team referrals and decisions, with consensus of opinion being vital
- Commitment to regular team meetings
- Free flow of information between team members
- Coordinated feedback and team evaluation, rather than a series of unrelated specialist assessments, to give people or patients/clients a sense of clarity and unity, leading to more successful uptake of team recommendations
- A flexible system to meet people's or patients'/clients' differing needs or priorities
- Access to balanced and unbiased information.

Carrying out the activities in Box 2.10 will help you to understand the characteristics of effective teamwork.

Becoming a nurse in the 21st century

The present education of nurses has been influenced by many factors, not least public expectation and scrutiny of what has gone before. The major changes have involved the educational outcomes at the point of registration. This section discusses a number of issues including pre-registration nursing programmes, the NMC outcomes and proficiencies, the role of the HCA and National Vocational Qualifications (NVQs).

Pre-registration nursing programmes

The new direction for the nursing profession, established in the wake of Project 2000, brought a profound

Table 2.2 Helpful and hindering roles in team working

Helpful roles	Hindering roles
Establishing: Helping to start the group along new paths by proposing tasks and goals, defining problems, helping set rules and contributing ideas by: • Getting started • Clarifying purpose • Defining goals • Maintaining direction	*Aggression*: Asserting personal dominance and attempting to get own way regardless of others by: • Criticizing • Attacking personality • Dominating • Name calling
Persuading: Requesting facts and relevant information on the problem. Seeking out expressions of feelings and values by: • Questioning • Encouraging and guiding responses, advocating • Developing alternatives	*Manipulation*: Responding to a problem rigidly and using stereotypical responses by: • Topic jumping • Masking statements as questions • Selective interpretation • Gate keeping
Committing: Helping to ensure that all members are part of the decision-making process by: • Facilitating involvement • Summarizing • Gaining commitment • Problem-solving	*Dependence*: Reacting to other people as authority figures, abdicating problem-solving to others, expecting others to lead the solution by: • Agreeing with everything • Avoiding decisions or closure through sarcasm • Seeking sympathy • Expressing futility, resignation or helplessness
Attending: Demonstrating a willingness to become involved by: • Listening • Showing an interest • Monitoring and observing • Taking notes or recording • Sharing responsibilities • Regular attendance at meetings • Exchanging ideas and suggestions	*Avoidance*: An emotional retreat in thought or actions by: • Withdrawing psychologically • Withdrawing physically • Reflecting boredom • Escaping the group

Adapted from Hersey & Blanchard (1988).

REFLECTIVE PRACTICE Box 2.10

Effective teamwork

Think about situations where you have observed members of the MDT working in your placement.

Student activities

- How is team coordination carried out?
- Who are the other team members?
- What are the team members' responsibilities in the delivery of care?
- To what extent do team members adopt helpful or hindering behaviours (see Table 2.2)?
- How do you think these behaviours may impact on patient/client care?

shift in ethos and culture. Following a review of nursing education, the UKCC (1999) recommended measures that would enable fitness for practice through better preparation of student nurses which was to be based on healthcare need. There was also a move to ensure that placement experience and mentors prepared competent practitioners who were able to provide safe care. This resulted in the development of proficiencies for pre-registration nursing programmes. Two major changes were:

- Supernumerary status for nursing students who are now considered to be students with important learning needs rather than part of the workforce
- Shifting from a focus on illness to the promotion of health and prevention of illness.

Nursing programmes now include a common foundation programme, which is followed by one of four branch programmes:

- Adult nursing
- Children's nursing
- Mental health nursing
- Learning disabilities nursing.

The NMC has a responsibility to ensure that registered nurses, midwives and specialist community public health nurses provide high standards of care to their patients and clients. To this end, the NMC (2004c) has set out CFP outcomes necessary for entry into a branch programme and the standard of proficiency that must be achieved prior to registration (Table 2.3). They are described under four domains:

- Professional and ethical practice
- Care delivery
- Care management
- Personal and professional development.

Common foundation programme
All nursing students undertake the same CFP. This is because all branches of nursing share common skills and knowledge. The CFP lasts for 1 year and the main areas of study are:

- Professional ethical and legal issues (see Chs 5–7)
- The theory and practice of nursing (most chapters)
- The context in which health and social care is delivered (see Ch. 3)
- Organizational structures and processes (see Ch. 3)
- Communication (see Ch. 9)
- Social and life sciences relevant to nursing (see Ch. 8 and later chapters)
- Frameworks for social care provision and care systems (see Ch. 3).

This book explores all these areas in sufficient depth to enable you to learn about them with examples that relate to each branch of nursing. The relevance to clinical nursing practice is reinforced throughout the CFP and half of the programme takes place in clinical settings. All students undertake placements that reflect nursing as it applies to the care of adults, children, people with mental health problems and those with learning disabilities. Before progressing to a branch programme, the NMC outcomes (NMC 2004c) (see Table 2.3) must have been met.

Branch programmes
Branch programmes last for 2 years and, like the CFP, are half theory and half practice. The theoretical subjects studied are the same as during the CFP, but they are applied to the different branch programmes and include more detailed knowledge that underpins the more specialized care provided by RNs. Before registration, students are required to demonstrate achievement of professional standards of proficiency (see Table 2.3) and complete a self-declaration of good health and good character (NMC 2004c).

Branches of nursing

The main differences between the current branches of nursing are explored below. While most nurses undertake only one branch of nursing, the patient/client boundaries are not mutually exclusive; there is therefore a need for all RNs to have an understanding of each of the branches. For example, both adult and children's nurses will encounter clients with learning disability when they access primary healthcare through GP surgeries or require admission to hospital, and mental health nurses may have clients with coexisting physical conditions such as diabetes, chronic bronchitis or leg ulcers.

Table 2.3 Standard 7 – First level nurses – nursing standards of education to achieve the NMC standards of proficiency

Standard of proficiency for entry to the register: professional and ethical practice
Manage oneself, one's practice, and that of others, in accordance with *The NMC code of professional conduct: standards for conduct, performance and ethics*, recognizing one's own abilities and limitations

Domain	Outcomes to be achieved for entry to the branch programme	Standards of proficiency for entry to the register: professional and ethical practice
Professional and ethical practice	*Discuss in an informed manner the implications of professional regulation for nursing practice* • Demonstrate a basic knowledge of professional regulation and self-regulation • Recognize and acknowledge the limitations of one's own abilities • Recognize situations that require referral to a registered practitioner *Demonstrate an awareness of The NMC Code of Professional Conduct: Standards for Conduct, Performance and Ethics* • Commit to the principle that the primary purpose of the registered nurse is to protect and serve society • Accept responsibility for one's own actions and decisions	• Practice in accordance with *The NMC Code of Professional Conduct: Standards for Conduct, Performance and Ethics* • Use professional standards of practice to self-assess performance • Consult with a registered nurse when nursing care requires expertise beyond one's own current scope of competence • Consult other healthcare professional when individual or group needs fall outside the scope of nursing practice • Identify unsafe practice and respond appropriately to ensure a safe outcome • Manage the delivery of care services within the sphere of one's own accountability

(Continued)

Table 2.3 *(Continued)*

Standard of proficiency for entry to the register: professional and ethical practice
Practise in accordance with an ethical and legal framework which ensures the primacy of patient and client interest and well-being and respects confidentiality

Domain	Outcomes to be achieved for entry to the branch programme	Standards of proficiency for entry to the register: professional and ethical practice
Professional and ethical practice	*Demonstrate an awareness of, and apply ethical principles to, nursing practice* • Demonstrate respect for patient and client confidentiality • Identify ethical issues in day-to-day practice. *Demonstrate an awareness of legislation relevant to nursing practice* • Identify key issues in relevant legislation relating to mental health, children, data protection, manual handling, and health and safety, etc.	• Demonstrate knowledge of legislation and health and social policy relevant to nursing practice • Ensure the confidentiality and security of written and verbal information acquired in a professional capacity • Demonstrate knowledge of contemporary ethical issues and their impact on nursing and healthcare • Manage the complexities arising from ethical and legal dilemmas • Act appropriately when seeking access to caring for patients and clients in their own homes

Standard of proficiency for entry to the register: professional and ethical practice
Practice in a fair and antidiscriminatory way, acknowledging the differences in beliefs and cultural practices of individuals of groups

Domain	Outcomes to be achieved for entry to the branch programme	Standards of proficiency for entry to the register: care delivery
Professional and ethical practice	*Demonstrate the importance of promoting equity in patient and client care by contributing to nursing care in a fair and antidiscriminatory way* • Demonstrate fairness and sensitivity when responding to patients, clients and groups from diverse circumstances • Recognize the needs of patients and clients whose lives are affected by disability, however manifest	• Maintain, support and acknowledge the rights of individuals or groups in the healthcare setting • Act to ensure that the rights of individuals and groups are not compromised • Respect the values, customs and beliefs of individuals and groups • Provide care which demonstrates sensitivity to the diversity of patients and clients

Standard of proficiency for entry to the register: care delivery
Engage in, develop and disengage from therapeutic relationships through the use of appropriate communication and interpersonal skills

Domain	Outcomes to be achieved for entry to the branch programme	Standards of proficiency for entry to the register: care delivery
Care delivery	*Discuss methods of, barriers to, and the boundaries of, effective communication and interpersonal relationships* • Recognize the effect of one's own values on interactions with patients and clients and their carers, families and friends • Utilize appropriate communication skills with patients and clients • Acknowledge the boundaries of a professional caring relationship *Demonstrate sensitivity when interacting with and providing information to patients and clients*	• Utilize a range of effective and appropriate communication and engagement skills • Maintain and, where appropriate, disengage from professional caring relationships that focus on meeting the patient's or client's needs within professional therapeutic boundaries

Standard of proficiency for entry to the register: care delivery
Create and utilize opportunities to promote the health and well-being of patients, clients and groups

Domain	Outcomes to be achieved for entry to the branch programme	Standards of proficiency for entry to the register: care delivery
Care delivery	*Contribute to enhancing the health and social well-being of patients and clients by understanding how, under the supervision of a registered practitioner, to:* • Contribute to the assessment of health needs • Identify opportunities for health promotion	• Consult with patients, clients and groups to identify their need and desire for health promotion advice • Provide relevant and current health information to patients, clients and groups in a form which facilitates their understanding and acknowledges

(Continued)

Table 2.3 (*Continued*)

Domain	Outcomes to be achieved for entry to the branch programme	Standards of proficiency for entry to the register: care delivery
	• Identify networks of health and social care services	choice/individual preference • Provide support and education in the development and/or maintenance of independent living skills • Seek specialist/expert advice as appropriate

Standard of proficiency for entry to the register: care delivery
Undertake and document a comprehensive, systematic and accurate nursing assessment of the physical, psychological, social and spiritual needs of patients, clients and communities

Domain	Outcomes to be achieved for entry to the branch programme	Standards of proficiency for entry to the register: care delivery
Care delivery	*Contribute to the development and documentation of nursing assessments by participating in comprehensive and systematic nursing assessment of the physical, psychological, social and spiritual needs of patients and clients* • Be aware of assessment strategies to guide the collection of data for assessing patients and clients and use assessment tools under guidance • Discuss the prioritization of care needs • Be aware of the need to reassess patients and clients as to their needs for nursing care	• Select valid and reliable assessment tools for the required purpose • Systematically collect data regarding the health and functional status of individuals, clients and communities through appropriate interaction, observation and measurement • Analyse and interpret data accurately to inform nursing care and take appropriate action

Standard of proficiency for entry to the register: care delivery
Formulate and document a plan of nursing care, where possible, in partnership with patients, clients, their carers and family and friends, within a framework of informed consent

Domain	Outcomes to be achieved for entry to the branch programme	Standards of proficiency for entry to the register: care delivery
Care delivery	*Contribute to the planning of nursing care, involving patients and clients and, where possible, their carers; demonstrate an understanding of helping patients and clients to make informed decisions* • Identify care needs based on the assessment of a patient or client • Participate in the negotiation and agreement of the care plan with the patient or client and with their carer, family and friends, as appropriate, under the supervision of a registered nurse • Inform patients and clients about intended nursing actions, respecting their right to participate in decisions about their care	• Establish priorities for care based on individual or group needs • Develop and document a care plan to achieve optimal health, habilitation and rehabilitation based on assessment and current nursing knowledge • Identify expected outcomes, including a time frame for achievement and/or review in consultation with patients, clients, their carers and family and friends and with members of the health and social care team.

Standard of proficiency for entry to the register: care delivery
Based on the best available evidence, apply knowledge and an appropriate repertoire of skills indicative of safe and effective nursing practice

Domain	Outcomes to be achieved for entry to the branch programme	Standards of proficiency for entry to the register: care delivery
Care delivery	*Contribute to the implementation of a programme of nursing care, designed and supervised by registered practitioners* • Undertake activities that are consistent with the care plan and within the limits of one's own abilities *Demonstrate evidence of a developing knowledge base with underpins safe and effective nursing practice*	• Ensure that current research findings and other evidence are incorporated in practice • Identify relevant changes in practice or new information and disseminate it to colleagues • Contribute to the application of a range of interventions which support and optomize the health and well-being of patients and clients

(*Continued*)

Table 2.3 *(Continued)*

Domain	Outcomes to be achieved for entry to the branch programme	Standards of proficiency for entry to the register: care delivery
	• Access and discuss research and other evidence in nursing and related disciplines • Identify examples of the use of evidence in planned nursing interventions *Demonstrate a range of essential nursing skills, under the supervision of a registered nurse, to meet individuals' needs, which include:* Maintaining dignity, privacy and confidentiality; effective communication and observational skills, including listening and taking physiological measurements; safety and health, including moving, and handling and infection control; essential first aid and emergency procedures; administration of medicines; emotional, physical and personal care, including meeting the need for comfort, nutrition and personal hygiene	• Demonstrate the safe application of the skills required to meet the needs of patients and clients within the current sphere and practice • Identify and respond to patients and clients' continuing learning and care needs • Engage with, and evaluate, the evidence base that underpins safe nursing practice

Standard of proficiency for entry to the register: care delivery
Provide a rationale for the nursing care delivered which takes account of social, cultural, spiritual, legal, political and economic influences

Domain	Outcomes to be achieved for entry to the branch programme	Standards of proficiency for entry to the register: care delivery
Care delivery		• Identify, collect and evaluate information to justify the effective utilization of resources to achieve planned outcomes of nursing care.

Standard of proficiency for entry to the register: care delivery
Evaluate and document the outcomes of nursing and other interventions

Domain	Outcomes to be achieved for entry to the branch programme	Standards of proficiency for entry to the register: care delivery
Care delivery	*Contribute to the evaluation of the appropriateness of nursing care delivered* • Demonstrate an awareness of the need to assess regularly a patient's or client's response to nursing interventions • Provide for a supervising registered practitioner, evaluative commentary and information on nursing care based on personal observations and actions • Contribute to the documentation of the outcomes of nursing interventions	• Collaborate with patients and clients and, when appropriate, additional carers to review and monitor the progress of individuals or groups towards planned outcomes • Analyse and revise expected outcomes, nursing interventions and priorities in accordance with changes in the individual's condition, needs or circumstances

Standard of proficiency for entry to the register: care delivery
Demonstrate sound clinical judgement across a range of differing professional and care delivery contexts

Domain	Outcomes to be achieved for entry to the branch programme	Standards of proficiency for entry to the register: care delivery
Care delivery	*Recognize situations in which agreed plans of nursing care no longer appear appropriate and refer these to an appropriate accountable practitioner* • Demonstrate the ability to discuss and accept care decisions • Accurately record observations made and communicate these to the relevant members of the health and social care team	• Use evidence-based knowledge from nursing and related disciplines to select and individualize nursing interventions • Demonstrate the ability to transfer skills and knowledge to a variety of circumstances and settings • Recognize the need for adaptation and adapt nursing practice to meet varying and unpredictable circumstances • Ensure that practice does not compromise the nurse's duty of care to individuals or the safety of the public

(Continued)

Table 2.3 *(Continued)*

Standard of proficiency for entry to the register: care management
Contribute to public protection by creating and maintaining a safe environment of care through the use of quality assurance and risk management strategies

Domain	Outcomes to be achieved for entry to the branch programme	Standards of proficiency for entry to the register: care management
Care management	*Contribute to the identification of actual and potential risks to patients, clients and their carers, to oneself and to others, and participate in measures to promote and ensure health and safety* • Understand and implement health and safety principles and policies • Recognize and report situations that are potentially unsafe for patients, clients, oneself and others	• Apply relevant principles to ensure the safe administration of therapeutic substances • Use appropriate risk assessment tools to identify actual and potential risks • Identify environmental hazards and eliminate and/or prevent where possible • Communicate safety concerns to a relevant authority • Manage risk to provide care which best meets the needs and interests of patients, clients and the public

Standard of proficiency for entry to the register: care management
Demonstrate knowledge of effective interprofessional working practices which respect and utilize the contributions of members of the health and social care team

Domain	Outcomes to be achieved for entry to the branch programme	Standards of proficiency for entry to the register: care management
Care management	*Demonstrate an understanding of the role of others by participating in interprofessional working practice* • Identify the roles of the members of the health and social care team • Work within the health and social care team to maintain and enhance integrated care	• Establish and maintain collaborative working relationships with members of the health and social care team and others • Participate with members of the health and social care team in decision-making concerning patients and clients • Review and evaluate care with members of the health and social care team and others

Standard of proficiency for entry to the register: care management
Delegate duties of others, as appropriate, ensuring that they are supervised and monitored

Domain	Outcomes to be achieved for entry to the branch programme	Standards of proficiency for entry to the register: care management
Care management		• Take into account the role and competence of staff when delegating work • Maintain one's own accountability and responsibility when delegating aspects of care to others • Demonstrate the ability to coordinate the delivery of nursing and health care

Standard of proficiency for entry to the register: care management
Demonstrate key skills

Domain	Outcomes to be achieved for entry to the branch programme	Standards of proficiency for entry to the register: care management
Care management	*Demonstrate literacy, numeracy and computer skills needed to record, enter, store, retrieve and organize data essential for care delivery*	• Literacy – interpret and present information in a comprehensible manner • Numeracy – accurately interpret numerical data and their significance for the safe delivery of care • Information technology and management – interpret and utilize data and technology, taking account of legal, ethical and safety considerations, in the delivery and enhancement of care • Problem-solving – demonstrate sound clinical decision-making which can be justified even when made on the basis of limited information

(Continued)

Table 2.3 *(Continued)*

Standard of proficiency for entry to the register: personal and professional development
Demonstrate a commitment to the need for continuing professional development and personal supervision activities in order to enhance knowledge, skills, values and attitudes needed for safe and effective nursing practice

Domain	Outcomes to be achieved for entry to the branch programme	Standards of proficiency for entry to the register: personal and professional development
Personal and professional development	*Demonstrate responsibility for one's own learning through the development of a portfolio of practice and recognize when further learning is required* • Identify specific learning needs and objectives • Begin to engage with, and interpret, the evidence base which underpins nursing practice *Acknowledge the importance of seeking supervision to develop safe and effective nursing practice*	• Identify one's own professional development needs by engaging in activities such as reflection in, and on, practice and lifelong learning • Develop a personal development plan which takes into account personal, professional and organizational needs • Share experiences with colleagues and patients and clients in order to identify the additional knowledge and skills needed to manage unfamiliar or professionally challenging situations • Take action to meet any identified knowledge and skills deficit likely to affect the delivery of care within the current sphere of practice

Standard of proficiency for entry to the register: personal and professional development
Enhance the professional development and safe practice of others through peer support, leadership, supervision and teaching

Domain	Outcomes to be achieved for entry to the branch programme	Standards of proficiency for entry to the register: personal and professional development
Personal and professional development		• Contribute to creating a climate conducive to learning • Contribute to the learning experiences and development of others by facilitating the mutual sharing of knowledge and experience • Demonstrate effective leadership in the establishment and maintenance of safe nursing practise

Reproduced with kind permission of the Nursing and Midwifery Council (2004).

Adult nursing

Adult nurses are primarily responsible for health promotion and providing holistic care for physically ill or injured adults with wide-ranging levels of dependency in both hospital and community settings. The focus is on the individual patient, rather than the condition from which they may be suffering; and the needs and anxieties that their condition may generate, including the pressures on their family and friends.

Adult nursing placements include care homes, hospital wards and specialist clinics, and community placements that may involve visiting people at home or attachments to health centres. Nurses play an increasingly prominent role in the provision of health-focused care in the community. Many hospital-based nurses are found in specialist areas such as intensive care, cancer care and care of older adults (Table 2.4). Adult nurses work with people over 18 years of ages who have acute (short-term) and chronic (long-term) conditions.

Despite the wide range of specialties, there are a number of features common to most adult nursing roles (Box 2.11). While this often includes physical care, it extends well beyond that, including counselling, advice and education that draws upon interpersonal and communication skills to address psychological, social and spiritual aspects of holistic care.

Most patients have specific problems but can eventually look forward to an independent future. The nurse's role is to offer support while it is needed and give people the skills, strength or knowledge that will help them to regain independence. Box 2.12 provides the opportunity to consider the types of health-related problems that people may experience as a result of sudden illness and change in independence.

Learning disability nursing

Health policy in the UK is explicitly directed at social inclusion and social justice for all citizens. This policy is clearly outlined in *Valuing People* (DH 2001) and *The Same as You?* (Scottish Executive Health Department 2000a). These documents state that people with learning disabilities should be respected and valued and afforded the same opportunities as others, as well as receiving additional support and services to meet their individual needs.

In Scotland the policy around promoting health and supporting inclusion for people with learning disabilities has developed considerably over recent years. As there are, as yet, no similar developments elsewhere in the UK, it is useful to examine how policy and practice in Scotland has been developing. *Caring for Scotland* is the strategy for nursing and midwifery in Scotland (Scottish Executive

Table 2.4 Some adult nursing specialties

Specialty	Focus of care
Palliative care (see Ch. 12)	Holistic relief of symptoms such as pain or breathlessness (rather than effecting a cure), support for patients and their families and friends. This is often, but not necessarily, for people with cancer
Accident and emergency nursing	Any presenting problem that requires urgent intervention
Women's health (gynaecology)	Women requiring health screening, family planning, sexual health advice and interventions involving the reproductive organs
Orthopaedics	Maximizing mobility and independence in people with bone problems such as fractures, congenital bone malformations
Older adults (gerontology)	Holistic approach to problems which are often multiple or specific conditions which tend to become increasingly common with age
Ophthalmic nursing	Problems affecting the eye and vision
Dermatology nursing	Conditions affecting the skin, which often affect body image (see Ch. 11)
Cancer nursing (oncology)	Helping people to cope with the diagnosis of and treatment for cancer and any related nursing problems
Rehabilitation (see Ch. 11)	Assisting people to achieve optimal functioning and reduce the risk of mortality/morbidity through health promotion
Cardiology (see Ch. 17)	Caring for people with heart disorders, supporting families with a child with a congenital heart defect, cardiac rehabilitation
Perioperative care (see Ch. 24)	Nursing care required before, during and after surgery

CRITICAL THINKING Box 2.11

Rehabilitation nursing

As a primary nurse (p. 49), Sandra is the RN responsible for every aspect of nursing care for a group of eight older adults on a rehabilitation ward, who are cared for in two bays of four beds, one male and one female. She directs the work of associate nurses (p. 49), who are less experienced and assist with care delivery. Sandra is accountable for patient care, i.e. she ensures that the care is of good quality and appropriate to patients' needs. Today Sandra's patients range in age from 69 to 84 and present a variety of nursing problems due to their underlying medical conditions:

- Zayan is unable to move one side and cannot speak coherently following a severe stroke. This means he is very dependent on nurses for all aspects of his care.
- Doris has swollen legs and becomes very breathless when she exerts herself due to heart failure. She finds it difficult to mobilize.
- Emrys is on the ward for his regular 2-week period of respite care so that his daughter who normally cares for him at home can have a break. He has slow movements, rigidity and a marked tremor due to Parkinson's disease. This means that he finds it difficult to turn over in bed, feed himself and walk to the lavatory.

Sandra begins her day by reading the notes made by the night staff about her patients' progress and reflecting on the care they have received. Next she visits each of the patients with the associate nurse, taking the care plans along with her. The purpose of the visit is to discuss the day's care with each patient and to agree the priorities that will meet their needs. Sandra knows from nursing research that it is good practice to involve patients and their families in decisions about their care (Bakalis & Watson 2005).

Student activities

- What do you think Sandra will discuss with her patients when she meets them?
- What do you think Sandra will be observing?

Health Department 2000b). This strategy outlined the intention of the Scottish Executive to undertake a review of the contribution of all nurses and midwives to the care and support of people with learning disabilities. *Promoting Health, Supporting Inclusion* was published by the Scottish Executive in 2002 and details the actions required from all nurses and midwives to improve the health and well-being of children, adults and older people with learning disabilities in Scotland. Recommendation 1 of *Promoting Health, Supporting Inclusion* invited NHS Health Scotland, Scotland's national health improvement organization, to undertake a strategic needs assessment of the health needs of children, adults and older people with learning disabilities. This comprehensive health needs assessment was published in 2004 and details the inequalities that require to be addressed strategically and locally in order to promote social justice for this group of Scottish citizens (NHS Health Scotland 2004). Thus it is evident that these health inequalities need to be redressed so that people with learning disabilities can indeed be included in our society in an equitable, respectful and dignified fashion.

There is some confusion regarding the use of the term learning disability, which can vary from country to country. The term learning disability has been adopted in the UK and is the one that users of services prefer. However, the terms intellectual disability and developmental disability are commonly used in other parts of the developed world. In the UK the term usually refers to a variety of disorders that adversely affects the acquisition, retention and understanding of new or complex information and often also the use of verbal or non-verbal communication. It has a lasting effect on development and results in a varying degree of support from others being required to cope with daily living (Gates & Wilberforce 2002).

REFLECTIVE PRACTICE Box 2.12

The impact of sudden illness or change in independence

Imagine you wake up one morning to find that you have lost all sensation and power in your dominant hand.

Student activities

- How would you feel?
- What impact would this have on your day?
- What usual activities would you have difficulty in doing by yourself?
- Would it change the contribution that you make to your family or household?
- What would you expect of the healthcare team?
- What would you expect of your family?
- What would you expect of the university?

The role of the nurse is to help people with a learning disability and their families to maintain and improve their lifestyles by promoting health, and to participate fully as equal members of society. The Quality Assurance Agency (QAA) for Higher Education (2002, p. 9) identifies that learning disability nurses:

> . . . work with people with a range of learning disabilities and with their families and significant others. Learning disability nurses' work is underpinned by the concepts of partnership, inclusion and advocacy. The role of the learning disability nurse, specifically is to assist and support people to become and remain healthy, to improve their competence and quality of life, and to fulfil their potential. Learning disability nurses work with people with a spectrum of needs and abilities in a wide variety of settings, often working collaboratively with professionals from a range of health and social care agencies. This support may take place in the National Health Service (NHS), voluntary or independent sector, or in the client's own home.

It can be seen then that the primary role of the learning disability nurse is in meeting the health needs of people with a learning disability. However, the role is wide-ranging and could also include helping people to develop their manual and recognition skills so that they can use kitchen equipment to make a pot of tea. In other instances, nurses may, with the rest of the MDT, be involved in underpinning people's efforts to find a job and bring up a family. It requires considerable sensitivity and skill to offer the best care to people with learning disabilities and their families without being intrusive.

The ultimate aim is to empower the individual to maximize their full potential. O'Brien (1981) describes this process as 'normalization' which includes five accomplishments:

- Community presence
- Community participation
- Making choices
- Ensuring competence
- Enhancing respect.

The distinctive contribution of learning disability nurses is their influence on behaviours and lifestyles that promote health and maximize well-being and independence for people with learning disabilities, their families and carers. Care takes place in a wide variety of settings: people's own homes, their family homes, community houses, residential care, schools, workplaces, leisure centres and healthcare facilities. Some nurses maintain this broad spread of activity, whereas others choose a specialist area such as supporting people with interactional challenges and complex needs education, or management of learning disability services.

The main challenge is meeting health needs since it is apparent that the health needs of people with learning disabilities are greater and more complex and often present differently from those of the general population. Some conditions occur more frequently than in the rest of the population. These include:

- Vision and hearing impairments (see Ch. 16)
- Mental health problems
- Gastro-oesophageal reflux disorder (GORD) (see Ch. 19)
- Epilepsy (see Ch. 16).

Other health needs are associated with particular groups, e.g. people with Down's syndrome are more prone to depression, thyroid function disorders, hearing impairment and dementia. It is obviously important that learning disability nurses have the ability to recognize these differing health needs but it is also apparent that all nurses require an awareness of these specific health needs in order to reduce intentional discrimination and enhance access to healthcare services (NHS Health Scotland 2004).

Learning disability nurses coordinate care and work with the whole family and other carers to befriend, teach, support, counsel and carry out therapeutic activities. They also make regular assessments of healthcare needs and ensure the availability of resources to meet them. In this field it is not only important for nurses to know how to care for the well-being of their clients but also to teach their families, friends and carers who provide regular care to do the same. Often this entails caring for a person who has seizures or epilepsy, incontinence (see Chs 20, 21) or a physical disability that has led to immobility (see Ch. 18) or sensory impairment.

The Scottish Human Services Trust works in partnership with organizations to help them become more responsive to the people they serve (Box 2.13). Their values of inclusion mirror those of 'person-centredness' (p. 47) and are considered appropriate for use in the health and social care of people with a learning disability. Box 2.14 provides the opportunity to consider the impact of this in relation to people with learning disabilities.

Using the information in Box 2.14, consider the realities of caring for John. It is frequently physically and psychologically demanding, particularly on parents and other carers. Breaks from physical caring will be few and liable to interruption at any time. Furthermore, there is the need to ensure that John does not become frustrated or depressed by the constraints and demands

Box 2.13 **Values of inclusion**

- Everyone is born in – we are all born as equal citizens and part of a community, we are only later excluded
- All means all – everyone capable of breathing, even if breathing requires support, is entitled to be included – no-one is too disabled to qualify
- Presence is a prerequisite – if people are physically excluded, they have to be physically included (presence being the first criterion for inclusion) – if you're not there, no-one will know you are missing
- In is not with – being there is necessary – but being with takes time and effort. A community is not merely a locality; it is also a network of connections and relationships. We have to help people to be part of and belong to communities, not just be lonely residents within them
- Everyone is ready – no-one has to pass a test or meet a set of criteria to be eligible – everyone is ready to be part of the community now and it is the community's task to find ways of including them
- Everyone needs support – and some need more support than others – no-one is fully independent and independence isn't our goal. We are working towards interdependence and differing degrees and kinds of support at different times
- Everyone can communicate – just because someone can't speak doesn't mean that they don't have anything to say – everyone can communicate and we have to work harder at hearing, seeing, understanding and feeling what people are communicating to us
- Everyone can contribute – each person has their own gifts and strengths – and each person has a unique contribution to make. Our task is to recognize, encourage and value each person's contribution
- Together we are better – we do not believe that the world would be a better place without disability in it. We are not dreaming of a world where all disabilities are cured and eradicated – we believe that diversity does bring strength and that we can all learn and grow by knowing one another.

Reproduced with kind permission of the Scottish Human Services Trust (2004).

REFLECTIVE PRACTICE Box 2.14

The impact of learning disability

John is a 25-year-old man who has complex needs that have affected both his intellectual and physical development. John uses non-verbal communication to convey his needs to his family and carers. John has a specially adapted wheelchair to aid his mobility and his house has specifically designed lifting equipment. On weekdays he attends a local centre for people with learning disabilities but, when at home, John spends much of his time in the lounge on a special chair, watching television or listening to music. John's physical comfort – which includes those things we take for granted such as bathing, shaving, using the lavatory, dressing and undressing – is carried out by his parents. He goes out for weekend trips with his parents in a car that is specially adapted to suit the purpose.

Both his parents have taken early retirement to look after John full-time as his physical needs have increased over the last 2 years. John's parents have had to adapt to their reduced income and become full-time carers, which has had an impact on their quality of life.

They have kept in touch with two couples that they have known for many years and meet up once a month for a meal at John's house with each couple contributing a course. Everyone looks forward to the meal but John's parents have to leave their guests to assist John prepare for bed.

Student activities

Talk to a learning disabilities nurse about:

- The difficulties experienced by families caring for a person such as John who has a learning disability.
- The nurse's role in supporting clients like John and his family.

placed on his life. Since it is difficult for John to travel, the family will hardly ever go away from home together, even to enjoy a meal out. Finally, John's parents may constantly worry about what will happen to John when they grow older and die; most parents of people with a learning disability live in fear of their children going into institutional care when they are no longer there to look after them. The learning disability nurse could help John's parents in a variety of ways, for example:

- Their fears could be fully explored
- A plan could be identified for how John may be prepared both now and in the future
- Respite care could be arranged
- Information from support organizations such as PAMIS could be provided (see Useful websites, p. 68).

In conclusion, the role of the learning disability nurse is built on developing equal partnerships with the people they work with so that the health needs of people with learning disabilities, their families and carers can be met in an effective, efficient and resourceful manner. Learning disability nurses treat people as unique, whole individuals with specific needs and desires. They practise in a sensitive and non-discriminatory manner to enable people to fulfil their needs and aspirations so that people with learning disabilities can truly be include within our society.

Mental health nursing

Mental health nurses care for people with mental health problems, also known as mental distress, in diverse settings in both the hospital and community. They play key roles in the promotion of good mental health and the prevention of mental health problems, provide care and interventions to people experiencing mental health problems and support people to develop strategies to enable them to work towards recovery. A major focus of the role of mental health nursing is promoting social inclusion and challenging stigma. To facilitate this, mental health nurses must practise in a way that is underpinned by a clear values base that is focused on delivering rights-based care. At the time of writing the publication of reviews of the role of mental health nursing in Scotland and England are set to influence further development of the profession (Box 2.15).

Everyone can experience distress at some time in their life, e.g. episodes of stress, anxiety or depression (see Ch. 11). At any given time, one adult in six suffers from some form of mental health problem (National Statistics Office 2004); in other words, mental health problems are as common as asthma.

Mental health nurses are at the forefront in providing the support required for people with mental health problems who need to access health services, working as part of multidisciplinary teams with other professionals such as GPs, psychiatrists, social workers and allied health professionals to coordinate and provide care. A wide range of other services, e.g. voluntary organizations, local government and housing agencies, may also be involved. In recent years, there has been a significant shift from hospitals to the community as the main setting for mental health care. Nurses work with people in their homes, in small residential units and in local health centres with considerable autonomy in how they plan and deliver care. Community psychiatric nurses (CPNs) (increasingly known as community mental health nurses) are key members of the MDT in mental health service provision. The one-to-one therapeutic relationships that mental health nurses form with their clients are at the heart of mental health nursing. Nursing interventions include providing social and physical care, and psychological and psychosocial interventions such as counselling and cognitive behavioural therapy, as well as working with other professional groups and the voluntary organizations involved in supporting people with mental health problems. Mental health nurses also have a role in assessing and managing individual risk, which requires sophisticated assessment skills.

Mental health nurses work with people of all ages and from a wide range of backgrounds, and mental health nursing provides opportunities to practise in diverse areas including older people's mental health, child and adolescent mental health services (CAMHS), forensic mental health services and acute inpatient care.

REFLECTIVE PRACTICE Box 2.15

The future for mental health nursing

In 2006 the Chief Nursing Officers in both Scotland and England launched reports (see Resources) of reviews of the future role of mental health nursing. While the reviews were conducted in both countries independently, and used different methods, they share many common messages about the future role of mental health nursing and make several recommendations for the future development of the profession.

Student activities

1. Access both reports and considers the key messages about:
   - The policy that sets out the future direction for mental health care and services
   - The role of mental health nursing
   - The future development of the profession.
2. You may also wish to reflect on the differences and similarities between the reports

[Resources: The full Scottish Review Report entitled *Rights, Relationships and Recovery*, a summarized version, and a 5-year Action Plan to support the development of the profession in Scotland. Online: www.scotland.gov.uk/Publications/2006/04/18164814/0; The English Report *From Values to Action*. Online: www.dh.gov.uk/PublicationsAndStatistics/Publications/PublicationsPolicyAndGuidance/PublicationsPolicyAndGuidanceArticle/fs/en?CONTENT_ID=4133839&chk=RJV7mg All available July 2006]

Children's nursing

Children's nurses are responsible for teaching families, providing support and helping families to make decisions in the best interest of their child. To do this, nurses need to develop partnerships with families and acknowledge that family members provide nursing care. Chevannes (1997) identified three stages of interaction when working in partnership with families:

- Family members should be encouraged to state the care needs as they see them
- The child and the carer in conjunction with the nurse should identify the types and patterns of care in relation to the child's needs
- The child, carer and nurse should all participate in devising care plans.

Some difficulties may be encountered, for example:

- Parents might be intimidated in a strange environment
- Language barriers may exist due to 'jargon' used by healthcare professionals (see Ch. 9)
- Parents may be reluctant to discuss the values and beliefs held in their culture and that stereotypical assumptions (see Ch. 1) may be formed about some families.

Children have different physical, psychological and social needs at different ages and developmental stages (see Ch. 8). Children's need for intervention by health professionals starts before conception and continues through adolescence and transitional care to adult services. The type of intervention required depends upon the particular health needs of the child and family at any given time. Children's nurses learn skills in caring for whole families, including grandparents, siblings, carers and friends. Skills in family-centred care also involve teaching (see Ch. 4) so that the nurse can teach families and empower them with knowledge and skills so that they can carry out almost any of nursing care the child requires.

Children's nurses in hospitals provide care and skilled observation and treatment. They involve parents at all times, helping them to cope with their fears and the trauma of sudden hospital admissions. Parents may be unsure that they have done everything they should have and whether they have called the doctor early enough. The children's nurse listens to these worries, explores issues with parents and provides information and health promotion advice as appropriate. Involving parents helps them to feel included in the nursing care and maintains their relationship with their child.

Children's nurses work in homes, schools and other community and hospital settings. They work in special schools for children with learning disabilities or may support children who have long-term health problems such as asthma, cystic fibrosis, diabetes or eczema and those with life-limiting conditions. This can be at home and in community, day care, hospice or hospital settings.

Nurses working with children in any setting must become vigilant, observant and attentive in order to identify vulnerable children, i.e. those at risk or potential risk from physical or emotional injury, abuse or neglect. Although children are generally best looked after by their families, the welfare of children is absolutely paramount and their needs are uppermost if there is conflict between those and carers/parental needs. Nurses have a responsibility to respect and promote the rights of the child and play an important role in child protection by reporting any suspicion of non-accidental injury, abuse or neglect and following local protocols for safeguarding children (see Chs 3, 6).

Roles of non-registered staff

Non-registered staff such as HCAs, clinical support workers, therapy assistants or nursing auxiliaries (see Ch. 3) work with registered nurses and other healthcare professionals, helping with treatment and looking after people's comfort and well-being. They are employed in many areas in both hospitals and the community. The nature of their role depends on the area in which they work, but it is important to note that the registered practitioner is accountable for the work of non-registered staff (including students, see Ch. 7).

HCAs on a hospital ward might make beds, take temperatures and help patients with washing, feeding and toileting. In clinics and high dependency areas some undertake more complex procedures, e.g. take blood, take observations, change dressings and manage intravenous infusions. In the community, e.g. health centres, care homes and schools, they might take blood samples, help those with complex needs with eating or going to the toilet or they may have first aid responsibilities.

National vocational qualifications

National vocational qualifications (NVQs) and Scottish vocational qualifications (SVQs) are methods of gaining academic credit through a combination of theory, work-based learning and assessment. Some NHS organizations and other employers have developed work-based training for clinical support workers that lead to the acquisition of NVQs/SVQs levels 2 and 3, which can provide entry into pre-registration nurse education. The main purpose of this development was to improve the skill mix in practice, to ensure clinical support workers are competent in the skills they are expected to carry out and to offer improved career opportunities. NVQs and SVQs are also available in many fields outside the healthcare sector.

Roles of the nurse

This section describes the generic roles of the nurse in clinical settings, as well as some specialist and advanced roles undertaken by nurses.

Generic roles for the experienced RN

Nurses working in clinical settings can fulfil roles that include:

- Managing a caseload
- Administering medications; some may also prescribe medication after further training
- Assessing, planning, implementing and evaluating care
- Documentation of care
- Liaison and coordination of care
- Discharge planning
- Managing a team.

Mentoring

It is expected that RNs will take on the role of mentoring student nurses about a year following registration (Box 2.16). They should receive support from nurse educators in carrying out this role. The NMC (2004d) outlined standards for mentors and mentorship that include:

- Establishing effective communication and working relationships based on mutual trust and respect
- Facilitation of learning by understanding students' learning needs and integrating learning from practice and educational settings
- Demonstrating the ability to assess practice
- Demonstrating safe and effective care and good relationships with patients/clients
- Ensuring effective learning experiences by contributing to quality assurance and audit
- Contributing to an environment in which change can be initiated and supported
- Applying research into practice.

This approach is based on a partnership between the student, mentor and university lecturer. Promoting this partnership approach encourages student nurses to do the same for the patients/clients for whom they are caring.

REFLECTIVE PRACTICE Box 2.16

The role of the mentor

After reading the standards for mentorship, reflect on your experience and answer the following questions.

Student activities

- What is the role of the mentor?
- What are my responsibilities as a student nurse?
- What is the role of the university when I am on placement?
- Discuss your thoughts with a fellow student and share your ideas.

Teaching

Nurses need to provide environments that are conducive to learning and be able to respond to the individual learning needs of colleagues, members of the public, patients/clients or carers. Different roles have evolved to support learning in practice settings; these include mentorship (see above), clinical teacher, practice educator, link lecturer and lecturer practitioner. These roles aim to bridge the theory–practice gap by closely linking theory and practice, and involve teaching students and staff, supporting ward managers, assessing competence in practice and contributing to education programmes. These teaching roles provide an opportunity for student nurses to be supported by experienced mentors and teachers, enabling them to reflect, learn and develop their practice and improve their level of confidence when interacting with patients/clients.

Lecturers who teach nursing in universities are normally RNs who have undertaken a teaching qualification recognized by the NMC. In addition to classroom teaching, they facilitate student-centred learning including reflective groups, provide support to personal students and act as link lecturers in practice placements. Many also undertake nursing research.

Clinical leadership

Clinical leaders are from any discipline within an organization; they are often team leaders but not necessarily line managers. While managers promote organizational structures, leaders promote the achievement of excellence in others (RCN 2006). However, in clinical nursing it is expected that a leader coordinates a team of healthcare professionals whose focus is ensuring that effective patient-centred care is delivered. The qualities required that are central to patient-centred leadership are:

- Learning to manage oneself
- Building and maintaining effective relationships with other staff
- Focus on patients/clients
- Internal and external networking to share good practice and to support each other in developing practice
- Increasing political awareness to influence both local and national policy.

Leadership is about setting direction, opening up possibilities, helping people achieve their potential, communicating and delivering; what people do as leaders is even more important than what they say (see Ch. 9). The Department of Health (2005) suggests that clinical leadership is about not knowing everything, reflecting on practice, harnessing the energy of the clinical team, stopping 'doing' and starting to be creative, making improvement part of everyday work and encouraging others to lead and improve. Leaders of improvement need to:

- Create a shared vision with their colleagues
- Align improvement with this vision
- Build a more receptive context for improvement
- Engage clinical colleagues
- Encourage and support communities for practice improvement
- Identify lessons learned.

Department of Health (2005)

Clinical nurse specialists

The clinical nurse specialist (CNS) has acquired extensive specialist knowledge about a specific area of nursing. CNSs work closely with doctors who specialize in the same area of healthcare and are involved in patient care, family and staff education and support. Many CNSs run clinics where they have a caseload of patients and often have full responsibility for making decisions about care. Some also prescribe and monitor the effects of medication (see Ch. 22). They often work across the hospital and community interface, following the patient pathway.

CNSs share their specialist knowledge with other nurses, help to ensure that national standards are put into practice locally and may contribute to developing care policies, e.g. management of breast cancer, learning disabilities, palliative care and aspects of children's nursing, pain management and mental health. National standards provide a consistent approach to the education of specialist nurses (UKCC 2001). These standards indicate that specialist practice involves exercising judgement, discretion and decision-making in clinical care in any area of healthcare delivery.

The CNS role has developed in some areas to provide outreach services where the CNS acts as a link between different areas on the patient pathway. For example, in critical care their role may be to enable early identification of patients whose conditions are deteriorating and require more specialist input, provide advice to ward nurses or to transfer seriously ill patients, e.g. to coronary care or intensive care units. Another example is outreach nurses who bridge the gap between community and hospital, providing support for children and/or adults with complex needs and their families/carers.

Nurse practitioners

A nurse practitioner is a registered nurse who has undertaken a specific course of study and who takes full clinical responsibility for clinical decisions based on systematic physical assessment, accurate diagnosis and the delivery of a wide range of treatment options. Doctors previously undertook most of these roles. The roles are diverse and can include pre-assessment to post-discharge follow-up in areas such as dermatology, stoma and breast care, accident and emergency, general practice and walk-in centres.

Nurse consultants

The nurse consultant is an expert practitioner who works with a specific group of patients or clients, influencing the quality of care through:

- Demonstrating expert practice
- Demonstrating professional leadership and consultancy
- Contributing to education, training and development
- Contributing to research and service development.

Expert practice includes both direct and indirect nursing practice, which must make up 50% of the nurse consultant role.

Professional leadership involves a variety of skills and processes that involve facilitating a culture of practice development that allows staff to become leaders themselves. The consultancy role encompasses not only giving advice and guidance but also developing the clinical skills and problem-solving abilities of nurses. Enhancing outcomes for patient care involves influencing clinical practice in any healthcare setting. This encompasses consultancy across traditional boundaries or care settings, interagency working, and partnership or community development in addition to the specialist area.

The education, training and development role aims to develop a culture for learning in practice and to maintain links with higher education.

The role of practice and service development, research and evaluation involves establishing a research culture (see Ch. 5). Nurse consultants are required to make a significant contribution to the strategic development of clinical governance (see Ch. 3) and in the promotion of clinical effectiveness in their area of practice.

The role is complex and its success is through the promotion of patient-centredness, development of teamwork and meeting service needs while demonstrating effective transformational leadership (Manley 2000).

The modern matron

The modern matron, sometimes known as the clinical nurse manager, was introduced to provide support to ward managers and to refocus attention on patient care. It was considered that 'the basics' had been lost in areas of nursing such as infection control, adequate food and drink for patients/clients, pressure area management, communication, dignity and compassion as ward managers and clinical leaders were spending more time dealing with management and paperwork. The role of the modern matron has three main functions:

- Providing leadership to professional and direct care staff within their group of wards in order to secure and assure the highest standards of clinical care
- Ensuring the availability of appropriate administrative and support services within their groups of wards
- Providing a visible, accessible and authoritative presence in ward settings to whom patients and their families can turn to for assistance, advice and support.

The role of the 'traditional' matron disappeared in the 1960s when formal management was introduced into the NHS. However, the security, stability and 'care focus' that the role had provided to both staff and patients was overlooked. The old-style matron was often considered to be a formidable character who held considerable authority and respect for both their knowledge and expertise from both patients and staff.

Modern matrons must have credibility and expertise and present themselves as figures of authority without imposing fear. The role is intermediary; patients can ask to speak to the matron if they have a complaint about their care or the standards of the ward. The matron is in a prime position to resolve complaints at a local level by providing feedback to ward staff.

Modern matrons need skills that include effective communication, mediation, influence, negotiation, understanding and experience of working on wards. In addition, the role requires sound clinical experience, the ability to monitor and measure the effectiveness of care, change management and an understanding of the dynamics between a distressed patient group and ward staff. As a result, the ward staff are supported in their role of caring for patients.

Nurses as researchers

At the heart of the drive to modernize the NHS is a commitment to the development of high quality, person-centred services that are evidence based. The vision for nursing in the 21st century is for all nurses to be able to both seek out evidence and apply it in their everyday practice, with an increasing number actively participating in research and practice development. All RNs are expected to have the ability to understand and implement research findings (see Ch. 5) but only a small number will become full-time researchers who will contribute to the development of nursing knowledge.

Summary

- Nursing does not exist in isolation; it changes in response to society and the political agenda of the day. This is what makes nursing an exciting and challenging career.
- Fundamental nursing beliefs include compassion, sensitivity and humanity.
- Nurses practise autonomously and in collaboration with others to ensure that individuals of all ages, groups and communities receive the nursing and healthcare that they require.
- Becoming a nurse provides an opportunity to help others, to enable people to cope with difficult life-changing situations and to provide an environment that allows people to learn about themselves, their health and the impact they have on those close to them.
- Nurses see people at the 'great times' in their lives, great happiness, great sadness and great strength.
- It may be here that we see each other at our most human; for us it is this chance to share with others that which is the essence of nursing.

Self test

1. Outline the contribution that Florence Nightingale has made to nursing.
2. How did Virginia Henderson define nursing?
3. How did World War 2 impact on nursing?
4. When did nurses gain registration?
5. Describe the channels of communication used in task allocation.
6. List four advantages of primary nursing.
7. What is the role of the modern matron?

Key words and phrases for literature searching

Accountability
Advanced practice
Community nursing
Florence Nightingale
History of nursing
Humanism
Mary Seacole
Modern matron
Nurse consultant
Nurse education
Nursing theory
Patient allocation
Person-centredness
Practice development
Primary nursing
Professional practice
Proficiency
Project 2000
RCN
Task allocation
Team nursing

Useful websites

Nursing and Midwifery Council	www.nmc-uk.org Available July 2006
PAMIS – *a Scottish organization that works with people with profound and multiple learning disabilities, their family and professionals who support them*	pamis@dundee.ac.uk
Royal British Nurses' Association/King's College London Archives Services	www.kcl.ac.uk/iss/archives/collect/10ro65-1.html Available July 2006
Royal College of Nursing Archive	www.rcn.org.uk/archives Available July 2006
Thoemmes Continuum: History of Nursing	www.continuumbooks.com Available July 2006
United Kingdom Centre for the History of Nursing and Midwifery	www.ukchnm.org Available July 2006

References

Adams A, Bond S, Hale CA 1998 Nursing organizational practice and its relationship with other features of ward organization and job satisfaction. Journal of Advanced Nursing 27:1212–1222

Adams F 1969 From Association to Union: professional organisation of asylum attendants 1869–1919. British Journal of Sociology 20:13, 18

Bakalis NA, Watson R 2005 Nurses decision-making in clinical practice. Nursing Standard 19(23):33–39

Baly ME 1995 Nursing and social change. 3rd edn. Routledge, London

Brooking JI, Ritter SA, Thomas BL (eds) 1992 A textbook of psychiatric and mental health nursing. Churchill Livingstone, Edinburgh

Carter B, Dearmun AK (eds) 1995 Child health care nursing: concepts, theory and practice. Blackwell, Oxford

Casey A 1988 A partnership with child and family. Senior Nurse 8(4):8–9

Chevannes M 1997 Nurses caring for families – issues in a multiracial society. Journal of Clinical Nursing 6(2):161–167

Chinn PL, Kramer MK 1995 Theory and nursing: a systematic approach. 4th edn. Mosby, St Louis

Davies C 1976 Experience of dependency and control in work: the case of nurses. Journal of Advanced Nursing 1:273–282

Department of Health 1997 The new NHS: modern, dependable. TSO, London

Department of Health 1998a A first class service: quality in the new NHS. DH, Leeds

Department of Health 1998b Smoking kills. A White Paper on tobacco. TSO, London

Department of Health 1998c Report of the Scientific Committee on Tobacco and Health. TSO, London

Department of Health 2000 The NHS plan: a plan for investment, a plan for reform. TSO, London

Department of Health 2001 Valuing people: a new strategy for learning disability for the 21st century, Cm 5086. TSO, London

Department of Health 2002 Developing key roles for nurses and midwives – a guide for managers. Online: www.dh.gov.uk/assetRoot/04/10/17/39/04101739.pdf Available July 2006

Department of Health 2004 Patient and public involvement in health: the evidence for policy implementation. Online: www.dh.gov.uk/assetRoot/04/08/23/34/04082334.pdf Available July 2006

Department of Health 2005 Improvement leaders' guides. Department of Health Publications, London

Department of Health 2006 Our health, our care, our say: a new direction for community services. Online: www.dh.gov.uk/assetRoot/04/12/74/59/04127459.pdf Available July 2006

Department of Health and Social Security 1972 Report on the Commission for Nursing (Briggs Report). HMSO, London

Dunphy LM, Winland-Brown JE 1998 The circle of caring: a transformative model of advanced practice nursing. Clinical Excellence for Nurse Practitioners 2(4): 241–247

Gates B, Wilberforce D 2002 The nature of learning disabilities. In: Gates B (ed) Learning disabilities: towards inclusion. 4th edn. Churchill Livingstone, Edinburgh, Ch. 1

Hart C 2004 Nurses and politics. Palgrave Macmillan, Basingstoke

Henderson V 1961 Basic principles of nursing care. International Council of Nurses, London

Hersey P, Blanchard KH 1988 Management of organisational behaviour. 5th edn. Prentice Hall, Englewood Cliffs, NJ

Jupp MR 1994 Management review of nursing systems. Journal of Nursing Management 2(2):57–64

Kamerman S, Khan B 1993 Home health visiting in Europe. Home Visiting 3(3):39–52

King I 1981 A theory of nursing: systems, concepts, process. Wiley, New York

Kitson AL 1996 Does nursing have a future? British Medical Journal 313(7072): 1647–1651

Lansdown R 1996 Children in hospital: a guide for family and carers. Oxford University Press, Oxford

Larsson G, Larsson BW 2003 Quality improvement measures based on patient data: some psychometric issues. International Journal of Nursing Practice 9:294–299

Makinen A, Kivimaki M, Elovainio M, Virtanen M 2003 Organisation of nursing care and stressful work characteristics. Journal of Advanced Nursing 43(2):197–205

Manley K 2000 Organisational culture and consultant nurse outcome. Part 2: nurse outcomes. Nursing Standard 14(37): 31, 34–39

Marriner Tomey A, Roper N, Logan W et al 2000 The Roper–Logan–Tierney model of nursing; based on activities of living. Churchill Livingstone, Edinburgh

McCormack B 2003 A conceptual framework for person-centred practice with older people. International Journal of Nursing Practice 9(3):202–209

Mental Capacity Act 2005 Online: www.opsi.gov.uk/acts/en2005/2005en09.htm and www.opsi.gov.uk/acts/acts2005/20050009.htm Available July 2006

Menzies I 1961 The functioning of social systems as a defence against anxiety. Tavistock, London

Ministry of Health 1959 The Platt report: a report on the welfare of children in hospital. HMSO, London

National Health Service and Community Care Act 1990 Online: www.opsi.gov.uk/acts/acts1990/Ukpga_19900019_en_1.htm Available July 2006

National Statistics Office 2004 Population estimates. Online: www.statistics.gov.uk/CCI/nugget.asp?ID=6 Available July 2006

Neuman B 1995 The Neuman systems model. Appleton & Lange Norwalk, Connecticut

NHS Executive 1999 Making a difference. Strengthening the nursing, midwifery and health visiting contribution to health and healthcare. HSC 1999/158. Department of Health, London

NHS Health Scotland 2004 People with learning disabilities in Scotland. The health needs assessment report. NHS Health Scotland, Edinburgh

Nolan P 2000 History of mental health nursing and psychiatry. In: Newell R, Gournay K (eds) Mental health nursing. Churchill Livingstone, Edinburgh

Norman I, Cowley S 1999 The changing nature of nursing. Blackwell, Oxford

Nursing and Midwifery Council 2004a The NMC code of professional conduct: standards for conduct, performance and ethics. NMC, London. Online: www.nmc-uk.org/aFrameDisplay.aspx?DocumentID=201 Available July 2006

Nursing and Midwifery Council 2004b Standards of proficiency of specialist community public health nurses. NMC, London. Online: www.nmc-uk.org/aFrameDisplay.aspx?DocumentID=324 Available July 2006

Nursing and Midwifery Council 2004c Standards of proficiency for pre-registration nursing education. NMC, London. Online: www.nmc-uk.org/aFrameDisplay.aspx?DocumentID=328 Available July 2006

Nursing and Midwifery Council 2004d Standards for the preparation of teachers of nurses, midwives and specialist community public health nurses. NMC, London. Online: www.nmc-uk.org/aFrameDisplay.aspx?DocumentID=325 Available July 2006 (under revision at time of publication)

O'Brien 1981 The principle of normalisation: a foundation for effective services. Campaign for People with Mental Handicaps, London

Orem D 1991 Self-care deficit theory. Sage, California

Parse RR 1987 Nursing science: major paradigms, theories and critiques. Saunders, Philadelphia

Paterson JG, Zderad LT 1988 Humanistic nursing. John Wiley & Sons, New York

Pearson A, Vaughan B, Fitzgerald M 1996 Nursing models for practice. 2nd edn. Butterworth-Heinemann, Oxford

Peplau HE 1952 Interpersonal relations in nursing: a conceptual framework of reference for psychodynamic nursing. Putman, New York

Quality Assurance Agency (QAA) for Higher Education 2002 Scottish subject benchmark statement. Nursing. Online: www.qaa.ac.uk/academicinfrastructure/benchmark/scottish/nursing.asp Available July 2006

Rowe H 1996 Multidisciplinary teamwork – myth or reality? Journal of Nursing Management 4:93–101

Roy C, Andrews HA 1999 The Roy adaptation model. Appleton & Lange, Stamford, Connecticut

Royal British Nurses' Association 2003 King's College London Archives Services – Summary Guide. Online: www.kcl.ac.uk/iss/archives/collect/10ro65-1.html Available July 2006

Royal College of Nursing 1984 Changing provision for sick children and diseases in childhood in Liverpool since 1850. RCN Bulletin 6. RCN, London

Royal College of Nursing 2006 RCN clinical leadership programme. RCN, London. Online: www.rcn.org.uk/resources/clinicalleadership Available July 2006

Salvage J 2002 Rethinking professionalism: the first step for patient focused care? Institute for Public Policy Research, London

Scottish Executive 2002 Promoting health, supporting inclusion. The national review of the contribution of all nurses and midwives to the care and support of people with learning disabilities. TSO, Edinburgh

Scottish Executive Health Department 2000a The same as you? A review of services for people with learning disability. TSO, Edinburgh

Scottish Executive Health Department 2000b Caring for Scotland. The strategy for nursing and midwifery in Scotland. TSO, Edinburgh

Scottish Executive Health Department 2003 Evaluating family health nursing through education and practice. Online: www.scotland.gov.uk/socialresearch Available July 2006

Scottish Executive Health Department 2005 Delivery for health. SEHD, Edinburgh

Scottish Human Services Trust 2004 Values of inclusion. Scottish Human Services Trust, Edinburgh. Online: www.shstrust.org.uk/values.htm Available July 2006

Selanders LC 1993 Florence Nightingale: an environmental adaptation theory. Sage, Newbury Park

Smith F 1995 Children's nursing in practice: the Nottingham model. Blackwell Science, Oxford

Sparrow S 1986 Primary nursing. Nursing Practice 1(3):142–148

Stein LI 1967 The doctor–nurse game. Archives of General Psychiatry 16(6): 699–703

The Scottish Office 1999 Towards a healthier Scotland: a White Paper on health. TSO, Edinburgh

UKCC 1985 Project 2000: a new preparation for practice. UKCC, London

UKCC 1999 Fitness for practice: The UKCC Commission for Nursing and Midwifery Education. UKCC, London

UKCC 2001 Standard for specialist education and practice. UKCC, London

Watson J 1988 Nursing: human science and human care: a theory of nursing. Appleton-Century-Crofts, Norwalk, Connecticut

Watt S, Mitchell R 1995 Historical perspectives. In: Carter B, Dearmun AK (eds) Child health care nursing concepts, theory and practice. Blackwell, Oxford

West M 1994 Effective teamwork. BPS Books, Leicester

West M, Field R 1995 Teamwork in primary care: perspectives from organisational psychology. Journal of Interprofessional Care 9(2):117–122

World Health Organization Europe 2000 EUR/00/5019309/1300074 The family health nurse: context, conceptual framework and curriculum. WHO Regional Office for Europe, Copenhagen

Further reading

Abel-Smith B 1960 A history of the nursing profession. Heinemann, London

Burkhardt MA, Nathaniel AK 2002 Ethics and issues in contemporary nursing. 2nd edn. Delmar, Clifton Park

D'Antonio P 1999 Revisiting and rethinking the rewriting of nursing history. Bulletin of the History of Medicine 73(2):268–290

Maggs C 1990 Nursing history: the state of the art. English Historical Review 105(416): 756–757

3

Health and social care delivery systems

Norrie Brown and Maureen MacMillan

Glossary terms

Audit
Clinical governance
Healthcare
Integrated care pathways
Intermediate care
Interprofessional working
Multiagency team
Multidisciplinary teams
Primary care
Quality assurance
Secondary care
Social care
Social services
Tertiary care

Learning outcomes

This chapter will help you:

- Begin to understand what is meant by health and social care provision and how it is organized
- Outline the structures of the National Health Service (NHS) in the United Kingdom and the key developments in the NHS since its inception
- Demonstrate an understanding of the multidisciplinary team (MDT) and multiagency working
- Begin to understand the framework and mechanisms for the provision of high quality health and social care.

Introduction

Health and social care provision in the UK is multifaceted in that it involves a variety of areas and is multidisciplinary because a number of different professional groups work together. It can also be described as being a multiagency enterprise since there are many organizations with different sources of funding involved in it. This means that it is a complex system and one that varies in the different countries that make up the UK. This chapter will concentrate on the structure of services provided in England as the largest member country. Where appropriate, some of the important variations that exist within the other three countries will be highlighted, but readers will need to consider how the service applies to where they live. Examples of how to locate or access information about local service provision are supplied.

When thinking about the NHS in the UK, consideration needs to be given as to why, when and how it was formed. This chapter outlines the answers to these questions as well as giving some idea of how the health of the general population is looked after, and how the health and social care structures are organized or arranged to prevent illness and to provide treatment and care for the vulnerable members of society.

The complexity of the NHS, its organization, structure and the various relationships between the many professionals that are necessary to deliver effective services is dynamic and are interesting areas to explore. Where appropriate, various aspects of health and social care are illustrated using community-based scenarios. The information and the understanding gained from this chapter will provide an underpinning for the content and learning that readers will achieve from other chapters in this book. This chapter provides an introduction to the history of the NHS and its current structure and function, health and social care provision, the services it offers and its funding, and multidisciplinary and multiagency working. The appropriate legislation which underpins the delivery of health and social care is discussed throughout. In addition, the chapter considers the provision of high quality health and social care, consumer involvement and the mechanisms that are put in place to positively influence the delivery of high quality care.

The structure, services provided and delivery of health and social care have undergone numerous changes over past decades in order to meet the developing needs of the UK population. It is important that the provision of health and social care is dynamic and able to respond as needs change. Readers should be aware that changes, both minor and major, are planned or being proposed or discussed. It is important that readers ensure that they are aware of changes to services as they happen. For example, the English White paper *Our Health, Our Care, Our Say: A New Direction for Community Services* will lead to profound changes in the way services are delivered, including moving resources from hospital care to spending more on care closer to home and on preventative services (Department of Health [DH] 2006).

Health and social care provision

In the period following World War 2 (1939–1945), the Welfare State (which arose from the Beveridge Report 1942) was created in the UK. This was seen as a blueprint for the state in playing a greater role in the removal of what Beveridge termed the 'five giant evils', namely:

- Disease
- Idleness
- Ignorance
- Squalor
- Want.

This was to be achieved through:

- The NHS
- Full employment
- State education up to 15 years of age
- Public housing
- The National Insurance and Assistance schemes in order to tackle 'want'.

These recommendations (Beveridge 1942) formed the basis of the Welfare State, which included the provision of health and social care in order to combat the 'five giants'.

The founding principle upon which the NHS was set up and continues to be underpinned is the provision of quality care that:

- Meets the needs of everyone
- Is free at the point of need
- Is based on a patient's clinical need, not their ability to pay.

However, since the formation of the NHS in 1948, it has failed to keep pace with changes in the health and social care needs of the population. These are still seen as challenges to be met by *The NHS Plan: A Plan for Investment, A Plan for Reform* (DH 2000). In 2003 the structure of the NHS and social care system in England was radically transformed in which:

- Greater choice was offered to all patients/clients and users of the services and were considered first
- Services were based on a clear framework of stated values
- National standards with mechanisms for independent inspection and regulation were followed
- A partnership of public, private and 'not for profit' organizations provided services, increasing involvement in decision-making by clinical teams
- The direction, production of resources, transformation and oversight of the whole system was led by the Department of Health (Merry 2003).

Since 1992, with the publication of the White Paper *The Health of the Nation: A Strategy for Health in England* (DH 1992), the government started to set targets for the health of the population in addition to targets for the provision of healthcare services (Macpherson 1998).

Brief history – changes since 1948

In order to understand the NHS and how it operates today, an awareness of the historical context of why and how the NHS came about is necessary (Box 3.1). This helps to make sense of where it is today as well as understanding why successive governments over the years have made some policy decisions. For example, in the early part of this century there was considerable media coverage about the creation of foundation hospitals in England. Important concerns for many politicians that were expressed at that time were, whatever changes to hospital provision took place, access to treatment should be free at the point of delivery and be based on patient/client need rather than an individual's ability to pay. An understanding of the historical context of NHS developments will help readers to understand that concerns about foundation hospitals were related to the fundamental principles of the NHS and led to much political discussion. Changes in the NHS are largely influenced by prevailing politics of the time.

Types of health and social care provision

The provision of health and social care services is divided into:

- Statutory
- Non-statutory
- Voluntary
- Charitable provision
- Private sector.

Statutory services are those controlled by Acts of Parliament (see Ch. 6). There are some aspects of care provision that are non-statutory, i.e. not governed by Acts of Parliament. In addition, certain supporting services are provided by voluntary agencies or charitable organizations, such as befriending schemes. A scheme such as this might, for example, involve a lonely older man living by himself having a volunteer drop in to see him on a regular basis to make sure that he is alright and that he does not become too isolated (Box 3.2, see p. 74).

Private hospitals, care homes and clinics also provide services to people who, in addition to paying taxes, choose to pay directly or indirectly through private health insurance for private healthcare services.

Box 3.1 **Key health and social care developments since 1948**

The structure of the NHS has been reformed on a number of occasions, with different structures operating in Scotland, Wales and Northern Ireland.

- 1948 – NHS inaugurated on 5 July and people rushed to use services
- 1949 – Patient demand for services outstripped supply and pushed costs to worrying levels
- 1952 – Prescription charges introduced
- 1956 – Guillebaud Inquiry Report defends the structure and costs of the NHS since the proportion of the gross domestic product (total value of goods and services produced in the country in a year) costs were falling
- 1957 – Royal Commission on mental illness asked for a single law to cover all mental illness, removal of the distinction between mental and physical illness and, where possible, the treatment of mental illness be provided in the community
- 1959 – New Mental Health Act (England) came into being and the treatment of mental illness to be provided in the community
- 1960 – Mental Health (Scotland) Act came into being
- 1962 – Porrit Report recommended the setting up of primary, secondary and tertiary structures with area boards set up to run the NHS
- 1964 – Salmon Report recommended setting up a new grading and pay structure for senior nurses (implemented in 1966)
- 1965 – Seebohm Committee established to review personal social services
- 1969 – Green Paper on reorganization of health and social services in Northern Ireland
- 1969 – Independent Hospital Advisory Service and the Scottish Hospital Advisory Service set up to review care and treatment in long-stay mental and mentally handicapped hospitals
- 1970 – Local authorities required to create single Social Service Departments by law
- 1973 – NHS Reorganization Act set up Area and District Health Authorities to run hospital and community health services, the public had participation through Community Health Councils and a Health Service Ombudsman was appointed
- 1976 – Publication of the report on the future of child health services; publication of *Priorities for Health and Personal Social Services in England* required that choices would have to be made in healthcare for economic reasons
- 1979 – Publication of *Patients First*, which proposed simplification of the NHS structure for healthcare decisions to be made as near to the point of delivery as possible
- 1980 – The Black Report *Inequalities in Health* (Black et al 1980) published (see Townsend & Davidson 1982)
- 1982 – Publication of *Care in Action*, which prioritized services for older people, people with learning disabilities and other deprived groups
- 1984 – Health and Social Security Act enacted tighter regulation for health and local authorities to oversee the private sector which was increasingly providing institutional care for elderly people
- 1986 – Cumberledge Report published and called for resources to be switched from hospitals to the community; the development of nurse practitioners; freedom for nurses to do some prescribing (legislated in 1992 by the Medicinal Products: Prescription by Nurses etc. Act) (see Chs 6, 22); the launch of Project 2000 introduced in 1988 (see Ch. 2).
- 1988 – Griffiths Report *Community Care: Agenda for Change* published. Proposed that local authorities should act as purchasing agents for community care; implemented in 1990
- 1989 – White Paper *Working with Patients* published
- 1990 – First Director of Research and Development in the NHS appointed, coinciding with the drive for greater application of evidence-based treatment
- 1991 – Citizens' charter enacted and became the start of hospital 'league tables'
- 1992 – White Paper *The Health of the Nation: A Strategy for Health in England* laid down 25 health policy targets; similar documents published in the other three countries of the UK
- 1992 – United Kingdom Central Council for Nursing, Midwifery and Health Visiting (UKCC) published *Guidelines for Professional Practice* – accelerated the switch from a hierarchical nursing profession to one based on autonomy (nurses being responsible for independent, competent practice)
- 1994 – The Audit Commission published *Finding a Place: A Review of Mental Health Services for Adults*, which identified the main challenge for the effective delivery of services as being managerial rather than clinical, and set out an action plan for all levels of the NHS
- 1997 – White Papers *The New NHS* (England), *Designed to Care* (Scotland) and *NHS Wales: Putting Patients First* published, with Scottish Parliament and Welsh Assembly assuming direct responsibility
- 1999 – White Paper *Learning Together* published and is the main strategy encompassing education, training and lifelong learning for all NHS Scotland staff
- 1999 – Report entitled *Fair shares for All* establishes formula for allocating funds to health boards in Scotland

- 1999 – White Paper *The Health Act* describes how the NHS will differ in each of the four nations of the UK and outlines powers to develop more partnerships between the NHS, local authorities and social services
- 1999 – White Paper *Saving Lives: Our Healthier Nation* published in England. Plans policies to improve health and reduce inequalities
- 2000 – White Paper *Our National Health: A Plan for Action, A Plan for Change* published, resulting in unified health boards in Scotland to deliver healthcare to meet a range of government priorities, e.g. tackling waiting times, access to and discharge from hospital
- 2000 – White paper *The NHS Plan: A Plan for Investment, A Plan for Reform* published
- 2001 – Publication of *Improving Health in Wales: A Plan for the NHS with its Partners* – a Welsh Assembly report outlining the long-term strategy for the NHS in Wales
- 2001 – *Quality and Fairness* strategy published to reconfigure hospital services in Northern Ireland and to make changes to the primary/secondary care interface
- 2003 – White Paper *Partnership for Care: Scotland's Health* sets out plans to abolish NHS Trusts
- 2003 – White Paper *Improving Health in Scotland: The Challenge* published – one of 44 action points calling for health improvement to become a feature of future public sector planning
- 2004 – White Paper *Choosing Health: Making Healthier Choices Easier* published in England.

[After Macpherson (1998), Merry (2005)]

The aforementioned dynamic nature of health and social care services is illustrated by the fact that many statutory, non-statutory, voluntary sector and private sector organizations are working together in increasing numbers in order to provide a range of services to meet the complex health and social care needs of a growing number of people.

The differences between the various types of service provision are outlined below.

Statutory services

Statutory services are those provided by virtue of laws made in Parliament (see Ch. 6) and which are funded, managed, run and evaluated by central government. This is carried out via the:

- Department of Health in London
- Scottish Parliament through the Scottish Executive Health Department in Edinburgh
- National Assembly of Wales via the NHS Directorate in Cardiff
- Department of Health, Social Services and Public Safety for the Northern Ireland Assembly in Belfast.

However, not all statutory services are delivered directly by government organizations or agencies, and not all services are delivered with staff and patients/clients on a face-to-face basis, e.g. telephone contact with NHS 24 in Scotland and NHS Direct in England. Many services are contracted out and delivered by non-statutory agencies. Examples of non-statutory agencies providing statutory services include:

- Magnetic resonance imaging (MRI) – the Department of Health have contracted Alliance Medical, a private company, to provide 120 000 scans in mobile MRI scanners; this was planned to boost the MRI scanning capacity by 15% (DH 2005a). As a result of this scheme, more than 25 000 patients have received MRI scans, dramatically reducing the average waiting time for scans in many parts of the country. In Huddersfield, for example, waiting times were cut from 38 to 8 weeks.
- Assertiveness outreach teams, such as the Tulip Outreach Team in London, are funded by health and social services, and cater for clients who are mainly black or Asian who may be homeless or at

REFLECTIVE PRACTICE Box 3.2

Suicide in older men

In a Royal College of Psychiatrists (RCP) press release (2004), Professor Snowdon reported that, in the UK, men in their mid-fifties are less likely to kill themselves than their fathers and grandfathers. However, suicide in older men is twice the rate in older women.

Student activities

1. Access the RCP press release and answer the following questions:
   - What reasons are thought to make older men want to take their own lives?
   - What are the reasons for men in their mid-fifties deciding not to take their own lives?
   - How has the suicide rate in men compared to women since the 1950s?
2. Find out what voluntary or charitable befriending services exist in your area.
3. Visit the MIND (mental health charity in England and Wales) website below and find out what suicide prevention strategies they suggest.

[Resources: MIND – www.mind.org.uk/Information/Factsheets/Suicide Available July 2006; Royal College of Psychiatrists 2004 Older men less likely than younger men to kill themselves (press release) – www.rcpsych.ac.uk/press/preleases/pr/pr_586.htm Available July 2006]

CRITICAL THINKING Box 3.3

Treatment centres

A relative who lives in England tells you she is having her cataract operation at last, and it will be done in one of the new treatment centres. She asks you if there is one near you and what you know about the centres.

Student activities

- Access the website below and find your nearest treatment centre.
- Find out what procedures are done.
- What are the core characteristics of these centres?

[Resource: www.dh.gov.uk/PolicyAndGuidance/OrganisationPolicy/SecondaryCare/TreatmentCentres]

CRITICAL THINKING Box 3.4

The NHS Plan . . . targets – waiting times for surgery

Target – Patients will be admitted for treatment within 18 weeks from referral by their General Practitioner (GP).

Alice, who has pain and reduced mobility due to arthritis, has been told that she will be put on the waiting list for a hip replacement but is likely to wait for at least 12 months for surgery.

Student activities

- How do think Alice and her family might feel about the delay?
- How would you feel if she was your mother?
- Find out the waiting time for hip replacement and other orthopaedic surgery in your locality.

risk of becoming homeless. Further information about the Tulip Mental Health Group (a consortium of voluntary and statutory groups) can be accessed at www.tulip.org.uk.

- Treatment centres – dedicated units offering safe, fast, pre-booked day and short-stay surgery and diagnostic procedures in specialities such as ophthalmology (e.g. cataract surgery) and orthopaedics (e.g. joint replacement surgery) (Box 3.3).

The NHS Plan (DH 2000) sets out various targets, e.g. reducing waiting times for operations, by which the government hopes to be able to claim that improvements in the nation's health and increased value for money have been achieved (Box 3.4).

Non-statutory services

Non-statutory services cater for specific client groups such as:

- People with mental health problems
- Frail older people
- People with human immunodeficiency virus (HIV) disease
- People with learning disabilities
- People who misuse alcohol.

These services include the provision of day centres, care homes, low-cost housing, carer support (e.g. those caring for someone with Alzheimer's disease), etc. The services offered can be physical care, psychological care, the provision of information and support, or a combination of all three. Another aspect of their activity may be to lobby for improved statutory services and some do this to great effect. Many of the organizations which provide these services, e.g. Sue Ryder Care and the Royal National Institute of the Blind (RNIB), are increasingly being involved in partnerships between the NHS and local authority Social Service Departments in response to government initiatives such as *Partnerships for Care* in Scotland (Scottish Executive 2003) and *The New NHS: Modern, Dependable* in England (DH 1997).

Voluntary or charitable provision

Many of the services provided by voluntary and consumer groups tend to be offered by self-help, disease-based or disease-focused groups. Examples of groups that provide support for carers and individuals include:

- Terrence Higgins Trust – HIV and AIDS
- National Osteoporosis Society – osteoporosis
- Scottish Association for Mental Health, MIND – mental health problems
- Marie Curie, Macmillan Cancer Support, Maggie's cancer centres in Scotland – cancer (see Ch. 12)
- Age Concern, Alzheimer's Scotland – older people and those with dementia.

As well as providing support and information for patients/clients and their families, these groups may also work to improve care and assistance provided by statutory services.

Private sector

Private healthcare is provided by private companies who have traditionally offered a range of mainly short-term hospital care. Increasingly, private healthcare providers also supply GP services (e.g. GP-Plus launched in Edinburgh in 1999) as well as health screening and elective surgery (e.g. cataract removal, termination of pregnancy and hip replacement). Some people see the growth in private healthcare provision as a means of replacing statutory health services due to the inability of the NHS to cope with demand for these services, e.g. termination of pregnancy. In addition to private companies, other providers include not-for-profit companies or provident associations, e.g. BUPA, which re-invest monies into services.

In England, and increasingly in Scotland and the other countries of the UK, where the statutory services are unable to deal with long waiting lists for hospital treatment, health authorities are allowed by government to send their patients to receive treatment in private sector hospitals. The demand for private healthcare services is not uniform across the UK. Scotland, Wales and Northern Ireland have fewer private sector hospital beds per head of population than in England. Interestingly, the Scottish Executive Health Department bought an underused private hospital in Glasgow in order to meet demand and to relieve the pressure on waiting list targets in Scotland. In 2001, the NHS in England took similar action by purchasing a private heart hospital in London. Some health authorities in England have also begun to send patients abroad for treatment as a way to meet waiting time targets set by central government.

Government policy forcefully states that the divisions that existed between the statutory and private sector health service providers should be brought to an end and 'so harness the capacity of private and voluntary providers to treat more NHS patients' (DH 2000, p. 96). This working relationship and changed approach to the provision of healthcare services is a radical departure from previous Labour Government policy but it is an acknowledgement that private sector healthcare provision does, indeed, meet many needs that the NHS is unable to, as well as officially recognizing the fact that NHS 'already spends over £1 billion each year on buying care and specialist services from hospitals, nursing homes and hospices run by private companies and charities' (DH 2000, p. 96). The changes outlined in *The NHS Plan* have been superseded by the *NHS Improvement Plan: Putting People at the Heart of Public Services* (DH 2004) which states, 'To support capacity and choice by 2008, independent sector providers will provide up to 15% of procedures on behalf of the NHS' (p. 10).

Box 3.5 outlines a situation in which various health and social care providers might have a contribution to make.

Alice has a set of needs that, by itself, the healthcare system is not able to meet. She has:

- Physical health needs – dealing with her arthritis, pain (may be affecting sleep, see Ch. 10), poor mobility (see Ch. 18), falls
- Social care needs – dealing with isolation and loneliness, shopping, cooking, lack of socializing, safety in relation to falls (see Ch. 13)
- Activities of living – dealing with personal hygiene and help with bathing (see Ch. 16), eating a balanced diet (see Ch. 19)
- Mental health needs – dealing with feelings of depression.

The hip replacement will take up to 12 months to be done. Meanwhile Alice, who is now feeling very vulnerable, has a variety needs that require to be met in order to maintain her dignity, improve her quality of life, prevent further deterioration of her mental state and prevent other health problems from developing. The health service has a statutory obligation to look after Alice's healthcare needs but not her social care needs. These have to be met by other organizations and agencies working independently and together.

Comparisons of the UK funding model with other systems

Levitt et al (1999) argue that a country's health and social care provision reflects the national priorities of that country in many ways. These may include historical circumstances to meet particular health needs; for example, malaria control versus a tuberculosis vaccination programme, compared with the latest portable bone scanner versus a community mental health nurse.

All governments have to make choices about financing healthcare (Box 3.6). They also spend more than they would like to and complain of waste and poor control, and all are concerned for the future. In 2005, for example, many Southern African countries were forced to make difficult choices between funding treatment for HIV/AIDS versus treatment for malaria; this is a particular concern when societies find it difficult to accept that a problem with HIV/AIDS actually exists. According to Levitt et al (1999), the funding arrangements for healthcare and social care vary markedly between countries. They go on

CRITICAL THINKING Box 3.5

Meeting Alice's needs

Alice, as you will remember, is on the waiting list for hip replacement surgery for arthritis (see Box 3.4, p. 75). Recently she has had a couple of falls at home. Her hip is causing her a great deal of pain and this, in turn, restricts her movement. She is unable to go to the shops or to do many things that she would normally do, but for the pain and fear of falling, such as having a bath, cooking and meeting friends. Alice tells her family that she is increasingly isolated and this is getting her down and making her feel depressed.

Student activities

- Think about Alice's needs in terms of activities of living, safety, physical health, mental health and social care needs.
- Discuss with your mentor how Alice's needs could be met and which service providers would be involved.

ETHICAL ISSUES Box 3.6

Difficult choices

Your aunt has a heart condition (irregular rhythm) and she is extremely distressed and worried about dying. The primary care trust (PCT) is unable to fund her non-urgent treatment in the current financial year because it has run out of money. The local newspaper published the story, which has since been picked up by the national newspapers who are calling for the Health Minister to put pressure on the PCT to re-examine its priorities.

Student activities

- Do you think this kind of media pressure is helpful?
- What do you think might happen to other services if the PCT bends to the pressure?
- If your aunt is treated more quickly because the PCT changes its mind, how might other patients/clients feel if they are also waiting for treatment?

to state that: 'In all developed countries there is a mix of state funding, insurance and direct payments . . . A major concern of all governments is to control costs whatever their methods of financing healthcare' (p. 241).

The UK opted for a direct payment system via general taxation by central government (Table 3.1). However, some people choose to pay private health insurance to augment their healthcare provision. This enables them to make choices about when, where and who will provide the healthcare service needed at a particular time. Being able to make such choices allows those individuals to be treated more quickly for non-urgent conditions as opposed to joining a waiting list.

The funding for social care also varies. In the UK, central government allocates the bulk of resources to local authorities with small amounts of additional funding coming from local taxation (council tax). However, central government and local authorities do not fund all social care. For example, a person who needs to go into a care home but has a certain level of financial resource will be required to pay in full or contribute to this service. A person living in a care home would, however, receive an allowance for nursing care that requires the services of a registered nurse. Where a person has limited money or savings, the local authority would pay the care home fees. People living in England who need assistance with personal care such as washing and dressing are required to pay for these personal services. The situation in Scotland is completely different, as the Scottish Executive finances the cost of personal care.

In 1949 the amount of money spent by the UK government on healthcare was estimated to be just under £10 billion (Yuen 2003). This compares to healthcare spending in 2004/2005, estimated at just over £67.4 billion, which is set to rise to £90 billion by the year 2007/2008 (DH 2004). Interestingly, spending on the health service in Scotland in 2004 was £7.8 billion for the treatment of five million people and is expected to rise to £9.3 billion in 2007/2008 – nearly as much as it cost for the whole of the UK when the health service was first started (Audit Scotland 2004).

The National Health Service

This part of the chapter focuses on how the NHS is structured in the four countries of the UK and functions of the various bodies within them.

The original aims of NHS (Ministry of Health 1946) were the promotion of a comprehensive health service designed to secure improvement in the:

- Physical and mental health of the people
- Prevention, diagnosis and treatment of illness.

Table 3.1 Comparison of the British funding model with other systems

Country	Total health expenditure as % of GDP* (approximate)	Taxation	Social insurance	Private insurance	Out of pocket payments
France	10%	Some revenues from tax on car insurance cover the deficit from social insurance	Majority of population covered by three occupational health insurance funds, split between employees and employer	People pay supplementary insurance What they pay is earnings related	Insurance covers some of costs of GP and medicines Exemptions apply to some people and for some medicines
Germany†	10%		Statutory Health Insurance (SHI) scheme for just over half population, remainder covered by retirement, accident and long-term care insurance	Private insurance Employer contributions	
US	13%	Taxation funds Medicaid and some Medicare, and general assistance Public hospitals supported by state and local taxes	Some social insurance contributions go towards funding of Medicare	Private insurance provided as fringe benefit to employees Participants in Medicare also pay for supplementary cover	Co-payments inpatient and primary care payable by the privately insured and Medicare participants
UK	7%	General central government tax funds NHS	Some general social insurance contributions used to fund NHS	Private insurance is used to supplement NHS cover	Charges for some medicines, dental care, eye care and some social care

*Yuen (2003); † Busse & Riesberg (2004).
GDP, gross domestic product.

These remain the aims of the NHS today and encompass care for the whole population (for all UK countries) from 'the cradle to the grave', providing services for acute and chronic (long-term conditions) illness in a variety of settings, such as hospitals, day hospitals, health centres, home care, walk-in centres, telemedicine (NHS Direct, NHS 24) and so on. However, the healthcare needs of the population when the NHS was first introduced were very different from the healthcare needs of today's population. Since its inception the structure of the NHS has changed and will continue to do so.

Structure and function of NHS

The structure of the NHS in England is the most complex in the UK. This is, in part, due to the population and the geographical size of the country. The NHS system is fundamentally divided into three tiers in the four countries (Figs 3.1, 3.2) but there are some differences in NHS structure between countries. Further information about these differences in structure, health and other policies and services is available from the appropriate government website (see 'Useful websites', p. 95). The three-tier system reflects the shift in government thinking, which aims to reduce centralization by devolving decision-making to the professionals who are delivering the services and the patients/clients receiving them.

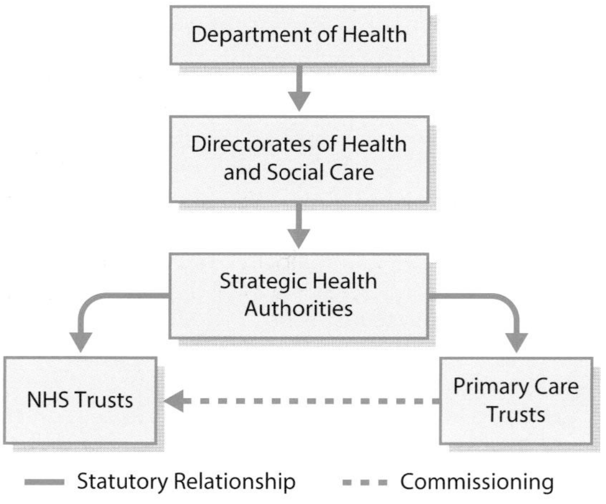

Fig. 3.1 The NHS in England 2004 (reproduced with permission from Merry 2004)

In England, the Department of Health is charged to ensure that the health of the population is looked after; if necessary, they bring Bills before Parliament to ensure that the appropriate legal framework is in place for meeting their responsibility. The Secretary of State and the health ministers within the Department of Health have the responsibility to ensure that the NHS, social care and public health services work together to meet the nation's health and social care needs.

The Secretary of State and health ministers are advised by a group of national clinical directors and key specialists covering the full range of health service provision, e.g. mental health, children, primary care, older people and cancer. These positions are mirrored in the other countries of the UK.

Central government, in its various forms, is the enacting, funding and driving force for provision of services. The government develops strategies and plans for the health of the nation, legislates as to how this will be done and provides the funding that enables various professional and non-professional groups to deliver services to the population.

The intermediaries between central government and those who deliver healthcare are the Strategic Health Authorities (SHAs) in England (Box 3.7), Health Boards in Scotland, Regional Health Authorities in Wales and Health and Social Services Boards in Northern Ireland. These bodies plan the delivery of services at a regional level. Currently in England the primary care trusts (PCTs) commission services from NHS Trusts and both PCTs and NHS Trusts provide healthcare directly to patients/clients in the community and hospital. NHS provision is divided into primary, secondary and tertiary care (see pp. 79–82), with various forms of intermediate care

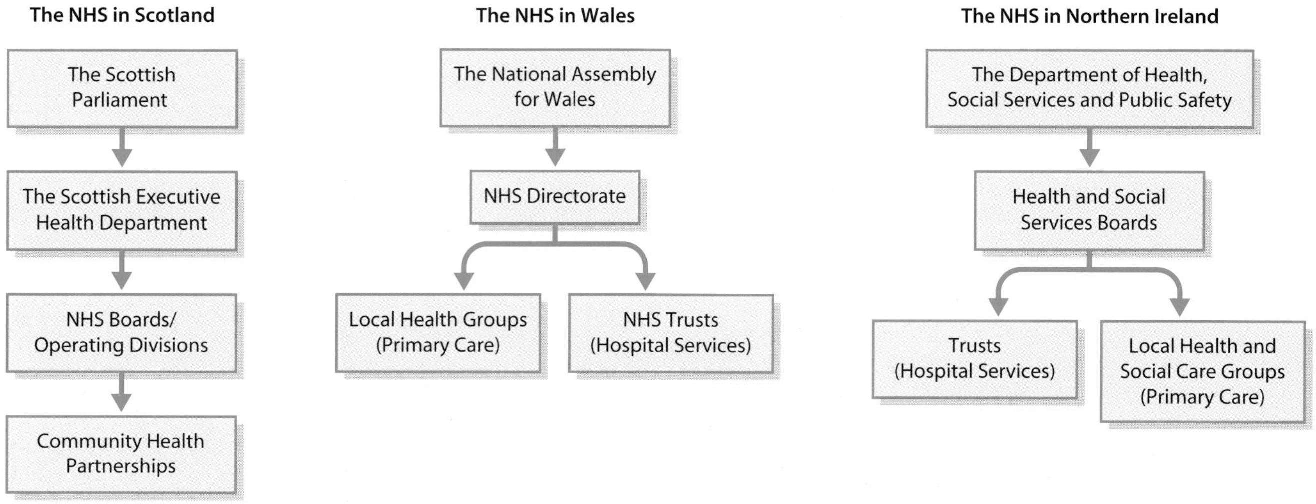

Fig. 3.2 The NHS in Scotland, Wales and Northern Ireland (reproduced with permission from Merry 2004)

used to bridge the gap between primary and secondary care.

Primary healthcare

PCTs and GPs and other members of the primary healthcare team provide a range of primary healthcare services directly to people living in the community. The PCTs also take lead responsibility for developing and sustaining partnerships with other agencies, including local authorities, voluntary organizations and private providers.

For most people in the UK their first contact with the health service, irrespective of where they live, has, up until relatively recently, been the GP. Traditionally, GPs and other healthcare professionals working from the same base, such as the GP's premises or a health centre, have provided most community-based primary healthcare services. The other healthcare professionals who may be part of the MDT working from health centres include:

- *Practice nurses* – their role includes the detection, assessment and management of conditions such as asthma and diabetes; health promotion clinics, travel health, immunizations, sexual and reproductive health; screening clinics including well women/men clinics, breast awareness, cervical cytology and preconception advice, etc.
- *Specialist community public health nurses* – including health visitors who promote health and prevent illness in the under 5s, school-aged children, mothers and older people (Box 3.8). In Scotland, family health nursing (generalist skills in public health and disease management) is being developed. School nurses with a specialist practice qualification and occupational health nurses may also be involved
- *Community practitioners* – district nurses, community mental health nurses, children's community nurses, learning disability nurses, link nurses and midwives (see Box 3.8)
- *Nurse practitioners* – patients/clients can choose to consult a nurse practitioner (and/or their GP) who will assess their healthcare needs, make a diagnosis, order investigations and provide treatment within their competence
- *Physiotherapists* – help to rehabilitate people who have suffered loss of physical function due to illness, injury or old age
- *Occupational therapists* – treat people who experience physical and mental health problems through the use of physical activities
- *Dietitians* – promote health and treat disease by applying nutritional science to improve people's diet and eating habits
- *Speech and language therapists* – work with a variety of people in order to assess and treat speech, language and communication problems and difficulty in swallowing
- *Osteopaths, chiropractics and other complementary and alternative medicine therapists* (see Ch. 10).

Dentists, dental hygienists, optometrists and podiatrists also provide primary healthcare services in the community.

The services offered by primary healthcare teams may also include health protection in schools, sexual health

Box 3.7

Strategic Health Authorities

There are currently 10 SHAs in England. This number was reduced from 28 to 10 in 2006. SHAs are responsible for developing strategic plans for improving local health services in specific geographical areas; for example, East of England SHA covers Norfolk, Suffolk, Cambridgeshire, Essex, Bedfordshire and Hertfordshire. SHAs are structurally located between the Department of Health and the primary and secondary providers. SHAs also negotiate and help to find solutions to local problems and make sure that local service providers are answerable for the services they provide and increase the capacity of local health services in order to extend services.

The SHAs are responsible for monitoring and measuring the performance of NHS Trusts and PCTs against government targets and for ensuring that the government's national priorities are integrated into the work of the PCTs and the NHS Trusts, thereby being concerned with primary healthcare and community services run by the PCTs and the acute hospital services run by the NHS Trusts.

Box 3.8

Core functions of community practitioners and health visitors

According to the Department of Health (2003) there are three core functions that underpin primary care nursing in the UK and six principles that run through all public health work.

Core functions

- First contact care: acute assessment, diagnosis, care, treatment and referral
- Chronic disease management, continuing care and rehabilitation
- Public health: health protection and promotion programmes that improve health and reduce inequalities.

Principles

- Knowing the health needs of the population
- Making sure services are accessible to those whose needs are greatest
- Working with others to do something about the wider determinants of health
- Getting local people involved in what you do
- Being aware of and ready to respond to infectious disease outbreaks and other threats to health
- Using evidence.

REFLECTIVE PRACTICE Box 3.9

Working with others to improve health

A community mental health nurse is interested in working with people who are experiencing mental distress and may offer services such as anxiety management, cognitive behaviour therapy for people who experience depression and group therapy sessions. In the health centre they may work with other community mental health nurses, e.g. in group work, but they may also work with other professionals such as psychiatrists, occupational therapists, art therapists, complementary therapists, alternative medicine practitioners and speech and language therapists.

Student activities

- Think about a patient/client you met during a placement who needed help from many different professionals.
- What worked well? What benefits occurred because different professionals were involved?
- Were there any problems, e.g. keeping everyone informed? Discuss these with your mentor.

EVIDENCE-BASED PRACTICE Box 3.10

Walk-in centres

Using a postal survey, face-to-face interviews and a focus group, Chapple et al (2001) sought to ascertain which groups would use walk-in centres, under which circumstances and to what extent these centres would meet their healthcare needs. In the abstract of the article, Chapple et al conclude that:

> Walk-in centres without GPs and with limited services will disappoint the public. It is important that walk-in centres are evaluated and attention paid to 'local voices' before additional money is allocated for such centres elsewhere.

According to Salisbury et al (2002), the key features of NHS walk-in centres are:

- Extended opening hours (usually 7 am to 10 pm daily)
- Walk-in access without the need for an appointment
- Convenient location
- Provision of information and treatment for minor conditions
- Health promotion, supporting people in caring for themselves
- Building on, not competing with or duplicating, existing services
- Maximizing the role of nurses using skill mix
- Nurses supported by clinical assessment software
- Good links with local general practices
- Services that meets the needs of their identified population.

Student activities

- Read the article by Chapple et al (2001). Why would certain groups use a walk-in-centre and other groups not?
- Read the article by Salisbury et al (2002) and consider how the findings from the Chapple et al study are linked to the key features of walk-in centres.
- Using Salisbury et al, find out which age groups were more likely to use a walk-in centre and at what times.
- Access the article by Jackson et al (2005) and compare their findings with Chapple et al's conclusion.

[References: Chapple A, Sibbald B, Rogers A, Roland M 2001 Citizens' expectations and likely use of a NHS Walk-in Centre: results of a survey and qualitative methods of research. Health Expectations 4(1):38–47; Salisbury C, Chalder M, Scott TM, Pope C, Moore L 2002 What is the role of walk-in centres in the NHS? British Medical Journal 324:399–402. Online: http://bmj.bmjjournals.com/cgi/content/full/324/7334/399 Available July 2006] [Resource: Jackson CJ, Dixon-Woods M, Hsu R, Kurinczuk JJ 2005 A qualitative study of choosing and using an NHS Walk-in Centre. Family Practice 22(3):269–274]

and prevention of teenage pregnancy; the prevention of falls in older people; nurse-led mobile outreach services to rural communities; working with homeless people; support for cardiac rehabilitation and Asian women with diabetes; heart disease prevention programmes, etc. Community mental health nurses often work in health centres to provide nursing interventions for people who may be experiencing mental distress, or what the NHS in England's website calls 'less complex and severe mental health problems. . .for example, depression, stress or anxiety' (NHS England 2005).

All of these services involve health visitors or community practitioners working with other healthcare professionals and thereby emphasize the important contribution of nurses in meeting a community's healthcare needs, developing services, improving health and reducing inequalities (Box 3.9).

Newer 'first access' routes

In response to the pressures on GP services and new GP contracts, different models and points of first access to healthcare services have been developed, particularly with 'out-of-hours' services. Increasingly, people's first contact with the NHS will be through a telephone health service – NHS Direct in England and NHS 24 in Scotland, or a walk-in centre.

For example, the telephone health services, NHS Direct and NHS 24, offer a 24-hour nurse-led telephone health information and advice service, with further information and advice available online (NHS Direct – www.nhsdirect.nhs.uk). These services provide a single access point to the NHS out-of-hours services.

The development of nurse-led walk-in centres (WICs) in England has also raised the profile of the work of nurses in community settings. Nurse-led WICs differ from health centres, which are led by GPs and nurses. No appointment is needed and WICs offer a quick, convenient way to access a range of NHS services, including free consultations, minor treatments, health information and advice on self-treatment. WICs have close links with local GPs, ensuring continuity of care for patients/clients (Box 3.10).

Intermediate care

The intermediate care service is the response by the Department of Health to the National Beds Inquiry consultation exercise which focused on services for older people, as they were the largest group of users of hospital services (DH 2001a). The consultation found that there were insufficient hospital beds in the right places in order to meet the needs of this group of patients.

Implementation of an intermediate care service would relieve pressure on acute hospital beds and reduce both the length of stay in hospital and hospital waiting times. The key elements of intermediate care services (DH 2001a, p. 12; HSC 2001/003) include:

- Non-appointment 'drop in' facilities
- Fast access to diagnostics and pathology, leading to more effective interventions
- Multidisciplinary teams focused on particular groups and conditions
- A mix of nurse-, therapist-, consultant- and GP-led services
- Fast access to acute settings where needed
- Access to non-acute inpatient settings where appropriate
- Timely discharge into appropriate settings.

Intermediate care is organized by the PCT and is designed to blur the gap between community care and hospital care (primary and secondary care services) with the intention of acute hospital-based health practitioners working in the community and vice versa. This means that the most appropriate staff in the most appropriate setting, e.g. community hospital, would provide patients/clients with 'seamless care'.

Examples of how intermediate care has been implemented include a Community Assessment, Rehabilitation and Treatment scheme in Rotherham, which is run by a MDT (comprising nurses, physiotherapists and occupational therapists) for patients who have been discharged from hospital after a period of acute care or who have not required hospital admission. Another service provided by the Bedfordshire and Luton Community Trust for early discharge from hospital provides rehabilitation for patients who have had a stroke, chest infection or bone surgery (Box 3.11).

CRITICAL THINKING Box 3.11

Intermediate care

Intermediate care has obvious advantages for both patients and the NHS. Patients can leave hospital sooner or their admission can be prevented by the timely intervention of a fast response specialist team at home.

Student activities

- Find out what intermediate care facilities/teams exist in your area.
- Consider the findings of the studies below and search the literature for further research articles about the efficacy of intermediate care.

[Resources: Green J, Young J, Forster A et al 2005 Effects of locality-based community hospital care on independence of older people needing rehabilitation: randomized controlled trial. British Medical Journal 331(7512):317–322; Young J, Robinson M, Chell S et al 2005 A whole system study of intermediate care services for older people. Age and Ageing 34(6):577–583]

Secondary and tertiary healthcare

Secondary healthcare provision centres on district general hospitals (DGHs) which provide services that include general medicine, surgery (other than specialist services), orthopaedics and child health, as well as midwifery services and some inpatient mental health services (see p. 82). DGHs also offer emergency care in Emergency Departments (also known as Accident and Emergency [A&E] Departments). Reasons for attending the Emergency Department include:

- Chest pain
- A fall resulting in a fracture
- After an accident
- Drug overdose.

Nurse-led minor injuries units attached to traditional Emergency Departments are increasingly available and offer specific services and reduced waiting times. People using the Emergency Department may be treated and discharged, given immediate treatment and admitted to a ward for further care, or transferred to a specialist unit.

Secondary healthcare is usually acute and can be either elective or emergency care and usually takes place in an NHS hospital. Elective care is planned specialist medical or surgical care, which usually follows referral from a primary or community health professional, most often the GP. Examples of elective care include a hip replacement operation or a course of chemotherapy for cancer. An elective care patient may be admitted either as an inpatient or a day case patient, or they may attend an outpatient clinic.

Increasingly, patients/clients are benefiting from quicker and more convenient elective services that include:

- Day surgery (see Ch. 24), where patients are treated and go home the same day if certain criteria are met. There has been an increase in the number of procedures that can be done in this way as the result of developments such as 'keyhole surgery'. The benefits to the patient are that they are able to recover at home and there is less disruption to their work and home life
- Treatment centres (see p. 75), run either by the NHS or the independent sector, offer patients fast, safe and streamlined surgery and diagnostic tests in several specialities, concentrating on orthopaedics and ophthalmology (eyes).

Other examples of secondary care services include specialist services for mental health, learning disability and older people.

Tertiary healthcare services are hospital-based services such as neurosurgery (brain surgery), cancer care, etc. for a patient/client with an unusual condition, or needing highly specialized treatments in a specialist centre such as a teaching hospital or regional centre.

NHS Trusts

Within each area served by the Strategic Health Authority there are several types of NHS Trust. These include:

- PCTs (see pp. 78, 81)
- Acute Trusts
- Foundation Trusts
- Mental Health Trusts
- Care Trusts
- Ambulance Trusts
- Special Health Authorities.

Acute Trusts

Acute Trusts run hospitals and have the responsibility for ensuring that hospitals provide high quality care and that public money is used efficiently. They also determine strategy for developing the hospital in order to improve services.

They employ a sizeable portion of the NHS workforce, including clinical staff (e.g. nurses, midwives, doctors, pharmacists, medical scientists, physiotherapists, radiographers, speech therapists, occupational therapists, psychologists, etc.) and non-clinical staff (e.g. managers, accountants, receptionists, secretarial staff, porters, cleaners, and maintenance, security and catering staff).

Some of the Acute Trusts are tertiary regional or national centres for more specialized care. Others are attached to universities and part of their role is to provide training for health professionals. Acute Trusts can provide services in the community; this may be provided in the person's home, clinics or health centres.

Foundation Trusts

These are NHS hospitals run by local managers, staff and members of the public, and are customized to meet the needs of the local population. Foundation Trusts have more freedom to spend money and to decide about how they will be run, and can also raise money from both the public and private sectors within borrowing limits. They have come to represent the government's commitment to decentralization of control of public services although they remain within the NHS. The numbers of Foundation Trusts in England are expected to increase.

Mental Health Trusts

Mental Health Trusts provide health and social care services for people with some mental health problems. Such services can be provided through GPs or other primary care services, and may include counselling or community and family support or general health screening. Mental Health Trusts and local authority Social Service Departments also provide more specialist services such as psychological therapies or services for people with severe mental health problems.

People with mental health problems may require care in the mental health unit (Psychiatric Unit) of the local DGH or in more specialist units such as regional secure units and special hospitals (e.g. Broadmoor). The type of services they provide include in-depth assessment such as that required by the courts, psychological therapies or specialized medical treatment for conditions that include severe anxiety problems or psychotic illness, e.g. schizophrenia.

In common with other mainstream health services, mental health services are also delivered in primary, secondary and tertiary settings. Modernization of mental health services was one of the government's key priorities (DH 2000). This set out a 10-year programme to improve standards of care; for example, to create an extra 500 secure beds in 2004; more than 320 24-hour staffed beds; 170 assertive outreach teams and access to mental health services 24 hours per day, 7 days per week for those individuals with complex mental health needs. The government's priority at this time was that people with severe and enduring mental health problems were provided with services that were more responsive to their needs.

Care Trusts

Care Trusts operate across both health and social care. They may provide a whole range of services including primary care, social care and mental health services. Care Trusts are formed when the local NHS and local authorities agree that working closely together is necessary or that it would benefit local care services. A Care Trust can include combinations of mental health, primary care and social care services, depending upon local need. Currently there are only very few Care Trusts but it is expected that others will be formed.

Ambulance Trusts

There are currently 12 Ambulance Trusts in England and they provide emergency access to healthcare, such as through paramedic first response vehicles or emergency ambulances staffed by paramedics. The number of Ambulance Trusts was reduced in 2006 through the merger of many existing Trusts. Requests (999 calls) for attendance of an ambulance are prioritized – the most urgent being when the condition of the person is life threatening. If necessary, the patient's condition is stabilized, e.g. intravenous fluid replacement, administration of 'clot busting' drugs (thrombolytics), before onward transport to an Emergency Department or specialist centre; this is usually by road but in urgent cases it might be by air ambulance. Ambulance Trusts are also responsible for transporting many patients to hospital for non-urgent treatment.

Special Health Authorities

Special Health Authorities such as NHS Blood and Transplant, National Patient Safety Agency, etc. provide services to the whole country. They are independent but can be subject to ministerial direction like other NHS bodies.

Box 3.12 **Children's Trusts**

Children's Trusts result from the legislation that followed the inquiry led by Lord Laming into the death of Victoria Climbié (Victoria Climbié Inquiry 2003) (see Ch. 6). The report highlighted many deficiencies in the communication and working arrangements between the various statutory and voluntary agencies – social services departments, Metropolitan police child protection teams, the NSPCC and hospital services.

Children's Trusts are part of the broader measures planned in the government initiative *Every Child Matters: Change for Children* (Department for Education and Skills [DfES] 2004). Children's Trusts were set up to remedy the deficiencies mentioned above and are intended to help local authorities, and their partners, to meet their statutory duties as set out in the Children Act 2004 (the legislative framework for the *Every Child Matters* programme) to cooperate and improve children's well-being. All local authorities in England are expected to have established Children's Trusts, or their equivalents, by 2008.

[Resources: Children Act 2004 – www.opsi.gov.uk/acts/acts2004/20040031.htm; Children Act 2004 (Explanatory notes) – www.opsi.gov.uk/acts/en2004/2004en31.htm; Victoria Climbié Inquiry – www.victoria-climbie-inquiry.org.uk]

Children's services

The structure of the health service aimed at meeting children's healthcare needs is also changing. Reasons for the changes are similar to those driving the changes in adult services and other services, and they too are commissioned and purchased by PCTs. Children's health services are aimed at meeting the diverse range of healthcare needs and providing a more integrated service between primary, secondary and community care organizations. Services generally focus on infants, children and young people under the age of 16.

Children's Trusts

Increasingly, services for children are integrated within Children's Trusts, which were established by the Children Act 2004 (see Ch. 6) (Box 3.12). Children's Trusts include input from local authority Children's Services Departments (created from the Education Department and Social Services Department), various healthcare services and other agencies such as the police. Most local authorities have a Children's Trust and it is the local authority that is the lead partner in this arrangement. By bringing these services together under one organizational structure it is hoped that children and families will receive a much better service more able to meet their needs (Box 3.13).

CRITICAL THINKING Box 3.13

Akasma – a little girl with complex needs

Akasma has a learning disability and additional physical problems. She has no verbal communication but is able to communicate with signs and a communication book. Akasma has difficulty eating solid food and is fed through a gastrostomy (see Ch. 19). Akasma's mobility is very limited and her family have a wheelchair for her. She needs help from community nurses, physiotherapist, occupational therapist, dietitian and speech and language therapist.

Prior to the inception of the Children's Trust, Akasma's mum had to make contact and negotiate with many professionals to have Akasma's needs assessed and access the services required to meet these needs. Looking after a child with complex health needs is very tiring and stressful, and having to talk with a range of professionals only added to the burden. Problems arose because the various professionals and helpers did not always communicate with each other and had very different approaches to the way that they delivered services.

Student activities

- How do you think the Children's Trust and other government initiatives could improve this family's experience of the services?
- Identify a Children's Trust in your area and find out what it does to support and protect vulnerable children and their families.
- Are there any examples of integrated children's services that operate in your area?

[Resource: DfES/DH 2004 NSF for children, young people and maternity services. Disabled children and young people and those with complex health needs (see 'Markers of Good Practice', p. 6). Online: www.dh.gov.uk/assetRoot/04/09/05/56/04090556.pdf Available July 2006]

The key integrated services within a Children's Trust include:

- Procedures for safeguarding all children, especially vulnerable children or children identified as being 'at risk'
- Assessment and services for children in need, such as family support
- Foster and residential care
- Adoption services
- Child care
- Early years education
- Education welfare service
- Special educational needs
- Educational psychology
- Youth services
- Community paediatric services
- Drug Action Teams
- Children's and Young People's Joint Commissioning Groups
- Teenage pregnancy coordinators

- Child and Adolescent Mental Health Services (CAMHS)
- Speech and language therapy, health visiting and occupational therapy services concerned with children and families
- Youth Offending Teams.

PCTs will be able to delegate functions to the Children's Trust, and are able to share funds with the local authority.

Other health services for children include 'ambulatory care centres'. These centres include facilities that provide day care procedures, assessment beds, general outpatients, minor accident and emergency services and community-based services.

Children in hospital

As for most people, where possible, the best place for children to be cared for is at home. However, children also require hospital treatment and the quality of care that they receive should be targeted to meet their needs – in hospital, their own home and the community. Action for Sick Children, a UK charity whose purpose is to ensure that sick children receive the best quality of care possible, drew up a document outlining the rights that children should be entitled to should they be admitted to hospital. The document developed by Action for Sick Children has been adopted as the Charter for Children in Hospital by the European Association for Children in Hospital (EACH) and sets out a number of good practices when caring for children in hospital. These are:

'• Children should be admitted to hospital only if the care they require cannot be equally well provided at home or on a day basis
- Children in hospital shall have the right to have their parents or parent substitute with them at all times
- Accommodation should be offered to all parents, and they should be helped and encouraged to stay. Parents should not need to incur additional costs or suffer loss of income. In order to share in the care of their child, parents should be kept informed in a manner appropriate to age and understanding. Steps should be taken to mitigate physical or emotional stress
- Children and parents shall have the right to be informed in a manner appropriate to age and understanding. Steps should be taken to mitigate physical or emotional stress
- Children and parents have the right to informed participation in all decisions involving their healthcare. Every child shall be protected from unnecessary medical treatment and investigation
- Children shall be cared for together with children who have the same developmental needs and shall not be admitted to adult wards. There should be no age restriction for visitors to children in hospital
- Children shall have full opportunity for play, recreation and education suited to their age and condition and shall be in an environment designed, furnished, staffed and equipped to meet their needs
- Children shall be cared for by staff whose training and skills enable them to respond to the physical, emotional and developmental needs of children and families
- Continuity of care should be ensured by the team caring for the children
- Children shall be treated with tact and understanding and their privacy shall be respected at all times' (EACH Charter http://each-for-sick-children.org/charter.htm).

Every Child Matters programme

The *Every Child Matters: Change for Children* (DfES 2004) is an approach aimed at promoting the well-being of every child (from birth to age 19 in England) whatever their background or circumstances. The Green Paper *Every Child Matters* (2003) acknowledges the past failings of the various agencies to protect vulnerable children and sets out policies to improve children's lives. The Green Paper states:

'There was broad agreement that five key outcomes really matter for children and young people's well-being:

- Being healthy: enjoying good physical and mental health and living a healthy lifestyle
- Staying safe: being protected from harm and neglect and growing up able to look after themselves
- Enjoying and achieving: getting the most out of life and developing broad skills for adulthood
- Making a positive contribution: to the community and to society and not engaging in anti-social or offending behaviour
- Economic well-being: overcoming socio-economic disadvantages to achieve their full potential in life.'

(*Every Child Matters*, p. 14, © Crown Copyright 2003)

Other innovations in children's well-being

Additional innovations in children's well-being include the Sure Start scheme, Diana Nursing Teams and DebRA Children's Nursing Service (Box 3.14).

The Sure Start scheme aims to ensure that children under 4 years of age who live in disadvantaged areas get the best start in life. It involves a number of different agencies working together to develop projects to support the physical, intellectual and emotional development of young children. Projects include working with and supporting parents and helping them with childcare, playing with their children, providing early years education in children's centres, etc. The Sure Start scheme is also seen as contributing to the *Every Child Matters: Change for Children* (DfES 2004) programme through:

- Health improvement for children and their families
- Decreasing crime and child poverty
- Helping parents to work and study
- Assisting lone parents back into work and training (DfES 2005).

Diana Nursing Teams were set up in 1999 by The Diana Memorial Committee. The teams provide specialist nursing care and practical help for very sick children and their families. In Scotland, the approach taken was to fund people to undertake community children's nursing programmes. One such Diana Nursing Team operates from Addenbrooke's Hospital in Cambridge. This is a nurse-led MDT and includes:

- Team leader
- Children's nurses and healthcare assistants
- Clinical psychologist
- Play specialist
- Occupational therapist
- Research coordinator and clerical/administrative support.

The team provides help for children and their families who have life-threatening or life-limiting conditions and who may need long periods of treatment, progressive conditions which may or may not be curable, and other severe medical conditions that can cause weakness and other complications (Cambridge University Hospitals NHS Foundation Trust 2005).

DebRA Children's Nursing Service is an example of a UK charitable organization that works on behalf of people who have the genetic skin blistering condition epidermolysis bullosa (EB). Parents whose children were affected by EB set up the charity. The aim of the nursing service is to offer specialist nursing care to families and health professionals with a particular focus on skin and wound care, feeding, pain relief, genetic counselling and working with St Thomas' Hospital in London to coordinate prenatal diagnosis.

REFLECTIVE PRACTICE Box 3.14

Innovations

A small selection of innovative schemes that improve the lives of children and their families are discussed here but many other 'ground breaking' schemes operate throughout the UK.

Student activities

- Find out what schemes operate in your area.
- Are there schemes that focus on special groups, e.g. children with a learning disability, children in the care of the local authority ('looked after children'), young people involved in crime or in substance misuse, etc.?

Social care provision

This part of the chapter outlines the structures and functions of some of the groups that provide social care. Historically, social care has not been a function or a responsibility of the healthcare system but of local government. These authorities organize the provision of social care under the auspices of social services departments (known as social work departments in Scotland). Many of the services offered by the social care sector nowadays are often the result of joint ventures between the health service, other statutory services, such as education and the criminal justice system, and non-statutory organizations and the voluntary sector (see p. 86 for examples of specific projects). Multidisciplinary and multiagency working is central to social care provision.

Structure and funding of social care provision

A diagrammatic representation of the structure and funding of social care provision is provided in Figure 3.3.

There is some confusion about what 'social care' means because some authors use the terms 'social care', 'social services' and 'social work' interchangeably, but they are, in fact, very different. Even when there is agreement as to what the different terms mean, the way in which services are delivered and by which organization may vary across the UK. As Alcock (2003, p. 97) explains:

> Social services is the generic term used to refer to the provision of both social care and social work and in particular the provision of this by public agencies to all those who might need such services within a defined area. For the most part, this is provided in the UK by departments or sections of local authorities although in Northern Ireland it is administered jointly with health services by

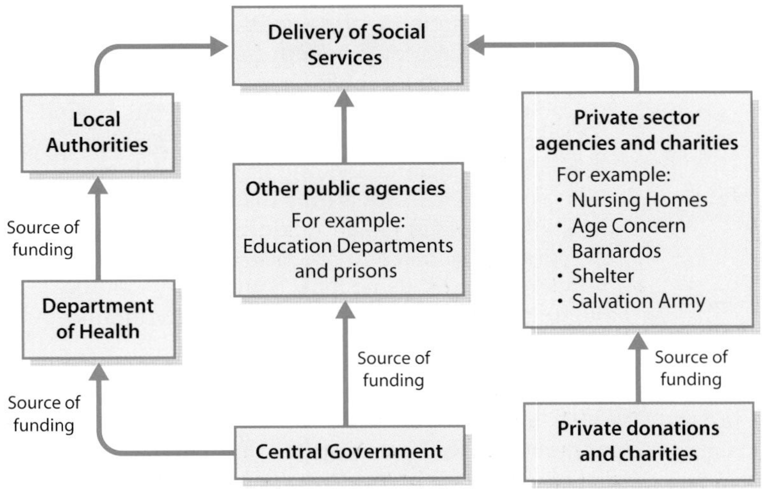

Fig. 3.3 The structure and funding of social care services

joint boards and trusts. All local authorities are required to provide such personal social services (PSS) and in general do so through a social services department (SSD), in Scotland called social work departments. Social services includes social care and social work but the term also generally encompasses a wider range of services provided for local people on an individual or community basis including community work, welfare rights advice and even financial support. Social services may also be provided by other agencies such as health service bodies or voluntary sector organizations.

Social care, specifically, is the term used to describe the support offered by society to sick, vulnerable or disabled people who are unable to provide fully for themselves (Alcock 2003). Social care is expanded on by Alcock (2003, p. 97) as:

> . . . the provision of individual support and attendance to vulnerable sick or disabled people who are unable to provide fully for themselves. The support is provided by other members of society, sometimes on an unpaid basis (generally by family members), sometimes on a paid basis by social care workers; paid workers may provide care at a person's home or in a residential establishment. Social care is, of course, provided to children but in this context the term is generally used to refer to the provision of support to adults.

Moreover, the Local Government Association and the Association of Directors of Social Services (2003) have challenged the traditional definition of social care that sees social care narrowly defined as just providing health and social services for vulnerable people. Both organizations present their 'vision for social care' as incorporating a wide range of services that includes what people say they want, e.g. independence, their own home, a decent income, social relationships, and to include housing, employment, leisure, regeneration and transport in the range of services that should be covered by a redefined understanding of social care as it relates to service provision for older people.

The vast amount of money spent on social care provision in the UK reflects the number of people employed in the sector and also the number of people who use the service, as well as the range of services required to meet the social care needs of vulnerable people. In England alone in the financial year 2004/2005 the breakdown was:

- Over 1.6 million people used social services
- 25 000 employers of social care staff (150 of these were local councils)
- Over 1 million people worked in social care services:
  - 600 000 employed by the private and voluntary sector
  - over 400 000 employed by local councils
- Over £14 billion of public money was invested in the social care sector

(After Platt 2004).

In addition, the vast majority of voluntary sector provision receives funding from public donations and charities (see Fig. 3.3).

According to the Commission for Social Care Inspection (2004, p. 1), in England social care covers:

> . . . all the different types of support that people may need in order to live as independently, safely and fully as possible. It covers a huge range of services including residential care homes, meals on wheels, fostering services and drop-in centres for disabled people. It doesn't include medical care, but many social care services operate alongside health services – such as where an older person returning home after a hospital stay may require nursing visits and help around the house and with shopping.

Social care provision by the voluntary sector

Voluntary sector organizations receive money from central government and local authorities for specific projects. For example:

- *Scottish Association for Mental Health* runs a horticultural training centre in Ayrshire to assist people who have experienced mental health problems to acquire skills and confidence needed to become independent. It works in collaboration with Jobcentre Plus Offices (integrated work and benefits services), social work departments and the NHS
- *SANE*, the mental health charity, works with local and health authorities to provide 'locally focused helpline support' to callers and information on local support networks. Also obtains feedback from service users so authorities can better target their services
- *Barnardo's* collaborates with Edinburgh's 'Working Together' Partnership (voluntary services, social work, education and health agencies) to keep children with their families and in their local school and community
- *Shelter*, a pressure group, campaigns to end homelessness and bad housing in the UK, and works to support homeless people move into suitable and permanent accommodation through its 'home-to-home' initiative with several local authorities
- *Mencap*, a charity for learning disabled people, provides long-term accommodation for those with a learning disability. For example, in Northern Ireland Mencap have a residential care home and several supported living schemes providing support and care in conjunction with social services and housing associations. Residents benefit from being with other people, sharing household chores, having their own bedroom, going on holiday and helping out around the houses. Mencap also has a National College (two sites in England and one in Wales) where young people with a learning disability can learn the skills they will need for adulthood, developing the personal, social and practical skills required for independence by using local community facilities and engaging in real-life working environments – shops, cafes, farms, etc.

Social work definition and roles

The International Association of Schools of Social Work (IASSW) and the International Federation of Social

REFLECTIVE PRACTICE Box 3.15

Key roles of social workers

All nurses in every setting will have contact with social workers as multidisciplinary and multiagency collaboration increases.

Student activities

- Reflect on your understanding of what social workers do in general.
- Access the websites below and check your understanding.
- Discuss with your mentor the specific roles that social workers perform in your area of practice.

[Resources: Skills for Care/TopssEngland 2002 The National Occupational Standards for Social Work (p. 12). Online: www.topssengland.net Available September 2006; A comprehensive view of the complex role of social workers – Social Work in Wales – is online at www.allwalesunit.gov Available July 2006]

Workers agreed a global definition of social work in 2001:

> The social work profession promotes social change, problem solving in human relationships and the empowerment and liberation of people to enhance well-being. Utilising theories of human behaviour and social systems, social work intervenes at the points where people interact with their environments. Principles of human rights and social justice are fundamental to social work.
>
> (IASSW 2005)

The British Association of Social Workers has adopted this definition.

The six key roles for social workers are identified by the National Occupational Standards for Social Work (Skills for care/TopssEngland 2002) (Box 3.15).

Social care workers

Social care may be provided by paid or unpaid members of society, e.g. social workers, social care workers, family members and significant others.

Social workers are employed by local authorities to identify adults or children who might be in need of individual support or protection as a result of their social or family circumstances and, where possible, aim to provide this support or, more generally, to assist their clients in securing support from other agencies. For their adult clients, social workers generally work in this enabling role. Social workers are professionally accountable for their practice. From April 2005 an individual is not entitled to use the title 'Social Worker' unless they are registered with one of the following four regulatory bodies:

- Social Care Council (England)
- Northern Ireland Social Care Council
- Care Council for Wales
- Scottish Social Services Council.

As outlined by the Scottish Social Services Council (2005), the four regulatory bodies have similar responsibilities, including:

- Protecting those who use social services
- Raising standards of practice in social services
- Strengthening and supporting the professionalism of the social service workforce
- Registering and regulating the conduct of social service workers.

As with registered nurses, social workers and other professionals are unable to meet all of the needs of their clients. Many social workers work as part of a team that may involve social care workers or support workers. Unlike social workers, support workers are not currently registered or regulated and work in many intermediate care services and social care settings, e.g. rehabilitation assistants, home care support workers and early discharge workers. A difficulty with the title 'support worker' is that there is no agreement on what the role means or entails. The diverse care settings in which support workers are employed, particularly in intermediate care, mean that their roles tend to vary according to the service and the setting. A parallel ambiguity exists with the definition and role of support workers in healthcare settings, where support worker is an umbrella term covering roles such as healthcare assistants, nursing auxiliaries, therapy assistants and clinical support workers (NHS Careers 2005).

Support workers are employed by a variety of statutory and non-statutory organizations. Examples include the following:

- The Alzheimer's Society employs carer support workers in Bedfordshire who provide one-to-one support for carers in their own homes by offering assistance with problems that may arise when caring for someone with dementia
- South West Yorkshire Mental Health NHS Trust employs family support workers to provide practical and emotional support to people who care for someone experiencing severe and enduring mental health problems
- Learndirect employs support workers across the UK working with families experiencing problems (e.g. drug misuse, partner in hospital or prison, etc.) by helping them to acquire parenting and home management skills, physical and emotional care and dealing with difficult behaviours.

Social care and vulnerable groups

Adult clients form the main groups that need social care, e.g. older people (47%), children (23%), people with learning disabilities (14%), people with a physical disability (7%), people with mental health needs (5%), 'central strategic' 1% and 'others' 3% (DH 2002).

Services for older people

Services offered for older people focus on caring for people in their own homes, promoting independence and reducing time spent in hospital. Of course, how independence is promoted and achieved depends upon the context in which people are being cared for, but it is vitally important that there is close collaboration between health and social care workers when delivering older people's services. This is particularly the case when services include homecare, meals provision, respite and day care and cleaning services. For many people, being able to look after themselves is fundamental to their independence, and having control and being able to make choices about how people look after themselves is crucial. The promotion of self-care is one way that social care staff and nurses can help people to maintain their independence and dignity.

Older people are the largest group of patients/clients using the NHS. According to *The NHS Plan* (DH 2000), people aged over 65 years account for two-thirds of hospital patients and 40% of emergency admissions. As was stated previously, many older people are in hospital inappropriately. *The NHS Plan* sets out a major package of investment to improve the standards of care and services for older people. Its four objectives are aimed at putting older people at the centre of service delivery. They are:

- Assure standards of care
- Extend access to services
- Promote independence
- Ensure fairness in funding.

A National Service Framework (NSF) for Older People, to be implemented through local health and social care partners, set standards for eight areas aimed at improving services for older people living at home, in care homes or hospitals (DH 2001b). The eight areas are:

- Tackling age discrimination
- Person-centred care
- Intermediate care
- Hospital care
- Strokes
- Falls
- Mental health problems of older age
- Promoting health and active life in older people.

Examples of how some of these standards are being met include:

- A Guide to Services for Older People in Thanet. This resulted from a partnership between social services, a community housing association, the district council and the primary care group (precursor of PCTs) (Standard 2 – Person-Centred Care)
- Employment of a full-time Stroke Prevention Service Advisor in Hull. The advisor visits clients at home and establishes a lifestyle programme for these clients by providing information and support so they can make lifestyle changes to avoid further strokes (Standard 5 – Strokes).

Services for children

Social workers collaborate with other professionals, within statutory frameworks, to safeguard all children and to identify vulnerable and 'at-risk' children. In England and Wales, local safeguarding children boards (LSCBs) – comprising local authorities, NHS bodies, the police and others – coordinate the activities of the various agencies to ensure that they work effectively to safeguard children.

An interagency child protection conference can place a child's name onto the child protection register if they decide that they are at continuing risk of significant harm such as injury, abuse or neglect. The confidential register is kept by the Social Services Department but is available to professionals involved in safeguarding children, e.g. social workers, health visitors, doctors, teachers, police officers, etc.

In most instances involving children, social workers have lead responsibility for undertaking assessment of children's needs as well as assessing their parents' ability to care for them. In the majority of cases children will remain at home with social services coordinating the plan and interventions to safeguard the child as well as setting out the respective roles and contributions of parents, family members, professionals and other agencies. They will, where necessary, support parents to increase their skills such as through parenting classes (see Sure Start, p. 84).

Sometimes, as a last resort, the child protection team will need to obtain a court order authorizing the removal of the child from the family home in order to safeguard their welfare. Where a child has been removed from home as part of a care order, the social worker ensures that appropriate arrangements are in place for the care of the child with their participation as well as that of other agencies, e.g. the police, school and health services, and the Children's Panel in Scotland. This partnership, wherever possible, will also involve the child's parents.

Social workers may also work with and support families who have a child with a physical disability in order to minimize the impact of the disability and help them to reach their potential to lead as full a life as possible. This may involve organizing short-term breaks with foster parents or, where necessary, care in a residential unit or helping with school and leisure activities, e.g. swimming, youth clubs, etc.

Services for people with a learning disability

The government estimated that there are 210 000 people with severe learning disabilities in England and about 1.2 million people with a mild or moderate disability (DH 2001c). Learning disability is defined in *Valuing People: A New Strategy for Learning Disability for the 21st Century* (DH 2001c) as the presence of:

'• A significantly reduced ability to understand new or complex information, to learn new skills (impaired intelligence), with
• A reduced ability to cope independently (impaired social functioning)
• Which started before adulthood, with a lasting effect on development.'

The equivalent publication in Scotland is *The same as you? A Review of Services for People with Learning Disabilities* (Scottish Executive 2000).

Services for people with learning disabilities in the UK have gradually moved from large hospitals into the community. The government's main aim for service provision for people with a learning disability is the promotion of independent living as part of their local communities (DH 2001c), e.g. the County Council joins with the local NHS and other statutory and voluntary agencies to form a Learning Disability/Difficulty Partnership Board in order to improve the services provided for people with learning disabilities. It is especially important to put the person at the centre of care planning so that they have both choice and control over what they do. These services may include:

- Supported living projects
- Access to training and employment or meaningful daytime activities
- Respite, living at home with supportive respite care, etc. (Box 3.16).

REFLECTIVE PRACTICE Box 3.16

Services for people with a learning disability

The Foundation for People with Learning Disabilities – a learning disability charity – aims to promote the rights, quality of life and opportunities for people with a learning disability and works with a variety of statutory and non-statutory bodies in order to:

- Conduct research and develop projects that promote social inclusion
- Support local communities and services to include those with a learning disability
- Improve services for people with a learning disability
- Share knowledge and information.

Student activities

- Reflect on how well the services provided by your local authority promote social inclusion.
- Select one area, e.g. daycare, and consider the degree of choice and control the person has over what is provided.
- Access the website below and find out how the organization works with people and local authorities to promote social inclusion.

[Resource: The Foundation for People with Learning Disabilities – www.learningdisabilities.org.uk/index.cfm Available July 2006]

Providing high quality health and social care – quality issues

This section focuses on how standards of care and quality of health and social care services are promoted and maintained. Some aspects of clinical governance, including benchmarks for best practice and integrated care pathways (ICPs), clinical guidelines, NSFs, the Healthcare Commission and patient/client involvement, are outlined.

The NHS Plan identified 10 core principles considered to be fundamental to modernizing and rebuilding the NHS. Principle 5 states, 'The NHS will work continuously to improve quality services and to minimise errors' (DH 2000). The issue of quality was not to be confined to clinical aspects of care but to patients'/clients' quality of life and their whole experience of the healthcare system. This was set up, not only to improve services at every level, but also to ensure that patients/clients, no matter where they live, have equal access to the best quality of care.

Figure 3.4 illustrates the relationship between the mechanisms that are thought to underpin and inform the improvement of quality in the NHS.

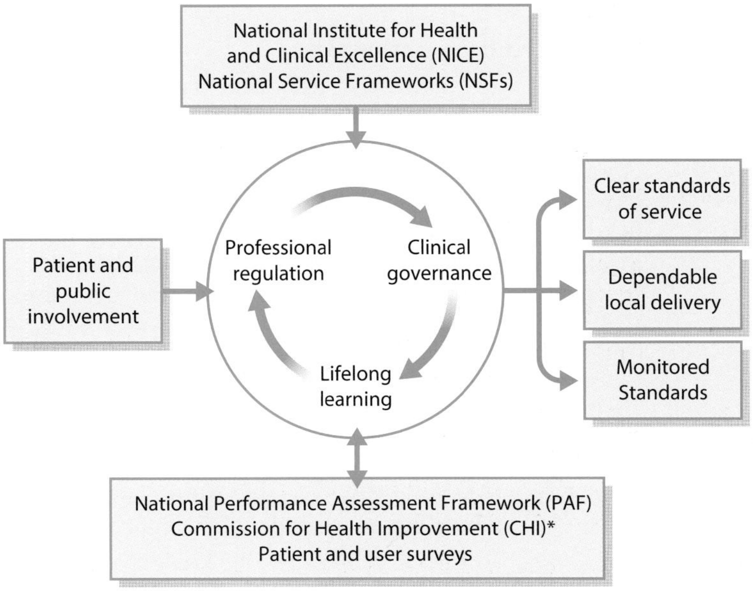

*Healthcare Commission has replaced the work of the CHI

Fig. 3.4 Delivering improved quality in the NHS

At the centre of care delivery are health professionals. A health professional's knowledge and skills must be adequately provided for during an initial period of preparation and be continuously updated throughout their careers. The various statutory regulatory bodies, such as the Nursing and Midwifery Council (NMC), are responsible for maintaining professional standards. For example, the NMC determines the level of competence and knowledge required to register as and practise as a nurse, midwife or specialist community public health nurse. They specify a pre-registration programme of education of a certain length that encompasses both theory and clinical practice. The NMC is also responsible for maintaining standards through Post-Registration Education and Practice (PREP) with the continuing professional development (CPD) and the PREP (Practice) standards (see Ch. 7). The quality of professional regulation is one of the factors that influence clinical governance.

Clinical governance

In order to provide high quality care and patient/client satisfaction, mechanisms, referred to as clinical governance, have been implemented. In common with the other countries of the UK, NHS Wales (2003, p. 207) defined clinical governance as:

> . . . a framework through which NHS organisations are accountable for continuously improving the quality of their services and safeguarding high standards of care by creating an environment in which excellence in clinical care will flourish. Any efficient organisation has a system for improving quality; clinical governance is the system in the NHS. Information from complaints is an important part of this framework.
>
> Many activities come under the umbrella of clinical governance: risk management, clinical audit, significant event audit, evidence-based practice, consulting skills, learning from complaints, involving patients and carers, and professional development.

Full coverage is beyond the scope of this chapter and readers are directed to Further reading (e.g. NHS Wales 2001) and to other chapters for specific components: Chapter 5, Audit, Evidence-based practice; Chapter 7, CPD; Chapter 9, Leadership; Chapter 13, Risk management.

Clinical governance is part of a Department of Health initiative that brings together professional regulation and lifelong learning in order to bring about improvements in the quality of the service provided.

According to Middleton and Roberts (2000, p. 16):

> In essence, clinical governance can be seen as a quality framework which can be used to coordinate disparate quality initiatives and the process of change.

Benchmarking

Benchmarking is used to compare an organization's care standards against those of an outside, but similar, organization, which is chosen especially for quality excellence. Benchmarking helps organizations to achieve ongoing improvements. It is a quality improvement tool that improves poor quality practice and allows organizations and practitioners to learn from each other and contributes to the effective use of resources.

Essence of Care (NHS Modernisation Agency 2003) provides benchmarks for best practice for health and social care practitioners in a number of areas such as self-care, etc. (Box 3.17).

REFLECTIVE PRACTICE Box 3.17

Benchmarks for best practice in self-care

- 'Patients are enabled to make choices about self-care and those choices are respected
- Patients' self-care abilities are continuously assessed and inform care management
- A comprehensive ongoing risk assessment is undertaken and all involved in management of self-care, including patients and/or carers, are aware of inherent risks and how these may most appropriately be addressed
- Patients and/or carers and advocates have the knowledge and skills to manage all aspects of self-care
- Patients and practitioners are working in partnership to establish their responsibilities in meeting self-care needs
- Patients and/or carers and advocates understand and can access the services that organizations can provide
- The environment promotes patients' ability to self-care
- Patients can access resources that enable them to meet their individual self-care needs
- Users participate in planning and evaluating services.'

(NHS Modernisation Agency 2003 Benchmarks for principles of self-care, pp. 1–2)

Student activities

- Consider the best practice benchmarks above.
- Think about a patient/client you met on placement and reflect on how much choice the person had, and to what extent they participated in planning and evaluating services.

Integrated care pathways

Integrated care pathways (ICPs) are documents which outline the care and treatment that a patient/client should receive from the first contact with health services until they leave that care (see Ch. 14). ICPs provide multidisciplinary outlines of anticipated care (care that professionals say patients/clients should get), placed in an appropriate timeframe, to help a patient with a specific condition, or set of symptoms, move progressively through a clinical experience to a positive outcome (Middleton et al 2001).

The development and use of ICPs can be viewed as a 'tool' that supports the implementation of clinical governance (Middleton & Roberts 2000).

ICPs assist healthcare professionals, managers and administrators to make the best used of limited resources but at the same time to provide high quality, timely, evidence-based best practice, and aims to have:

- 'The right people
- Doing the right things

> **CRITICAL THINKING** Box 3.18
>
> ### Integrated care pathways
>
> Examples of ICPs include improvement of the documentation for older patients/clients with complex health needs on an inpatient assessment unit (Brett & Schofield 2002), developing urinary incontinence pathways (Bayliss & Salter 2004) and the treatment of adult drug misusers (NHS National Treatment Agency for Substance Abuse [NTA] 2005).
>
> The NTA (2005) suggests that care pathways should be agreed between and with local providers and contain a number of elements, including:
>
> '• Definition of the client group served
> • Eligibility criteria (including priority groups).'
>
> **Student activities**
>
> - Access the NTA website.
> - Note what the NTA says about the main elements of an ICP and compare this with the elements outlined in Bayliss and Salter (2004).
>
> [References: Bayliss V, Salter L 2004 Pathways for evidence-based continence care. Nursing Standard 19(9):45–51; Brett W, Schofield J 2002 Integrated care pathways for patients with complex needs. Nursing Standard 16(4):36–40; Resource: NHS National Treatment Agency for Substance Abuse 2005 Models of care for the treatment of adult drug misusers. 5. Integrated care pathways. Online: www.nta.nhs.uk/publications/mocsummary/section5.htm Available July 2006]

- In the right order
- At the right time
- In the right place
- With the right outcome
- All with the attention to the patient experience.'

(National Library for Health 2006).

ICPs are used in many settings for people with very different conditions (Box 3.18).

Improving quality and promoting excellence

The treatment and care that patients/clients receive from health and social care professionals should be justified in terms of its effectiveness and efficiency and be based on the best available evidence (see Ch. 5). The standards to be achieved are set by the National Institute for Health and Clinical Excellence (NICE) and the NSFs. Also outlined is the role of the Healthcare Commission and patient surveys in quality improvement.

Clinical guidelines

NICE is charged with promoting clinical excellence and the effective use of available resources in the NHS. It is also responsible for the development and dissemination of guidelines for the management of a range of diseases, the most appropriate interventions to treat that disease or condition, measuring the effectiveness of those interventions and for ensuring that this guidance is shared with professionals. For example, clinical guidelines have been produced by NICE for the treatment of schizophrenia, infection control, head injury (children and adults) and eating disorders. Guidelines are protocols for clinicians to ensure that they are providing the best and most appropriate treatment/care to patients/clients. Guidelines may suggest a treatment pathway and offer a range of options which clinicians can take depending on the signs, symptoms, test results and the patient's wishes. The guidance offers advice on how to assess and treat a patient's disease or condition. The protocols may also contain information that clinicians can offer to patients/clients and their relatives.

The guidelines from NICE are not compulsory but there is an expectation that the NHS will accept the advice the guidelines offer; if it is not, then practitioners are advised to write an explanation in the patient's records.

The Healthcare Commission includes a range of NICE appraisals of treatments and technologies (including drugs) in its clinical governance monitoring of the NHS in England and Wales. The system for assuring quality of services in Scotland has similarities to England and Wales, but there are some differences. NICE guidelines are also used in Scotland and Northern Ireland. However, in Scotland, the Scottish Intercollegiate Guidelines Network (SIGN) also has an important role in quality assurance by reducing differences in clinical effectiveness and clinical outcomes by developing and disseminating Scottish national guidelines.

NICE is a Special Health Authority (see p. 82), whereas SIGN is a non-statutory autonomous body attached to an umbrella organization, NHS Quality Improvement Scotland (NHS QIS). NHS QIS develops and monitors the implementation of clinical standards (Box 3.19, see p. 92).

National Service Frameworks

According to the Department of Health, in England the NSFs are in place in order to:

- Set national standards and identify key interventions for a defined service or care group
- Put in place strategies to support implementation
- Establish ways to ensure progress within an agreed timescale
- Form one of a range of measures to raise quality and decrease variations in service, introduced in *The New NHS* (DH 1997) and *A First Class Service* (DH 1998). *The NHS Plan* re-emphasized the role of NSFs as drivers in delivering the modernization agenda (DH 2000).

A rolling programme of NSFs, started in 1988, includes coronary heart disease, cancer, mental health, older people, diabetes, long-term conditions, renal services, and children, young people and maternity services.

There are five components to each NSF:

- National standards set by NICE and synthesized and validated by an External Reference Group (ERG)

Box 3.19 **NHS Quality Improvement Scotland**

Scotland has one main body for clinical effectiveness – NHS Quality Improvement Scotland (NHS QIS), a special health board established by the Scottish Executive in 2003. NHS QIS works with the Scottish Intercollegiate Guidelines Network (SIGN), the Scottish Medicines Consortium (SMC – clinical and cost effectiveness of medicines) and the Scottish Health Council (SHC – set up to involve patients/clients in decisions about health services, share best practice, involve and help patients/clients feedback to health boards).

NHS QIS state that their role is to:

'• Provide clear advice and guidance to NHSScotland on effective clinical practice, in order that changes can be made to the benefit of patients/clients. Our advice and guidance is based on a thorough review of the evidence available
- Set clinical and non-clinical standards of care to help improve performance and set targets for continuous service improvement. Such standards show the public the level of care they can expect
- Review and monitor the performance of NHSScotland to determine how well NHS services are performing against the targets that we have set. Instances of serious service failure within NHSScotland will also be investigated by NHS QIS and recommendations made to prevent their reoccurrence
- Support and encourage NHSScotland staff in improving services through running development programmes, publishing best practice statements and organising conferences and events that will aid the sharing of best practice
- Promote patient safety by learning from past experiences and putting arrangements in place that will ensure that patients/clients are safe at all times.'

NHS QIS is also an umbrella for several other organizations that work to improve the quality of healthcare in Scotland.

[From NHS Quality Improvement Scotland (2005)]

- Interventions and evidence base (each standard is based on rigorously assessed research and expert opinion, including the views of service users and carers)
- Service models (possible ways in which to deliver care to patients/clients at a local level)
- Examples of good practice, e.g. in the NSF for Mental Health (Box 3.20) the campaign by the Royal College of Psychiatrists to reduce the stigma surrounding mental health problems via an educational initiative
- Measuring progress.

Box 3.20 **NSF for Mental Health. Modern Standards and Service Models**

The NSF for Mental Health (DH 1999a) is for adults up to 65 years of age. It has seven standards covering five areas and each of the seven standards is stated with the rationale for its inclusion, the service models specifically aimed to achieve it, the standards by which it will be assessed and those with the responsibility to achieve it.

The five areas are:

- Health promotion and stigma
- Primary care and access to specialist services
- Needs of those with severe and enduring mental illness
- Carers' needs
- Suicide reduction.

The seven standards are:

- Standard 1 – addresses mental health promotion and the discrimination and social exclusion associated with mental health problems
- Standards 2 and 3 – cover primary care and access to services for anyone who may have a mental health problem
- Standards 4 and 5 – cover effective services for people with severe mental illness
- Standard 6 – relates to individuals who care for people with mental health problems
- Standard 7 – draws together the action necessary to achieve the target to reduce suicides as set out in *Saving Lives: Our Healthier Nation* (DH 1999b).

[References: Department of Health 1999a National Service Framework for mental health. Modern standards and service models. TSO, London; Department of Health 1999b Saving lives: our healthier nation. TSO, London; Resource: Department of Health 2006 National service frameworks (NSFs). Online: www.dh.gov.uk/PolicyAndGuidance/HealthAndSocialCareTopics/fs/en#4804536 Available July 2006]

Healthcare Commission

The Healthcare Commission is a statutory body set up in England to scrutinize the quality of healthcare and public health. The Healthcare Commission promotes quality improvement in both the NHS and independent sector. For example, at the time of writing they are consulting on a *Draft 3-year Strategic Plan for Adults with Learning Disabilities 2006–2009*, with a view to promoting improvement to the health and healthcare of adults with learning disabilities.

The Healthcare Commission is independent of the NHS and its main functions are to:

- Assess the management, provision and quality of NHS healthcare and public health services
- Review the performance of each NHS Trust and award an annual performance rating

CRITICAL THINKING Box 3.21

NHS surveys

Patient/client involvement is a key theme in government thinking and policy. Patient surveys are one way of finding out what people think about services.

Student activities

- Visit the survey website at www.nhssurveys.org Available July 2006.
- Locate a survey that relates to your area of practice and discuss the key findings with your placement mentor.

- Regulate the independent healthcare sector through registration, annual inspection, monitoring complaints and enforcement
- Publish information about the state of healthcare
- Consider complaints about NHS organizations that the organizations themselves have not resolved
- Promote the coordination of reviews and assessments carried out by the Commission and others
- Carry out investigations of serious failures in the provision of healthcare.

The Healthcare Commission takes active steps to reduce inequalities in health and improve people's access to and experience of healthcare by promoting human rights and diversity. The Commission also works closely with the Mental Health Act Commission (not Scotland), making sure that there is adequate and effective protection of patients/clients who are detained under the Mental Health Act (see Ch. 6).

Performance Assessment Framework and National Patient Surveys

In line with the government's commitment to making information about the quality of healthcare services available to the public, the Performance Assessment Framework (PAF) has been put in place. This approach looks further than the economic evaluation by assessing six areas, namely: health improvement, access to healthcare, efficiency, delivery of healthcare, health outcome and patient and carer satisfaction (DH 2005b).

A series of National Patient Surveys (NPSs) (Box 3.21) have been carried out and include:

- Outpatients and Accident & Emergency Departments in Acute and Specialist Trusts
- Patients/clients in PCTs
- Service users in Mental Health Trusts.

There is an expectation that the survey results will require action by Trusts. An example of some of the conclusions from the NPS on patient experience of outpatient departments indicated that 7% more patients were being seen within 3 months for their first appointment than in a previous survey conducted in 2003, and highlighted the need for better and improved communication between staff and patients/clients, particularly in relation to tests, treatment and danger signals to look out for.

Patient/client involvement

The involvement of patients/clients and the public was set out as fundamental to *The New NHS* (DH 1997) as a means of further enhancing quality of care provided by the NHS. Other core values were to make the NHS more responsive to the public's healthcare needs and their expectations, and to make the NHS more open and accountable to the public. Therefore, services would be delivered by means of a public partnership with the service providers, e.g. the public would be involved in decision-making and monitoring processes, service planning, etc.

An additional independent, public 'arm's length body', the Commission for Patient and Public Involvement in Health (CPPIH), was established in 2003 in order to:

- Set up, fund, staff and performance manage Patient and Public Involvement Forums (PPI Forums)
- Appoint all members of PPI Forums
- Set quality standards for and issue guidance to PPI Forums
- Submit reports to the Secretary of State for Health on how PPI was working
- Report on issues about the safety or welfare of patients/clients to the appropriate national bodies
- Conduct national reviews of services from patients' perspectives via data collected and collated from PPI Forums.

Patient and Public Involvement Forums

Currently, there is a PPI Forum for every NHS Trust and PCT in England. They are made up of local people and have new powers. The forums take an active role in health-related decision-making within their communities. PPI Forums are key to raising awareness of the needs and views of patients/clients and the public, and placing them at the centre of health services. They have a number of primary roles, which include:

- Obtaining views from local communities about health services
- Making reports and recommendations on the range and day-to-day delivery of health services
- Influencing the design of and access to NHS services
- Providing advice and information to patients/clients and their carers about services
- Working together with other PPI Forums to share experiences and to address common issues.

PPI forums provide an independent voice for patients/clients and members of the public. Primary care PPI Forums monitor and review the services commissioned from NHS Trusts. At the time of writing further changes in PPI structures are planned.

Other patient/public involvement structures

Other structures for patient and public involvement include the Patient Advice and Liaison Services (PALS), Independent Complaints Advocacy Service (ICAS) and Overview and Scrutiny Committees (OSCs).

Patient Advice and Liaison Services

PALs, as the name suggests, have as a major part of their role the responsibility to provide information and advice that patients/clients need when they use NHS services (see Ch. 5). For example, when problems do arise, the PALs team liaises and works with NHS staff, organizations and support groups and, if there is no resolution to the identified problem, patients/clients will be supported to make formal complaints to appropriate service managers. Further information about the core functions of PALs can be obtained at www.dh.gov.uk/assetRoot/04/06/67/50/04066750.doc.

Independent Complaints Advocacy Service

ICAS is funded by the NHS but operates independently. If patients/clients or members of the public want to make a formal complaint about an aspect of the service, the role of ICAS is to provide independent support and to act as advocates on their behalf, or to help them work through the processes and procedures involved in making a complaint in order to achieve their desired outcome.

Overview and Scrutiny Committees

OSCs were set up in local authorities to look at health service changes, health inequalities and ongoing operation and planning of health services in their local areas rather than how services are delivered or how services match government targets (Merry 2005). These committees are empowered to invite senior health staff to provide information and to explain how local needs are being addressed. This is thought to encourage openness and transparency in discussions about how local health and health services are being developed.

Summary

- Knowledge of the history, policies and legislation underpinning the NHS and health and social care provision, and how they are organized is crucial for practitioners to understand how important it is for both the NHS and social care to be dynamic in order to meet changing needs.
- An understanding of the evolving professional roles within health and social care allows nurses to work collaboratively and effectively with other professionals in the MDT and in multiagency working (statutory and non-statutory agencies).
- Nurses also need a good understanding of the complexity of the current systems of organization and funding arrangements in order to have flexible working relationships with other professionals, volunteers and service users.
- Holistic care depends on nurses having a greater awareness of the complex needs of patients/clients, families and other carers.
- Holistic care depends on the commitment of nurses to plan and deliver services by working together in MDTs and with many agencies. Multiagency working is vital for holistic care of all the population but especially so for vulnerable groups that include children, people with mental health problems or learning disabilities and older people.
- The frameworks and mechanisms for ensuring high quality care are important in guaranteeing improvements in the patient's/client's or carer's experience. Experience of a quality healthcare system is dependent upon all those involved having a voice in how, where and when care is delivered and developed and by whom.

Self test

1. When did the Welfare State come into being?
2. What were the giants that the Welfare State tried to combat?
3. What is the difference between a statutory and a non-statutory health/social care service?
4. List some of the professionals who form the primary healthcare team.
5. Outline some of the services an older person can expect to receive from social services to remain independent in their own home.
6. List some of the ways in which the quality of health and social care is promoted and maintained.

Key words and phrases for literature searching

Audit	National Health Service
Clinical guidelines	NHS Trusts
Frameworks	Policy
Funding	Private sector
Governance	Quality
Healthcare	Social care
Levels of care	Social work
Multiagency working	Statutory services
Multidisciplinary teams	

Useful websites

Action for Sick Children	www.actionforsickchildren.org Available July 2006
Age Concern *(fact and information sheets about health)*	http://www.ageconcern.org.uk/AgeConcern/6CAE34D017DD4279A805B52B6C3548E7.asp Available July 2006
Commission for Social Care Inspection	www.csci.gov.uk Available July 2006
Department of Health	www.dh.gov.uk Available July 2006
Department of Health, Social Services and Public Safety (Northern Ireland)	www.dhsspsni.gov.uk Available July 2006
Devolved administrations in Northern Ireland, Scotland and Wales	www.direct.gov.uk/QuickFind/LocalCouncils/LocalCouncilArticle/fs/en?CONTENT_ID=4007758&chk=6AB2yM Available July 2006
Direct Government – Caring for someone	www.direct.gov.uk/Audiences/CaringForSomeone/fs/en Available July 2006
Healthcare Commission	www.healthcarecommission.org.uk Available July 2006
National Audit Office	www.nao.gov.uk Available July 2006
National Institute for Health and Clinical Excellence	www.nice.org.uk Available July 2006
NHS Direct, Best Treatments	www.besttreatments.co.uk/btuk/conditions/8620.html Available July 2006
NHS Modernisation Agency	www.wise.nhs.uk/cmswise/default.htm Available July 2006
NHS Quality Improvement Scotland	www.nhshealthquality.org Available July 2006
NHS structure:	
England	www.nhs.uk/England/AboutTheNhs/Default.cmsx Available July 2006
Northern Ireland	www.n-i.nhs.uk Available July 2006
Scotland	www.show.scot.nhs.uk Available July 2006
Wales	www.abpi.org.uk/wales/wales_nhs.asp Available July 2006
NHS Surveys	www.nhssurveys.org Available July 2006

References

Alcock P 2003 Social policy in the UK. 2nd edn. Palgrave, Basingstoke

Association of Directors of Social Services 2003 All our tomorrows: inverting the triangle of care. Online: www.adss.org.uk/publications/other/alltomtext.pdf Available July 2006

Audit Scotland 2004 An overview of the performance of the NHS in Scotland. Online: www.audit-scotland.gov.uk/publications/pdf/2004/04or01ag.pdf Available July 2006

Beveridge W 1942 Report on social insurance and allied services, Cm 6404. HMSO, London

Black D, Morris J, Smith C, Townsend P 1980 Inequalities in health: a report of a research working group (Black Report). Department of Health and Social Security, London

Busse R, Riesberg A 2004 Healthcare systems in transition: Germany. WHO Regional Office for Europe on behalf of the European Observatory on Health Systems and Policies, Copenhagen. Online: www.observatory.dk Available September 2006

Cambridge University Hospitals NHS Foundation Trust 2005 Children's Community Nursing Teams (the Acute Team and the Diana Team). Online: www.addenbrookes.org.uk/orgs Available September 2006

Commission for Social Care Inspection (CSCI) 2004 Social care factsheet: exploding the myths about social care. CSCI, London

Department for Education and Skills (DfES) 2004 Every child matters: change for children. Online: www.dfes.gov.uk or www.everychildmatters.gov.uk Available July 2006

Department for Education and Skills (DfES) (updated 2005) Every child matters. Sure Start. Online: www.dfes.gov.uk or www.everychildmatters.gov.uk Available July 2006

Department of Health (DH) 1992 The health of the nation: a strategy for health in England. HMSO, London

Department of Health (DH) 1997 The new NHS: modern, dependable. TSO, London

Department of Health (DH) 1998 A first class service: quality in the new NHS. DH, Leeds

Department of Health (DH) 2000 The NHS plan: a plan for investment, a plan for reform. TSO, London

Department of Health (DH) 2001a Shaping the future NHS: long term planning for hospitals and related services. Response to the consultation exercise on the findings of the National Beds Inquiry. Online: www.dh.gov.uk/PublicationsAndStatistics Available September 2006

Department of Health (DH) 2001b National Service Framework for older people. Online: www.dh.gov.uk/PublicationsAndStatistics/Publications/PublicationsPolicyAndGuidance/PublicationsPolicyAndGuidance Article/fs/en?CONTENT_ID=4003066&chk=wg3bg0 Available July 2006
Department of Health (DH) 2001c Valuing people: a new strategy for learning disability for the 21st century, Cm 5086. TSO, London
Department of Health (DH) 2002 Statistical bulletin: personal social services current expenditure in England: 1999–2000. Online: www.dh.gov.uk Available July 2006
Department of Health (DH) 2003 Liberating the public health talents of community practitioners and health visitors. TSO, London
Department of Health (DH) 2004 NHS improvement plan: putting people at the heart of public services, Cm 6268. TSO, London
Department of Health (DH) 2005a Statutory services delivered by private bodies: MRI scans. Online: www.dh.gov.uk/PublicationsAndStatistics/PressReleases/PressReleasesLibrary/fs/en Available July 2006
Department of Health (DH) 2005b Quality and performance in the NHS performance assessment framework. Online: www.dh.gov.uk/PublicationsAndStatistics/Publications/PublicationsPolicyAndGuidance/PublicationsPolicyAndGuidanceArticle/fs/en?CONTENT_ID=4007174&chk=HqpSut Available July 2006
Department of Health (DH) 2006 Our health, our care, our say: a new direction for community services. Online: www.dh.gov.uk/PolicyAndGuidance/OrganisationPolicy/Modernisation/OurHealthOurCareOurSay/fs/en Available July 2006
Green Paper 2003 Every child matters. Online: www.dfes.gov.uk or www.everychildmatters.gov.uk Available July 2006
HSC 2001/003: Implementing the NHS plan: developing services following the National Beds Inquiry. Online: www.dh.gov.uk/PublicationsAndStatistics/LettersAndCirculars/HealthServiceCirculars/HealthServiceCircularsArticle/fs/en?CONTENT_ID=4004783&chk=a41Hau Available July 2006
IASSW 2005 International definition of social work. Online: www.iassw-aiets.org
Levitt R, Wall A, Appelby J 1999 The reorganized National Health Service. Chapman & Hall, London
Macpherson G (ed) 1998 Our NHS: a celebration of 50 years. BMJ Books, London
Merry P (ed) 2003 Wellard's NHS Handbook (2003–4). JMH Publishing, Wadhurst
Merry P (ed) 2004 Wellard's NHS handbook (2004–5). JMH Publishing, Wadhurst
Merry P (ed) 2005 Wellard's NHS handbook (2005–6). JMH Publishing, Wadhurst
Middleton S, Roberts A (eds) 2000 Integrated care pathways. A practical approach to implementation. Butterworth Heinemann, Oxford
Middleton S, Barnett J, Reeves D 2001 What is an integrated care pathway? Online. Available: www.evidence-based-medicine.co.uk/what_is_series.html
Ministry of Health 1946 National Health Service Act. HMSO, London
National Library for Health 2006 About integrated care pathways. Online: www.library.nhs.uk/pathways Available July 2006
NHS Careers 2005 The NHS team – career options. Online. Available: www.nhscareers.nhs.uk
NHS England 2005 Authorities and Trusts. Online: www.nhs.uk/england/default.aspx Available September 2006
NHS Modernisation Agency 2003 Essence of care: patient-focused benchmarks for clinical governance. Online: www.modern.nhs.uk/home/key/docs/Essence%20of%20Care.pdf Available July 2006
NHS Quality Improvement Scotland 2005 Improving the quality of care and treatment delivered by NHSScotland. Online: www.nhshealthquality.org Available July 2006
NHS Wales 2003 Improving health in Wales. Complaints in the NHS. A guide to handling complaints in Wales. Online. Available: www.wales.nhs.uk/documents/nhs-complaints-guide.pdf Available July 2006
Platt D 2004 The care revolution. Regulating for outcomes: ensuring user focused regulation. Speech given at the ECCA Conference 24/9/04, Commission for Social Care Inspection
Scottish Executive 2000 The same as you? A review of services for people with learning disabilities. Online: www.scotland.gov.uk/ldsr/docs/tsay-00.asp Available July 2006
Scottish Executive 2003 Partnerships for care: Scotland's Health White Paper. TSO, Edinburgh
Scottish Social Services Council 2005 Social workers registration guide. Online. Available: www.sssc.uk.com
Skills for Care/TopssEngland 2002 The national occupational standards for social work. Online: www.topssengland.net/view.asp?id=140 Available July 2006
Townsend P, Davidson N (eds) 1982 Inequalities in health: the Black Report. Penguin, Harmondsworth
Yuen P 2003 OHE compendium of health statistics, 2003–2004, 15th edn. Office of Health Economics, London

Further reading

Baggott R 2000 Public health: policy and politics. Palgrave, Basingstoke
McMurray A 2003 Community health and wellness: a sociological approach. 2nd edn. Elsevier, Sydney
NHS Wales 2001 Improving health in Wales. Clinical governance – a toolkit for clinical teams. Online: www.wales.nhs.uk/publications/clin-gov-toolkit-e.pdf Available September 2006
Peckham S, Exworthy M 2003 Primary care in the UK: policy, organization and management. Palgrave, Basingstoke
Watkins D, Edwards J, Gastrell P 2003 Community health nursing: frameworks for practice. 2nd edn. Baillière Tindall, Edinburgh
Watson NA, Wilkinson C (eds) 2001 Nursing in primary care: a handbook for students. Palgrave, Basingstoke
Watterson A (ed) 2003 Public health in practice. Palgrave, Basingstoke

SECTION 2

Professional practice

Learning and teaching

4

Morag Gray

Glossary terms

Asperger's syndrome
Autism
Dyslexia
Learning
Learning outcomes
Learning strategy
Learning style
Learning theories
Motivation
Reflection

Learning outcomes

This chapter will help you:

- Outline the major theories of learning
- Describe the factors associated with the learning process
- Recall three different reflective models
- Write aims and SMART learning outcomes
- Summarize the key components of successful teaching.

Introduction

Nursing programmes aim to provide safe, knowledgeable, skilful and caring practitioners who are able to provide effective evidence-based care (see Ch. 5). Nursing students take on the role of learner at both university and in placements. In placements, mentors are involved in formal and informal teaching and learning experiences with students and patients/clients. From an early stage you will be involved in informal and simple patient/client teaching activities, assuming the role of teacher while the patient/client becomes the learner. It is therefore important to understand the processes of teaching and learning from both learner and teacher perspectives to maximize both your own learning and that of the people in your care.

'Learning is the process whereby knowledge is created through the transformation of experience' (Kolb 1984, p. 38). Learning is all about educating oneself to think, as well as appreciating the importance of reflecting on that thinking in order to learn. Individuals learn and behave in different ways as a result of their educational experiences. The result of learning is commonly seen as a relatively permanent change in behaviour.

Theories of learning

There are different theories of learning, none of which has gained universal acceptance, and these are discussed in this section.

Behaviourism

Behaviourism as a theory of learning was dominant in the 1960s. Its origins lie with the Russian psychologist, Pavlov, and the American behavioural psychologist, Skinner.

Classical conditioning is the type of learning made famous by Pavlov's experiments with dogs where Pavlov found that if he rang a bell and at the same time fed the dogs, the dogs began to associate the sound of the bell with food. Eventually the dogs would salivate when they heard the bell despite not receiving food. This is called a 'conditioned response'.

Skinner's experimental work involved rats, pigeons and latterly humans. Skinner found that rats or pigeons placed within a cage-like box containing a food tray and a lever to release food would demonstrate trial and error behaviour until the lever was pressed. Over time, the animal learned the connection between pressing the lever and the release of food. Skinner's work led to what is known as 'operant conditioning', by which a new behaviour can be taught assuming that rewards are related to the learner producing successive approximations to the desired behaviours.

Behaviourists assert that memory is the result of strengthening of associations between a stimulus and a response. It therefore follows, according to behaviourists, that almost all kinds of learning can be described and explained in terms of the gradual learning of stimulus and response. A stimulus is equivalent to an event, person or thing in an environment, whereas a response is something that the learner does. The theory of stimulus–response in learning is most useful in providing advice regarding how to teach simple knowledge and skills, and has also made a valuable contribution to training programmes for people who have a learning disability (Bastable 2003).

Any event that increases the probability of a piece of behaviour being displayed by the learner is called a 'reinforcer'. Skinner proposed that by providing reinforcement to an individual in a particular situation displaying certain behaviour, they would be more likely to display this behaviour again when in a similar set of stimulus conditions. For example, when training an animal to perform particular tasks, the teacher looks for behaviour consistent with what is desired and positively reinforces that until the animal displays the desired behaviour. This technique is called 'shaping'. Following shaping, prompting or guiding, or 'chaining' can be commenced.

Once each component of a task has been learned, the steps have to be joined together into a sequence so that completion of the first step becomes a stimulus signalling the second step, and so on. Backward chaining can also be useful, particularly when teaching children and people with a learning disability (Box 4.1).

The learner is presented with a task with all the steps completed except the last one, which they must complete and the process of completion then reinforces the behaviour. In this way, the individual gains instant satisfaction of completing the task and is more likely to have a positive learning experience. In this type of learning it is important to use social reinforcement along with praise for completing the task because social approval is very powerful. Social reinforcers include non-verbal communication such as smiling, eye contact, winking, physical contact such as a hug or pat on the back, nodding or clapping (see Ch. 9). Social reinforcement can be particularly effective with children and young people and to some adults when given by people whose opinions are valued or respected (Box 4.2). It is vital that any form of social reinforcement is:

- Sincere and non-ambiguous
- Clear about the specific behaviour being praised.

These Skinnerian techniques are reputed to be most effective in teaching social skills. They can also be used to decrease the occurrence of undesirable behaviours. To summarize, behaviour which is rewarded is likely to be repeated; conversely, behaviour which is ignored is likely to fade.

Box 4.1 Using backward chaining in teaching

Goal: John will put his trousers on.

The technique involves breaking down the task or skill to be learned into small manageable steps. For example, teaching John how to put on trousers with an elasticated waist could be broken down as follows.

1. Pick up trousers by waistband.
2. Lower trousers and lift up leg.
3. Put left leg into left trouser hole.
4. Put right leg into right trouser hole.
5. Pull trousers up to knees.
6. Stand and pull trousers to waist

To use backward chaining, the teaching sequences would start with step 6. The teacher would carry out steps 1–5 for John and then get him to do step 6 himself.

On completion of step 5, John would be asked to put his hands on the sides of his trousers with his thumbs inside the waistband. Then, while guiding John's hands, the teacher asks him to pull his trousers up. On completion of the task, praise is given by saying, e.g. 'That's great, you pulled your trousers up!'

Once John has learned step 6, he would then start at step 5 and so on until he is able to complete all six steps by himself.

REFLECTIVE PRACTICE Box 4.2

Social reinforcement

Student activities

- Reflect on a situation when you received some personal social reinforcement. What made this situation special or significant to you?
- Think also of a situation where you felt you had done something well but for some reason you did not receive any praise or social reinforcement. What effect(s) did this have on you?

Another strategy to use in order to reduce behavioural problems is positive programming. LaVigna and Donnellan (1986) suggest this is the preferred strategy and provide an example of an individual who hits staff. Firstly, this behaviour needs to be seen within the context of the setting so that a judgement can be made as to whether it is inappropriate. Assuming it is, the reason for such behaviour needs to be identified. In this case, the individual hits staff when he's engaged in an activity that he does not enjoy and hits out to signal that he wants a break. Using the positive programming strategy, the individual is provided with a card that says 'Break' and told that when he shows this to staff, they will allow him a 5-minute break before resuming the activity.

Cognitive theories of learning

Cognition relates to the mental processes involved in thinking, perceiving, problem-solving and remembering. The mainstay of cognitive theory is that thinking and reasoning play a major part in how people learn. Reinforcement is not an automatic process but rather the learner realizes the benefits of adopting certain behaviours. Through paying attention, the learner selectively observes and extracts what they perceive as valuable components of behaviour. Proponents of cognitive theory argue that people learn from experience, by 'doing', and that this learning is then inserted into their framework of existing knowledge. The act of doing involves repeated practice and the provision of reinforcement or rewards encourages further learning.

Gestalt learning theory is a form of cognitive theory that emphasizes that it is important to view the whole when learning rather than taking a reductionist approach which involves looking at small parts that make up the whole. For example, when teaching a skill it is best to demonstrate the whole procedure at normal speed so that the learner can gain a holistic view of what is expected. Thereafter, the skill is usually broken down into its component parts in order to learn. The aim is that, with practice, the learner will be able to perform the whole skill competently.

Another form of cognitive theory is the assimilation theory developed by Ausubel et al (1978). It is aptly named because it emphasizes the importance of integrating new knowledge with existing knowledge. Just before the preface of Ausubel et al's (1978) book is an often-cited quotation by Ausubel:

> If I had to reduce all of educational psychology to just one principle, I would say this: the most important single factor influencing learning is what the learner already knows. Ascertain this and teach him accordingly.

Humanistic theories of learning

These emerged in the 1950s and 1960s from individuals such as Abraham Maslow and Carl Rogers. Both Maslow and Rogers rejected the behaviourist theory that human beings were unthinking and can be shaped and programmed by patterns of rewards and punishments. Instead they focused on people's potential, believing that humans strive to reach the highest possible level of achievement.

Maslow (1954) is best known for developing the hierarchy of needs which is important in respect to learning as these needs play an important role in motivation. The hierarchy is usually presented as a pyramid with the most basic needs (physiological) at the base. The key aspect of Maslow's work is that, before someone can learn effectively, their most basic needs must be met. For example, if people are hungry, thirsty or in pain they are unlikely to be able to concentrate in order to learn. The next layer in the pyramid relates to safety needs. If learners' physiological needs are met but they fear for their physical or psychological safety, then their learning will be impeded.

The third layer relates to the need to belong and be loved. Even if the previous two levels are met, if a learner feels excluded from a group, this will affect their learning because their belonging and love needs will not be met. The fourth layer relates to esteem. Despite having their belonging and love needs met, if they perhaps ask a question and someone ridicules them for asking a silly question, then that too will affect their learning as their self-esteem needs would not be met. Individual self-esteem needs can be met through recognition, acceptance, praise and a belief that others acknowledge their worth. The final layer in the pyramid is called self-actualization. This, according to Maslow, is the highest form of achievement where the learner achieves their full potential.

Rogers (1994) argues that human beings have a natural potential for learning, which is most significant when what is to be learned is perceived as relevant and the learner is active in the process. Furthermore, Rogers argues that self-concept and self-esteem are necessary during any learning experience. The most lasting form of learning, according to Rogers, is that which involves the learner being self-directed. In other words, the self-directed learner is motivated to explore a topic at their own pace and in their own time and relishes the experience of being independent and creative. If, however, learning involves a change in someone's behaviour or is viewed as a threat to how they organize themselves or to the way they live, it is often resisted. That is why, for example, attempts to change one's eating habits or sedentary behaviour can be very difficult to achieve.

Rogers (1994) developed 'client-centred therapy' in which he aimed to provide his clients with the knowledge and skills necessary to find their own solutions to their problems rather than being told what they should do. Roger's work led to what we know today as student-centred learning. This involves the teacher being the facilitator of learning: guiding students on how to learn, fostering their enthusiasm, initiative and responsibility, and providing them with a variety of learning experiences through which they can discover and learn. Student-centred learning is defined by Cannon (2000, p. 2) as 'ways of thinking about learning and teaching that emphasize student responsibility for such activities as planning learning, interacting with teachers and other students, researching and assessing learning'. It also encourages the use of group learning so that, as well as having peer support, students also learn about working in teams (Bastable 2003). Learning how to work effectively as a team member is a fundamental skill for all healthcare professionals.

Andragogy

Malcolm Knowles coined the term 'andragogy' at the end of the 1980s to differentiate it from 'pedagogy'. Pedagogy, in its strictest sense, relates to how children learn. The word pedagogy is derived from the Greek words *paid*, meaning child, and *agogus*, meaning leader of, and therefore pedagogy literally means the art and science of teaching children. Pedagogy involves:

- The teacher as the expert
- Learners being dependent on the teacher for the transmission of knowledge
- Learners being ready when they are told what they have to learn
- External motivation for learning led by the teacher (Knowles et al 1998).

Andragogy is about how adults learn. Knowles et al (1998) argue that adults learn best when they are involved in doing something or are active in the process. In short, andragogy reflects a student-centred approach to learning. Being active in the learning process facilitates the formation of meaning and provides depth to understanding. Knowles identified certain characteristics in respect to adult learning. Adults need to know why they should be learning something and how it will be beneficial to their work or other facets of their lives. Adults' approach to learning is more problem-solving in nature as opposed to subject-centred. Adults prefer to take charge of their own learning or, in other words, to be self-directive and responsible. Adults use their varied life experience as a rich resource for learning and connect any new learning to their existing knowledge and experience. When planning any educational activity involving adults, it should be underpinned by adult learning principles (Box 4.3).

In relation to the principles of adult learning, or andragogy, the models of experiential learning by Kolb (1984) and Race (1993) are now explored.

Box 4.3 **Summary of adult learning principles**

- Establish an effective learning climate, where learners can feel safe and comfortable expressing themselves
- Involve learners in planning of appropriate methods and curricular content
- Involve learners in diagnosing their own learning needs – this will help trigger internal motivation
- Encourage learners to formulate their own learning outcomes – this gives them more control of their learning
- Encourage learners to identify resources and devise strategies for using the resources to achieve their learning outcomes
- Support learners in carrying out their learning plans
- Involve learners in making judgements on their own learning – this can develop their skills of critical reflection.

[From Kaufman (2003, p. 213)]

Kolb's experiential learning cycle

Kolb (1984) presented a model of learning consisting of four phases, known as Kolb's experiential learning cycle (Fig. 4.1). The cycle is based on the premise that people learn much more effectively when they are encouraged to be active in the process. Kolb suggests that learning results from two things: the way an individual perceives and the way the individual processes what they perceive. Kolb (1984) suggested that learning styles are composed of a combination of the four phases in his experiential learning cycle. He stated that individuals perceive either through concrete experience or through more abstract concepts and that they process information in one of two ways: through active experimentation or through reflective observation.

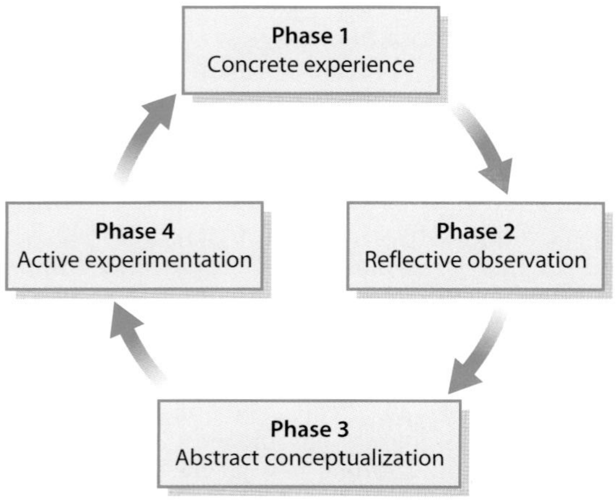

Fig. 4.1 Kolb's experiential learning cycle (reproduced from Kolb 1984)

Concrete experience

This phase starts with a concrete experience in that the individual begins by doing something. During the concrete experience, learners are actively involved and tend to rely on their feelings rather than using a systematic approach to problems or situations. According to Mills (2002) during concrete experience individuals use all five senses: sight, smell, touch, taste and hearing in order to deal with the obvious, i.e. the here and now.

Reflective observation

During this phase the learner requires to take time out to consider, or reflect, on what has happened during the concrete (or doing) phase. The learner relies on objectivity and careful consideration to search for meaning by studying things from a variety of different perspectives and asking questions (Bastable 2003).

Abstract conceptualization

This phase involves trying to make sense of what has happened. It involves individuals visualizing, using their imagination and conceiving ideas to move beyond the obvious to uncover the more subtle implications (Mills 2002). The learner makes comparisons between what they have done and what they have reflected upon, and draws on their existing knowledge. Learners may draw on theories, models and previous observations and experiences. During abstract conceptualization, learners tend to rely more on logic and ideas in regard to problems or situations rather than on their feelings (Bastable 2003).

CRITICAL THINKING — Box 4.4

Learning to ride a bicycle

Student activities

- Access the following website and follow the example of learning to ride a bicycle: www.humanoptions.com/natural.html.
- Having read the example, think about any skill that you have recently learned using the process described in how to learn to ride a bicycle.
- Think about a nursing skill you have recently learned, or are still learning, following this process.

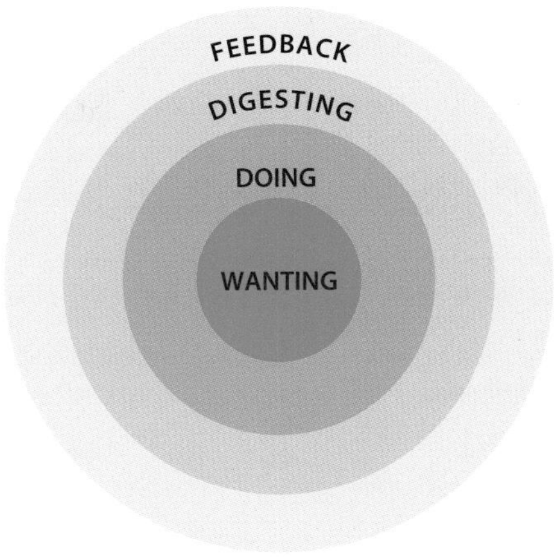

Fig. 4.2 Race's ripples model (reproduced with permission from Race 1993)

Active experimentation

This is the final phase of the cycle where the learner considers what they have learned and how they are going to implement it into practice. In other words, they place what they have learned into context so that it is both meaningful and useful to them (Bastable 2003).

Summary

The above way of thinking about learning follows the principle that learning is continuous, as people continually test out new ideas in practice and adjust their ideas and behaviour in light of their experience. Kolb highlighted two particular aspects:

- The use of 'here and now' experiences to test ideas
- The use of feedback to change practices and theories.

At this point it may be useful to think about an example (Box 4.4).

Race's ripples model

Race, a British educationalist, presented his alternative experiential model of learning in 1993. This model is also based on experiential learning – or 'learning by doing' – and reflects Kolb's view that by receiving feedback from others and reflecting on one's learning is of paramount importance to the learning experience. Race's model consists of four elements (Fig. 4.2), which together constitute successful learning. Race's model differs from Kolb's because, rather than using a cycle, Race's model involves four processes that interact with one another rather like ripples on a pond.

Wanting

This is the central process and lies at the heart of the model. Race believes that wanting or needing to learn is crucial to the internal motivation that drives the learner in the first place. Motivation ripples out from the heart of the model into the surrounding layers.

Doing

From wanting or needing to learn the next process is doing, which corresponds with the belief that adults learn best by doing or being active in the process.

Digesting

This has parallels with the second stage in Kolb's cycle as both involve the learner reflecting on their experience in order to make sense of it and developing a sense of ownership.

Feedback

The fourth process is feedback. Receiving timely feedback is viewed as essential since it is important to the quality of the learning experience to see both the results of one's learning and to obtain feedback from others regarding how effective it was. According to Race's model, feedback is as crucial as the central process of needing and wanting.

Summary

Figure 4.2 suggests that motivation ripples outwards in successive layers, with positive feedback sending the ripples back towards the centre; this in turn has a positive effect on needing and wanting. The position of feedback on the outside ring of the model symbolizes the fact that feedback is gained from external sources (teachers, peers, self-assessment) and needing and wanting are derived internally. In between these two are 'doing' and 'digesting', both of which are influenced by internally generated needing and wanting as well as by externally generated feedback.

Now carry out the activities in Box 4.5.

CRITICAL THINKING — Box 4.5

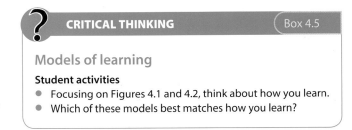

Models of learning

Student activities

- Focusing on Figures 4.1 and 4.2, think about how you learn.
- Which of these models best matches how you learn?

The learning process

People have a tendency to adopt ways of learning with which they feel most comfortable. These are known

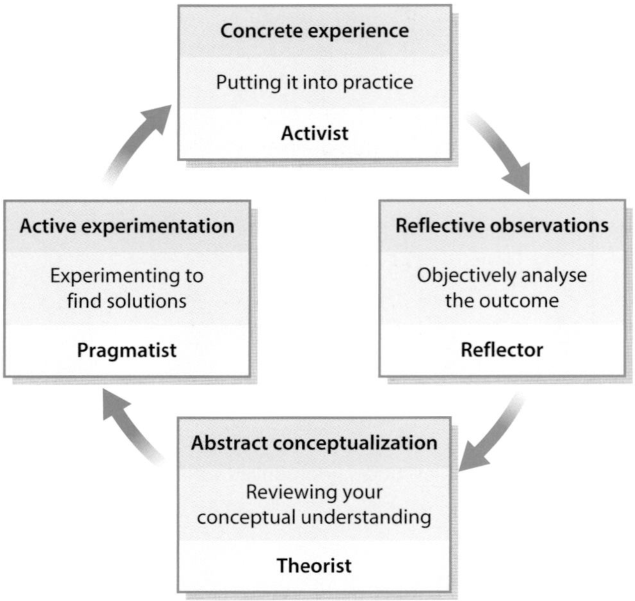

Fig. 4.3 Honey and Mumford's learning styles (reproduced from Honey & Mumford 1992)

as learning styles, which are explored at the beginning of the section. Thereafter, approaches to learning and reflection are discussed.

Learning styles

The term 'learning styles' refers to the way in which individuals choose to learn. According to Bastable (2003), learning style models are based on the idea that certain characteristics of learning styles are biological in origin, while others are developed as a result of environmental influences. Different people have different learning needs and bring their own individual knowledge, experience and resources to the learning process and learn in different ways. It is important to be aware of the differing learning styles because it is recognized that people learn better and more quickly when teaching methods match their preferred learning style. When someone learns successfully, their self-esteem increases, which in turn has a positive effect on their learning. Honey and Mumford (1992) built on Kolb's work and identified four learning styles or learning preferences that individuals naturally prefer to use: activists, reflectors, theorists and pragmatists (Fig. 4.3). You should consider the activity in Box 4.6 as you read the remainder of this section about learning styles.

CRITICAL THINKING Box 4.6

Your learning styles

Many people have a combination of characteristics from different learning styles rather than having characteristics from only one.

No one learning style is better or worse than another and learning styles change over time.

Student activity

As you read about the different learning styles, think about whether you have some or all of the characteristics of each.

Activists

People who prefer doing things and involving themselves fully in new experiences are referred to as activists. They enjoy the concrete experience and have the following characteristics:

- Open-mindedness
- 'Try anything once', usually without any planning
- Learn best when being 'thrown into things' and enjoy working alongside others in order to solve a problem
- Learn least well from passive activities such as reading, watching or listening
- Prefer activities that have a short lifespan
- Get bored with repetition and resist replaying past events in their minds, preferring instead to live in the present.

Reflectors

Reflectors prefer to reflect and observe. They tend to collect information, sift through it thoroughly, look at the issues from a range of perspectives and, not surprisingly, can be slow to make decisions or come to any conclusions. They have the following characteristics:

- Cautiousness, postponing making decisions or definitive conclusions as long as possible; however, when they do so their decisions are usually soundly based on what they have learned
- Learn best when they are able to stand back, listen and observe
- Learn least well when rushed into things with insufficient information or time to plan.

Theorists

People who prefer to focus on trying to understand reasons, ideas and relationships are called theorists and ask the question 'What?'. They enjoy using their logic and ideas (rather than their feelings) in order to understand situations and problems (abstract conceptualization) and have the following characteristics:

- Tendency not be to happy until they have an understanding of what underpins their observations
- Tendency to be perfectionists and need to know the underlying principles and theories to ensure that any actions are based on logic rather than subjectivity or ambiguity
- Learn best when they can use a theory, model, framework or other system
- Learn least well when they are asked to engage in activities which are unstructured, ambiguous and/or lack depth.

Table 4.1 Characteristics of surface, strategic and deep learning approaches (after Ramsden 1988)

Surface	Strategic	Deep
Intention to reproduce, memorize	Aware of learning context	Intention to understand
Passive approach	Active approach	Active approach
Rely on rote learning	Actively seeking information re-assessment requirements	Looking for meaning Interacts actively with content
Driven by fear of failure	Extrinsic motivation	Intrinsic motivation
Not looking for relationships between ideas	Competitiveness and self-confidence Driven by hope for success	Relating ideas to previous knowledge/real life Examines evidence critically Intrinsic motivation

Pragmatists

Those who are receptive to new ideas and like to try things out to see if they work are called pragmatists. They enjoy active experimentation and usually have the following characteristics:

- Enjoyment of experimentation and problem-solving
- Very practical
- Prefer to work quickly, avoid delays and progress things that interest them
- Respond well to problems and challenges
- Learn best when there is an obvious link between the subject matter and their current job
- Learn least well when there are no immediate benefits or rewards from the activity.

Deep, strategic and surface learning

Another facet to learning styles is the depth of effort to which learners exert themselves. Different intentions lead to contrasting study strategies and learning experiences. People do not usually just adopt one approach but rather, based on the circumstances, choose the approach that most suits a particular set of circumstances. Using deep or strategic approaches is associated with a better quality of learning (Table 4.1).

Deep approach to learning

This approach is generally expected of learners studying at university. Students who adopt a deep approach to their learning study with the aim of deriving meaning from what they learn, and then compare that meaning to previous experiences and ideas. Such students are intrinsically motivated to learn successfully about the subject area and, as a result, the deep approach to learning is associated with long-term success (Kirby et al 2003). The same applies to patients or clients who learn about their illnesses or conditions, as those who adopt a deep approach are likely to access the Internet to obtain information and question healthcare professionals in order to clarify their understanding.

REFLECTIVE PRACTICE Box 4.7

Your approaches to learning

Student activities

- Think of your own experiences as a student. Can you identify examples of when you engaged in deep, strategic and surface learning?
- How useful was each type of learning for your understanding of the subject?
- What were the reasons for engaging in each type of learning? (see Table 4.1).

Strategic approach to learning

The intention of learners using this approach is to achieve the highest possible grades. Learners take a strategic (sometimes called achieving) approach to maximize their marks or grades by systematically managing the time and effort they put into their study. These learners, often motivated by competition, are alert to what the assessment criteria and requirements are and often gear their work towards the perceived preferences of lecturers.

Surface approach to learning

The intention in this approach is to cope with course requirements. Learners adopting this approach are primarily motivated by a fear of failing to meet course requirements. They study without reflecting on either what they are doing or why they are doing it. They treat each aspect of learning as an unrelated bit of knowledge, which in turn makes it difficult to make sense of new ideas. Learners try to 'suss out' what the teacher wants and aim to provide this by concentrating solely on assessment requirements and routinely memorizing facts and procedures. Learners using a surface approach rarely achieve understanding and it is therefore not surprising that this approach is associated with poor academic performance.

Summary

Before reading on, you should carry out the activities in Box 4.7. When overloaded with coursework it is likely that a strategic approach will be taken. If the subject matter is compulsory but boring, a surface approach may be taken in order to meet minimum requirements. Where there is an intrinsic interest in the subject matter, such as when a client or patient wishes to learn about a health problem, then a deep approach is more likely to be taken.

Reflection

Essentially reflection is an active, conscious act in which an individual examines their experiences, beliefs, values, behaviour and knowledge that leads to a new understanding and appreciation of the situation which prompted the reflective process (Boud et al 1985). It is a process that involves looking beyond the immediate situation and delving below the surface in order to provide care relevant to the particular context of the patient or client. Stepping back in this way informs practice, creates learning and brings new meaning. From that understanding, judgements can be made on how to ensure one's practice is based firmly on evidence.

Dewey (1933) initially brought the idea of reflection to nurses' attention. In the 1980s, Schon's work highlighted the central role of reflection in professional practice, predominantly in teaching and nursing (Foster & Greenwood 1998). Schon (1983) described reflection as having two constituents:

- Reflection-in-action, which is generated from an experience and involves thinking about what one is doing while actually doing it
- Reflection-on-action that occurs when the practitioner considers aspects of their practice afterwards.

Greenwood (1993) added a third dimension to reflective practice – 'reflection-before-action'. Greenwood argued that reflection-before-action was important as it related to practitioners reflecting about what they intended to do before they actually did it and in this way minimize the risk of making errors.

Reflection is therefore the process of examining and thinking about what we do within the context of the world around us. Reflection is more than just describing what we do or an event that occurred. It goes beyond that to thinking about why we do things, whether they have gone as intended, why they did or did not go well and/or why and how we might do things differently the next time.

Purpose of reflection

Being a reflective practitioner is essential to being a nurse and, indeed, is an expected outcome of all healthcare programmes. Reflection facilitates understanding of both oneself and others within the context of practice and encourages thinking about practice. Nursing students must learn about the importance of reflection as a way of linking theory to practice. The emphasis placed on the process mirrors the value placed upon reflection for the profession as a whole. There are a number of ways to encourage the use and development of the skills of reflection. These include regular reflective group sessions with peers and academic staff, keeping a reflective journal, log or diary, and incorporating reflection within written assessments.

Johns (1999) began an article about reflection with the following:

> A.A. Milne commenced *Winnie-the-Pooh* with the story of Edward Bear being dragged downstairs behind Christopher Robin bumping on the back of his head. Milne noted that as far as Edward Bear knew, it was the only way of coming downstairs, although it sometimes felt there was another way: 'If only he could stop bumping for a moment and think about it.' Taking the analogy further, the moment of reflection begins when the bumping stops and it is possible to stand back and think.

Models of reflection

There are several models of reflection and three are considered below. They all contain the same principles but are differentiated by the level of detail they provide.

Gibbs' reflective cycle

Gibbs (1988) presented a reflective cycle as a way of providing structure for practitioners to follow when reflecting. It consists of six sequential steps, beginning with the description of an event through to producing an action plan for future practice (Fig. 4.4A).

Atkins and Murphy's framework for reflection

Atkins and Murphy presented the framework for their reflective model in 1993 (Fig. 4.4B) and is more detailed than Gibbs' model. This model emphasizes the skills used in the reflective process, namely:

- Self-awareness (see Ch. 9)
- Description
- Critical analysis
- Synthesis
- Evaluation (see p. 109).

When using Atkins and Murphy's model it is important to recognize that the first step of awareness of uncomfortable feelings and thoughts can be stimulated by positive as well as negative experiences. For example, during a teaching session it becomes apparent that evidence demonstrates that an aspect of care you have been performing in practice is no longer appropriate. The experience is positive in that the teaching session involved disseminating up-to-date good practice, but it also produced uncomfortable feelings as the evidence supporting the new practice was more than 6 months old and in that time you have been practising unaware of the new evidence.

The final step in Atkins and Murphy's model is also action as in all reflective models. Finishing a reflective account with an action plan is a fundamental premise because, as a practice-based profession, nursing is about seeking to learn from experience in order to improve practice.

LEARN framework for reflection

The College of Nurses of Ontario, Canada (1996) developed this framework. It is presented as a cyclical process containing the five steps that should occur during the

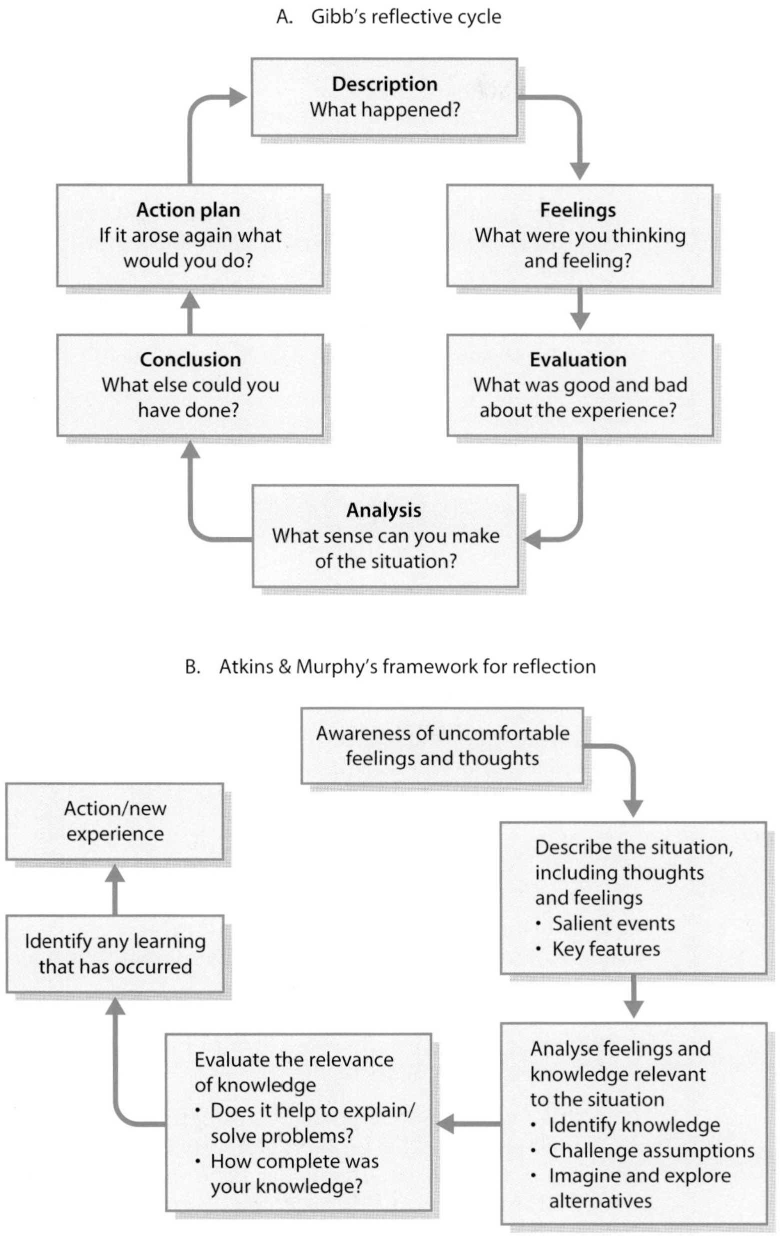

Fig. 4.4 Models of reflection. **A** Gibb's reflective cycle (reproduced from Gibbs 1988). **B** Atkins and Murphy's framework for reflection (reproduced from Atkins & Murphy 1993. The work is also available from www.glos.ac.uk)

process of reflection. LEARN is an acronym for these five steps (see Box 4.8).

The process of reflection

Brown et al (2003) suggest the following as triggers or stimuli for reflection:

- Something that went really well
- A crisis
- An uncomfortable situation
- A situation where what usually works did not work
- An occasion when the usual explanation did not suffice, prompting the need for a new one.

You should now carry out the activities in Box 4.9. The trigger or stimulus for reflection is often referred to as a critical incident. A critical incident is defined as an event that has an impact or significant effect on your learning or practice. Analysing critical incidents is a useful way of gaining an understanding of the dimensions of your role and interactions with patients/clients and other healthcare professionals.

Reflection begins with choosing an incident that represents an issue that warrants further exploration for any of the reasons listed above. The first step involves the nurse/practitioner becoming self-aware, accepting that there may be other ways of thinking about or practising nursing, and being honest about how a significant event affected them as an individual and the impact that this had within the practice setting. This is important for linking theory to practice.

The next step is description, where the individual comprehensively describes verbally and/or in writing all components of the significant event, constantly bearing in mind the importance of maintaining confidentiality

REFLECTIVE PRACTICE Box 4.8

Using the LEARN framework

Step 1 **L**ook back at an experience or event that has happened in your practice recently. Review it in your mind as if you were watching a video.

Step 2 **E**laborate and describe, verbally or in writing, what happened during the event. How did you feel and how do you think others felt? What were the outcomes? Were you surprised by what happened during the event or did it turn out as you expected?

Step 3 **A**nalyse the outcomes. Review why the event turned out the way it did. Why did you feel or react the way you did and why did others feel/react the way they did? If the event or outcomes were not what you expected, consider how you could improve on them next time. This is an opportunity to really question your beliefs and assumptions, and ask yourself what the experience reveals about what you value. It is also a great time to ask for feedback from others.

Step 4 **R**evise your approach based on your review of the event and decide how, or if, you will change your approach. This might involve asking others for ideas for dealing with the situation next time or how to work on a learning need. With your new learning, you may decide to try a new approach, learn more about the subject, or decide that you handled the situation very well.

Step 5 **N**ew trial. Put your new approach into action. This may require anticipating or creating a situation in which you can then try out your new approach.

[Reproduced with permission from the College of Nurses of Ontario]

Student activity

Think of a scenario or an incident which you have either observed or been involved in while on practice placement and work through it using the five steps of the LEARN framework.

(NMC 2004; see also Ch. 7). The incident should be described by including where and when it happened, what actually happened in detail (who did what, said what, etc.) and your own thoughts and feelings during and after the incident.

This is followed by broadening and deepening your understanding by exploring existing knowledge and theories that influenced what happened in the significant event, and exploring and challenging your assumptions. Probe the incident by answering the following questions:

- Why was the incident significant to me?
- Why do I view the incident in that way?
- Why was this incident particularly effective/ineffective?
- What assumptions have I made about the problem, patient(s)/client(s) or colleagues?

REFLECTIVE PRACTICE Box 4.9

Identifying an incident to reflect on

Student activities

- Recall a situation where you witnessed a patient being taught something. It could be a child being taught how to use an inhaler or a person being taught about their medication.
- Write down the key elements of the situation and consider the five triggers or stimuli described in the text.
- Which of these best describes your chosen situation?

REFLECTIVE PRACTICE Box 4.10

Reflecting on your practice

Student activities

- Using the notes you made for Box 4.8, work though the incident or situation using the steps described in the text.
- Write down your thoughts at each stage. You may find looking at Figures 4.3 and 4.4 and Box 4.11 useful to guide your reflection.

- How else could I interpret the incident?
- What other action(s) could have been taken that may have been more helpful?
- What have I learned from this process?
- What can I do to improve my own or others' practice in light of this process?

In this phase new knowledge is integrated with existing knowledge to solve problems creatively and predict consequences. It is usually at this stage that the process identified in the above steps is written up using relevant literature to support assertions, judgements and conclusions (Box 4.10).

When writing up a critical incident analysis or a reflective account, the first person (I) is used rather than the third person which is normally used in academic writing. Use of the third person provides distance from both the incident and the reflective process, which is inappropriate when the focus should be on the individual person's journey. It is essential that written reflective accounts abide by The NMC *Code of Professional Conduct: Standards for Conduct, Performance and Ethics* (2004) and protect individual anonymity and confidentiality in relation to those involved in any incidents or events (Box 4.11).

Once written, it is useful to share your reflective analysis with others as this facilitates learning from others' perspectives, allowing further exploration to be undertaken as appropriate. It is also good practice to further reflect on the process of sharing your analysis with others (Box 4.12).

Box 4.11

Maintaining confidentiality in reflective accounts

'On an early shift in the third week of my surgical placement I watched Staff Nurse Robin Hood (*pseudonym*) teaching a patient called John Smith (*pseudonym*) how to change his colostomy bag. The way that Robin explained the procedure to John was very clear and as John had been encouraged to watch how his bag was changed since his operation the whole teaching process seemed to go well. Robin was very careful to explain each step to John, emphasizing particular points such as the importance of cleaning and drying the skin surrounding the stoma, making sure that there were no wrinkles in the adhesive dressing around the stoma and ensuring that the bag was securely fastened. I really thought the way that Robin stressed the importance of listening for the bag clicking into place was especially useful as that is one of the points that I always find reassuring when I change a colostomy bag.'

In longer reflective accounts or coursework, this may be achieved by inserting the following near the beginning: 'In order to maintain confidentiality (NMC 2004) all the names of those involved have been replaced with pseudonyms.'

REFLECTIVE PRACTICE Box 4.12

Sharing your reflective experience

Student activities

Now that you have finished writing up your reflective account, share it with a colleague and then ask yourself the following questions:

- Was I able to justify my interpretation of the event successfully?
- Was I asked to consider new perspectives?
- If so, what did consideration of these additional perspectives reveal?

Did the outcome change your judgement?

The final step in the reflective cycle is evaluation, where a judgement takes place in order to develop a new perspective on the critical incident or significant event. The new perspective is developed from the broadening and deepening of understanding and the acknowledgement of how the individual would adopt different practices in the future. The cycle ends with the development of an action plan including specific learning outcomes (see Box 4.20, p. 117) for future development. Burns and Bulman (2000) suggest practical tips to assist in the process of reflection (Box 4.13).

Box 4.13

Practical tips for reflection

1. Use a reflective model (e.g. Gibbs 1998) – stick it on your notice board above your desk where you study; refer to it as you work on your first jottings.
2. Get something down on paper as early as possible, not necessarily something academic or part of assessed work, but something you can check out with your mentor in the first instance.
3. Keeping a reflective diary is helpful for some people – write down what happened and why, what did I learn and what would I do next time?
4. Look back over your diary – use it to inform your academic work.
5. Make sure you fix up an early meeting with your mentor and keep it! Check your mentor knows what is expected of both of you.
6. Develop a repertoire of practice to draw on, store up experiences that you could use later in your reflective work, e.g. by making notes, jotting things down, so that important experiences are not lost.
7. Get to know your mentor, and use learning opportunities and experiences for writing reflective accounts.
8. If you can, get to know your tutor, make the most of any individual or group opportunities to get feedback.
9. Write down some notes on your reflection(s), then leave them for a while (about 2 days). When you re-read your reflective notes you may find it easier to engage in more critical reflection. Ensure that your writing does not reveal any confidential details.
10. If you are using a model or framework, refer to it and ensure all stages are covered in order to complete your analysis.
11. Go deep, not wide in your analysis.
12. Live with the lack of perfection – realize you won't always achieve the ideal, just do what you can to the best of your ability.

[From Burns & Bulman (2001, p. 35)]

Factors influencing learning

There are a number of factors that influence learning. These include motivation and readiness to learn, difficulties people may have in the process of learning and the environment in which learning takes place.

Motivation

Motivation influences what people do (if there is a choice), how long they do something and how well they do it. Motivation is a key factor in successful learning and is a central feature in most theories of learning. Without motivation learning does not take place, as we need to be motivated enough to pay attention while learning. There are two sources of motivation:

- Internal
- External.

Internal, or intrinsic, motivation arises from within the individual and is made up of personal factors that make them want to learn. Internal motivation is longer lasting and more self-directive than external motivation. This is because praise or concrete reward or incentive must be provided repeatedly to reinforce external motivation (see 'Behaviourism', p. 99). For individuals who are externally motivated, the desire to learn is secondary to the reward gained from learning. According to Knowles et al (1998), adults' motivation to learn is largely internally generated through self-esteem, quality of life and job satisfaction. Adults who are motivated to seek out learning experiences do so primarily because they have a use for the knowledge or skill being sought.

Since motivation is essential to learning it is important to be aware of the factors that enhance and diminish it, since there are many barriers to motivation. Factors that enhance and sustain motivation include a warm and accepting learning environment, incentives such as praise, feedback and knowledge of one's progress, and the way in which learning materials are organized. As can be seen from Box 4.14, the factors associated with diminishing motivation are more numerous than those which enhance it. The best way, therefore, to motivate adult learners is to enhance their reasons for learning and decrease the barriers.

When thinking of motivation related to patient/client education, additional barriers must also be considered. The individual's perception of their state of health can shape their motivation to learn as can their stage of development (Ch. 8) and ability to understand (Ch. 9). Confusion, pain, lack of sleep, noise, interruptions or lack of privacy can interfere with a patient's/client's ability to concentrate and therefore learn. The nurse as teacher who is insensitive to people's cultural, spiritual and/or social needs can also diminish motivation to learn (Box 4.15).

REFLECTIVE PRACTICE Box 4.14

Motivators: your study habits

Barriers to motivation

- High levels of anxiety
- Sensory deficits
- Low literacy
- Fatigue
- Inability to concentrate
- Poor past learning experiences
- Stress
- Lack of time
- Lack of money
- Lack of child-care facilities
- Low self-confidence
- Poor learning environment, e.g. inadequate lighting, heating and acoustics
- Being told that the subject matter is difficult and/or hard to understand
- Assessments that are too easy or too hard
- Pace either too fast or too slow
- Lack of feedback on progress

[Adapted from Reece & Walker 1994]

Student activities

1. Think about an occasion when a learning experience went well and identify factors that may have led to this.
2. Thinking about your usual study habits and routines, identify:
   - Barriers that may impede your learning
   - Strategies you could employ to reduce them.

Readiness to learn

'Readiness to learn' means that a learner is receptive and wants to engage in the learning process. In other words, they are motivated and able to learn. This is usually signalled by the learner asking a question and is crucial to the learning process – if an individual is not alert and motivated, learning will not occur. Nurses need to be alert for these signals, or cues, from their patients/clients. Coates (1999, p. 75) presents four groups of factors affecting readiness to learn:

- Physical factors including pain, fatigue, sensory deprivation
- Psychological factors such as motivation, attitude, emotional response to illness
- Intellectual factors including literacy and ability to understand
- Socioeconomic/cultural factors such as ethnicity, religious beliefs, health beliefs (see Ch. 1), family roles/relationships, support structures, financial concerns, home environment.

Readiness to learn influences the timing of useful teaching. Patients/clients are generally more receptive to information about their illness shortly after diagnosis or prior to treatment and want information that is immediate and personally relevant (Bastable 2003). There are a number of ways in which relevant information can be imparted and at a time when readiness to learn is often at its highest. For example:

- Patients attending a pre-admission clinic before planned surgery (see Ch. 24)
- Children having nutritional support at home
- People with a learning disability attending the GP or accessing screening procedures (see Ch. 1).

Bastable (2003) presents four types of readiness to learn and uses the acronym PEEK to describe these:

- **P**hysical readiness
- **E**motional readiness

REFLECTIVE PRACTICE Box 4.15

Motivators: patients and clients

Student activities

1. Reflect on patient/client teaching that you have seen carried out in your placement and:
   - Identify factors used to motivate patients/clients
   - Identify potential barriers to their motivation
   - Identify the extent to which learning activities integrate people's cultural, spiritual and social needs
   - Discuss your findings with your mentor.
2. Think about how the following scenarios could affect the individual's motivation to learn about their health problem.
   - Ian Fraser who is in pain and remains anxious following his recent myocardial infarction (heart attack)
   - Harriet Harrison who is suffering from postnatal depression following the birth of her second baby
   - Jennifer King (aged 8) who has recently been diagnosed with diabetes and is frightened about learning how to give herself injections
   - Sam Donaldson who has a learning disability and needs to learn how and when to wash his hands.

- **E**xperiential readiness
- **K**nowledge readiness.

All of these should be considered as they can have an adverse effect on the degree to which learning will take place.

Assessment of physical readiness is important, especially when the proposed learning requires physical strength or capability. For example, learning to walk with crutches requires physical strength and coordination, learning to inject a drug requires fine motor skills and good vision. Children or people with a learning disability who are learning to do up buttons also need fine motor coordination. Learning also requires the individual to be alert and have enough energy to concentrate (Bastable 2003).

Emotional readiness relates to a number of areas. For example, a little anxiety can motivate learning but undue levels are counterproductive. If patients/clients are scared or anxious about something they have to learn, this must be managed before learning can begin. For example, learning to self-administer injections may produce fear because of the necessity to inflict pain on oneself. Furthermore, fear and/or anxiety may cause patients or clients to deny the existence of their illness, which severely limits their readiness to learn. Emotional readiness also extends to students and 'fear of the unknown' often causes them anxiety. Despite mentors orientating nursing students into a new placement, students' high anxiety levels may mean that although they are listening to what is being said, they may be unable to hear what is actually being said.

Experiential readiness is related to individuals' past learning experiences and whether these have been positive or negative. Someone who has had previous poor learning experiences is unlikely to be motivated or willing to risk trying to acquire new knowledge or skills. According to Bastable (2003), experiential readiness involves the level of aspiration, past coping skills, cultural background and motivation.

Knowledge readiness relates to the individual's current knowledge, their level of learning capability and their learning style. It is important to establish the individual's knowledge base, as teaching what is already known is boring, demotivating and can be construed as insulting. Teaching should move from the known to the unknown. For example, when teaching a patient about their diabetes and the need for insulin, the nurse could ask them whether they already know that many people with diabetes require insulin. If is the case, moving from the known to the unknown could be explaining that the reason why insulin must be injected is because it is broken down and digested if taken orally and therefore would not work if given in tablet form.

Cognitive ability should be assessed because factors such as developmental stage, illness, dementia or learning disability can impair this to an extent that explanations need to be broken down into simple and smaller steps with frequent repetition built in. Simple language should be used. Including pictorial information can enhance understanding and convey meaning more readily. Nurses must seek ways to help individuals with a learning disability overcome any problems with processing of information (see below).

Individuals disadvantaged when considering information needs

Consideration requires to be given to people with particular needs, e.g. those who use wheelchairs, those with visual or hearing impairments (see Ch. 16), those with mental distress or illness, and those with learning disabilities. With a little thought, the needs of people with such difficulties can often be easily met. For example:

- For those who use wheelchairs, having leaflets and posters at an accessible height may be sufficient
- Those with a visual impairment may benefit from audiotapes with appropriate information or Braille sheets
- Access to videos or written information for those with hearing impairment.

Computers are another learning tool that can be used for many people, particularly since technology permits accessibility, i.e. the ability to access material regardless of a person's needs. They can be used in various ways such as accessing the Internet to find information and sending email messages to experts so that individual questions can be answered.

People who have problems in learning

There are a variety of problems that may impinge on how individuals learn. These include people with visual and/or hearing impairment, with mobility problems and those with mental health problems, e.g. dementia. Others may be those with:

- Dyslexia, which involves a range of abilities and/or a variety of problems that may affect several aspects of learning including reading, spelling, writing and numbers
- Autism, a lifelong condition that impinges on how an individual communicates with and relates to others
- Asperger's syndrome, which is a form of autism.

Chapter 2 describes what learning disability nursing involves. In relation to teaching and learning, it is important to realize that many individuals with learning difficulties have average or above average intelligence. In fact, Albert Einstein, Richard Branson and Tom Cruise are among those known to have had problems with learning. So having a learning difficulty or problem does not mean a person cannot learn, it just means that they learn differently. Gates and Wilberforce (2003, p. 7) cite the Department of Health's (2001) definition of the term learning disability, which is accepted to mean:

> A significantly reduced ability to understand new or complex information, to learn new skills (impaired intelligence), with a reduced ability to cope independently (impaired social functioning) which started before adulthood, with a lasting effect on development.

It is important to recognize that people with learning disabilities form a very diverse group (Gates & Wilberforce 2003) and can have a number of problems such as difficulty in solving practical and abstract problems, difficulty in conceptualizing patterns and difficulty in communication generally. Having one or more of these difficulties means that such people acquire knowledge and skills more slowly than other people. Not surprisingly, feelings of frustration can emerge. However, being taught different learning strategies can help people learn more effectively, e.g. using pictorial instructions on cards or a computer screen to illustrate the key steps in the task to be learned. Good teaching practices should meet most of the disparate needs of all learners, including those with disabilities, whether these are caused by physical problems, dyslexia or learning disability (Doyle & Robson 2002).

Now read the information in Box 4.16 and carry out the activity at the bottom.

CRITICAL THINKING Box 4.16

Language and reading difficulties

Language difficulty

Sheena has an expressive language difficulty. She has difficulty with expressing herself clearly and precisely because she finds it difficult to know which words are appropriate and how sentences should be structured. She also has problems copying from whiteboards, overheads and PowerPoint slides, and with note-taking, handwriting and spelling. To help Sheena she should be:

- Allowed to use a word processor with a spelling checker
- Encouraged to use specialist advice and guidance
- Given both written and verbal instructions
- Allowed to tape-record lectures or let someone take notes for her (a scribe).

Reading difficulty

Fred has dyslexia. This causes him difficulty with decoding unfamiliar words, understanding what he reads, knowing the meaning of words read, and maintaining an efficient rate of reading. To help Fred, he should be encouraged to:

- Skim read the chapter before actually reading it to get an idea of its structure and content
- Use different coloured pens to highlight main points or definitions
- Stop at the end of each page to check his understanding of what he has just read
- Read aloud parts that he finds particularly difficult and ask when he needs help or advice about meaning.

Student activities

- There is a client with dyslexia in your placement. Using the World Wide Web, find out what services are available to help.
- Find out about the support available for students with learning difficulties at your university.

[Resource: http://technet.gtcc.cc.nc.us/services/das/classroom_accommodations.html Available July 2006]

The learning environment

Regardless of where learning takes place – at university, in placements, clinics or day centres – creating a supportive environment is essential to successful learning. A supportive or conducive learning environment:

- Is free from physical or psychological harm
- Encourages mutual trust, respect and helpfulness
- Allows active participation and a questioning approach
- Is free from intimidation or rejection
- Is high in acceptable challenge
- Takes differing learning styles and cultural and ethnic origins into account.

Anxiety has a direct bearing on an individual's ability to learn as, physiologically, the stress response limits 'the available nutrients for learning. This limits the connections between neurones resulting in slow thinking and depressed learning. Even short spans of stress will destroy a learner's ability to distinguish between important and unimportant information' (Dwyer 2001, p. 313). A conducive learning environment includes acquaintance of group members and this is why many courses start with ice-breaking exercises. Over time, the peer group develops cohesion in which each member begins to feel secure and knows that their contributions will be valued.

In applying Maslow's hierarchy of needs to the educational environment (see p. 101), Hutchinson (2003) explains that an individual's physical needs must be met first. Being in a cold or overheated room, sitting for long periods without adequate breaks or struggling to hear because of background noise all impinge on the ability to relax and pay attention. In terms of safety, Hutchinson (2003) points out that all those involved in teaching need to ensure that the learning environment is safe enough for learners to feel able to voice concerns or ask questions. Fostering mutual respect and acknowledging that learners' self-esteem and pride can be injured through humiliation and lack of sensitivity can enhance the latter. Mutual respect also falls into Maslow's belonging level by ensuring that all learners have their voice heard and their presence acknowledged. Additionally it is important to include and consult learners about planned and actual learning experiences. Self-esteem needs are met by providing feedback to make them feel valued. As Hutchinson (2003, p. 811) states, 'praise, words of appreciation, and constructive rather than destructive criticism are important. It can take many positive moments to build self-esteem, but just one unkind and thoughtless comment to destroy it.'

Stuart (2003) identifies four categories that make up what is often a complex learning environment, namely:

- People
- Learning opportunities and experiences
- Staff commitment to teaching and learning
- Material resources.

At university, academic staff are responsible for creating a good learning environment and many institutions use a personal tutor system where a named lecturer guides and supports learners through their programme by providing feedback on draft assignments and one-to-one discussions regarding their personal and professional development.

In practice settings, ward managers, members of the multidisciplinary team and mentors are responsible for creating and fostering a supportive learning environment. Mentors play a pivotal role in supervising, supporting, facilitating and assessing students' learning. In addition, healthcare assistants, patients/clients and their carers and families can also be sources from which to learn. An effective mentor is a good role model who has the ability to enhance the learning experience by being approachable, planning a variety of different learning experiences and maximizing learning opportunities. They appreciate the need to provide detailed feedback on how their mentee is progressing and offer guidance and support to improve their practice (Gray & Smith 2000). The same characteristics apply to any teaching, including that involving patients and clients.

Role models

Children are eager to find role models to copy or imitate, usually their parents. They watch them closely and follow their example. Role models (see Ch. 8) are also important to nursing and other healthcare students, as it is from them that students learn how to socialize into their profession. Nurses/healthcare workers tend to choose professional role models on the basis of their clinical skills, personality and teaching ability. From role models nursing students learn both appropriate and inappropriate behaviours, as role models can be good or poor. A good role model is someone a student can look up to, value and admire what they do and say, and may wish to emulate. A good role model is someone who demonstrates professionalism in all aspects of their practice whereas a poor role model does not. Nurses may think that they will only learn from good role models but by reflecting on what makes someone a good or poor role model means that students can learn from both. Negative role models can have unfortunate damaging effects as, rather than demonstrating good practice to nursing students, they exhibit poor practice. Inexperienced nursing students may not be knowledgeable enough to discriminate between what is safe and unsafe practice and therefore inadvertently learn poor practice (Box 4.17).

> **REFLECTIVE PRACTICE** — Box 4.17
>
> **Role models**
>
> **Student activities**
>
> Think of three people who you would identify as either good or less effective role models:
>
> - What characteristics do they have?
> - What makes them a good role model?
> - If they are a less effective role model, why did you identify them in this way?

It is important to note that individuals do not deliberately choose to be role models. Healthcare professionals are role models, good or bad, at all times because others are constantly watching them and forming opinions. Not only are students observed by qualified healthcare professionals but also by other students, patients/clients, carers and their relatives and friends. Nurses are also expected to be role models in terms of pursuing healthy lifestyles, promoting health and wellness and, in time, implementing health promotion strategies. Nurses can also learn from patients/clients and carers as role models as they can inspire them in many different ways. Learning from people with longstanding health problems can be very valuable, as they often know more about their conditions than many healthcare professionals.

Summary

In terms of the learning environment, learning opportunities and experiences are paramount in learners achieving their learning outcomes. As well as academic and placement staff ensuring that there are appropriate learning opportunities and experiences available, learners also have a responsibility to take maximum advantage of the opportunities afforded to them.

Teaching and learning methods

There are different teaching and learning methods that include mass instruction, individualized and group methods. The method used impacts on the effectiveness of learning and retention of information. The more active people are in the learning process, the better the learning, which means that experiential learning is the most effective method. A variety of teaching and learning methods are discussed in this section, including action learning, problem-based learning and the use of portfolios.

Mass instruction methods

These include lectures using a variety of learning technologies such as PowerPoint, videos, patient information leaflets and posters. These methods do not encourage an active approach from participants. Lectures are only 5% effective as a teaching method while reading is 10% effective and a video or poster is 20% effective (Wood 2004).

Individualized methods

These include directed study such as computer-assisted learning, reflection, portfolios, workbooks, demonstrations, flexible learning materials and patient information leaflets. These methods encourage a more active approach from participants and are therefore more effective. Demonstrations are about 30% effective while practice by doing is around 75% effective (Wood 2004).

Group methods

These include reflective group sessions, group work, self-help groups, action learning (see below), problem-based learning (see below), tutorials and seminars. Again these methods require active participation. Wood (2004) states that discussion groups are about 50% effective in terms of the learning process.

Role of teacher

Student nurses will be involved in using these methods both to teach others (peers and patients) and as active participants. The teaching role is the most active of all and this is reflected in the effectiveness of teaching others (90% effective) as a way of improving one's own learning (Wood 2004).

Action learning

Action learning describes a way of learning in which a group of people set about solving a problem. It involves learning in small cooperative groups, usually referred to as action learning sets. McGill and Beaty (1995, p. 11) define action learning as 'a process of learning and reflection that happens with the support of a group or "set" of colleagues working with real problems with the intention of getting things done'. In other words, learners work together in a group to solve a real-life problem and reflect upon the actual actions required.

The fundamental premise of action learning sets is to work together on solving real-life issues and/or problems by learning from others and reflecting on the process. The emphasis on 'real-life' problems means that adult learners working in an action learning set bring their own problems to the learning set and work together on how these can be solved. There is no one correct answer or solution, so the task is to develop a workable solution for a particular context. Action learning is based on a number of educational beliefs:

- Adults normally work better in groups
- The experience of working together in a supportive and constructive environment is beneficial
- Adults are capable of solving their own problems.

Through team working individuals learn from each other by respecting different perceptions, perspectives, experiences and knowledge bases, all of which are harnessed in developing a solution to a problem or critical incident. Action learning is used to encourage team working in solving work-based problems, finding resources, preparing presentations and placement-related activities (Box 4.18).

Box 4.18 Principles of action learning

- An action learning set is normally composed of between four and six members who remain together as a supportive group and meet regularly until the end of the action learning set
- Every member takes their turn in presenting their work related to the problem and being questioned by the others. The nature of the questioning should be open ended and inquisitorial, and intended to encourage reflection. An action plan is then prepared for the next meeting
- The action learning set has an experienced advisor who establishes the ground rules about how members work together, with particular emphasis on confidentiality and the importance of building trust.

Problem-based learning

Problem-based learning (PBL) has its origins in medical education at McMaster University School of Medicine in Canada. Its use is widespread in a variety of disciplines, including nursing (Rideout 2001). PBL is a learning and teaching strategy that promotes learning by encouraging learners to actively engage with others to analyse and solve problems – a fundamental skill required of all healthcare professionals.

PBL is a student-centred approach to learning that develops thinking and reflective skills with the aim of facilitating deep learning which is relevant to practice (Wilkie & Burns 2003). PBL involves active learning and develops team-working skills. It also requires students to solve problems, make decisions and explain new information gained to others, all of which facilitate a deep approach to learning.

The teacher, acting as a facilitator, introduces a problem-based scenario to learners without any previous teaching input or study. Working in small groups of 5–10, learners attempt to solve the problem(s) by suggesting a number of possible hypotheses and in doing so realize that their

Box 4.19 Seven steps to problem-solving

1. Identify and define the problem
2. Obtain all the facts
3. Determine a number of workable solutions
4. Evaluate each solution for workability
5. Select the action that appears to be the most practical
6. Implement the selected solution
7. Evaluate the results.

[From Rideout (2001)]

knowledge base is insufficient to solve or explain how the problem can be solved. This leads to learners identifying areas for further learning and collecting material to build the necessary knowledge and evidence base in order to solve the problem. Learners work though the problem in a systematic way and then reflect on both the content and the process so that they can meet the learning outcomes associated with the allocated problem scenario (Rideout 2001). Box 4.19 contains seven steps to solving a problem that can be used in any context, not just in PBL.

Portfolios

Tillema et al (2000, p. 270) define a portfolio as 'a purposeful collection of learning examples collected over a period of time and gives visible and detailed evidence of a person's competence. It serves as a tool to highlight progression in competence development under the control and responsibility of the person involved'. A portfolio can be used for a variety of purposes such as to:

- Value practical experience as a source of learning
- Encourage reflective practice
- Provide a storehouse for information about and evidence of experience, learning and achievements
- Encourage personal and professional development (McMullan et al 2003).

Portfolios are a means by which learners accumulate evidence to demonstrate achievement of learning outcomes and/or competencies. As evidence is collected, a portfolio represents an individual's learning, progress and achievement over a period of time. Portfolios encourage personal and professional development by the use of reflection, self-assessment, evidence of attainment of specific learning outcomes and competencies, and action plans for future learning. Reflection (see p. 106) is central to the learning processes involved in constructing and maintaining portfolios.

Having a portfolio to complete encourages deep learning, as the learner is required to actively engage in understanding the learning outcome and then compile evidence that demonstrates its achievement. Since portfolios are situated within practice, they encourage learners to make links between practice and its underpinning theory (Scholes et al 2004).

Portfolios provide a vehicle for discussion between learners and their mentor/tutor and, as such, are useful for monitoring progression. As a learner you should keep copies of all feedback from coursework and practice placements in your portfolio. Ensure that you read this through carefully before meeting with your personal tutor and/or mentor so that you can discuss the positive aspects of feedback and also those highlighted as requiring further development. Reflecting on your feedback, as well as the discussion with your tutor and/or mentor, should underpin your action plan to meet your personal learning needs. Portfolios are also the basis of Post-registration Education and Practice (PREP) and provide evidence of achieving both personal and specific professional learning outcomes.

The process of teaching

The following is common to all teaching methods/activities so while reading this section it is important to bear in mind that the information relates to readers in the roles of both student and teacher of others. This section explores what teaching includes and the steps involved.

Nursing students are often required to give presentations to their peers as part of their coursework. The rationale for this is that when preparing to teach others, teachers engage with the material very effectively and consequently their own learning becomes more in-depth and longer lasting. Likewise when students are involved in teaching patients, clients and/or carers they find that through the preparation required for the teaching session they also develop their knowledge of the subject matter.

Teaching is about passing on information, communicating, informing and instructing. Telling is not teaching. Teaching is usually perceived as a planned structured activity based on aims and learning outcomes (see p. 116), designed to bring about an increase or improvement in a person's knowledge, skill or attitude on the subject.

Patient/client education is the 'planned combinations of learning activities designed to assist people who are having or have had experience with illness or disease in making changes in their behaviour conducive to health' (Coates 1999). Patients or clients often need to be taught skills and/or knowledge to help them maintain optimum health (health promotion, see Ch. 1), prevent disease, manage illness and/or facilitate their independence. According to Bastable (2003), patient/client education has the potential to:

- Increase patient/client satisfaction with the nursing care delivered
- Improve quality of life
- Ensure continuity of care
- Reduce anxiety so that patients/clients know what to expect
- Effectively reduce the incidence and onset of complications associated with illness
- Promote agreement with treatment plans and help people make informed choices about treatment
- Maximize independence in performing everyday activities

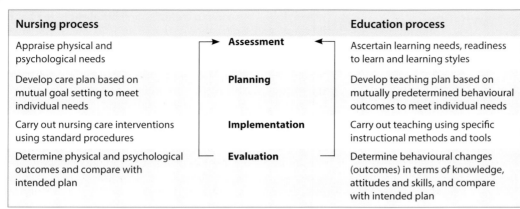

Table 4.2 Nursing process and education process in parallel (from Bastable 2003)

Nursing process		Education process
Appraise physical and psychological needs	**Assessment**	Ascertain learning needs, readiness to learn and learning styles
Develop care plan based on mutual goal setting to meet individual needs	**Planning**	Develop teaching plan based on mutually predetermined behavioural outcomes to meet individual needs
Carry out nursing care interventions using standard procedures	**Implementation**	Carry out teaching using specific instructional methods and tools
Determine physical and psychological outcomes and compare with intended plan	**Evaluation**	Determine behavioural changes (outcomes) in terms of knowledge, attitudes and skills, and compare with intended plan

- Energize and empower patients/clients as they become actively engaged in planning their own care, which in turn provides them with a sense of control.

The last bullet point above relates to information giving so that patients/clients can make informed decisions or give informed consent (see Ch. 6). Consent is normally prefixed by the word 'informed' and it is this which ensures that an individual who, before giving their informed consent, must:

- Have the relevant information
- Understand the information
- Be able to understand the probabilities and/or complications with any procedures and treatments being explained/suggested
- Be able to understand alternative choices to treatments/therapies being suggested
- Be mentally competent (see Ch. 6)
- Consent voluntarily.

Conflicts and challenges in giving information can arise for a number of reasons. Timing of information giving is important. Giving it too early can mean that key messages are forgotten and giving it too late can lead to individuals not having enough opportunity to reflect upon the information given and ask further questions for clarification. The Department of Health has key documents on the topic of consent (see 'Useful websites', p. 121).

Just as nurses assess, plan, implement and evaluate their care using the nursing process (see Ch. 14), the same stages apply to teaching. Bastable (2003) draws parallels between the process of education and the nursing process. The headings used in Table 4.2 are used to underpin discussion of the teaching process below.

Assessment

Before setting out to 'teach' someone, it is essential to identify what the person/patient/client or groups of peers/patients/clients (hereafter referred to as learners):

- Needs to know
- What they already know
- Their readiness to learn (p. 110)
- Their preferred learning style (p. 104).

Assessment of learners' needs prevents unnecessary repetition of known material and saves time and energy for all parties. In order to teach, it is essential to read around the topic area including all the up-to-date literature and evidence (see Ch. 5 for literature searching and sources of evidence). Once what the learners already know has been established, assessment of what should be taught can begin.

Planning

The purpose of this phase is to plan what, how and when the intended teaching will take place. Following assessment, it will be evident what is already known and what remains to be taught. Knowing what to teach is not enough and planning will identify which particular elements of the topic are essential to teach and those that are interesting, but not essential. Writing aims and learning outcomes helps in deciding what is essential and what is not. The nature of the learning outcomes provides the basis of deciding which teaching methods are most appropriate to use.

Consideration needs to be given to creating a motivating learning environment (see p. 112). To achieve this, it is important to involve learners in setting their own learning outcomes when possible and to ensure that the outcomes are at the appropriate level so they move learners to a higher level of understanding.

Aims and learning outcomes

> If there are no aims or learning outcomes, it is very difficult to focus one's learning or indeed provide evidence that any learning has actually occurred. In other words, 'if you don't know where you are going, any bus will do'.
>
> Cowan (2003, p. 33)

Aims attempt to provide shape and direction to teaching and learning. They are general statements representing an ideal, or aspiration, and illustrate the overall purpose of a course. Learning outcomes should be clear, specific and contained within one sentence. Their purposes are to:

- Allow the learner to know what is expected of them
- Help the teacher define what has to be taught

Table 4.3 Examples of levels within the cognitive domain

Domain level	Verbs associated with domain level	Example used in practice: On completion of the placement students should be able to:
Knowledge	Define, recall, identify, list, describe, draw, record	Recall knowledge and skills of assessment and its relation to planning, implementing and evaluating care
Comprehension	Describe, rephrase, explain, recognize, discuss, sort, rearrange, differentiate, estimate, conclude	Discuss barriers to communication within the assessment process
Application	Apply, generalize, demonstrate, illustrate, practise, relate, choose, develop, organize, use, transfer	Demonstrate a holistic approach to the assessment of patients and clients
Analysis (see below)	Analyse, distinguish, calculate, detect, deduce, classify, discriminate, categorize, test, inspect	Analyse the psychological and development needs of the sick child
Synthesis (see below)	Relate, produce, construct, organize, document, design, plan, propose, specify, derive, synthesize	Document the outcomes of nursing and other interventions relating to a patient or client with complex needs
Evaluation (see p. 119)	Judge, argue, justify, evaluate, assess, decide, compare, appraise, validate, select	Evaluate the role of the nurse within the multidisciplinary team context when caring for patients/clients with complex needs

- Assist the assessor by providing a means of deciding if the learner has met them.

Bloom (1964) proposed three main areas, also called domains, which are helpful in writing learning outcomes:

- The cognitive domain, concerned with knowledge and thinking
- The affective domain, which is concerned with feelings and attitudes
- The psychomotor domain that refers to manual, manipulative skills.

Each of these domains is further broken down into a hierarchy with the simplest ones at the bottom. For example, the cognitive domain begins with knowledge and then moves upward to comprehension, application, analysis and ends with synthesis. This means that once knowledge of a topic is acquired, the individual can apply that knowledge by examining the relationship between elements and functions. Analysis is the next level that involves considering the context in which the topic area is being analysed, identifying and challenging assumptions by exploring alternatives and then making a judgement. Synthesis occurs when the findings from analysis are used to make suggestions or recommendations (Gopee 2002). An example of each level is given in Table 4.3.

Effectively written learning outcomes must be unambiguous and should be SMART (Box 4.20). Chapter 14 identifies the need to be able to write SMART goals as part of the nursing process. Once SMART learning outcomes have been written, the next step is to devise a teaching (or lesson) plan.

Box 4.20 **Smart learning outcomes**

S: **s**pecific
M: **m**easurable – so that there is evidence that they have been achieved
A: **a**ction-orientated – verbs should lead or drive them
R: **r**elevant – both in terms of the nature and the reason for them
T: **t**ime-restricted – so that that there is a target date for successful completion.

Example

By the end of this module you should be able to:

- Collaborate with others in the multidisciplinary team to ensure continuity of care.

Teaching plans

The purpose of these is to provide a guide so that nothing is missed out under the pressure of delivery. Writing the content clearly on cards, using colour to highlight keywords or important points can be helpful as is identifying those parts of the plan that could be omitted if required. For example, essential information could be in one colour and less important information in another. However it is best to use only two or three colours otherwise, rather than helping key points to stand out, it could cause more confusion.

Consideration should be given to a number of factors when planning a teaching session. These include the:

- Method of presentation that will best suit the subject matter
- Length of time
- Number of participants
- Learning environment
- Time of day
- Resources available (Oliver & Endersby 1994).

A teaching plan can be constructed using the following headings: content, teacher activity, learner activity, audiovisual aids, time.

Teaching or lesson planning involves three main stages:

- Collecting, selecting and preparing relevant subject matter
- Preparing material and planning methods to be used
- Checking and rehearsing.

These stages are discussed below.

Collecting, selecting and preparing relevant material

Once the learners' existing knowledge has been assessed (p. 116), the topic areas that form the content of the teaching session are collected, prioritized and prepared. This stage involves searching the literature and evidence databases, collecting appropriate materials (such as already available patient information leaflets or compiling reference lists) and preparing notes.

Preparing material and planning methods to be used

The learning outcomes should be used to determine which teaching methods are appropriate. If, for example, one of the learning outcomes used the verb 'debate', then it would be appropriate to use a debate as part of the teaching session. Depending on the time allocated for the teaching session, a number of activities should be planned in order to maintain the learners' attention. It is recommended that there is a change of activity every 15–20 minutes and more frequently when children or people with a learning disability are involved. The learning outcomes will guide decisions on appropriate content and level.

The structure of the lesson should be planned in a logical sequence with reference to the following maxims:

- Move from the simple to the complex
- Move from the known to the unknown
- Move from concrete to abstract
- Provide examples to explain the principles
- Use principles to explain examples
- Emphasize the relevance of practice to theory.

Your teaching plan should also contain:

- Breaks in the presentation of new material when learners' understanding is assessed, and discussed further if necessary, before moving on to the next point
- A summary of the main points, showing links with future teaching sessions (if any) and, if appropriate, references for further study
- Prepared overheads or a PowerPoint presentation to signpost important points.

Implementation

The introduction to any teaching session should demonstrate the significance and relevance of what is to be learned. An explanation of the purpose of the lesson, its relationship to previous teaching sessions (if any), an outline structure of the teaching session and the learning outcomes for the session should all be provided as this creates shared meaning and an early rapport with the learners. Whatever teaching method is used, it is essential that through a warm and accepting learning environment, key points or issues are communicated by speaking clearly, using pauses and ensuring the pace is not too fast. The teacher should continually gauge their audience's understanding by observing their non-verbal reactions and repeating or re-phrasing as necessary.

Effective teaching depends on two interlocking factors: explanations and questions. Learning how to ask questions (see also Ch. 9) and give explanations requires practice. Hints on how to use questions and give effective explanations can be found in Box 4.21.

Teaching and learning clinical/practical skills

'To be skilled is to be able to perform a learned activity well and at will' (Cottrell 2001, p. 9). Skilled behaviour has to be learned and must be practised, e.g. learning to ride a bicycle (see Box 4.4, p. 103). What is learned in a skill is the selection of correct movements, at the right time and in the correct order. Tips for teaching a practical skill are as follows:

- Ensure you can perform the skill well yourself
- Reflect on how you were taught the skill and work out each important step involved in it
- Identify cues or signals such as those that can be seen, heard, felt, smelt or tasted, e.g. when teaching a patient how to assemble a piece of equipment, say: 'When you hear a clicking sound, you know that the syringe is primed'
- Personalize the teaching of skills to individuals or small groups
- When demonstrating or guiding someone through a skill, keep spoken sentences short and use terminology that is understood by learner
- If the learner is unfamiliar with the skill, demonstrate it at normal speed first and then again more slowly, emphasizing the importance of accuracy rather than speed
- A good sequence to adopt is: demonstration, explanation, then demonstration again
- Allow learners to practise on their own and avoid interrupting them unless they require help or guidance
- Be careful about pointing out incorrect technique to a learner. Never use sarcasm or let your comments be overheard by others (see 'Feedback', p. 120)
- Encourage the learner by commenting positively on their progress and how well they are doing
- Encourage the learner to practise as much as possible and then to teach someone else
- The time between practice sessions should be short as skill levels decline, information can be forgotten and motivation can be lost.

A skilled performance has the following characteristics:

- Precision – it is accurate
- Smoothness
- Timing – fast or slow as appropriate

Box 4.21 **How to use questions and give effective explanations**

Using questions
- Restrict the use of closed questions (see Ch. 9) to establish the facts or baseline knowledge, e.g. What? When? How many?
- Use open or clarifying/probing questions in all other circumstances, e.g. What are the options? What if?
- Allow adequate time for students to give a response – don't speak too soon
- Follow a poor answer with another question
- Resist the temptation to answer the learners' questions – use counter questions instead
- Be non-confrontational – you don't need to be threatening to be challenging.

Logical steps to provide clear and effective explanations
- Consider the issue or topic to be explained and assess your own knowledge. Revise as appropriate. Assess the likely existing knowledge base of the learner(s)
- Plan, prepare and structure the explanation so as to give a clear and straightforward picture of the topic
- Pitch the explanation at the right level, based on an assessment of learning needs
- Transmit the explanation in a series of statements or bite-size chunks
- During transmission:
  - assess learners' understanding by observing non-verbal cues and asking if they have any questions or points they would like clarified
  - maintain eye contact to establish a rapport and observe learners' reaction to components of the explanation
- Speak clearly, use pauses and appropriate pace
- Summarize periodically, 'so far, we've covered...', and again at the end by asking learners to sum up what they have heard. This is a powerful way of assessing their understanding
- Conclude the explanation by restating the key messages.

[From Spencer (2003)]

- Obvious confidence
- Efficiency – economical in effort
- Ease – fluent
- Adaptability – it meets individual needs of patients/clients
- Sensitivity – obtains maximum information from cues given by the patient, e.g. discomfort or anxiety, and takes appropriate actions to avoid unnecessary distress
- Anticipation – allows quick and appropriate response to any eventuality.

Evaluation

In this last phase, the teacher needs to decide whether the teaching plan has been effective and achieved what it set out to do, i.e. have the learning outcomes been achieved? This judgement uses the reflective cycle to assess one's performance and asking the learner(s) for feedback on the teaching session. Reflecting on the outcomes of evaluation is the basis for improving your practice as a teacher.

A judgement is made about how the learner has progressed in their learning including, if appropriate, how well they have assimilated learning a new skill. This can be assessed by asking the learner questions that test their knowledge and then observing them performing the skill. Having undertaken evaluation, it is then essential to give feedback.

Box 4.22 **Giving feedback**

Feedback should:
- Use clear unambiguous language
- Be specific, honest and personalized
- Be given in a way that respects the individuality and worth of learners
- Be given as soon as possible to provide the highest motivational impact
- Be delivered in a quiet and private setting
- Comment positively on good things
- Use the feedback sandwich technique: good news, not so good news and then good news.

When giving good news:
- Tell the learner what was good/right and why.

When giving not so good news:
- Be honest and constructive
- Be specific, kind and non-judgemental
- Tell the learner what was poor/wrong and why
- Inform the learner how they can improve their performance next time.

After giving feedback, the mentor should work with the learner to devise an action plan for areas requiring improvement.

Giving feedback

Learning is an active process which requires feedback for the learner to know how effective their learning has been. As well as providing information about how well a learner has performed, feedback should also identify areas for further improvement. Moreover, feedback can be motivating.

Feedback must be specific rather than general. It should be immediate and contain details of what was good about the performance and which elements require further practice and attention. A rationale for the latter should always be provided. It is also a good idea to ask the learner to evaluate their own performance so that they develop the ability to make judgements about their performance. The quality of the feedback is important, as praise is motivating and can encourage the learner to try to do better the next time. Although giving feedback on both positive and negative aspects of a performance is important, the manner in which this is done is probably even more important. The key factors are listed in Box 4.22 (p. 119).

Summary

- There are three major theories of learning: behaviourism, cognitive theory and humanism.
- Andragogy and experiential learning are the preferred ways of learning for adults.
- Pedagogy describes how children learn.
- The learning process is associated with four main learning styles and deep, strategic and surface approaches.
- Reflective models provide a basis for learning the skills of reflection.
- Learning outcomes must be unambiguous and should be specific, measurable, action-orientated, relevant and time-restricted.
- The key components of successful learning and teaching are that:
  - we learn best by doing
  - without readiness, learning is inefficient and may be harmful
  - motivation is essential
  - responses need immediate reinforcement
  - meaningful content is learned most easily and retained for longer
  - a conducive environment is necessary
  - deep learning is most successful.

Self test

1. Which learning approach is associated with the best academic achievement?
   a. Deep
   b. Strategic
   c. Surface
   d. Exterior.

2. Which of the following is associated with the humanistic theory of learning?
   a. Gestalt
   b. Pavlov
   c. Skinner
   d. Maslow.

3. The most effective teaching method to facilitate learning is:
   a. Lectures
   b. Discussion group
   c. Practice by doing
   d. Teaching others.

4. Which of the following statements characterizes an adult learner?
   a. Relies on others to decide what is important to be learned
   b. Expects what they are learning to be immediately useful
   c. Accepts the information being presented at face value
   d. Has little or no experience upon which to draw.

5. Which of the following assists learning?
   a. Being sent on a course
   b. Motivation
   c. Noisy environment
   d. Being hungry or thirsty.

6. Feedback on learning should be given:
   a. As soon as possible after the learning event
   b. In front of others
   c. Only in written format
   d. Only when something has been done correctly.

Key words and phrases for literature searching

Learning
Learning outcomes
Learning styles
Learning theories
Patient education
Teaching

Useful websites

British Dyslexia Association	www.bdadyslexia.org.uk/ Available July 2006
Informed consent	www.dh.gov.uk/PolicyAndGuidance/HealthAndSocialCareTopics/Consent/ConsentGeneralInformation/fs/en Available July 2006
Learning styles	www.support4learning.org.uk/sites/support4learning/education/learning_styles.cfm Available July 2006
Sense UK (*charity that provides services to support individuals with sensory impairment*)	www.sense.org.uk Available July 2006

References

Atkins S, Murphy K 1993 Reflection: a review of the literature. Journal of Advanced Nursing 18(8):1188–1192

Ausubel DP, Novack JD, Hanesian H 1978 Educational psychology: a cognitive view. 2nd edn. Holt, Rinehart and Winston, New York

Bastable SB 2003 Nurse as educator. 2nd edn. Jones & Bartlett, Boston

Bloom BS 1964 Taxonomy of educational objectives. McKay, New York

Boud D, Keogh T, Walker D 1985 Reflection, turning experience into learning. Billing, Worcester

Brown G, Esdaile SA, Ryan SE 2003 Becoming an advanced healthcare practitioner. Butterworth Heinemann, Edinburgh

Burns S, Bulman C (eds) 2000 Students' perspectives on reflective practice. In: Reflective practice in nursing. 2nd edn. Blackwell Science, Oxford, Chapter 6

Cannon R 2000 Guide to support: the implementation of learning and teaching plan Year 2000. ACUE, The University of Adelaide. Online: www.adelaide.edu.au/clpd/materia/leap/leapinto/StudentCentredLearning.pdf Available September 2006

Coates VE 1999 Education for patients and clients. Routledge, London

College of Nurses Ontario 1996 The LEARN model of reflection. College of Nurses, Ontario

Cottrell S 2001 Teaching study skills and supporting learning. Palgrave, New York

Cowan J 2003 Assessment for learning: giving timely and effective feedback. Exchange 4:33
Department of Health 2001 Valuing people: a new strategy for learning disability for the 21st Century. Cm5086. TSO, London
Dewey J 1933 How we think. Heath & Co., Lexington, DC
Doyle C, Robson K 2002 Accessible curricula: good practice for all. University of Wales Institute, Cardiff. Online: http://www.ltsn.ac.uk/application.asp?app=resources.asp&process=full_record&section=generic&id=128 Available June 2006
Dwyer B 2001 Successful training strategies for the twenty-first century: using recent research on learning to provide effective training strategies. International Journal of Educational Management 15(6): 312–318
Foster J, Greenwood J 1998 Reflection: a challenging innovation for nurses. Contemporary Nurse 7(4):165–172
Gates B, Wilberforce D 2003 The nature of learning disabilities. In: Gates B (ed) Learning disabilities. 4th edn. Churchill Livingstone, London, Chapter 1
Gibbs G 1988 Learning by doing. Further Education Unit, Sheffield
Gopee N 2002 Demonstrating critical analysis in academic assignments. Nursing Standard 16(35):45–52
Gray MA, Smith LN 2000 The qualities of an effective mentor from the student nurses' perspective: findings from a longitudinal qualitative study. Journal of Advanced Nursing 32(6):1542–1549
Greenwood J 1993 The apparent desensitisation of student nurses during their professional socialisation: a cognitive perspective. Journal of Advanced Nursing 18(9):1471–1479
Honey P, Mumford A 1992 The manual of learning styles. 3rd edn. Peter Honey, Maidenhead
Hutchinson L 2003 Educational environment. British Journal of Medicine 326(7393): 810–812
Johns C 1999 Reflection as empowerment? Nursing Inquiry 6(4):241–249
Kaufman DM 2003 Applying educational theory in practice. British Medical Journal 326:213–215
Kirby JR, Knapper CK, Evans CJ et al 2003 Approaches to learning at work and workplace climate. International Journal of Training and Development 7(1):31–52
Knowles MS, Holton EF, Swanson RA 1998 The adult learner: the definitive classic in adult education and human resource development. Gulf Publishing, Houston, TX
Kolb D A 1984 Experiential learning: experience as the source of learning and development. Prentice Hall, Englewood Cliffs, NJ
LaVigna GW, Donnellan AM 1986 Alternatives to punishment: solving behavior problems with non-aversive strategies. Irvington, New York
Maslow A 1954 Motivation and personality. Harper and Row, New York
McGill I, Beaty L 1995 Action learning – a guide for professional, management and educational development. Kogan Page, London
McMullan M, Endacott R, Gray M et al 2003 Portfolios and the assessment of competence: a review of the literature. Journal of Advanced Nursing 41(3): 283–294
Mills DW 2002 Applying what we know: student learning styles. Online: http://www.csrnet.org/csrnet/articles/student-learning-styles.html Available July 2006
Nursing and Midwifery Council 2004 The NMC code of professional conduct: standards for conduct, performance and ethics. NMC, London
Oliver R, Endersby C 1994 Teaching and assessing nurses: a handbook for preceptors. Baillière Tindall, London
Race P 1993 How does learning happen best? Online: www.londonmet.ac.uk/deliberations/effective-learning/happen Available July 2006
Ramsden P 1988 Improving learning – new perspectives. Nichols Publishing, New York
Reece I, Walker S 1994 A practical guide to teaching, training and learning. 2nd edn. Business Education, Sunderland
Rideout E 2001 Transforming nursing education through problem-based learning. Jones and Bartlett, Boston
Rogers CR 1994 Freedom to learn. 3rd edn. Merrill, New York
Scholes J, Webb C, Gray M et al 2004 Making portfolios work in practice. Journal of Advanced Nursing 46(6):595–603
Schon D 1983 The reflective practitioner: how professionals think in action. Basic Books, New York
Spencer J 2003 Learning and teaching in the clinical environment. British Medical Journal 326:591–594
Stuart CC 2003 Assessment, supervision and support in clinical practice. Churchill Livingstone, Edinburgh
Tillema HH, Kessels JWM, Meijers F 2000 Competencies as building blocks for integrating assessment with instruction in vocational education: a case from the Netherlands. Assessment and Evaluation in Higher Education 25(3):265–278
Wilkie K, Burns I 2003 Problem-based learning: a handbook for nurses. Palgrave Macmillan, Houndmills
Wood EJ 2004 Problem-based learning: exploring knowledge of how people learn to promote effective learning. Bioscience Education E-journal Online: http://bio.ltsn.ac.uk/journal/vol3/beej-3-5.htm Available July 2006

Further reading

Braungart MM, Braungart RG 2003 Applying learning theories to healthcare practice. In: Bastable SB (ed) Nurse as educator. 2nd edn. Jones and Bartlett, Boston, Chapter 3
Coates VE 1999 Education for patients and clients. Routledge, London
Gould B, Masters H 2004 Learning to make sense: the use of critical incident analysis in facilitated reflective groups of mental health student nurses. Learning in Health and Social Care 3(2):53–63
Heidari F, Galvin K 2002 Action learning groups: can they help students develop their knowledge and skills? Nurse Education in Practice 3(1):49–55
Mayer KF 2002 The process of obtaining informed patient consent. Nursing Times 98(31):30–31
Somerville D 2004 A practical approach to promote reflective practice within nursing. Nursing Times 100(12):42–45

5

Evidence-based practice and research

Maria Grant, Michelle Howarth and Rosie Kneafsey

Glossary terms

Bibliographic database

Evidence-based practice

Free text term

Hierarchy of evidence

Indexing term

Literature review

Qualitative research

Quantitative research

Search strategy

Learning outcomes

This chapter will help you:

- Understand the concept of evidence-based practice
- Discuss how evidence is used in practice
- Use information technology (IT) skills to perform a basic search for evidence using bibliographic databases
- Evaluate research evidence
- Reflect on own practice and identify evidence gaps
- Use problem-solving skills to work with peers/colleagues to identify how evidence could be used in own area of practice.

Introduction

The term 'evidence-based practice' (EBP) has been used synonymously with 'evidence-based medicine' or 'evidence-based healthcare' or 'evidence-based care' in the National Health Service (NHS) since the early 1990s. While many practitioners may have heard about EBP, it has been defined in many ways and has left practitioners uncertain about its meaning (French 2002). Despite this ambiguity, EBP plays a pivotal role in the NHS Modernisation Agenda (DH 1997) through the National Institute for Health and Clinical Excellence (NICE) and National Service Frameworks (NSFs). But what does the practitioner think about EBP? Can all practitioners really claim that their practice is evidence based? On what evidence are clinical decisions based?

These questions will be explored in this chapter through the use of themed activity boxes and issues for reflection that will guide you through the maze of EBP, what it means and how it is used in healthcare practice.

This chapter covers the main components of EBP and encourages you to reflect on your own practice and clinical decision-making. EBP is an idea that is used in all branches of nursing. You will be encouraged to relate the chapter text to your own branch of nursing. You will be directed to locate and appraise evidence relating to a chosen topic area within your practice to develop your understanding of EBP.

What is evidence-based practice?

Evidence-based medicine originated in the fields of medicine and epidemiology. Initial ideas about evidence-based medicine were first thought of by Archie Cochrane in 1972. Cochrane believed that many healthcare interventions were ineffective and that practitioners were heavily influenced by custom and tradition rather than new information gained from research (Stevens et al 2001). It was recognized that this could mean that practices that were ineffective or outdated were still being used despite evidence being available about better ways to treat patients or provide healthcare. Later, in 1991, Sir Michael Peckham suggested that it remained a serious problem (DH 1991). As such, the NHS Modernisation Agenda set out a 10-year plan to standardize and improve the NHS (DH 1997). Central to this plan was an emphasis on evidence-based practice and 'clinically effective care' that is now accepted as the cornerstone of modern healthcare.

EBP is now promoted in many Department of Health documents and through the Clinical Governance agenda. The *Making a Difference* document (DH 1999a) emphasized the need for reliable and robust evidence to underpin nursing, midwifery and health visiting. A similar strategy is promoted within *Saving Lives: Our Healthier Nation* (DH 1999b), which clearly advocates the need to implement EBP to improve services that promote public health. The importance of EBP is also reflected in many professional regulatory standards. For example, the Nursing and Midwifery Council (NMC) *The NMC Code of professional conduct: standards for conduct, performance and ethics* Section 6.5, clearly states the need for nurses, midwives and specialist community public health nurses to maintain their professional knowledge and competence to deliver care which is 'based on current evidence, best practice and, where applicable, validated research when it is available' (NMC 2004, p. 10). Cox and Reyes-Hughes (2001) consider that EBP has a pivotal role in clinical effectiveness and argue that it is the main driver for clinically effective practitioners. If practitioners are unaware of the effectiveness of an intervention, how then can they claim to be clinically effective?

Defining EBP

Several definitions of EBP exist and, initially, the concept of EBP was applied to medicine in the early 1990s (Box 5.1). Practitioners may find that they prefer one definition as opposed to another, or may find that they do not really have a preference. In each case, the important issue is that practitioners develop an understanding of evidence-based care and are able to question their own practice and the types of evidence used to underpin this.

All of the definitions in Box 5.1 identify research evidence as the 'best' evidence. Others, however, have broadened this to include types of evidence other than research. For example, the Royal College of Nursing (1996) suggests that audit, client feedback and expertise can all provide evidence. While all of the definitions advocate the use of evidence to support decision-making, there is an assumption that evidence is easily used in everyday practice. However, this process is not always easy. To help practitioners underpin their practice with evidence, a series of steps have been developed. These steps reflect models of evidence-based practice to help practitioners ensure that their practice is evidence based and include:

- Questioning practice
- Refining the question into a workable search question
- Finding the evidence
- Appraising the evidence
- Implementing the evidence
- Evaluating or auditing practice.

These steps will be explored in greater depth throughout this chapter.

As EBP has evolved, a variety of descriptive terms have been generated to describe it, based on the context of its use. You may hear the terms 'evidence-based medicine' or 'evidence-based healthcare' or 'evidence-based practice' cited frequently and used interchangeably. While there is some debate about the relationships between these terms, they are all very similar in their meaning which is about improving the quality of practice, reducing risk to clients, aiding decision-making and helping the allocation of resources.

As all these terms may be confusing, this chapter refers to evidence-based care as a term that relates to evidence-based medicine, healthcare and practice.

In conjunction with or in the absence of research evidence, other types of evidence are used to promote effective practice. EBP promotes clinical effectiveness (Cox & Reyes-Hughes 2001) by ensuring that practitioners facilitate care that is safe, effective and based on 'best' available evidence.

Box 5.1 Definitions of evidence-based practice

Sackett et al (1996, p. 71) suggest that evidence-based medicine is 'the conscientious, explicit and judicious use of current best available evidence about the care of individual patients. The practice of evidence based medicine means integrating individual clinical experience with the best available external evidence from systematic research.'

Muir Gray (1997, p. xi) advocates a similar definition when he stated that evidence-based medicine is about 'making decisions about a group of patients and/or populations and basing such decisions on careful appraisal of the best evidence available'.

On a more practical level, White (1997, p. 175) advises that evidence-based practice is 'a method of problem-solving which involves identifying the clinical problem, searching the literature, evaluating the research evidence and deciding on the intervention'.

The EBP cycle

The process of EBP always starts with a question about practice, the answer to which will guide the practitioner and reveal whether their current practice is evidence based (Fig. 5.1). The practitioner may then audit their practice and re-visit the original practice question. This cycle of events ensures that up-to-date practices are carried out and good standards of clinical practice are maintained.

Questioning practice

The first step towards EBP is the ability of practitioners to question their own practice. To do this, practitioners will need to identify *why* they make decisions in a particular way and acknowledge what or who has informed the decision. Often, practitioners may not take the time to think about *why* and *how* they made a decision and, all too often, these are based on ritual and custom rather than a reliable evidence base. All practitioners need to consider what decisions they are making and what evidence is being used to support such decisions. In order to make effective clinical decisions in practice, practitioners

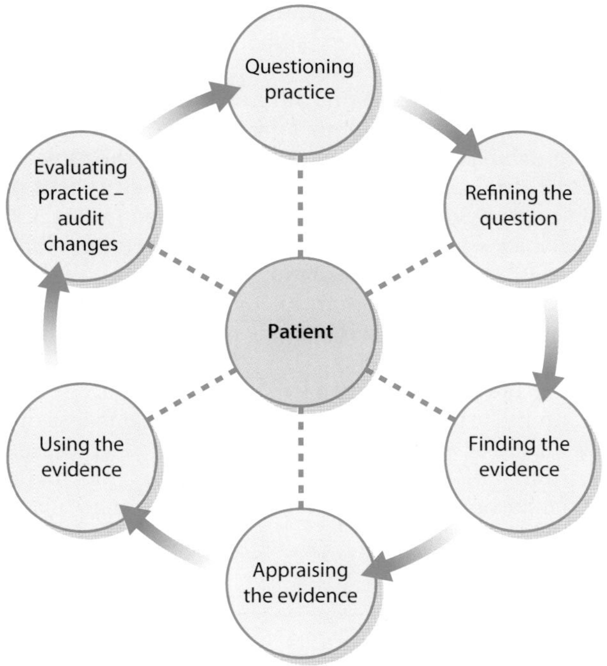

Fig. 5.1 The evidence-based practice cycle

need to be able to ask questions about the care or treatment they are providing (Box 5.2).

Now consider the material in Box 5.2. Here we can see that Staff Nurse Dyer now questions the type of dressings she applies. By questioning her practice, Staff Nurse Dyer is influencing the care she gives and clinical decisions she makes as a result. Questioning practice involves thinking about the appropriateness of the care being provided, e.g. Is it the right treatment? How do practitioners know that treatment works? How do different treatments compare? Is the treatment cost effective?

> **EVIDENCE-BASED PRACTICE** Box 5.2
>
> ### Effective decision-making and questioning practice
>
> **Effective decision-making**
>
> Sister Robbins asks Staff Nurse Dyer to redress a person's wound using Brand A as a dressing. Staff Nurse Dyer does not question the Sister as to her choice of dressings and follows Sister Robbins instructions and applies Brand A to the person's wound.
>
> Although Staff Nurse Dyer has provided care to the person by applying Brand A to their wound, they have not made a clinical decision. In this example, Sister Robbins made the decision and Staff Nurse Dyer followed the order.
>
> **Questioning practice**
>
> Later on that week, Staff Nurse Dyer observes Staff Nurse Flynn applying a different dressing to the same person's wound. Staff Nurse Dyer begins to wonder which dressing is best for the person and starts to question her own practice.
>
> This later example highlights how questions about practice are identified. Staff Nurse Dyer now questions the type of dressings she applies. By questioning her practice, Staff Nurse Dyer is influencing the care she gives and the clinical decisions she makes as a result.
>
> **Student activity**
>
> Think about a recent decision you have made in practice:
>
> - What was the decision?
> - How did you make the decision?
> - What/who influenced your decision? For example, was your decision based on any of the following types of evidence: research; guidelines; tradition; intuition; experience; advice from your mentor, colleagues, peers, qualified staff; ritual practice?

Refining the question into a workable search question

If decisions are based on tradition or ritual then there is a need to think about finding out if there is more reliable evidence to support decisions about practice. To accomplish this, it is useful to formulate a structured question to guide the search for evidence. Formulating workable questions is discussed in the searching for evidence section (pp. 127–128).

Finding the evidence

Once the question has been formulated, the next step is to find the evidence. This will involve using electronic databases such as MEDLINE and CINAHL. Finding evidence can be difficult and there is a need to practise in order to develop the skills needed to search effectively on databases.

Appraising the evidence

When the evidence has been located, practitioners then need to make sense of it. A range of guidelines has been designed to help practitioners make sense of the evidence and decide whether it is robust and believable. Guidelines for appraising evidence are explained later in the chapter.

Implementing the evidence

Following appraisal of the evidence, and once the practitioner is satisfied that the evidence is reliable and trustworthy, they then need to think about how to use this evidence in practice. Implementing evidence-based findings is no easy task, but with support from qualified staff and through reading this chapter, students should be able to make comprehensive plans to help them include the evidence in their practice.

Evaluating or auditing practice

Finally, once practitioners have introduced the evidence into practice, there is a need to reflect on and audit their work and whether it is safe and effective for the patient or client under their care. This may involve other colleagues and professionals who observed their actions.

Practitioners may find that they need to continually audit their practice to ensure that it is based on 'best' evidence. For example, practitioners may need to return to the original practice question and refine it, or they may discover that there is a gap in evidence. Whatever the situation, the important message is to be able to continually improve practice by questioning the decisions that practitioners make about a patient's or client's care needs.

Literature searching

A crucial way of finding out what is the best practice for a clinical situation is to discover what has been written about it in the literature. This means that practitioners need to be able to carry out a search of the literature and a review of the evidence (NHS Executive 1996).

There are numerous reasons for conducting a literature search. Searching and reviewing the literature identify whether previous studies or audits have been carried out in relation to the topic of interest or whether practice guidelines exist. This might be important if practitioners wish to make changes in practice, as it may be possible to read about how other practitioners improved their practice – both what they did and how they did it. It may also help to highlight potential problems or difficulties that might be encountered during the process of practice innovation (NHS Executive 1996). Determining what the literature identifies provides an opportunity for practitioners to incorporate new knowledge into their decision-making.

A dramatic rise in the amount of scientific literature published has resulted in the need to ensure that practitioners have the skills to find the literature they need (Palmer & Brice 1999). Typically practitioners lack the required skills and find it hard to search the literature efficiently. This has implications for practice as it means that it may not be based on current evidence despite it being available.

This section will provide an introduction to the basic principles and practice of searching for literature and evidence for practice. This will include exploring:

- Sources of literature
- Developing a search question
- Searching databases.

Sources of literature

There are many different sources of information available including books, the Internet, journals and professional organizations. Some will provide examples of original research while others – often referred to as evidence-based sources – will often provide an up-to-date review of the evidence available in a particular area. In both cases it is necessary to undertake an appraisal of the quality of the information presented (see p. 137).

The reason for choosing to use one source over another will depend on the type of information the practitioner wants to find. The following gives a brief overview of some of the key resources that can be used in a search for literature.

Bibliographic/electronic databases

Databases gather together and index large numbers of articles within specific subject areas, e.g. nursing, social sciences. There are many different databases available and they focus on different topic areas. Choosing a particular database(s) to search will depend on the topic area and the databases to which the University or school provides access. Some useful sources are listed in Box 5.3.

Databases may also distinguish between including examples of primary research projects and literature reviews (reviews of research). By searching a database systematically, practitioners can retrieve a list of references of relevant articles. Normally, the full text of the article is not provided and a trip to the library is needed to look up the article in a journal. Although databases often look different, they can usually be searched in the same way, and use similar formats to provide information, e.g. the author, title, journal source and often an abstract

Box 5.3 Useful databases

AMED – Allied and Alternative Medicine indexes physiotherapy, occupational therapy, rehabilitation, podiatry and complementary medicine articles from 1985 onwards.

BNI – British Nursing Index focusing primarily on British journals. Indexes nursing and midwifery articles from 1985 onwards.

CINAHL – Cumulative Index of Nursing and Allied Health Literature. A nursing and allied health disciplines database, including physiotherapy and health education. It indexes articles from 1983 onwards, and has a strong US focus.

Cochrane Library – A 'virtual library' or collection of databases that provide a starting point for accessing systematic reviews. These reviews are primarily concerned with the effectiveness of interventions and therefore concentrate on using randomized controlled trials (RCTs) as their foundation. The Cochrane Library includes:

- Cochrane Database of Systematic Reviews (CDSR)
- Database of Abstracts of Reviews of Effects (DARE), a collection of systematic reviews which include studies other than RCTs
- Cochrane Central Register for Controlled Trials (CENTRAL).
- NHS Economic Evaluation Database
- Health Technology Assessment reports

MEDLINE – A general biomedical database which covers international literature on medicine, allied health, biological and psychological sciences and humanities. It indexes articles from 1966 onwards. Research has suggested that for the majority of nursing queries, MEDLINE is likely to retrieve a higher number of relevant (and often unique) references (Okuma 1994, Brazier & Begley 1996, Brand-de Heer 2001).

(a clear and concise summary of the study design, results and implications for practice) of the article.

This information enables practitioners to find the full version of the article in the library. If the local library does not stock the required journal, it is usually possible to request the article using the interlibrary loan system. You will probably need to pay a small fee and the library will then request a photocopy of the article from another library.

Books

This group of resources includes textbooks and encyclopaedias. They are useful for obtaining background information and will generally provide a standard account of a specific subject area. They are good for obtaining a distinct piece of information, but can take a long time to get into print. This means that the information they contain is not always/necessarily up-to-date.

The Internet

The Internet provides a way of accessing information and resources in a variety of formats. These can include web pages that provide information, to web pages that provide access to resources such as bibliographic databases. The quality of websites is sometimes difficult to assess, so a good place to start is to use a gateway service. A gateway service is usually subject specific and provides access to quality-assessed websites. An example of a gateway service is the National Library for Health (NLH; www.library.nhs.uk) which provides access to a wide range of health-related services including an index of UK national clinical guidelines. Other examples are included in the list of Useful websites at the end of the chapter.

Journals and newsletters

Published at regular intervals, journals are a useful resource in obtaining the full text versions of primary research projects and articles on practice development, e.g. *Nursing Times*. More recently, journals have also begun to summarize or make evaluations of original pieces of research. Some adopt quite a formal or structured approach to providing information, e.g. *Evidence-Based Nursing* or *Effective Health Care* bulletins (www.york.ac.uk/inst/crd/ehcb.htm), whereas others are more informal, e.g. Bandolier (www.jr2.ox.ac.uk/bandolier).

Some journal sources are more reputable than others because they publish articles that have been peer reviewed. Peer review means that the articles have been sent for evaluation and comment by experts in the area before being accepted for publication, e.g. *Journal of Advanced Nursing*, *Journal of Learning Disabilities*. Journals are becoming increasingly available online either via a local library or information service, or via commercial ventures such as PubMed Central (www.pubmedcentral.nih.gov). PubMed Central represents one of a growing number of services which provide free and unrestricted access to a full text digital archive of life sciences journal literature, in this instance, provided by the US National Library for Medicine.

Reports

Like books, reports can be good for obtaining an overview of a subject area. They are often produced by government departments, e.g. Department of Health; professional organizations, e.g. Royal College of Nursing; universities and other statutory and voluntary organizations, e.g. Joseph Rowntree Foundation.

Developing a search question

Before beginning to search for literature, it is important to first think through what information is needed. An important step is developing a search question. A focused search question helps to ensure that the search for literature is structured and time is used efficiently. If the search question is vague, too many references are likely to be retrieved from a database search and the question will not be answered.

A useful framework to help in structuring a search question is the PICO acronym (Richardson et al 1995) (Box 5.4). The PICO acronym helps the practitioner to identify key elements of the search question, and each letter represents a different element:

- 'P' represents the **p**atient or **p**roblem under consideration
- 'I' represents the **i**ntervention or treatment under consideration

CRITICAL THINKING Box 5.4

Structuring a search question using PICO

Read the information about John and his questions about cranberry juice.

You are on placement with a practice nurse running a 'well man' clinic. John is 72 years of age and is waiting to go into hospital for prostate surgery. He has been suffering from recurrent urinary tract infections (UTIs) and has read that cranberry juice is really good at preventing UTIs. He asks about the effectiveness of cranberry juice. The nurse tells John that she is unsure but will make some enquiries and discuss the findings with him.

Student activity

Use the PICO acronym to plan the ideas you would use to search for information to answer John's question.

PICO acronym	Search idea identified using PICO
P: Patient or population	
I: Intervention	
C: Comparison	
O: Outcome	

You will probably have identified search ideas similar to the following:

- Patient/population = urinary tract infections
- Intervention = cranberry juice
- Comparison = water
- Outcome = reduced levels of infection.

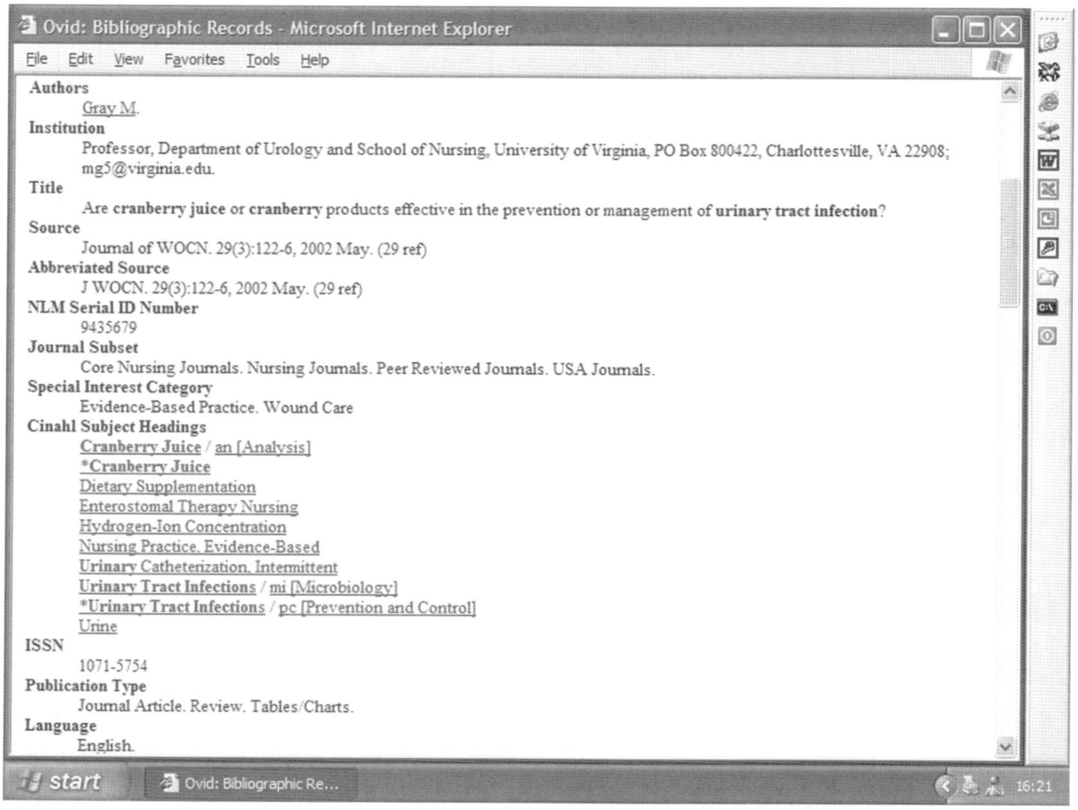

Fig. 5.2 A typical database record (reproduced by kind permission of OVID Technologies)

- 'C' represents the **c**omparison intervention or treatment under consideration
- 'O' represents the clinical **o**utcome(s) of interest.

Once the key elements of the search question have been identified, the next step is to organize these elements in order of importance. When starting a literature search, it is probable that only two search areas will be needed. However, by having a clear idea of the whole topic area before starting to search, it will be easier to add a third or even a fourth element to the search strategy, and narrow down the type of information being retrieved, without getting sidetracked.

Once there is a clear idea what the search question is, it is then necessary to decide on the most appropriate place to look for the information. Depending on the type of information needed, this might include some or all of the following:

- Reading books
- Contacting subject specialists
- Visiting recommended websites via gateway services (pp. 144 and 145)
- Searching electronic/bibliographic databases if examples of up-to-date research studies are needed.

Searching databases

Searching a database can seem daunting but there are a number of steps that, if followed, will make this process easier and more successful. It is sensible to ask the librarian for help in getting started.

The way databases present information can often look quite different, but there are some basic ways of searching which are common to all. The examples used here are from the CINAHL database via the OVID search interface, but a typical database record will include the name of the author, the title of the article, the source of the article, i.e. which journal is it published in, and a list of indexing terms or subject headings (Fig. 5.2).

The reason for the search will determine how comprehensive or complete the coverage of the database search will be. Practitioners who are changing practice once qualified or undertaking a thorough review of the literature for a dissertation will need to find as much information on a topic as possible. However, when searching for a couple of references to support an argument in an assignment, it probably will not matter if you miss a few papers. In both instances, the best place to start is by searching using the databases list of indexing terms.

Indexing terms

Indexing terms are also called MESH headings, subject headings, thesaurus terms or descriptors, but they all mean basically the same thing. These indexing terms are split into subject areas and are organized within a hierarchy (Fig. 5.3).

The most precise indexing terms – which are assigned by the database producer – are given to describe the content of each article. Using John's request for information on the effectiveness of cranberry juice in preventing urinary tract infections as an example, every article

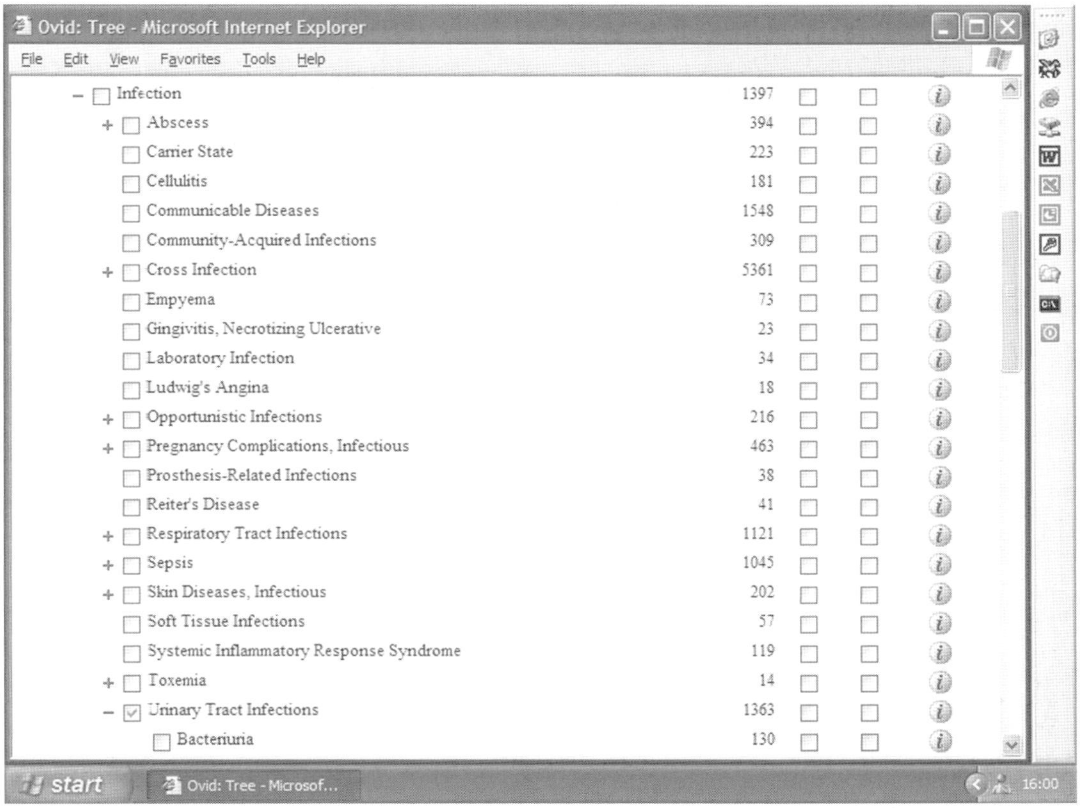

Fig. 5.3 Indexing terms are organized in a hierarchy (reproduced by kind permission of OVID Technologies)

that mentions urinary tract infections would be given the indexing term 'Urinary Tract Infection'. It does not matter which specific words have been used to describe the idea/topic because if they were discussing infections of the urinary tract, they will be indexed using 'Urinary Tract Infection'. However, if the search is for bacteriuria (bacteria in the urine), then the specific indexing term 'bacteriuria' is used because the broader indexing term of 'Urinary Tract Infection' would not retrieve articles discussing this specific area of interest within the category of urinary tract infections.

It is useful to find out which indexing term is likely to be assigned to the idea/topic being searched for because this can make it easier to search for relevant articles.

While using indexing terms can produce a more accurate search, it may initially take some time to identify the most appropriate indexing terms to use. Most databases will have an option that allows the user to ask for the most likely indexing term in the subject area to be suggested. This feature is sometimes called mapping, when the database makes a 'best guess' at suggesting which term(s) will be helpful. If available, it is a good idea to check the description of the indexing term to make sure it means what you think it does (Box 5.5, p. 130).

Although a database will often provide an opportunity to search for more than one term at a time, it is usually a good idea to search for each term separately. In this way, if an indexing term is not working as expected, e.g. it is retrieving irrelevant information, it is much quicker to exclude it from the search than having to retype the terms that are to be kept.

It is important to bear in mind that each database will have a slightly different set of indexing terms, so it is necessary to check the list of terms each time a search is started on a new database.

Free text terms

If it is necessary to undertake a more thorough literature search, e.g. for a final year project, this will probably need to use a combination of indexing terms searching with free text searching.

Free text searching is the development of a list of words, or free text search terms, that describe each component of the search question in more detail. For example, this might be a list that includes alternative spellings (including Americanisms), plurals, synonyms and abbreviations (Box 5.6, p. 130).

Free text searching will help ensure the retrieval of the maximum possible literature on a topic area, and will compensate for any mistakes by the database producers in missing or misapplied indexing terms. It is important to remember that as well as increasing the number of potentially relevant articles retrieved, there is also the possibility that it will increase the number of potentially irrelevant references too. In both instances there is a need to allow extra time to read through the retrieved abstracts.

Combining your search terms

Once the indexing terms for the subject area (and any free text terms for an extended search) have been identified,

CRITICAL THINKING — Box 5.5

Identifying indexing terms on a database

Access a database of your choice and identify the indexing terms for the four main elements of the PICO acronym (you might want to have another look at Box 5.4, p. 127).

PICO acronym	Search idea identified using PICO	Indexing term identified on database
P: Patient or population	Urinary tract infection	
I: Intervention	Cranberry juice	
C: Comparison	Water	
O: Outcome	Reduced levels of infection	

If you searched on the CINAHL database, you will probably have identified the following indexing terms:

- Patient/population = Urinary Tract Infections/
- Intervention = Cranberry Juice/
- Outcome = Systematic Review/.

There does not appear to be a suitable indexing term for water, so you may wish to consider using free text searching (see p. 129)

CRITICAL THINKING — Box 5.6

Developing a list of free text search terms

Add as many synonyms, alternative spellings, Americanisms, plurals or abbreviations to each of the elements of the PICO acronym below (you might want to have another look at Boxes 5.4 and 5.5).

PICO acronym	Search idea identified using PICO	Indexing term identified on database	Free text terms
P: Patient or population	Urinary tract infection	Urinary Tract Infections/	
I: Intervention	Cranberry juice	Cranberry Juice/	
C: Comparison	Water	–	
O: Outcome	Reduced levels of infection	Systematic review/	

You will probably have identified a range of free text search terms similar to the following:

- Patient/population = urinary tract infection, urinary tract infections, UTI, UTIs
- Intervention = cranberries, cranberry, cranberry juices
- Comparison = drinking water, H_2O, water
- Outcome = randomized controlled trial, randomized controlled trials, RCT, RCTs, systematic review, systematic reviews.

Note: When free text searching, the database will search for a precise match of the term typed in, so be sure that the spelling is correct.

it is necessary to link the words together using the 'AND' and 'OR' functions of the database. These are known as the 'Boolean Operators'.

When searching within a topic/indexing term it is necessary to use the 'OR' Boolean operator. 'OR' enables the user to search for a range of alternative ways of describing an idea/topic, so that any one of a number of indexing or free text terms may appear. Using the urinary tract infection as an example, the 'OR' Boolean operator will enable a search for any combination of indexing or free text search terms, e.g. 'Urinary Tract Infections/' or 'UTI' (Fig. 5.4A). An easy way to remember how to use the 'OR' Boolean operator is the mnemonic 'OR is more' (Palmer & Brice 1999).

Users may worry if, at this stage, they seem to be retrieving too much information. However, when all indexing terms are combined together using the 'AND' Boolean operator, the numbers will quickly decrease.

Once the indexing terms have been combined for each idea/topic, users then need to search for articles where both ideas appear, e.g. where cranberry juice is mentioned in the same article as urinary tract infection. In order to do this, the 'AND' Boolean operator is used (Fig. 5.4B).

A third Boolean operator – the 'NOT' Boolean operator – enables users to exclude papers that mention a particular topic/word (Fig. 5.4C). While this may initially appear to be a good thing, there is a distinct possibility that users could inadvertently exclude potentially relevant papers.

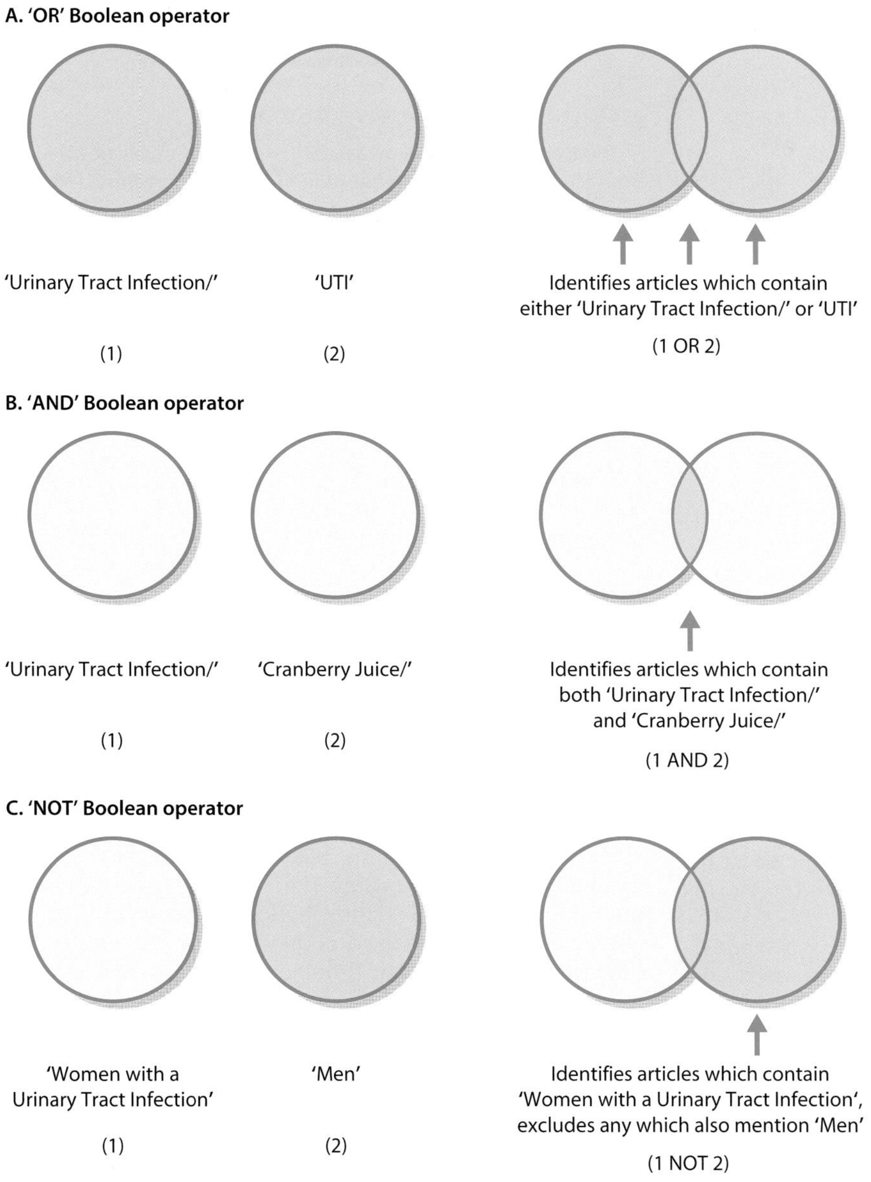
A. 'OR' Boolean operator
'Urinary Tract Infection/'
(1)
'UTI'
(2)
Identifies articles which contain either 'Urinary Tract Infection/' or 'UTI'
(1 OR 2)
B. 'AND' Boolean operator
'Urinary Tract Infection/'
(1)
'Cranberry Juice/'
(2)
Identifies articles which contain both 'Urinary Tract Infection/' and 'Cranberry Juice/'
(1 AND 2)
C. 'NOT' Boolean operator
'Women with a Urinary Tract Infection'
(1)
'Men'
(2)
Identifies articles which contain 'Women with a Urinary Tract Infection', excludes any which also mention 'Men'
(1 NOT 2)

Fig. 5.4 Boolean operators: **A**. 'OR' Boolean operator. **B**. 'AND' Boolean operator. **C**. 'NOT' Boolean operator

You are advised to use the 'NOT' Boolean operator with extreme caution . . . if at all.

A more effective way of reducing the number of papers retrieved is to add a further element to the search strategy (remember the four elements using PICO, but only starting by searching on the two most important ones) or by adding limits such as date range, publication type, e.g. review/systematic review, or language, e.g. English.

The aim of searching is to start off with a selection of references, sometimes called a 'sensitive' search, and then narrow the search down until the number of references is reduced to those that will be useful, sometimes called a 'precise' or 'specific' search.

Once the search is completed, it is important to make a note of the search strategy. It is good practice to include this in any assignment or report. If it is necessary to return to the search at a later date, it will also mean that there is no need to try to remember which search terms were used.

Sources of knowledge to support evidence-based practice

During the process of providing care, nurses and others must make a wide range of decisions. These decisions have important effects on the person's and family's experience of care, and the outcomes of healthcare interventions. Nurses may also be involved in assisting people to make decisions about their own care, such as whether to consent to a particular treatment or not. For nurses to be able to make safe and effective clinical decisions, they must draw on a range of different sources of knowledge. These sources provide a guide for practice and may include:

- The nurse's own experience
- Guidance from an experienced or trusted colleague
- A recent research article
- A practice protocol.

These different sources of knowledge can be defined as types of 'evidence' underpinning practice.

What is meant by 'evidence'?

Everyone uses evidence from a variety of sources, both in their daily personal lives and in professional practice. However, what constitutes 'evidence' has been debated for many years and is rooted in philosophy. Subsequently, as individuals, people will probably perceive evidence as meaning many different things.

Different types of evidence include the information gained from tradition and ritual, experience, intuition, authorities and experts, patients and families, research, audit and guidelines.

Tradition and ritual

Large parts of daily life are based on trusted traditions and rituals learnt from others during childhood. Traditions and rituals allow people to undertake activities with little thought or consideration as to the reasons why – they provide structure to everyday life (Walsh & Ford 1989). The process of learning traditions and rituals by observing the actions and activities of peers continues from childhood into adulthood and into the world of employment.

As such, learning traditions and rituals is a central means of transmitting knowledge and is important in nursing as students learn to 'become' nurses (Parahoo 1997). This is known as the process of occupational socialization, e.g. learning the 'ward routine' (Melia 1984). Students or practitioners learn from effective colleagues who practise safely and on the basis of best evidence. This can be a very useful means of sharing knowledge and good practice. However, relying on traditional knowledge may also lead to the transmission of outdated information and practice, putting both nurses and clients at risk. The moving and handling of patients provides a pertinent example. While many manual handling techniques are considered unsafe, such as the drag lift, outdated and dangerous practices remain widely used (National Back Pain Association 1998) (Box 5.7).

REFLECTIVE PRACTICE Box 5.7

Questioning your own practice

Think about and reflect on a recent example of ritualistic care, which has caused you to question the nursing care provided.

Student activities

- Try to identify the aspect of nursing care that was different from that given elsewhere or contradicted what you have learnt during your course.
- Write a brief account of the issue and identify what may have led to a ritualistic approach to care.

Experience

Practitioners use their own or the experiences of others to inform decisions they make about nursing practice. After experiencing an event, the memory of this is stored and is ready to draw upon in similar circumstance in the future. Practitioners may also discuss experiences with colleagues, thus passing their experiential knowledge on to others. However, while experience brings confidence and the ability to use professional judgement (Rolfe 2002), there is also a risk that experiential knowledge is based on a limited range of events or practice situations to which practitioners have been exposed. As such, practitioners may be unaware of new or different practices or treatments, or recommendations from research (Parahoo 1997).

Intuition

Intuition is defined as a way of knowing and behaving that is not based on rational or conscious reasoning (Parahoo 1997). While many nurses explain the importance of intuition in their nursing care, it is difficult to define exactly what it is. In addition, it is also easy to dismiss another person's intuition. For example, Polgar and Thomas (1995) describe the activities of the 19th century physician, Ignaz Semmelweis, who noted the high levels of maternal deaths at his hospital and suspected that medical students attending the mortuary were spreading infection via their hands. Unfortunately, while handwashing is now recognized as the cornerstone of effective infection control, at that time Semmelweis and his intuition were ignored and dismissed.

Authorities and experts

Often, practices in healthcare and nursing are determined by the knowledge and opinions of those members of the healthcare team in positions of authority. Knowledge is considered true because the person who states it has authority or is considered an expert. While experts may well possess high levels of knowledge in relation to best practice, at times conflicts may arise when one expert or person in authority holds differing views or opinions from another. It is also possible for experts to hold misplaced views or be biased in some way, as demonstrated in the example of the now discredited 'expert evidence' given in criminal proceedings linked with sudden infant death syndrome.

Service users and their families

During the process of providing individualized care, it is important to ascertain the views of people and their families. In this way, it is possible to work in partnership with them to tailor care and treatment to individual needs. This is an important aspect of evidence-based healthcare because it recognizes that people can be, and often are, the experts in their own care. As such, they should be able to make choices and decisions about what happens to them. Although this is a very important source

EVIDENCE-BASED PRACTICE Box 5.8

User involvement and empowerment

Visit either the Patient Advice Liaison Services (PALS) website at www.dh.gov.uk or the Strategies for Living website at www.mentalhealth.org.uk. Read the overview.

Student activities

- What are the key aims and objectives of PALS or the Strategies for Living?
- How do you think this initiative promotes user involvement and empowerment?
- Find out about the involvement and empowerment of children (visit www.actionforsickchildren.org and www.nelh.nhs.uk/childhealth).

EVIDENCE-BASED PRACTICE Box 5.9

Benchmarking

Locate information about the *Essence of Care: Patient Focused Benchmarking for Health Care Practitioners* via the Department of Health website (www.dh.gov.uk).

Student activities

- What are the key objectives of *Essence of Care*?
- How many benchmarks are included?
- Are there any benchmarking groups/activity in your organization?

of knowledge upon which to base nursing care, people often feel that they are not involved enough in their own care and are not asked about what services they think should be offered by the NHS. The Department of Health now recognize that service users should have more say in the care that they receive and the types of health service research carried out. In order to ensure that patients' views are listened to, NHS Trusts have expert patient groups and Patient Advice Liaison Services (PALS). Increasingly, in the field of mental health and learning disabilities, service users are taking the lead in defining what they see as the areas that should be researched and designing and conducting their own research. An example of this is the Strategies for Living Project, by the Mental Health Foundation, which intends to support service user-led research throughout the UK (Box 5.8).

Research studies

While other sources of knowledge constitute important aspects of the evidence base, knowledge derived from research is crucial to evidence-based practice. This is because, unlike other forms of knowing, research is a systematic approach to generating knowledge using well-established methods (Parahoo 1997, Hamer & Collinson 1999). While there are many different types and ways of carrying out research, the main aim of nursing research is to improve the quality of care and to enable effective clinical decision-making (Parahoo 1997). For example, research can tell practitioners what treatments work best or why they may not be so effective. Research can also help practitioners to find out about how people feel and experience things. For example, research can tell practitioners which drugs are effective in treating high blood pressure and also how people may feel about having a chronic condition or a learning disability.

Audit

Many aspects of nursing care are influenced by the results of audit, which students may come across during their clinical placements, e.g. audits of the use of pressure-relieving mattresses, the incidence of pressure ulcers or the occurrence of aggressive or violent behaviour. The *Essence of Care* document (DH 2001a) is an important nursing audit tool currently being used in many NHS Trusts (Box 5.9)

Essentially, clinical audit involves measuring an aspect of practice (such as how often nutritional assessments are carried out, see Ch. 19) and comparing it to agreed standards for best practice. Clinical audit can provide knowledge about nursing care and highlight where improvements are needed. Audit is an important link within the evidence-based practice cycle as, without it, it is not possible to state whether the right practice is actually occurring (Garland & Corfield 1999).

Guidelines

Practitioners may also use guidelines as a source of knowledge from which to base care that they provide. Guidelines are written after the best available evidence, from research and/or clinical expertise (where research evidence is lacking), and client views have been gathered and scrutinized. This evidence is then used to set a standard for best practice in relation to a particular treatment or aspect of care. By setting out recommended standards of practice, guidelines can thus help practitioners to provide the most effective care possible (Thomas & Hotchkiss 2002). For example, a guideline for the assessment and prevention of pressure ulcers has been produced by NICE. In Scotland the Scottish Intercollegiate Guidelines Network (SIGN) and NHS Quality Improvement Scotland (NHSQIS) produce guidelines (Box 5.10, p. 134). Guidelines can also be used as the standard against which to assess the quality of care during the audit process (Joyce 1999) and may be a way of eliminating variations in clinical practice that exist in different parts of the country.

Knowledge is thus derived from many different sources and, used in combination, can ensure that the care and treatment provided is as effective as possible (Box 5.11, p. 134).

Best evidence

As already stated, evidence-based care is an essential component of clinical effectiveness. To help make decisions about the most suitable treatments, interventions or services to provide, the best available evidence must

EVIDENCE-BASED PRACTICE Box 5.10

Guidelines

Locate a practice guideline associated with the management of obesity in children, or pressure ulcer management, which you have come across during your clinical placements.

Student activity

Either

- Visit the SIGN website (www.sign.ac.uk) and locate the guideline about the management of obesity in children and young people. Compare and contrast the guidelines for any similarities or differences.

Or

- Visit the NICE website (www.nice.org.uk) and locate the latest guideline about pressure ulcer assessment and prevention. Compare and contrast the guidelines for any similarities or differences.

CRITICAL THINKING Box 5.11

Types of evidence

Read the information about Mrs Kaur and Staff Nurse Smith's decision about Mrs Kaur's care.

Mrs Kaur is a 73-year-old lady who has an infected venous leg ulcer and is due to have her dressings changed today by Staff Nurse Smith. After removing the dressing, Staff Nurse Smith observes that the ulcer appears to have worsened. She asks Mrs Kaur what she thinks about the ulcer who agrees that it does look worse. Mrs Kaur also states that she has been in more pain recently. Staff Nurse Smith is concerned that the ulcer has become worse and begins to plan a course of action. After some thought, Staff Nurse Smith remembers that she has used another type of dressing on a venous ulcer in very similar circumstances. She decides to discuss this with her colleague and, with Mrs Kaur's consent, invites her colleague to review the ulcer. Staff Nurse Smith and her colleague look at the tissue viability guidelines and hospital protocol for the management of venous leg ulcers. After some discussion, Staff Nurse Smith made a decision to contact the tissue viability nurse for an opinion.

Student activity

Identify the different types of evidence used by Staff Nurse Smith.

You probably included the following types of evidence:

- Mrs Kaur's opinion
- Colleague's opinion
- Expert opinion (tissue viability nurse)
- Her own experience
- Guidelines
- Hospital protocols.

Through your reflection, you may have thought of other types of 'evidence'. For example, you may have attended a lecture, spoken with your personal tutor or attended a conference. What is important is that you develop the skills needed to differentiate between good or 'best' evidence and bad evidence.

be sought out. These sources of evidence must demonstrate the effectiveness of the intervention (Box 5.12). The notion of 'best' evidence is controversial and tensions exist between different beliefs about what constitutes 'best' evidence. Some argue that experimental research that demonstrates the effectiveness of an intervention is the best evidence; however, others disagree, viewing other types of evidence as more informative for certain clinical situations (Cox & Reyes-Hughes 2001).

A number of hierarchies now exist, enabling different types of research and evidence to be graded or ranked according to their ability to predict effectiveness, remove bias and control confounders and provide more confidence in the reliability of the findings (see pp. 140–141 for further information). One such hierarchy is described by Thompson and Cullum (1999) where the highest level of evidence is a systematic review of several high-quality randomized controlled trials (RCTs), through various grades to expert opinion, which is the lowest level in the hierarchy.

Experimental research such as RCTs is seen by many as the 'highest standard' of evidence because the findings are thought to be more valid and reliable than that of non-experimental descriptive research and other evidence.

In general, research is viewed by many as the most important source of knowledge for practice. It is a large topic area and the next section provides an introduction to some of the key aspects.

Overview of the research process

In order to carry out research correctly, certain rules and logical steps need to be followed. This is known as the 'research process' that is often viewed as cyclical in nature, rather than linear (Fig. 5.5).

When research projects are reported in academic journals and reports, they will often describe the research process followed. For the reader, this is important as it makes it clear how the research was carried out. It should also provide enough detail for readers to decide whether the project followed the proper rules or research process.

There are many different forms of research evidence and although there are exceptions, research can be defined broadly as quantitative or qualitative in nature.

Quantitative research

Quantitative research is described as the logical collection of numerical data under controlled conditions that uses statistics to analyse the data. This type of research is based on the belief that the world, events and phenomena are governed by laws that can be uncovered by measuring and counting and searching for correlations between different phenomena (Parahoo 1997). For example, this type of research might try to find out about

EVIDENCE-BASED PRACTICE Box 5.12

Use of evidence

Student activities

- Visit the Department of Health website (www.dh.gov.uk) and locate a National Service Framework that is relevant to your area of practice. How is evidence described and presented?
- Locate another NICE guideline through the NICE website (www.nice.org.uk) and try to identify the hierarchy of evidence used to develop the guideline. Write down how the evidence has been graded and how this is presented in the guideline.
- You may have noticed similarities in the way that evidence is presented in these and other guidelines that use similar hierarchies to underpin their guideline development.

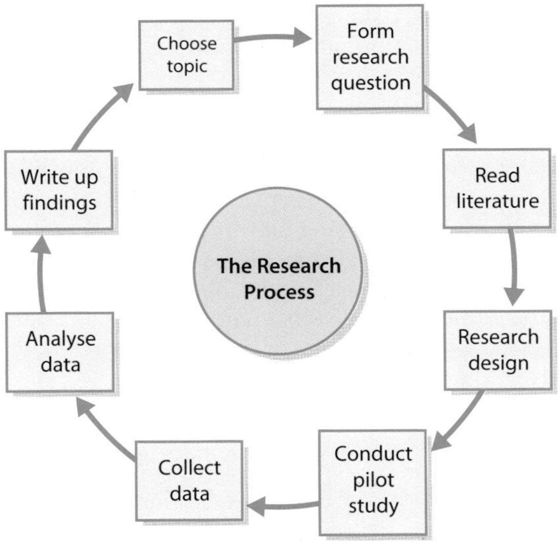

Fig. 5.5 The research process

'cause and effect' – i.e. does A + B = C? It often (but not always) involves the testing of hypotheses through objective measurements and observations to see whether the hypothesis is supported or rejected.

Qualitative research

Qualitative research can be defined as the logical collection of subjective data that often include narrative or observational materials without additional researcher control. This type of research assumes that the complexity of everyday life cannot be reduced to numbers as much meaning could be lost. It is also accepted that there is never simply one reality – that there will always be different experiences and perspectives. There is no attempt to control the environment in which data are being collected, as the aim is to understand events, as they unfold, from the perspective of those people experiencing them (Craig & Smyth 2002).

Quantitative and qualitative research in nursing

Both approaches to research are needed within nursing, as many research questions require the measurement of objective facts to inform the development of clinical practice. However, much nursing work cannot be broken down into measurable parts without the meaning of that phenomenon being lost. The focus of qualitative research is on the individuality of human experience that fits closely with the purpose of nursing.

Often, a particular research topic or research question will require a combination of quantitative and qualitative research. This allows for a more complete understanding of the particular phenomenon to be gained. For example, back injuries in nurses and moving and handling practices have been explored using both quantitative surveys and qualitative interview and observational studies. Box 5.13 (see p. 136) shows the contrasting approaches and types of information gained by two studies. In other cases, a combination (or 'mixed method') approach might also be used within one project. For example, a study exploring the role of the nurse in the rehabilitation setting used a combination of semi-structured interviews with nurses and clients and other members of the multidisciplinary team. This study also observed nursing practice and used client records and a questionnaire survey to ascertain data about the role of the nurse in rehabilitation (Long et al 2002).

Different types of research design

In order to begin collecting data to answer a research question, a plan or research design must be decided upon. The research design sets out whether the research approach will be quantitative or qualitative, how data will be collected (data collection tools), where/who data will be collected from (the sampling strategy or sample) and how data will be analysed (Parahoo 1997). Different research questions require that different research designs be used. For example, if the researcher were trying to find out about the effectiveness of a treatment (e.g. does drug A work better than drug B?), it would be most appropriate to use an experimental design such as a randomized controlled trial. Alternatively, if the researcher were seeking to understand people's thoughts and feelings, a qualitative approach would be used. It is important that the researcher chooses the best research design to answer the research question. There are many different research designs but some examples include:

- Systematic review
- Randomized controlled trial
- Survey
- Qualitative (ethnography, grounded theory and phenomenology).

For a fuller explanation of the many different research designs, data collection tools and sampling strategies, it is important to consult a more in-depth research text (see Further reading).

> **Box 5.13 Research relating to nursing, back pain and moving and handling**
>
> It was long recognized anecdotally that many nurses suffered from back injuries. However, the full extent of the problem was unclear as it had not been systematically investigated. As such, it was important to try to quantify and measure the size of the problem. To do this, a number of surveys were undertaken by different researchers. A particularly important one was a questionnaire survey of 4000 nurses. The results of this survey were influential as it was found that one in four nurses took time off with back injury and one in three currently had a back injury. The data were used further to try to estimate the size of the problem in relation to the qualified nursing population as a whole. Alarmingly, it was suggested that 27 000 nurses could potentially be suffering from back injury and 72 000 may have had time off as a result (Seacombe & Ball 1992).
>
> The high rates of back injury in nurses have been largely blamed on the practice of manually handling patients. Numerous researchers have examined nurses' moving and handling practices, looking at how nurses handle people and why they approach this activity in the way that they do, especially in light of the 1992 European Union regulations on the manual handling of loads (Health and Safety Executive 1992). Many of these studies have used qualitative approaches, choosing to collect data through interviews with participants. Kane and Parahoo (1994) looked at how student nurses learned about moving and handling. They interviewed 16 nurses, asking – among other questions – whether they would move a client with a staff nurse if she opted to use an unsafe lift; eight students would have conformed to the staff nurse's decision. This type of research can thus shed light on people's experiences, behaviours and attitudes.

Sampling strategy

When a study is conducted, it is not usually possible to collect information from every single person so desired because the total target population is too large. For example, in a study on the factors causing heart disease, it would not be possible (due to costs and time constraints) to contact every single person in the UK with heart disease to complete a lifestyle survey. It is therefore necessary to target a smaller number of people from within this total population. This is known as the sample (defined as a subset of the target population).

- In quantitative research, the goal of sampling is to gain access to a representative sample of the target population. This makes it possible to then make generalizations from the sample population to the population as a whole.
- In qualitative research, the goals of sampling are different. The purpose is to recruit people who are most likely to be able to contribute to an understanding of the phenomenon being studied. Although the emphasis on qualitative research is not on generalizability, if the respondents within the sample are known to be 'typical' or 'atypical', then the findings from the sample may be used to throw light on other similar phenomena.

Like the large number of research designs that may be selected, there are also different ways of sampling that will depend on the nature of the research design. Readers may come across a range of sampling approaches (Parahoo 1997) but further reading will be required to explore these aspects further.

Types of data collection

In the same way that there are a range of research designs and approaches to sampling, there are also a variety of ways of collecting data. These include techniques such as observation, questionnaires, documentary analysis and interviews.

Observation

Observation focuses on the researcher 'seeing' and perhaps experiencing what happens in a particular context by watching, documenting and then analysing events of interest. The researcher may either take part in the activities being observed (participant observation) or may 'sit at the sidelines' at a distance (non-participant observation). Box 5.14 includes material from observation during a study of the nurse's role.

Questionnaires

Questionnaires are a common way of collecting data and consist of a preset list of written questions to be answered, either in writing or verbally, by the respondent. For examples of different types of question used in questionnaires, see Blaxter et al (1998) in Further reading.

Documents

Documents may also be a useful source of data. Examples of documents include patient care records, policy documents, historical documents archived in a library, census statistics and reports, company annual reports and institutional documents.

Interviews

Interviews involve talking with and listening to people, asking questions and discussing issues with them. Interviews may be structured or unstructured and can be undertaken face to face or over the telephone. They may occur on a one-to-one basis or may be conducted as a focus group with up to eight people.

Ethical issues and research

All research projects raise ethical issues whether they involve direct contact with people or the use of

Box 5.14 **The nurse's role – observations of a staff nurse working on a rheumatology rehabilitation ward**

Listening
About the effect of illness on the client's life
Empathizing – *'No one has spoken to me like this before'*

Explaining and preparing
What to expect – *'You will be fully assessed by all members of the MDT* (multidisciplinary team), *the physio, the OT* (occupational therapist), *the podiatrist, the doctors'*
'You can ask anything you like . . .'

Educating
'Continue with exercise, but don't overdo activity on your legs'
Side-effects of drugs; benefits of medication (e.g. on sleep pattern); suggesting more regular use of pain killers
'I've never really discussed any pain relief with anyone. No one takes it seriously, they just back off and make you feel like you are whinging'
Staff nurse queries if they have ever been in touch with a self-help group . . . explained the value (information about new treatments new ideas, education, mutual support), help in applying the TENS machine

Offering choice
'Do you want a shower or a wash in your room?'

Asking
About possible link-up with practice nurse (to assist in pain control)

Reassuring
'Doctor will be around this morning' – after a painful night

Referring
To physio; to welfare rights officer to help with re-employment and OT; passing on information (to doctor, pharmacist).

[From Long et al (2001). Examples reproduced with kind permission from the Nursing and Midwifery Council.]

documentary evidence. To ensure that ethical issues are fully addressed, the plans for all research projects in health and social care must be submitted to Research Ethics and Governance Committees for review prior to the project being carried out. In addition, nurses conducting their own research, assisting other researchers or caring for people involved in research studies, need to do all that they can to ensure that the research they are involved with is of the highest standards.

ETHICAL ISSUES Box 5.15

Informed consent in research

Imagine you are a research nurse responsible for recruiting people into a study.

Student activities

- What information would people need in order to give informed consent to their inclusion in the research study?
- How would you ensure that people understood what they were agreeing to do?
- How would you take account of a research participant who is unable to consent due to age, mental distress, learning disability, dementia or who is unconscious?

A number of key ethical principles must be considered in relation to research. The first is the principle of 'respect for persons' (see Ch. 7). This means that researchers must protect individuals from harm and protect their autonomy. Research participants must be able to make informed choices and decisions about what happens to them, such as whether or not to take part in research. Thus, researchers must ensure that informed consent is gained prior to including anyone in a study (Box 5.15) (see Chs 6, 7).

In some situations, individuals may be unable to make an informed decision to take part in a study due to illness, age or conscious level. Special measures must be taken in this situation. Confidentiality must also be ensured in order to protect the dignity of people taking part in research. This means that, for example, personal information, or views expressed by respondents, or photographic images must be stored safely to comply with the 1998 Data Protection Act (DH 1998). Effective ways of protecting and disguising the identity of participants must also be devised, as respondents should be assured of anonymity (Royal College of Nursing Research Society 2003).

Appraisal of the evidence

The ability to identify good quality evidence requires the development of critical appraisal skills. Practitioners need these skills in order to differentiate weaker evidence from stronger (Box 5.16, p. 138). This involves developing a critical awareness that will enable practitioners to read, digest and understand the evidence.

This section provides an introduction to the process of critical appraisal and an example of an appraised article. Once practitioners become familiar with the appraisal process they find that their skills will advance and develop over time.

Critical awareness

While many practitioners are able to read the findings from a research paper, most may have problems evaluating the relevance of the findings for their own

EVIDENCE-BASED PRACTICE Box 5.16

Evidence on the effectiveness of cranberry juice

Refer to Boxes 5.4–5.6 (pp. 127 and 130) based on 'John' and the use of cranberry juice. You need to think about this scenario and the idea of clinical effectiveness and the EBP cycle (see Fig. 5.1).

Student activities

- Read the evidence you previously located on cranberry juice.
- Identify two 'types' of evidence, e.g. an RCT, a qualitative study or a guideline, which you think may help you to provide evidence-based care for John.

practice (Avis 1994). Often, people will read the abstract, introduction, findings and conclusions of a research paper, while ignoring the section on research methods. Unfortunately, by ignoring the methods section of the article, it is possible that vital details that provide insight into the strengths or weaknesses of a paper will be missed. This is important when considering the application of findings to practice.

Box 5.17 provides an overview of how important details could be missed. This example highlighted the need for Staff Nurse Brown to read the article in full. Because she did not read the research methods section, she was unable to answer Staff Nurse Sanchez's questions about the sample size and variables which may have significantly influenced the findings of the study. For example, it is known that smoking increases the risk of breast cancer. If any of the women smoked in either group, then this could have influenced the findings. For example, in this case, soya acts as the control variable: women in the non-soya diet group may have smoked more than the women in the soya group which would have led to an increased risk in developing breast cancer irrespective of whether they consumed soya in their diet. Smoking is therefore a confounding variable that should have been taken into account.

CRITICAL THINKING Box 5.17

The challenges of critically appraising research

Read the example below.

Staff Nurse Brown: 'I read an article yesterday which said that eating soya products is good for you'.

Staff Nurse Sanchez: 'Yeah... Really, what did it say?'

Staff Nurse Brown: 'Well, it said that something found in soya can help to prevent breast cancer.'

Staff Nurse Sanchez: 'So how did they come up with that conclusion?'

Staff Nurse Brown: 'Oh easy really, they compared the diet of a group of women who had breast cancer with the diet of a group of women who didn't have breast cancer and the findings showed that the women who didn't have breast cancer ate more soya products.'

Staff Nurse Sanchez: 'But how many women did they look at?'

Staff Nurse Brown: 'Erm... I think about 100.'

Staff Nurse Sanchez: 'Well, did any of the women smoke?'

Staff Nurse Brown: 'Oh, I'm not sure, I think I missed that bit out – it was a lengthy article.'

Student activities

- What problems does this example highlight?
- Why did Staff Nurse Sanchez ask how many women were in the study and whether any of the women smoked?
- What other details about the paper would you need to know before deciding whether you can trust the findings?
- Think about other confounding variables that could be associated with breast cancer.

Components of critical awareness

According to Hamer and Collinson (1999), to develop a critical awareness practitioners need to be able to reflect on their practice and identify questions about their own or others' practice in a non-biased way. Finding and then appraising evidence to answer their question is part of the evidence-based cycle. Appraising evidence is not just about identifying a paper's flaws, but determining the value or otherwise of the paper to their area of practice. To illustrate this, Box 5.18 includes an extract from a journal club meeting through which practitioners appraised and discussed a paper.

Newman and Roberts (2002, p. 87) suggest that the purpose of critical appraisal 'is to decide whether the quality of a research study is good enough for the results it provides to be used to answer a question posed by a healthcare practitioner or patient'. So, to summarize, critical appraisal empowers practitioners to identify quality evidence and make sense of the evidence in terms of its relevance to the question posed and the individual's practice.

Strategies to develop critical appraisal skills

The development of an evidence-based culture within the NHS is being supported by the government's modernization agenda. This has involved the introduction of clinical governance, NSFs, NICE and other guidelines used to help standardize care. As part of this, it is also recognized that NHS staff such as nurses, midwives and health visitors need better critical appraisal skills (DH 1997) to enable them to use evidence in practice. One way of developing practitioners' appraisal skills is through the use of journal clubs. Journal clubs are an ideal way to develop appraisal skills in a friendly and supportive atmosphere. Journal clubs have expanded and there are now online journal clubs as well as local clubs (see 'Useful websites', pp. 144–145).

Box 5.18 Extract from a journal club meeting

Barrett et al (2002) used a transparently designed RCT to examine the effectiveness of Echinacea for early treatment of the common cold. Initially, it was thought that the trial addressed a clearly focused issue in terms of the population studied, intervention used and outcome measurements. However, following appraisal, concerns were raised about the pharmacological preparation of the intervention, the representativeness of the sample and the validity of the outcomes measured.

Appraisal

Anecdotally, it is argued that Echinacea is effective in the treatment of colds for a compromised population, e.g. people who are immunosuppressed or frail older people. The population of healthy students under study in this trial used self-reported symptoms as outcome measures. This raised some concerns about the nature of the outcome measures used and the aims of this trial.

In relation to the self-report outcome measures, the group felt that there was too much variation; however, it was also argued that this might be the only way to measure cold outcomes. It was noted that some of the sample took other non-protocol medication although this was accounted for in the statistical analysis as one of the potential confounders.

The paper was well presented and utilized clear graphs to describe some of the findings which were thought to be useful. Some ambiguous statements were made in the paper which required clarification, e.g. the authors stated that 'nearly all' the participants rather than the number of participants. The group felt that the number of subjects needed to be clear when discussing the analysis of the data.

Outcome

The discussion above demonstrates some of the key attributes outlined by Hamer and Collinson (1999). The group used critical appraisal guidelines to appraise the paper and, as a result, key questions about the research design were asked. This resulted in some aspects of the paper being scrutinized more carefully and an informed decision made about the trustworthiness and appropriateness of the paper to their own areas of practice.

[Based on Barrett et al (2002)]

Developing critical appraisal skills

Critical appraisal skills are essential to the delivery of EBP and a variety of critical appraisal tools have been designed to help the reader decide on the quality of research papers (Box 5.19). These appraisal tools usually take the form of a series of questions that the reader needs to ask of the paper.

EVIDENCE-BASED PRACTICE Box 5.19

What evidence and how to appraise it?

Look at the evidence on cranberry juice you have already located (see Box 5.16).

Student activities

- What type of evidence have you located (e.g. a systematic review, RCT, guideline)?
- How are you going to make sense of the evidence?
- What tools or guidelines will you use to appraise the evidence?
- Obtain copies of two of the critical appraisal guidelines listed in Box 5.20 and, using one of the research papers you located on cranberry juice, compare and contrast the critical appraisal guidelines. Make a list of any similarities or differences.

Box 5.20 Examples of critical appraisal tools and guidelines

- Crombie I 1996 The pocket guide to critical appraisal. BMJ Publishing Group, London
- Public Health Resource Unit, Milton Keynes Primary Care NHS Trust 2003 CASP appraisal tools 2003. Online: www.phru.nhs.uk/learning/casp.htm Available July 2006
- Health Care Practice Research and Development Unit, University of Salford 2003 Assessment tools. Online: www.fhsc.salford.ac.uk/hcprdu/critical-appraisal.htm Available July 2006
- Thompson C 1999 Questioning evidence: its validity and importance. Nursing Times Learning Curve 3(4):4–6
- School of Health and Related Research, University of Sheffield 2003 Netting the evidence. Online: www.shef.ac.uk/~scharr/ir/netting Available July 2006

Crombie (1996) recommended that checklists/tools be used to review a paper or evidence to help identify its value. He suggested that this would assist in detecting any flaws in the paper, question its credibility and trustworthiness, and identify the potential impact on the area of practice. Critical appraisal should focus on ascertaining the value of the paper to an area of practice, rather than on rubbishing papers. A number of other tools/guidelines have been developed to help with the process of critical appraisal (Box 5.20). Some of these are available online and can be downloaded free of charge.

Questions to ask when critically appraising a research paper

The first and perhaps most crucial stage in the process of critical appraisal is that of identifying a clear research

Box 5.21 **Questions to consider when reading a research paper**

Interest?
Is it of interest? This can usually be discovered through reading the title and abstract.

Reason?
The reason why the study was done can be identified in the introduction.

How?
To ascertain how the study was done, it is necessary to read the methods section. This will explain the methodological approach to the study and rationale for the approach.

Findings?
The results section should clearly highlight the key findings and present any raw data.

Implications?
What are the implications of the study? These are normally outlined in the discussion section. The discussion section may draw on previous literature to highlight any similarities or differences between the study findings and existing literature.

Finally, what else was of interest?
As healthcare practitioners are constantly developing their skills and knowledge they may learn something unexpected from the study that could inform their practice.

question. If this is related to the stages in the evidence-based cycle, it becomes clear why this is so important. If the question is not clear at the outset, then the rest of the research process may be confusing to the reader.

There needs to be a good reason for undertaking a study and it needs to be transparent to the reader. Some would argue that if a study has been done before, then why repeat it? Others believe that it is unethical to repeat a study which has already been done or which has already demonstrated the effectiveness of an intervention. Greenhalgh (1997) argued that the reader needs to know what type of study has been done and whether the research design was appropriate to meet the study aims. The research process stages need to be transparent throughout the paper to enable the reader to understand and make full use of the findings. If the design used was inappropriate, then this may lead to confusing findings that do not address the aims of the study.

Crombie (1996) suggests that research papers are organized into four main sections. This includes the introduction, methods used, results gained and discussion of findings. There are also other questions that the practitioner needs to consider (Crombie 1996) (Box 5.21).

Thompson (1999) provides another example of an appraisal tool that uses 11 questions to guide the practitioner through a research paper. The questions are loosely based on the research process and prompt the reader to ask specific questions about the process (Box 5.22).

CRITICAL THINKING Box 5.22

Critically appraise a research article

Select an appraisal tool and apply it to your articles about cranberry juice. This will help you appraise your article in a systematic way. You may like to do this with a colleague and compare your answers, as well as evaluating the strengths and weaknesses of the two papers you appraised.

Box 5.23 **Points to look out for in qualitative research**

- Is there a description of the researchers' relationship and role with the research participants?
- Was the methodology used appropriate for the study?
- Did the authors provide any extracts from the interviews/focus groups/observation data to support their analysis?
- Is there any evidence of other literature used to support the researchers' findings?
- How were the data analysed?

Appraising different research designs

When appraising different research designs, it is important to identify the stages of the research process carried out by the researcher. As stated earlier, the research process should be transparent. Without this it will not be possible to make sense of the paper, which could limit the application of the findings to practice. In all cases the paper must be relevant to the practice issue. Practitioners need to ask questions that include:

- Will the paper help practice?
- How will it help?
- How will they know that it will help?

In conjunction with appraising the research process within research papers, there are specific details of each research design that should be sought. In each instance, readers need to look for evidence that the author has considered the methodology chosen and the rigour the researcher has applied to the methodology. This next section briefly explores four different research designs and highlights key points that should be considered when appraising these designs.

Appraising qualitative research (Box 5.23)

Qualitative research attempts to explore the meanings and experiences of individuals or groups about a particular topic. For example, practitioners may have read about mood disorders and understand the effects and treatment. But what is it like to have depression? Only those who have suffered with the condition will be

Box 5.24 Points to look out for in systematic reviews

- How many reviewers were involved? (There should be at least two.)
- How comprehensive was the search strategy?
- Were all the relevant databases searched?
- What were the inclusion and exclusion criteria?
- Were all the studies incorporated in the review similar?
- Were English and non-English articles included?
- How did the reviewers assess the quality of the research studies included in the review?

Box 5.25 Points to look out for in RCTs

- Was there a robust randomization procedure?
- Were the researchers and subjects 'blind'? (meaning that neither the researcher nor the research subject knew whether they were in the experimental group or the control group). This helps to reduce bias, e.g. preventing the researcher from entering healthier subjects into the experimental group
- Was everyone who entered the trial followed up and accounted for? It may be that some subjects left the trial for a variety of reasons. It is important to know what happened to the subjects
- Were the groups treated equally? Unequal treatment may have a significant impact on the findings.

Box 5.26 Points to look for in survey designs

- What was the length of the questionnaire? Was it too long?
- What types of question were included in the questionnaire?
- How was the questionnaire analysed?
- What was the response rate? (Questionnaires are notorious for their poor response rates; sometimes less than 10% are returned.)
- Who were the sample population?

REFLECTIVE PRACTICE Box 5.27

Experiences of completing a survey

Reflect on an experience where you have completed a questionnaire, e.g. as part of market research or a satisfaction questionnaire about a service.

- What type of questions did the questionnaire use?
- How were they structured?
- Did you complete and return the questionnaire?
- What factors helped you to decide to complete the questionnaire or not?

able to describe their experiences. Qualitative research provides an ideal method to explore these thoughts and feelings and helps gain insight into the experiences of people. In order to obtain the rich, in-depth data required to explore perceptions and feelings, the researcher becomes the data collection tool. In relation to qualitative work, the role of the researcher is important and should be clearly described, as their role is pivotal in the collection of data and analysis of the findings.

Appraising systematic reviews (Box 5.24)

Systematic reviews are conducted by following a series of logical steps and bring together the results of several studies on a single topic to provide an overall conclusion. Droogan and Cullum (1998, p. 14) state that 'systematic reviews reduce large quantities of research into key findings in a reliable way and offer a means of enabling healthcare professionals to keep abreast of research'.

In a systematic review, research evidence about a specific topic is located through a comprehensive search strategy. The evidence located is then appraised using validated appraisal tools and, finally, credible reviewers will summarize the findings for the reader. Strict inclusion and exclusion criteria are normally used to help the reviewers decide on the best sort of papers to be included in the review. Systematic reviews embrace international literature, including published and non-published work, and may take up to 2 years to complete. They are, therefore, considered to be a very valuable form of evidence. Systematic reviews of quantitative research (RCTs in particular) are designated as the 'gold standard' of evidence within the hierarchy of evidence. This is reflected in many guidelines currently in use, e.g. the *National Service Framework for Older People* (DH 2001b, pp. 14–15).

Appraising randomized controlled trials (Box 5.25)

Randomized controlled trials (RCTs) are an important quantitative method and are another type of evidence considered to be valuable. In establishing cause and effect of treatments, they attempt to manipulate variables within a control and an experimental group. As a result, they reduce researcher bias, introduce control and limit the confounding variables. Many believe that RCTs are a good type of evidence because they are reliable and it is often possible to generalize from the findings if the study is well designed.

Appraising survey designs (Box 5.26)

Surveys (quantitative method) are large-scale questionnaires of a selected population. They can provide details about the demographic make-up of a population or trends in terms of lifestyles. For example, a survey may be used to provide data about how many people smoked in a geographical area.

An example of a survey that you may have been involved with is the Census. This is undertaken every 10 years by the government to find out about the population's lifestyle status. Surveys use questionnaires to elicit details about a population. Short, closed-ended questions are usually used to uncover a variety of details from the respondent (Box 5.27, p. 141).

Putting evidence into practice

There are important reasons for ensuring that the best evidence is used in practice. Firstly, it is a crucial way of ensuring that people get the treatments and services that are most effective and will have the best health outcomes. EBP is also an essential way of ensuring that the public funding that supports the NHS is used wisely and that the treatments and services offered are cost effective. Together these factors lead to the provision of clinically effective care. Clinical effectiveness can be defined as 'the extent to which specific clinical interventions, when deployed in the field for a particular patient or population, do what they are intended to do. That is, maintain or improve health and secure the greatest possible health gain from the resources available' (NHS Executive 1996, p. 2).

Many people are responsible for ensuring that research and other forms of evidence are used in practice. This includes practitioners, managers, researchers, educators and service users. For practitioners, there is a professional responsibility for using the best evidence in practice and to ensure accountability in their practice (NMC 2002) (see Ch. 7). As such, nurses must attempt to keep up to date with developments within their field in order to fulfil the continuing professional development requirements for periodic registration (see Ch. 7). By using the right evidence in practice, practitioners can be more confident in the care that they deliver and the clinical decisions that they make, thus enhancing their clinical accountability (Joyce 1999).

In order to support practitioners in using evidence in practice, managers must also develop supportive structures within organizations to promote a culture where evidence is valued and to enable practice to be changed in light of evidence (Le May 1999). They must base decisions about, for example, services, staffing and treatments on the best available evidence.

Researchers have an important role in generating new knowledge and evidence for practice. However, they must be able to share this information with the practitioners who need to use it. This is dissemination and is usually done by publishing research findings within professional journals.

Educators may work with both practitioners and researchers and can help to teach the principles of EBP and support practice development. They may also be involved in research projects.

Finally, but importantly, service users also have a role in ensuring that evidence is used in practice. It is important that service users do ask about the best treatment or care options that are available and are able to challenge practices that they are concerned about.

Challenges to the use of evidence in practice

Unfortunately, despite the vast amount of evidence now available, there are many challenges to using it in practice. In many areas of the NHS, decisions are made on the basis of custom and practice that can lead to outdated or ineffective treatment and care being offered. For example, despite evidence to suggest a shorter fasting time for some types of surgery, people are still fasted preoperatively for too long. This type of practice does not use research to support or change practice. This is often described as the 'research–practice gap'.

There are many reasons for the failure to use research in practice. These often relate to the attitudes of practitioners who may be satisfied with routine practices. However, organizational pressures, a lack of managerial support and educational deficiencies can also inhibit practice development (Joyce 1999). In other cases there is a lack of high quality research to guide practice. This means that practitioners have no option but to follow their own experience. The quality of research evidence may also cause problems as different research studies often provide different results that may be conflicting or confusing (Joyce 1999). Research studies may be small scale, methodologically flawed or produce findings that are difficult to implement. It is also a problem when research seems irrelevant to practitioners who would have asked different research questions had they been involved in the design of the research. More recently, it has been recognized that a lack of structure or systematic approach to the research agenda has made it difficult to use evidence in practice.

Other challenges arise from practitioners' lack of time, poor access to libraries and inadequate literature searching and critical appraisal skills.

Overcoming the challenges is essential to improving care and service delivery. The most important approach is to improve the communication or dissemination of research findings. Unfortunately, while publication in academic and professional journals is the usual approach to sharing research information, this type of dissemination remains relatively ineffective and does not necessarily lead to changes in practice.

Earlam et al (2000) proposed a framework relating to the EBP cycle to consider when planning making changes in practice (Box 5.28).

Using systematic reviews

Systematic reviews of particular topics aim to collate evidence into a more usable form. Different studies on the same topic can produce conflicting results, making it problematic to use the information. Combining the results of studies results in clearer implications that are easier to put into practice.

Box 5.28 **Framework for planning changes in practice**

- *Let people know*: It is important to consider the method for disseminating the evidence. Useful lines of communication may be easily identified such as use of the Trust Intranet, Trust newsletter, ward meetings, leaflets and posters. Discussion with staff will help them decide on how best the evidence will be suited to the local population
- *Getting people to take on the change*: It is vital that staff are encouraged to accept a change and fully understand why change is needed. This may be achieved through workshops or study days or information leaflets
- *Test out the change*: It may be useful to pilot any change in practice in a small area and involve enthusiastic staff
- *Audit any differences in practice*: Monitoring and evaluating is the final step in the EBP cycle. Auditing the change plays an important part of the process and provides evidence of whether the change has been effective.

[Based on Earlam et al (2000)]

The use of guidelines and integrated care pathways

Similarly, clinical guidelines and integrated care pathways (ICPs) pull together evidence and set out what services and treatments people should receive (see Chs 3, 14). ICPs are designed to guide practitioners through a predicted 'patient journey'. Guidelines have been used for many years in the NHS, e.g. guidelines for routine antenatal care.

By providing service users with information of what care they should expect to receive, the previously passive patient–practitioner relationship becomes more active and equal. By providing service users with access to information, it is hoped that they will be more empowered to take responsibility for their own care. However, it is also important to remember that not all guidelines/ICPs are reliable and evidence based and the following key points should be considered before using one:

- Are the statements referenced?
- Are the references current?
- When was the guideline/ICP written?
- When is it due for review?
- Who wrote the guideline/ICP?
- Is it clear and free of jargon?

All of these points should be present in a guideline so that practitioners can be reassured of the guideline's evidence base and reliability (Box 5.29)

Role of government policy

Government policy has influenced practice through national strategies that can also encourage the use of evidence in practice. For example, the NSFs illustrate how government is attempting to get evidence into practice. By using evidence to support each NSF, the government is expecting practitioners to use the NSFs to support and guide their practice. Another example that illustrates this is NICE (see p. 144). NICE produces guidelines that are disseminated to Chief Executives and other Trust Board members for implementation in each Trust, thereby ensuring parity between NHS organizations across the country and ending the practice of 'post code prescribing'.

To ensure that NICE guidelines and the NSFs are based on the best type of evidence, the NHS Research and Development funding targets specific priority areas for the NHS. This approach ensures that important gaps in the evidence base can be appropriately investigated through research and, using this new information, more informed decisions can be made (Benton 1999).

CRITICAL THINKING Box 5.29

Integrated care pathways (ICPs)

- Find an ICP used in your clinical placement
- Visit www.library.nhs.uk and locate the care pathways database (this provides up-to-date information and contact details for ICPs that have been developed and those being piloted)
- Identify an ICP that covers the same condition as the ICP from your clinical placement
- Compare and contrast the two ICPs and discuss your findings with your mentor/personal tutor.

Implementing evidence

Although important, providing access to information is not usually enough to bring about the use of evidence in practice. Normally, specific strategies focusing on implementing evidence are needed and a range of approaches is most successful (Needham 2000). Earlam et al (2000) suggest that there are potentially three layers to implementation that should be considered. These are:

- *The individual*: Practitioners will also need access to post-registration education in relation to research, EBP, literature searching and critical appraisal.
- *The team*: Journal clubs and research interest groups may be part of this approach and will provide practitioners with an opportunity to discuss evidence and develop their knowledge of research and critical appraisal skills.
- *The organization*: Involves each NHS Trust having a local plan or strategy for the implementation of research, development and EBP. Local audit and guideline development may also help to foster a culture of EBP.

Earlam et al (2000) suggest that each layer needs to be addressed to enable changes in practice to be made successfully. The practice environment needs to be supportive of these elements and value the activities that will promote all stages of the EBP cycle.

Summary

- EBP acts as a bridge between different types of evidence and nursing practice.
- By promoting the uptake and implementation of research and other types of evidence, high standards of effective practice in healthcare are supported. Models and guidance have been developed to sustain the use of research.
- EBP is viewed as a means to challenge outdated, ritualistic practices by encouraging practitioners to be more questioning of their work and care delivery.
- Research is a valuable form of evidence that can be used to support, improve and develop practice. There are a number of steps to the research process including locating the evidence. At first, the prospect of conducting a literature search can be quite daunting. However, it is a skill that develops over time and, with practice, your abilities to search for literature will improve.
- Once practitioners have located some relevant research they then learn to appraise the evidence critically. When reading a research paper, each step should be made transparent so that it is possible to judge the value of the study. EBP relies on the availability of good quality evidence to improve practice. To ensure the implementation of good evidence in practice, practitioners need critical appraisal skills that help the reader to make sense of research evidence. By using a validated tool or guide, the reader can work through a research paper in a systematic way to judge the credibility and value of research papers.
- While practitioners may question their practice, find and appraise evidence, practice will not change unless evidence is effectively implemented. This requires the involvement of the individual practitioner, the nursing team and the organization.

Self test

1. Write a definition of the phrase 'evidence-based practice'.
2. Outline the stages of the evidence-based practice cycle.
3. List the different types of evidence discussed in this chapter.
4. List some of the common healthcare databases.
5. What is PICO and what does it stand for?
6. Why are critical appraisal skills important?
7. Describe the major difference between qualitative and quantitative research methodologies.
8. List four different research designs described in this chapter.

Key words and phrases for literature searching

Evidence-based practice	Qualitative
Literature review	Quantitative

Useful websites

Action for Sick Children	http://actionforsickchildren.org Available July 2006
Allied Journal Club	www.alliedjournalclub.com Available July 2006
Bandolier	www.jr2.ox.ac.uk/bandolier Available July 2006
Clinical Journal Club on the Web	www.journalclub.org/index.php Available July 2006
Cochrane Library	www.cochrane.co.uk Available July 2006
Effective Health Care Bulletins	www.york.ac.uk/inst/crd/ehcb.htm Available July 2006
Mental Health Foundation	www.mentalhealth.org.uk Available July 2006
National Library for Health (NLH) – *provides access to a wide range of health related services including an index of UK national clinical guidelines*	www.library.nhs.uk Available July 2006
National Institute for Health and Clinical Excellence (NICE) – *develops clinical guidelines, undertakes appraisals and provides*	www.nice.org.uk Available July 2006

Useful websites

other clinical guidance for the NHS for England and Wales	
NHS Centre for Reviews and Dissemination	www.york.ac.uk/inst/crd Available July 2006
NHS Quality Improvement Scotland (NHSQIS) – *sets standards, monitors performance, provides advice, best practice statements, guidance and support on clinical effectiveness and improvement for the NHS in Scotland*	www.nhshealthquality.org Available July 2006
Nursing, Midwifery and Allied Health Professionals (NMAP) – *a gateway service*	http://nmap.ac.uk Available July 2006
Online Medical Networked Information (OMNI) – *a health and biomedical gateway service*	http://omni.ac.uk Available July 2006
Scottish Intercollegiate Guidelines Network (SIGN)	www.sign.ac.uk Available July 2006
SOSIG – *a social sciences gateway service*	www.sosig.ac.uk Available July 2006

References

Avis M 1994 Reading research critically I. An introduction to appraisal: designs and objectives. Journal of Clinical Nursing 3:227–234

Barrett BP, Brown RL, Locken K et al 2002 Treatment of the common cold with unrefined Echinacea. Annals of Internal Medicine 137(12):939–946

Benton D 1999 Clinical effectiveness. In: Hamer S, Collinson G (eds) Achieving evidence-based practice: a handbook for practitioners. Baillière Tindall, London

Blaxter L, Hughes C, Tight M 1998 How to research. Open University Press, Buckingham

Brand-de Heer DL 2001 A comparison of the coverage of clinical medicine provided by PASCAL, BIOMED and MEDLINE. Health Information and Libraries Journal 18(2):110–116

Brazier H, Begley CM 1996 Selecting a database for literature searches in nursing: MEDLINE or CINAHL? Journal of Advanced Nursing 24:868–875

Cox CL, Reyes-Hughes A 2001 Clinical effectiveness in practice. Palgrave, Basingstoke

Craig JV, Smyth R (eds) 2002 The evidence based practice manual for nurses. Churchill Livingstone, London, Ch. 6

Crombie IK 1996 The pocket guide to critical appraisal. BMJ Publishing Group, London

Department of Health 1991 Research for health: a research and development strategy for the NHS. Research and Development Division, Department of Health, London

Department of Health 1997 The new NHS: modern and dependable. TSO, London

Department of Health 1998 Data protection act. Department of Health, London

Department of Health 1999a Making a difference: strengthening the nursing, midwifery and health visiting contribution to health and healthcare. Department of Health, London

Department of Health 1999b Saving lives: our healthier nation. A contract for health. TSO, London

Department of Health 2001a The essence of care: patient focused benchmarking for health care practitioners. Department of Health, London

Department of Health 2001b National service framework for older people. Department of Health, London

Droogan J, Cullum N 1998 Systematic reviews in nursing. International Journal of Nursing Studies 35:13–22

Earlam S, Brecker N, Vaughan B 2000 Cascading evidence into practice. King's Fund, London

French P 2002 What is the evidence on evidence-based nursing? An epistemological concern. Journal of Advanced Nursing 37(3):250–257

Garland G, Corfield F 1999 Audit. In: Hamer S, Collinson G (eds) Achieving evidence-based practice: a handbook for practitioners. Baillière Tindall, London

Greenhalgh T 1997 How to read a paper: getting your bearings (deciding what the paper is about). British Medical Journal 315:243–246

Hamer S, Collinson G (eds) 1999 Achieving evidence-based practice: a handbook for practitioners. Baillière Tindall, London, Ch. 1

Health and Safety Executive 1992 Manual handling operations: regulations and guidance on regulations. HMSO, London

Joyce L 1999 Development of practice. In: Hamer S, Collinson G (eds) Achieving evidence-based practice: a handbook for practitioners. Baillière Tindall, London

Kane M, Parahoo K 1994 Lifting: why nurses follow bad practice. Nursing Standard 8(25):34–38

Le May A 1999 Evidence-based practice. Nursing Times Clinical Monographs No. 1. Nursing Times Books, London

Long AF, Kneafsey R, Ryan J et al 2001 Researching professional education. Team working in rehabilitation: exploring the role of the nurse. English Nursing Board, London

Long AF, Kneafsey R, Ryan J et al 2002 The role of the nurse within the multi-professional rehabilitation team. Journal of Advanced Nursing 37(1):70–78

Melia K 1984 Student nurses' construction of occupational socialization. Sociology of Health and Illness 6(2):132–150

Muir Gray JA 1997 Evidence-based healthcare: how to make health policy and management decisions. Churchill Livingstone, London

National Back Pain Association 1998 The guide to the handling of patients: introducing a safer handling policy. Supplement to the 4th edition. National Back Pain Association, Teddington

National Institute for Clinical Excellence 2001 Pressure ulcer risk assessment and prevention. NICE, London

Needham G 2000 Research and practice: making a difference. In: Gomm R, Needham G (eds) Using evidence in health and social care. Sage Publications, London

Newman M, Roberts T 2002 Critical appraisal 1: is the quality of the study good enough for you to use the findings? In: Craig JV Smyth R (eds) The evidence based practice manual for nurses. Churchill Livingstone, Edinburgh

NHS Executive 1996 Achieving effective practice: a clinical effectiveness and research information pack for nurses, midwives and health visitors. NHS Executive, Leeds

Nursing and Midwifery Council 2004 The NMC code of professional conduct: standards for conduct, performance and ethics. NMC, London

Okuma E 1994 Selecting CD-ROM databases for nursing students: a comparison of MEDLINE and the Cumulative Index to Nursing and Allied Health Literature (CINAHL). Bulletin of the Medical Library Association 82(1):25–29

Palmer J, Brice A 1999 Information sourcing. In: Hamer S, Collinson G (eds) Achieving

evidence-based practice: a handbook for practitioners. Baillière Tindall, London
Parahoo K 1997 Nursing research: principles, processes and issues. Palgrave, Basingstoke
Polgar S, Thomas S 1995 Introduction to research in the health sciences. Churchill Livingstone, London
Richardson WS, Wilson MC, Nishikawa J et al 1995 The well built clinical question: a key to evidence based decisions. ACP Journal Club 123(2):A12–13
Rolfe G 2002 Reflective practice: where now? Nurse Education in Practice 2:21–29
Royal College of Nursing 1996 Clinical effectiveness: a Royal College of Nursing guide. Royal College of Nursing. Cited in: Cox CL, Reyes-Hughes A 2001 Clinical effectiveness in practice. Palgrave, Basingstoke
Royal College of Nursing Research Society 2003 The Royal College of Nursing Research Society: nurses and research ethics. Nurse Researcher 11(1):7–19
Sackett DL, Rosenberg WMC, Gray JAM et al 1996 Evidence based medicine: what it is and what it isn't. British Medical Journal 312:71–72
Seacombe I, Ball J 1992 Back injured nurses: a profile. Discussion paper for the Royal College of Nursing, Institute of Manpower Services, London
Stevens A, Abrams K, Brazier J et al 2001 The advanced handbook of methods in evidence based healthcare. Sage Publications, London
Thomas L, Hotchkiss R 2002 Evidence based guidelines. In: Craig JV, Smyth R (eds) The evidence based practice manual for nurses. Churchill Livingstone, London
Thompson C 1999 Questioning evidence: its validity and importance. Nursing Times Learning Curve 3(4):4–6
Thompson C, Cullum N 1999 Examining evidence: an overview, Nursing Times Learning Curve 3(1):7–9
Walsh M, Ford P 1989 Nursing rituals: research and rational actions. Butterworth-Heinemann, Oxford
White S 1997 Evidence-based practice and nursing: the new panacea? British Journal of Nursing 6:175–177

Further reading

Blaxter L, Hughes C, Tight M 1998 How to research. Open University Press, Buckingham
Brettle A, Grant MJ 2004 Finding the evidence for practice: a workbook for health professionals. Churchill Livingstone, Edinburgh
Evans D 2003 Hierarchy of evidence: a framework for ranking evidence evaluating healthcare interventions. Journal of Clinical Nursing 12:77–84
Smith P, James T, Lorentzon M, Pope R 2003 Shaping the facts of evidence-based nursing and health care. Churchill Livingstone, Edinburgh
Tarling M, Crofts L 2002 The essential researcher's handbook. 2nd edn. Baillière Tindall, Edinburgh

6 Legal issues that impact on nursing practice

Sherri Ogston-Tuck

Glossary terms

Civil law

Confidentiality

Criminal law

Duty of care

Informed consent

Negligence

Trespass against the person

Vicarious liability

Learning outcomes

This chapter will help you to:

- Outline legal frameworks and systems of law
- Develop an understanding of legislation relevant to nursing
- Understand the legal responsibilities and obligations integral to nursing
- Describe some of the legal issues that apply to particular areas of nursing.

Introduction

This chapter provides an overview of the law as it pertains to nursing. Issues that affect all branches of nursing are discussed as well as how legislation and the law influence specific branches. The law varies across the UK and the emphasis here is on the law in England and Wales. Readers should always be aware of the situation in their part of the UK.

It is important that nurses are aware of how the law affects nursing and always consider it in their day-to-day practice. Often it is only when something 'goes wrong' that nurses consider the law.

It is important to emphasize, however, that the law and nursing practice are subject to constant change. Often, the changes affecting nursing practice are the result of research and evidence-based practice (see Ch. 5). Legislation is not static and changes arise from new cases and current issues in society. The development and interpretation of law and its relationship to nursing and healthcare must always be considered. Professional and ethical issues pertain to this and it is important for nurses to think about how changes may influence practice. In addition, significant changes affecting patient rights, changes within the NHS and government initiatives must also be considered in relation to the law, to the practitioner and to the patient/client.

The law is a specialist area with its own language but it is highly relevant to nurses and their practice. All practitioners should maintain knowledge of and adherence to the law as it is important to standards and expectations of practice, patient/client outcomes and public well-being.

The law is discussed with the aim of providing a better understanding of relevant terminology and various systems of law related to nursing. This includes a brief discussion of the legal frameworks in England and Wales. Although differences in the law and legal systems in Scotland and Northern Ireland exist, it is worth remembering that there are common areas (Tingle & Cribb 2003). Important legislation related to different branches of nursing is reviewed.

Legal frameworks

A country's system of justice reflects its morals, history and politics. UK law and the structures within it have developed over hundreds of years. Terms, titles and legislation and systems of law all stem from the past and from tradition. An understanding of the law is necessary in order to meet standards of practice, ethical and professional responsibilities, and more importantly because the law represents society's judgement on these standards.

Types and sources of law

The legal system within the UK is divided into two divisions: public and private law. Public law is concerned with preserving the order of society whereas private law is concerned chiefly with disputes between individuals (Dimond 1995). The law is further divided into:

- *Criminal law* – deals with actions/behaviour regarded as wrong. Criminal offences relate to people and property and result in a prosecution and, if the defendant is convicted, usually results in punishment (discharge, fine, community penalty or a custodial sentence). The burden of proof in criminal cases means that the prosecution must prove the facts 'beyond reasonable doubt'.
- *Civil law* – deals with the conduct and conflicts between people. A person (the claimant) who has suffered a perceived wrong can seek redress by bringing an action or claim in the civil courts. The claim may be settled with an award of financial compensation or damages, or an order (injunction) banning an unlawful act or an order that requires some action. The burden of proof in civil cases is lower; the claimant must prove the facts 'on a balance of probabilities'.

The difference between criminal and civil law is reflected in the courts and procedures, and the sanctions which may be applied. For example, most criminal cases are heard in the Magistrates' court with serious or complex cases heard in the Crown court. The Crown Prosecution Service or another prosecuting body brings the case against the defendant. Civil cases are between the claimant and another person or organization and are heard in the County court or the High court depending on the amount of damages or degree of harm.

The law is derived from:

- Legislation, statute law – Acts of Parliament
- Case or common law – judge-made, which set precedents for future cases
- European Community law.

European Community law is binding on UK courts. Decisions made by the European Court of Justice may be directly binding on English courts.

Acts of Parliament

Most English law is in the form of Acts of Parliament (statutes). An Act of Parliament is primary legislation, e.g. the Disability Discrimination Act 2005. Statutory instruments (subordinate or secondary legislation) made under delegated powers provide the regulations needed to implement a particular Act.

An Act results from a Bill (a draft proposal). Proposals for legislative changes may be contained in government White Papers. Consultation papers, sometimes called Green Papers, which set out government proposals and seek comments from interested parties, including the public, may precede these. There is no requirement for there to be a White or Green Paper before a Bill is introduced into Parliament.

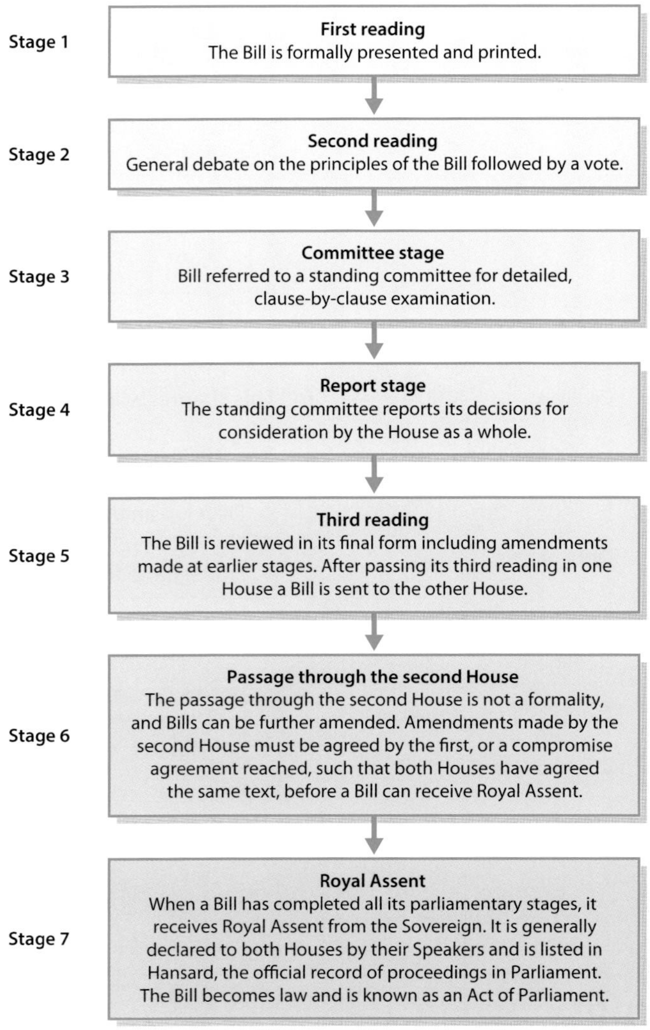
Stage 1
First reading
The Bill is formally presented and printed.
Stage 2
Second reading
General debate on the principles of the Bill followed by a vote.
Stage 3
Committee stage
Bill referred to a standing committee for detailed, clause-by-clause examination.
Stage 4
Report stage
The standing committee reports its decisions for consideration by the House as a whole.
Stage 5
Third reading
The Bill is reviewed in its final form including amendments made at earlier stages. After passing its third reading in one House a Bill is sent to the other House.
Stage 6
Passage through the second House
The passage through the second House is not a formality, and Bills can be further amended. Amendments made by the second House must be agreed by the first, or a compromise agreement reached, such that both Houses have agreed the same text, before a Bill can receive Royal Assent.
Stage 7
Royal Assent
When a Bill has completed all its parliamentary stages, it receives Royal Assent from the Sovereign. It is generally declared to both Houses by their Speakers and is listed in Hansard, the official record of proceedings in Parliament. The Bill becomes law and is known as an Act of Parliament.

Fig. 6.1 How a bill becomes law

The draft proposal or Bill is introduced into either the House of Commons (the elected Lower house) or the House of Lords or Upper house (currently an unelected body). The procedure of passing a Bill is similar in both Houses, and has seven stages (Fig. 6.1). If both Houses vote for the proposal then the Bill is ready to become an Act; however, it only becomes law after receiving Royal Assent.

The law undergoes constant reform in the courts as established principles are interpreted, clarified or reapplied to meet new circumstances; laws become outdated, new policies require new laws, or new laws are needed to ensure that the UK complies with international or European Law, e.g. The Human Rights Act 1998 (see pp. 150 and 151).

Case or common law – judge-made law

Case law or judge-made law predates statute; however, common law rules may be regarded as secondary because

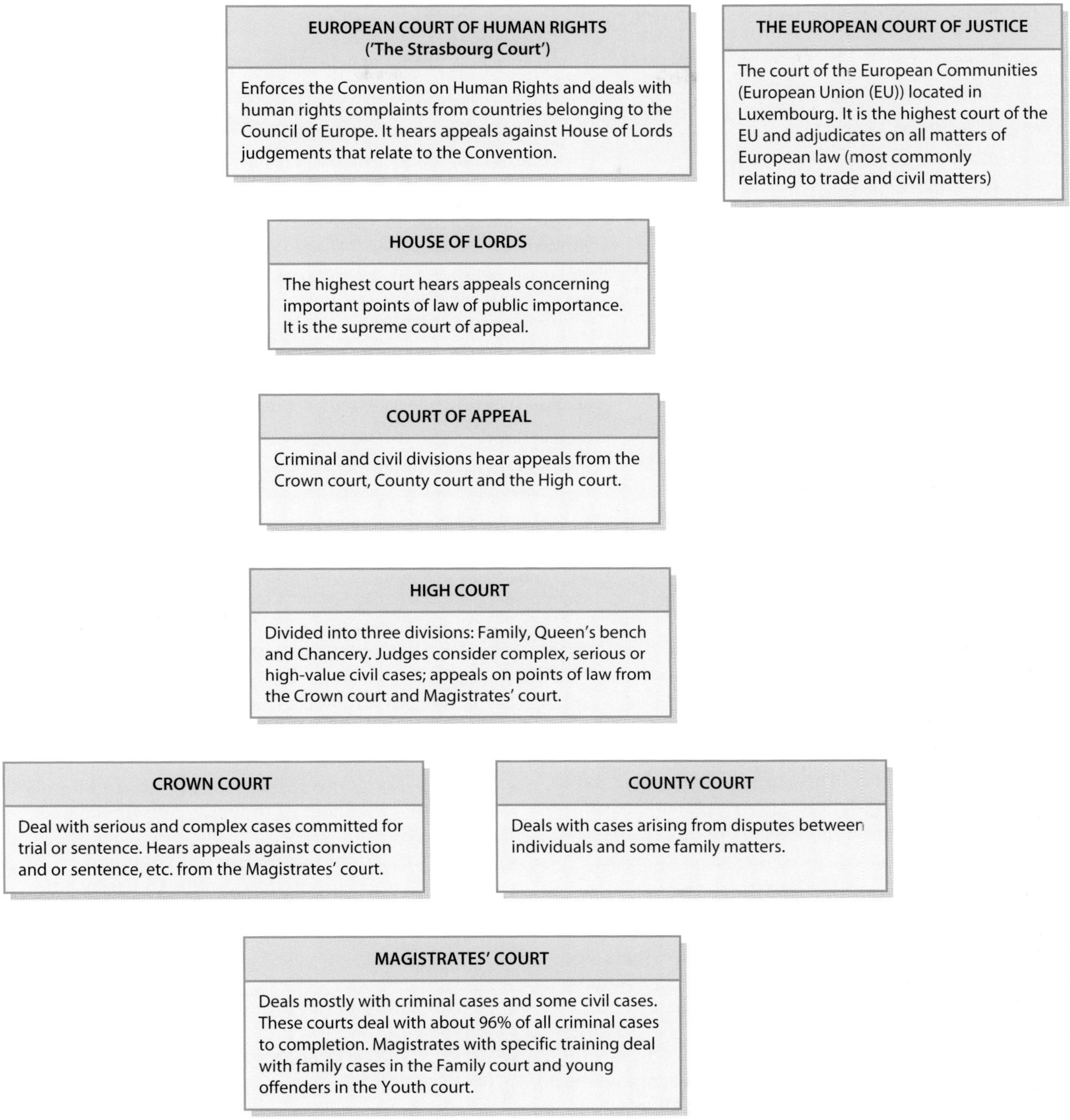
EUROPEAN COURT OF HUMAN RIGHTS ('The Strasbourg Court')
Enforces the Convention on Human Rights and deals with human rights complaints from countries belonging to the Council of Europe. It hears appeals against House of Lords judgements that relate to the Convention.
THE EUROPEAN COURT OF JUSTICE
The court of the European Communities (European Union (EU)) located in Luxembourg. It is the highest court of the EU and adjudicates on all matters of European law (most commonly relating to trade and civil matters)
HOUSE OF LORDS
The highest court hears appeals concerning important points of law of public importance. It is the supreme court of appeal.
COURT OF APPEAL
Criminal and civil divisions hear appeals from the Crown court, County court and the High court.
HIGH COURT
Divided into three divisions: Family, Queen's bench and Chancery. Judges consider complex, serious or high-value civil cases; appeals on points of law from the Crown court and Magistrates' court.
CROWN COURT
Deal with serious and complex cases committed for trial or sentence. Hears appeals against conviction and or sentence, etc. from the Magistrates' court.
COUNTY COURT
Deals with cases arising from disputes between individuals and some family matters.
MAGISTRATES' COURT
Deals mostly with criminal cases and some civil cases. These courts deal with about 96% of all criminal cases to completion. Magistrates with specific training deal with family cases in the Family court and young offenders in the Youth court.

Fig. 6.2 The court system (England and Wales)

of the many statutes that now exist. The rules in case law are derived from legal principles laid down by judges over many years. Nevertheless, case law still remains an important source of law, particularly in negligence cases (see pp. 155–157). Case law is subject to a system of precedent where the earlier decisions made by a higher court mean that a lower court must follow their decision. Rulings of the House of Lords (the highest court) are binding on all lower courts, whereas those of the Court of Appeal are generally binding on lower courts (McHale & Tingle 2001) (see Fig. 6.2).

Court system in England and Wales

The hierarchy of the court system (criminal and civil proceedings) in England and Wales is outlined in Figure 6.2.

Important legislation for nursing

There are many diverse Acts of Parliament relevant to nursing. Although detailed discussion of every Act is beyond the scope of this book, Table 6.1 (see p. 152) outlines some important Acts and sources of information.

Table 6.1 Important legislation for nursing (England and Wales)

Act of Parliament	Where to access the Act or Explanatory notes
Access to Health Records Act 1990	www.opsi.gov.uk/acts/acts1990/Ukpga_19900023_en_1.htm Available July 2006
Children Act 1989 (see pp. 152 and 158)	www.opsi.gov.uk/acts/acts1989/Ukpga_19890041_en_1.htm Available July 2006
Children Act 2004 (see p. 152)	www.opsi.gov.uk/acts/en2004/2004en31.htm Available July 2006
Data Protection Act 1998 (DPA) (see p. 152)	www.opsi.gov.uk/acts/acts1998/19980029.htm Available July 2006
Disability Discrimination Act 2005	www.opsi.gov.uk/acts/acts2005/20050013.htm Available July 2006 www.opsi.gov.uk/acts/en2005/2005en13.htm Available July 2006
Freedom of Information Act 2000	www.opsi.gov.uk/acts/acts2000/20000036.htm Available July 2006 www.informationcommissioner.gov.uk/eventual.aspx?id=33 Available July 2006 www.opsi.gov.uk/acts/en2000/2000en36.htm Available July 2006 www.foi.nhs.uk/act_home.html Available July 2006
Health and Safety at Work Act 1974 (see Ch. 13)	Health and Safety Executive – www.hse.gov.uk Available July 2006
Health and Social Care Act 2001	www.opsi.gov.uk/acts/en2001/2001en15.htm Available July 2006
Human Rights Act 1998 (HRA) (see below and p. 151)	www.opsi.gov.uk/acts/acts1998/19980042.htm Available July 2006
Human Tissue Act 2004 (see p. 161)	www.opsi.gov.uk/acts/en2004/2004en30.htm Available July 2006 www.uktransplant.org.uk Available July 2006
Medicinal Products: Prescription by Nurse Act 1992 (see Ch. 22)	www.uk-legislation.hmso.gov.uk/acts/acts1992/Ukpga_19920028_en_1.htm Available July 2006
Mental Capacity Act 2005 (see pp. 160 and 161)	www.opsi.gov.uk/acts/en2005/2005en09.htm Available July 2006 www.opsi.gov.uk/acts/acts2005/20050009.htm Available July 2006
Mental Health Act 1983 (MHA) (see pp. 151 and 152)	www.direct.gov.uk/DisabledPeople/HealthAndSupport/YourRightsInHealth/HealthRightsArticles/fs/en?CONTENT_ID=4014771&chk=jVhUS1 Available July 2006
Public Interest Disclosure Act 1998	www.opsi.gov.uk/acts/acts1998/19980023.htm Available July 2006

However, some – such as The Human Rights Act 1998 and The Children Act 2004, both of which have far-reaching effects – are discussed here in more detail, or covered later in the chapter.

The Human Rights Act

The Human Rights Act (HRA 1998) is wide ranging and promises that the state will respect the rights and freedoms of individuals. Human rights are very much a part of everyday life – as citizens, professionals, patients and clients (McHale & Gallagher 2004). Nurses need to be aware of the potential implications of the Act for their practice and care provision. The HRA 1998 applies to children (a person under the age of 18) as well as adults.

The HRA 1998, which became law in 2000, incorporates the rights and freedoms guaranteed under the European Convention on Human Rights (the Convention). The Convention was drafted following World War 2 and the UK was one of the first countries to sign up in 1953. In total, 45 countries signed and these make up the Council of Europe. The Convention confers a number of rights on people (Tingle & Cribb 2003). It is divided into schedules, which are further divided into articles. These are:

- Article 2 – Right to life
- Article 3 – Prohibition of torture
- Article 4 – Prohibition of slavery and forced labour
- Article 5 – Right to liberty and security
- Article 6 – Right to a fair trial
- Article 7 – No punishment without lawful authority
- Article 8 – Right to respect for private and family life
- Article 9 – Freedom of thought, conscience and religion
- Article 10 – Right to freedom of expression
- Article 11 – Freedom of assembly and association
- Article 12 – Right to marry and found a family
- Article 14 – Prohibition of discrimination

as well as

- Article 1 of the First Protocol – Protection of property
- Article 2 of the First Protocol – Right to education
- Article 3 of the First Protocol – Right to free elections (right to vote).

Since the HRA 1998 came into effect in 2000, English courts deciding on a matter connected with one of the rights must, as far as applicable, have regard to decisions made by the Strasbourg Court (McHale & Tingle 2001). In addition, new legislation must also comply. It also means that all public bodies must act in accordance with the Convention, including the healthcare system (Tingle & Cribb 2003).

It is worthwhile considering how some HRA Articles impact on nursing practice (Box 6.1). Nurses act as advocates for their patients/clients, to safeguard standards of care and to speak out where the patient/client may be at risk. The Nursing and Midwifery Council (NMC) *code of professional conduct: standards for conduct, performance and ethics* (NMC 2004) already requires registrants to bring any circumstances that may compromise

REFLECTIVE PRACTICE Box 6.1

The Human Rights Act and nursing practice

- Bob, aged 82, has advanced lung and brain cancer, and has been unconscious for 24 hours. Following consultation with Bob's family and the care team it is decided that he will not be resuscitated
- Shelagh is 5 years old and has a learning disability. She screams and kicks out when the nurses try to give her oral drugs to control seizures. One nurse usually holds Shelagh on her lap while another nurse administers the drug
- Madge has been told that she must lose weight before she can have hip surgery
- Francis has severe dementia and lives in a care home. His family visit and find him dressed in clothes that are not his and discover that he has outdoor shoes on, but no socks.

Student activities

- Reflect on the scenarios above and consider which Articles are relevant.
- Think about a situation you have encountered in placement where an Article(s) of the HRA was pertinent to patient/client outcomes. Discuss these with your mentor.

[Resource: Study Guide. Human Rights Act 1998, 2nd edn – www.humanrights.gov.uk/pdf/act/act-studyguide.pdf]

CRITICAL THINKING Box 6.2

Mental distress

Sam is wandering in and out of the local pub and the takeaway. It is a busy Saturday evening and he is increasingly agitated and distressed by the noise, traffic and unfamiliar people. The pub landlord calls the police when Sam starts shouting at people having a meal. The police officer, who knows Sam well, is worried about his distressed state and, also noticing that he has a head wound, summons an ambulance. When Sam arrives at the Emergency Department accompanied by the police officer he is very distressed and will not allow the staff near him. The charge nurse fears for Sam's safety. The duty psychiatrist is asked to come to the department to assess Sam.

Student activities

- Think about the feelings of the people who witnessed Sam's distressed state.
- How would you have felt if you had been in the pub when Sam came in?
- Speak to a mental health nurse and find out what provisions of the current mental health legislation in your part of the UK can be used by the psychiatrist to both help and protect Sam in the short term.

patient/client care and safety to the attention of an appropriate authority. Article 2 reinforces this professional obligation.

Article 2 has clear implications for decisions regarding withholding and/or withdrawing of life-preserving or life-saving treatment. It must be clear, however, that there will always be challenges with regard to non-resuscitation orders and demands for more aggressive treatments for people with serious illness.

Article 3 states that no one shall be subject to torture or inhumane degrading treatment or punishment. Inhumane treatment is deemed to be any treatment that causes intense physical and mental suffering.

Mental health legislation

In England and Wales the Mental Health Act (MHA) 1983 (Department of Health [DH] 1983) currently makes provision for the compulsory detention and treatment in hospital of those with a mental disorder. It is important to remember that many people with mental health problems are in hospital as voluntary or informal patients, i.e. not detained there under any provision of the MHA. Following consultation on updating the MHA 1983, including a draft Mental Health Bill 2004, the Government announced in 2006 that a shorter Bill would amend the 1983 Act.

The Mental Health (Care and Treatment) (Scotland) Act 2003 is the legal authority for mental health services in Scotland. Unlike the Scottish Mental Health Act (1984), the new Act is rights-based and underpinned by a set of guiding principles. These help to set the tone of the Act and guide its interpretation. As a general rule, anyone who takes any action under the Act has to take account of the principles (see www.nes.scot.nhs.uk/mha).

At the time of writing an independent review of mental health and learning disability (law, policy and provisions) is in progress in Northern Ireland (see www.rmhldni.gov.uk).

It is important to remember that mental health issues and mental health legislation can affect anyone and involves all areas of healthcare (Box 6.2).

The MHA 1983 (Section 1, p. 2) describes four categories of mental disorder:

- *Mental illness* (not defined)
- *Severe mental impairment*: 'A state of arrested or incomplete development of mind which includes severe impairment of intelligence and social functioning and is associated with abnormally aggressive or seriously irresponsible conduct on the part of the person concerned'
- *Mental impairment*: 'A state of arrested or incomplete development of mind (not amounting to a severe mental impairment) which includes significant impairment of intelligence and social functioning and is associated with abnormally aggressive or seriously irresponsible conduct on the part of the person concerned'
- *Psychopathic disorder*: 'A persistent disorder or disability of mind (whether or not including significant impairment of intelligence) which results in abnormally aggressive or seriously irresponsible conduct on the part of the person concerned.'

Conditions generally accepted as falling under the category of 'mental illnesses' include schizophrenia and mood disorders (depression and manic behaviour). Most admissions under the MHA 1983 requiring the category of mental disorder to be specified are admissions of people with a diagnosis of a 'mental illness'.

The Children Act 2004 and child protection

The Children Act 2004 is an important piece of legislation in the protection and welfare of children. The impetus for this legislation was the death of Victoria Climbié and the subsequent inquiry into the circumstances of her death chaired by Lord Laming (Box 6.3). Background to the Children Act 2004 can be accessed at the Department for Education and Skills (DfES) website (www.dfes.gov.uk/publications/childrenactreport); this includes:

- Children Act 1989
- Children Act Report 2002
- Children Act Report 2003
- Green paper *Every Child Matters* 2003 (see Ch. 3)
- Children Act 2004.

The report into the death of Victoria Climbié urged major reforms of children's services. The Children Act 2004 (and subsequent Regulations) provides the legislation for wide-ranging strategies for improving children's lives including the appointment of a Children's Commissioner.

REFLECTIVE PRACTICE Box 6.3

Safeguarding children

Victoria Climbié was abused, neglected and tortured to death by her great-aunt and the woman's boyfriend. Both were convicted of murder and sentenced to life imprisonment.

The police, health professionals and social services all had contact with Victoria while she was being abused. A public inquiry chaired by Lord Laming exposed a picture of incompetence and error at every level. Lord Laming promised to make recommendations to ensure such a tragedy never happens again.

Student activities

- Access the Victoria Climbié Inquiry website and reflect on the failings that allowed the abuse to continue and ultimately Victoria's death.
- Consider the recommendations and discuss them with your mentor.
- Find out what services/protocols are in place in your area for safeguarding children.

[Resources: BBC – news.bbc.co.uk/1/hi/in_depth/uk/2002/victoria_climbie_inquiry/default.stm; Victoria Climbié Inquiry – www.victoria-climbie-inquiry.org.uk; England: Department for Education and Skills – www.everychildmatters.gov.uk/socialcare; Northern Ireland: Department of Health, Social Services and Public Safety – www.dhsspsni.gov.uk/index/health_and_social_services/child_care/child_protection/child_protection_links.htm; Scotland: Scottish Executive – www.scotland.gov.uk/Topics/People/Young-People/children-families/17834/10227; Wales: All Wales Unit – www.allwalesunit.gov.uk All available July 2006]

The Act deals with the services which all children use, and the services needed by children who have additional needs (DfES website 2005) (see Ch. 3). The Act aims to ensure that the planning, commissioning and delivery of children's services are integrated. Other aims include improving multidisciplinary working, preventing duplication, integrating inspection procedures and increasing accountability (DfES website 2005). The legislation allows local authorities flexibility in the ways they provide children's services.

Where healthcare professionals suspect that a child may be neglected or abused by parents/carers or others, they have a clear duty to act. The action taken will be determined by the immediacy for protection, treatment or care. NHS Trusts etc. and local authorities have child protection policies that must be followed by healthcare professionals and others working with children (see Box 6.3). Nurses should note the NMC position on the matter of confidentiality in child protection matters: 'Where there is an issue of child protection, you must act at all times in accordance with national and local policies' (NMC 2004, Clause 5.4, p. 9).

Data Protection Act 1998

The provisions of the Data Protection Act (DPA) 1998 are designed to balance the right of individuals to privacy and the rights of those people/organizations who have valid reasons for holding and using personal data, such as healthcare professionals. The DPA provides people with some rights about data held about them but also sets out certain duties/obligations for the people/organizations that collect, hold and process such information.

Nurses have a responsibility to protect data as most manage, or will manage, personal information about people (see also 'Documentation and record keeping', p. 154, and 'Confidentiality', p. 157). The DPA sets out eight principles of good practice, e.g. data held must be accurate. Readers requiring more information are directed to the *Data Protection Act Factsheet* produced by the Information Commissioner (2005).

It is also important to be aware of the patient's/client's rights in relation to personal information held about them, how it is managed and how they can request access to it (see Access to Health Records Act 1990, Table 6.1). The DPA, the HRA 1998 (see pp. 150 and 151) and the Freedom of Information Act 2000 (see Table 6.1) are interlinked.

Legal concepts integral to nursing

This section considers legal concepts that are important for nurses, including safeguards for practice, duty of care, negligence, consent, etc. Nurses are accountable for their actions and omissions (see Ch. 7). Registered nurses remain accountable even when acting on the instructions of another practitioner such as when administering drugs prescribed by a doctor. The nurse has responsibilities even where a doctor has made the original mistake. Nurses must always challenge lack of clarity, errors or discrepancy in a drug prescription or other treatment.

There are four arenas of accountability relating to the nurse's duty of care and negligence, etc. These are:

- To the nurse's employer
- Professional accountability to the NMC
- Civil law
- Criminal law.

All four arenas are discussed more fully in this section (see pp. 155–157).

Safeguards for practice

There are various safeguards that protect both patients/clients and the nurses accountable for planning and providing care. Several of these, such as statutory regulation, professional indemnity insurance, documentation and record keeping, are discussed below.

Statutory regulation (see Ch. 7 for detailed coverage)

Health professionals are subject to statutory regulation, e.g. the General Medical Council (GMC) regulates doctors; the Health Professions Council (HPC) currently regulates 13 professions including dietitians, physiotherapists, etc. The Nursing and Midwifery Council (NMC) is the regulating body in the UK for nurses, midwives and specialist community public health nurses. At the time of writing, wide-ranging reviews of non-medical and medical professional regulation are due to report. It is likely that the number and functions of regulatory bodies will change. The purpose of statutory regulation is to ensure standards of care and practice and to provide protection for the public. The NMC regulates the profession and maintains a register of practitioners (Box 6.4). When a practitioner seeks employment the employer would ensure the practitioner is registered with the NMC as well as requiring a satisfactory Criminal Records Bureau check.

The law protects the title of registered nurse, midwife, etc. and it is a criminal offence to use the title without being registered with the NMC.

REFLECTIVE PRACTICE Box 6.4

Fitness to practise

Registered practitioners must be 'fit to practise', meaning that they meet standards for safe practice and work within guidelines of professional and safe practice.

Student activities

- Visit the NMC website and review the *Fitness to Practise* document (www.nmc-uk.org/(e1zplgrmpf4rem45uwvrmy55)/aSection.aspx?SectionID=7).
- Reflect on the reason(s) why a practitioner may be considered 'unfit to practise'.

The NMC *Code of professional conduct: standards for conduct, performance and ethics* (NMC 2004) (see Ch. 7) has two key functions: to inform the profession of the standard of professional conduct of registered practitioners, and to inform the public, other professionals and employers of those standards and conduct expected of professionals.

For student nurses, their training and education must include essential placement hours and core skills. These are mandatory requirements for professional registration and must be achieved by student nurses before registration. Once a nurse qualifies, the NMC continues to monitor professional development and education as a requirement for periodic registration (see Ch. 7).

The NMC provides guidance for clinical experience to student nurses (see Ch. 7). For example, student nurses must always introduce and identify themselves as students, as some patients/clients may not wish to be cared for by a student nurse. If the patient/client asks the student nurse to leave they must do so (NMC 2005a). Although student nurses are not accountable professionally to the NMC until they become registered, they can be called to account by the law or their college or university for any actions or omissions (NMC 2005a).

Contracts of employment

Employees are protected by a contract of employment but have responsibilities to the employer to fulfil their contractual obligations. Thus, the nurse's employer would have the expectation that the nurse acts in accordance with that contract, e.g. keeping confidential information secure. In an employment contract, boundaries or limitations of practice are clearly stated and responsibilities identified. It is important to be aware of how the employer and the practitioner interpret it. A job description should provide clear expectations of the practitioner and identify functions expected within that role. Contracts also protect the employer. For example, if a nurse were to practise outside their job description or contract, their employer may not accept liability for any negligent acts or omissions (see p. 155).

Direct liability is where the employer is at fault; indirect or vicarious liability is when the practitioner is at fault. Some employers accept the liability (see below) but others may not.

When disputes arise between employee and employer they may be referred to an industrial tribunal. These hear unfair dismissal, discrimination and other cases in relation to statutory employment rights as well as some breach of contract actions.

Professional indemnity insurance

The NMC recommends that registrants have professional indemnity in the event of a claim for negligence: 'Some employers accept vicarious liability for negligent acts and/or omissions of their employees' (NMC 2004, Clause 9.2, p. 12). However, this cover does not include actions outside work. Registrants working independently will need to obtain their own insurance cover. As some agency work may not be covered by insurance, registrants should check their insurance status and if necessary obtain cover through a professional organization or trade union, such as the Royal College of Nursing (RCN). It is important for practitioners to be aware of professional responsibilities and boundaries, and have an appreciation for the law.

Conscientious objection

Healthcare professionals, patients or their family may have a conscientious objection to a particular clinical procedure, e.g. termination of pregnancy. Nurses may object to their participation in abortion on religious or cultural grounds. The Abortion Act 1967 gives the nurse the right to refuse to be involved in these clinical procedures. However, the statutory right of conscientious objection does not extend to those persons more remotely connected to the abortion process (McHale & Tingle 2001). The NMC (2004, Clause 2.5, p. 5) states that:

> You must report to a relevant person or authority at the earliest possible time any conscientious objection that may be relevant to your professional practice and that you must continue to provide care to the best of your ability until alternative arrangements are implemented.

Policies, procedures and guidelines

In addition to the guidance provided by The NMC *Code of professional conduct: standards for conduct, performance and ethics* (NMC 2004), nurses have access to national guidelines and local policies, procedures and practice guidelines produced by their employer (see Ch. 5). Nurses must also consider how the law affects professional guidelines, practice and patient/client outcomes.

Documentation and record keeping

Proper documentation is a fundamental aspect of recording what nurses do and how they decide on a particular course of action. There is a saying that 'if nursing care is not written down then it did not happen'. As nursing records can be used in evidence in a variety of settings, including professional conduct hearings and courts, what is documented and how care is documented are extremely important (Box 6.5). Full and accurate records can protect the nurse if allegations of poor or negligent care are made. The NMC publication *Guidelines for Records and Record Keeping* (NMC 2005b) offers guidance and all nurses should be familiar with its contents. In addition, the Access to Health Records Act 1990 ensures that records are accurate and used appropriately by those to whom they relate and others, such as nurses and the multidisciplinary team (MDT).

The interpretation of what is written may be quite different from its intended meaning. The example in Box 6.5 may be viewed as uncaring or judgemental. It may be seen as lacking professionalism. Sparse detail and abbreviations can make the meaning unclear and open to misinterpretation if used in a court of law. Information needs to be accurate, measurable, quantifiable and qualitative. For example, '++' portrays none of these. Documentation is a means of recording data about a patient/client, which the MDT may share. Documentation that lacks clarity or meaning is dangerous and fails to achieve what it was intended to do.

REFLECTIVE PRACTICE Box 6.5

Documentation and record keeping

Sean's folder is kept at the end of his bed. It contains his drug chart, observation record, nursing progress notes and care plan. Sean's records of previous admissions, tests and doctors' notes are kept in a different folder near the nurses' station.

He can access the folder at his bedside quite easily and he does so, reading through the nurses' notes. One entry reads:

02.00 – Pt not sleeping well. Pt c/o of breathlessness throughout the night and appeared anxious. Assisted pt ++ and repositioned many times.

R. Louis Staff Nurse

04.00 – Pt spent most of the night in an upright position.

R. Louis Staff Nurse

06.00 – Still c/o of difficulty . Pt using inhalers ++ with little effect.

Oxygen therapy remains at 2 L per min and breathing remains poor. Doctor aware and for reassessment later today.

R. Louis Staff Nurse

Student activities

- Reflect on whether the nursing notes outline the care given in sufficient detail.
- Consider how Sean or a court might interpret this information.
- Discuss with your mentor the pros and cons of having patient/client notes by the bedside and accessible.

REFLECTIVE PRACTICE Box 6.6

Reporting incidents/accidents

Reflect on an incident or accident that occurred while on placement. Who completed the incident form, when was it completed and what information was recorded?

Student activities

- Access the incident form used in your clinical area.
- Consider what information needs to be recorded on the form and the questions that are asked.
- Discuss with your mentor what other documentation is required following a clinical incident and where other documentation regarding the incident must be recorded.

Reporting incidents/accidents (see Ch. 13)

Following any clinical incident – whether it is a drug error, verbal abuse or violence, or accident or injury to a patient/client, staff, visitor or member of the public – it is essential that this be reported and documented (Box 6.6). Importantly, 'near misses' should also be reported and documented.

A statement is a formal account and record of an incident or sequence of events. It is prepared by the person(s) involved, e.g. the staff nurse who witnessed the incident or was involved in the event. As an incident form has limited space to record an event, the facts should be accurate and concise. All NHS organizations will have a protocol and forms for the reporting of clinical incidents (see Ch. 13).

In the case of litigation, records of this nature are used when presenting the facts in court and referred to in an investigation. Often, this may take months and therefore accurate documentation at the time of an incident is crucial.

In addition, some incidents, e.g. an injury lasting more than 3 days or a work-related disease, must be reported to the Health and Safety Executive under Reporting of Incidents, Diseases and Dangerous Occurrences Regulations (RIDDOR) (see Ch. 13).

Duty of care and negligence

Nurses have a duty of care to patients/clients and visitors. This is the legal obligation to take reasonable care to avoid causing a person harm.

In addition, duty of care extends to off duty times. The NMC (2004, Clause 8.5, p. 11) states:

> In an emergency, in or outside the work setting, you have a professional duty to provide care. The care provided would be judged against what could reasonably be expected from someone with your knowledge, skills and abilities when placed in those particular circumstances.

Once a nurse volunteers to help in an emergency, then a duty of care is assumed.

Nurses also have contractual obligations to their employer and a professional duty to safeguard the patient/client and standards of practice.

Negligence

Negligence is an act with any element of carelessness or lack of regard resulting in injury, harm or loss. It is any act or omission that falls short of a standard to be expected from 'the reasonable man'. Negligence can result in a civil claim for compensation or in a criminal prosecution. Duty of care is an essential element in negligence claims (Box 6.7). There are three civil wrongs or torts, which must be proven for a successful claim of negligence. They are:

- A duty of care is owed
- The duty of care is breached
- The breach must have caused damage.

It is estimated that hundreds of thousands of patients are harmed each year by medical errors (National Patient Safety Agency [NPSA] 2005). However, according to the NHS Litigation Authority (NHSLA) in 2004–2005 they received 5609 claims of clinical negligence and 3766 claims of non-clinical negligence against NHS bodies (NHSLA 2005). These figures represent a reduction in claims from the previous year; clinical negligence claims for 2003–2004 were 6251, with 3819 claims of non-clinical negligence (NHSLA 2005).

? CRITICAL THINKING Box 6.7

Staff nurse Sue

Sue is a qualified nurse working a night shift in a nursing home. There are two care assistants working with Sue and a more senior nurse in charge of the home. The floor Sue is responsible for has several residents with dementia. The floor is busy and Sue is changing a dressing when she hears Joan, a resident in the next room, cry out several times.

Darren, one of the care assistants, comes in with a query and Sue asks him to check on Joan while she finishes the dressing. Meanwhile, Joan has attempted to get out of bed, falls and hits her head on the floor.

Later, an incident report (see p. 154) is completed. Joan suffered a minor head injury with swelling over one eye. Her family are informed and visit the next day. The family make a complaint about the nursing care, which eventually results in a claim for negligence.

Student activities

- Identify the acts and omissions leading up to the incident.
- Although Sue delegated responsibility to the care assistant, consider her accountability.
- Consider the three civil wrongs/torts in this case.
- How could the situation have been avoided?

Interestingly, very few clinical claims actually reach the courts, as most are either abandoned by the claimant (38.01%) or settled out of court (43.1%) (NHSLA 2005). In an analysis of all the clinical claims handled by the NHSLA since 1995, 1.97% settled in court in favour of the patient (including claims brought on behalf of children), 0.5% of those going to court found in favour of the NHS with 16.42% still not resolved (NHSLA 2005).

If a nurse has been negligent, generally it is the employer, i.e. the NHS Trust, that will be sued but a claim may also be brought against the nurse. Most claims for clinical negligence since 1995 have been in the specialities of surgery and obstetrics and gynaecology, with nursing having the smallest number of claims. If the practitioner is self-employed, personal indemnity insurance is necessary, as they would be personally liable for their actions and omissions (see pp. 153–154).

It is essential that nurses recognize their accountability. It should be emphasized that being accountable for acts, omissions and outcomes means that nurses must consider the consequences of everything they do in relation to patient/client care.

Following an incident that results in an official complaint from the patient/client or family, the NHS Trust will initiate a full and thorough investigation. A negligence claim is a lengthy process, whereby witnesses, the claimant and anyone else involved are questioned and investigated. The information is compiled such that statements given represent oral testimony of the events that occurred. Legal advice would be necessary during this process.

As mentioned earlier, there are four arenas in which nurses may be accountable and answerable for their acts and omissions: to their employer, to the NMC, in a civil court and in a criminal court. In some cases, the nurse will be answerable in all four arenas, e.g. in the event of a patient's death caused by a drug error.

Accountability to employer

Where negligence has occurred and harm caused because the nurse failed to follow reasonable instruction, guidelines or protocols, the employer has the right to take disciplinary action against the employee. For example, a staff nurse failed to check the patency of an intravenous (i.v.) cannula prior to starting an i.v. infusion containing an antibiotic. Within 15 minutes the patient complained of pain and burning at the site. The staff nurse said that this sometimes happened and not to worry. The patient continued to have pain and told another nurse who looked at their arm. The i.v. fluid containing the antibiotic had infiltrated into the tissues ('tissuing') (see Ch. 19). Fortuitously, no tissue damage had occurred.

The incident was reported and investigated and it was found that the staff nurse had not followed local guidelines for the administration of i.v. antibiotics. The patient eventually made an official complaint.

The staff nurse was required by his employer to undertake further training in i.v. therapy and drug administration and to work under direct supervision until considered to be competent. The patient and their family received an apology from the NHS Trust and were informed of the remedial action. They were satisfied and decided not to take legal action.

Should a qualified nurse fail to practise safely or work within stated guidelines and protocols, their employer may require a period of supervised practice, action plans, training, counselling, disciplinary procedures such as oral or written warnings, and possibly suspension or dismissal. They may also make a report to the NMC.

Professional accountability to the NMC

If a nurse is accused of misconduct, such as an action/omission that is found to be negligent, or they are convicted of certain criminal offences, they will be reported to the NMC. The NMC reviews the information surrounding the allegation and informs the individual of the allegation made. An Investigating Committee decides whether there is a case to answer and also decides if interim suspension or interim conditions of practice are justified. If the Investigating Committee decides there is no case to answer the case is closed. On the other hand, if there is a case to answer it will be referred to the Conduct and Competence Committee (CCC) or to the Health Committee if the nurse is considered unfit to practise by virtue of their physical or mental health. The standard of proof required by the CCC is the criminal standard, but it is likely to become the civil standard. If the CCC finds the facts proven they may, depending on the degree of unfit practice and risk to the public, decide to:

- Take no further action
- Remove or suspend the nurse from the register
- Impose conditions of practice or a caution.

Civil accountability

Nurses may encounter the civil courts in relation to negligence claims or trespass against the person (any interference with the person's bodily integrity and liberty, including assault and battery, see p. 157) or other civil wrongs that the patient/client might suffer. When a patient/client suffers harm as a result of clinical negligence, they or the family can bring an action (claim) for negligence and compensation for the harm. In order to succeed in the claim, the three civil wrongs/torts must be met (see p. 155). The law recognizes duty of care between the patient and the nurse. When determining a breach in duty of care, the nurse's conduct would be compared with what the ordinarily skilled nurse in that speciality would have done in the same circumstances, and what precautions would have been taken to avoid harm from known risks. Judges use the Bolam test when determining whether a nurse or other health professional has been negligent.

The Bolam test is a rule not only of substantive law in defining what amounts to adequate care, but is also used to determine standards of care. It is also a rule of evidence, indicating how a court determines whether adequate care has been given (Tingle & Cribb 2003). In determining the 'legal standard' of care, advice would be sought by lawyers acting for the nurse/NHS Trust, etc. and the claimant. If the case goes to court an 'expert opinion' is given by an expert witness. The judge would draw conclusions based on this standard of professional practice. It is important to note that the courts are more testing of expert evidence than in 1957.

These legal principles stem from the case of Bolam v Friern HMC [1957] 2 All ER 118 where a doctor administered electroconvulsive therapy to Mr Bolam without anaesthetic or muscle relaxants, resulting in Mr Bolam's jaw being fractured. The judge, Mr Justice McNair, stated:

> The test is the standard of the ordinary skilled man exercising and professing to have that special skill. A man need not possess the highest expert skill . . . it is sufficient if he exercises the ordinary skill of an ordinary competent man exercising that particular art. . . . a doctor is not guilty of negligence if he has acted in accordance with a practice accepted as proper by a responsible body of medical men skilled in that particular art. . . . Putting it the other way round, a doctor is not negligent if he is acting in accordance with such a practice, merely because there is a body of opinion that takes a contrary view.

His comments later became known as the 'Bolam test', which also applies to nurses and other health professionals.

Various systems exist where defended cases of negligence can be fast tracked according to the size of the claim. However, at the time of writing, an NHS Redress Scheme is proposed, whereby certain cases involving errors with hospital care can be concluded without litigation. This is dependent upon the NHS Redress Bill becoming law. In addition, a Compensation Bill has been introduced in the House of Lords; it considers the regulation of claims management and an aspect of the law of negligence (for further information, see Government Bills 2005/06, available online at www.commonsleader.gov.uk/output/Page944.asp).

Criminal accountability

Criminal law is concerned with intent, i.e. the person intended to commit the crime, or was reckless or negligent about the consequences of their actions. The nurse is answerable to a criminal court when there is an allegation that a crime has been committed, e.g. when a grossly negligent act by a nurse results in a patient's death. In such a case the nurse could be charged with manslaughter (unlawful killing of a human being where premeditation is absent) and face imprisonment. It is this type of situation that could result in the nurse being answerable in all four arenas of accountability, i.e. dismissal, action by the NMC, a civil claim as well as the criminal charge. For example, a nurse administers a drug (already drawn up in a syringe and left at the patient's bedside) without further checking or verification, and as a result the patient dies. The drug was for oral administration and led to the patient's death when given intravenously.

REFLECTIVE PRACTICE Box 6.8

Idle chatter

Two nurses are discussing a patient/client in the canteen. At surrounding tables there are other members of staff, visitors, patients and outside contractors.

The nurses' conversation, which is loud enough for others to hear, centres on a patient's long history of mental health problems.

Student activities

- What might be the consequences of other people overhearing the conversation?
- Reflect on how you would feel if you were a relative or patient/client overhearing the conversation.

[Resources: Data Protection Act 1998, the Human Rights Act 1998 (see pp. 150–151); The *NMC code of professional conduct: standards for conduct, performance and ethics* (NMC 2004, Clause 5, pp. 8–9)]

Confidentiality

Confidential information is limited to those who use it and access it, and their use must be legitimate. Nurses are responsible for protecting the confidentiality and security of the patient's/client's personal and health information (see Ch. 7). However, nurses may be required to provide information, e.g. if required by law, order of the court, if it is in the public interest or when child protection is involved. As outlined in *Confidentiality: NHS Code of Practice* (DH 2003, p. 7):

> Patient information is generally held under legal and ethical obligations of confidentiality. Information provided in confidence should not be used or disclosed in a form that might identify a patient without his or her consent, *and*
>
> A duty of confidentiality arises when one person discloses information to another (e.g. patient to clinician) in circumstances where it is reasonable to expect that the information will be held in confidence. It –
>
> - Is a legal obligation that is derived from case law
> - Is a requirement established within professional codes of conduct
> - Must be included within NHS employment contracts as a specific requirement linked to disciplinary procedures.

All written and electronic information about patients/clients must be stored securely and access limited, e.g. by password, to the care team. Confidentiality applies to written and electronic records and verbal information (Box 6.8).

Patient/client records contain a great deal of information that might identify the person, including:

- Name
- Hospital number
- Date of birth
- Address/contact details
- Marital status
- GP and address
- Place of work/occupation
- Next of kin/contact details.

In addition, records also reveal information about the person's health, lifestyle, current and past medical conditions and other confidential information.

Nurses should always 'seek patients' and clients' wishes regarding the sharing of information with their family and others' (NMC 2004, p. 9). When it is not possible to obtain permission, such as with children, some people with mental health problems and some people with learning disabilities, the nurse will need to discuss the situation with colleagues.

Breaches in confidentiality are potentially very harmful to patients/clients and families. Unauthorized or inadvertent disclosure can lead to disciplinary action by the employer or action by the regulatory body for professional misconduct (see p. 156).

Consent

Consent for care or treatment is a very important legal issue in nursing practice. It is vital that the person consents before any treatment, care, examination or assessment. It is the absolute right of an adult competent patient to give or withhold consent and in doing this prevents physical contact becoming a civil or criminal actionable wrong, namely trespass against the person, which includes assault and battery.

Assault is an attempt or offer of unlawful contact wherein the person is put in fear of violence or unlawful force. Battery is defined as unlawful contact or touching.

Very often a patient/client may give 'implied' consent, e.g. by rolling up their sleeve for blood pressure recording. However, patients still require information and explanation, such as the reason for carrying out the task, and the implications of it should be made clear to the patient/client. In some instances, such as prior to an injection, verbal consent is appropriate; however, in other instances written consent will be necessary, e.g. prior to an examination, invasive procedure or surgery.

There are three criteria needed to satisfy 'valid' consent: capacity, voluntarily, informed. A person must be able to understand the information to make a decision. They must be able to weigh up the information, and consider the consequence of having or not having the procedure. However, sometimes further information or explanation may be needed. A person may be competent to make some decisions even if they are not competent to make others. It is important to remember that obtaining consent is a continuing process, not a one-off event (DH 2001).

In order that consent is legally binding and compelling (or valid), the patient/client has to be given the information they require to make a conscientious decision, whereby they may accept or refuse treatment. They must not be forced, coerced or tricked into making the decision, nor should other professionals or institutional pressures or family or friends influence them. Consent is voluntary and the patient/client can change their mind at any time or withdraw their consent at any time.

What is sufficient information? The patient/client must always be informed of the risks involved in the proposed procedure so that they have an opportunity to avoid or reduce these risks. Thus the patient/client needs to understand in broad terms, in a language they can understand, the nature and purpose of the procedure. The person who will be carrying out the procedure usually obtains consent but registered nurses who have had special training may obtain consent in certain circumstances.

In all cases, patients/clients should be provided with sufficient information in order to make a decision. This should include the benefits and the risks, e.g. drug side effects. They should be informed of any alternative treatments or therapies. If the patient/client is not offered as much information as they need to make a decision, and in a form they can understand, then their consent may not be valid (DH 2001). In the case of Chester v Afshar [2004] 4 All ER 587 (HL) the surgeon had failed to tell a woman of a 1–2% inherent risk (i.e. a risk regardless of the surgeon's skill) of an adverse result from the operation. The claimant conceded that she would have gone ahead with the operation but would have delayed her decision in order to give it more thought. The House of Lords judgement was that the surgeon had violated the patient's right to make an informed decision. If the claimant had been fully informed of the risk, she would have still have had the same operation under identical conditions and performed by the same surgeon but on an occasion when the randomly occurring risk would probably not have happened (adapted from Tingle J, Wheat K, Readers in Law, Nottingham Trent University, Foster C, Barrister, London, 10 February 2006, personal electronic mail).

Consent in children

Children should always be consulted (subject to age and understanding) and kept informed about what is planned. The Children Act 1989 ensures children's wishes and feelings are taken into account.

The age of consent to medical treatment varies across the UK:

> ... In relation to obtaining consent for a child, the involvement of those with parental responsibility in the consent procedure is usually necessary, but will depend on the age and understanding of the child. If the child is under the age of 16 in England and Wales, 12 in Scotland and 17 in Northern Ireland, you must be aware of legislation and local protocols relating to consent.
>
> (NMC 2004, Clause 3.9, p. 7)

There are three key points in relation to age of children that need to be emphasized. They are:

- At 16 a young person can be treated as an adult and can be presumed to have capacity to decide
- Under the age of 16 children may have capacity to decide, depending on their ability to understand what is involved
- Where a competent child refuses treatment, a person with parental responsibility or the court may authorize investigation or treatment which is in the child's best interests.

Maturity is a key factor and older children can have the maturity and capacity to make important decisions about their own medical treatment whereas others may not have reached that level of maturity at the same age. It is imperative that professionals assess maturity and the individual's capacity to understand issues surrounding the proposed treatment and risks.

An important ruling regarding the competence of a child to consent to treatment is the Gillick competence (Box 6.9). In Gillick v West Norfolk and Wisbech Area Health Authority [1985] 3 All ER 402 (HL) the House of Lords ruled that a child under 16 years of age can give legally effective consent to medical treatment if they have achieved 'sufficient maturity and intelligence to enable him to understand fully what is proposed'. The test laid down in Gillick requires that the health professional must assess whether the particular child is competent to consent to a particular treatment (McHale & Tingle 2001).

Two important considerations – the child's best interests and whether they have the mental capacity to exercise their rights responsibly – restrict children's rights. Striking a balance between these two principles depends on the individual child and the situation.

In caring for children, the main priority for the nurse is to obtain valid consent from the appropriate person, i.e. the child or the person with parental responsibility. Usually this is the mother or father of very young children. However, this may not be possible, if for example a child is injured at school, in which case consent may be obtained from the teacher or child minder. The teacher would have the right to do what is 'reasonable in all circumstances' in safeguarding or promoting the child's welfare (McHale & Tingle 2001). This is further complicated by whether the treatment is in the child's best interests. Parental consent does not cover whatever treatment the parents believe

CRITICAL THINKING Box 6.9

Gillick competence: Fraser guidelines

It is considered good practice for doctors and other health professionals to follow the criteria outlined by Lord Fraser in 1985, in the House of Lords' ruling in the case of Gillick v West Norfolk and Wisbech Health Authority. The Fraser guidelines (DH 2004, p. 4) are:

- The young person understands the health professional's advice
- The health professional cannot persuade the young person to inform his or her parents or allow the doctor to inform the parents that he or she is seeking contraceptive advice
- The young person is very likely to begin or continue having intercourse with or without contraceptive treatment
- Unless he or she receives contraceptive advice or treatment, the young person's physical or mental health or both are likely to suffer
- The young person's best interests require the health professional to give contraceptive advice, treatment or both without parental consent.

Young people under the age of 16 often seek sexual health advice from a school nurse. This may include requests for emergency contraception or information about abortion.

Student activity
Ask a school nurse how they assess a young person's competence before supplying/prescribing emergency contraception.

[Resource: Department of Health (DH) 2004 Best practice guidance for doctors and other health professionals on the provision of advice and treatment to young people under 16 on contraception, sexual and reproductive health – www.dh.gov.uk/assetRoot/04/08/69/14/04086914.pdf Available September 2006]

to be in their child's best interests and any treatment is ultimately dependent upon the healthcare professional's assessment of what is appropriate for the child.

The law makes a distinction between a child's right to consent to treatment and to refuse treatment. Refusal of treatment is a complex area. According to McHale and Tingle (2001, p. 117):

> At present, even if a Gillick competent child refuses medical treatment it appears that his or her parents may override the refusal. Even so, the court in Re W ([1992] 3 WLR 758) suggested that before a major surgical procedure is undertaken on a child against the child's will, it will be desirable for the issue to be referred to the court. The court will then determine what is in the child's best interests, taking into account the child's expressed wishes and the strength of the child's beliefs.

Parents and/or children may refuse consent for treatment. For example, a parent refuses consent and the child is unable due to critical illness. Consideration of the child's best interests is vital. In this instance healthcare professionals should hesitate before giving treatment and consider the potential outcomes of giving the treatment or of withholding treatment. Often it is the urgency of the child's condition that dictates justification for treatment without parental consent. For example, if the child is bleeding to death, then it is justifiable to treat, even in the face of parental opposition (McHale & Tingle 2001). In some cases the courts make the decision.

In other circumstances, refusal may be from both the parent and child, e.g. where the child and family are refusing a blood transfusion according to the teaching of their religion (Jehovah's Witness). In such a situation the outcomes and consequence of refusal must be made clear to both the child and parents. The dilemma for health professionals is if that refusal could lead to the death of that child. Authorization for treatment would be dependent upon the court's decision.

Consent – people with learning disability or fluctuating mental capacity

There are situations where capacity may be in doubt. For example, a patient/client may not understand what they have been told or they may appear confused. The nurse may need to assess if the patient/client is capable of making a particular decision. This can be especially difficult in some patients/clients who have a learning disability or suffer from fluctuating mental capacity.

In the case of Re C [1994] All ER 819 the court upheld the right of a man with serious mental health problems to prevent amputation of his gangrenous foot in the future without his written consent. Thorpe. J. proposed a three-question test to establish if the patient/client possessed capacity. The three questions asked were:

- Did the patient comprehend the information given?
- Did patient believe it?
- Had the patient weighed up the information, balancing needs and risks, before reaching a decision?

(McHale & Tingle 2001).

A difficulty with the test used in Re C arises because capacity is dependent upon the information given (Grubb 1994). For example, a nurse provides a patient/client with complex information about a procedure requiring consent. If the information includes medical terms, the patient may not understand the information given. However, if the patient/client is given a clear, simple explanation about the same procedure, in non-technical language that they can understand, then they may have possessed the necessary capacity to consent.

Nurses must carefully consider what they say and how it is said. The views of the patient/client and their relatives/carers are equally important in assessing the person's capacity to understand and give consent. In addition, awareness that the patient may have the capacity to make one decision, but at the same time is incapable of making another, has led to the conclusion that such a test for capacity should be decision specific.

Providing care for someone with a learning disability may present some difficulties (Box 6.10).

REFLECTIVE PRACTICE Box 6.10

The 'Bournewood' case

A man, aged 40 years, was unable to speak and had limited understanding. He had a history of self-harming behaviour and frequent outbursts of agitation. For over 30 years the man was cared for in an NHS hospital.

He was discharged on a trial basis but after an incident where he became agitated with self-harming behaviour he was detained in hospital under the MHA 1983. Because the man was compliant and did not resist admission, he was admitted as an informal patient (see p. 151) in his own best interests under the common law principle of necessity.

Legal action was commenced to secure his discharge from hospital. This was unsuccessful in the High Court but later the Court of Appeal held that the man had been unlawfully detained, and that because of the MHA 1983 the common law principle of necessity could not be used to detain someone for treatment for a mental health disorder. The man was formally detained under the MHA 1983 and later discharged.

The House of Lords overturned the Court of Appeal's judgment and the case was taken to the European Court of Human Rights. This Court found that there had been a violation of Articles 5(1) Right to Liberty and 5(4) Right to Security.

Student activities

- Reflect on the decision of the European Court of Human Rights.
- Discuss with your mentor how this judgement affects your area of practice.

[Resource: Department of Health 2005 'Bournewood' consultation. The approach to be taken in response to the judgment of the European Court of Human Rights in the 'Bournewood' case – www.dh.gov.uk Available July 2006]

REFLECTIVE PRACTICE Box 6.11

Refusal of medical treatment

In the case of Ms B v An NHS Trust it was clear to all concerned that she would die once treatment ceased. The implications for other refusals of treatment are not always so clear-cut.

Student activities

- Locate information about other cases, such as Re MB [1997] 2 FLR 426 (McHale & Tingle 2001, pp. 93, 198–200). Consider the events in this case.
- Compare the case of MB with that of Ms B and discuss it with your mentor.

[Resource: BBC 22 March 2002 Q & A: Right-to-die decision – http://news.bbc.co.uk/1/hi/health/1887286.stm Available July 2006]

The case described in Box 6.10 has important implications for the organizations and the people involved in the treatment and care of individuals who lack capacity to consent to treatment. The man's rights had not been breached simply because he was admitted to hospital in his best interests rather than under the MHA 1983, but because procedural safeguards surrounding his admission had failed to protect him.

The recommendations from this case included proper assessments of those incapacitated and unable to make such decisions, alternatives to hospital or residential admissions, and that appropriate information be given to patients, family and carers.

The Mental Capacity Act

The Mental Capacity Act 2005 provides a statutory framework for decision-making on behalf of adults (see Table 6.1), thus protecting vulnerable adults and their carers, and professionals. In Scotland, the Adults with Incapacity (Scotland) Act 2000 fulfils a similar function.

The Mental Capacity Act 2005 has a long history, which started with a Law Commission Report (number 231) (Mental Incapacity) in 1995, followed by a lengthy consultation, a draft Mental Incapacity Bill in 2003 and eventually a renamed Mental Capacity Bill in 2004, which became law in 2005.

The Act applies to adults who lose mental capacity, e.g. due to dementia in later life and to people who lack mental capacity due to conditions present at birth, e.g. some forms of learning disability. The Act governs decisions about welfare and health, financial matters and participation in research. It also includes a new scheme for lasting power of attorney, which may include health-related decisions. It makes clear who can take decisions in which situations and how they should go about this. It starts from the fundamental premise that a person has capacity and that all practical steps must be taken to help the person make a decision.

Right to refuse treatment

A competent adult patient has an absolute right to refuse or withdraw from treatment or change their mind about treatment. Their decision must be respected, even if it results in death; for example, the case of Ms B v An NHS Trust [2002] 2 All ER 449 in which Dame Elizabeth Butler-Sloss made the judgement that Ms B had the necessary mental capacity to refuse treatment, which in this case meant switching off the ventilator and allowing her to die (Box 6.11).

One way in which patients/clients can maintain control or choice in decisions about their health or life or circumstance (when their mental capacity is altered) is through the use of advance directives (referred to as an advance decision to refuse treatment in the Mental Capacity Act 2005).

Advance directive

An advance directive is a legally binding statement prepared in advance by a competent adult before they lose the mental capacity to make decisions. It allows the person to give or withhold consent at a point where their lack of capacity would normally exclude them (Tingle & Cribb 2003). An advance directive specifies the person's

CRITICAL THINKING Box 6.12

Advance directives

There is sometimes confusion about what an advance directive can do and the criteria that must be met for it to be valid.

Student activities

Visit the Age Concern website below and find answers to the following questions:

- What are the criteria required for a valid advance directive?
- How many witnesses are required and who should not witness it?
- Can a person refuse basic nursing care in an advance directive?
- Who should know that the advance directive exists?

[Resource: Age Concern 2005 Advance statements, advance directives and living wills – www.ageconcern.org.uk/AgeConcern/Documents/IS5_1005.pdf]

wish to refuse some or all medical treatment and the circumstances when the refusal would apply (Box 6.12).

Advance directives must be clearly drafted, with full understanding of their implications, and cover circumstances which may occur (Tingle & Cribb 2003). They are subject to restrictive interpretation:

- The person must have had the capacity at the time of making the statement
- Only clear refusals of specified treatment may be upheld
- If there is any doubt about the validity of the advance directive, a declaration may be obtained or treatment given in line with the best interests of the patient.

An advance directive can provide a useful guide as to what treatment should not be given and in what circumstances. It is vital, however, to note that such a document does not authorize an action that is unlawful, such as euthanasia. The Mental Capacity Act 2005 sets out rules about advance directives to refuse treatment (see p. 160) and will become the legal authority for advance directives in 2007. Many uncertainties surround their use, e.g. a person's circumstances can change after the advance directive has been written. In some cases, years may pass before it is revisited (often at the time of illness/injury) and thus the validity of competence at the time of its writing may be questioned. Lack of specificity can present problems for healthcare professionals. The provision of lasting power of attorney may offer some resolutions (see 'The Mental Capacity Act 2005', p. 160).

End-of-life issues

End-of-life issues – including withholding/withdrawing treatment and 'do not attempt resuscitation' (DNAR), also called 'do not resuscitate' (DNR), orders – present healthcare professionals with legal, ethical and professional issues to resolve. Although detailed coverage is beyond the scope of this chapter, it is important that nurses are aware of the issues (see also Chs 7, 12, 17). While it is likely that nursing students will encounter some of these situations, they will not be directly involved in decision-making but should take the opportunity to observe and discuss the issues that arise with their mentor. Box 6.13 provides suggestions for sources of information about some of these issues.

Box 6.13 **End-of-life issues, information sources**

Specific sources

1. Withholding or withdrawing treatment:
   - Airedale NHS Trust v Bland [1993] 1 All ER 821 – the landmark case concerning Anthony Bland who was left in a permanent vegetative state (PVS) following the Hillsborough disaster. Artificial feeding was not in the best interests of the patient and could be withdrawn.
2. Assisted dying and euthanasia:
   - Assisted Dying for the Terminally Ill Bill (HL), reintroduced into Parliament in November 2005 – www.publications.parliament.uk/pa/Id200506/Idbills/036/2006036.htm Available July 2006
   - Royal College of Nursing (2004) confirms opposition to Assisted Dying Bill and calls for improved palliative care. RCN press release – www.rcn.org.uk/news/display.php?ID=1255&area=Press Available July 2006
   - Judgements – The Queen on the Application of Mrs Dianne Pretty (Appellant) v Director of Public Prosecutions (Respondent) and Secretary of State for the Home Department (Interested Party) 29 November 2001 – www.parliament.the-stationery-office.co.uk/ Available July 2006
3. Organ donation and transplant:
   - Human Tissue Act – www.opsi.gov.uk/acts/en2004/2004en30.htm Available July 2006
   - UK Transplant – www.uktransplant.org.uk. Available July 2006
4. Do not attempt resuscitation orders:
   - A joint statement from the British Medical Association, the Resuscitation Council (UK) and the Royal College of Nursing 2002 – www.bma.org.uk/ap.nsf/Content/cardioresus Available July 2006

General sources

- Garwood-Gowers A, Tingle J, Wheat K 2005 Contemporary issues in healthcare and ethics. Butterworth-Heinemann, Oxford
- Johnstone MJ 2005 Bioethics. A nursing perspective. 4th edn. Churchill Livingstone, Edinburgh
- UK Clinical Ethics Network – www.ethics-network.org.uk/Ethics/ethics.htm Available July 2006

Summary

- The law is constantly evolving and it is essential for practitioners to be aware of new developments.
- Duty of care and accountability for practice are central responsibilities for nurses in every discipline.
- Nurses are accountable to their employer, the statutory regulating body (NMC) and the criminal and civil courts.
- Clinical negligence claims and other litigation are important to nurses and their practice.
- Complex issues that include consent to treatment, refusal or withdrawal of treatment and mental capacity affect all nurses.

Self test

1. What are the sources of law in the UK?
2. Why is the Human Rights Act so important to nurses?
3. What is duty of care?
4. Name the four arenas of accountability for nurses.
5. Which of the following is essential for valid consent?
   a. It is written
   b. It is implied
   c. It is obtained by carers
   d. It is voluntary.
6. What is an advance directive?

Key words and phrases for literature searching

Civil law	Duty of care
Confidentiality	Legislation
Consent	Liability
Criminal law	Negligence

Useful websites

Department of Health	www.dh.gov.uk Available July 2006
Health and Safety Executive	www.hse.gov.uk Available July 2006
Law Commission	www.lawcom.gov.uk Available July 2006
Nursing and Midwifery Council	www.nmc-uk.org Available July 2006
Office of Public Sector Information (*source for legislation throughout the UK*)	www.opsi.gov.uk Available July 2006

References

Department of Health (DH) 1983 Mental Health Act. HMSO, London

Department of Health (DH) 2001 12 Key points on consent: the law in England. HMSO, London

Department of Health (DH) 2003 Confidentiality: NHS code of practice. Online: www.dh.gov.uk/PublicationsAndStatistics/Publications/PublicationsPolicyAndGuidance/PublicationsPolicyAndGuidanceArticle/fs/en?CONTENT_ID=4069253&chk=jftKB%2B Available July 2006

Dimond B 1995 Legal aspects of nursing. 2nd edn. Prentice Hall, London

Grubb A 1994 cited in McHale J, Tingle J 2001 Law and nursing. 2nd edn. Butterworth-Heinemann, Edinburgh

Information Commissioner 2005 Data Protection Act Factsheet. Online: www.informationcommissioner.gov.uk/eventual.aspx?id=34 Available July 2006

McHale J, Gallagher A 2004 Nursing and human rights. Butterworth-Heinemann, Edinburgh

McHale J, Tingle J 2001 Law and nursing. 2nd edn. Butterworth-Heinemann, Edinburgh

NHSLA 2005 Key facts. Online: www.nhsla.com/home.htm Available July 2006

NPSA 2005 Annual review 04/05. Online: www.npsa.nhs.uk/web/display?contentId=4331 Available July 2006

Nursing and Midwifery Council (NMC) 2004 Code of professional conduct: standards for conduct, performance and ethics. NMC, London

Nursing and Midwifery Council (NMC) 2005a Students – guidance on clinical experience. Online. Available: www.nmc-uk.org

Nursing and Midwifery Council (NMC) 2005b Guidelines for records and record keeping. NMC, London

The Mental Health (Care and Treatment) (Scotland) Act 2003 Online: www.scotland.gov.uk/Publications/2003/11/18547/29201 Available July 2006

Tingle J, Cribb A 2003 Nursing law and ethics. 2nd edn. Blackwell, Oxford

Further reading

Butterworth C 2005 Ongoing consent to care for older people in care homes. Nursing Standard. 19(20):40–5.

Children's Legal Centre 2005 Working with young people: legal responsibility and liability. 6th edn. Children's Legal Centre, Colchester

Dimond B 2005 Legal aspects of nursing. 4th edn. Pearson, Harlow

Hutchinson C 2005 Addressing issues related to adult patients who lack the capacity to give consent. Nursing Standard 16(19):47–53

Martin J 2005 Clinical negligence and patient compensation. Nursing Standard 19(25):35–39

McInroy A 2005 Blood transfusions and Jehovah's Witnesses: the legal and ethical issues. British Journal of Nursing 14(5):270–274

Pearce L 2005 Good counsel. Nursing Standard 19(24):17–18

7

The *NMC Code of conduct* and applied ethical principles

Dorothy Horsburgh

Glossary terms

Accountability
Autonomy
Beneficence
Code of conduct
Confidentiality
Consequentialist ethics
Deontological ethics
Ethics
Justice
Morals
Non-maleficence
Respect for persons
Virtue ethics

Learning outcomes

This chapter will help you:

- Outline the role of the Nursing and Midwifery Council (NMC) in protecting the public within the UK
- Demonstrate a knowledge of the NMC's *Code of professional conduct: standards for conduct, performance and ethics*
- Discuss the relationship between students of nursing and the NMC
- Discuss, in an informed manner, the implications of professional regulation for nursing practice
- Demonstrate an awareness of, and apply ethical principles and theories to, nursing practice
- Identify, and reflect upon, ethical issues in everyday nursing practice.

(Adapted from NMC 2005a)

Introduction

Registered nurses (RNs) practise in a variety of care settings and provide care for individuals who have a wide range of needs. Nursing students receive a generic preparation for practice for the first 12 months of their 3-year programme. By the end of this period they are required to have achieved specified outcomes (NMC 2005a) in order to progress to their chosen Branch Programme, during which they specialize in caring for people in one of the following areas:

- Adults who have physical health problems
- People who have mental health problems
- Child health
- People who have learning disabilities.

People who require nursing care are in a vulnerable position by virtue of the problems for which they require assistance. It is therefore important that they are afforded protection and the purpose of this chapter is to describe and discuss the ways in which protection is provided and some of the challenges that student nurses and registered practitioners may encounter in their everyday practice. This chapter should be read in conjunction with Chapter 6, which deals specifically with legal issues and nursing. The focus of this chapter is the requirements that the statutory regulatory body (NMC) has of registered nurses and the implications for nursing students. The focus is also upon the ethical and moral issues that are integral to nursing practice.

The role of the Nursing and Midwifery Council

Protection of the public

Since 1919, when the Nurses' Registration Act was passed, public protection has been provided by a statutory body, originally named the General Nursing Council (GNC). Changes in policy and in the statutory regulatory body's remit over time resulted in replacement of the General Nursing Council by the United Kingdom Central Council (UKCC) in 1992. The Nursing and Midwifery Council (NMC) has fulfilled this role since 2002.

Quality assurance of educational programmes

The NMC has a UK-wide remit for the quality assurance of educational programmes that lead to registration as a nurse, midwife or health visitor and all other recordable NMC qualifications, e.g. specialist practitioner. There are national differences in UK health and education policy and provision, and therefore the NMC has service level agreements with relevant bodies to deliver its educational quality assurance framework. This is carried by:

- 'Visitors' representing the NMC in England
- NHS Education Scotland (NES)
- Health Professions Wales (HPW)
- The Northern Ireland Practice and Education Council for Nursing and Midwifery (NIPEC).

Further information relating to the remit of the above, and general and specific information about the NMC, can be found at www.nmc-uk.org.

Registration of students as qualified practitioners

Protection of the public has remained a constant feature of the regulatory body and this function includes regulation of the preparation for practice of students and the criteria for their registration as qualified practitioners. Students are required, on successful completion of their pre-registration programme, to provide a self-declaration of good health and good character. This declaration must be supported by the registered nurse (whose name has been notified to the NMC) responsible for the overall direction of the students' educational programme at the approved educational institution. This person must also verify students' attainment of the theoretical and practical competencies required for registration (NMC 2005a, p. 10).

Register of practitioners

A central role of the NMC is maintenance of a register of practitioners and supervision of their subsequent practice. Periodic re-registration of practitioners requires evidence of the individual's continuing fitness to practise, which includes ongoing professional development. The NMC's requirements in relation to post-registration education and practice (PREP) are set out in *The PREP Handbook* (NMC 2005b).

The Nursing and Midwifery Council's Register

In 2004 the NMC replaced a complex 15-part register with a simplified three-part register:

- Nurses – this has separate parts for specialisms in Adult Nursing, Mental Health Nursing, Child Nursing and Learning Disability Nursing. There is a second level part for existing enrolled nurses, but this is closed to new applicants.
- Midwives
- Specialist community public health nurses.

Post-registration education and practice

The purpose of PREP is to ensure the best possible provision of care for patients by ensuring that all registered practitioners update and develop their practice. The PREP requirements are professional standards, set by the NMC and required by law for renewal of registration. There are two separate PREP standards, one of which relates to continuing professional development (CPD), which the NMC identifies as a key component of clinical governance. Clinical governance essentially means that the quality of nursing care that people receive should be of an equally acceptable standard, in all care settings in the UK, rather than allowing for variation from one area to another. The second PREP standard relates to the minimum number of hours for which practitioners must have worked, by virtue of their registration, during the previous 5 years.

To fulfil PREP requirements practitioners identify their own learning needs and the activities by which these may best be met. They are required to document these activities and to produce this record (see Ch. 4) if required to do so by the NMC.

Fitness to practise

Allegations made against practitioners of misconduct or unfitness to practise (e.g. due to ill health or drug misuse) are investigated by the NMC and, if these are upheld, action is taken. Depending on the nature of the offence the practitioner may be reprimanded, or alternatively their name may be removed from the register, thus removing their right to practise as a nurse. If unfitness to practice due to ill health is found to be the case, then treatment may be necessary before the person can continue to practise. The NMC also provides advice for nurses in relation to standards of professional practice (NMC 2002a).

Provision of information

The NMC publishes documents, on a wide variety of aspects of professional practice. These are reviewed and updated on a regular basis, following consultation with practitioners and other interested groups.

It provides the UK public (including practitioners, employers and clients) with information about the standards that are expected of all registered nurses and midwives. The purpose of these documents is to establish the standards expected of practitioners by the statutory body that act as benchmarks against which nursing practice may be measured. The aim of this is to ensure that a satisfactory standard of care is provided and, where necessary, enhanced.

NMC expectations of nursing students

Nursing students are not professionally accountable during their preparation for practice: the individual accountable for the consequences of their actions and omissions is the registered practitioner with whom they work. This person is usually referred to as a mentor or preceptor and will have undergone preparation for this role. The expectations of nursing students are set out in *An NMC Guide for Students of Nursing and Midwifery* (NMC 2002b). Students are not, however, absolved from being called to account for the consequences of their actions and omissions by their university and/or the law. As the purpose of the NMC's guidance to students is to prepare them for practice as registered practitioners, the following section will describe and discuss the *Code of Professional Conduct: Standards for Conduct, Performance and Ethics* (NMC 2004) with which registered nurses must comply. Examination of the *Code of Professional Conduct* will place in context the subsequent discussion of the NMC's guidance to students. Implications for students in practice placements will then be discussed using practical examples to highlight relevant points. The *Code of Professional Conduct* is not intended to provide practitioners with specific answers to each and every situation, but to set out the overall standards with which their practice must comply.

The *Code of professional conduct*

While the *Code of professional conduct: standards for conduct, performance and ethics* (NMC 2004) applies to registered nurses and not students, it is a good idea to obtain a copy now, if you have not already done so. It is important that, by the point of registration, you have understood and internalized the elements of the Code and their relevance to your future practice. Your university should be able to provide a copy or, alternatively, copies may be obtained from the Publications Department of the NMC (see 'Useful websites', p. 180).

The purpose of the *Code of professional conduct* (NMC 2004) is to:

- inform the professions [nursing and midwifery] of the standard of professional conduct required of them in the exercise of their professional accountability and practice
- inform the public, other professions and employers of the standard of professional conduct that they can expect of a registered practitioner.

Registered nurses are expected to:

- Provide protection and support for the health of individual patients and clients
- Protect and support the health of the wider community
- Act (whether at work or not) in a way that justifies the trust and confidence placed in them by the public
- Uphold and enhance the reputation of the nursing profession.

Registered nurses are individually accountable for their actions and omissions, independent of the advice, directions, actions or omissions of other professionals. In addition to professional accountability, registered nurses are legally accountable for their practice (see Ch. 6). The lines of accountability, and the implications of these for practitioners, will be discussed later in this chapter.

In caring for patients and clients, the NMC (2004) identifies the requirements of the practitioner (Box 7.1).

Box 7.1 NMC requirements of practitioners

In caring for patients and clients, you must:

- Respect the patient or client as an individual
- Obtain consent before you give any treatment or care
- Protect confidential information
- Cooperate with others in the team
- Maintain your professional knowledge and competence
- Be trustworthy
- Act to identify and minimize risk to patients and clients.

[From NMC (2004)]

Respecting the patient or client as an individual

This involves ensuring that the patient or client is consulted in all aspects of their care and that their preferences, wherever possible, are taken into account. Care provision should be of an equally high standard for all patients irrespective of:

- Gender
- Age
- Race
- Ability
- Sexual orientation
- Socioeconomic status
- Lifestyle
- Cultural, religious or political beliefs.

Any conscientious objection to providing care, e.g. an objection to providing care for a person who is to undergo termination of pregnancy, must be reported at the earliest opportunity to the appropriate person (e.g. line manager) and, until alternative arrangements are made, the nurse should continue to provide care.

Appropriate boundaries must be maintained between nurses and their patients or clients, i.e. avoidance of overlap between professional and personal relationships, and care must always focus on the needs of patients or clients (Ch. 9).

Obtaining consent before giving treatment or care

Patients and clients should be provided with the information required in order to give what is termed 'informed consent' (Chs 6, 24). If the capacity of the patient or client to understand, retain and act upon information is questionable, then alternative arrangements will need to be made (see Ch. 6). For example, an individual may be granted power of attorney to make decisions on behalf of a patient/client.

Protecting confidential information

Information about patients or clients must be treated as confidential and used only for the purposes for which it has been provided, i.e. provision of healthcare. Patients and clients may assume that information about them will be shared among relevant members of the healthcare team, but disclosure of information outwith the care team, including provision of information to relatives or friends of the patient or client, should only be carried out with the patient or client's consent (see p. 165).

Cooperating with others in the team

The team includes the patient or client and their family and/or friends, as well as informal carers and professional providers of health and social care. It may also include workers in the independent and voluntary sectors. Nurses are expected to work along with these people in provision of care, including maintenance of healthcare records and communication of relevant information to other team members. Registered nurses, even while working within a team, remain individually accountable for their own actions.

Maintaining professional knowledge and competence

This is closely linked with the earlier section in this chapter on post-registration education and practice. In addition to maintaining knowledge and competence, nurses must recognize their limitations and only undertake practice in which they are competent.

Being trustworthy

This involves behaving in a way that upholds the reputation of the nursing profession. It is important to realize that this relates not only to behaviour while at work, but at all times, and includes behaviour that is not directly related to professional practice.

The NMC also emphasizes that registration must not be used to promote commercial products or services, e.g. a particular type of wound dressing or drug. Any potential conflict of interest between a nurse's ability to provide impartial care and a financial interest must be brought, by the nurse, to the attention of their employer and/or the NMC to protect patient care.

Acting to identify and minimize risk to patients and clients

If nurses consider that the environment for patient or client care is unsafe then they must report this to a senior person, both verbally and in writing. Examples of an unsafe environment include not only the physical surroundings, but also staffing levels and competence of practitioners. It includes any concern that a nurse has about the fitness to practise, for whatever reason, of another member of the care team.

Even outwith work, nurses have a professional obligation to provide care in an emergency situation. The standard of care provided is that which could reasonably be expected of a nurse with equivalent experience, placed in similar circumstances.

While the readers of this book are nursing students, not registered practitioners, it is necessary that they are aware of the standards with which they will be expected to comply on completion of their educational programme.

While the requirements of the *Code of Professional Conduct* (NMC 2004) may, at first sight, appear to be clear, unambiguous and uncontestable, it will be seen that challenges for practitioners in practice may arise in relation to them all.

Implications of the *Code of professional conduct* for nursing students

As nursing is a practice-based occupation, placements that provide students with first-hand experience of nursing care are a vital component in preparation for becoming registered practitioners. During placements students should work only under the direct supervision of a registered nurse (RN). This does not mean that the RN requires to be physically present at all times, but it does entail that the RN should be aware, at all times, of the student's location and activities. The RN is accountable for the consequences of the actions and omissions of the student and is therefore required to be conversant with the students' programme and their stage within it.

One element of the *Code of Professional Conduct* reminds RNs that they 'have a duty to facilitate students of nursing and others to develop their competence' (NMC 2004, clause 6.4). RNs are therefore under an obligation to teach and supervise students, while students have a responsibility to develop the stipulated proficiencies prior to being registered as a nurse (NMC 2005a, Table 2.3). This includes ensuring that the care that students provide does not exceed their current level of understanding and competence. If students consider that they are requested or required to carry out activities for which they are unprepared, then this should be identified, at the time, to their mentor or to the RN who is in charge of the placement. It is also advisable for students to notify a member of the teaching staff from their educational institution. The fact that students are not professionally accountable to the NMC does not mean that they are unaccountable to their higher education institution (whose recommendation to the NMC is a prerequisite for their registration) or to the law.

Patients and clients are at the centre of healthcare and their wishes must be respected at all times. Students should identify their status, if the client does not already know this, in order that the latter may indicate acceptance or refusal of their care provision. (Indeed, it is a criminal offence for individuals to represent themselves falsely and knowingly as registered nurses.) If a patient or client refuses care from students, or asks them to leave while care is being carried out, then students must comply with this. While the majority of patients and clients accept that students' participation in nursing care is an integral component of their preparation for practice as an RN, respect for the rights of the patient/client overrides students' rights to knowledge and experience (NMC 2002b, p. 4). Similarly, if a patient, client or their friends or family voice disquiet at any aspect of care, students should refer this immediately to their mentor or the RN in charge of the placement at the time. Students should also be familiar with the local policy for documenting concerns or complaints, as there may be some variation in the specific procedure within different areas of practice.

Confidentiality

Patients and clients provide information that is frequently of 'a sensitive nature', as defined by the Data Protection Act (HM Government 1998a). Patients and clients therefore need to be assured that information provided is not divulged, other than for the purpose for which it was supplied, i.e. their healthcare. If, for example, students describe the care provision for a specific patient/client within a written assignment, then they must ensure that patient/client and placement details are anonymized, e.g. by using a pseudonym. Students must also avoid talking about patients/clients when their conversation may be overheard and, if discussing patient/client care in, for example, a reflective session in their educational establishment, then they need to take the same measures to protect confidentiality.

Access to patient and client records

Access to patient/client records should be in relation only to the need to implement effective care and local policies and practices on handling and storage of records must be adhered to (Ch. 6). Documentation by students of care that they have provided should be carried out under supervision of an RN and the RN should countersign the student's signature. The NMC has advice within the *Code of professional conduct* (NMC 2004) specific to confidentiality and a document providing guidelines for records and record keeping (NMC 2005c), with which students should familiarize themselves.

Confidentiality in practice

Maintaining confidentiality of information provided by patients/clients is not always clear-cut, as the following situation illustrates.

The situation outlined in Box 7.2 illustrates a number of points, one of which is the importance of ensuring that patients and clients are made aware of a student's status. Students are frequently involved in direct, and often intimate, care provision and thus may be viewed by patients/clients as approachable and someone in whom they may confide information that they might be more hesitant to reveal to qualified staff. As can be seen in the situation

ETHICAL ISSUES Box 7.2

Maintaining confidentiality?

You are undertaking a placement in a surgical ward. It is suspected by the qualified staff that Katie, a 37-year-old patient who has been admitted to the ward via the Accident and Emergency Unit, has sustained injuries that are non-accidental and the nature of which preclude their having been self-inflicted. While you are assisting Katie to carry out personal hygiene, she tells you that her partner was the perpetrator. She emphasizes that this information should not be passed on to anyone else.

Student activities

- What should you, as a student, do in this situation?
- Write down the reasons for your answer.

described in Box 7.2, this degree of intimacy may place students in a difficult position. On the one hand, there is a requirement to maintain confidentiality and to accede to individual wishes (NMC 2004); on the other hand, there is the need to ensure that qualified staff have access to all information that is relevant to a patient's/client's care.

It is useful to refer at this point to the *Code of professional conduct*, which addresses issues related to confidentiality (NMC 2004, clause 5). This points out that, as it is impractical to obtain consent on each occasion that information sharing is required, it is important that patients/clients are made aware, when their care commences, that some information may need to be shared with other members of the care team. It is not clear, in the scenario, whether Katie was given this information in advance of her contact with the student. In situations in which information may need to be disclosed outwith the immediate care team, the person's consent should be obtained. If consent is withheld, disclosure is only justifiable when:

- It is required by a law or order of a court
- It is believed by those involved in the patient's/client's care that divulging information is in the wider public interest, i.e. to prevent harm to the patient/client or to a third party
- There is an issue of child protection, in which case action must be taken in accordance with national and local policies.

For the student, the answer is that they should explain to Katie that the information provided cannot be kept confidential. The student is not in a position in which non-disclosure of the information would be justifiable, as it is the responsibility of students to ensure that information relevant to patients'/clients' current and future care is passed to their mentor or to the RN in charge of the placement at the time. However, this situation also raises the issue that, when an assurance of confidentiality cannot be provided to a patient or client, they should be informed of this and of the rationale for the decision.

For the RN to whom this information is divulged, there is an obligation to discuss its implications with other members of the care team, as it may impact upon the patient's/client's current and future care requirements. It is also important to document the information in their notes (NMC 2005c). In relation to divulgence of the information beyond the immediate care team who are responsible for the patient's/client's welfare, the position is less clear. It might be argued that information should be passed to the police, for example, in order to investigate the allegations made and to provide protection for the patient/client from further harm. However, Katie is an adult and there is no indication within the scenario that she lacks the mental capacity (Ch. 6) to make her own decisions.

Qualified staff might discuss the situation and the potential consequences for Katie of reporting, or not reporting, the matter to the police, but if she refuses to make a statement then there is little that the staff can do. Respecting Katie's wishes may cause disquiet among staff as to the possibility that future harm may result, but this may not be a justification for interference. Indeed, it is difficult to predict the outcomes of actions and omissions and reporting of the incident could, at least in Katie's view, have the potential to create further problems.

It would probably be the case that the staff would discuss with Katie the possibility that she could, at a future date, bring a charge against her partner and that documentation of her current condition and care would be available should she wish to call upon it. Staff might also provide Katie with information about sources of support, both formal and informal (e.g. family, workplace colleagues, Samaritans, Women's refuge, police), which she could draw on if she chose to do so.

Katie's situation presents a dilemma to staff, i.e. it is a problem that does not have a clear-cut solution. Whichever action, or inaction, the staff consider most appropriate is likely to cause them disquiet at the time and on subsequent reflection.

If a child is involved there is no room for debate. If Katie had divulged that her partner was abusing her 12-year-old child, then the situation would be quite different, as is made clear by the *Code of professional conduct* (NMC 2004, clause 5.4) and the law (see Ch. 6). In such circumstances it would be explained to the woman that, as the welfare of a child was in question, the information would have to be reported to Social Services in order that they could investigate the situation.

Ethical principles

Having discussed the situation in Box 7.2 in general terms, it is now useful to examine it further, in order to identify the principles underpinning the decisions that might be made. The ethical principles that will be identified are sometimes referred to as being prima facie. The phrase means 'at first sight', i.e. each principle should be respected 'at first sight' but, in the light of the situation, another principle might need to take precedence. For example, autonomy (the right to make one's own decisions) appears, at first sight, to be one that should be respected, but there may be circumstances in which another principle would override it. This will be identified in the discussion that follows.

Autonomy and justice

Within Western societies, great importance is placed on autonomy. The word autonomy literally means to be 'self-governing', but clearly within society there are limits upon the degree to which one may exercise autonomy. For example, it is usually accepted that the right of one individual to exercise autonomy should not interfere with the rights of other individuals to exercise their autonomy. The right of one person to hold regular noisy parties would interfere with the rights of others to have a peaceful night's sleep. The right of one person to drive recklessly interferes with the rights of other individuals to use the roads in safety. In situations such as reckless driving and breach of the peace, society usually places legal penalties upon those who infringe or threaten the rights of others. So, autonomy may be exercised, provided that harm is not caused to others in the process.

In Katie's situation, exercise of autonomy in refusing to report the injuries to the police does not directly appear to interfere with the rights of others. (Indeed, were the staff to ignore the patient's wishes and report the matter to the police, a prosecution would be unlikely, in the absence of the victim's cooperation.) Were the welfare of a child involved, the patient's 'autonomy' could, and should, be overruled, as the patient is not able to make a decision that would place a child at risk of continuing abuse.

Non-maleficence and beneficence

The reason that staff who might wish to intervene on the woman's behalf would probably put forward would be the desire to prevent harm to the patient (an idea known as non-maleficence) and to act in the patient's best interest (known as beneficence). There is also the problem that consequences of actions or omissions are difficult to predict: anticipated harms or benefits may not materialize in reality. Identification of 'best interests' can also be problematic, as the attitudes, values and beliefs that individuals bring to any situation will influence the decisions that they make (Ch. 1). Actions that nursing staff may consider to be in patients' best interests are not necessarily ones with which patients would agree. A respect for patients, the importance of which is emphasized by the *Code of professional conduct* (NMC 2004), indicates that staff should comply with patients' wishes when these are clearly expressed and when the patient has the legal capacity to make decisions (Ch. 6).

Client autonomy in healthcare is not always straightforward, as the right to autonomy is usually based on a person having insight into the consequences of their actions or omissions. (One would not consider a small child to be autonomous, for example, in their desire to run across a busy road to reach the park. Interference would be considered not only justifiable, but mandatory.) In order to be autonomous therefore, patients need to be provided with the information upon which to base their decisions and be able to understand, retain and act

REFLECTIVE PRACTICE Box 7.3

Too many patients and too few staff

In a busy placement there are several patients who need assistance to eat and drink, but only a few staff on duty. Some patients will therefore have to wait longer than others for their meal that may be cold by the time they receive it.

Student activities

Identify a practice placement in which several patients or clients required help with an activity of living, e.g. washing, dressing, eating, bathing, and:

- Identify how staff decided which patient or client should be cared for first.
- Consider whether these decisions were based on the needs of individual patients or clients, or on the number of staff available to assist.

upon it. In Katie's situation if the available options were discussed with her along with the possible outcomes of each, this would facilitate an autonomous decision.

In summary, the four principles that were used in the discussion above are:

- *Autonomy* (the ability to make one's own decisions): This is linked to another principle, respect for persons, which means that even in the absence of the ability to make an informed decision, the individual is at the centre of the decision-making process
- *Justice*: A person has the right to refuse to take the matter further, but equally has a right to protection from the law, should they wish to avail themselves of it
- *Non-maleficence* (prevention of harm)
- *Beneficence* (creation of benefit).

While Katie's situation created a problem that is unlikely to be encountered on a daily basis, there are many problems that nurses can encounter on a regular, if not everyday, basis (Box 7.3). While this is not a 'life and death' issue, decisions made by staff will have an impact on patients' quality of life.

The ethical and moral dimensions of nursing practice

The nature of healthcare provision is such that decisions made and the treatment and care provided, or withheld, may alter the duration and quality of the lives of the individuals who experience it. The relationship of nursing to health and well-being (Ch. 1) provides it with a moral dimension such that it is usually impossible to identify some elements of its practice as morally significant and others as morally neutral. It might be thought, for example, that measuring a patient's blood pressure is a psychomotor skill that is morally neutral, but the nurse's ability to measure and record the blood pressure accurately has the potential to affect the patient's health and well-being and this is morally significant. All decisions and actions taken (or omitted) in relation to client care are closely connected to their beneficial, or harmful, effects upon the client. While some aspects of nursing are in themselves technical, competence or lack of it has an effect upon the client's welfare. If nursing practice is accepted as having a highly significant moral dimension, then evaluation of nursing care quality involves moral reasoning processes in order to arrive at moral judgements. In Box 7.3 where staff shortages prevented all patients being provided with the help needed to eat and drink simultaneously, the decisions made about whom to assist, and when, were not only technical, but also moral in nature. It is now useful to examine the concepts of ethics and morals and their implications for nurses.

Ethics and morals

Ethics and morals are terms that are frequently used interchangeably. When differentiating between the two, the term ethics is usually taken to refer to the study of morals, whereas morality relates to people's behaviour.

Ethics and morals are sometimes viewed as something to which we resort in time of crisis, but it is arguable that morality is not one single dimension of life within society but is essential for society to function successfully. Thompson et al (2000, p. 258) argue that 'moral judgement, decision and action are as natural a part of living and doing as breathing. We all grow up in some sort of moral community.' They stress that not all moral decision-making is associated with drama and crisis and that 'most of us develop remarkable skill in making rapid moral assessment of the problems facing us in the practical situations in our lives and in taking the appropriate decisions' (p. 256). Thompson et al (2006, p. 3) argue that moral choice is an integral, and inescapable, part of everyday life and a focus on life and death dilemmas clouds the fact that the majority of moral issues faced by nurses are encountered in daily practice.

Downie and Calman (1994, p. 12) argue that:

> It is misleading to think that there are clinical discussions or professional decisions and occasionally also separate moral decisions. Rather, our argument will be that *all* clinical or professional decisions have a moral dimension to them, for morality, like attitudes, is all-pervasive. Moreover, since morality is all-pervasive it cannot be compartmentalized and it is therefore impossible to separate the moral decisions of someone in a professional capacity or role from the moral decisions of that same individual in a private capacity.

Downie and Calman (1994, pp. 15–16) also state that:

> *morality is inescapable.* The point is that living together with other people requires that we acknowledge certain actions to be right or just or compassionate, and others to be wrong or unjust or inconsiderate. Without some agreement on what we ought to do, and what we must not do, there could be no social harmony and co-operation . . .we may not be conscious of the moral nature of our actions precisely because morality is an inescapable part of our lives.

ETHICAL ISSUES Box 7.4

Allocation of resources

It is sometimes argued that individuals whose health problems can be perceived as 'self-inflicted' should not have the same entitlement to treatment as others. One example is that of cigarette smokers.

Student activities

Do you consider that smokers should have the same rights to treatment as non-smokers?

- Take 5–10 minutes to explain your answer.
- Then, take another 5–10 minutes to identify counter-arguments to the ones that you have put forward.

You could also carry out this exercise through discussion with others.

The notion that it is impossible to demarcate clearly between the work and private life of a registered nurse is one that is made clear in the *Code of Professional Conduct* (NMC 2004, clause 8.5), which emphasizes that registered nurses have a professional duty to provide care, in an emergency situation, within or outwith their work setting.

Having said that ethics and morals are central to nursing practice, it is the case that problems or dilemmas can, and do, occur. A dilemma is, by definition, a situation to which there is no solution and action taken will be with the purpose of creating the least harm. More common than dilemmas are problems, to which solutions may be found, although these solutions may not be without complexity.

Ethical theories

Ethical theories are sometimes used within the UK in relation to healthcare provision and these will now be described and discussed in the light of a particular situation. In the situation outlined earlier, Katie, who had been abused, was central to the discussion illustrating the application of ethical principles. Now carry out the activities in Box 7.4 that relate to decisions that may be made in relation to allocation of healthcare resources.

The responses and reasons that people provided to the activities in Box 7.4 will vary, but it is useful to identify and discuss some of the most commonly used arguments in favour of, and against, the equal entitlement of cigarette smokers to treatment.

In your own discussion you may well have arguments that are additional to those listed in Box 7.5 although those in the box are often used to support arguments for, or against, equal access to healthcare treatment for cigarette smokers. It can be seen that the issue of whether or not cigarette smokers should enjoy equal access to treatment as non-smokers is not a clear-cut and straightforward issue.

It is important, in nursing practice, to be able to identify arguments for, and against, a particular course of action and to analyse which of the arguments appear to be the most compelling and why. So, the activity in Box 7.4 was intended to be useful in relation to the *process* of identifying arguments for, and against, a particular viewpoint, as well as in relation to the *product*, in this case compiling a list of arguments. Reflection *on* practice (Ch. 4) also involves this type of activity. Over time, and with experience, reflection *in* practice enables practitioners to analyse and evaluate situations at the time that they occur, thus enabling the practitioner to be reflexive, in addition to reflective. This is a skill that will develop throughout the students' educational programme and further development will continue following registration. Events that facilitate reflective and reflexive practice are those in which practitioners explicitly identify *why* a particular situation proceeded well or badly in relation to its component parts.

Practitioners also need to identify their own attitudes, beliefs and values. In the arguments for, and against, equal access to treatment for cigarette smokers, it is likely that your personal attitudes, beliefs and values, rather than a notion of 'objective' judgements, may have come into play initially. These may have been clearly evident in your replies, or may have been implicit in the reasons provided for the response.

Some of the arguments outlined in Box 7.5 will now be examined to identify some of the ethical theories that underpin them.

Consequentialist ethics

One argument put forward in Box 7.5 was that, when health resources are finite, they should be allocated in a manner that will create the greatest health benefit for the greatest number of people. This type of thinking is 'consequentialist' and one form of consequentialism, called 'utilitarianism', was proposed by a UK lawyer, Jeremy Bentham (1748–1832). His theory was further developed and refined by John Stuart Mill (1806–1873). Bentham used the term 'happiness', but this was later redefined by Mill as 'benefit', and, whereas Bentham's focus was clearly upon the good of the majority, Mill also advocated tolerance for minority beliefs and lifestyles.

The utilitarian theory of deploying resources to provide the greatest benefit for the greatest number of individuals frequently underpins UK government policy, both at central and local levels (Box 7.6). It is a consequentialist theory because the focus is on the consequences of action or inaction: the methods taken to achieve the desired consequences (i.e. the greatest benefit for the greatest number of individuals) are deemed to be morally right or wrong insofar as they facilitate, or inhibit, attainment of benefits. (This type of theory is sometimes also referred to as 'teleological', i.e. derived from the Greek *teleos*, meaning 'end'.) For example, if cigarette smokers are less likely than non-smokers to benefit from a particular treatment, and resources to provide that treatment are limited, then the treatment should be available to those who will benefit most, i.e. the non-smokers.

Box 7.5 **Arguments for, and against, equal entitlement of smokers to treatment**

Arguments for equal entitlement of smokers to treatment

- Decisions about treatment should be made according to an individual's need
- Healthcare workers should provide care for people who require it, not make value judgements about lifestyle or behaviours
- Each individual is equally important – cannot deem some people to be more 'deserving' of treatment than others
- Cigarettes contain addictive substances – smokers should be recognized as having an addiction and receive help to overcome this, not censure
- If an individual stops smoking they may have many years of life ahead
- Outcomes are unpredictable: a person who smokes may outlive a non-smoker
- Cigarette smokers, over their lifetime, generate significant government revenue [excise duty and VAT in the UK comprise approximately 80% of the cost of 20 cigarettes (ASH 2002)]
- Cigarette smokers claim less state benefits in the UK, in the long term, than non-smokers. 50% of smokers die prematurely, losing an average 8 years of life (Edwards 2004), and therefore receive less pension benefit and are less likely to require long-term care in old age
- Cigarette smoking is a legal activity
- Criteria for designating an illness as 'self-inflicted' are problematic, e.g. sports injuries may be 'self-inflicted' and many people's lifestyle has, to a greater or lesser extent, contributed to their health problems

Arguments against equal entitlement of smokers to treatment

- Healthcare resources are limited, therefore decisions have to be made about their allocation
- Scarce resources should be allocated to areas where they can provide the greatest healthcare benefit for the greatest number of individuals: cigarette smokers are less likely to benefit from many treatments than non-smokers and may be at greater risk of development of complications of treatment, e.g. a greater likelihood of chest infection following anaesthesia
- If cigarette smokers are treated, but continue to smoke, the benefits of specialized treatment may be minimal, or of short duration
- Cigarette smoking is a matter of individual choice, therefore healthcare problems that arise as a result of cigarette smoking are self-inflicted
- Cigarette smoking has been recognized for many years as being harmful: individuals who smoke are aware of the risks that they take
- It is unjust to those who care for their own health if cigarette smokers have equal, or preferential, access to treatment
- Treating cigarette smokers on the same basis as those who do not smoke provides official endorsement of cigarette smoking, or at least no incentive for individuals to stop smoking

ETHICAL ISSUES Box 7.6

Utilitarian approaches

Student activity

Identify what you consider to be the strengths and limitations of allocating scarce health resources where they will create the greatest benefit for the greatest number of individuals.

Strengths and limitations of a utilitarian approach

Some of the arguments in favour of a utilitarian approach are that it is the only feasible way in which to cater for the healthcare needs of a large, and fairly diverse, population. The impossibility of addressing the needs of every individual within a country means that policy makers have to adopt a 'broad brush' approach and aim to create the greatest benefits for the greatest number of people. Adoption of this strategy is intended to ensure that the health needs of the majority of the population are addressed.

Unpredictability of outcomes

One problem with a utilitarian approach is that it is based on the ability to identify the actions, or inactions, that will ensure beneficial outcomes. (It is important to recognize that 'inactions' as well as 'actions' have consequences, e.g. if a decision is made *not* to treat a patient – 'inaction' – then this will have consequences, as will providing treatment – 'action'.) In reality it is often difficult to predict what the outcomes of actions and/or inactions will be. If the intended action is to provide treatment so that an individual will have many more years of a healthy life, then not only may the action itself fail to achieve this end, but also the unpredictability of life may result in an individual dying of another, possibly unrelated, cause. For example, if a non-smoker is treated in preference to a smoker, on the grounds that they are likely to achieve a greater long-term health benefit, it is possible that the non-smoker may die from another cause within a year of treatment, whereas the smoker may survive for many years. So, the unpredictability of actions, inactions and outcomes is one factor that may be used to criticize a utilitarian approach to resource allocation.

What counts as 'benefit'?

Another concern about the implications of consequentialist theories is that they may encourage a simplified view of 'benefits' as equating neatly with 'years of life'. This is a quantitative approach (see Ch. 5), in which the numbers of survivors and length of their survival are important. It may also be argued that quality of life may be of equal importance as length of life. For example, treating non-smokers who have certain forms of heart disease may provide them with many years of health, whereas treating smokers with similar problems may enable them to mobilize outdoors, as opposed to being housebound and this may improve their quality of life, even if only for a relatively short time.

Are numbers all that count?

Another limitation of consequentialist theories is that individuals who suffer from a relatively rare health problem, or one that is not considered to be a healthcare priority, may be unable to access treatment if resources have been geared towards provision of treatment for the majority. For example, relatively few individuals require a liver transplant, whereas many people have heart disease or cancer, or know of someone with these problems.

Does the end result justify the means?

The fact that consequentialist theories focus on results and not the actions and inactions that are necessary to create these may be deemed unacceptable, at least in some instances. It may be considered that the actions and inactions are, in themselves, of moral importance. For example, it may be anticipated that telling a patient the truth about an unfavourable diagnosis and prognosis will create distress for that patient, for their friends and relatives and for the care team. A consequentialist might argue that, if creation of the greatest benefit for the greatest number of people will be achieved by telling a lie, then that is the morally correct thing to do. It is the end result, or consequence, that is of moral importance and not the means used to achieve it. An alternative viewpoint is that there is something about telling the truth, or telling a lie, that is morally right or wrong in itself, independent of the consequences.

Taking consequentialism to extremes might (at least in theory) entail that, in the case of a person who was in need of healthcare, but who was without friends or relatives and who wished to die, it would not only be acceptable, but desirable, for that person to die. This would free up the resources that would be used in their care for the care of others and thus maximize benefits for the greatest number of people.

Rule utilitarianism

One way to circumvent the potential problem outlined in the previous paragraph is to refine the theory. Rule utilitarianism states that, rather than deciding in individual instances what will create the greatest benefit for the greatest number, the 'rule' should be implementation of actions (or inactions) that it is anticipated will, if adopted by society as a whole, create the greatest benefit for the majority. It might then be argued that it would not create the greatest benefit for society as a whole if a culture were promoted in which the lives of individuals were held in low regard.

Consequentialist ethics: summary

There are many arguments in favour of, and against, a consequentialist approach to ethics, a few of which have been identified here. Overall, its charm may lie in its relative simplicity. It contains no spiritual or religious elements and relies on identification of factors that will create the largest net benefit for the greatest number of individuals. However, the relative simplicity of the theory may be a shortcoming when it encounters the complexity of individuals' needs for care and determination of what comprises a 'benefit'. The difficulty in predicting outcomes is also problematic, as is the idea that actions and inactions are, in themselves, neutral and are morally relevant only in respect of their results. For further reading about utilitarianism, see Thompson et al (2006) and the Further reading section at the end of this chapter.

Deontological ethics

Some of the arguments for, and against, smokers' equal access to treatment use justifications that are not dependent upon intended consequences. One example is the idea that treatment decisions should be made on the basis of individual need and that healthcare workers have a duty to provide care regardless of an individual's lifestyle or behaviours. This argument is evident in the *code of professional conduct* (NMC 2004, clauses 2.1 and 2.2) which emphasizes the importance of respecting the patient or client as an individual. This type of argument proposes that actions and/or inactions are morally acceptable or unacceptable in themselves, independent of their anticipated or actual consequences. This type of argument is termed 'deontological'.

Deontology is derived from the Greek words *deon*, meaning 'duty' and *logos*, meaning 'science' or 'study of'. A deontological theory specifies moral requirements and moral prohibitions. The *code of professional conduct* (NMC 2004) is an example of a deontological code. The *code* does not refer at any point to the maximization of benefits for the greatest number of patients, nor does it refer to the end result justifying the means by which it was attained. Rather, the *code* specifies the duties of registered nurses, including their duty of care to all patients as individuals.

Kant (1724–1804) developed deontological theory, including the concept of the categorical imperative. Basically, this involves asking oneself whether, if one's proposed action (or inaction) were to be implemented by people universally, would it be morally acceptable? For example, if a person considered telling a lie, they should first consider whether, if this practice were universal, the result would be acceptable. It is likely that, while an individual might consider that their own action (in this instance telling a lie) in a specific situation might be acceptable, they might also realize that, if such action were adopted universally, chaos would ensue, as no individual would be able to place trust in another. If individuals decide to behave in a manner that would be acceptable if it was universally practised, then they are acting in accordance with a categorical imperative. A deontological approach to truth telling would be that telling the truth, or a lie, is of moral importance, *in itself*, as an action, rather than solely in terms of its consequence. The individual's intentions are also important, e.g. that the intention of an individual in carrying out a particular action was fulfilment of a duty.

While the *code of professional conduct* (NMC 2004) is a secular, or non-religious, document, and while a deontologist may be agnostic or atheist, the majority of religions can be classed as deontological, i.e. a religion usually requires that its adherents behave in specific ways, which are deemed to be right or wrong *in themselves*, as opposed to right or wrong in relation to their beneficial or deleterious consequences.

Areas of potential conflict

One area of potential conflict may be readily identified from the fact that deontologists may have a variety of backgrounds: their commonality lies in the requirement, duty or obligation to behave in particular ways. One person's idea of duty may vary considerably from, and indeed may be diametrically opposed to, that of another individual, if they have a different set of deontological beliefs. In relation to termination of pregnancy, for example, individuals who believe strongly in the right of women to decide whether to continue with, or terminate, a pregnancy, may express a deontological belief that healthcare workers have a duty to provide termination of pregnancy on demand. On the other hand, individuals who are strongly against termination of pregnancy may base their belief on a perceived duty to preserve human life, or potential human life, at all costs. This example shows that deontologists may hold diametrically opposed views, although they share in common the belief that individuals have certain obligations or duties, with which they must comply.

Virtue ethics

A theory of ethical behaviour, originally expounded by Aristotle in the 4th century BC and developed more recently by Macintyre (1981), concerns the role of the virtues. A virtue is a character trait that is perceived as socially valuable and a moral virtue is one which is morally valuable (Beauchamp & Childress 2001). Virtue theorists consider that morality, rather than being the domain of ivory-tower academics, is a practical skill that is exercised on a daily basis. If children are socialized into behaving in a morally acceptable manner in relation to others, then this should become habitual practice over time. Within this theory humans are perceived as social in nature, but individuals require to practise certain behaviours or virtues on a regular basis in order to maintain them. It is insufficient only to know what is right: it is necessary to put that knowledge into practice (Ch. 1). The concept of moderation in behaviour is important and individuals must take responsibility for their voluntary actions. Thompson et al (2006, p. 302) explain that Aristotle's system of ethics requires both intellectual and moral virtues (Fig. 7.1).

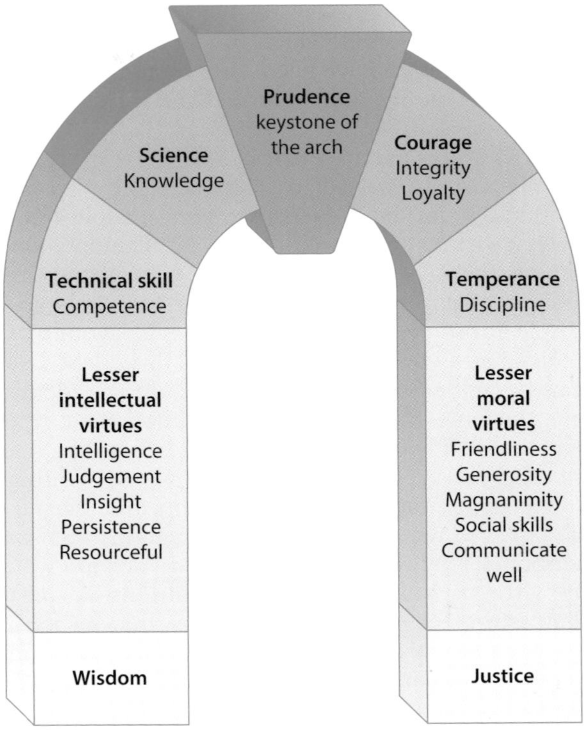

Fig. 7.1 Symbolic representation of Aristotle's view of the relationship between prudence and the intellectual and moral values (reproduced with permission from Thompson et al 2006)

Intellectual and moral virtues

The intellectual virtues are those that relate to skill in decision-making and problem-solving, while moral virtues are character traits (or habits) that are prerequisites for an individual to be reliable, effective and efficient in action. The keystone (see Fig. 7.1) that links and binds the intellectual and moral virtues together is the quality of prudence, which may also be referred to as practical wisdom. Thompson et al (2006, p. 308–309) argue that 'situation ethics' is needed, as this actively acknowledges the importance of the 'specifics' of particular situations, rather than, as some ethical theories require, attempting to develop principles that are universal in application and that may be applied to any situation. Consequentialist and duty-based approaches to ethics are viewed as attempting to force unique events to comply with an inappropriate general framework for action. Neo (i.e. modern versions of) Aristotelianism, or virtue ethics, draws to some extent on the traditions of Christian ethics in its requirement to consider each situation as being unique, comprised as it is of individuals. Individuals are not identical to one another and they all have needs that should be addressed in an understanding, individualized and caring manner.

Concerns about virtue ethics

Concerns are also raised in relation to the idea of virtue ethics. It can be argued that some people find the idea that virtues can be cultivated in all individuals to be impossible. The qualities deemed to be virtues might also lack consensus amongst the population at large. For example, for some people, intellectual endeavour may be perceived as a virtue, while for others this is not valued. It can be argued that, even if practice of the identified virtues becomes habitual over time, situations may arise in which individuals abandon virtuous behaviour, at least temporarily. For example, in response to continuing severe staff shortages, which complaints to management have failed to rectify, a normally thoughtful and caring practitioner may find that their capacity, or motivation, to be virtuous has diminished, or is absent. For virtues to flourish, it is important to recognize that responsibility is not solely that of the individual: the environment also needs to be one in which the qualities deemed to be virtues are promoted and prevailing conditions are such that they may flourish.

Constraints on ethical behaviour

Indeed, it may be argued in relation to any ethical theory that, while some behaviours may be those for which individuals (sometimes referred to as 'agents') are directly responsible, the structures within which individuals operate (in both work and domestic settings) may inhibit, or facilitate, moral conduct. This interaction between an individual (the agent) and the structures within which they live and work should not be underestimated as a determinant of people's ability to behave morally.

Ethical theories: summary

The previous section outlined three ethical theories that are of relevance to UK healthcare provision. More detailed explanation and discussion of ethical theories is provided by Thompson et al (2006) and others in the Further reading section at the end of this chapter.

Power: its use and abuse

Power has a variety of definitions, but most include the notions of command, authority, control and the ability to influence events and produce effects. The nature of healthcare is that those who seek it are usually, due to their need for assistance, in a situation in which their ability to exert power is limited. Students may not consider themselves to be powerful players within the healthcare team, but the position of patients or clients who require assistance places them in a position of vulnerability in relation to all who provide their care. The abuses of power reported by the media tend to be those that are extreme in nature, e.g. the case of Harold Shipman, an English GP, convicted in 2000 for the murder of over 200 of his patients. It is important to remember that many decisions in everyday nursing practice are not those of life and death, but of care quality, and relate to treating patients and clients as individuals who are entitled to respect. Now consider the scenario outlined in Box 7.7.

CRITICAL THINKING — Box 7.7

An abuse of power?

John is a student undertaking his first practice placement in a community house for adults who have learning disabilities. He had no experience of care settings before starting his university programme 4 months ago. One of the residents, Alex, who has a moderately severe learning disability and is overweight, asks John for sugar in his tea. John is about to comply when one of the care workers shouts across the dining room that Alex is 'not allowed sugar' as he is on a diet. Alex protests loudly and swears at the care worker, who replies that, unless Alex 'behaves', he will have to return to his room.

Student activities

- Take a few minutes to discuss the above situation with others, or to jot down your own thoughts about what should be done in this situation. In particular, identify what action, if any, John should take.
- Write down a rationale for your ideas, perhaps by reference to bioethical principles, or to an ethical theory.

An abuse of power?

Individual reactions to the scenario in Box 7.7 will vary, but some relevant points are identified below:

- It is not a 'life or death' situation
- Alex is not subjected to physical abuse
- Care workers may exert considerable influence and control (power) over clients
- Alex is subjected to misuse of power
- Alex's autonomy is disregarded, i.e. his right to make his own decisions
- Alex's 'capacity' (Ch. 6) to make his own decisions is unknown

but

- the care worker's action (shouting, rather than speaking discreetly with Alex) is abusive.

In this short scenario, and with no direct knowledge of the people concerned, it is impossible to place the situation in context and to understand the individuals' motivations for their actions. However, the fact that Alex is in a position of vulnerability as he needs care does not mean that he should be placed in a position where decisions are made on his behalf, without prior consultation and agreement. It also does not mean that he should be subjected to what might be classified as a form of emotional abuse, i.e. humiliation in front of other residents and threats of removal to his room.

On reflection then, while it may be that the care worker acted in what she perceived to be the resident's best interest, and it is the case that beneficence is a prima facie ethical principle (i.e. a principle that, at 'first sight' should be respected), it may still be argued that it was unacceptable to take the action that she did, as her actions interfered with John's autonomy, which is another prima facie ethical principle. An individual's autonomy in relation to health issues usually overrides beneficence by others (for exceptions to this, see Ch. 6). It may also be argued that the resident's 'best interest' was not served by the way that the care worker handled the situation.

What should John do in this situation? Although students are not professionally accountable to the NMC, it may be argued that, as a future registered nurse, John should have the residents' interests as his main concern and take some action to protect these. There are several options available to John:

- Confront the care worker (within or outwith the dining room) and tell her that he found her action unacceptable
- Discuss the situation with his mentor, or person in charge of the placement, at the time
- Contact the university to express his concerns
- Do nothing because, as a new student, John might be uncertain as to what constitutes acceptable or unacceptable practice. Even if John did feel that this was poor practice, he might feel unable to complain, for fear of repercussions during the remainder of his placement. He could reassure himself that the resident had not suffered physical abuse and that, as a student, he was not in a position to alter practice or have a complaint upheld
- Do nothing because John is aware that he has to work closely with the care worker and her colleagues for the remainder of his placement and does not wish to make himself unpopular. Additionally, John knows that he has to achieve a satisfactory placement assessment and does not wish to jeopardize this.

Of the above, while John does not perhaps have a legal or professional obligation to report the incident, it may be argued that he does have a moral obligation to do so. Alex is a vulnerable individual who has received treatment that appears to be detrimental to his emotional, although not physical, well-being. If there are valid reasons for the care worker's response to the resident, then these should be made clear. John could perhaps approach the care worker and ask why she had spoken to Alex in the way that she did. An alternative would be for John to request clarification from his mentor or the person in charge of the placement. Formalized care policies, guidelines and procedures provide a benchmark for staff, clients and other interested parties against which the quality of care delivery may be measured. They clarify acceptable and unacceptable staff behaviours and would have been a helpful resource for John.

If John failed to receive a satisfactory explanation from staff within the unit, or from the presence of policies, guidelines or procedures, he could then contact his university in order that the incident be explored with the Link Lecturer. John could also make a written complaint about the care worker's behaviour which would then be the subject of official investigation (Ch. 3).

Such action may be termed 'whistleblowing' by the media. The Public Disclosure at Work Act (HM Government 1998b) provides legal protection for employees who divulge unacceptable work practices (Ch. 6). Students are not employees of the management of placement areas and cannot therefore be subject to their disciplinary processes and procedures, but they are subject to those of their higher educational establishment. Registered nurses are provided with legal protection by the Act (HM Government 1998b) if they disclose unacceptable practice(s) although this does not prevent potential censure of that individual by colleagues for having divulged unacceptable practice(s).

John, as a student, may feel that it is difficult to raise concerns about poor, or unacceptable, practice within a placement area for fear of intimidation by staff (this concern may also be experienced by registered practitioners). The Royal College of Nursing (RCN 2000a) has issued guidance in relation to bullying and harassment at work and also a specific guide for students (RCN 2002b) to enable them to deal with these issues, should they arise.

The situation above showed that power does not reside solely in the management team in healthcare settings. People who provide direct care for patients and clients wield a considerable amount of power over their well-being and abuse of this power does not necessarily manifest as the flagrant forms of abuse that are likely to make news headlines. The example also illustrated that students who witness what they consider may be unacceptable practice may be uncertain about how to proceed in making a formal complaint. Advice should, in those instances, be sought from the sources identified in the previous section.

Vulnerable groups

The most vulnerable members of society are likely to become the victims of abuse, both in institutional and domestic settings. These include:

- Children – *Working Together to Safeguard Children* (DH 1999) and the government's Green Paper *Every Child Matters* (HM Government 2003) provide much useful information
- Women
- Individuals who have a learning disability
- Individuals who have a limited ability to speak or express themselves
- Individuals who have a mental health problem
- Older adults, especially those who are physically and psychologically frail
- Non-English speakers
- Asylum seekers
- Individuals without legal authority to be in the UK.

Some client groups are more vulnerable to abuse than others, including individuals who receive ongoing (as opposed to short-term) care, those who have a limited ability to articulate or whose reports of abuse are unlikely to be heeded, e.g. if they receive few visitors in whom they could confide, are potential victims for abuse.

Box 7.8 **Categories of abuse**

- *Physical*: Including inappropriate restriction of an individual's liberty of movement and misuse of medication, e.g. sedation
- *Sexual*: Including sexual acts to which the vulnerable person was unable to provide consent, was not in a position to consent, e.g. due to being below the age of consent or due to incapacity, or was under pressure to consent
- *Psychological*: Including threats, humiliation, controlling, isolation
- *Financial*: Including exploitation and pressure to behave in certain ways
- *Neglect*: Failure to provide appropriate care and attention or access to services
- *Discriminatory*: Including that on grounds of race, sex, disability, sexual orientation, religious or cultural belief.

[Adapted from DH 2000]

The NMC provides guidelines for practitioners working with people who have mental health problems and learning disabilities (NMC 2002c) and, additionally, guidelines to provide advice on practitioner–client relationships and the prevention of abuse (NMC 2002d).

'At-risk' care settings

Abuse within care settings may be classified in a number of ways (Box 7.8) and is more likely to occur in certain circumstances (Wardhaugh & Wilding 1998). Care settings and management styles that may result in poor, or unacceptable, practice include the following:

- Institutions isolated from the community at large
- Minimal preparation of care staff for practice
- Minimal ongoing support and supervision of care staff
- Devaluation by management of care staff's work.

In these circumstances clients may be perceived as units of work, rather than as individuals with individual needs. Care areas without clear lines of accountability or policies and procedures that do not clearly state acceptable (and unacceptable) staff behaviours facilitate, or at least do not inhibit, care that is of poor quality or could be categorized as abuse.

As identified above, some client groups are more vulnerable to abuse than others. Further examples in care settings include those who:

- Receive ongoing (rather than short-term) care
- Have a limited ability to articulate
- Are unlikely to be heeded if they report abuse, e.g. have few visitors in whom they can confide.

Use of restraint

The forcible restraint of individuals within care settings is controversial. The scenario in Box 7.9 describes a situation that relates to care of a child, but the principles can be generalized to care of patients and clients of varying ages and with diverse needs.

CRITICAL THINKING Box 7.9

Restraint of a child

Anna is a student undertaking a placement within a children's hospital. She is involved, under the supervision of her mentor, in carrying out a variety of procedures for young children, but is uneasy about the use of restraint to ensure that the children remain still and by the distress that this causes some of the children. Anna wonders whether this use of restraint is justifiable.

Student activity

Identify the grounds on which you would consider restraint of a child to be ethically justifiable.

The United Nations *Convention on the Rights of the Child* was based on the premise that children have an active contribution to make within society (United Nations [UN] 1989). Collins (1999) points out that the restraint of children was, until recently, considered to be acceptable practice and uncontroversial. Restraint continues to be used by either a parent or carer during immunization by injection, venepuncture and lumbar puncture. Gray (2002) suggests that the effect of the UN Convention, UK legislation and societal changes in the perception of the role of children within society has resulted in an unfavourable view of restraint, which is now more widely considered to be an outdated practice. Pederson and Harbury (1995) identified that time constraints, coupled with a lack of knowledge of distraction techniques, was one reason provided to justify the use of restraint. A survey carried out by Robinson and Collier (1997) suggested that paediatric nurses perceived restraint as a quick and easy means of ensuring that procedures were completed quickly and safely (although 69% of respondents did identify that restraint was a major cause of distress to children). Collins (1999) suggested that use of restraint resulted from nurses' lack of understanding of the efficacy of using distraction and relaxation as a means of reducing pain and distress in children undergoing procedures. Gay (1991) had earlier described the use of dolls to provide a visual demonstration to children of the procedure that they were about to undergo and also identified that providing an opportunity for children, where possible, to handle real or modified equipment reduced their anxiety levels.

The Royal College of Nursing (RCN 1999) published guidelines that placed emphasis upon prior explanations to the child about procedures and the use of alternatives to restraint, e.g. distraction, wherever possible. The RCN also identified the need for development and implementation of policies and procedures that specified:

- Permissible methods of restraint
- Situations in which their use was acceptable
- The documentation required.

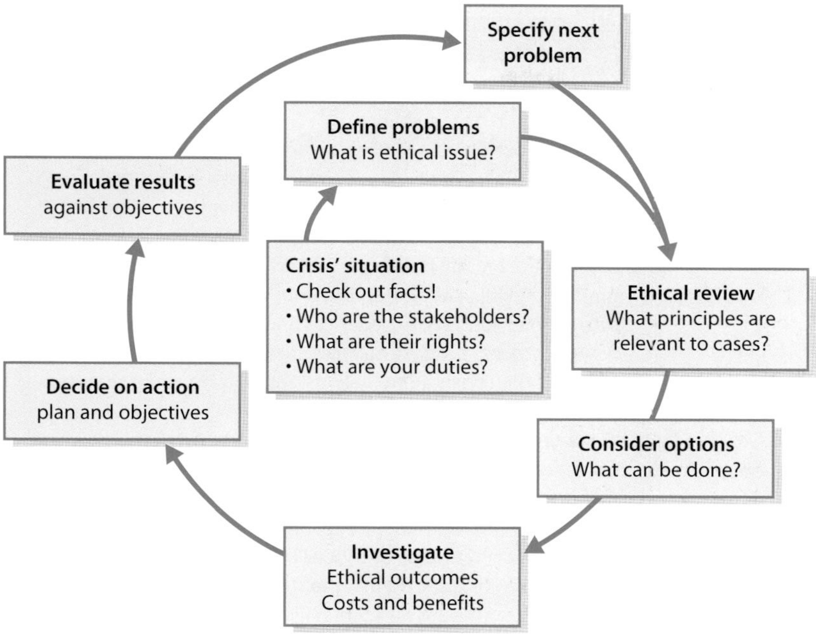

Fig. 7.2 The DECIDE model for ethical decision-making (reproduced with permission from Thompson et al 2006)

The minimum amount of restraint necessary should be used, for the shortest duration possible, accompanied by clear explanations to the child as to what is happening. Ongoing discussion among staff of issues surrounding child restraint and a procedure for registering any disquiet should be clearly explained. Documentation is required (NMC 2005c) of the need for restraint, the method used, its duration and any discernible effect on the child.

It may be seen from the above that the disquiet that Anna experienced in the situation outlined in Box 7.9 was justified. It may be that the situations in which Anna witnessed (and perhaps participated in) the restraint of children were those in which the actions of staff were justified, but it is important that restraint is not carried out without reflection on, and in, practice and that an evidence base is used to support the rationale for its use (see Chs 4, 5). If practices that appear to cause patients or clients distress are implemented, it is of particular importance that the rationale for these is explained and that potential alternatives are explored.

Ethical frameworks and models

Reflecting on, and in, practice can be structured (Ch. 4). In relation to ethical problems or dilemmas, frameworks or models may also be used to reach decisions in specific situations. There are a number of frameworks that may be used to explore ethically sensitive situations. One example is Seedhouse's (1988) 'ethical grid' and another is that of Brown et al (1992). The DECIDE model (Thompson et al 2006, p. 323) will be used to explore the situation in Box 7.11.

The DECIDE model

The authors of the DECIDE model (Thompson et al 2006, p. 323) (Fig. 7.2) advocate that, in a crisis situation (originally defined in Greek as a 'decision time'), a structured series of questions can be used to assist ethical problem-solving. These are shown in Box 7.10. The first step is to verify the facts, then identify the 'stakeholders' (i.e. those who are interested parties in the situation). The rights of the stakeholders are then established, as are the duties of other parties in relation to fulfilment of these.

Following this initial process, it is important to define the problem and to identify the relevant ethical issue(s). Once this has been established, a review to identify the ethically relevant principles is carried out and then the available options are considered. Investigation of the options explores their potential outcomes and the costs and benefits attached to each. The action that is deemed most appropriate is then decided upon, implemented and subsequently evaluated for its effectiveness, or otherwise, in solving, or at least alleviating, the problem.

The DECIDE model in practice

The following discussion illustrates the issues that may arise from the activities in Box 7.11 and, because the scenario is brief, there is limited information on which to base a discussion. It is not intended to provide the 'ideal' answer. The steps of the DECIDE model are each considered in turn using the framework in Box 7.10.

Defining the problem(s)

The first step is to verify the facts, which are:

- Tom has a mental health problem
- Tom lives in a community house with support

Box 7.10 **The DECIDE model**

D – Define the problem(s)
What are the key facts of the case? Who is involved? What are their rights, your duties? What is the main ethical problem to be addressed?

E – Ethical review
What ethical principles have a bearing on the case and which principle or principles should be given priority in making your decision?

C – Consider the options
What options do you have in the situation? What alternative courses of action? What help, means and methods do you need to use?

I – Investigate outcomes
Given each available option, what consequences are likely to follow from each course of action open to you? Which is the most ethical thing to do?

D – Decide on action
Having chosen the best available option, determine a specific action plan, set clear objectives and then act decisively and effectively

E – Evaluate results
Having initiated a course of action, monitor how things progress, and when concluded, assess carefully whether or not you achieved your goals

[From Thompson et al 2006, p. 324]

ETHICAL ISSUES Box 7.11

Whose rights?

Tom is a young man who has a diagnosis of schizophrenia. He has been in hospital on two occasions when his experiences have been causing him distress. He now lives in a community house with support from a residential care worker and a community mental health nurse. Tom takes medication as prescribed which alleviates, but does not eradicate, some of his distressing thoughts, experiences and feelings. These include hearing voices (auditory hallucinations) that mock and frighten him, and the consequent feelings of suspicion and uneasiness cause him considerable distress.

Some of the residents in the neighbourhood raised objections when the proposal for the community house was put forward 2 years ago because they were under the misapprehension that people who had mental health problems might display antisocial behaviour. Tom has, on several occasions, shouted in the street in response to the distress caused by his auditory hallucinations. Tom's feelings of mistrust understandably worsen when people stare at and talk about him. Neighbours are worried about his shouting, believing it is directed at them, and complain that it has become unsafe for their children to walk, or play, outdoors because of Tom's behaviour.

Student activities

- Write down, or discuss with others, your perspective on the above scenario.
- Explain the reasons that support your views.

This scenario provides limited information and there is no personal knowledge of the individuals involved. However, with the information available:

- Imagine that you are the registered nurse responsible for Tom's care and use the DECIDE model to explore the scenario, either on your own, or with others.

- Tom takes medication as prescribed
- The medication controls Tom's symptoms, but does not eradicate them
- Tom's symptoms include auditory hallucinations and feelings of paranoia which he finds distressing
- Tom is sometimes verbally aggressive to people who stare at him or talk about him
- Some of the people who live near the community house objected to its existence at the planning stage
- Some of the neighbours find Tom's behaviour threatening.

The stakeholders are Tom, the neighbours who complained that Tom's behaviour was threatening, Tom's support workers (including yourself as the registered nurse), his psychiatrist and, in a wider sense, possibly other individuals who have mental health problems, and all other members of society.

The rights of all the stakeholders appear to be those of freedom (autonomy) to live their lives within society. Your duty, as the registered nurse responsible for Tom's care, is to act to ensure that Tom's best interests are served (NMC 2004). You do, however, also have a duty to take action if you consider that Tom's behaviour presents an actual threat to others. You have a duty to comply with your contract of employment.

The next step is to define the problem and, as the problem is not only practical (e.g. accompanying Tom to the shops) but also has implications for Tom's future health, freedom and well-being (and also has implications for the perceived freedom of some of the neighbours and their children), it appears to be an ethical problem.

Ethical review

The next stage of the model is to review the ethical elements. These appear to be those of competing rights, i.e. Tom's right to move around freely and not to be prescribed medication to the point where the side-effects (including lethargy and drowsiness) would impede this right. The principles involved are:

- Preventing harm to Tom: non-maleficence
- Acting to preserve his best interests: beneficence
- Preserving his autonomy as much as is possible without it interfering with the autonomy of others
- Justice.

Unless Tom is being held under an appropriate section of the Mental Health Act (see Further reading and Ch. 6) he is entitled to freedom of movement. The ethical review would include acknowledgement of your duty as the registered nurse responsible for Tom's care to uphold his best interests and to act as his advocate if required to do so.

The rights of the neighbours to be free from harassment are also important within the ethical review, but it is not clear that there is an *actual* threat to their well-being. Their negative perception of Tom's behaviour may be based on a lack of knowledge about the nature of his illness and this may be fuelled by negative and inaccurate media representations of people who have a mental health problem (DH 2003).

Consider and investigate options

The next two stages in the DECIDE model (see Fig. 7.2) are identification of the options available and investigation of what would constitute ethically acceptable outcomes, including the costs and benefits of each. The options in this case appear to be:

- To do nothing and hope that, over time, the neighbours will accept that Tom's behaviour does not constitute a threat. This does not, however, seem ethically acceptable, as the neighbours will remain uneasy and Tom's feelings of worry and isolation will probably be reinforced by the neighbours' behaviour
- Request that the psychiatrist increase Tom's medication in an attempt to reduce his symptoms to a 'socially acceptable' level. However, as this might increase deleterious side-effects and constitute a form of chemical restraint, this does not seem an ethically justifiable solution
- Encourage Tom to remain indoors. This also seems ethically unjustifiable as it attempts to restrict Tom's freedom of movement
- Arrange to discuss the situation with the concerned neighbours to allow them to express their concerns and allow you to explain Tom's behaviour. This seems ethically justifiable, but there is the problem of ensuring that your duty of patient confidentiality is maintained (NMC 2004). It might be possible to carry out such a discussion so long as no specific details about Tom or his particular mental health problem were divulged. It might be possible to seek Tom's permission to divulge information, but dependent upon the severity of his problems there might be the issue of whether he is in a position to provide informed consent (Ch. 6) to this request.

Your duty, as the registered nurse responsible for Tom's care, is to act to ensure that Tom's best interests are served (NMC 2004) and to act as his advocate if required to do so. The term advocacy has its origins in the judicial system and retains rather a confrontational association. An advocate is an individual who speaks on behalf of another, either in response to a request from that person or because their position in relation to the other person may require them to do so. The position of registered nurses in relation to their clients, so far as the *Code of Professional Conduct* (NMC 2004) is concerned, is that the nurse should support the client's best interests and this may be assumed to include advocacy, if required. There are arguments for, and against, registered nurses adopting advocacy roles in relation to their clients (see Ch. 6). It may be argued, for example, that independent advocates (i.e. those who have no other formal input into the client's care) are better placed to act purely in accordance with the client's known, or assumed, wishes.

CRITICAL THINKING Box 7.12

The DECIDE model in practice

Student activities

- Identify and reflect on a situation from your own practice placement experience in which a problem was present.
- Use the DECIDE model to work through the actions that either were, or might have been, carried out in that situation.

Decide on action

The next stage is to decide on action, in conjunction with Tom, and to compile a plan and identify objectives. The investigation indicated that the best action might be to speak with Tom in an attempt to explore how he understands and feels about the situation and to speak with the neighbours, ensuring that specific details of Tom's condition were not discussed, thus maintaining client confidentiality. Reassuring the neighbours that Tom did not present a risk to their safety would be important and they might wish advice as to how best to interact with Tom when they meet. With Tom's permission, it might be useful for him to meet with the neighbours, accompanied by an independent advocate.

The intended objectives, or outcomes, would be:

- That Tom's symptoms would not be exacerbated by the neighbours' negative reactions towards him
- That the neighbours' anxieties would be alleviated and that their attitude towards Tom (and perhaps the presence of the community house) would be more positive.

Evaluate results

The final stage of the DECIDE model (see Fig. 7.2) is an evaluation of the effectiveness of the action taken. This may be measured against the objectives that were identified during the decision stage, so those who worked with Tom, Tom himself and the neighbours would be able to provide feedback as to whether the intended objectives had been fully, or partially, met. (There is a further step in the DECIDE model, which is to specify the next problem; whether another problem would arise would remain to be seen.)

While the above scenario was used to demonstrate application of the DECIDE model (Thompson et al 2006, p. 323), the framework it provides is relevant across a wide range of healthcare settings and for individuals with varying needs. Box 7.12 provides an opportunity for you to reflect on a situation within your own practice.

Summary

This chapter provides:

- An introduction to the role of the NMC and the guidance it provides for nursing students and registered practitioners.
- An overview of fundamental ethical principles, theories and frameworks.
- Discussions of some everyday ethical issues that may arise in nursing practice using branch-specific scenarios to highlight them. The underpinning themes can be generalized to a variety of care settings and to clients with diverse needs.
- A basis for further understanding of professional and ethical issues that may arise during nursing programmes and following registration.

Self test

1. State three functions of the Nursing and Midwifery Council.
2. Identify the NMC document that is central to the practice of registered nurses.
3. Identify the NMC publication that is most relevant to you, as a nursing student.
4. Identify the purpose of the *Code of professional conduct: standards for conduct, performance and ethics.*
5. Write a short definition of the following terms:
   a. Ethics
   b. Morals.
6. Write a short definition of the following terms:
   a. Non-maleficence
   b. Beneficence
   c. Autonomy
   d. Respect for persons
   e. Justice.

Key words and phrases for literature searching

Nursing and Midwifery Council
Ethics
Morals
Nursing practice
Students

Useful websites

Children's rights	www.crae.org.uk Available July 2006
Nursing and Midwifery Council	www.nmc-uk.org Available July 2006

References

ASH (Action on Smoking and Health) 2002 Basic facts: Three – Taxation. Online: www.ash.org.uk/html/factsheets Available July 2006

Beauchamp TL, Childress JF 2001 Principles of biomedical ethics. 5th edn. Oxford University Press, Oxford

Brown JM, Kitson AL, McKnight TJ 1992 Challenges in caring: explorations in nursing and ethics. Chapman & Hall, London

Collins P 1999 Restraining children for painful procedures. Paediatric Nursing 11(3):14–16

Department of Health 1999 Working together to safeguard children. Online: http://www.dh.gov.uk/assetRoot/04/07/58/24/04075824.pdf Available July 2006

Department of Health 2000 No secrets: guidance on developing and implementing multi-agency policies and procedures to protect vulnerable adults from abuse. TSO, London

Department of Health 2003 Attitudes to mental illness 2003: Report. Online: www.dh.gov.uk/assetRoot/04/07/91/16/0479116.pdf Available July 2006

Downie RS, Calman KC 1994 Healthy respect: ethics in health care. 2nd edn. Oxford University Press, Oxford

Edwards R 2004 The problem of tobacco smoking. British Medical Journal 328: 217–219

Gay J 1991 Caring for children in A&E. Paediatric Nursing 3(7):21–23

Gray J 2002 Conscious sedation of children in A&E. Emergency Nurse 9(8):26–31

HM Government 1998a Data Protection Act. TSO, London

HM Government 1998b Public Disclosure at Work Act. TSO, London

HM Government 2003 Green Paper. Every child matters. TSO, London. Online: www.dfes.gov.uk/everychildmatters Available July 2006

Macintyre A 1981 After virtue. 2nd edn. Notre Dame University Press, Notre Dame

Nursing and Midwifery Council 2002a Professional advice from the NMC. NMC, London

Nursing and Midwifery Council 2002b An NMC guide for students of nursing and midwifery. NMC, London

Nursing and Midwifery Council 2002c Guidelines for mental health and learning disabilities nursing. NMC, London

Nursing and Midwifery Council 2002d Practitioner–client relationships and the prevention of abuse. NMC, London

Nursing and Midwifery Council 2004 Code of professional conduct: standards for conduct, performance and ethics. NMC, London

Nursing and Midwifery Council 2005a Standards of proficiency for pre-registration nursing education. NMC, London

Nursing and Midwifery Council 2005b The PREP handbook. NMC, London

Nursing and Midwifery Council 2005c Guidelines for records and record keeping. NMC, London

Pederson C, Harbury B 1995 Nurses' use of nonpharmacologic techniques with hospitalized children. Issues in Comprehensive Pediatric Nursing 18: 91–109

Robinson S, Collier J 1997 Holding children still for procedures. Paediatric Nursing 9(4):12–14

Royal College of Nursing 1999 Restraining, holding still and containing children: guidance for good practice. RCN, London

Royal College of Nursing 2000a Dealing with harassment and bullying at work: a guide for RCN members. RCN, London

Royal College of Nursing 2002b Dealing with bullying and harassment: a guide for nursing students. RCN, London

Seedhouse D 1988 Ethics: the heart of health care. Wiley, Chichester

Thompson IE, Melia KM, Boyd KM 2000 Nursing ethics. 4th edn. Churchill Livingstone, Edinburgh

Thompson IE, Melia KM, Boyd KM, Horsburgh D 2006 Nursing ethics, 5th edn. Churchill Livingstone, Edinburgh

United Nations 1989 The United Nations convention on the rights of the child. CRDU, London

Wardhaugh J, Wilding P 1998 Towards an explanation of the corruption of care. In: Allott M, Robb M (eds) Understanding health and social care: an introductory reader. Sage, London

Further reading

Allott M, Robb M (eds) 1998 Understanding health and social care: an introductory reader. Sage, London

Beauchamp TL, Childress JF 2001 Principles of biomedical ethics. 5th edn. Oxford University Press, Oxford

Downie RS, Calman KC 1994 Healthy respect: ethics in health care. 2nd edn. Oxford University Press, Oxford

HM Government 1983 Mental Health Act. TSO, London (currently under review)

HM Government 1986 Mental Health (Northern Ireland) Order. TSO, London

HM Government 2004 Mental Health (Amendment) (Northern Ireland) Order. TSO, London

Nursing and Midwifery Council 2002 Supporting nurses and midwives through lifelong learning. NMC, London

Scottish Executive 2003 Mental Health (Care and Treatment) (Scotland) Act. TSO, Edinburgh

SECTION 3

Nursing and lifespan implications

8

The human lifespan and its effect on selecting nursing interventions

David Tait

Glossary terms

Culture

Family

Milestones

Motivation

Normalization

Psychology

Roles

Socialization

Sociology

Learning outcomes

This chapter will help you:

- Develop an awareness of psychological and sociological aspects affecting development
- Describe the main stages and processes of human development through the lifespan in relation to theoretical frameworks
- Outline the main stages of physical development and milestones
- Describe psychosocial development and the emergence of self and self-concept, cognitive and moral development and emotional attachment
- Discuss the main points of psychosexual development, personality and social integration
- Begin to appreciate the relevance of these events and frameworks for nursing practice.

Introduction

This chapter aims to provide an overview of the multifaceted process of development that occurs throughout a person's life. It begins with an outline of two social sciences, psychology and sociology, with explanation of contrasting approaches to both, which recur throughout. Key topics from each subject are explored, namely motivation, culture, socialization and family. Physical development is described from conception through infancy and childhood milestones, adolescence and adulthood to old age. Psychosocial development covers the emergence of the self-concept, cognition and morality, emotional attachment and separation, aspects of sexuality and personality, and social integration. Implications of this subject matter for student nurses and nursing practice are highlighted as they arise, i.e. why it is important for all nurses to be aware of patients' developmental issues when planning and implementing their care.

Psychology and sociology related to development and nursing

This section outlines the psychological and sociological theories, approaches, frameworks and important topics such as motivation and culture required for understanding developmental processes.

What is psychology?

Gross (2001) has described how psychologists seem to provoke three typical reactions in others. These are:

- Concern that they should be careful what they say or do in their presence, as if psychologists are 'mind-readers'. Although not literally true, psychologists, and indeed nurses, do interpret body language to infer what a person is thinking or feeling (see Ch. 9).
- A misconception that psychologists' work relates largely to emotionally distressed or mentally ill clients. This probably represents confusion of psychology with psychiatry, the branch of medicine specializing in such conditions, although clinical psychologists do contribute to therapies, e.g. in assisting people to cope with anxiety (see Ch. 11).
- Puzzlement about what exactly a psychologist does; this is understandable, as psychology is a wide-ranging field of diverse origins that overlaps with other subjects such as sociology (see p. 189 onwards).

The word psychology is a composite of the Greek term *psyche*, which refers to the ancient view of the soul, spirit or mind, and *logos*, which means discourse or intellectual debate, a then-favoured method of pursuing investigation or study. Thus, in modern terms, it can be taken to mean 'the study of the mind', or of mental processes, and it is clearly useful for nurses to understand what is going on in a patient's/client's mind and the resulting consequences, i.e. patient behaviour.

The father of psychology is usually identified as Wilhelm Wundt who, in 1879, initiated scientific research into the mind. Wundt aimed to study perceptual discrimination of sensory input, e.g. vision under controlled conditions, and so develop an understanding of what he termed the 'elements of consciousness', building blocks of the mind. He felt able to investigate discernible differences in intensity and quality of stimuli, and so begin to describe the structure of the human mind – termed the 'structuralist' approach to psychology.

William James likened Wundt's method to trying to understand a house by contemplating its individual bricks, and considered that the 'whole' mind as an integrated entity was of more significance than the sum of its parts, inspiring the Gestalt viewpoint, which gained currency from the 1920s. James was more interested in what the mind could *do* and what it is *for*, i.e. the 'functionalist' approach. This focuses on studying thoughts and emotions, and how they help people to survive in their environment. From these early origins, this hybrid discipline branched into at least three distinct schools or approaches – psychodynamic, behaviourist and humanistic.

Psychodynamic approach (see pp. 212, 214 and 218)

This stemmed from the publications of Sigmund Freud from the 1890s onwards. Essentially, this emphasized the importance of unconscious processes in emotions and behaviours. Freud developed a therapeutic approach called 'psychoanalysis', designed to gain access to the unconscious mind using means such as hypnosis, tranquillizing medication and dream analysis.

Behaviourist approach

By the early 1900s, American academics such as J.B. Watson had become increasingly critical of the subjective methods used by Freud and Wundt. They argued that mental events were inaccessible to and therefore inappropriate for scientific investigation. It was argued that psychologists should concentrate on dispassionately and accurately observing outward behaviour, for example responses to experimentally controlled stimuli. Much of the behaviourists' focus was on studies of animal learning, which they viewed as taking two forms:

- Classical conditioning – a process of passively associating things that seem to be linked in time and place, e.g. Pavlov's dogs learning that the sound of a bell signified imminent food.
- Operant conditioning – noting the consequences of one's actions, e.g. behaviour being 'reinforced', or strengthened, by its gaining rewards or weakened by ensuing punishment.

This approach assumed the validity of comparisons between humans and animals, and that environmental factors can and could be used to determine or 'shape' an individual's behaviour, just as animals can be trained to perform skills beyond their normal repertoire. Psychologists could thus devise methods of engineering people's behaviour in 'desirable' directions by means of 'conditioning' programmes. Behaviourism held sway in psychology until after World War 2, when its emphasis on animal observation and scientific rigour began to be questioned.

Humanistic approach

A new school of psychologists, including Abraham Maslow and Carl Rogers, then emerged as a 'third force' in this subject. The humanists focused on aspects of purely human experience, such as free will and self-fulfilment. Their methods of enquiry were subjective and person-centred, such as interview and self-report. Offshoots included therapeutic self-help groups and learner-directed educational approaches. Humanism emphasizes the positive potential in people and the importance of fostering appropriate individual choices in maximizing each person's well-being and life satisfaction.

Applying psychological approaches to health

The three approaches can be exemplified with reference to a health issue such as smoking, as follows.

- The psychodynamic approach would propose unconscious processes as the underlying cause, such as fearful or guilty thoughts generating nervous tension, which tobacco may alleviate. Smoking might also be considered a form of oral pleasure or a by-product of self-destructive instinct (see pp. 187 and 214). To assist smoking cessation, underlying conflicts or urges should be brought to awareness, so they can be consciously addressed and resolved. 'Orality' might be satisfied by other means, e.g. chewing gum, with added nicotine initially.
- Behaviourists would assume that smoking is a learned behaviour, a habit created by consistent associations, including routine and reward. This might include automatic 'lighting up' at certain times of day or under particular circumstances, for example after meals or when feeling stressed or bored, gaining periodic 'escape' from a hospital environment, and to feel 'grown-up' or sophisticated. It also gives the smoker's fingers something to do when fidgety. This perspective would aim to facilitate 'unlearning' of these associations, e.g. by suggesting changes of daily routine and use of non-smoking facilities. Health promotion campaigns in the UK have emphasized that tobacco smoke odorizes clothes and hair and that those who quit have regained 'a mind of their own'. Smokers being inconvenienced, e.g. being forced to go outside health service premises to smoke, verbally admonished or refused surgery until they stop would be examples of 'punishment', a form of operant conditioning.
- Humanists would presume that smokers are aware of positive benefits that they derive from tobacco – a reality often ignored by health promoters. For example, relaxing activities such as reading or drinking alcohol may be enhanced by tobacco smoking, and might be a relatively affordable

pleasure for people who are socioeconomically disadvantaged. The client would be respectfully encouraged to review their choice to smoke, perhaps by comparing the benefits gained from smoking with those they would obtain from stopping, e.g. greater stamina, fitness, longevity, disposable income and attractiveness. Humanists might also try to harness smokers' inherent respect for people by highlighting adverse effects they may impose on others, e.g. unpleasant smells, respiratory irritation or even permanent harm from secondary smoke – especially in the case of young children.

Motivation

Motivation is the underlying cause of actions. Without it people would be inert and not function. It provides individuals with the stamina and focus required to perform their activities.

Essentially then, motivation is used to explain behaviour. Without apparent explanation, behaviour may appear to be fruitless, perplexing or dangerously unpredictable. Nurses need to understand what happens in their environment, including the actions of others, not only to be able to predict eventualities but also to plan their own behaviour and interventions appropriately. Box 8.1 provides an opportunity to consider the motivation to become a nurse.

REFLECTIVE PRACTICE Box 8.1

Motivation to become a nurse

Think about your reasons for becoming a nurse. It may be useful to compare your reasons with those of colleagues, and note any that are different from your own.

Student activities

- Try to compile a list of several distinct motives. Possible reasons might include wanting to care for others, to work with and help people, or professional career aspirations.
- Consider why other people may have different reasons for becoming a nurse.
- Read the text outlining theories/approaches of motivation (p. 187–189). Then return to your original motives for becoming a nurse and try to relate them to the motivation theories outlined.

The 'instincts' theory of motivation

Early psychologists studied animals and compared their behaviour with that of humans, who were viewed as the most evolved and complex members of the animal kingdom.

Consider the question, 'What makes cats hunt, birds sing and monkeys climb?' The usual response is their respective 'instincts'. The next question to address is, 'What is meant by the term instinct?' A reasonable answer might be a complex, unlearned behaviour pattern, i.e. more than a single reflex, specific to a species, which is elicited by a specific stimulus or 'releaser', e.g. a mouse appearing in front of a cat. The word derives from the Greek to 'impel' or 'instigate'.

'Acting on instinct' is often used to describe automatic behaviour, such as using touch to comfort a distressed patient. However, many consider that there are no evident instincts in humans, as it can be argued that even seemingly natural characteristics such as associating with others, sexual desire, masculine aggression, parenting and intuition all involve some process of learning and are not always present.

Early attempts by William McDougall to explain all human behaviour in terms of instincts foundered on two problems. Firstly, because of the complexity and variability of human behaviour, his approach with 800 separate instincts was unconvincing in explaining why humans differ from each other so widely in preferences and responses, as only some humans hunt, sing and climb, and very few enjoy all three. Second, this approach was criticized for its lack of explanatory value, because it led to a circular argument. The question, 'What makes humans act in certain ways?' would prompt the answer 'instincts'. To the follow-up query, 'What are instincts?', MacDougall's response might have been 'things we naturally possess that make us act in those ways'.

Freud proposed that just two instincts motivated behaviour:

- Eros – the 'life-force' promoting survival, sexuality and creativity. Examples may include people whose desire to live helps to 'carry them through' illness against medical predictions; patients who tolerate prolonged, unpleasant and expensive fertility treatment; and individuals whose engagement with work or their 'art' may be at the expense of their health.
- Thanatos – this is the polar opposite and generates destructive impulses; in its most extreme expression, a 'death wish'. It may be evident in risk-taking behaviours, e.g. participating in dangerous sports or unsafe sexual practices, using recreational drugs, deliberate self-harm or suicide attempts, or vicariously in the appeal of action movies.

Behaviourist theories of motivation

In the 1950s, Lorenz demonstrated that newly hatched goslings follow the first large moving object, whether either himself or an inanimate figure that they are exposed to in a critical period during their early days of life – thought to be an instinctive releaser normally allowing them to be led to the relative safety of water. Subsequently they were described as behaviourally attached to or 'imprinted on' this initial figure as their particular, if experimentally odd, 'Mother Goose'.

It is possible to suggest examples of critical periods, releasers or imprinting in human development. For instance, there is considerable evidence that language acquisition (see Ch. 9) and 'healthy' personality development – socialization (pp. 194–195) and attachment (pp. 212–214) – are dependent on exposure to normal human society in the first 4 years of life. Parental feelings and caring skills may be experienced or 'released' for the first time after

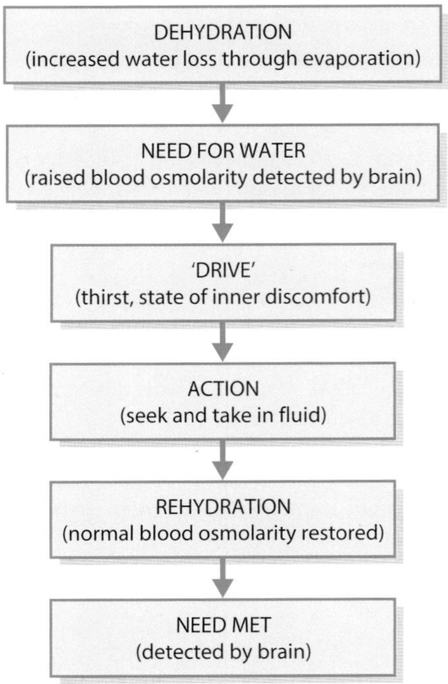

Fig. 8.1 An example of a drive

> **Box 8.2 Maslow's hierarchy of human needs**
>
> **7 Self-actualization**
> Achieving one's personal aspirations and potential
>
> ***6 Aesthetic needs**
> Beauty in one's surroundings; an ordered environment
>
> ***5 Cognitive needs**
> Knowledge and understanding, curiosity and exploration; search for meaning
>
> **4 Esteem needs**
> Being valued by others and oneself; a sense of personal worth and competence
>
> **3 Love and belongingness (affiliation) needs**
> Giving and receiving affection; trust and acceptance of others, being part of a group
>
> **2 Safety needs**
> Both physical preservation and psychological composure
>
> **1 Physiological needs**
> Homeostatic necessities required for bodily survival
>
> * Omitted in some descriptions.

having one's own child and, in some cases, following a parent into nursing may be considered to be an example of imprinting.

Drive theory

Clark Hull argued that all behaviour was impelled by 'drives', hypothetical internal states arising from 'needs'. Figure 8.1 shows how this approach can be used to explain increased fluid intake on a hot day, essentially a homeostatic mechanism (Ch. 19).

Hull's theory explains biological or 'primary' needs relating to homeostasis, such as hunger, thirst and sleep, but seems less convincing when proposing 'secondary' drives to explain the wider range of human pursuits, e.g. intellectual or social activities.

Nonetheless, the terms 'drive' or 'driven' are often used conversationally with regard to motivation, and Hull's framework accords well with the experience that it is sometimes better to want or pursue something than to attain it.

Humanistic approach to motivation

Humanists believe that people are unique in possessing a rich mental life, including free choice of action, dreams and personal goals, rendering behaviourist comparisons with other species futile.

Maslow proposed a 'hierarchy of needs' to explain human behaviour. Although this originally comprised five levels of need, two more levels have since been added. Note that some descriptions omit levels 5 and 6 shown in the 7-level adaptation (Box 8.2). The goal at the highest tier of the hierarchy is individual fulfilment or self-actualization, but this can normally only be attained following prior satisfaction of lower levels of need. The hierarchy of needs can be represented as a pyramid with self-actualization at the apex and the physiological needs at its base (see Atkinson et al 2000).

Examples of how nurses may help patients/clients to meet needs at each level include:

- *Physiological needs*: Assisting people in relation to nutritional and fluid intake (Ch. 19), breathing (Ch. 17), temperature regulation (Ch. 14), rest and sleep (Ch. 10) and elimination (Chs 20, 21). They may also extend to other nursing activities such as providing advice on sexual matters, e.g. family planning, as reproduction was viewed as basic need.
- *Safety needs*: These include maintaining physical safety, e.g. against environmental hazards such as protecting people from falls, traffic during outings or scalding liquids (Ch. 13) and infection (Ch. 15). Psychological aspects of care include offering explanation or reassurance in advance of investigations/treatments to increase patient cooperation and reduce fear of the unknown (Chs 9, 11), providing some consistency in daily routine and minimizing or responding to pain (Ch. 23).
- *Affiliation or belongingness needs*: Enabling people to feel loved and not alone, for example by encouraging visits from family members, passing on telephone messages, displaying greetings cards, celebrating their birthdays, organizing social activities with other patients/clients where appropriate and establishing a sound nurse–patient/client relationship (Ch. 9).
- *Esteem needs*: Nurses should always show a respectful manner towards patients/clients, recognize their achievements, e.g. progress in rehabilitation (Ch. 11); counter self-deprecation, e.g. in depression; reinforce

positive aspects of their self-image (Chs 9, 11) and help them to feel fresh and 'look their best' (Ch. 16).

- *Cognitive needs*: Provide patients/clients with the prerequisite knowledge and skills to optimize self-care (Chs 3, 11) and prevent relapse, keep them informed of developments and facilitate active mental occupation, e.g. via reading materials, crosswords, television, liaising with occupational therapists or employment training services (see Ch. 4).
- *Aesthetic needs*: May relate to the patient's/client's appearance, e.g. the nurse may help a patient/client to select matching clothes, organize a hairdresser or beautician. Nurses may be involved in maximizing the attractiveness of care surroundings, for example by tidying bedding, minimizing unpleasant odours, arranging flowers and by recognizing important festivals for patients/clients such as by putting up Christmas decorations or helping clients to celebrate Diwali (Deepavali), the Hindu festival of light, in which people exchange presents, light their homes and have fireworks.
- *Self-actualization*: A person's goals and possibilities may be heavily constrained by ill-health or disability. For some patients, being able to walk again after an accident, or to return to home or work after treatment, may be the major aspiration. Other specific ambitions might be a relatively independent existence in the community for a person with a learning disability (also called intellectual disability), or in mental health, where recovery is not simply the absence of symptoms. It is based on hope, involvement, participation, inclusion, meaning, purpose, control and self-management, meaningful activity, employment, maintaining social networks and activities when distressed and having the chance to contribute, or give back, in some way. The nurse may contribute to the requisite therapeutic relationship, skills provision and support network, enabling the client to attain their individual aims.

Maslow's concept of self-actualization is embodied in *peak experiences*, cherishable moments of ecstatic happiness when everything seems to 'gel' and feels right, and a person's essential current ambition is fulfilled. He considered that all humans were capable of these, although they are usually infrequent and some may occur 'once in a lifetime'.

There are, however, exceptions to the hierarchical structure of lower needs always being fulfilled before higher needs. It is possible to identify valid exceptions to Maslow's order of priorities. For instance:

- Fasting before anaesthesia places safety (level 2) before eating and drinking (level 1)
- People may pursue higher needs such as social activities, sport, career and creativity (levels 3–5) at the expense of their physical health or safety (levels 1–2)
- A terminally ill patient may waive analgesia (level 2) in order to keep their mind clear for crucial decisions such as testamentary amendments (level 7).

What is sociology?

Definitions vary, and often reveal the standpoint of the writer. Macrosociology emphasizes the study of society overall, while microsociology focuses on the interactions of individuals within it. All degrees of magnification in between these extremes are possible, for instance when studying groups within society. Health workers can be considered through the one-to-one dealings of individual nurses with their patients/clients, the functioning of ward teams or types/grades of nurses, the profession as a whole, or the entire NHS workforce.

The focus could enlarge further to cover people in Britain, Westerners or, indeed, all mankind. Sociology can therefore be defined as the study of societies, their component groups and individual interactions.

However, all sociologists would agree that people cannot be understood as individuals in a vacuum; to be human is to be social. People arise from social groups and from within society, and are part of its fabric during their lifespan. In effect, people are society, i.e. each person is equivalent to a brick within the building and society is 'within each person', as contact with others in society shapes each person. Because of this, nurses can only understand others and themselves by appreciating this social dimension common to all people.

Several sociologists' views have been particularly influential over the 19th and 20th centuries; an outline is provided in Box 8.3 (see p. 190).

Conflict approaches

These consider society as characterized by competition between antagonistic groups, each in pursuit of opposing interests. These include:

- Marxists stressing economic disparity in Western societies
- Feminists protesting against male domination over wealth and social institutions, e.g. family life, Parliament or the over-representation of males in senior healthcare posts.

Conflict perspectives characteristically argue the need for radical revision or overthrow of society's attitudes, institutions and general way of life.

Microsociological approach

This focuses on the individuals and groups whose daily interactions comprise society's life, e.g. how nurses behave towards patients/clients and their colleagues, the experiences of student nurses in clinical areas or whether nursing is a 'profession'. Such studies view people as entering social situations with pre-existing ideas about themselves, others and the situation, e.g. their relative status and expected actions, and this subjective perspective largely determines their interpersonal behaviour. Members of a society possess shared meanings in the use of symbols such as language, gestures and other non-verbal behaviour including dress, focus on which is often termed 'symbolic interactionism' (see Ch. 9).

Box 8.3 **Influential sociologists**

Auguste Comte
During the 19th century the French 'Father of Sociology' was positive that his 'Queen of Sciences' would establish truths about recently urbanized, 'industrial' society and so be able to prescribe remedies for its human difficulties. This gave him the confidence to dub himself the 'Great Priest of Humanity' and his optimistic outlook has been shared by many of his successors.

Karl Marx
Marx was particularly conscious of the extreme economic inequalities within newly industrialized mid-19th century society. He predicted that the masses of employed workers – 'the proletariat' – would come to realize their exploitation and the need to wrest ownership of factories and land, the source of societal wealth, from their employers, the capitalist minority. The post-revolutionary sharing of society's 'means of production' would inaugurate an era of classless, socialist utopia.

Max Weber
Weber modified Marx's economic 'conflict' interpretation of society by focusing more narrowly and deeply on the perspectives and interactions of individuals and groups within society. For example, he noted the diversity of skills, status and aspirations within the working class, which Marx had tended to treat as a homogeneous mass. Weber also emphasized the usefulness of greater subjectivity within sociology, empathy being a prerequisite to understanding the shared meanings in human interactions – *verstehen*. An example of this approach would be to consider the many possible factors contributing to the anxiety experienced by a patient newly admitted to hospital.

Emile Durkheim
Comparative study between societies was Durkheim's hallmark. He used newly accumulated data on populations, such as census information, to make deductions about the actions, thoughts and feelings of individuals. In particular he came to view suicide as a reflection of the circumstances, expectations and laws of the groups, organizations and society to which one belongs, rather than a purely private, individual act. It is only possible to understand phenomena such as 'suicide bombings' by taking their social context into account.

Park, Cooley and Mead
In the United States, the 19th and early 20th centuries saw huge expansion of industrial cities, which together with mass immigration led to many social problems such as crime, ghetto squalor and intergroup hostility. Robert Park and his colleagues used the city of Chicago as a laboratory for research 'in the field', while Charles Cooley and G.H. Mead worked on the social interactions of key significance in childhood development (see the 'self', pp. 204–207).

Talcott Parsons
During the 20th century Parsons formulated a comprehensive theory of society as a functioning entity, with each individual, group and organization playing its part or 'role' to make the system work and deriving benefits in return for their contribution. This represents an alternative macrosociological ('big picture') structuralist perspective or viewpoint to that of Marx on societal study, looking at society as a single, whole entity. Parson's 'structural functionalist' or 'consensus' approach views society as a harmonious arrangement wherein people basically agree on fundamental operational principles. This enables society to operate or function effectively. Each member works to benefit society, and in return active membership benefits each member, e.g. nurses provide health care, while potential patients transport them to work or provide food for them.

Why is sociology relevant to nursing?

Consider the following quotation:

> No man is an island, entire of itself ... any man's death diminishes me because I am involved in mankind; and therefore never send to know for whom the bell tolls, it tolls for thee.
>
> John Donne 1624

The excerpt from this 17th century poet's meditation compares a man's death to a clod of earth being washed into the sea. It emphasizes how inextricably each person is bound up with other members of their society and its groups, even if the person is not conscious of this communality in their individual day-to-day pursuits and concerns. It is reminiscent of the sociobiological explanation of why people are inclined to help others – the cardinal function of nursing. Due to a common evolutionary ancestry, this argues that all humans are genetically related to each other, so that assisting others to survive helps preserve some of their own genes.

Knowledge of sociology helps nurses to understand the behaviours of patients/clients, families and colleagues. For example, a patient's/client's outward distress is automatically attributed to physical pain, or else fear regarding the experience or findings of an operation (Box 8.4). In other words, physical or psychological factors specific to the individual tend to be the initial assumption.

However, patients'/clients' concerns often arise from a wider social context, such as worries about family members, employment or even care of pets. A patient/client might be more concerned about being forbidden to move

CRITICAL THINKING Box 8.4

Michael

Michael is recovering from surgery, which has been technically successful. Despite having received appropriate information and nursing care to maximize his physical comfort, he remains restless, tearful and frequently demands nursing attention.

Student activities

- Consider why Michael might be reacting in this way.
- Discuss the scenario with your mentor.

REFLECTIVE PRACTICE Box 8.5

Adjusting to new nursing environments

All student nurses encounter unfamiliar settings at the beginning of new placements, which can provoke anxiety.

Student activities

- What is involved, for example, in settling into a new clinical environment?
- What social rules have to be learned, and why?
- What behaviours are appropriately 'automatic' and how does this vary according to your role there?

heavy items at work after back surgery and the effects on their livelihood and self-worth than about any transient postoperative pain or discomfort. Health professionals rarely gain such insights from case notes or superficial encounters with the patient/client; they often emerge only when imparted in the context of a trusting relationship with the patient/client, which takes time and effort to develop (see Ch. 9).

Sociology provides insights into aspects of the nurse's own culture and, by logical extension, into different cultures, particularly significant with the increasing cultural diversity of British society. Examples of this include the social practices specific to some members of minority groups. A patient/client or their relatives may be upset or feel offended if an otherwise caring environment fails to accommodate their cultural norms such as food preferences, consultation of their spouse or prayer requirements.

This awareness can also be turned to enhancing the nurse's self-understanding, for instance by analysis of their own social experience (Box 8.5).

The layout, titles and respective roles of new colleagues, in addition to the names and needs of the current patients/clients, must all be learned. The management style of the charge nurse on any day may be important, for example whether the use of first name terms is mutually acceptable and how strict time constraints are for completing tasks or meal breaks. Appropriate use of initiative has to be gauged through experience, and may be quite different for a nurse in a student role compared with their concurrent part-time or former auxiliary role, perhaps in the same environment. Understanding the dynamics of this process may help to diminish the stress of the new placement.

Sociology can also shed light on larger scale social issues, possible remedial strategies and insight into the effectiveness of these measures, e.g. by performing research and analyzing its findings (see Ch. 5). Approaches include compiling and analysing quantitative data, e.g. the incidence of teenage pregnancy, and qualitative measures such as surveying attitudes, e.g. to binge drinking or unprotected sex.

Whatever their focus and theoretical standpoint, it would be hoped that social scientists would provide insightful appraisal of social realities to at least complement those offered by religions and secular common sense.

CRITICAL THINKING Box 8.6

Is commonsense all we need?

Read the statements below and decide whether they are true or false.

- A long and healthy life results from inheriting a sound constitution.
- Older people are repositories of wisdom and are consequently viewed with universal respect.
- The provision of a high quality, effective educational system that is accessible to all would result in the disappearance of social inequalities.

Student activities

- Discuss the statements with your mentor or a fellow student and decide why your true/false decision is important.
- Consider the sociological aspects of each statement and their relevance to nursing.

Common sense and sociology

Nurses need to consider how sociology can enhance commonsense thinking (Box 8.6). Further discussion of sociology and commonsense is available in Further reading (e.g. Giddens 1989).

Perhaps the best way to ensure a long life is to pick healthy parents, as longevity or brevity tends to run in families. However, although genes play a role in determining susceptibility to many diseases, environmental factors appear to contribute equally as significantly. This explains the close association between health and wealth, apparent in the significantly raised incidence of nearly all serious disease categories among the poorest sections of society (Townsend & Whitehead 1990) (see Ch. 1). Relevant factors include quality of housing, diet, occupation, leisure activities and, more controversially, healthcare provision. Thus a person's family environment may have much more significance to health than their genes.

Regarding the second statement, most older adults retain their mental vigour with only around 5% of those over 65, and 20% of those over 80 years of age, exhibiting dementia (Alzheimer's Society 2006). They undoubtedly represent stores of accumulated knowledge and skills, distilled into wisdom by a lifetime's reflection on their experience. Despite this, older adults in Western society have been typically viewed as a redundant group who are an economic burden on the productive section of society. They tend to be functionally marginalized, i.e. excluded from the social mainstream in, for example, occupation and leisure, rationed in resources such as facilities and benefits, and viewed not with respect but in a derogatory manner, ranging from well-meaning pity to outright contempt, some of the many expressions of ageism.

Although education is often regarded as the key to universal achievement and equality, there is much to suggest that the Western system tends to perpetuate and cement inequalities. Middle-class children tend to achieve more and better qualifications than their working class counterparts, perhaps in part because their parents provide better preparation, encouragement and facilities, but also because they seem to relate more easily to teachers and their style of communication. This disparity is accentuated by other social factors that predominate in the working class such as early pressure to earn, widely varying facilities even within the state system and peer group behaviours. Thus children from affluent backgrounds are more likely to progress directly to full-time higher education and from there to better paid jobs, often in their parents' professions.

Culture

Take a moment to think of what the term 'culture' means to you. Common responses include normal patterns of behaviour within one's country, including eating, drinking and speech, and 'lofty' forms of social expression such as art, music and literature.

Culture can be defined as the way of life of a society – a group of people who share a distinct identity, often within a circumscribed locality. Components of a culture include beliefs, values and norms.

It is, however, important to remember that the components of culture typically change within a society over time, allowing it to gradually adapt to changing circumstances and evolve. An example of this is the insistence in the late 19th and early 20th century that student or 'probationer' nurses were all female and would attend Christian services each Sunday, stay within the nurses' home when not on duty and leave the profession once married (see Ch. 2). This is quite different to experiences of student nurses in the 21st century.

Beliefs

These are factual ideas such as religious beliefs about whether there is one God, or more, or none. Some beliefs may involve lifestyle issues, e.g. a nutritional belief about what is good or bad to eat, or how it should be prepared, which varies hugely between societies, as does the acceptability of alcohol. Traditional cultures may revere people who see visions and hear divine voices, whereas in Western cultures a psychiatrist is likely to be consulted.

Box 8.7 Types of norm

- *Folkways*: Common conventions whose original rationale is obscure, e.g. throwing rice at newly-weds symbolizes fertility, buying and decorating a Christmas tree, or referring to mundane events such as time of rising from and going to bed. Non-adherence tends to be condoned or viewed as harmless eccentricity.
- *Customs*: More universal traditions, whose original sense is apparent, e.g. shaking hands, singing national anthems, giving presents at weddings and birthdays. Non-adherence may cause offence.
- *Mores*: Strict regulations governing conduct, or 'thou shalt nots', which may be formalized in legislation (see Ch. 6), with punitive sanctions for transgression. Mores range from disapproval of theft – in some cultures this is punished by surgical limb amputation, while motoring offences such as driving just over the speed limit may result in a fixed penalty fine – to *taboos*, which are totally prohibited activities such as cannibalism, incest and paedophilia.
- *Rules*: Specific guidelines that vary from informal local instructions to written policies or codes of professional conduct, such as that published by the NMC (2004).

Values

These are broad guidelines for activities, conveying what principles a society deems valuable or worth preserving. In the West, freedom of speech, occupation and choice of partner is highly prized, which may conflict with values such as patriotism, equality of wealth and respect for older people, which are more esteemed in other societies. Values tend to be more absolute than beliefs, i.e. are subscribed to whole-heartedly or not at all, so that optimizing 'health' may either govern one's lifestyle fully or not at all. The sanctity of life, i.e. that life is precious and should not be taken intentionally, is another value central to healthcare but not to all human situations.

Norms

These are more specific behavioural expectations relevant to particular circumstances, equivalent to everyday 'do's' and 'don'ts'. For instance, personal greetings such as tongue protrusion are expected in Maori ceremonies but not at social gatherings in the Western world, there are occasions where polite versus familiar speech is expected, eating etiquette including table manners and fashionable attire. Conformity increases the likelihood of social acceptance and success, e.g. belching is rarely appreciated at formal dinners in the UK, and often mirrors the underpinning value, e.g. paying for goods reflects honesty or adhering to nursing advice suggests that a patient/client values health. Norms are in turn often subdivided into folkways, customs, mores and rules (Box 8.7).

Cultural universals

As well as the foregoing components, some elements of culture are common to all societies. For example language, both verbal and non-verbal, enables interpersonal communication (see Ch. 9). Mutual understanding of the spoken and written word can give members of a society a unique communal currency, especially if fluency is restricted to small populations, e.g. the Celtic tongues in the UK.

Facial expressions conveying universal emotions such as joy, sorrow, fear and surprise are recognized across cultural groups, but conventions governing the meaning of gestures and acceptable degrees of interpersonal touch and distance vary widely. Other aspects probably common to all cultures, past and present, include:

- Religious ceremonies
- Communal buildings and housing
- Money and property
- Art forms including graphics, music and dance
- Humour
- Jewellery and dress
- Exchange of gifts
- Courtship and marriage
- Specific dietary and hygiene-related practices (Chs 16, 19).

Cultural bias and relativism

Comparing the different practices and underpinning belief systems of different cultures tends to encourage people to favour those of their own society. There are many possible reasons for this bias. These include respect for those people who have nurtured them, greater familiarity with their own ways and boosting group self-esteem through criticizing foreign behaviours. However, in a culturally diverse society, this may lead to intergroup hostility and discrimination, resulting in unequal treatment, not least in healthcare settings. Thus it is important to remain aware of this tendency, and to try to accept these differences as indicators of the distinctiveness of a particular group rather considering whether they are better or worse than one's own experiences. Aspects of Western culture, which might strike an outsider as different or unusual, are considered in Box 8.8.

REFLECTIVE PRACTICE Box 8.8

Some characteristics of Western culture

- Preoccupation with material goods
- Working hours that leave little time for family life or require delegation of child care to strangers
- Pursuit of individual success
- Contraception and abortion practices
- Consumption of convenience food and alcohol
- Ideal of thin women
- Interest in spectator sports
- Pampering of pet animals
- Frank expression of sexuality
- Media portrayal of violence
- Feeling compelled to observe festive seasonal customs, such as buying Easter eggs, although not attending an Easter church service
- Variety of political opinions and their free expression

Student activities

- Think about your views on the ideas above.
- Find out about the views of a patient/client and/or a friend from a different background.

REFLECTIVE PRACTICE Box 8.9

Culture shock

Think about a time when you became part of a new subculture, for example starting a new school, meeting your partner's family or starting your nursing course.

Student activities

- What aspects of the new subculture made you feel anxious?
- Were there any similarities with the stressors associated with admission to hospital or a care home (see p. 194)?
- What helped to reduce the anxieties (e.g. printed information about your course sent before you started)?
- Reflect on the extent to which you have observed nurses help people to overcome some of the practices within a care setting that may contribute to culture shock

Subcultures

Individuals within a society form groups that have their own distinctive views and practices. These variations inside a culture give rise to subcultures – effectively 'cultures within a culture'. A common example is youth culture, as young people have typical values, beliefs and norms such as a code of conduct in relation to dress, speech and musical taste. These may vary markedly from those of older adults who comprise the influential majority and so the cultural yardstick of society. Other 'variant' subcultures include those of minority ethnic groups, students and healthcare professionals. Some subcultures overtly refuse to comply with existing laws in a society, and are termed 'deviant' subcultures, such as criminal gangs. 'Counter-cultures' are antagonistic towards the prevailing dominant culture, although they may not break any of its legal statutes, e.g. travelling people, self-sufficient smallholders and pacifist campaigners in the UK (Giddens 2001).

Culture shock

This is the term given to the sense of disorientation experienced when exposed to an unaccustomed culture or subculture. Varying degrees of this occur when on holiday abroad, when entering a new workplace or setting (Box 8.9). Admission to hospital or to a care home may provoke anxiety. The possible stressors (see Ch. 11) associated with the hospital/care home subculture might include:

- Strange language, e.g. technical terms used by staff
- Changes in norms, e.g. having to follow instructions regarding what and when to eat and drink, go to bed/arise, taking medication, undergoing investigations, wearing nightclothes during the day, undressing in front of strangers, restrictions on where one may go
- Questioning values, reappraising priorities, e.g. health over pleasure, one's occupation and its pressures
- Threats to composure, e.g. facing the real prospect of one's own mortality, religious practices being compromised
- Tolerating other people's behaviour, e.g. noisy staff, visitors and patients
- Challenged preferences, e.g. channel on a communal television, self-disclosure expected by other residents.

CRITICAL THINKING Box 8.10

Cultural awareness in nursing practice

You are helping the registered nurse (RN) to admit a client who is anxious about being admitted to the unit. The RN asks the client for his Christian name and is surprised when he challenges her by saying that he is Muslim.

Student activities

- Find out about Muslim naming systems.
- Find out the policy for asking about names on your next placement.
- Choose a religion/culture that you are unfamiliar with and identify the usual practices in relation to some of the activities described in this section.

[Resource: BBC (Religion and Ethics) – www.bbc.co.uk/worldservice/people/features/world_religions/index.shtml Available July 2006]

Culture and healthcare (see Ch. 1)

A profound interconnection exists between these two. People from different cultures may have conflicting ideas about what constitutes health or illness, for example the diagnostic criteria for mental health problems such as schizophrenia differ enormously between Western and Eastern perspectives, and studies have shown wide cultural variations regarding pain tolerance (see Ch. 23), risk-taking behaviours, e.g. use of cannabis by Rastafarians, and unsafe sexual behaviours and the spread of the human immunodeficiency virus (HIV) in sub-Saharan Africa.

Nurses have to be sensitive to the cultural expectations of individual patients/clients and families, without making stereotypical assumptions, if they are to deliver holistic care (Box 8.10). This may involve aspects that include:

- *Health beliefs* (see Ch. 1).
- *Naming systems*: For example, most Sikh names comprise a personal name, a gender designation (Singh for males and Kaur for females) and a last/family name. Avoid offence by using the terms 'first name' rather than 'Christian name' and 'last/family name' instead of 'surname'.
- *Assessment interview* (see Ch. 14): Some groups are patriarchal and the father of the family may expect to answer questions and make decisions, or at least be present at interviews, concerning his wife or children. Nurses must be guided by clause 3 of The NMC *Code of professional conduct: standards for conduct, performance and ethics* (2004), which deals with consent to treatment or care (see Ch. 7).
- *Dietary considerations* (see Ch. 19): Proscriptions exist such as avoidance of pork by Jews and Muslims, and beef by Sikhs and Hindus; many sects are entirely vegetarian; vegans do not eat any animal products including eggs and dairy products; Mormons avoid caffeine and alcohol. Foods may be prescribed, e.g. Moslems require Halal meat obtained from animals slaughtered in accordance with Islamic law; Jews require Kosher food, which conforms to and is prepared according to the laws of Judaism. Religious fasting may be observed, such as Muslims during Ramadan. However, patients/clients may be exempt from fasting restrictions due to their age or medical condition; younger ones especially may not adhere to orthodox practices.
- *Dignity*: Members of several cultural/religious groups are concerned with maintaining modesty and would be particularly unhappy to wear revealing hospital gowns, sharing ward areas, bathing facilities and lavatories with or being nursed by the opposite sex.
- *Personal hygiene/elimination* (see Chs 16, 20, 21): Hindus and Muslims prefer to wash using running water, and to wash after elimination rather than use lavatory tissue. Strict Muslims must wash before prayers. They use their left hand for 'dirtier' areas and the right hand for handling food. Women may wish to wash their whole bodies at each personal hygiene intervention during menstruation.
- *Medical interventions*: Blood transfusions and permanent tissue transplants are not permitted by Jehovah's Witnesses; Christian Scientists deny sickness as a reality and may refuse any treatment beyond prayer, even for a sick child; Hindu women may object to vaginal examinations; Chinese patients/clients may prefer traditional, e.g. herbal remedies and acupuncture (see Ch. 10), options to those of Western medicine.
- *Family planning*: Many religions, including Buddhism and Roman Catholicism, disapprove of artificial birth control and termination of pregnancy. Many cultures such as in China and India have a preference for male babies.
- *Palliative care* (see Ch. 12).

Socialization

This is the process whereby a society transmits its culture (or group its subculture) to its future members. As a

REFLECTIVE PRACTICE Box 8.11

Personal experience of socialization

Think back to an episode when you learned something from a parent or person close to you, from the mass media and from a RN while on placement.

Student activities

- Reflect on the agents of socialization in each case and your relationship with them and the feelings that coloured the experience.
- How did these feelings differ between the three examples and how did this affect your learning?

Note: You may find that feelings significantly colour such recollections. As socialization is an interpersonal process, it often imparts learning in a profound and emotional manner.

Box 8.12 **Rights and responsibilities related to the role of student nurses**

Possible rights

- Paid a bursary/salary, no tuition fees
- To be educated
- To receive free uniforms where appropriate
- A safe and healthy environment in which to work and study
- Supernumerary status in placements

Possible responsibilities

- Attend classes and placements
- Apply oneself adequately to studies
- Meet assignment deadlines
- Be presentable when on duty
- Conduct oneself professionally

result, individuals acquire the knowledge and skills that allow them to function socially, leading to personal and communal success. Socialization is usually described in two phases: primary and secondary (Box 8.11).

Socialization is a two-way process throughout, with the novice challenging the 'mentor' by asking questions and proposing alternatives, so that becoming a parent involves learning from interactions with one's children, and the same give-and-take occurs during grandparenting.

Primary socialization

This occurs in early childhood, and the main 'agents' are usually close family members. The preschool child acquires fundamental skills relating to interaction with others including speech, gesture and appropriate behaviour, and self-care, e.g. continence, dressing, feeding. In addition, attitudes including moral and religious beliefs are transmitted. On occasions, teaching can be formal, or deliberate, such as instruction on tying shoelaces. At other times, it may be imparted unconsciously, or informally, as when a child overhears their parent's private opinion about something. Because of the initial and personal nature of this process, primary socialization often carries profound emotional undertones, and may cement lifelong memories and bonds.

Secondary socialization

This refers to cultural transmission that occurs from entering school, and continues throughout life. It equips the growing person to survive and prosper outwith the family environment; its agents include teachers, peers (equals such as friends and fellow students), work supervisors and colleagues, and the mass media, e.g. authors, journalists and broadcasters.

The term tertiary or 'professional' socialization (see p. 207) is sometimes used in relation to the acquisition of knowledge, skills and attitudes required in performing high-level occupations such as nursing.

Roles

Functionalist sociology pictures socialization as gearing individuals to fulfil roles, which are social positions involving expected behaviours. Each person typically performs several roles, usually focusing on one at a time, including some that are:

- Familial, e.g. daughter, mother, grandmother, sister, aunt
- Occupational, e.g. nurse, doctor, domestic assistant
- Miscellaneous, sometimes temporary ones such as patient, client or customer.

It can be seen that many roles have reciprocal partners, in that one to some extent defines the other, so that it is hard to imagine the traditional role of nurse or doctor without someone filling the role of patient/client.

Each role can be viewed as beneficial to other members of society but also to the performer; although every role has its duties or obligations, it also confers rights and privileges if carried out adequately (Box 8.12).

Thus society can be viewed as a symbiotic community, each role-bearer contributing to its smooth running, and in turn receiving rewards such as healthcare when sick. Parsons extended this framework to formulate the 'sick role', which people could legitimately adopt when ill, as in such circumstances they could not fully perform their normal roles (see Ch. 1). As with all roles, this conferred rights and privileges, provided the sick person fulfilled certain duties and obligations.

Role conflict

Fulfilling several roles can be a tricky balancing act and sometimes 'role conflict' is inevitable. It occurs where the demands of fulfilling one role impairs the performance of another, such as family commitments undermining focus on study or nursing duties (Box 8.13, p. 196).

Often domestic commitments detract from energy and available time for family relationships, study and other work. Caring for dependent older relatives can also

REFLECTIVE PRACTICE Box 8.13

Potential role conflict

Student Nurse Sarah has two children of school age. Her husband is in full-time employment, and Sarah works as a care assistant two days a week to supplement the family income.

Student activities

- What roles does Sarah fulfil?
- What competing pressures are there likely to be for her attention?
- Consider ways in which she might minimize her current role conflict.

REFLECTIVE PRACTICE Box 8.14

What 'family' means

Although a term used in everyday speech, it is not easy to agree on a universally acceptable or concise definition of 'family'.

Student activities

- What does the term 'family' mean to you?
- Do you know other families with features different from your own?
- Reflect on the ways in which the family in Western society has changed over the 20th century. It may be interesting to seek the views of people from previous generations.

have a significant impact on a person's own parenting, work and personal life.

The family

A person's understanding of the term 'family' pervades the way in which they view the world. This is evident in the use of terms such as 'Father Time' and 'Mother Earth'. Political parties vie to be the 'party of the family' and espouse 'family values', and the family is often regarded as the basic unit, or even a microcosm of society (Box 8.14).

The term 'family' means different things to different people, but the common associations it raises are emotions such as love and affection, or possibly mixed or negative ones, personal closeness, intimacy and shared experiences, communal housing, financial support, advice, the roles mentioned earlier and caring for one another.

Although people can have different family experiences, a general definition is 'a group of people, bound by kinship ties, who live together, share resources and who look after each other in times of need'. All societies have some form of family unit that performs – although some would say controls – essential functions including the reproduction, economics and socialization of its members.

Family structures

Family structures vary widely both between and within cultures. Common variants include:

- *Nuclear family*: Two adults, a man and a woman living in a household with their biological children.
- *Extended family*: Three or more related generations living in close proximity, including indirect relatives such as cousins, aunts and uncles.
- *Reconstituted family*: Two adults who regroup with children from their current and previous relationships.
- *One-, single- or lone-parent family*: One parent living with their biological children.
- *Gay-parent family*: Where a gay or lesbian person, often with their partner, brings up a child.
- *Polygamy*: A man or woman with several concurrent spouses. This is illegal in Western societies, and usually refers to a man openly living with more than one 'wife'. It is sometimes culturally sanctioned to facilitate procreation.
- *Commune/Kibbutzim*: An arrangement common in Israel where unrelated people share living facilities and cooperate to produce food/income and provide mutual care, e.g. of offspring (Haralambos & Holborn 2005).

In addition to its universality and pivotal position in society, the family has received much consideration as either an integral part of healthcare provision or a contributing factor to many physical and mental health problems.

There are many ways in which the family may be significant for an individual's health and healthcare, both positively and negatively. These include transmitting 'healthy genes' or those producing abnormal conditions; providing the emotional climate surrounding child-rearing and adult interactions, e.g. loving care or forms of abuse. Communication patterns may be supportive or disruptive to mental health, and family income is usually crucial in determining material comfort. Links between wealth and health are well documented (Ch. 1); lifestyle choices such as diet, smoking and exercise are often influenced by domestic attitudes. Close relatives may be understanding of, or intolerant of, certain conditions, e.g. learning disabilities, mental health problems, substance misuse or HIV infection. Family dynamics may involve either mutual devotion to or guilt at not shouldering the burden of a family member's care needs. Relatives may also disagree with care decisions, e.g. prolonging active treatment or disclosing poor prognosis, and place great value on customs required for a loved one's care or treatment (Denny & Earle 2005).

As with individuals and the culture in which they exist, the family does not remain static but continuously evolves to adapt to changing pressures and circumstances. In many ways it represents a mirror of society at any given time, reflecting its development, limitations and current challenges, its successes and its shortcomings.

Trends in family structures

Considerable changes in family structure have taken place over the last few decades.

Some examples of these trends, as suggested by Abercrombie and Warde (2005), and which do not necessarily apply to all social groups or countries, include the following:

- Divorce has become more common and death before retirement age is now a less common cause of family disruption.
- Cohabitation of unmarried adults is widely accepted, as are children born out of wedlock.
- The extended and, more recently, nuclear arrangements have become less common than reconstituted, one-parent, and gay-parent families.
- Choice of partner is now less subject to constraint.
- The average number of children per family is generally fewer in the UK, but their survival rate is higher.
- The importance of wider kinship groups, e.g. 'clans' and mothers' networks, has diminished and the family unit is more home-centred or 'privatized'.
- Male status and power ('patriarchy') has been eroded, with more legal rights, work opportunities and economic independence for women; domestic roles are more symmetrical, with both genders contributing to housework, childcare and decision-making.
- Families tend to be more geographically mobile, often prompted by employment opportunities. This potentially removes them from supportive networks, such as grandparents for childcare.
- More people are following a single lifestyle for longer; women tend to have children later in life, with an increasing proportion choosing to remain childless.

Development across the lifespan

As late as Victorian times, children were viewed as small adults, pre-programmed for adult knowledge and behaviour to emerge with passing years. This view, which implies the importance of natural growth in physical size and strength, changed with greater awareness of child exploitation and misery, e.g. in the novels of Charles Dickens. Protective legislation began to confer rights on children, such as education. Prior to 1833, under nines could work up to 12 hours a day in factories. Only after the Education Act of 1870 did attendance at school become compulsory for most children until age 13 in the UK; the leaving age became 15 only after World War 2 and 16 years in 1972. Another factor in reappraising childhood was the increasing scientific interest in the process of adaptation that followed Darwin's publications on evolution. From the early 1900s, much enquiry focused on how the individual's concept of 'self' was formed, parallel with Freud's contemporary ideas on unconscious processes being formative in adult sexual and personality patterns. The latter was to inspire Erikson's model of a person integrating socially through their resolution of a series of 'personal crises'. The middle part of the 20th century saw much investigation of how cognitive, moral and emotional maturity is acquired, such as through the work of Piaget, Kohlberg and Bowlby.

This section outlines the important stages of physical and psychosocial development throughout the lifespan. Factors affecting development and their potential significance to health are briefly considered. Developmental milestones from birth to school age are introduced, and the Denver II (1990), a developmental screening test (previously known as the DDST), is included (pp. 202–203). Detailed discussion of the developmental milestones is beyond the scope of this book and readers requiring more information should consult Further reading (e.g. Hockenberry et al 2002).

Physical development

This section outlines how the body grows and develops before birth and then through the stages commonly identified thereafter, namely infancy, childhood, adolescence, adulthood, middle and old age. Chapter 14 provides further information about monitoring children's growth in height and weight gain.

Various hormones influence growth and development throughout the lifespan, such as those that stimulate growth during infancy and those that initiate the events of puberty. Some examples are outlined in Table 8.1 (see p. 198).

Conception to birth

Almost every month following the establishment of menstrual cycles during puberty until the menopause (cessation of menstrual cycles), a non-pregnant woman ovulates or releases usually a single oocyte, or egg, from one of two ovaries. However, the frequency of ovulation decreases some years before the menopause. The oocyte enters the uterine tube, where it may be fertilized by one of the millions of spermatozoa or sperm deposited into the vagina by her sexual partner. The nucleus of the oocyte and that of the spermatozoon (the gametes) each has 23 chromosomes (the genetic material), so that when they merge forming a zygote at conception or fertilization, the normal human complement of 46 chromosomes per cell is usually restored. Thus an individual receives half of their genes from each of their parents.

After 24–36 hours, the first cell division occurs, and mitosis continues rapidly. Within 3 days a cluster of cells is formed, about the size of a pinhead. During the second week, the cluster of developing cells implants into the specially prepared lining of the uterus known as the decidua, which will provide nourishment until the development of the placenta. The term embryo is used from the early developmental stages until the eighth week of pregnancy (gestation). Thereafter, until birth it is known as a fetus.

The cluster of cells continues to develop and will eventually differentiate into all the specialized cells of the human body. Occurring alongside these events are the processes that result in the formation of two protective membranes, the chorion and amnion that enclose the embryo/fetus, the umbilical cord and the placenta. The amnion contains the amniotic fluid in which the developing fetus floats throughout pregnancy. The placenta,

Table 8.1 Hormones affecting growth and development (after Hinchliff et al 1996)

Hormone	Source	Effects
Growth hormone (GH)	Anterior pituitary gland	Stimulates growth in many tissues, e.g. bone and skeletal muscle Stimulates protein synthesis Cell growth and repair
Thyroid hormones	Thyroid gland	Needed for normal development of central nervous system Deficiency during early childhood results in small stature and impaired mental development and learning disability
Parathyroid hormone with vitamin D and the hormone calcitonin secreted by the thyroid gland	Parathyroid glands	Bone growth and formation
Insulin	Pancreas	Glucose uptake Inhibits protein breakdown and stimulates protein synthesis
Glucagon	Pancreas	Glucose usage Rapid rise in blood glucose level
Glucocorticoids, e.g. cortisol (see also Ch. 11)	Adrenal glands (cortex)	Regulates tissue growth Excess during periods of growth inhibits growth in height
Oestrogen	Ovaries	Female secondary sexual characteristics Female body fat distribution Bone density
Testosterone	Testes	Male secondary sexual characteristics Widespread anabolic effects on many body (somatic) tissues to produce male physique

which has close contact with maternal blood vessels in the uterus, delivers oxygen and nutrients to and removes waste from the fetus through blood vessels in the umbilical cord via the adapted fetal circulation of vessels and shunts that mostly bypasses the lungs and gastro-intestinal tract. These adaptations are normally reversed soon after birth.

During the early weeks after implantation, all the organ systems start to develop, so that a heart beat, lungs and limbs are detectable within 4 weeks, and the eyes, ears, nose and mouth as well as rudimentary digits can be visualized after 8 weeks of pregnancy. At this early stage, the embryo is particularly vulnerable to adverse factors such as toxins and microorganisms, and these may have major effects on developing organs, e.g. the rubella virus may cause heart defects and deafness.

There are many possible causes of learning disabilities, either genetic (hereditary) or environmental (Fig. 8.2), which can occur during different stages of development. These include:

- Preconceptual, e.g. pre-existing conditions in the mother
- Prenatal, e.g. Down's syndrome (Box 8.15), exposure to microorganisms such as cytomegalovirus (CMV) or maternal alcohol misuse
- Perinatal, e.g. insufficient oxygen or brain injury during birth
- Postnatal, e.g. meningitis, brain injury and social deprivation (Watson 2002).

From the end of the second month to the end of pregnancy (usually 40 weeks) the fetus grows from 2.5 cm in length and 7 g in weight to around 50 cm and over 3500 g. Sex can be ascertained after 3 months, while development of the brain, lungs and heart make viability possible from about 24 weeks of gestation (Bee & Boyd 2004). Detailed

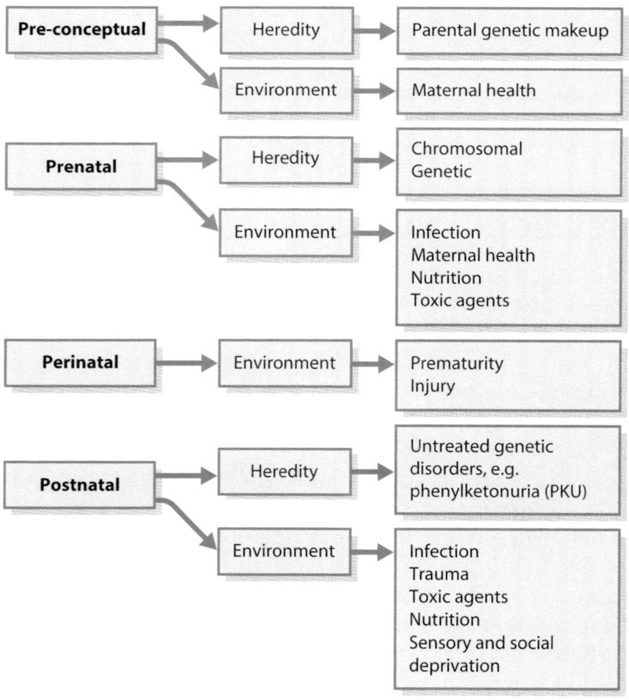

Fig. 8.2 Factors causing learning disabilities by timing (adapted from Gates 2002 with permission)

CRITICAL THINKING Box 8.15

Down's syndrome

A friend and her partner are planning to have a baby and she asks you what causes Down's syndrome and the risk of having a baby with Down's syndrome. She also asks what diagnostic tests are available during pregnancy.

Student activities

- Use the websites below to find answers to your friend's questions.
- Arrange to talk with a learning disability nurse about the degree to which Down's syndrome may affect individual people.

[Resources: Down's Syndrome Association – www.downs-syndrome.org.uk; Down's Syndrome Scotland – www.dsscotland.org.uk; UK National Screening Committee: Down's Syndrome Screening Programme NHS – www.screening.nhs.uk/downs/home.htm All available July 2006]

information about fetal development can be found in Further reading (e.g. Chamley et al 2005).

Infancy (0–12 months) (see also 'Developmental milestones', pp. 201–203)

Although infants typically lose some weight in the days immediately following birth, once feeding and digestive processes are established, growth is extremely rapid, with up to 0.5 kg being gained per week, so that birth weight is doubled on average by the age of 18 weeks. Similarly, an infant can increase in length by 1 cm over a single week during this stage.

The first teeth start to erupt around 6 months of age (see Ch. 16); a delay in the eruption of teeth may be an indicator of other developmental problems.

Motor strength and coordination also steadily advance during infancy. The head is disproportionately large, and requires a steadying hand to support it in the neonatal period (first 28 days). However, by 8–12 weeks, the infant's neck muscles are able to prevent the head lolling backwards, and by 9–12 months the infant can sit and latterly stand unaided.

Mobility also increases: by 3–6 months, the infant should be able to roll over, crawl by 6–9 months and some infants can walk well by 12 months.

Childhood (1–10 years)

The rate of growth slows, but by the age of 2–3 years, children attain half their adult height, although less than one-fifth of their healthy adult weight.

During the preschool period, up to 5 years of age, there are continuing increases in size and strength, accompanied by apparently boundless energy, and punctuated by the appearance of skilled behaviours such as doing up buttons (see also 'Developmental milestones', pp. 201–203).

For further detail of growth during childhood the reader is referred to Further reading (e.g. Montague et al 2005).

Box 8.16 **Secondary sexual characteristics**

Both sexes

- Growth and development of external genitalia
- Maturation of gametes (oocytes or spermatozoa)
- Larynx enlarges, deepening voice, especially of males
- Appearance of body hair – axillary, leg and pubic areas
- Sebaceous glands become active, which may cause greasy skin and acne
- 'Musky' body odour from the effect of sex hormones on apocrine sweat glands

Females

- Breasts develop and pelvis widens
- Subcutaneous fat redistributed
- Onset of menstruation: the first period or menarche occurs between 11 and 14 years, dependent on reaching a critical body mass

Males

- Increased muscle bulk and shoulder girth
- Penile erections
- Nocturnal emission of semen
- Facial hair

Adolescence (11–18 years)

During adolescence, the period between the onset of puberty and adulthood, further growth spurts are stimulated by the sex hormones oestrogen and testosterone (see Table 8.1). These episodes of sudden growth may pose challenges in relation to coordination of a typically gangling frame. At the same time, self-consciousness is further increased by the appearance of secondary sexual characteristics (Box 8.16) with inherent and unavoidable challenges to self-image (see p. 201).

Younger adulthood (18–40 years)

Early in this stage, most people reach their maximum height, because the epiphyseal plates (cartilage) of long bones become bone (ossify), thus preventing further growth in stature. However, growth in height may cease earlier in young women. It is important to maximize bone density during the teens and twenties (Box 8.17, p. 200). Bone mass peaks during the late twenties but after 35–40 years of age it starts to decline. Not only are individuals now at their peak of skeletal muscle bulk and physical strength, speed and athletic potential, but the cardiovascular system also possesses its maximum oxygen-carrying capacity and immune responses are at their peak, so that young adults recover quickly from exercise, injury and illness. Brain mass and sensory powers are similarly at their highest point, resulting in optimal ability to discriminate stimuli.

The middle years (40–65 years)

Most adults in Western society can currently look forward to living well into their seventies or eighties, owing to

HEALTH PROMOTION Box 8.17

Eating disorders and bone density

Eating disorders such as anorexia and bulimia nervosa can have far-reaching consequences for bone health. Apart from an inadequate intake of the nutrients needed for bone growth and density (e.g. calcium, vitamin D, protein, etc.), there are other issues for young women with eating disorders. Those with a very low body weight may stop having periods and the lack of oestrogen puts them at risk of loss of bone density, which may never be rectified even if they gain weight and their periods return. This may also occur when young women exercise excessively with or without an eating disorder. Loss of bone density or a failure to reach peak density increases the risk of osteoporosis (see Ch. 18).

[Resource: National Osteoporosis Society – www.nos.org.uk Available July 2006]

reduced mortality from disease, occupational accidents, etc. compared with past generations (see Ch. 1). By the mid-forties there are usually detectable, but not serious, signs of decline in all body systems (Box 8.18).

Even into their fifties, however, many people consider themselves healthy and if no longer in their physical prime, not far short of their best in terms of intellectual and social functioning – their 'prime of life'.

Older adulthood

Beyond the relative physical and functional plateau that extends from young adulthood to middle-age, individuals must progressively adapt to the more obvious changes that accompany ageing, often exaggerations of those which start to appear in the middle years.

As indicated by Mader (2000), physical aspects include:

- Skin changes, e.g. reduced tone, wrinkles, dryness, widespread pigmentation with 'age spots' and slower healing
- Marked hair loss in both sexes

Box 8.18 Changes in body systems in middle years

The integumentary system

- Skin may sag; wrinkles ('crow's feet') develop around eyes and mouth
- Pigmentation becomes patchy and there is an increased risk of skin cancer through the cumulative effects of sun damage over many years
- Hair may become grey and thins in both sexes. In men there may be typical male pattern baldness, although this can happen much earlier.

The senses

- Thickening and reduced elasticity of the lens of the eye results in problems with near vision (presbyopia), where the person eventually needs to hold a book at arm's length. It is corrected with reading or bifocal spectacles
- Slow adjustment to changes in light intensity
- Hearing changes with an inability to hear sounds at the extremes of pitch. This may be apparent only on audiometric testing
- Sensitivity to touch and pain diminishes, although tolerance of discomfort may be lowered.

Cardiovascular and respiratory systems

- The power of cardiac muscle contraction is reduced
- Arterial walls lose elasticity
- The lumen of arteries may be reduced by hard fatty deposits (atherosclerosis), which raises blood pressure and significantly increases the risk of heart attacks and strokes (see Ch. 17). This is the commonest serious health problem in this age group
- Elasticity in the lungs and lower air passages also diminishes, although resultant breathlessness is only usually noticed during unaccustomed exercise.

Body weight in middle years

- Individuals tend to gain weight steadily from as early as their late twenties until their mid-fifties. It is not a consequence of middle age as such, but a result of reduced physical activity while continuing to have the same or greater food intake. Women have a greater tendency to increase their weight at this time, with fat accumulating over the hips and lower abdomen – 'middle-age spread' – whereas men tend to accumulate fat over the abdomen above the waist.
- For both sexes in Western society, obesity is of special concern for those in middle adulthood, being linked to type 2 diabetes mellitus, hypertension, cardiovascular complications and some cancers (see Ch. 19).

The reproductive system

- While sexual appetite (libido) usually persists, alterations in function become evident
- Usually between the ages of 45 and 55 years, most women experience the climacteric, including the menopause (cessation of menstruation), ending natural fertility. This can cause variable emotional and physical symptoms including mood fluctuations, headaches, insomnia and 'hot flushes'. The vagina tends to become smaller and its secretions decrease. This can make intercourse uncomfortable, although sexual interest may increase at this time
- Men tend to find penile erection slower and less reliable from middle-age onwards, with slower and less forceful attainment of orgasm.

- Loss of height, about 1.2 cm per 20 adult years due to vertebral curvature and intervertebral disc compression/erosion
- Reduced bone mass with increased risk of fracture, especially in women, due to postmenopausal absence of oestrogen; however, men experience these problems at a later age
- Usually inconsequential, but progressive loss of neurones.

Functional aspects typically include more troublesome reductions in:

- Sensory acuity with obvious visual and hearing loss (Ch. 16)
- Muscle strength and speed of movement, joint flexibility (Ch. 18)
- Organ efficiency, e.g. kidney function is reduced by 50% at 75 years of age.

However, although the incidence of illness and disability does increase with age, most older people, especially those under 75 years, are healthy and independent. They retain their mental faculties and continue to enjoy life, especially if they can reconcile themselves to adapting to their relative limitations. Although the proportion of older people in Western society is increasing, health-related factors such as diet, housing, technological and medical advances may allow their prospects to be brighter than for previous generations.

Developmental milestones

Human development is often thought of as a process involving the achievement of competencies or 'milestones', i.e. the ability to perform tasks that society expects of its members at a given point of their lives. Such competencies are progressively acquired during physical maturation (increasing age, size, strength and coordination) and through opportunities for practice. Development is therefore viewed as a complex interplay of biological, environmental and social factors.

The usual way of assessing an infant's/child's developmental progress is to compare their behaviours with those displayed by the majority of their contemporaries. Following detailed studies, abilities have been organized into comparative grids, for example the Denver II (1990) (Fig. 8.3), which divides infant's/children's milestones into four categories:

- Personal/social – relating to other people and self-care
- Fine motor – adaptive: concerning vision and use of the hands
- Language – responding to and using speech
- Gross motor – maintaining posture and moving head/limbs/whole body.

Cross-comparison can establish whether a particular infant/child has attained a series of milestones established as typical for their age. This is a matter of concern to many parents, but it should be appreciated that compiling 'average' scores involves rating some children as showing behaviour relatively early or late. Significance is only really attached to this if all related behaviours or overall progress follows the same pattern. Additionally, it is common for children to be advanced in some abilities and delayed in others, and for boys and girls to develop at slightly different rates (Box 8.19, p. 204).

Psychosocial development

This refers to the psychological and sociological perspectives on the process of development. The stages are considered by age group.

Infancy and childhood

The main issues relating to infancy are considered under self-concept and attachment below.

Early in childhood, preschool milestones must be attained, a process that may in some instances occur naturally, but in others such milestones are awaited anxiously and require greater facilitation. By the age of 5, children are required to attend school, mix with peers and accept direction from unrelated adults (see 'Socialization', p. 195), an experience that can initially prove traumatic.

As mentioned above, young children possess enormous energy (to be expended in a shorter day than their parents'/carers' reserves) as well as steadily increasing bodily strength and frame size. Awareness of this potential power, constrained by restrictions imposed by adults and accentuated by intense emotions, can lead to behavioural problems. These range from the tantrums of the 'terrible twos' to destructive rages, scuffles and vandalism in school years. Such features can be pronounced in the behaviour of some young people with learning disabilities, whose psychological resources may be overstretched at times by the demands of normalization, i.e. adapting to the myriad stresses of life lived within mainstream society. In these situations it is important that parents/carers consider what is being communicated or how the environment can be adapted.

Adolescence

The physical changes during puberty generate psychosocial challenges for the adolescent, who must come to terms with new experiences, including:

- Sexual desires, fantasies and awareness of/or decisions about sexual orientation (see also p. 217)
- Intensification of peer relationships
- Impending autonomy from their parents
- Establishing a personal identity
- Feelings of ambivalence towards these processes.

All this is accompanied by concurrent cognitive, e.g. scholastic, and ethical developments that will be considered later. Teenagers tend to be acutely aware of their bodily appearance and hygiene (taking much time over self-care), and concerned about issues of modesty and privacy, relevant to those nursing them. By the late teenage years many individuals have reached their highpoint in terms of physical suppleness, speed and reproductive ability, but outlets for these may be limited and external constraints resented.

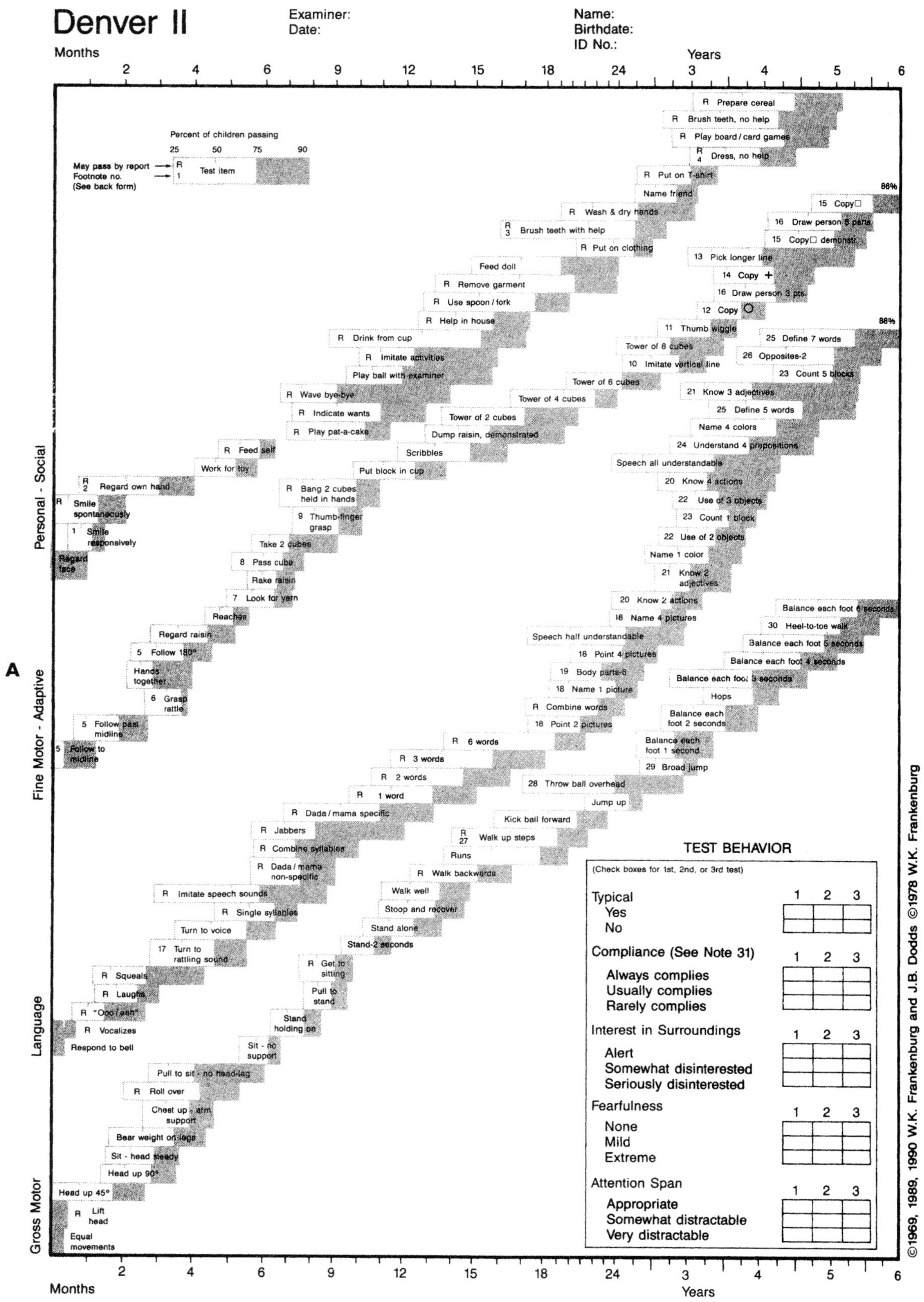

Fig. 8.3 The Denver II (1990) Developmental rating scale. Copyright 1969, 1989, 1990. WK Frankenburg and JB Dodds; copyright 1978 WK Frankenburg (reproduced by kind permission of Denver Developmental Materials Inc.)

DIRECTIONS FOR ADMINISTRATION

1. Try to get child to smile by smiling, talking or waving. Do not touch him/her.
2. Child must stare at hand several seconds.
3. Parent may help guide toothbrush and put toothpaste on brush.
4. Child does not have to be able to tie shoes or button/zip in the back.
5. Move yarn slowly in an arc from one side to the other, about 8" above child's face.
6. Pass if child grasps rattle when it is touched to the backs or tips of fingers.
7. Pass if child tries to see where yarn went. Yarn should be dropped quickly from sight from tester's hand without arm movement.
8. Child must transfer cube from hand to hand without help of body, mouth, or table.
9. Pass if child picks up raisin with any part of thumb and finger.
10. Line can vary only 30 degrees or less from tester's line.
11. Make a fist with thumb pointing upward and wiggle only the thumb. Pass if child imitates and does not move any fingers other than the thumb.

12. Pass any enclosed form. Fail continuous round motions.
13. Which line is longer? (Not bigger.) Turn paper upside down and repeat. (pass 3 of 3 or 5 of 6)
14. Pass any lines crossing near midpoint.
15. Have child copy first. If failed, demonstrate.

When giving items 12, 14, and 15, do not name the forms. Do not demonstrate 12 and 14.

16. When scoring, each pair (2 arms, 2 legs, etc.) counts as one part.
17. Place one cube in cup and shake gently near child's ear, but out of sight. Repeat for other ear.
18. Point to picture and have child name it. (No credit is given for sounds only.) If less than 4 pictures are named correctly, have child point to picture as each is named by tester.

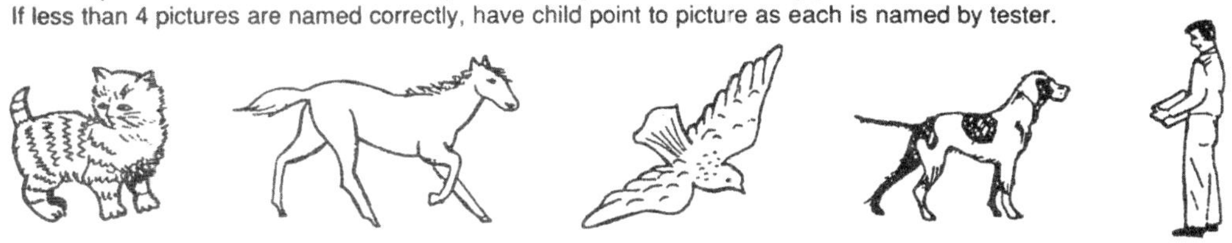

B

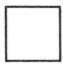

19. Using doll, tell child: Show me the nose, eyes, ears, mouth, hands, feet, tummy, hair. Pass 6 of 8.
20. Using pictures, ask child: Which one flies?... says meow?... talks?... barks?... gallops? Pass 2 of 5, 4 of 5.
21. Ask child: What do you do when you are cold?... tired?... hungry? Pass 2 of 3, 3 of 3.
22. Ask child: What do you do with a cup? What is a chair used for? What is a pencil used for? Action words must be included in answers.
23. Pass if child correctly places <u>and</u> says how many blocks are on paper. (1, 5).
24. Tell child: Put block **on** table; **under** table; **in front of** me, **behind** me. Pass 4 of 4. (Do not help child by pointing, moving head or eyes.)
25. Ask child: What is a ball?... lake?... desk?... house?... banana?... curtain?... fence?... ceiling? Pass if defined in terms of use, shape, what it is made of, or general category (such as banana is fruit, not just yellow). Pass 5 of 8, 7 of 8.
26. Ask child: If a horse is big, a mouse is __? If fire is hot, ice is __? If the sun shines during the day, the moon shines during the __? Pass 2 of 3.
27. Child may use wall or rail only, not person. May not crawl.
28. Child must throw ball overhand 3 feet to within arm's reach of tester.
29. Child must perform standing broad jump over width of test sheet (8 1/2 inches).
30. Tell child to walk forward, heel within 1 inch of toe. Tester may demonstrate. Child must walk 4 consecutive steps.
31. In the second year, half of normal children are non-compliant.

OBSERVATIONS:

Fig. 8.3 *(Continued)*

REFLECTIVE PRACTICE Box 8.19

Developmental assessment

In order to detect problems at an early stage, it is important to assess the progress of infants and children in attaining certain milestones, such as smiling or building a tower of bricks.

Student activities

- Think about infants/children you have met on placement or those in your own family and reflect on their progress using the four categories of Denver II.
- Ask you mentor or a specialist community public health nurse (health visitor) what physical criteria are assessed in infants/children aged 0–5 years, starting with the Apgar scoring system (heart rate, respiratory effort, muscle tone, reflex irritability and colour) performed immediately after birth.

REFLECTIVE PRACTICE Box 8.20

Self-consciousness and nursing

Feeling self-conscious is an uncomfortable but universal experience.

Student activities

- Think of two instances where you have felt self-conscious in nursing practice.
- Consider how the resulting discomfort might be reduced.

Young adulthood

This phase is usually considered to begin around 20 years of age, although attainment of adulthood may be culturally defined in various ways, for example:

- Reaching an age milestone, e.g. 18 or 21 years
- Related legal entitlements, e.g. being allowed to purchase alcohol, enter certain occupations such as nursing, or have sexual intercourse
- Social events such as leaving home, attending university or getting married.

The nervous system functions at its peak, resulting in optimal ability to detect and memorize information, and to solve problems. Physical attractiveness is often regarded as most striking at this time. Consequently, self-confidence may simultaneously expand. While each of these attributes may gradually diminish from the age of 26 onwards, factors such as experience, reasoning ability and motivation may more than compensate.

The middle years

A common psychological challenge for women in their mid-forties to fifties is the 'empty nest syndrome', having to adjust to their children entering young adulthood and leaving home. This can prompt women to re-enter the labour market or restart their career, which, not uncommonly, coincides with marital separation or divorce. Career opportunities can, however, be offset by the need to provide care for older relatives. Childless women also come to the realization that they are now unlikely to have a child.

Male awareness of sexual difficulties, occupational and relationship stagnation, perhaps compared with their spouse's new lease of life, and of approaching mortality can combine to precipitate the 'male menopause', either expressed in introverted self-doubt or the purchase of a Harley–Davidson motorcycle.

Older adulthood

Psychological aspects of old age are well documented (Gross 2001). These may include diminished ability to solve new problems, memorize and retrieve information. As all of the above changes seem to be negative and relate to loss, perhaps it is unsurprising that depression is relatively common in older adults, and the prospect of ageing may be ignored, dreaded or defused through humour.

Retirement can also be a rewarding period where the person has more time to devote to relationships, e.g. with partners, children, grandchildren and friends, hobbies and part-time or voluntary work. Lifestyles associated with contentment in old age vary between authorities, for instance the contrast between 'disengagement' and 'activity' models (Gross 2001).

The 'self' and 'self-concept'

These terms are often used interchangeably when examining how people think about themselves, and consider their own nature and actions. This process is also referred to as 'self-awareness' or 'self-consciousness'. It might be viewed as a straightforward, natural part of a person's existence, but the 'self' is a complex notion, unique to human beings, which they have to develop and continuously modify throughout their lives. It involves forming the ability to take the role of subject and object, observer and observed, at the same time. Self-consciousness is particularly intense when a person is especially aware of being viewed as an object, for example suddenly finding themselves in front of a group of 'spectators', such as when arriving late for a class (Box 8.20).

Possible instances might include:

- Entering a new nursing environment. Try to arrange a prior orientation visit when the area is 'quiet' or in the company of another student.
- Patients/clients often feel like objects when being examined, treated or having nursing procedures performed. Try to maximize their privacy and dignity, and engage them in natural conversation where possible.

The self can be conceived as comprising three interrelated elements: self-image, self-esteem and ideal self.

CRITICAL THINKING Box 8.21

The TST

One way of investigating a person's self-image would be to ask people to describe themselves. Kuhn and McPartland in their 'twenty statements test' (TST) used this approach in 1954.

Student activity

- Write down 20 different responses to the question, 'Who am I?', i.e. 'I am . . . . . .' etc.
  The answers may fall into three main categories: personality traits, roles and factual.

Note: There are no right or wrong answers.

Self-image

The first of these is effectively the impression people hold of them, and includes how they think that they appear outwardly to others and the kind of person that they believe they are (Box 8.21).

Personality traits

These are adjectives that allow people to subjectively describe their mental processes such as thoughts and feelings, or their behaviour. Examples might include 'I am. . . *kind, caring, practical, hard working*, which are all good characteristics for a nurse, *outgoing* or *shy*. Sometimes these can be grouped to form a so-called personality 'type', for example traits such as 'shy and retiring', 'thoughtful', 'serious' and 'cautious' may combine to constitute an *introvert*, contrasting descriptions such as 'sociable', 'lively', 'fun-loving' and 'impulsive' relating to the opposite *extrovert* type (Eysenck 2000). Eysenck (senior)'s, other main distinctions were between:

- '*neurotic*' – anxious, emotionally variable, versus '*stable*', calm, consistent, and
- '*tough-minded*' – hard-headed, ruthless, versus '*tender-minded*', sensitive, empathetic types.

Trait and type approaches to self-description are commonly used in everyday language as well as in psychological research, and imply that aspects of the self are relatively fixed once established, and can be compared and contrasted between individuals, e.g. colleagues or clients.

Roles (see pp. 195–196)

Such answers may include familial roles such as 'mother', 'daughter', 'aunt' or 'sister', or occupational ones such as 'student', 'nurse' or 'doctor'. Also common may be statements of religious identity, e.g. 'I am a 'Christian' or 'Muslim'.

Factual

Factual matters include gender, marital status and age (perhaps commoner if the respondent is towards the extremes of lifespan). Literal answers are characteristic of younger age groups, for instance children under 8 years tend to answer the TST in terms of activities, e.g. 'I am *playing*', ' . . . *at school*', or even ' . . . *talking to you*!' Between 8 years and adolescence, answers usually revolve around facts such as their:

- Name, e.g. 'I am Sandra'
- Sex, e.g. 'I am a girl'
- Size, e.g. 'I am tall'
- Nationality
- Age
- Preferences, e.g. 'I am keen on music', or 'I am going to be a nurse'
- Performance, e.g. 'I am good at football/sums/playing the piano'

(Miell 1990).

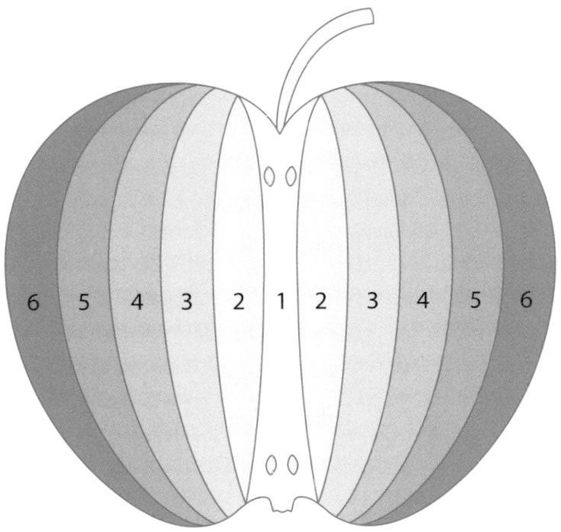

1 = 'core' self
2–6 = increasingly 'peripheral' selves

Fig. 8.4 A concentric representation of the self

The relative importance of a person's TST answers can be gauged by asking them to rank each in order of importance. This then enables the construction of a concentric model of the self-image (Fig. 8.4), with the central one representing the most important self-descriptor and the true 'core- self', compared with the progressively less important 'peripheral- selves' outside this.

Physical characteristics, such as size or appearance, form part of the 'bodily self', or 'body image', and may appear in response to the TST if perceived to be a particularly significant part of the outward self. The bodily self also includes sensations such as hunger, thirst, satiety, warmth, cold, pleasure and pain – common preoccupations during ill-health, and which help to direct conscious awareness towards survival-related actions. It also covers anatomical components (body structure), which might be automatically regarded as an, or indeed *the* essential part of people's living selves, although they lose parts of it without concern, as when cutting their hair and nails. Possession of bodily parts or even fluids can be an ambivalent matter, e.g. when considering donating or receiving organs or blood.

However, there will be circumstances where an adolescent or adult patient/client would particularly fixate on the bodily self when responding to the TST. For example, chronic pain, preoccupation with weight in anorexia nervosa or obesity, disfiguring burns, paralysis, loss of continence, breast removal or stoma-forming surgery, and depression may engender self-loathing.

Self-esteem

The ability to evaluate their self-image leads people to examine the second component of the self – their 'self-esteem'. This is how people feel about the image they hold of themselves, the degree to which it pleases or displeases them, and whether they take pride in or feel shame towards it. Thus people can run a range of emotions when appraising themselves, from conceit to despair with all points between these extremes, and these judgements vary with time, their behaviour and circumstances. This self-evaluation may be directed at specific aspects of the self, for instance appearance, thoughts about issues or other people, emotions such as desires, or actions that have been performed. Alternatively, it may be a 'global' amalgamation of such detailed appraisals, generating an overall estimation of self-value at a given moment.

Self-esteem is enormously influenced by the culture to which people belong. Western culture is often said to value material wealth and individual attainment. Thus an individual member of this society is likely to have their self-esteem bolstered by financial security, ownership of impressive clothes, house and car, academic qualifications and a high status job, many of which can be contingent on each other. Absence of such indicators of personal success is liable to lower a person's self-esteem, unless they belong to a non-materialistic subculture, e.g. a religious organization or an anti-capitalist protest group, from which they may derive a quite different yardstick of personal worth.

Self-esteem clearly has a major bearing on emotional well-being and so is integral to personal happiness. If people aim to be personally fulfilled and happy, this seems to imply a potentially aspirational element to the self-concept. If self-image represents the 'person' that people consider themselves to be, sometimes termed the 'actual self', it may not be all they would like to be or could be. The wished-for improved version was termed the 'ideal self' by Rogers (see p. 184). Another way of tackling the problem of lowered self-esteem is to avoid exacerbating factors. People often evaluate their self-image by comparing themselves with others. If inappropriately successful figures are chosen for reference purposes, it is likely that disappointment will ensue, for example, comparing one's physical attractiveness with that of a film star or one's material success with a millionaire. Similarly, a student nurse is liable to feel inferior in poise and skills to an experienced registered nurse.

William James suggested a formula akin to:

$$\text{Self-esteem} = \frac{\text{success}}{\text{ambitions}}$$

In other words, the higher their expectations, the more likely they are to exceed the person's achievements, and the likelier they are to be disappointed. This indicates some need to be realistic in personal targets, e.g. the goals negotiated with a patient/client for their rehabilitation, although equally it could be argued that without aspirations people are unlikely to improve themselves or achieve anything significant in their lives. Rearranging the formula gives:

$$\text{success} = \text{self-esteem} \times \text{ambitions}.$$

Therefore, harbouring high self-regard and goals is likely to make people more successful, so that a positive view of the present and future self may be conducive to generating good fortune, e.g. in a student's nursing career aims.

Development of the self

As people are not born with an intact, innate self-concept, how is it formed? Piaget (p. 207) proposed that the infant below the age of 6 months is egocentric or self-centred in that they are unaware that a world separate from themselves actually exists. It takes at least a further year to create an understanding of the reality of the surrounding environment, including the people within it. Work on object permanence (see p. 208) suggests that young children only develop a consistent interest in (which implies a concept of) absent things and people, i.e. the 'not self', by about 18 months. Furthermore, research by Lewis and Brooks-Gunn in the late 1970s suggested that only above this age do children recognize their own image, for instance in a photograph or their reflection in a mirror, as distinct from images of other children of the same age.

This work followed up findings by Gallup in the early 1970s on primates, which found that only higher apes seemed able to develop similar self-recognition, and only then if they had been exposed previously and early in life to other members of their own species. This usually occurs naturally, and seems essential to future social functioning such as mating and parenting (see attachment, pp. 212–214). On the basis of his results, Gallup asserted that the self is 'a social structure, and arises through social experience'. In other words, humans at least begin to form their self-image through being reared by other humans, and gradually recognize their form as similar to those of the children and adults they see around them, until they can conceive their own physical boundaries and appearance towards the end of their second year of life.

From early infancy, children naturally interact with those around them, initially exchanging gaze and facial expressions like smiling with their mother, then during their second year beginning to use recognizable words of their 'mother tongue'. Such symbols, along with gestures such as waving, provide the means of communicating shared meanings during interpersonal interactions, the basis for what is termed the 'social interactionist' perspective, initiated by George Herbert Mead in the 1930s. Mead developed the observations made in the 1890s by William James on the linguistic distinction between the terms 'I' and 'me' – both in this context sometimes given the prefix 'the'. The first-person pronoun 'I' is used to denote the self as the subject of the act of thought, speech or behaviour. James likened this to a knowing but hidden observer, almost like an ever-alert motion camera, placed within what he termed a person's 'stream of consciousness'. This 'I' might be equivalent to the essential 'core- self' referred to earlier, a secret entity in some ways, unattainable even to its owner.

On the other hand, the pronoun 'me' refers to the self when viewed or treated as an object, and amounts to what in a person is outwardly observable, such as their physical appearance, clothes (e.g. when you ask another person whether a new coat is 'me' or 'not me'), overt behaviour and even reputation. This use of 'me' in speech has already been noted in relation to the bodily image, and its evaluation is much affected by social influences such as the perceived or anticipated opinions of others. Thus the 'me' may be modified in order to maximize one's self-esteem, and it is the 'I' in this framework that makes these judgements and decisions.

Although fully understanding the social interactionist argument with its peculiar linguistic interrelations is challenging, it suggests that once consistently mastering the use of the terms 'I' and 'me', the child must be displaying awareness of the parallel existence of both 'self' and others, and how their standpoint and those of other people interacts.

As well as through the acquisition of language skills, Mead contended that the self-concept developed by means of assuming roles. He described three stages of his own conception of 'primary socialization' (see p. 195) during which this occurred. In the initial preparatory stage, the young child can be seen closely imitating parental actions, such as washing dishes and vacuum cleaning. At this time, the child is very sensitive to parental feedback, whether encouraging or disapproving, and internalizes their judgements (Miell 1990).

In the second stage, play often involves the re-enactment of adult behaviour when the child is alone, frequently accompanied by a commentary conveying previously expressed parental attitudes, such as praise or criticism of what a toy is being made to do.

Finally, by participating in relatively formal games, the older child has to adhere to rules established by others. To be successful, the child must learn to take the viewpoint of others, both on their side and in opposition, for instance in cards or ball games, in order to anticipate what the others are likely to do. Thus, through each stage, the child engages more and more with the viewpoints of other people, developing the power of empathy. Eventually they are able to appreciate the typical perspective of those within their culture, for example what the average person might think of their thoughts, appearance and behaviour (Cooley's looking-glass 'self'). Mead termed this adoption of the 'role of the generalized other', and this ability provides a yardstick against which to evaluate one's self or a virtual mirror to reflect one's self-image as viewed by others. This limitless source of socially grounded feedback enables the person to subtly and continuously modify and refine their 'selves' throughout life, both in later interactions with the agents of secondary socialization (p. 195) and in moments of solitary 'self-reflection'.

Refinement of self in adulthood occurs during 'professional' or 'tertiary' socialization, whereby people acquire the knowledge, skills and attitudes peculiar to an occupational role (p. 195). Goffman (1971) described the process of assuming the behavioural component of such a role in terms of taking part in a drama. Initially an actor may feel not entirely natural in a part, and uncertain about how convincingly they can fulfil a well-established role, just as a student might that of 'nurse'. A professional 'mask' is self-consciously adopted to begin with, and feedback gained on performance from observers, e.g. mentor. Aspects of performance can be modified until the person feels confident about fulfilling the role's requirements and can routinely 'play' it naturally.

To summarize, the 'self' is an elusive and vague concept. It comprises psychological and physical components that are interrelated. People develop their self-concept in the course of continuing social experience, through their interactions with others. Their view of themselves is much influenced by the culture in which they exist, and the reactions to them of the people they encounter, both real and imagined. The self-concept is fluid; they can adapt their 'selves' to varying situations, such as behaving quite differently in professional and domestic roles. Lastly, because of the tendency to constantly evaluate the self-image, which generates conscious self-esteem, the self-concept is crucial in determining a person's emotional well-being – it is intrinsic to their inner contentment.

Cognitive (intellectual) development

The most influential researcher in this field has been the Swiss psychologist Jean Piaget (1896–1980) who worked on the development of early intelligence tests. These instruments implicitly assume that intelligence is an attribute determined at birth, or early in life, and unchanging thereafter, and that it can be estimated through standardized questions. Rather than taking this usual focus, Piaget became fascinated with children's typically incorrect answers to items beyond their chronological ability. He felt that these yielded unique insights, as they reflected the characteristic, if immature, ways in which children think. Consequently, he devised a series of tests specifically designed to shed light on intellectual processes at different ages.

Piaget believed that human understanding of reality was not inborn, but had to be actively 'discovered' through interactions with the real, outside world, the child effectively learning as a scientist would. In other words, intelligence 'evolves', just like the characteristics of a species in response to environmental challenges, ensuring survival and success. Initially, reflexes ('automatic' responses) suffice in these interactions, so that the infant can both derive nourishment from its mother's breast or a bottle teat and investigate objects such as toys through automatic sucking and licking. A psychologically comforting state of 'equilibrium' results through being able to 'accommodate' or successfully respond to every encountered challenge by existing strategies – 'schemata' (singular schema) are the building blocks of Piagetian intelligence. However, the growing infant comes to find sucking and licking less successful in dealing with solid food or unpleasant-tasting objects that they handle, resulting in inner dissatisfaction or 'disequilibrium'. This

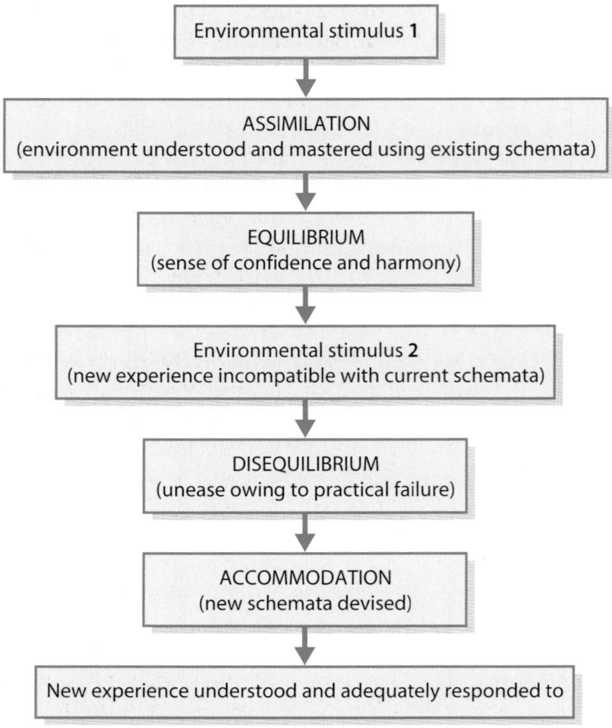

Fig. 8.5 Piaget's adaptation model of the development of intelligence

necessitates the formation of new strategies, such as biting and chewing food, scrutinizing and fingering objects, better suited to new challenges – the process of 'accommodation'. According to Piaget, this continuous process, known as 'equilibration', of employing old schemata until they fail and then replacing them with new, more suitable ones characterizes adaptation, and so intellectual development, throughout life (Fig. 8.5).

Assimilation allows people to practise recently acquired skills, e.g. in nursing, until they achieve routine competence in them. Accommodation enables people to formulate innovative approaches towards solving new problems. Both processes are thus complementary and integral to lifelong learning and the development of the mastery that characterizes the expert nurse.

An everyday example might be being offered chopsticks for the first time in a Chinese restaurant, where a person might try them, especially if everyone else around does. Assimilation would involve trying to use the sticks as a blunt spoon, attempting to scoop the food up with them. Much of it, especially the rice and sauce, will fall before it reaches their mouth, creating embarrassment and frustration (*disequilibrium*). With practice, the person learns to move each chopstick separately, allowing the tips to grasp food securely (*accommodation*). Success makes the person feel competent and appeases their hunger (*equilibrium*). Feeding dependent patients also involves new strategies, such as prior consideration of comfort, hygiene and dignity, then asking them in what sequence or mixtures they would like their food, when they might like a drink and observing repeatedly when their mouth is empty. All of these strategies occur automatically when people can feed themselves (adapted from Napier University Module booklet 2, 1997, 2001).

Piaget's four stages of cognitive development

Piaget contended that children invariably progress through four consecutive stages en route to acquiring an adult intellect. Each stage has its own characteristic schemata, way of thinking or intelligence.

Piaget envisaged intellectual development as proceeding continuously through the stages, driven but also limited by accumulating experience and biological maturation. His ideas have received considerable cross-cultural confirmation, although a number of studies have suggested the need for revision of the details.

Criticisms have been directed at:

- The questioning method adopted in his studies, which may affect children's answers
- The age parameters accorded to the stages, generally now thought to underestimate children's abilities
- The proposed end-goal of cognitive development, as some authorities regard this as continuing to develop throughout life.

Sensorimotor stage (0–2 years)

This stage is so-named as the infant's 'thinking' appears limited to sensing events and objects, and reacting to them by muscular movements, e.g. reaching for rattles, crying if wet. As a result, sensorimotor intelligence is 'practical', as the infant is reacting only to circumstances and objects that are evident to them. It takes some months for the infant to show awareness of absent things, such as searching for objects that are hidden or made to disappear, even if they witness their disappearance. This convinced Piaget that 'object permanence', i.e. that people and objects have an independent and permanent existence of their own, separate from the infant, has to be developed through experience. Piaget described the infant yet to acquire this notion as in a state of pure 'egocentrism'.

By about 18 months, the child starts to use symbols to represent absent people and objects, such as words, imitative behaviour and toys. Thus they will ask for Mum or a favourite cuddly toy by name, re-enact behaviour previously exhibited by a parent or sibling ('deferred imitation') and use a building brick as if it were a car in representational or 'make-believe' play.

Preoperational stage (2–7 years)

The child continues to improve in use of language and other symbols, but tends to be convinced, and confused, by how things outwardly appear rather than by operating on the basis of logic, i.e. logical 'operations' do not yet characterize thought. Thus during the first 2 years of this stage, the 'preconceptual' substage, the child focuses or 'centres' on one striking aspect of an object to the exclusion of other relevancies. So adult males of similar age and appearance may be indiscriminately called Daddy, and four-legged animals of a certain size, from cats to Shetland ponies may be called 'doggies'. Inanimate objects

HEALTH PROMOTION Box 8.22

Safety in play – choosing the right toy

Toy manufacturers typically specify if their products are unsuitable for children less than 3 years of age, as small components may cause choking (see Ch. 17).

Student activities

- Consider the manufacturer's warning in the context of what you know about developmental milestones achieved between 0 and 3 years (see p. 201).
- Why would Piaget have deemed 3 years as a significant watershed?

that move, like the sun and moon, cars or footballs are viewed as living.

By 4 years of age, the child progresses to the 'intuitive' substage, where some logic is present but intuitive thought, relying on what feels right, make cross-classification or 'class-inclusion' tasks difficult. An example is the comparison of toy cows, e.g. either white or black in colour. Identifying the more numerous colour is easy, but these are also thought to outnumber the total number of toy cows. However, this might be due to the lack of practical relevance of the task to a small child. In the 1970s, Donaldson showed children the cows with some standing and others on their side, which were said to be 'sleeping'. It seemed easy for them then to judge that 'all' cows outnumbered 'sleeping' cows.

Before 7 years of age, the child still displays egocentrism, but in a lesser form than in the sensorimotor stage, equivalent here to a relative inability to see a situation from anyone else's standpoint. For instance, the child will know if they have a brother, can tell you this brother's name, yet may insist their brother does not have a brother or sister of his own. Children who should by age be markedly egocentric can sometimes perform empathetic skills such as 'talking down' to and selecting suitable toys for 2 year olds, which inexperienced adults might find difficult (Box 8.22), or understanding that keeping a secret means that others are excluded from this knowledge.

Concrete operational stage (7–11 years)

After entering this stage, children become able to solve previously tricky logical operations such as 'conservation tasks'. For example, they can be confronted with two identical short, broad tumblers, and invited to judge when both are filled with milk to the same level. The content of one of these is then poured into a taller glass as the child watches. The child is then asked if there is now the same in it as in the other original broad tumbler, or whether there is less or more. Piaget thought that the essential indicator of attaining this stage was to agree that they were the same. By focusing on more than one feature simultaneously, 'decentring', one can understand that height compensates for breadth so that milk transferred to a different-shaped container conserves its volume and its physical identity, despite its changed appearance. Preoperational children insist that the tall glass has more even if they agree that none was spilled in transfer. Other measures of conservation ability relate to substance and number.

One criticism of this research questions the significance of the word *more* – for a child below 7 years, does the term simply mean receiving a higher level of milk or juice in a glass, suggesting that the preoperational immaturity may be linguistic rather than logical? Another relates to the method of questioning and the power relationship between experimenter and respondent. How might a child interpret an adult repeating the question, 'Are both the same or does one have more?' after rearranging the test items? Perhaps a child might feel that they should ignore what is logically correct, maybe suspecting some magical trickery, or that they should change their answer to the question second time around, as this is what the grown-up presumably expects if asking it twice.

Finally, relative terms such as *big*, *bigger* and *biggest*, previously used interchangeably, are employed appropriately from now on, allowing accurate verbal comparison between two or more objects. The stage gets its name from the observation that the newly characteristic logical strategies are reliably used only when the components of the problem can be seen and perhaps touched, i.e. they have a *concrete* presence.

Formal operational stage (11–15+ years)

This refers to the ability to follow the *form* or theoretical outline of a problem when remote from its physical reality or lacking a concrete context. Examples include following verbal or written instructions rather than observing then imitating someone showing you how to do something, or being able to delay implementation of new learning. Comparing two absent objects such as people described independently of one another becomes straightforward, e.g. 'if John is taller than Mary, and Jim is smaller than Mary, is Jim or John the tallest?' – a transitivity test, requiring correct use of relative terms.

Logic can now thus be applied in an abstract way, making future practical applications easier, since general principles can be applied to many different situations, as in linking nursing theory to subsequent practice settings. The contrast between formal and concrete operational thinking is akin to that between insight and behavioural or social learning (Ch. 4). However, there is some doubt if all or even most adults are able to function consistently at this level, as adults may persist in using unsuitable trial and error or observational approaches to tasks that could be solved by creative, abstract thinking, sometimes with frustrating results. For example, when setting up unfamiliar equipment, some people push buttons randomly or ask another's opinion, rather than consulting the instructions.

Hypothetical thinking enables consideration of (im)possibilities, e.g. science fiction, surreal humour and alternative courses of action, which leads to some of the conflicts that typify adolescence, including friction with elders, personal identity crises and vacillation over career choice.

HEALTH PROMOTION Box 8.23

Health promotion for different stages of cognitive development

Nurses in all areas of practice have an important health-promoting role. However, effective health-promoting initiatives require careful planning, which considers the person's/group's stage of cognitive development.

Student activities

- Think about an area of health promotion relevant to your branch of nursing, e.g. healthy eating, relaxation and stress reduction, dental care, hand hygiene, etc.
- Plan a series of health-promoting activities appropriate for each of Piaget's stages.
- How would you modify your approach for an adult with a learning disability?

[Resource: Department of Health 2006 Essence of care. Patient-focused benchmarking for health care practitioners. Online: www.dh.gov.uk/PublicationsAndStatistics/Publications/PublicationsPolicyAndGuidance/PublicationsPolicyAndGuidanceArticle/fs/en?CONTENT_ID=4005475&chk=A0A4iz Available July 2006]

Formal operational thought requires attainment of the highest level of thinking in Piaget's model. People with learning (intellectual) disabilities may have particular difficulty using and relating to formal operational thinking, as it requires intellectual ability at the level of secondary school age. Thus they may benefit more from practical demonstrations and supervised experience, e.g. in living skills and health promotion, compared with more abstract methods such as verbal or written explanation (Box 8.23).

Box 8.24 provides an opportunity to consider what children can do, and relates practical observations to Piaget's four stages.

CRITICAL THINKING Box 8.24

What can children do?

A series of practical, age-related activities are provided for you to use.

3–15 months
Hide a toy behind a cushion. Observe if the child tries to search behind it. If they do, move it behind an adjacent cushion. Usually this occurs from about 8 months, but the child is easily 'fooled' if the hiding place is discreetly changed, and will not persist with their search until into their second year.

2–3 years
Find out whether the child can consistently distinguish between different animals, perhaps using a picture book or visiting a zoo.

4–5 years
See if the child can play hide-and-seek, a game that requires participants to imagine where others would conceal themselves to avoid detection.

6–8 years
Try out the liquid conservation test; can the child 'conserve' or not?

9–14 years
Ask the young person, 'What would happen if people could fly?' In the concrete operational phase this is either considered seriously or answered in a literal manner, e.g. 'That would be fun', 'Where would our wings be attached' or 'Don't be silly'. Those at the formal operations stage are likely to be flippant, and suggest 'You could sleep longer before school' or 'It might save fossil fuels'. In other words, the answers reflect the differences between the literal reaction of children to science fiction and fantasy, viewing supernatural powers as something to emulate, and adults' intrigue with the interesting notions involved and their possible ethical ramifications.

Student activities

- Observe the abilities of children that you know (e.g. in a nursery placement or within your family) in relation to the practical activities.
- Consider their abilities in relation to Piaget's stages.

Alternative theories of intellectual development

Jerome Bruner studied the changing ways in which the child represents the world. Initially in the 'enactive' stage this is through actions, such as motor responses, akin to Piaget's sensorimotor stage. Then in the 'iconic' stage, formation of mental images becomes paramount, roughly equivalent to the preoccupation with appearances in Piaget's preoperational stage. Finally, around 7 years of age, the 'symbolic' stage commences, in which use of and growing sophistication of language directs thought and its development. Piaget preferred to regard changes in use of language as reflecting rather than engineering an individual's cognitive advances. Research, e.g. deaf children whose language skills are typically delayed more than their thinking abilities, tends to support his opinion.

In the 1930s, Lev Vygotsky had also argued the importance of inner speech or verbal thought in development. He considered that this and other forms of social activity were instrumental in encouraging problem solving and self-sufficiency. For example, an adult may tutor a child in a task such as putting on clothing through either general advice or specific prompts, providing the 'apprentice' with the 'scaffolding' of another's experience, so accelerating mastery. Student nurses can similarly benefit from the practical expertise passed on by mentors. Cultural learning is similarly imparted between generations by interpersonal means (p. 195), and people's most highly developed cognitive skills tend to relate directly to those valued by the society to which they belong (Gross 2001).

CRITICAL THINKING Box 8.25

A moral dilemma

Somewhere in Europe, a woman was dying from cancer. One drug might save her, newly discovered by a pharmacist working in the same town. The pharmacist was charging 10 times what the drug cost him to make. The sick woman's husband, Heinz, went everywhere he knew to borrow the money needed to purchase the medication, but he could gather only about half of the cost. He told the pharmacist that his wife was dying and asked him to sell it for less or let him pay later, but the answer was a firm 'no'. Heinz became desperate and broke in to steal the drug for his wife.

Student activities

- Consider whether Heinz's actions were right or wrong.
- Justify your reasons.

Box 8.26 **Kohlberg's stages of moral development**

I Preconventional morality
Stage 1 – Moral behaviour is what goes unpunished by authority
Stage 2 – Moral acts are those that are rewarded

II Conventional morality
Stage 3 – Moral behaviour is that which would please most other people
Stage 4 – Moral acts consist of performing one's public duty

III Post-conventional morality
Stage 5 – Moral behaviour adheres to democratic laws, where applicable
Stage 6 – Moral behaviour is purely a matter of individual conscience

Table 8.2 Rationale at various levels of moral development for Heinz scenario (see Box 8.25)

Stage	For stealing the drug	Against stealing the drug
1	Heinz may not be caught or convicted	Heinz is the likely suspect and will probably be imprisoned
2	Heinz's wife and family will love him for his devotion	Heinz may face a fine he can't afford or lose his job for being convicted
3	A public outcry would follow in support of him	Significant others whom Heinz respects may disapprove of his actions
4	Heinz would be fulfilling his duty of care to his wife	Flouting the law may generally erode its social authority
5	A legal test-case could follow, resulting in a change in the law	Technically theft is illegal, no matter what an individual's motive behind it
6	The principle of respecting life takes precedence over property	The pharmacist's rights have been infringed, and future research deterred

Cognitive approaches to moral development

As with intellect, cognitive approaches regard morality as developing progressively and consciously during childhood and adolescence through a predictable succession of stages, each as distinctive as those relating to other forms of thought.

In Piaget's view, 5–9 year olds conceive morality as an absolute system of rules and sanctions directed by higher adult authorities, 'external' morality, demanding one-sided respect, to whom obedience is a virtue in itself, termed 'moral realism'. Those over 10 years increasingly feel more constrained by their own principles of right and wrong, 'internal' morality, which evolve through respectful mutual negotiation. Thus lying to an adult is viewed as no worse than doing so to a peer. Understanding and respecting the viewpoints of others becomes an ethical prerequisite of trusting social relationships, 'moral relativism'. Piaget considered that these qualitative moral changes result from, and so lag behind, the cognitive transformations, e.g. the ability to decentre and reduced egocentrism, which typify the attainment of operational thought.

Kohlberg's work

In the mid 1950s, Lawrence Kohlberg designed nine scenarios involving moral dilemmas, i.e. problems involving at least two ethical principles that are impossible to resolve completely satisfactorily (see Ch. 7). The most famous of these is provided in Box 8.25.

What interested Kohlberg was the rationale given for favouring one course of action over another. Analysis of his subjects' responses led him to formulate a theory that individuals can progress through three levels of moral development, each comprising two substages and, like Piaget's types of morality, contingent on preceding intellectual advances (Box 8.26).

Either basic response to Heinz's and to the other dilemmas that Kohlberg devised, i.e. whether Heinz should or should not have stolen the drug, can be fitted into Box 8.26, depending on the reasoning given for the judgement, allowing the respondent's stage of moral development to be inferred. Some examples are provided in Table 8.2.

Kohlberg reported that only 20% of adults are governed by 'post-conventional' morality and just 10–15% operate on the most advanced level. This finding may be related to the limited proportion of adults who consistently demonstrate Piaget's stage of formal operational thought. As well as advancing through cumulative reasoning ability, Kohlberg thought that morality developed alongside biological maturation and practical challenges inevitable in new social experiences. His work has received criticism on the basis of his research methods (seen as both subjective and abstract) and his implicit assumptions, e.g. that 'Western liberal' morality is superior to a 'traditional conservative' standpoint. However, it is generally regarded as the best explanation of how a child's pragmatic sense of right and wrong potentially progresses to more generalized ethical codes of adulthood.

Alternative theories of moral development

The cognitive approach of Piaget and Kohlberg is often accused of ignoring the emotional component in moral development. This is integral to some of the alternative approaches to moral development discussed below.

Freudian psychodynamic theory and moral development

Freud proposed that control of innate, amoral impulses from infancy until around 4 years of age is tempered by assessing 'what can be got away with'. At around 5 years of age, the conscience emerges out of identification with the words and deeds of one's same-sex parent and internalizing his or her values. The self is punished for the 'should-nots' it commits, engendering guilt, while fulfilling moral obligations generates feelings of self-satisfaction and pride. Conscience thus comes to replace parental authority as an internal moral watchdog. Freud contended that sexual and aggressive impulses, which cannot be expressed, are forced out of conscious awareness (see defence mechanisms, pp. 215–216, and Ch. 11).

Behaviourism (conditioning)

Eysenck suggested that people typically learn from childhood to connect wrongdoing with punishment through memory of past associations; thereafter even anticipated or pondered misdeeds may arouse negative emotions such as fear and guilt. Similarly, good deeds may be associated with rewards such as praise and the pleasant feelings of self-congratulation that follow. Thus moral behaviour is usually 'reinforced' and becomes predominant.

Social observational learning theory

In the 1960s, Bandura emphasized the significance of other individuals, known as 'models', that people observe from childhood onwards and whose behaviour they come to emulate. These include relatives such as parents or siblings, acquaintances, sporting champions, celebrities and even fictional characters in various entertainment media. Factors influencing the likelihood of such 'modelling' include perceived similarities between observer and model, e.g. gender, age, ethnicity, culture, considerations of status and personal qualities, and whether the model's behaviour has beneficial consequences.

Development of interpersonal bonds

This process occurs with particular intensity during preschool childhood, the nature of the experience being of possibly lifelong significance. Formation of such bonds is often referred to as 'attachment' (see Ch. 9). Their severance, whether temporary or permanent, is known as 'separation'.

Infants tend to receive adult attention from the outset due to their natural attractiveness and the curiosity they arouse, as well as any parenting instinct they may evoke. By 6 weeks of age infants will smile at human faces, then after 3 months seem able to distinguish familiar ones from those of strangers, becoming increasingly uncomfortable in the presence of the latter. They engage in active exchanges of expression, such as mutual gazing for continuous 20-second periods and reciprocal smiling, and seem able to detect differing moods in others through facial scrutiny, e.g. they appear perplexed if mother maintains a blank expression.

By 6 or 7 months of age, it has been held that children start to form a lasting emotional bond or attachment to one specific adult, usually the natural mother. Increasing attachment may develop until the child is nearly 3 years old (Bowlby 1988). This is apparent from the child attending to and seeking attention from this figure, and craving constant physical closeness to them. The toddler typically shows distress on separation and relief when reunited. Accordingly, Bowlby described attachment behaviour as the child's 'first love affair'.

In the 1950s, it was suggested that infants become attached to the person who feeds them, i.e. they are essentially motivated by the need to secure nourishment. As the child has to rely on its mother to satisfy primary drives (see p. 188) such as hunger and thirst, it develops a secondary drive for this servicing figure.

However, Harlow's work with infant Rhesus monkeys who had been separated from their mothers and other monkeys at birth suggested otherwise. They preferred to cling to a cloth-covered contraption which rocked soothingly as a base rather than a wire 'mother' that contained their milk-feeding bottle, suggesting warmth and comforting physical contact to be the more powerful attraction.

In the next decade, it was argued that the attachment figure is the person who usually responds to the human infant's behaviour in general and who is the main provider of stimulation. This might sometimes be the father, who perhaps returning from daytime occupational absence, and having little to do with feeding or comforting, becomes the child's preferred playmate, the intense nature of his stimulating interactions, e.g. energetic games or bedtime story-reading, proving important in attaching his child to him. As the child grows older, it may develop multiple attachments, e.g. to grandparents, aunts and uncles, older siblings, neighbours and nursery carers, facilitating substitution for maternal absences with a minimum of emotional upset.

The significance of attachment

It could be that fear of strangers, some of whom might be ill-intentioned, and of isolation from the dependable adult that provides care has significant survival value to a vulnerable youngster. The latter also acts as a safe base from which to explore other things, places and people, so paving the way for future detachment and self-sufficiency.

Bowlby believed that continuous, individual loving care in early childhood was a prerequisite for developing interpersonal trust and fulfilling emotional relationships in adulthood. It is therefore crucial to a person's future social competence, happiness and mental health, as important to the latter as nutrients are to physical health.

Reactions to separation from the attachment figure

In the 1950s, filmed evidence from research by James and Joyce Robertson on the distressed behaviour of hospitalized children startled many professionals involved in childcare (Box 8.27).

Subsequently, Bowlby described three behavioural stages exhibited by children in these circumstances:

- *Protest*: The child cries and fights to cling onto the departing mother. After separation has occurred, intermittent distress is evident.
- *Despair*: After a week or so, the child becomes apathetic and inconsolably sad, possibly blaming himself for his mother's absence; her future return is seemingly no longer anticipated.
- *Detachment*: Later, the child begins to respond again to others, such as nursing staff. When reunited with his mother, he may reject her and take considerable time to relearn the original loving, trusting bond with her.

The behavioural stages are reminiscent of those described in various models of loss and bereavement (see Ch. 12) and suggest that separation from the mother can be an emotionally traumatic experience for a preschool child. Bowlby used the term maternal deprivation to convey the effects of prolonged such separation, but this has been criticized for implying that only the mother is important in childhood attachment processes. Some specific situations where the implications of attachment are likely to be significant are discussed below.

Looked-after children, fostering and adoption

There has been concern about the effects of institutional care on orphans and whether children really need to form attachments to foster or adoptive parents early in life. In 1978, Tizard and Hodges observed that 4-year-olds cared for in institutions were over-friendly towards strangers and more 'clingy' towards carers. These children, however, seemed unselective and superficial in their attachments, displaying little emotion when staff members left (possibly a self-protection response following repeated separation or loss experiences) and quarrelsome with their peers (Hayes 2000). It was also reported that adopted children seemed to fare better scholastically and emotionally than those returned to their biological parents, although socioeconomic factors may partially account for this (Thomson & Meggitt 1997). Other studies suggest that adopted adolescents display significantly more adjustment and behavioural problems, unless adoption had occurred in infancy (Santrock 2004), and offer some support for Bowlby's theory.

REFLECTIVE PRACTICE Box 8.27

Separation anxiety

You may observe this occurring with your own children or during a nursery placement. Think of occasions when parents leave their children in the care of unrelated adults, for instance at nurseries or in hospital.

Student activities

- Did you witness any of the signs of separation anxiety?
- Do children react any differently to separation from their fathers, compared with their mothers?
- Does it make a difference if other carers are familiar to the child?

Working mothers

Dr Benjamin Spock expressed influential concerns in the 1950s that children might be damaged if deprived of essential continuous mothering. However, many children may benefit from the stimulation provided by substitute carers and other children in nurseries. Moreover, their mothers' psychological as well as financial well-being may be significantly enhanced through working outside the home, through adult social contact and occupational stimulation. It may be observed that preschool children can form multiple attachments, including those with regular carers at nursery or child-minders, but they still show an obvious emotional preference for their returning parent.

Hospitalization

Separation due to hospitalization is stressful for both child and parents, whichever is the patient/client. Separation can occur in a wide variety of circumstances and hospitals now have a range of measures to minimize its psychological impact (Box 8.28, p. 214).

Parental loss by death or divorce (see Ch. 12)

Bowlby's theory would predict no difference in children's emotional reaction to loss of a parent through death, parental break-up or abandonment, as all are essentially permanent separations from an attachment figure.

There have been suggestions that divorce increases the likelihood of antisocial behaviour, particularly in boys, as does separation from both parents, but only if this is preceded by prolonged and severe marital disharmony. This has led to the conclusion that amicable parting of parents is preferable for their children's mental well-being than continuing marital strife (Hayes 2000). There are also well-established links between parental loss in childhood and depression (along with increased risk of divorce) in adulthood (McLeod 1991).

CRITICAL THINKING Box 8.28

Reducing the effects of separation for parent and child in hospital

There is no disputing that separation due to hospitalization causes distress for children and their parents.

Student activities

1. Choose circumstances that are relevant to your area of nursing, for example:
   - Full-term neonates
   - Premature babies requiring special or intensive care
   - Young children under 5 years
   - Mothers who have been admitted for treatment
   - Palliative care.
2. Find out what strategies are in place within your particular area of practice to reduce the negative effects of parent–child separation.

[Resources: Action for Sick Children – www.actionforsickchildren.org Available July 2006; Chapter 11, e.g. Table 11.5]

Variations in the attachment process

Ainsworth et al (1978) distinguished between:

- *Secure attachment* (characterizing about two-thirds of children): The child uses the mother as a base for exploring or playing, returning periodically for comforting contact. Brief separations are tolerated and reunions joyful.
- *Insecure avoidant attachment*: Mother is avoided or ignored on returning, comfort from others being equally acceptable.
- *Insecure ambivalent attachment*: Maternal departure distresses the child, who then rejects physical contact with its reappearing mother.

Secure attachment has been linked to social assurance and emotional balance, and regarded as a kind of psychological 'immune system' for future mental resilience (Holmes 2001). Other factors such as later life experiences and family stressors are, however, likely to be significant, and insecure attachment does not invariably foreshadow future psychological problems.

The nature of the attachment relationship appears to stem partly from the parent's approach. If it is consistently loving, responsive and sensitive, the secure pattern is likely to follow. If neglectful, critical or abusive, the insecure forms seem likelier. The child itself may also influence it, e.g. an unwell child tends to demand more parental interventions, and the young child's personality may also be significant. Thomas and Chess (1977) described three types of infant temperament or natural predisposition:

- Easy (the most common) – the child is typically predictable, cheery and unfussy
- Difficult – the opposite of easy
- Slow to warm up – the child is wary of new situations, but usually contented once familiarized.

Such early characteristics do not seem to be reliably reflected in a child's adult personality. Parents may also vary in their preferences regarding their child's temperament. A mother who lacks confidence might be reassured about her competence by an easy infant, while one domineered as a child herself may welcome the assertive behaviour of a difficult baby.

Culture and genetics may also be of significance. Chinese infants appear much more restrained, calm and easily soothed than Caucasian ones. This could reflect inherited characteristics or the value placed by the Chinese culture on self-control. Chinese–American parents are reported as less likely than those of other North American racial groups to encourage their infants' smiling and vocalizing, or independent play (Bernstein et al 2003). Such factors are likely in turn to influence the nature of the attachment process.

Freud's psychodynamic theory

Sigmund Freud (1856–1939) worked for most of his life in Vienna, first as a neurologist, then a psychiatrist, publishing numerous works to explain his treatment, known as psychoanalysis, and its underpinning psychodynamic theory. The latter viewed mental life as much influenced by continuous interplay between three active and largely unconscious structures, namely the:

- Id
- Ego
- Superego.

The id comprises the inborn source of a person's mental energy, generated by two antagonistic inherited instincts, Eros and Thanatos (p. 187). Eros represents the positive life-drive, whose energy, the libido, impels behaviour conducive to survival and reproduction. As meeting such needs is associated with self-gratification, the id has been described as operating via the 'pleasure principle'. The opposing Thanatos initiates negative impulses such as aggressive and self-destructive behaviour. Infants are regarded as functioning via pure id.

The ego develops in response to experience of real world constraints, as the child finds their demands increasingly unmet by reflex activity or the intervention of others. Practical strategies have to be devised to satisfy id impulses in accordance with parental expectations and social rules. As it leads to compromise to gain an individual's end, the ego operates on the 'reality principle', i.e. what actions a person is likely to get away with.

Growing exposure to and identification with the values of parents and significant others promotes their adoption or internalization as the system of ethical principles known as the superego, effectively one's conscience (p. 212). This then compels the ego to obey the dictates of conscience and act in accordance with the new governing 'morality principle'.

A person's basic wants (id), practical options (ego) and moral considerations (superego) often conflict, causing a build-up of tension in the 'pressure cooker' of the unconscious (mind). Squeezed between the incessant demands of the id below and the inhibitions of the superego above

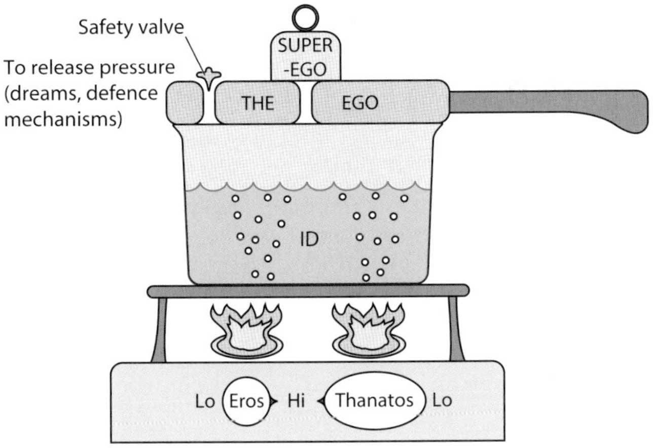

Fig. 8.6 'Pressure-cooker' model of unconscious mental structures

(Fig. 8.6), the ego has to formulate an interminable series of behavioural compromises. Freud suggested that the outcome determines each person's personality and mental health.

Safety valves

In order to protect the ego from being overwhelmed, Freud suggested that two principal methods of pressure (steam) release develop: dreaming and defence mechanisms.

Dreaming is a disguised method of expressing often-unacceptable desires, or wish-fulfilment. Intense fears can also be enacted during sleep, although the true meaning of the experience is concealed from the dreamer by the rich symbolism involved as well as loss of recall on awakening. Interpretation of dreams became a major tool of psychoanalysis.

Defence mechanisms are a series of unconscious tactics by which the ego can prevent unpleasant emotions from troubling the conscious mind. Each involves self-deception and distortion of reality, and can at best provide temporary respite rather than a true solution to the underlying problem (see Ch. 11 for more information about defence mechanisms in stress and coping). Some of the main defence mechanisms are:

- Repression – unpalatable memories or emotions are prevented from entering consciousness, but still leave an uncomfortable tinge, a state of 'unblissful unawareness'. This mechanism is the basis for all the others, which therefore also each carry discomfiting emotional undertones.
- Denial – unpleasant realities are driven out of awareness and ignored, allowing the person to function normally but within a 'fool's paradise'.
- Reaction formation – attitudes completely opposite to those unconsciously held are expressed, reminiscent of Shakespeare's 'methinks thou dost protest too much'.
- Displacement – emotions are redirected from their actual target towards a safer, innocent recipient such as 'slaying the messenger' of bad news.
- Rationalization – constructing a logical explanation to justify unacceptable actions, then believing one's own argument, claiming 'I have good reason'.
- Intellectualization – minimizing the anxiety in a situation by appraising it in abstract, objective terms, focusing on 'logic in adversity'.
- Projection – perceiving undesirable qualities or motives in others that you possess yourself, a case of 'the pot calling the kettle black'.
- Identification – characteristics, even if unpleasant or threatening, of other acquaintances are incorporated into one's own behaviour, a case of 'if you can't beat them, join them'.
- Sublimation – unacceptable impulses are energetically channelled into socially approved pursuits.

Even if repressed out of conscious awareness, covert thoughts and impulses may occasionally surface in the form of slips of the tongue known as 'Freudian slips'; memory lapses, e.g. of unwanted events or responsibilities; or physical mishaps, e.g. damaging disliked objects, all of which suggest to Freudians that there is no such thing as an innocent accident.

However, if the lid is kept too firmly on unconscious turmoil, the energy of the suppressed anxieties may be converted into emotional and physical ailments (previously known as psychosomatic). Box 8.29 (see p. 216) provides an opportunity to identify the defence mechanism operating in a series of scenarios.

Psychosexual personality development

Freud believed that personality developed through a series of consecutive stages, each distinguished by the part of the body affording most contemporary stimulation and resultant pleasure. Particularly controversial, especially at the turn of the 19th century, was his contention that the stage-related gratification was sexual in nature, even in infants. Either insufficient or excessive enjoyment within a stage could result in fixation there – remaining preoccupied with or continuing to indulge in the pursuits characterizing that period. This could be manifest in related traits and activities during adulthood. Such primitive vestiges could become particularly pronounced during stressful episodes, when the individual might dramatically revert, or regress, displaying strikingly immature behaviour. According to Freud, there are five stages: oral, anal, phallic, latent and genital.

Oral stage (0–24 months)

This reflects Piaget's sensorimotor intelligence (see p. 208) and is subdivided into two phases:

- An initial *passive* phase, when the mouth's principal activity is sucking, either feeding at the breast or bottle, or, outwith meals, at grasped objects.
- A later *active* phase, coinciding with the emergence of the first teeth from around 6 months, arming the infant with the ability to bite as well as chew. Attempts at speaking become increasingly distinct during this period.

CRITICAL THINKING Box 8.29

Which defence mechanism?

Scenarios

- The consultant made some critical remarks to the ward sister about inaccuracies on patients' charts. Shortly after, sister shouted at a student nurse for being a few minutes late on duty.
- The staff nurse said that she didn't mind that someone else had been chosen for promotion, as she had just wanted the interview experience.
- On unexpectedly failing his exam, Mike told his parents that they should accept it philosophically, and view it as a mind-broadening experience for their son.
- Karen had been told that the two charge nurses loathed each other, but did not believe this, as they always seemed very polite to each other.
- The student took a long time to feel at ease in her ward placement. Later she discovered that she had been a patient there as a small child.
- Dr Jones was terminally ill with breast cancer. She had ignored a suspicious lump for a year.
- During the coffee-break with her fellow nurses, Julia denounced their absent colleagues as terrible gossips.
- Joanna worked as a theatre nurse and had two main hobbies, gardening and pottery.
- Eric knew that he worked with insensitive colleagues. He was taken aback when his girlfriend complained that she found him increasingly brusque.

Student activities

- Consider the scenarios and identify which defence mechanism is probably present.
- Discuss your findings with a fellow student and decide which mechanisms, if any, can be used to explain scenarios in your own practice.

Freud regarded weaning to be the main goal by the end of the oral stage, and the most common problems as resulting from either early cessation of or protracted breastfeeding.

The effects of fixation in the 'passive oral' personality may result in behaviours such as being dependent (like an infant), demanding (wailing for attention), greedy or gluttonous, breast-obsessed and displaying sucking behaviours, e.g. smoking, imbibing alcohol to excess, pen- or thumb-sucking, with regression to this if highly stressed.

In the 'active oral' personality the effects may include talkative, prone to sarcasm or abusive outbursts, as if the mouth is used as a weapon, as well as gum chewing, pencil nibbling or nail biting if anxious.

Anal stage (2–3 years)

The focus changes to the process and structures of elimination, particularly of faeces. This stage also comprises two substages:

- An initial *expulsive* phase, when satisfaction and parental praise is derived from expelling excrement.
- Later, parents try to encourage continence, and praise and the child's pleasure are related to retaining excrement until appropriate opportunities for voiding, the *retentive* phase.

Routine continence is the main goal by the end of the anal stage. Toilet training can become a frustrating and ambivalent process for all concerned, with difficulties resulting from both prolonged incontinence and rigid, authoritarian supervision (see Chs 20, 21).

The effects of fixation early on, an 'expulsive anal' personality, may be characterized by a person who is untidy, messy, wasteful, generous, unpunctual, prone to coarseness and vulgarity in speech and humour.

If fixation is later, a 'retentive anal' personality results, and the person may be fastidious, hygiene obsessed, methodical, perfectionist, obsessive, restrained, miserly and obstinate.

Phallic stage (4–5 years)

The child now becomes fascinated with genitalia, their own and those of other people, leading to curiosity about the mechanism of reproduction as well as genital fondling. Adult disapproval often follows, complicated by increasing attraction to the opposite sex parent and hostility to that of the same sex. Freud termed this gravitation the 'Oedipus complex' in boys and the 'Electra complex' in girls.

The main goal is that the 'mummy's boy' and 'daddy's girl' complexes resolve naturally through gradual acceptance of and identification with the same sex parent. Common problems are continued sexual inwardness and parental preoccupation.

The effects of fixation may include a lifelong worship of one's opposite sex parent and choosing love partners by their resemblance to that figure; a competitive, ambitious and boastful nature, demonstrating an unconscious need to surpass the same sex parent. Narcissism, the preoccupation with one's own attractiveness and flirtatiousness, may reflect the self-directed and abstract nature of sexual impulses inherited from this stage, and another vestige may be difficulties relating to authority figures.

Latent stage (6–11 years)

This is the temporary submersion of preceding sexual preoccupations into unconscious undercurrents. The child appears immersed in their hobbies and school activities. Playmates are typically of the same sex, and revulsion is commonly expressed at any exhibitions of affection, nudity or sexual passion that they may encounter, e.g. on television or between parents.

The focus switches to scholastic and sporting prowess (see stage 4 of Erikson's model below).

The effects of fixation include adult immersion in work, study or pastimes, sexual coldness or indifference to the presence of the opposite sex.

Genital stage (12 years and above)

With the onset of puberty, sexual impulses reappear in a more conscious and urgent form, requiring satisfaction

Table 8.3 Erikson's stages of psychosocial development (after Gross 2001)

Stage	Approximate age range	Significant others
1. *Basic trust versus mistrust* Infants develop awareness of how sensitively and consistently their needs for nourishment, comfort and stimulation are met, and thus whether or not the world seems to be a safe, predictable and welcoming place	0–1 year	Mother-figure, main care providers
2. *Autonomy versus shame and doubt* Toddlers develop a sense of individual 'self' and increasing muscular power, and often wish to exercise choice and do things for themselves. Adults may feel obliged to intervene at times, e.g. for reasons of safety or efficiency, and children may feel ashamed at failed initiatives or doubt their abilities, e.g. when struggling with toilet training	2–3 years	Parents, child-minders, nursery staff
3. *Initiative versus guilt* Preschool children ask probing questions of adults to deepen their understanding, participate imaginatively in games and are boldly energetic. Such independent actions bolster self-confidence, but this may be shaken if adults show disapproval of the enquiries, or criticize play as silly or dangerous, resulting in self-censure and guilt	4–6 years	As in previous stage, teachers latterly
4. *Industry versus inferiority* Primary school children are keen to learn, to make things and see how they work. Their self-esteem depends largely on their ability to fulfil set tasks in comparison with their peers' performance. Opportunities, guidance and encouragement are crucial, as a sense of failure results from perceived underachievement	7–12 years	Teachers, friends, parents
5. *Identity versus role confusion* Adolescents begin to formulate a concept of who they are in relation to society, including their intended occupational and sexual preferences – their cultural, work and sexual identities. They engage with and either commit to or reject ideologies, e.g. political and moral. Inability to emerge with clear roles and values can result in anger or apathy, and lack of future direction	13–19 years	School 'chums', boyfriend, girlfriend, mentors Ambivalent towards parents
6. *Intimacy versus isolation* Young adults build on their new identity to seek proximity and share interests and feelings with others, in the workplace and through committed sexual relationships. Isolation may result from fear of self-revelation or inability to select or obtain rewarding employment or partners	20–30 years	Colleagues, employers, lovers, spouse/partner
7. *Generativity versus stagnation* In middle adulthood, the main concern is to care for and raise children, benefit others with your experience and/or be productive at rewarding work or art and craft, so making a contribution to society. If denied these outlets, middle-age can feel empty and wasted	31–50s	Children and partner, customers or clients, mentees
8. *Ego integrity versus despair* Mature adulthood is seen as a phase for reflection on one's life cycle, which should be seen as having had a meaningful pattern and having been useful, despite inevitable adverse experiences. This allows the person to anticipate death with dignified acceptance and composure. An unsatisfactory life review focuses on failures and missed opportunities, fear of dying and a futile wish for sufficient time to start anew	50s onwards	Oneself and all humanity

in intimate relationships and eventually through physical intercourse. This urge remains throughout adult life, and Freud envisaged its ultimate fulfilment in the form of enduring monogamous love. Equally conventional was Freud's view of males, both in social and sexual roles, as naturally aggressive, adventurous and dominant compared with female passivity, maternalism and domesticity.

The main goal is physical love and reproduction; in this stage fixation is desirable. However, earlier fixations can interfere with this goal.

Criticisms and benefits of the psychodynamic approach

Criticisms of Freud's approach included a lack of scientific basis and subjectivity. Another criticism was directed at its pessimism about human nature, as being at core irrational, hedonistic and destructive, and irresponsibility in focusing on childhood sexuality, a charge whose intensity surprised Freud. In addition, it may offend modern sensibilities as inherently sexist and viewing males as behaviourally and anatomically superior.

However, the benefits of Freud's approach may include:

- Greater tolerance of sexuality, e.g. its open discussion and idiosyncratic expressions.
- Increased understanding and acceptance of people suffering from mental dysfunction; anxiety, his clinical focus, is a universal experience.
- The emergence of gentler, 'talking' treatments for mental disorders; Freudian psychoanalysis is the forerunner of modern psychotherapy.
- The enrichment of Western language and thought, as many of the terms and notions above are now part of cultural heritage.

REFLECTIVE PRACTICE Box 8.30

Erikson's stages applied to nursing

Erikson suggested that people needed to make sense of and resolve typical challenges at whatever 'stage' of life they are.

Student activities

- Reflect on current issues and concerns in your personal life. Are they similar to those suggested by Erikson for your age group?
- Discuss with your mentor how Erikson's stages can be applied in your area of practice.

Erikson's stage theory of psychosocial development

In the 1950s, Erik Erikson explored the relationship between psychological and social development. He produced a framework in which personal development occurs via a natural series of eight stages, each dominated by a major issue or crisis presented by the social environment (Table 8.3, see p. 217). If the child, adolescent or adult resolves the contemporary challenge positively, then a sound foundation is established for progression to later stages, and a healthy personality and functioning are more likely. However, a relatively maladaptive response will result in poor resolution of the issue, psychological problems and diminished ability to cope with later crises. Erikson suggested that it is possible to rectify inadequate confrontation of an issue retrospectively, even if another stage's time parameters are the ideal point at which to resolve that crisis (Box 8.30). Conversely, previously gained ground can be lost once chronologically beyond a stage, e.g. to lose as well as regain trust in life during adulthood.

Summary

- An understanding of the major psychological and sociological concepts relevant to the human lifespan is important for nurses in all areas of practice.
- The contrasting approaches to psychology and sociology each yields useful insights into individual and social behaviour.
- Considering motivation assists nurses to understand the behaviour of others and to meet their needs.
- Culture, socialization and family are significant factors in health.
- Physical development relates not only to increasing size and strength over the lifespan, but also to the changing function of body systems. This affects a person's ability to function in a social context.
- Both genetic and environmental (including social) factors are important in development.
- Psychosocial development encompasses advances in self-perception, thought, morality and personality.
- Both conscious and unconscious processes may be significant in development and health.
- Aspects of development may be envisaged as a necessary progression through a series of age-related stages.

Self test

1. Match each motive with the appropriate psychological approach:

(i) self-actualization	(a) psychodynamic
(ii) self-destruction	(b) behaviourism
(iii) drive	(c) humanism

2. Parsons related societal privileges to fulfilling obligations in:
   a. Role theory
   b. Subcultures
   c. Secondary socialization.

3. What type of family comprises two adults who live together with children from their present and previous relationships?

4. At what age would you expect most children to be able to:
   a. Walk up steps
   b. Utter their first recognizable word
   c. Wash and dry their hands
   d. Draw a recognizable human figure.

5. A deficiency of the growth-related hormone thyroxine during infancy may lead to:
   a. Weight loss
   b. Reduced bone density
   c. Learning (intellectual) disabilities.

6. Which of the following generally accompany normal ageing:
   a. Skin pigmentation
   b. Reduction in height
   c. Diminished sensory acuity
   d. Less efficient kidney function
   e. Dementia.

7. Piaget termed devising new strategies to adapt to unaccustomed problems as:
   a. Assimilation
   b. Accommodation
   c. Equilibration.

8. Adult moral judgements are dependent on attaining what level of thought?

9. According to Bowlby, what is the critical time period for forming emotional bonds in infancy?

10. The genital stage of Freud's psychosexual scheme is chronologically attained during which of Erikson's psychosocial stages?

Key words and phrases for literature searching

Adaptation
Ageing/aging
Attachment
Behaviourism
Cognitive
Conditioning
Culture
Development
Developmental milestone
Erikson
Family
Freud
Growth
Humanist
Intellectual
Intelligence
Kohlberg
Motivation
Normalization
Norms
Piaget
Psychodynamic
Psychology
Psychosexual
Psychosocial
Role
Self
Separation
Socialization
Sociology
Values

Useful websites

BBC UK History	www.bbc.co.uk/history/timelines/britain/vic_indust_growth.shtml Available July 2006
Scottish Recovery Network	www.scottishrecovery.net/content Available July 2006
US National Library of Health MedlinePlus Medical Encyclopedia – *provides information of developmental milestones at different ages*	www.nlm.nih.gov/medlineplus/ency/encyclopedia_D-Di.htm Available July 2006

References

Abercrombie N, Warde A 2005 Contemporary British society. 3rd edn. Polity Press, Cambridge

Ainsworth MDS, Blehar M, Waters E, Wall S 1978 Patterns of attachment: a psychological study of the strange situation. Erlbaum, Hillsdale, NJ

Alzheimer's Society 2006 Facts about dementia. Online: www.alzheimers.org.uk/Facts_about_dementia/Statistics/index.htm Available July 2006

Atkinson RL, Atkinson RC, Smith EE, Bem DJ, Nolen-Hoeksema SN 2000 Hilgard's introduction to psychology. 13th edn. Harcourt, Fort Worth, TX, p. 471

Bee H, Boyd D 2004 The developing child. 10th edn. Allyn & Bacon/Pearson Education, Boston

Bernstein D, Penner LA, Clarke-Stewart A, Roy EJ 2003 Psychology. 6th edn. Houghton Mifflin, Boston

Bowlby J 1988 A secure base: clinical applications of attachment theory. Routledge, London

Denny E, Earle S 2005 Sociology for nurses. Polity Press, Cambridge

Denver Developmental Materials Inc 1990 The Denver scale II. Denver Developmental Materials, Denver

Eysenck MW 2000 Psychology – a student's handbook. Psychology Press, Hove

Frankenburg WK, Dodds JB, Archer P et al 1990 The Denver II (developmental rating scale). Denver Developmental Materials, Denver

Gates B (ed) 2002 Learning disabilities: toward inclusion. 4th edn. Churchill Livingstone, Edinburgh

Giddens A 2001 Sociology. 4th edn. Polity Press, Cambridge

Goffman E 1971 The presentation of self in everyday life. Penguin, London

Gross RD 2001 Psychology: the science of mind and behaviour. 5th edn. Hodder and Stoughton, London

Hayes N 2000 Foundations of psychology. 3rd edn. Thomson, London

Haralambos M, Holborn M 2005 Sociology: themes and perspectives. Harper Collins, London

Hinchliff SM, Montague SE, Watson R 1996 Physiology for nursing practice. 2nd edn. Baillière Tindall, London

Holmes J 2001 The search for the secure base. Brunner-Routlege, Hove

Mader SS 2000 Human biology. 6th edn. McGraw-Hill, Boston

McLeod JD 1991 Childhood parental loss and adult depression. Journal of Health and Social Behaviour 32(3):205–220

Miell D 1990 The self and the social world. In: Roth I (ed) Introduction to psychology, Vol. 1. Open University Press, Milton Keynes, Chapter 2

Napier University 1997, 2001 The individual, family and society: Module booklet 2. Faculty of Health and Life Sciences, Edinburgh

Nursing and Midwifery Council 2004 Code of professional conduct: standards for conduct, performance and ethics. NMC, London

Santrock JW 2004 Life-span development. 9th edn. McGraw-Hill, New York

Thomas A, Chess S 1977 Temperament and development. Brunner and Mazel, New York

Thomson H, Meggitt C 1997 Human growth and development for health and social care. Hodder and Stoughton, London

Tizard B, Hodges J 1978 The effect of early institutional rearing on the development of 8-year-old children. Journal of Child Psychology and Psychiatry 19:99–118

Townsend P, Whitehead M 1990 Inequalities in health: the Black report/the health divide. Penguin, London

Watson D 2002 Causes and manifestations of learning disabilities. In: Gates B (ed) Learning disabilities: toward inclusion. 4th edn. Churchill Livingstone, Edinburgh, Chapter 2

Further reading

Brooker C 1998 Human structure and function. 2nd edn. Mosby, London

Chamley C, Carson P, Randall D, Sandwell WM 2005 Developmental anatomy and physiology of children. A practical approach. Churchill Livingstone, Edinburgh

Denny E, Earle S 2005 Sociology for nurses. Polity Press, Cambridge

Durkin K 2001 Developmental social psychology. In: Hewstone M, Strobe W (eds) Introduction to social psychology: a European perspective. 3rd edn. Blackwell, Oxford

Giddens A 1989 Sociology. Polity Press, Cambridge

Hockenberry MJ, Wilson D, Winkelstein ML, Kline N 2002 Wong's nursing care of infants and children. 7th edn. Mosby, St Louis, Chapter 7

Holmes J 1993 John Bowlby and attachment theory. Routledge, London

Light P, Oates J 1990 The development of children's understanding. In: Roth I (ed) Introduction to psychology, Vol. 1. Open University Press, Milton Keynes, Chapter 3

Montague SE, Watson R, Herbert R 2005 Physiology for nursing practice. 3rd edn. Baillière Tindall, Edinburgh

Thompson T, Mathias P (eds) 2000 Lyttle's mental health and disorder. 3rd edn. Baillière Tindall, Edinburgh

9

Relationship, helping and communication skills

Naomi Sharples

Glossary terms

Body language

Communication

Empathy

Interpersonal skills

Language

Listening

Positive regard

Relationships

Self-awareness

Values

Learning outcomes

This chapter will help you to:

- Discuss what is meant by communication
- Outline the development of language
- Describe the use of language
- Outline interpersonal communication skills
- Describe nursing relationships, therapeutic and professional
- Recognize, minimize or overcome communication barriers
- Start to develop the skill of breaking bad news.

Introduction

This chapter explores how knowledge of communication, language and interpersonal skills can enhance professional nursing practice and nursing relationships. Such knowledge and skills are relevant to all the other chapters of the book. This chapter considers how people understand language and communication and presents various frameworks and activities for the reader to practise with the aim of developing their interpersonal skills and thus the quality of the care and positive relationships and interactions they are able to engage in with patients/clients/children, carers and colleagues.

Well-developed interpersonal and communication skills are considered essential for all nurses, regardless of where they work. This is evidenced by the addition of benchmarks for best practice in communication to the original eight sets of benchmarks in the *Essence of Care* document (NHS Modernisation Agency 2003). Nurses need to be critical of their communication skills in the care environment and need to be able to provide evidence of how they actually meet the information, communication and linguistic needs of patients, clients, children, families and carers (Box 9.1).

REFLECTIVE PRACTICE Box 9.1

Benchmarks for communication

Agreed patient-focused outcome (NHS Modernisation Agency 2003):

'Patients and carers experience effective communication sensitive to their individual needs and preferences, which promotes high quality care for the patient.'

Student activities

- Think about the statement above. What does it mean for your nursing practice?
- Consider how you know what to say and how to talk with people who may be distressed or angry or deeply sad.
- Access the *Essence of Care* document and read the 11 benchmarks for best practice in communication. Discuss them with your mentor.

[Resource: NHS Modernisation Agency 2003 Essence of care: patient-focused benchmarks for clinical governance – www.modern.nhs.uk/home/key/docs/Essence%20of%20Care.pdf Available July 2006]

There is a focus on a number of skills and techniques that will enhance the nurse's ability to deliver care within the context of a positive and empowering communication environment. Developing communication skills takes practice, as does any nursing skill, but with practice comes the ability to quickly develop working and therapeutic relationships, thus enhancing people's experience of healthcare.

The primary aim of this chapter is to enable the reader to recognize when communication is appropriate and also how to improve communicative and interpersonal skills. Most of the time people manage communication and relationships correctly; however, because these aspects of language are so innate, people often resort to habitual ways of being with people. Often these habits will be appropriate but they can also create problems that may result in difficulties in interacting effectively with people. For example, a nurse may offend or possibly damage relationships with patients/clients/children, carers and colleagues. There is a great need for nurses to consider exactly what they say to people, how they say it and how this affects them.

If nurses are serious about good interpersonal skills they may start to feel a little anxious about communication if they are not sure about saying or doing the right thing. Feeling unsure is good, as it indicates that nurses are starting to think carefully and more critically about what they say to people, how they relate to them and how this affects their experience of health professionals.

Another aim of the chapter is to bring readers out of the unconscious competence zone and for them to work within the conscious competence and conscious incompetence areas. The zones of learning and experience are:

- *Unconscious competence*: People do not think about what they are saying – they just open their mouth and speak and more often than not it is right
- *Conscious competence*: People know what they are going to say, why they are going to say it and what result they want
- *Conscious incompetence*: People will be aware of what they do not know about communication and interpersonal skills – 'they know what they don't know'
- *Unconscious incompetence*: People do not know what they do not know, e.g. meeting someone who speaks a different language, a language they have no knowledge of or the skills to understand or express ideas.

There is considerable debate about the origin of this model, which can be found at www.businessballs.com.

Focusing on Gibbs' (1988) reflective model (see Ch. 4) will also encourage nurses to consider more deeply their thoughts, feelings and behaviours; it will bring communication to the forefront of the mind and, by so doing, move understanding from an innate level – an unconscious competence level – to a more considered consciously competent level.

Good communication offers pathways into relationships between individuals and ultimately the ability to effectively care for people. Caring for someone entails looking after their needs on many different levels – from physical needs to emotional support, from information giving to working in partnership. Caring is a deeply held value for nurses and, to communicate this care, nurses must show concern, attention, empathy and respect, and focus on people's needs.

Communication theory

People are 'wired' to communicate, to develop language, reason, empathy and even storytelling skills. Parents and main carers are innately skilled in developing the language ability of their children; people have the capability and importantly the motivation to match the communication needs of other people in various situations and from diverse cultures, social strata and backgrounds. Pinker (1994) suggests that people are born with the ability and the language faculty to understand any natural language. This faculty is like no other learning experience: it does not require conscious effort and exceeds all other notions of learning theory – all it needs is to be stimulated by a language environment.

Despite these innate abilities, people still make errors when communicating with others; some errors are small, such as 'pacifically speaking' rather than 'specifically speaking', but others are more serious. Practitioners who assume that the patient/client/child cannot understand what is being said in their presence may cause them anxiety or fear, and can create feelings of hostility.

Models for communication

A number of models are outlined below. These include Lasswell's model, the blueprint of behaviour model and a model derived from Shannon and Weaver's model.

Lasswell's model of communication

In 1948 Lasswell devised a very effective model of the communication process which can be used for any communication interaction (Fiske 1993). In daily life almost everything involves communication – from nursing handover to lectures, conversations with family to addressing a conference, from singing a nursery rhyme to a child to seeing a live band perform. Lasswell's model looks at communication as a process that has an effect on (influences) the receiver's behaviour to some degree (Fig. 9.1).

Box 9.2 explores some of the questions associated with the components of Lasswell's model.

Lasswell's model provides information about the communication process. However, to 'understand how to understand' this process and how people make choices in this process, it is important to consider the influences on people's perception of the world. For example, the design of buildings communicates a message. Hospitals may communicate clinical specialities, care, security and cleanliness, or quite the opposite (Box 9.3).

Blueprint of behaviour model

The neurolinguistic programming (NLP) model showing the blueprint of behaviour is a useful tool in appreciating how people understand the world around them, how this influences the way the person will communicate and therefore how others may respond to them (Fig. 9.2, see p. 224).

Everyone has unique life experiences that influence the way they understand the world. The senses are also unique: people see, hear, smell, touch and taste in ways that are particular to them. The language used and understood is also unique to and influenced by background, social class, education, family, spirituality and cultural heritage. Given so many individual distinctions, it is the predisposition to communicate that enables people to create such effective connections with others.

However, language, senses, experiences, beliefs and values can act as filters that affect the way people interpret and internalize external stimuli and this determines the way people communicate and behave with others. The term 'filter' represents the physiological and neurological processes that act on information as it comes through the senses and into language, values and belief systems. Filtered external stimuli are internally represented and understood by each individual in a different

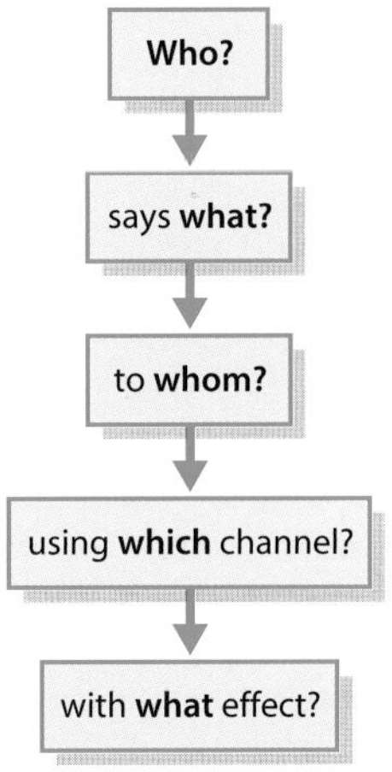

Fig. 9.1 Lasswell's model of communication

REFLECTIVE PRACTICE Box 9.3

What does the care setting communicate?

Consider a clinical environment that you are familiar with and look at it using Lasswell's model.

Student activities

- What is the environment communicating?
- Consider the effect on the people who work in the environment or those who live or visit the area.
- Identify specific units such as an intensive care unit for babies, or for people in mental distress – what do they communicate?

CRITICAL THINKING Box 9.2

Exploring Lasswell's model

Who?

Who is sending the message? Is it a friend, patient/client or someone trying to sell something? What are their language and communication skills? What is my relationship with this person? What is their agenda, their ultimate objective in communicating?

What?

What is the message they are sending? Does it relate to me? What knowledge will help me to understand the message and respond appropriately?

To whom?

To whom are they sending the message? Is it to me alone, or are millions of people receiving this message through an advertisement on television, or hundreds of people who work at a particular hospital?

Which channel?

Which channel of communication are they using – visual media, gestural/visual, spoken/hearing, light, sound, vibration, touch, smell, taste? Channels are as flexible as the senses – smells often communicate deep memories for people, and sounds (e.g. music, speech, rhythms) can influence people's emotional states, both positively and negatively. People tend to have a stronger preference for receiving information either visually, through their auditory channel (see p. 224), or kinaesthetically, through touch or feelings. Usually people prefer a mix of channels and media: the more access to information they have through a variety of media, the more likely they are to understand the message and to remember it.

With what effect?

All communication has an effect on the parties involved. The effect for a nurse may be to respond appropriately to clients' needs, to help a small child to accept a medical procedure or to encourage a client to make an informed choice about their health needs. In a wider context the communication may influence people to buy a new sofa, to eat in a certain restaurant or to develop a political opinion.

Student activities

- Choose a recent communication and use Lasswell's model to analyse how it happened and its effects.
- Using the questions posed above as a starting point, what other questions may have been relevant?

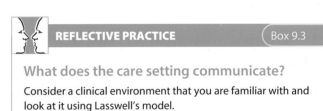

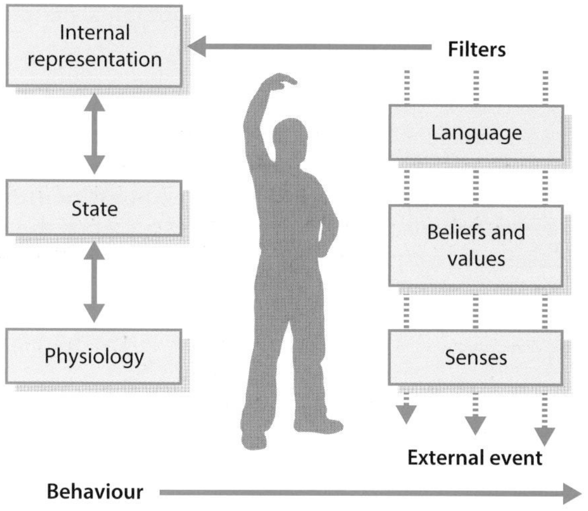

Fig. 9.2 Blueprint for behaviour

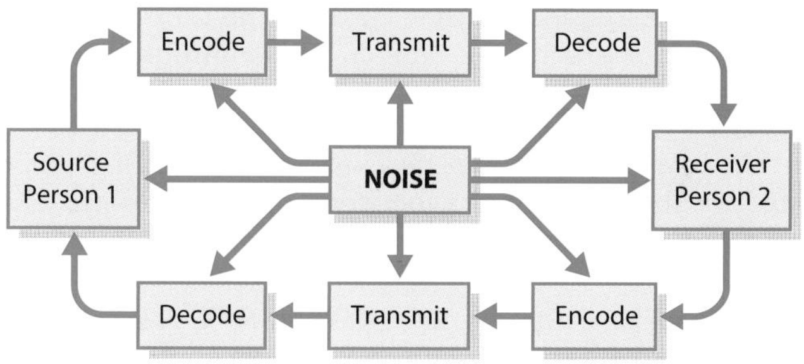

Fig. 9.3 Communication model derived from Shannon and Weaver's model

way. These representations influence emotions, which in turn influence the language used and people's subsequent behaviour.

Understanding how these filters create accessible or inaccessible pathways between individuals and groups enables nurses to be clear and creative in communicating often vital information to patients/clients, carers and colleagues.

A model derived from Shannon and Weaver's model

A simple communication model, derived from Shannon and Weaver's model (Fiske 1993), provides a description of the communication process between two people (Fig. 9.3): person 1 encodes, creates their message and transmits it to person 2 who decodes the message for meaning, and encodes or creates a response, which is transmitted to person 1 to decode and understand.

It would be useful to consider this model while at the same time keeping the blueprint of behaviour model in mind. It helps to build a picture of the factors that affect:

- People individually
- The communication process between people
- The communication process between people and their environment.

Communication process – getting the message across

Most people have a preference for either the auditory or the visual channel for sending and receiving messages (see p. 223), but choosing the most appropriate channel is vital for effective communication.

For example, the sender thinks of an idea which will have been triggered by an internal or external event. The thought/message is encoded into words in the brain; the message is then transmitted from the brain to the structures involved in voice production (e.g. larynx, tongue, palate and lips), to the outside world and the listener. The listener picks up the sound through the ears and the sound is transmitted along the vestibulocochlear (auditory) nerves to the brain. There it is decoded and understood by the listener who will react to the message and feed back to the sender.

At any point in this sequence noise can influence the quality of the message. A noise could be environmental interference, such as a noisy environment where people are competing to be heard, or clinical equipment beeping and buzzing. It may be that the person is experiencing pain and is concentrating on this rather than on the person speaking.

Other major influences on the communication process in care settings are language differences, anxiety, fear and anger. People who are experiencing extremes of emotions are not in a position to fully understand a message, e.g. a distressed relative in the Emergency Department. People who have mental distress or are experiencing hallucinations find that their ability to comprehend others can be limited.

Noise changes the message. To understand how it has been changed the sender relies on the listener's feedback or a change in behaviour to check if the message has been understood. In a situation where the message is clear and understood, the sender may not need to go further. If the message was not understood, the sender takes the responsibility for adjusting the message and possibly the channel chosen to transmit the message in an attempt to succeed in communicating their idea (Box 9.4).

Acknowledging potential noise in the communication process enables the nurse to adjust the message accordingly. Thus the nurse is 'accommodating' the communication rather than 'diverging' from the needs of the other person (see p. 230).

Similar, but more complex skills are needed in specific situations. For example, when nurses communicate with a person with a learning disability the communication is determined by the nurse's knowledge of the person and their linguistic and cognitive ability. Carers, friends, family and speech and language therapists (SLTs) often inform this knowledge (Box 9.5).

Language

Earlier sections have emphasized that each person has a different blueprint of behaviour with unique challenges,

REFLECTIVE PRACTICE Box 9.4

Getting the message across

The feedback from a patient/client was to tap their ear, shake their head and shrug their shoulders. The nurse may think that they have not heard the message:

- By quickly analysing the message – the sender feels it was clear
- The situation – the message was in context
- Possible noise factors – these were at an acceptable level.

By ruling out many possibilities, the nurse may conclude that the person is deaf or hard of hearing. If the nurse has sign language skills and encodes the message in sign, the visual channel can be used to transmit the message through hand shapes, facial expressions and body movement. The patient/client receives and understands the message via the visual channel. Feedback could be a smile and thumbs up.

Student activities

Think about a situation from clinical practice where the listener did not hear your spoken message:

- How did you know the listener had not heard?
- What other communication channels did you consider?
- How might you have communicated with the person?

the ability to change, to develop and, in the case of the senses, to deteriorate. Choices in communication are dependent on many factors, one of the most important of which is language.

All human languages comprise words or signs, sounds, visual movement, rules, grammar, vocabulary, knowledge of meaning and creativity. All languages are complex and based on a finite number of sounds or hand shapes, if it is a sign language. All languages provide the users with the ability to produce an infinite number of sentences (Crystal 1999).

Many people feel that language is a complicated and difficult subject with hidden depth and unseen trickery that make the idea of learning a new language unattainable. Babies and children learning their first language do not have these anxieties; they usually have a natural curiosity that supports language acquisition. Play is an important component in the processes involved in language development. Depending on a child's age and stage of development, one of the main sources of communication with children is through play (see pp. 226–227).

Language development in children

Language development is vital for a child to progress from a point where they are unable to express thoughts, feeling or behaviours to one where they can express abstract thoughts, complex emotions, describe intricate behaviours and develop engaging relationships with others (Box 9.6, see p. 226).

Box 9.5 **People with learning disabilities – assessing communication difficulties**

Children and adults with a learning disability may face greater challenges in acquiring language. These difficulties not only relate to their cognitive development but also to the physical problems that coincide with some developmental differences. They may have problems with articulation, expressive language or receptive language (see pp. 227–228).

Structured assessments by the multidisciplinary team (MDT), comprising audiologist, SLT, ophthalmologist and physiotherapist, are therefore vital to this client group.

The assessments focus on:

- Hearing and communication skills – hearing loss is more common for people with learning disabilities (see Ch. 16)
- Assessment of oral cavity, larynx, pharynx and nasal cavity to ascertain if there are any anomalies that would preclude speech development, or the ability to produce sound or factors affecting the quality of the sound
- Vision is also crucial to language learning and needs to be assessed regularly
- Gross and fine motor movement ability will also have an impact on their ability to use gesture, sign language or to vocalize
- Cognitive impairments are also assessed by the SLT to discover if there is a neurological basis for any problems the client maybe experiencing.

Following the assessments, the MDT plans interventions with the client, family and carers to facilitate the client's move towards communicative competence. These are evaluated and the plan reviewed on a regular basis.

Examples of interventions could include:

- Naming games, completing the sentence games
- Mouth and tongue exercises
- Voice practice and breathing exercises
- Listening games, rhythm games, sound identification games
- Social skill development to enhance interpersonal communication skills
- Advice to family/carers about the best method of communication, e.g. signing, or some other communication aid.

Box 9.7 (see p. 226) provides an opportunity to reflect on a situation involving communication with a child.

Children who are denied access to a language environment have problems acquiring language. 'Feral' children or children who experience severe neglect are confounded by the complexity of language rules and social relationships, particularly if they are not discovered until later childhood. It appears that, if not appropriately

Box 9.6 Normal early language development

- *Newborn babies* cry, scream, coo and whimper, alerting parents/carers that they are hungry, cold, want contact or are content. This is the prelinguistic phase (before true language).
- *At 3 months* the palate and pharynx begin to develop; before this age they are unable to create speech sounds.
- *Around 6 months* babies start to 'babble'. This is where they learn to differentiate true language sounds from those that will not be needed. Deaf babies 'babble' with their hands forming the hand shapes that are some of the finite set of shapes they will use. Babies start to practise the articulation of words later in this stage. Although babies cannot use words, they listen intently, watch people's faces and imitate mouth movements, shapes and voice intonation. This communication and language stimulation is imperative for the child's development (Boysson-Bardies 1999).
- *Between 7 and 12 months* babies babble with more clarity, particularly certain sounds that move easily into fundamental words, e.g. 'mama', 'dada'. Such words and sounds help to develop the speech muscles. Infants develop one-word skills, focusing this development on the things/people around them, e.g. 'mama', 'no', 'up'. Mostly the words have a naming function, show an emotion or give a command (Fromkin & Rodman 1997).
- *In their second year* children begin to form two-word sentences. These often contain more information than people may at first think. For example, 'cat dirty' could be describing the cat's fur or that the cat has done something dirty. The child can put two concepts together that when 'translated' mean more than the words alone. This reinforces the fact that babies and young children can understand and conceptualize at a level beyond their ability to articulate. As the child develops, so their ability to form sentences increases and they begin to develop the rules of language.
- *From 3 to 7 years* children continue to develop skills in the complex rules of grammar and word usage. By the age of 7 most children have developed understanding and skill in most of the language rules that they will need for their future.

stimulated, nerve pathways become obsolete and children have problems developing and using the more complex language rules.

Play as a communication tool

Most people can recollect the games they played with other children and adults as they grew up. Remembering imaginary stories that were re-enacted, games with rules, games with songs and deep attachments to favourite toys can give a sense of happiness. Play is crucial to language development, understanding relationships and developing an understanding of 'self' and how the 'self' relates to the outside world.

In all societies children have a drive to play. Essentially play enables the child to make sense of the world around them, the relationships with others, the meaning of idea, and to develop language and strategies to enable them to function in their society.

Play is of vital importance for children who are either in receipt of healthcare or for children who are trying to understand and come to terms with illness, disability and death (see Ch. 12) in their family. Nurses can provide enhanced support for children by their ability to utilize play in the child–nurse relationship.

Babies use 'practice' play to understand their movements and sensations. Play is vital in developing control over gross and fine motor movements to start interacting with the world. This involves grasping, taking objects to the mouth, pulling, hitting, clapping, pushing, grabbing and moving objects, fitting one inside the other, delighting in the movement of the objects and the interaction and responses of parental figures. Babies continue with the trial and error approach to affecting change on objects in their environment, e.g. rolling balls away by pushing or discovering that hard objects make louder noises than soft objects.

During the second year children continue to develop by using play to explore more complex ideas, e.g. learning

REFLECTIVE PRACTICE Box 9.7

Communicating with children

Think of a child that you have spent time with in a caring capacity.

Student activities

Using Gibbs' (1988) model of reflection, consider the following questions:

- What were you doing? What was the child doing? How old were they? Who was present? What were they doing? What were you saying? What was the child communicating?
- What did you do to ensure the child understood you? How did you speak to the child? How did you know that the child understood you, what evidence did you perceive? What effect did the communication have on the child's behaviour? What effect did their communication have on your behaviour? What would you do differently next time to enhance the communication?
- What do you need to know to enhance your communication with children? How will you obtain that information? How will you know that accessing and understanding the information has changed your behaviour?

Table 9.1 Therapeutic play – uses in healthcare

Aim	Process
Distracting the child from a procedure they may find upsetting or painful	Identifying the type of play appropriate to the age of the child, the nurse will use play to focus the child's concentration away from the procedure
To give information	The nurse will use toys and other media such as paints, modelling materials, online games and specifically designed dolls to inform the child about their health
Play as a 'normal' child function, which promotes physical and psychological development	Nurses and play therapists will use play to create a sense of normality for children in situations that are not normal Play can be a valuable coping strategy for children to use
To assess a child's development	Specialist practitioners use play as an assessment tool to ascertain the child's stage of development, thus identifying any deficits in the child's cognitive, linguistic, emotional or physical development All nurses should be able to identify any obvious differences in the age of a child and their level of play, language and social interactions
To encourage the child to express their fears and wishes	Provide toys and creative materials to assist a child in expressing their thoughts without the child having to resort to language Children need space and time to develop their understanding and the language of new or emotionally difficult issues and toys provide this opportunity
To assist the child's parents in their appreciation of how the child understands their situation	Involve parents in the child's play and help parents to understand the concepts the child is working on Help parents link the play themes to the child's situation so that they can support the child in this process

to feed themselves by pretend feeding of adults or toys. Adults actively encourage pretend play but their interactions are often triggered and controlled by the child who leads the play. This play encourages person-to-person interactions; it helps the child to modify behaviour according to the reactions of others. It also enables the child to practise social skills such as turn taking, waiting, requesting, constructing and destructing scenarios.

Preschool children delight in 'rough and tumble' using large pieces of furniture or nursery props to design sets for play. This play is vital for the development of coordination, muscle development, playing with others, fighting battles against good and evil. This helps children understand a wider range of emotions and strategies for life.

From the age of about 4 years children start to understand games with rules; these games have a number of ways to support the development of the person. All games for two or more players require communication and language skills. They develop the child's understanding of competition, fair play, choosing a team, working together and developing a defensive or offensive strategy to win. The child develops a sense of what it means to belong to a group, and how to form and work in a group. Games with rules can be a major part in developing a child's self-esteem and self-awareness, and understanding their own skills and limitations.

Pretend play allows the child to develop and practise life skills. Children use the scenarios around them to develop their meaning of the world. Children will role-play scenes from family interactions, taking on the role of carer or healer, and developing skills in looking after others. They will also use information from wider cultural roles, from the media and current characters such as Postman Pat or an action hero/heroine. Objects are used to trigger play, e.g. dressing-up boxes can provide an infinite range of possibilities. Children can use pretend play to work through conflict situations, negotiate results and stage the scenarios so that they can understand or impose their views and wishes on the events.

Nurses and play specialists utilize play with children in a number of ways, such as in relation to painful or invasive interventions. Play becomes the communication vehicle for identified aims for the child's care (Table 9.1).

Adults also play, and many care environments, e.g. mental health units, provide facilities for play, e.g. board games, pool or table tennis. Play with adults has a number of benefits; it:

- Alleviates boredom
- Motivates activity to help people to stay mobile and fit
- Provides distractions
- Develops teamwork between clients and staff
- Develops rapport
- Shows people aspects of their life other than illness or distress
- Provides a sense of achievement
- Develops the concepts of sharing and empowerment.

Developmental problems – receptive and expressive language

Developmental problems of language may affect reception and/or expression of language.

Children who have hearing loss have problems developing language because they cannot receive sound information in a meaningful way. It is crucial to provide access to language for the child in a mode that is accessible. Children with a useful residual level of hearing may be helped by hearing aids or a cochlear implant depending on the cause of the hearing loss. These children develop speech, comprehension and expression by relying on aids and lipreading. For children from signing families, or for children whose residual hearing is not at a level that would facilitate understanding, sign language is preferable. Children who learn to sign from an early age follow the same developmental process as children learning speech.

Children who are deaf–blind face immense challenges in learning language. SLTs, parents/carers, educators and support groups such as Sense (www.sense.org.uk) support their language development very closely.

Children with cerebral palsy may have difficulties in speech production (expression) due to lack of muscle control. Nurses need to be aware that people with cerebral palsy may take longer to express themselves; people who are familiar with their speech may be helpful in understanding the person. However, it is important to be aware that family members acting as interpreter may be neither wanted nor appropriate (see pp. 247, 248–249).

Children with a cleft palate and/or cleft lip may also experience difficulty in speech production. Cleft palate is an abnormal opening in the palate that connects the nasal and oral cavities; this may also involve the upper lip. Most cleft palate problems are swiftly and effectively rectified by early surgery but input from specialist dental/orthodontic services and an SLT may be needed.

Language styles and influences

The way people communicate with others depends on a number of influences that are usually subconscious. Nurses will find it useful to understand why they speak to people the way they do and how this is dependent on the situation, the people they are communicating with and the background of everyone involved.

Formality

Consider the following statements:

- 'Wow, work was hard today, one man was really ill, but he's on the mend now.'
- 'It has been a busy day. Mr Clark has been taken off the ventilator and is breathing independently.'
- 'On the thirteenth of May between 10.00 and 10.45 hours Staff Nurse Elliot and I worked with Mr Clark ensuring he could breathe independently of the ventilator. I then proceeded to write up the account of the intervention in Mr Clark's notes.'

The same person spoke each sentence but in different situations, at home with his partner, during shift handover and in a court of law. It is obvious which statement was used in each situation, but what is it about the sentence that fits the context in which it is spoken? The level of formality in each situation determines the level of formality in the language used.

The first sentence suggests an informal setting, a friendship or relationship with a person not involved in the speaker's work life. Not a great deal of factual information is given because of confidentiality (see Ch. 6). Social information is provided to inform the listener of the speaker's feelings.

The second sentence is more formal, the context supports increased information about the patient rather than the member of staff. The sentence does suggest some informality initially, which can have a positive effect on team and individual connections, though it moves quickly on to deal with the pertinent issue of care.

The final sentence is very formal, there is a high degree of clarity, and more words are used to provide detailed information. There are no feelings expressed at all. People would certainly find it odd if people spoke in this way on a daily basis; it is highly structured and by the absence of emotional information it lacks any social use and could estrange the listener. In a court situation, however, the facts of the matter are of ultimate importance and feelings are not relevant in this context. In each example the situation determines the language style used.

The people within the situation also determine the language used. For example:

- 'Pick those up . . . clever girl . . . That's it. Ah, good girl.'
- 'Please could you pick those books up, thanks.'
- 'I want all those books picked up and put away, immediately.'

One person is speaking to a small child of about 2 years old, another is speaking to a colleague and the third is speaking to an adult who has annoyed them considerably. How do people know?

- When speaking to young children people adjust the number of words and the amount of information given in each sentence. They also give words of encouragement.
- The second sentence is quite neutral, clear information prefixed and ended by pleasantries. The formality is reduced a little by the use of 'thanks' rather than 'thank you'.
- The final sentence is very different in tone. It is one sentence containing three commands. There are no pleasantries and suggests either that the speaker is annoyed or is in a position of authority.

Clearly, reading the statements above requires some degree of guesswork because it is not possible to hear or see the speaker. Different tones, facial expressions and gestures could change the meanings completely.

Age

Age has an interesting influence on language; people may speak to older people in the same 'singsong' style

CRITICAL THINKING Box 9.8

Stefan

Stefan, who is 79 years old and has dementia, lives in a care home. It is nearly lunchtime and Stefan is very agitated about his house keys. Stefan's carer is keen to take him to the lavatory before lunch. Stefan is frantically searching the drawers in his bedroom. The carer says: 'Come on Stefan, don't be silly. The house was sold years ago. You lunch is getting cold. Come on, there's a good boy.'

Student activities

- Using the *Essence of Care* (NHS Modernisation Agency 2003) benchmarks for best practice in communication, think about the scenario involving Stefan, or a similar experience in a placement.
- Compare the carer's communication against the benchmark statements and identify areas for change.

using short encouraging sentences that they would use with children. This can sound patronizing and does not respect the life experience the older person brings to the situation. However, when people are caring for individuals who may not be able to respond on the same level as the carer, the carer may inappropriately resort to language that reinforces a care relationship that the carer can understand. This tendency is neither appropriate nor useful to the client. Caring in a way that is respectful and dignified for older people is a high level skill that requires nurses who are particularly skilled in communication (Box 9.8).

People with learning and physical disabilities, and mental distress

People with learning and physical disabilities also face similar situations. Again, carers must cope with a complex communication situation and sometimes, rather than adjust their language to suit a person with cognitive difficulties in an age-appropriate way, they resort to speaking to the individual as if the person was a child. These limitations in carers' communication skills must be addressed, as they disempower the person they are working with.

Such influences on the interaction are based on fundamental differences that include the:

- Background of the speaker
- Person addressed, and their cognitive and perceptual ability
- Age of the person listening
- Situation in which the exchange is taking place.

Nurses who work with people with learning disabilities or with children, or nurses who work in more than one language, show skills in 'convergence' (see below).

CONSIDER THE LANGUAGE USED BY THE CLIENT

BSL — SSE — Spoken English

THEN CONSIDER ISSUES OF AGE

Child — Adolescent — Adult

THEN CONSIDER THE SITUATION

Informal — Therapeutic — Formal

THEN CONSIDER THE COGNITIVE ABILITIES OF THE CLIENT

Cognitive difficulties — Average intelligence — High intelligence

THEN CONSIDER THE CLIENT'S MENTAL STATE

Extreme distress — Distress — Well

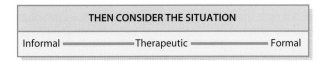

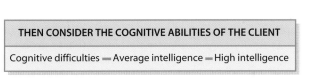

Fig. 9.4 Considerations in communications to meet clients' needs

They develop skills in talking to each individual in a way that meets their communication and cognitive level.

Another example of this can be found in services for deaf people with mental health problems. Some specialist mental health nurses work with deaf people in services where clients may use British Sign Language (BSL), Sign-Supported English (SSE; a variation of BSL) and speech. Figure 9.4 represents a cline for these languages and language variations and other considerations such as distress.

Nurses move up and down each cline depending on the communication needs of the person with whom they are engaging. By doing this, they match the communication needs of the clients to provide as full access to communication as possible, given the skills and limitations of the nurse and the client. The nurse and the client accommodate to the needs of each other in this fluid situation – remember that clients also have the innate skill to match the needs of the nurse. Typically in settings where more than one language is used, clients do assist nurses and other professionals in understanding their [the client's] language. This puts the client in an empowered position, thus giving respect to and acknowledgement of their language skills.

In addition to the considerations on the cline, nurses consider issues of gender, social background, education experience, family connections, spirituality and culture.

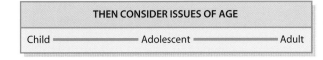

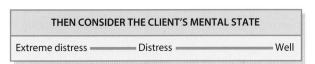

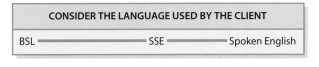

This creates a very complex communication situation where highly skilled communicators are essential.

Accommodating and diverging in communication

People usually accommodate to the communication needs of others quite naturally (Fromkin & Rodman 1997). When travelling abroad with little or no knowledge of the language, people reduce conversation to more simple sentences, use clear pronunciation, and increase the use of gesture to emphasize the point. As already discussed, when talking to small children people adjust language to suit their needs, speaking in simpler terms, using fewer key concepts per sentence, and breaking down communication into chunks that the child can more readily access. When speaking to a person to whom they relate well, people 'converge' and start speaking in a similar manner. This is evident by similar use of vocabulary, pronunciation, conversation tempo and often an accent or dialect change to accommodate the other person.

Nurses accommodate to the needs of patients/clients/carers when they explain complex therapies. They speak in non-technical terms and use less jargon to enable the other party to understand. Where the nurse speaks Hindi and Punjabi and the client speaks Gujarat and Punjabi the client and the nurse will accommodate each other by using Punjabi even though it may not be either person's preferred language.

On occasion, people do not accommodate to the needs of the listener – they 'diverge'. Divergence often occurs when the:

- Speaker is not skilled at understanding the needs of others
- Other person has upset them
- Person is making a political statement
- Person aspires to a higher social class or intellectual status
- Person wants to show a difference in backgrounds (Holmes 2001).

There are numerous examples of speech divergence in healthcare. For instance, a healthcare professional provides technical information to the patient/client very quickly while moving in the opposite direction, thus disempowering the patient/client. It requires assertiveness and confidence to challenge the speaker, something that people in hospital may lack due to their illness, anxiety or because they may feel in a subordinate position (see Ch. 7).

It is clear that converging often creates an effective communication environment whereas diverging creates difference. However, people can use divergence to assist people to change their level of formality or informality to help them to adjust to the needs of the situation. When people converge too much it can sound patronizing. Where a patient/client is relying on the nurse to make them feel confident in the therapeutic process it is useful to use technical terms and to support the client with an explanation of the meaning of each term.

Interpersonal communication skills

Interpersonal communication can be divided into verbal, signed and non-verbal. This section outlines verbal and non-verbal communication and listening skills. In addition, common courtesy, which is key to all forms of interpersonal communication, is considered.

People represent their world in different ways and have different preferences in the way they access information about their world. People tend to use a visual system, an auditory system or a kinaesthetic system. Some people like to 'see' what people are saying, some like to 'hear' a good idea and some like to 'feel' a sense of what is going on.

When communicating with patients/clients it is useful to be able to use their preferred representational system because this will enable them to access the information with less effort. Initially this may seem rather complicated, but by looking at the words that may suit people it will be easier to understand and practise.

In order to recognize someone's representational system it is necessary to listen to the words they use to describe their world, perhaps by asking them to talk about something that they have enjoyed, e.g. their favourite place. Listening for the 'describing' words the client uses will provide clues about their preference for one or two systems or all three (Table 9.2).

Common courtesy

That nurses adhere to the norms of common courtesy is the wish of most patients/clients and carers. People tend to identify issues to complain about when they feel

Table 9.2
Representational word systems

Representational system	Examples of words used	Possible responses
Visual	'I see the idea'	'Does that give you a clearer view of things?'
Auditory	'That rings a bell'	'I heard that you wanted to sound out the options'
Kinaesthetic	'I have a bad feeling about this drug'	'How would you feel about taking a similar drug?'

others are being rude to them. The number of such complaints is increasing. The signs of courtesy include:

- Paying attention to people when the nurse is with them or when they request the nurse's attention
- Being civil to a person, treating them with respect, behaving towards them as a valued human being
- Being polite, which is essential to developing a rapport with people; for example, saying please and thank you, not rushing people, smiling, and using the person's preferred name all help to ensure the person feels a sense of their importance in the process.

Consideration for others also depicts courtesy. Considering the other person in all dealings with them sounds obvious, but unfortunately people feel that nurses do not always show consideration. This could be not listening to requests, rushing their bathing routine or not considering individual preferences, e.g. in food, cosmetics, clothing, etc. This all shows a lack of consideration for the person.

The signs of common courtesy are clearly identified although they are sometimes difficult to achieve due to the resources allocated, the emotional context in which nurses work and the barriers to communication that must be overcome (see pp. 245–249). However, being able to identify what elements of courtesy people expect as users, consumers and stakeholders in the healthcare system allows nurses to identify their strengths and limitations from which to develop improved skills and sensitivity.

Verbal communication

Spoken words are arbitrary representations of ideas that have been agreed by people who use a language. In other words, they are an agreed sound or group of sounds that we know, representing a thing or an action. Without such agreement on the meaning, the words would be nonsensical or idiosyncratic, understood only by the person who produced them. As such they would not be useful to others though they may hold a great deal of significance for the person who created the sound. Verbal communication usually has written equivalents to the words produced, although some languages do not.

Nurses employ various verbal communication strategies to develop relationships, seek and understand information, provide feedback to others and to demonstrate professional compassion and self-awareness. Some strategies are outlined below. It is useful for nurses to recognize when they use these strategies naturally, before developing their skills further.

Strategies – questioning with good intentions

People use positive intentions when questioning others. This helps them to show courtesy (see above) and respect and this develops trust; therefore they get the correct information in a short space of time with 'ecology', i.e. without damaging the relationship environment.

Open questions

Open questions are used to gain information about people, their feelings, their beliefs and values, their perceptions and wishes. Open questions usually begin with a 'What . . .? Who . . .? How . . .? When . . .? Where . . .?'. To help people accept these questions nurses can also use a softener such as 'It would be good to know how. . .'. Open questions 'open up' the listener's mind to answers that they can give, information that they hold. Softeners, however, may be so gentle that it becomes a closed question, e.g. 'Please could you tell me when . . .'. It is so easy to respond 'no' to this very polite request.

Closed questions

Closed questions are used when specific information is needed quickly or if there are other limitations causing barriers, e.g. the client is distressed. Closed questions are those to which the person can answer 'yes' or 'no', e.g. 'Do you like soap on your face? ', 'Are you unhappy?'. It may be the nurse's intention to gather more information than purely a 'yes' or 'no'. It can be very frustrating trying to get beyond the yes/no responses unless the speaker considers what they are going to ask and what strategy they will use to enhance the information given. Closed questions can be opened by leaving the end of the sentence unfinished, e.g. 'Are you unhappy . . . or . . .?'. This is a useful strategy when the client/child/carer really does not want a lengthy conversation but the nurse needs to open a way for further discussion.

Funnelling

Funnelling is a strategy used firstly to obtain general information then to narrow the information down to an agreement or clear conclusion.

Summarizing

This is a strategy whereby the listener summarizes information given by the speaker. The purpose of summarizing is to check the listener's understanding at the same time as acknowledging what has been said, thus showing that the listener has heard.

Paraphrasing

This strategy is similar to summarizing but with more use of the listener's own words. This often helps the listener get the information straight in their own mind.

Clarifying

This enables the listener to present the information back to the speaker then to question if this is what they heard. It is also useful for the speaker to identify with their own thoughts coming from another source; sometimes it sounds or feels different, thus providing another perspective.

Feedback

Feedback provides the listener with acknowledgement of their performance. It can reinforce the behaviour so that it is more likely to happen again and it helps to motivate people through the knowledge that their behaviour was appropriate.

Box 9.9 (see p. 232) provides an example of some of the strategies discussed above.

NURSING SKILLS Box 9.9

Verbal communication strategies

Occupational therapist (OT) – 'Ghedi has been out with the student to the sports centre. He relaxed once he knew that he could choose a time that was set aside for people new to the gym. He said that he was happy to attend about twice a week, so he bought a 6-month off-peak pass. It was really reasonable; I have one they really are worth the money. Anyway he went to his first session, Tai Chi, then back for lunch. He says he feels confident and relaxed and he really does look it too.'

Summarizing

Keyworker – 'Oh, thanks for that information, so [*in summary*], he's got his membership, will be attending at off-peak times, he had his first session of Tai Chi and he is feeling confident and relaxed. Great.'

Paraphrasing

Keyworker – 'OK, so Ghedi has been out, joined the sports centre, paid for 6 months off-peak and has already started to use the facilities. He's fine with this and feeling confident'.

Clarifying

Keyworker –'OK [*let me get this clear*], Ghedi has been out this morning to the sports centre, got an off-peak membership, he is feeling better because he knows this is a quieter time and he has already been to his first Tai Chi class and feels fine about the arrangements?'

Feedback

Keyworker –'That's great news. I hope the student will be going with Ghedi again soon as this is so important to him.'

Assertive communication

The skill of assertiveness is important to nurses. Assertiveness enables people to be honest with themselves and in their relationships with others. Assertiveness helps to enhance relationships, avoid power games and is a vehicle for clear outcomes. Hargie (1996) details four elements of assertive communication:

- *Content* – where the rights of the people involved are embedded gently in the statement. This could be done using an explanation, empathy for the listener, praise for the listener, an apology for the consequence for the listener or a compromise that is favourable to both people
- *Covert elements* – where the speaker is able to recognize their rights and the rights of the listener in the communication process. These include respect, expressing feelings, having your own priorities, being able to say 'no', being able to make mistakes and choosing to say nothing (see Further reading suggestions, e.g. Holland & Ward 1997)
- *Process* – concerned with how a person expresses themselves assertively. Is their body language (see Non-verbal communication below), intonation (see p. 248) and choice of language reflective of a confident assertive person? Are the processes that make up communication congruent, in keeping with what is being said? The process also involves managing the setting so that people are not embarrassed, or the 'noise' levels are kept to a minimum (see pp. 246–247). Increasing the likelihood of assertive communication happening again involves feedback to the listener to show that their accomplishment is appreciated
- *The non-verbal cues* – gesture, touch, proxemics and posture – also need to reflect confidence, regard and respect for self and others (see below and pp. 233–234).

Negotiation and delegation

These are areas that depend on assertive communication. Negotiation is the process where people come together with their own ideas, discuss their ideas and agree on an outcome that is acceptable to both parties. It could be as simple as negotiating a change in the off duty, e.g.

> Nurse A asks Nurse B to change a duty on Wednesday because she needs the morning off. Nurse B agrees if Nurse A will do the same for her next Sunday. They agree and the plan is negotiated.

Delegation is another way of getting things done. Delegation often occurs between people of different authority, for example:

> Staff Nurse A: 'Andrew, Ms Wilkinson's medicines are ready to be picked up. Please could you go over for them?'

Staff Nurse A has delegated the task of collecting the prescription from pharmacy to Andrew, a first year student nurse. When delegating to another person it is imperative to be polite, assertive and clear. Offering information to support the request allows the other person to understand why they are being asked to perform a task. Delegation is reliant on a number of issues:

- Can the person accept the delegated task? Do they have the right level of knowledge, experience, skills, responsibility or status?
- Is it the right time to delegate this task to this individual?
- Are you delegating because you have left something too late? If so, how will the timeframe for completion affect this person?
- Does the situation allow for the task to be delegated?

Non-verbal communication

Non-verbal communication is that part of communication that is not reliant on words. As approximately 60% of communication is non-verbal, non-verbal skills are essential for effective communication. It is clear that people determine a great deal of meaning from aspects of communication other than words. People who are blind or partially sighted generally place more emphasis on the intonation of a person's voice to pick up the non-verbal messages (see Ch. 16). Argyle (1994) suggested that non-verbal communication was made up of:

- Accent
- Bodily contact

- Direction of gaze
- Emotive tone in speech
- Facial and gestural movements
- Physical appearance
- Posture
- Proximity
- Speech errors
- Timing of speech.

This chapter focuses on gesture, touch, proxemics and posture. Paralinguistic issues, i.e. the voiced aspects of non-verbal behaviour, for instance guggles, are discussed later (see pp. 235, 238).

Gesture

Gesture is a crucial aspect of non-verbal communication. Some psychologists and linguists suggest that early humans used gesture before they used spoken or signed language (Armstrong et al 1996). Gestures can be classified into categories of increasing complexity.

Universal gestures that are understand by most people include opening arms and eyes wide to suggest bigness; furrowed brows, pursed lips, drawing body inwards and moving index fingers together would suggest smallness. Subtler gestures include a cupped hand to the mouth to indicate a drink, or a single upwards gesture of the hand with palm facing upwards suggests that someone stand up.

Certain gestures are recognized as specific to a language community, such as the 'OK' gesture with thumb and index finger touching to make a circle with the other fingers raised. However, it is important to be aware that some gestures that are acceptable in one community are possibly offensive in another. For example, the 'OK' gesture is offensive in Brazil. Each language community shares an understanding of its own group of gestures.

Touch

This is a complex and intricate communication subject and often difficult to tackle. Children tend to be touched more than adults. Interestingly, babies and young children who are not touched do not thrive as well as those who are (Hargie 1996).

Touch for many people is an essential aspect of their working lives. Nurses in particular must learn how to touch people in a professional context without causing embarrassment or concern to the patient/client. In addition, nurses must ensure their own safety. Nurses use two clear types of touch: first and often the most intimate type is the necessary touch nurses use when attending to people's physical needs and during other nursing interventions; the second type is the touch that communicates a feeling or a meaning, such as, 'I am here to care for you' or 'It will feel better soon'. Everyone has a very personal view about touch, when it is appropriate and when not. People from different cultures will touch each other according to their accepted norms.

It is suggested that a well-timed touch on the shoulder or hand can help a person in distress to feel comforted, or feel the care of another person, which creates a sense of trust. Touch in this scenario is thought to encourage the person's cathartic release by communicating that you are right with them in the moment, close to them and sharing their feelings. This affirms their sense of self; it respects their distress and shows the nurse's commitment to their needs.

There is also a view that touch can block an emotional release. The use of touch when someone is crying, for example, is a means to stop them crying rather than conveying the message that crying is fine and to be encouraged. If this were the case the nurse would be communicating a need to control the patient's/client's emotions for the nurse's benefit, rather than it being a positive patient/client-centred intervention.

Touch is more appropriate in some clinical settings than in others. Understanding what is acceptable in each area is important and nurses can learn much from each other (Box 9.10). As a student new to a client group it is useful to know how people deal with the patients'/clients' emotions. Also crucial is an understanding of common courtesy (see pp. 230–231) and the social norms of the patients/clients and carers who are most likely to attend the clinical setting. Nurses need to be able to consider this information while at the same time working with the emotional needs of the people in their care (Varcarolis 1998).

It is vital that nurses also recognize their own feelings around touch (Box 9.11).

REFLECTIVE PRACTICE Box 9.10

Appropriate touch – learning from others

Nurses who are consciously competent in respecting a client's dignity will more readily engage their trust, and therefore be more likely to be able to work therapeutically and less likely to cause offence. Think about occasions when you worked with registered nurses who perform the most intimate of procedures while maintaining the dignity of the patient/client.

Student activities

- How did the nurse behave in relation to touch?
- What did they say to the patient/client?
- How do you think the patient/client felt?

REFLECTIVE PRACTICE Box 9.11

Feelings about touch

Spend some time thinking about your feelings with regard to being touched and touching others.

Student activities

- What is your norm?
- How does that fit in with the clinical environment?
- Could you leave yourself or others open to the risk of inappropriate touch or at risk of feeling alone and isolated when in distress?

Proxemics

Proxemics is a fascinating area of communication because people have very different views about their own personal space; how close people like to be to others and how close they like others to be to them can be very complex and bound by personal rules.

Boundaries enable people to feel comfortable in their environment. Some boundaries are fixed, such as walls and rooms within buildings; others are semi-fixed, such as the seating in the health centre or seating arrangements in a dining room and the location of the television. These arrangements are an indication of where to sit, where to eat and which way to face. Fixed and semi-fixed boundaries can help or hinder communication between people.

The other type of boundary is the informal space between people. This space is fluid and is utilized in different ways for different messages and in different settings.

The person listening will be aware of the distance between themselves and the speaker and vice versa. There are clear cultural differences in the distance people accept between each other.

Knowingly intruding into someone's personal space can be very intimidating for the listener. This approach is used to interrogate or bully people, resulting in their disempowerment. It may be necessary to gently remind colleagues or children or clients that their comfort zone may be smaller than that of other people. Some people are so at ease with another person that they may use them as a 'human prop' when recounting a story. To re-enact a story they may talk to the listener and relate to them physically as if they were there at the time to show the listener the gravity of the situation, the humour or the distress. Some people are happy to be human props but others find it disconcerting and embarrassing because it focuses attention directly on them.

Posture

How a person holds their body in relation to other people and in relation to the fixed and semi-fixed boundaries communicates a great deal about what they are feeling and thinking. Posture sends a very clear message; for example, leaning forward indicates interest and respect for the other person. On the other hand, despite looking at the other person, a lack of interest is portrayed if the listener's body is orientated towards the door, and sitting back in the chair with feet turned towards the door suggests they would rather be somewhere else.

How a person filters the information provided by the external event will affect their thoughts, feelings and behaviours; therefore their posture is a mirror of their inner beliefs (see p. 235).

When a nurse wants to create a sense of confidence they walk into the situation with their head held high, at a moderate pace, and do not slouch because they recognize that this would convey a message that is unsuitable.

People will look at the nurse's posture and decide very quickly whether they like them or not and whether they can be trusted or not. Where clients have poor short-term memory and have difficulty remembering people's faces, names or roles it is imperative to use posture that is confident and respectful because the client has to make continual assessments of people to see if they ought to trust them or not.

Once people have made a judgement it is difficult to convince them otherwise. This may seem a little harsh but it is a survival technique that has helped people to function in social settings for thousands of years.

Listening skills

How do people know that they are really listening to someone, or that someone is really listening to them? Many nurses claim to be good listeners, because in the clinical environment to suggest otherwise is almost as bad as saying they are poor nurses.

People often know when someone is not listening to them; they feel ignored, undervalued, frustrated and disempowered. Not listening to the other person can seriously affect the relationship. In a nurse–patient/client relationship the outcome of not listening to a client can result in their choices being reduced, e.g. not eating their choice of food, the nurse not understanding their fears and anxieties, the potential for misdiagnosis and ultimately ineffective or even harmful treatment. If nurses fail to listen to colleagues, not only is vital information missed but it can also affect the colleagues' motivation, trust, self-esteem and skills.

There are a number of reasons for listening and different types of listening skills are needed. Wolvin and Coakley (1985) identified four types of listening:

- *To comprehend in order to understand information*: When listening for understanding the focus is on main topics, ideas and data. In the clinical setting it is used during ward rounds and handovers, for receiving information from patients/clients, etc.
- *To appreciate sound, to feel relaxed or at ease*: This includes listening to music on headphones or in a Snoezelen room (see Ch. 11), listening to a meditation tape, listening to recordings of 'sounds of nature' in order to relax. . .all for pleasure, meditation or well-being
- *To evaluate information, when the speaker wants to persuade or to influence behaviour*: This may include evaluating information from a drug company representative, wound care advisors and continence nurses, and to weigh up points in team meetings
- *To empathize where the focus is on the speaker rather than the listener*: In this situation the aim is to listen to patients/clients etc. who need to talk/express themselves in order to alleviate stress, to problem-solve or to release tensions. This type of listening is a therapeutic skill that practitioners must acquire.

Characteristics of good listening

Good listening skills are vital to rapport and empathy, which are discussed later (see pp. 237–238). The following characteristics of good listening are based on English

CRITICAL THINKING Box 9.12

Mirroring

Watch an experienced nurse and patient/client or a couple who are getting on well.

Student activity

Observe their posture, their mannerisms, their tempo or timing of their movements. See if you can notice how much the listener is mirroring the speaker. For example, do they have similar facial expressions, gestures, posture and movements?

speaking Western cultural norms. People from different linguistic and cultural groups have different norms of communicative behaviour (see pp. 247–248).

Appropriate eye contact

Appropriate eye contact is where the person listening looks at the person who is speaking. They blink just after the speaker blinks or when they are ending a sentence. The listener's blink rate matches that of the speaker and corresponds with their head nods of encouragement. The eye gaze is generally soft, slightly heavy lidded as opposed to staring and hard (eyes slightly wider than usual denotes some muscular tension). However, the listener's gaze also mirrors the verbal and non-verbal expressions of the speaker.

Mirroring

When engaged in listening, people naturally find themselves 'mirroring' the speaker's posture. This does not mean copying their every movement as if playing a game; instead the listener may be leaning slightly in the same direction, tapping their pen at the same time the speaker is tapping their foot, folding one arm across the body as the speaker folds both arms (Box 9.12).

This behaviour is a natural sign for the speaker that the listener is with them, acknowledging their mood, recognizing their feelings and trying to understand them. This behaviour increases rapport between the speaker and listener and encourages the process to continue.

Nurses and other healthcare professionals often need to develop trust and rapport quickly in order to work effectively with people. Being aware of their skills in mirroring another person is vital in enhancing the therapeutic or professional relationship (see pp. 236–245).

Guggles

Guggles are the sounds (non-words) uttered when listening, e.g. 'mmmms', 'ahs', hmm'. These affirm the speaker's point, agree with them and confirm their view or idea. To do this, guggles rely heavily on intonation and tunes (see p. 248). The use of guggles by the listener encourages the speaker to continue by providing evidence that the listener is listening (Box 9.13).

REFLECTIVE PRACTICE Box 9.13

Skills that encourage and discourage conversation

Next time you are listening to a friend telling you a story (one that is not too sensitive), listen to your own guggles.

Student activities

- Gently increase the number of guggles you use. What difference does it make to your friend's storytelling?
- If you gently reduce the number of guggles so that you hardly express any, how does this affect the storytelling?
- If you increase them a little more, does this make any difference?
- How many guggles become too many and stop your friend telling the story because they feel uncomfortable?
- Tell your friend what you having been doing, apologize and ask them how it made them feel.
- Think about the experience with your friend and consider how you will use it to improve your listening skills with patients/clients.

Active listening

Nurses and others often highlight active listening as an essential skill, as the term implies a requirement for energy and concentration on the part of the nurse. The aim is to enhance the quality of the therapeutic relationship and to facilitate problem-solving by being with the speaker on a social, psychological and emotional level (Egan 1998). In active listening, the listener:

- Listens to the speaker, bearing in mind the context of the speaker's message with regard to their background, life experience and current situation
- Attends to the speaker's non-verbal behaviours
- Listens and understands the speaker's message
- Listens for inconsistencies in the message and incongruence between what is being said and the speaker's non-verbal behaviour.

Active listening requires the practitioner to understand:

- How and why people communicate the way they do
- What language they are likely to use
- How a person's non-verbal communication provides information about the message.

Nursing relationships

The first half of this chapter has provided the knowledge and encouragement needed to develop skills in a variety of components that create a good communicator. This section draws upon this learning for enhancing communication in a variety of relationships with different outcomes.

The types of relationship that people connect with on a day-to-day basis are intimate, social, professional and therapeutic. In this section the focus is on the therapeutic and professional relationships that nurses experience and how these relate to care and health outcomes.

Therapeutic relationships

Nurses have therapeutic relationships with the patients/clients/children, families and carers they work with. The therapies they offer cover a wide range of interventions from an adult nurse providing education about insulin therapy to mental health nurses providing cognitive behavioural therapy. Interventions also include assisting people and children with the activities, e.g. eating and drinking, in ways that maintain the individual's independence, dignity and health. An essential component that underpins all nursing interventions, from daily living needs to sophisticated procedures, is the 'therapeutic relationship' (Box 9.14).

This relationship is the foundation on which the nurse and patient/client can work together to identify issues that are affecting the patient/client and that require change. The therapeutic relationship facilitates the patient/client to move from their current state of ill health, distress or need to their desired state of maximum attainable health, well-being and strength. Where patients/clients are unlikely to achieve full health, the therapeutic relationship is used to assist reconciliation, alleviate stress and provide solace and support.

The therapeutic relationship relies on specific components being in place, including rapport, empathy, trust, genuineness, warmth and positive regard (see pp. 237–239). The therapeutic relationship requires the nurse to have active listening skills and proficient interpersonal skills (see pp. 234–235). It is also vital for the practitioner to know their own values and beliefs and how these can produce filters that may affect their resourcefulness.

Skills that develop 'connectedness', the emotional connection between two people, are great; however, the nurse also needs to develop a range of communication strategies. This may sound quite manipulative and in the wrong hands good communication skills can be devastating if the aim of the strategy is to gain at the expense of another person. An excellent example of good communication skills in the wrong hands is the stereotypical 'cold-calling sales person'. When developing relationships and communication strategies it is necessary to reflect on the desired outcome and decide whether it is ethically and morally correct.

Box 9.14 The therapeutic relationship

Who
- Nurses and other health professionals.

Who may
- Provide a specific health-related service.

Who will
- Have skills to maximize the personal exploration and health of the patient/client
- Use strategies to underpin these skills
- Focus on the patient's/client's needs
- Be led by the patient's/client's issues
- Develop problem-solving capacity in the patient/client
- Evaluate the change in the patient/client to identify progress towards maximum health.

Who don't
- Work outside contractual boundaries
- Relate on an intimate or social level with the client
- Need the client to like them
- Expect mutual appreciation to occur.

Attributes of a nurse–patient/client relationship

Not all nurse–patient/client relationships are the in-depth type utilized by nurses who work in learning disability or mental health settings. The focus of nursing relationships is to bring about change in a person's health or facilitate an optimum quality of life. Sometimes this is about empowering the person to do this independently; on other occasions the nurse will be undertaking a nursing intervention for a client. There are some attributes common to all nurse–patient/client relationships that are also witnessed in nurse–family/carer relationships.

Being there

O'Brien (2000) suggests that patients/clients like the nurse to 'be there' for them. This appears a simple task but it is an intense and emotionally powerful task to do for someone. Being there is being present for the patient/client when needed. This need will sometimes leave the nurse feeling exhausted because they have given so much emotionally (see Ch. 11) and may occur while the nurse is supporting the patient/client in and through their distress.

Self-disclosure

O'Brien (2000) also found that, in developing and sustaining a nurse–patient/client relationship, the nurse needed to give the client some information about him/herself. This was to show humanity and put the two people on an equal footing. The more people share with another person, the closer they can feel to them, thus increasing rapport.

Patients/clients sometimes think that they are the only ones who are having difficulties; by some self-disclosure the patient/client is able to see that others share their difficulties. This also validates their feelings and provides perspective for the problem.

It is also easy to disclose too much information, particularly when nurses have developed a good rapport with the patient/client or carer. Having good rapport (see pp. 237–238) enables nurses to feel comfortable with the other person and to discuss things not usually discussed. This can be damaging to the nurse and to the patient/client if the information shared can be used to make the other person feel vulnerable in any way.

Being concerned

Being concerned enhances the nurse–patient/client relationship (O'Brien 2000). Nurses develop a protective feeling towards the people they work with while at the same time recognizing the need for the patient/client to make their own decisions about their lives and their health. Nurses were clear that their role was to offer choice and alternatives to facilitate the patient/client in problem-solving.

Trust

Trusting another person is sometimes hard and at other times easy. Some people automatically trust medical professionals because they believe they are in a position of expert knowledge and power, and are caring. In trusting someone, people tend to expect certain behaviours. For example, they want the person to be:

- Honest and not to lie
- Kindly and not to be cruel
- Consistent in their behaviour towards them so that they 'know where they stand'
- True to their word – if they say they are going to do something and they do, then people will trust them to be true to them again.

Trust is hard to win and very easy to lose, and regaining lost trust is very difficult. Losing trust is best avoided by giving time, energy, concern and regard to everyone involved.

Being 'as if'

It would be naïve to assume that nurses will never be challenged by wanting to ignore the person, to snap at a patient/client or child who appears overly demanding, to wish that the patient's/client's family would realize that the nurse has other people to look after, or that they feel like crying too. At the most challenging times nurses who manage to maintain their professionalism tend to use clear strategies for dealing with the situation. Some strategies to maintain a professional profile include:

- Wearing a uniform or clearly defined work clothes helps to give some identity to the task – 'in these clothes I am first and foremost a nurse'. A uniform/work clothes provides some distance
- Recognizing a colleague who would manage well in this challenging situation. Identify how they would be behaving and copy this behaviour
- Disassociating from the emotions of the situation by thinking of something less upsetting. Breathe deeply; do something to take your mind off the upset for a few seconds, re-engage as a resource for the person
- Seeing the situation in a scientific way or as a service provider can reduce the emotional labour involved.

Whatever the strategy chosen, it is important to remain outwardly congruent (outward behaviour should be true to the situation) or others may construe that the nurse does not care.

Empathy

Empathy is when a person puts themselves in the other person's position, attempting to understand the world as they see it. Empathy is an emotional response to another person's situation; people often describe feeling a physical sensation in their abdomen or chest when they see someone in a bad emotional or physical state.

It is not uncommon for people to want to laugh if they see or hear others laughing, yawn when they see others yawning and cry when others are upset. They are 'wired' to echo the movements and the expressed emotions of others. By doing this people feel the same physical feeling, have thoughts that relate to the feeling and behave in ways that relate to the thoughts and feelings. People can influence others with their happy mood or bad temper. Emotions are 'catching' because people have a tendency to automatically empathize. Other people's movements also influence people, e.g. by making chewing movements while feeding a child or nodding at a conversation on television.

For some people empathizing does not come easily. These people are naturally self-orientated. This does not mean they are self-centred, it means they are more internally focused. People with autism and Asperger's syndrome have challenges in empathizing because they have a limited 'theory of mind'. This constrains their ability to understand that they and other people have thoughts, feelings and behaviours, which results in serious limitations in their social and communicative competence.

Another result is the chaos that people with autism feel with regard to other people's behaviour that can look random and bewildering to them. Some people with autism will go through life without social connections or needing to be with others, preferring the calm of their own world, routines and structures. Other individuals can be aware that there is a difference in the way they relate to others. This realization of poor psychological connectedness can be challenging and confusing and can result in an increased sense of difference for the individual.

Children with autism show this lack of psychological connectedness with those around them and also in their play; they do not role-play because they cannot attribute behaviours, thought and feelings to the toys. The inability to imitate others such as playing 'mum' or 'teacher' stifles the child's development in attributing roles to people, standing in other people's shoes and seeing the world through their eyes, i.e. empathizing (Box 9.15, see p. 238).

Rapport

Rapport is the connection between two people, where they talk on the same 'wavelength', share the same humour and share in each other's pain and sorrow. Couples, family members and lifelong friends often hold deep rapport.

Rapport plays a significant part in developing a therapeutic relationship but this does not mean that without rapport nurses cannot facilitate change in people's health. However, rapport promotes productive relationships and thereby better outcomes for all.

Table 9.3 (see p. 238) outlines the different levels of rapport.

The third level is often associated with being deeply attached to someone. Although most people have the opportunity to feel this depth of closeness during their lives, others are less fortunate. This level of rapport is not appropriate for a nurse to share with a patient/

client or carer. Feeling this close to someone negates any possibility of a professional therapeutic relationship, as the nurse would not be a resource for the patient/client/child or carer. Nurses who share this level of rapport with people they work for can experience immense stress, destroy professional trust and can seriously affect the health of the patient/client (see 'Boundaries are healthy', pp. 240–241).

A working level of rapport gives power to each person in the relationship; it gives the nurse room to provide the correct care within the limitations of their role and responsibilities and encourages them to refer to another person when necessary. The professional alliance that is formed respects the participants for the skills and knowledge they bring to the situation. Importantly, people remain independent of each other; they do not merge into one entity.

Rapport is easier between individuals who share similar life experiences, values, belief systems and language. This is because trust comes easier in these situations. In developing rapport and empathy with patients/clients and carers it is important to realize that people relate to each other on very different levels and to different degrees depending on their circumstances and their ability to comprehend others. Some people have difficulty in understanding how to relate to other people in a healthy way. These difficulties in relating to others may be due to anxiety, anger, confusion or poor relational skills.

CRITICAL THINKING Box 9.15

Toby

7-year-old Toby has autism. He is extremely distressed, having fallen and hit his head. Toby needs to attend the Emergency Department, but his mother, who is also very upset, feels that there is no possibility of Toby cooperating with a visit to hospital. Toby is clinging desperately to his red lorry, looking straight ahead and avoiding contact with his mum.

Student activities

- Think of ways in which you could communicate the need for Toby to go to hospital to Toby (use Lasswell's model and provide a rationale for each possibility).
- How would you help his mother to assist in the situation? How would you show empathy to her?

Facilitating change

In the therapeutic relationship nurses are trusted to assist change in patients/clients and carers by facilitating the understanding of information. They are also entrusted with the task of helping a person involved in this health process to move from the current state A to the desired state B (Fig. 9.5).

Essential communication and interpersonal skills underpin facilitation. Box 9.16 considers the nurse–patient/client relationship in different settings. A patient/client is unable to move from A to B if they cannot relate to the nurse, i.e. if rapport, trust, the nurse's concern and the nurse's skills in 'being there' for the client are not evident. Nor will they move from A to B if the nurse does not have the communication strategies to be a resourceful facilitator.

Table 9.3 Levels of rapport

Level of rapport	Description	Who
Level 1	No rapport	Strangers who have just met. They neither need to know each other nor want to
	The beginnings of a connection	People who have spent a little time together and are exploring common ground
Level 2	A connection creating good communication	People are making the effort to understand each other socially, professionally Finding out about each other and using interpersonal skills to express ideas, needs, to investigate and gather evidence either on a social or professional level; this might be from meeting someone for the first time and realizing you both enjoy the same music Sales people may have excellent communication skills and are adept at creating rapport at speed because that is when you are most likely to purchase their product You could be working with a family who are being educated regarding the health of their child who has a long-term illness
	Good connection, good communication, mutual feelings of relating well	The people involved are actively listening to each other, good eye contact, personal space is within 3 metres
Level 3	Excellent connection, relaxed, easy communication, parties sense a physical closeness	People involved feel the other person really knows them, feels they can share everything, almost as if the other person automatically knows what they are thinking They can pre-empt the other person's next move

It is clear that all the scenarios provide different levels of contact between nurse and patient/client/carer, all of which require different levels of relationship building. No one way fits all and nurses have to accept that while they continue to value good interpersonal communication skills and strategies, not all nurse–patient/client/carer relationships need to be in-depth to be resourceful but it is vital that some are.

Positive regard

Positive regard is the ability to hold and convey feelings for other people that are not based on negative beliefs about the person. Having positive regard for patients/clients, carers, parents and colleagues enables the nurse to approach others with positive intentions towards them. Maintaining positive regard for people can help nurses manage their thoughts, feelings and behaviours even in situations where the other person may be behaving in a way that is not appropriate.

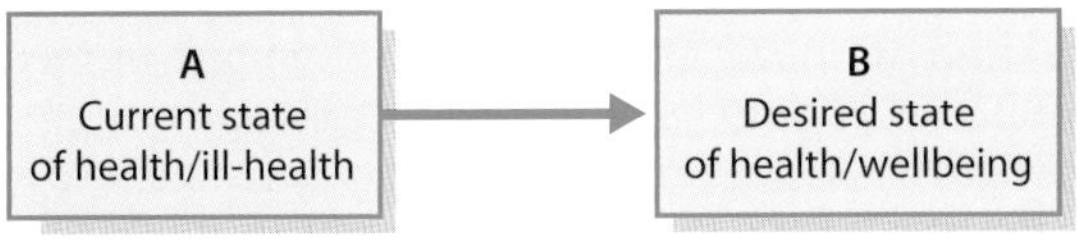

Fig. 9.5 Facilitating change from the current state to the desired state

Attachment

People learn how to relate to others from the attachments they develop as children (see Ch. 8). These attachments focus on principal caregivers and result in the ability to relate to themselves and to others. Where they have strong, nurturing, encouraging and fulfilling relationships with others they are confident in their skills and developing abilities, which is expressed through their mental well-being. Environments without emotional sustenance, encouragement, love or stability can result in people having emotional problems and an impoverished sense of mental well-being, thus creating people who experience vulnerability and dysfunctional relationships.

Nurses meet people who are in extreme situations – people who are frightened, ill, angry and anxious, whose ability to deal with their current crisis is based on their mental and physical well-being, which by the very fact that they are seeing a nurse could be compromised. Therefore it is reasonable to suggest that nurses work with people who have difficulty with relationships, whether this is situational and transient or long-term and embedded in the thoughts, feelings and behaviours of the individual.

Not all nurses have high levels of mental well-being nor have they experienced positive nurturing upbringings in secure and loving environments as this is clearly not plausible, nor should it be a prerequisite for the profession. What is important is that nurses understand themselves and the positive and negative experiences that contribute to their current ability to relate to others, to develop insight and to be resourceful for the people they work for and with (Box 9.17).

CRITICAL THINKING Box 9.16

Nurse–patient/client relationship and care delivery

1. Emily is key nurse to 8-year-old Imran who has leukaemia and his parents Rahil and Muntasir Ahmed. Imran's parents are always with him and are fully involved with the team in providing his care. Imran will need long-term care, both at home and in hospital.
2. Simon is running the 'walk in clinic' at the GP surgery and has just met Mr Desai who has come to the clinic with a suspected dislocated shoulder following a fall.
3. Ali is a student nurse on a community placement that caters for people with moderate to severe learning disabilities. He is working closely with his mentor and Paul who is experiencing a particularly distressing time due to his parents' divorce. Paul resorts to obsessional behaviours as a coping mechanism for his feelings of anxiety; these behaviours only emerge in times of severe stress.

Student activities

In each case consider:

- What opportunities does the nurse have to develop a nurse–patient relationship with the patients/clients/families?
- What level of rapport could be developed between the nurse and the family?
- How will the nurse develop the patient's/client's/family's trust in them?

REFLECTIVE PRACTICE Box 9.17

Mapping relationships

Consider for a moment your own ability to relate to others.

Student activities

On a piece of paper, draw yourself in the centre and add your current social network. This may include family members, friends, colleagues and pets. Consider each person individually:

- How long have you known them?
- How often do you see them?
- How close are you?
- What could you tell them?
- What areas of your life do they not access?
- How well do they know you?

Now draw another map of your social network from 5 years ago and repeat the questions. Are you surprised at any differences? How do feel about the way your network has developed? Is there anything you would change? If so, how would you go about changing things and why?

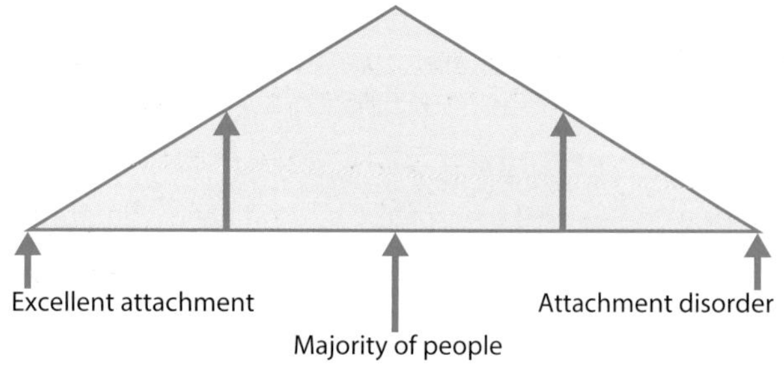

Fig. 9.6 Attachment continuum

Some children have families that are highly nurturing and safe, with the potential to be resilient to emotional challenges. Most people have families that experience the ups and downs of emotions, love, loss and nurturing with some resilience to these challenges. A few people with little innate resilience to emotional challenges experience the most challenging of environments and these people may develop attachment disorders. It is clear that whether it is an issue of physical illness, developmental need or mental well-being, nurses can be involved with people at all stages on this attachment continuum (Fig. 9.6). Mental health nurses will be more involved with people with attachment problems and emotional distress, depression and behavioural disturbances because of the clear link between these issues and challenges to mental health.

Nurses provide care for others, i.e. they are caregivers. This is a very powerful position to be in because of the responsibility given to the nurse while the patient is in need. For people who have experienced good attachment there is little to do other than reinforce their sense of emotional well-being through being there for them, being concerned for their care and health outcomes, and being skilled in the delivery of that care. For people who have experienced more negative attachments and who do not express a sense of well-being, nurses must realize that their actions can have considerable impact on the patient/client and carer as they take on the role of caregiver. Nurses need to develop skills in areas that include:

- Expressing roles and responsibility within clear boundaries
- Expressing positive regard that is ethical (see Ch. 7)
- Teamworking, both inter- and multiprofessional
- Providing a consistent, fair and equitable approach to patients/clients and carers
- Communicating clearly to everyone involved
- Being curious and learning from others
- Being creative and flexible to find appropriate solutions to needs
- Recognizing their own need to be needed or to care and ensuring that the motivation to satisfy this need does not disempower others.

The points above are a guide to skills that are useful in providing services for all and particularly for people with more complex relationship needs. With this in mind, consider the nurse who feels special because they are the only person who can work with or care for a patient/client, or who a patient/client wants near them. This nurse should reflect on their own need to feel needed, to feel special and how the patient/client may be fulfilling these needs and why this may lead to an unhelpful service for the patient/client. Student nurses are often able to spend more time with patients/clients and carers and so can find that they develop strong attachments. Hopefully, with the issues raised above, nurses will be able to develop their resourcefulness further, thus protecting themselves and the people they work with from emotional stress or harm.

Boundaries are healthy

Boundaries are useful and positive rules that enhance resourceful relationships to improve health outcomes. Some nurses find the correct level of boundary between themselves and patients/clients easy to judge, whereas others find it more challenging and many nurses can remember experiences where they 'got it wrong'.

Boundaries begin to develop as soon as the nurse meets the patient/client or carer and explains their role and responsibilities. A clear and concise explanation gives information about what the nurse does, thus enabling the patient/client or carer to begin to develop a picture of why each healthcare professional is involved and, crucially, how they, the patient/client or carer will be involved in the process.

On one level the public needs to know the roles, responsibilities and level of involvement they can expect from healthcare practitioners, as outlined above. At a deeper level nurses are enhancing the ability to be in a resourceful position for the people they work with. Boundaries enable nurses to maintain a professional commitment to the public; nurses are resources who offer healthcare, expertise and skills to facilitate change in ways that would be difficult if they became 'friends' with the people they work with. Professional and therapeutic boundaries are safety nets for the protection of everyone involved.

Boundaries also provide clarity for professionals. People working in healthcare often find themselves working across professional boundaries; nurses may overlap with occupational therapists (OTs) or social workers in the same way as they may overlap with traditional nursing roles. For example, supporting people in their own homes with developing independence skills could be facilitated by a nurse, an OT or a social worker, particularly when they work in multidisciplinary teams (MDTs) such as assertive outreach teams or home treatment teams in community mental health services (see Ch. 3).

These teams function with clear communication systems and full understanding of each member's roles and responsibilities, skills, specific training and the therapeutic relationships they have with the patients/clients. Of primary importance to such teams is the consistent engagement of difficult-to-engage clients rather than individual professionals being territorial about their traditional roles. The client is paramount; the clinician's skills support the patient/client and each other through enhanced teamwork and communication.

Boundaries sometimes go wrong by being unclear, breached, ignored, too stringent or, more seriously, abused. Unclear boundaries do not provide the supportive structure needed for clinicians to deliver the service required. Moreover, lack of clarity disempowers the patient/client and carer because they do not have the information required to be fully involved in their care. Unclear boundaries can lead to breaches of professional conduct (see Ch. 7), including over-involvement or abuse by either the care provider or the person receiving care.

Professionals who are unclear about each other's roles create confusion, which can lead to breakdown in communication and service delivery. This means that patients/clients and carers suffer. Unclear professional boundaries can lead to missing information, which can have extremely serious consequences such as role confusion, misdiagnosis, incomplete risk assessments or poor care and health outcomes.

Stages of the therapeutic relationship

The stages of the therapeutic relationship identified in Varcarolis (1998) are:

- Preorientation
- Orientation
- Working
- Termination

Preorientation stage

This occurs prior to communicating with the patient/client. It is crucial at this stage for the nurse to recognize their beliefs and values regarding the person and their family. This requires the nurse to be mindful of the values and beliefs they hold. Understanding how their blueprint of behaviour may differ from the other person's and how this may affect the therapeutic relationship is important. With this knowledge the nurse can monitor their own behaviour, working towards better understanding and acceptance for other people.

This stage allows the nurse to find out information from the patient's/client's notes, the MDT and possibly family members. This information can enhance the communication between nurse and patient/client at the initial meetings. It may also enable the nurse to make informed choices regarding the need to provide immediate care and to manage risk.

Orientation stage

This stage of the relationship can take time. It provides the opportunity to establish roles and responsibilities, boundaries and trust. It is at this critical point that the nurse will discuss confidentiality (see this page and p. 242), times and regularity of meetings, and arrangements for informing each other should it be necessary to cancel a meeting. An important feature of this discussion is for the nurse to have the confidence to talk with the patient/client about how the sessions/meetings will end once the patient/client is ready to move on.

Working stage

During the working stage of the relationship the nurse enables the patient/client to safely:

- Explore current issues impacting on their lives
- Establish well-formed goals
- Develop problem-solving skills to address the issues
- Identify behaviours that are resistant to change and to facilitate shifts in these behaviours
- Provide a safe place for the client to try out new behaviours and beliefs
- Evaluate progress according to the patient's/client's journey
- Redefine patient/client goals as movement occurs.

Termination stage

With a clear understanding of goals identified and resolved in the working stage, termination of the relationship is a necessary and therapeutic point of the relationship. Termination may also need to occur if the patient/client and nurse are 'stuck' and one or other does not have the resources to move the relationship forward.

It is at this stage that the patient/client and the nurse can reflect on the journey they have both taken. Sharing the feelings that termination arouses in the nurse is valuable to the patient/client. Not only does it teach each person how they can cope with a relationship ending, it gives respect to the patient/client.

Working in partnership with families – confidentiality

Confidentiality is an important concept for nurses (see Chs 6 and 7). The Nursing and Midwifery Council (NMC) (2004, Clause 5, p. 8) provides a clear statement: 'As a registered nurse, midwife or specialist community public health nurse, you must protect confidential information.'

The principle of confidentiality is to protect individuals from indiscriminate disclosure and divulgence of their personal information. All people have the right to privacy and to personal information to be protected by the professionals who work with them.

Nurses build relationships on trust, ensuring patients/clients develop trust and so enhance the ability to work therapeutically. Nurses ask people to give very intimate and detailed information as part of the nursing process (see Ch. 14). People need to know that the information they give to health professionals is safe from improper disclosure:

> If the patient or client withholds consent, or if consent cannot be obtained for whatever reason, disclosures may be made only where:
>
> - they can be justified in the public interest (usually where disclosure is essential to protect the patient or client or someone else from the risk of significant harm)
> - they are required by law or by order of a court.
>
> Where there is an issue of child protection, you must act at all times in accordance with national and local policies.
>
> NMC (2004, Clauses 5.3, 5.4, p. 9)

Nurses who breach confidentiality are liable to disciplinary action from their employer, action by the regulatory body that could result in their removal from the professional register and ultimately legal action from the patient/client or carer (see Ch. 6).

Nurses have a duty to inform patients/clients and carers of their responsibilities regarding maintaining and possibly breaching confidence. Nurses may initially find this a difficult topic to discuss with someone who has come to them for 'help'. However, having the confidence to clearly outline your role as a nurse and the boundaries of that role shows the client respect and honesty, which should help in developing the nurse–patient/client relationship.

Nurses do need to judge whether they should explain the full details of when they would be required to breach confidentiality. For example, a community nurse working to support an adult newly diagnosed with diabetes may find it unnecessary to discuss 'abuse' or 'serious offences'. However, it is acceptable to outline roles, responsibilities and boundaries in a clear and informative manner.

Breaking bad news

It is a particularly daunting prospect to tell someone something that they would class as 'bad news'. Breaking bad news often focuses on informing people about serious illness or death. However, just as with the experience of pain, 'bad news' is very individual to the person receiving it, e.g. a patient/client being told that their partner has phoned to say they missed the bus and cannot visit today may consider this to be 'bad news'. Therefore, it is useful to assume that, because people have different blueprints of behaviour and different internal maps of the world, it is impossible to know how the person will react to news.

Most patients/clients, carers and parents want to know the truth, even the bad news. Breaking bad news to a child is very dependent on their age, stage of development and the wishes and involvement of the parents. People with cognitive and communication difficulties, people who speak another language and people in distress need nurses to be sensitive to their communication needs.

In breaking bad news to a client with a cognitive disability, the nurse needs to be aware of the person's cognitive level and their concept of illness or death, and it is important that the person is told straight away in terms they can understand, i.e. provided with information that is as meaningful as possible. This is not considered to be patronizing, as it provides the information needed to build their understanding of issues.

Registered nurses who give bad news will use their interpersonal skills, rapport and empathy. They will be aware of their verbal and non-verbal communication. They will use skills to match the other person's communication by converging, matching vocabulary, pace and loudness, and being congruent to the message (Kurtz et al 2004). Feedback skills are used by the speaker to ensure that the message has been decoded and understood, to ensure their communication has the desired outcome. Again, having a communication model in mind will help the nurse focus on the communication act and outcome.

Different strategies for breaking bad news have been developed and most follow a set pattern (Box 9.18) which provides assistance to the nurse and the right level of information to the listener. These strategies can be tailored to all clients, carers and children by adapting your language and interpersonal skills in accordance with their communication needs.

Professional relationships

The primary purpose of a professional relationship is to work with other professionals in order to fulfil the needs of the core task, i.e. patient/client care. The components of a professional relationship centre around the professional skills the participants bring to the relationship so that the core task can be met. Professional relationships are enhanced through:

- Understanding roles and responsibilities
- Defined boundaries where appropriate
- Clear communication strategies
- Openness and honesty
- Trust
- Responsibility and accountability accepted by each professional for their area of work.

Communication and care coordination within the MDT

It is important to recognize that, despite each person's professional independence, they also relate to each other as members of a team. This enhances the unity, effectiveness and efficiency of the team and meets the individual need for belonging. Most, though not all, people find this relationship positive (Mullins 1995). Members of the team relate along a number of dimensions including power, status, liking, communication, roles and leadership (see pp. 243–244) (Buchanan & Huczynski 2004). All the dimensions are communicated through non-verbal, verbal and other communication strategies.

Communication within MDTs requires clear management and facilitation on a number of levels, including the:

- Environmental level
- Skills and capabilities level
- Beliefs and values level
- Identity level
- Vision or mission level (Hall 2000).

Communication within MDTs also requires systems and assertive control and the flexibility to respond to changes. The information should go through as few people as possible to avoid the possibility of distortion (Guirdham 2002).

Nurses empower the MDT and their profession by clearly explaining their roles, responsibilities and professional boundaries to facilitate joint working that provides efficient, effective, evidence-based care (see Ch. 5).

Box 9.18 **Strategies for breaking bad news**

Preparation
- See the person as soon as possible
- Reduce the levels of external 'noise' and possible interruptions
- Use a comfortable/neutral setting
- Organize family or friend support
- Know the correct background information
- Check your own feelings regarding the information – another nurse may be the correct person to give the information.

Starting off
- Gather information about what has happened recently and what information is already known
- Assess the emotions, thoughts and feelings of the person to decide where to start the discussion, how to pitch it and how much information to give
- Outline the need for discussion and a possible process and ask the permission of the person
- Find out how much information the person wants to know.

Presenting the information
- Present information clearly. Know what is to be said and the communication outcome
- Present the information in understandable 'chunks', remembering the 'noise' created by stress and distress
- If possible, get clarification that the person has understood
- Be gentle, empathic and acknowledge the person's feelings
- Use accessible language and use silence to enable the person to digest the information
- Be aware of the person's responses. Be attentive to their verbal/non-verbal language that provides clues to their inner feelings, thus enabling the nurse to adapt communication and relational skills.

Provide support and clarify next steps
- Have a support plan ready for the person, e.g. specialized support resources, family members, nurses, GP, social workers, counsellors
- Explain clearly what will happen next
- 'Chunk' the information on support and next steps into understandable parts; support with written or pictorial information as appropriate
- Give clear timeframes where appropriate, though for some illnesses this could be difficult
- Allow for the person to look for the best possible outcome in the information and gently encourage them to focus on the information given.

Leadership

There is much literature that discusses the need for good quality leaders in all areas of healthcare and particularly in nursing. Leaders are identified as those who influence the behaviour of others (Mullins 1995). Nurses as team leaders enable the people they lead to care for patients/clients and carers by:

- Being aware of their needs
- Listening to their views
- Hearing their concerns
- Being able to access their knowledge of their health status.

Team leaders also have to focus on the broader information sources and strategies that inform their practice and that of the nursing team they lead. It is little surprise that nurses in this position can spend over 80% of their time in communicating.

Leadership behaviours

For nurses, their approach to leading will depend on the situation they find themselves in, the individuals and teams around them and the tasks that are required. This author proposes that nurses have a responsibility to evaluate and develop their emotional intelligence skills (see p. 244), as it is these skills that enhance relationships and the care environment and are also strongly suggestive of good leadership. Before looking more closely at emotional intelligence, it is appropriate to consider some styles of leadership. All the styles described below are appropriate in healthcare but when they are utilized depends significantly on the situation.

The plethora of leadership approaches can be daunting when nurses begin to explore the subject. Research by Binney et al (2005) shows leadership has three main elements:

- Leadership occurs between people, i.e. it is a social interactive process that facilitates links between people in organizations
- A leader's behaviour is shaped by the context in which they find themselves leading; as the situation/environment changes, so does the leader's behaviour
- Leaders are most effective when they take their skills to a situation, for the benefit of the individuals, groups and task, when they can relate to others as real people with emotional and cognitive intelligence and life experience that they can draw upon for the benefit of those around them.

It is useful to recognize what types of leadership behaviour are suitable in what situation. In accepting that there is a continuum of leadership behaviour that moves from high levels of control by the leader to high levels of freedom for those who are led, it can provide a framework for nurses to identify effective leaders and also assess their own leadership skills. This continuum in often described

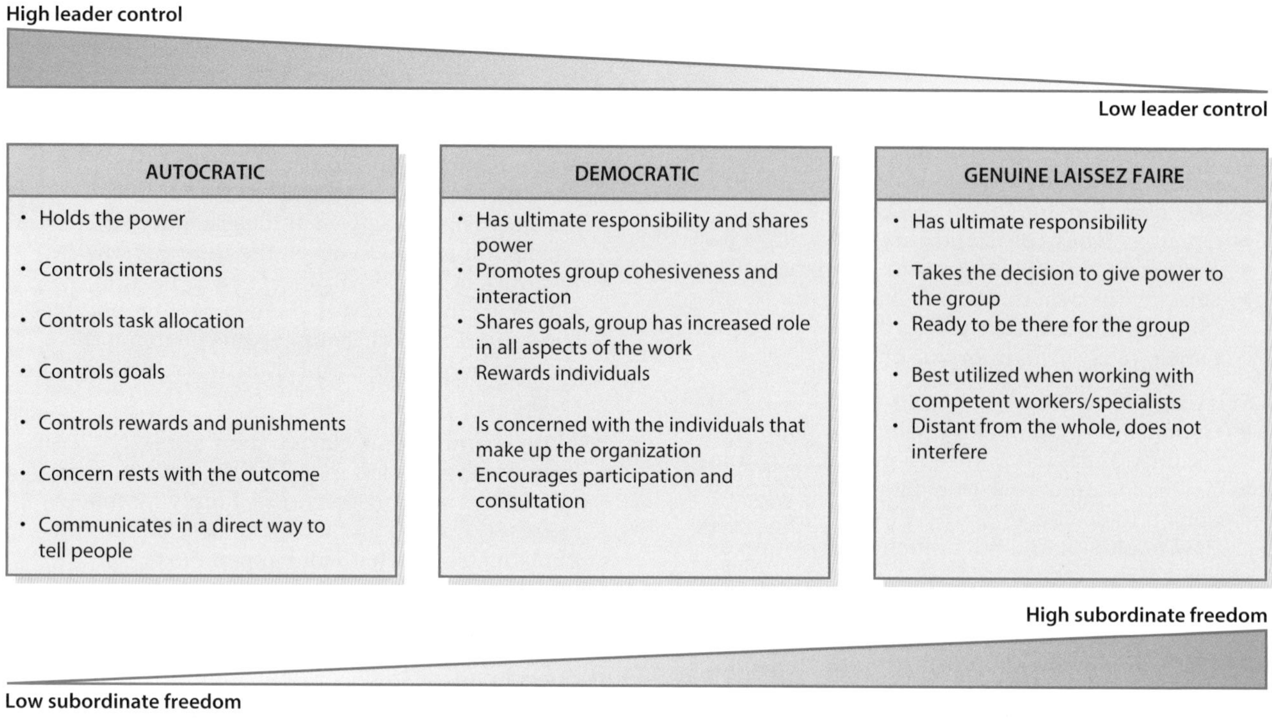
High leader control
Low leader control
AUTOCRATIC
• Holds the power
• Controls interactions
• Controls task allocation
• Controls goals
• Controls rewards and punishments
• Concern rests with the outcome
• Communicates in a direct way to tell people
DEMOCRATIC
• Has ultimate responsibility and shares power
• Promotes group cohesiveness and interaction
• Shares goals, group has increased role in all aspects of the work
• Rewards individuals
• Is concerned with the individuals that make up the organization
• Encourages participation and consultation
GENUINE LAISSEZ FAIRE
• Has ultimate responsibility
• Takes the decision to give power to the group
• Ready to be there for the group
• Best utilized when working with competent workers/specialists
• Distant from the whole, does not interfere
High subordinate freedom
Low subordinate freedom

Fig. 9.7 Leadership styles

in terms of three leadership styles identified by Lewin et al (1939) (Fig. 9.7):

- Autocratic
- Democratic
- Laissez faire.

Adair (1998) focuses leadership action in three interlinked areas: the task, the team and the individual. Communication and interpersonal competence of the leader are key to their ability to lead individuals as a team to achieve the task.

Emotional intelligence

Pre-1990 there was an assumption that intellect or 'rational' intelligence was fundamental to good working relationships and leadership. However, it is now thought that the intellect that is centred on understanding emotions (personal and other people's emotions) and how these affect other people can enhance working relationships and leadership outcomes.

Emotional intelligence is encapsulated by the way people communicate, the language they use and the non-verbal cues they utilize. Emotional intelligence is made up of a number of skills:

- Self-awareness, insight
- Managing own emotions
- Being aware of personal motivators and what motivates others
- Being able to empathize with others, being perceptive to the emotions of others
- Interpersonal skills in developing rapport, to persuade, to influence others.

Effective leaders have higher levels of emotional intelligence than leaders who are less effective (Goleman 1997).

Promoting quality and standards

Nurse team leaders develop over time; they evolve skills that shape people and services. But when is a leader a leader? Is a leader always the person in charge? Are those in responsible positions always leaders?

All nurses, including students, need the communication skills to influence the behaviour of others, e.g. educating patients/clients, children and carers about all aspects of their health. They also need to influence the behaviour of their colleagues. Nurses use leadership skills to inform, teach and support colleagues and also to challenge each other's practice. The ability to gracefully challenge other people's behaviour in a way that is clear, informative and respectful is an essential aspect of delivering quality interventions and services (Box 9.19).

Relationships with families and main carers

Relationships with main carers and families are as important as the ones with patients/clients. As discussed above, nurses facilitate good relationships with carers by clearly describing their roles, responsibilities and boundaries.

Good relationships with families/carers are vital for the health outcomes of the patient/client. They are also important in ensuring that families/carers are supported in their caring role. Caring for carers has been a low priority for some nurses. However, carers' needs are increasingly being addressed through support and lobbying from carer organizations, government initiatives, e.g. National

CRITICAL THINKING Box 9.19

Promoting quality care – challenging poor practice

- A child has knocked their drink over the floor. The team leader witnesses the accident and sees a colleague ignore the child and walk straight past the mess on the floor. The team leader asks politely if they could fetch another drink and clear up the spillage but their colleague says it's not their job and walks off. . .
- The key nurse has written a comprehensive care plan with the client, detailing their relaxation exercise programme and how they will request support from staff should they need it. The plan has been communicated clearly to the team. When the key nurse returns next day the client is upset because the nurse on duty during the evening refused to help with the relaxation exercise despite having time to do so. The client cannot see the point of 'working in partnership' if this is what happens. The key nurse checks the nursing notes where it clearly states that the client had not asked to practise the relaxation exercises. . .
- A student is talking to a resident when they over hear another resident's daughter asking a colleague why her mother's clothes have not been changed for 4 days despite obvious food stains. Your colleague shrugs and says: 'If you have a complaint you better write to the home manager.'

Student activities

Discuss the scenarios with your mentor:

- Discuss what the nurse observing the poor practice/behaviour should do to safeguard the child/client/resident.
- How should the nurse challenge a colleague's practice and behaviour in a way that ensures the problem is not repeated while maintaining their colleague's sense of dignity and showing respect for the individual?

CRITICAL THINKING Box 9.20

Colin and Jeanette

Colin is the main carer to his daughter Jeanette who is a young woman of 20 with a moderate learning disability. Jeanette has been admitted for abdominal surgery and Colin is very worried about her reaction to hospital. He states that, although he is tired from increased physical caring, he would like to stay with Jeanette so that he knows she is settled, comfortable and not anxious. He explains that when Jeanette is anxious she can quickly become depressed and very introverted, which sometimes results in self-harming behaviour as a coping mechanism.

The nurse admitting Jeanette recognizes that Colin is the expert regarding Jeanette's physical and emotional needs, but realizes that Colin is tired and as main carer he also has substantial needs.

Student activities

- What communication and interpersonal skills would you utilize in meeting Colin's needs?
- What dilemmas exist for the nurses supporting and caring for Colin and Jeanette?
- Outline a possible mutually agreeable plan for Colin, which meets both his and Jeanette's needs.

Service Frameworks, *Essence of Care* (NHS Modernisation Agency 2003), and patient involvement bodies (see Ch. 3).

Working with carers enhances the experience of patients/clients. Good support is far reaching and makes a positive difference to people's lives. Any working involvement requires effective interpersonal skills and good communication strategies and systems. For example, the scenario in Box 9.20 requires tact, commitment, courtesy, empathy, rapport, matching language, and understanding how the nurse's and carer's beliefs and values may influence their actions.

Barriers to communication

Effective communication skills and strategies are clearly important for nurses. However, it is recognized that such skills are not always evident and nurses do not always communicate well with patients/clients, carers and colleagues. This generalization is reason for concern. The barriers to effective communication outlined in this section will help nurses to understand the challenges, how these impact on practice and possible strategies to overcome them.

Task-orientated culture

Nurses work in busy environments; they have to complete a specific amount of work in a day and work with a variety of other professionals, patients/clients and carers. The roles are hard, challenging and tiring. There is a culture to get the work done, to 'do the diary', make appointments, make beds, meet physical needs and ensure that record keeping is up to date. Some nurses still consider colleagues who spend time talking with patients/clients to be avoiding the 'real' work and lazy.

People like to 'fit in' to the dominant culture and do not want to be outside the group. Nurses and students who might have been confident in spending time with patients/clients in an area where this was valued, when faced with a task-orientated culture have the dilemma of fitting into the group or being outside the group and spending time engaging with clients.

Self-awareness skills

Self-awareness involves exploration of thoughts, feelings and behaviours. It includes an understanding of how internal and external events influence people and how they behave. The more nurses search within themselves for meaning and understanding, the better they understand their skills and limitations and how their responses can affect others. The more nurses understand themselves, the more they develop. The concept of self-awareness suggests that people are always able to learn, develop and improve. Some people are very self-aware; they clearly understand how they are affected by internal and external stimuli and know how their response may affect people around them. Other people lack this level of understanding of self and, as a result, they do not know the likely effects on others and this can be a barrier to effective communication.

Nurses are strongly encouraged to work within their limitations. When people work beyond their competence through lack of self-awareness, mistakes occur and people can suffer. Most nurses can recall an occasion where communication was impeded by lack of self-awareness, e.g. by people not listening properly or by looking at a problem from their own point of view.

Nurses may feel that concentrating too much on 'what to say' makes it more difficult to say anything, let alone the 'right thing'; this can cause people to be concerned about what and how they say things. This is indicative of developing self-awareness, which is positive and helps the nurse become a more reflective and concerned communicator.

What influences people's knowledge about themselves to make them more self-aware? People are influenced by their beliefs and values: those who are internally motivated will only accept feedback on their behaviour from people whom they hold in high regard; others do not rely on their own internal beliefs but instead like to know other people's opinions about their thoughts and behaviours. People who are either entirely internally motivated or entirely externally motivated will limit the influences on their development. A mixture of both approaches is the most reasonable way to develop knowledge about self and others.

People are products of their life experiences, senses and language environments, as these aspects have formed their value and belief systems. There continue to be influences in life that provide feedback to deepen self-awareness, if people are open to development.

People gain information to support self-awareness from:

- Social links and friendships
- Emotional lives
- Close relationships
- Spiritual and ethical beliefs
- Financial concerns/control
- Current job role and career aspirations
- What meanings they place on words of value such as love, life, happiness, honour, care, professionalism, etc.

People continue to be shaped by information that enables an increasing self-awareness and ability to empathize and develop rapport with others. The knowledge people gain through reflection and meaningful self-questioning allows them to develop a wider perspective of life (Box 9.21). Limited knowledge of themselves and others means that they are unable to contribute effectively.

REFLECTIVE PRACTICE Box 9.21

Self-questioning skills

In order to develop self-questioning skills, you can try layering your questions around the themes (see bullet-pointed list, this page) known to influence people's lives. To begin the layering process, ask yourself simple questions around the meaning of the words you chose to use and 'listen' to the answers. You will find a natural focus for your next question, as part of your answer will lead to another meaningful question. For example:

- *My career, what does my career mean to me?* My career means that I am part of a profession.
- *What does being in a profession mean to me?* It means that I have a responsibility to enact my roles and responsibilities in a way that respects nursing as an art.
- *What does the term 'the art of nursing' mean to me?* The art of nursing is about the relationship nurses have with patients/clients and families that promote care giving.

Student activities

- *What does the relationship nurses have with their patients and families mean to you?*

When questioning yourself, get used to asking the question using the words you have just 'heard' from the last answer. This strategy of reflection will help you develop your reflective skills when dealing with patients/clients and carers, as reflection enhances the therapeutic relationship.

Internal noise

Shannon and Weaver's model (see Fig. 9.3, p. 224) refers to internal 'noise'. Fear and anxiety can affect the person's ability to hear what the nurse is saying. People with feelings of fear and anger can find it difficult to hear. Illness, pain and distress can alter a person's thought processes. For example, if a client is experiencing visual or auditory hallucinations, they can find it very difficult to concentrate on what the carer is communicating because their brain is already occupied with other stimuli.

Reducing the cause of the anxiety, distress, anger, pain or visual/auditory hallucination would be the first step to improving communication. This can be achieved in a number of ways and it is for the patient/client and nurse to choose which is likely to be most effective. Ways of reducing internal 'noise' include:

- Choose a quiet environment if possible
- Deal firstly with the issue that is foremost in the patient's/client's mind before embarking on the nurse's topic
- Ask the patient/client when it would be good for them to talk. Do not assume that you as the nurse are always wanted or the patient/client is always in a position to be with you
- Are you choosing a particularly difficult time to discuss an issue? Consider what is happening for the patient/client at the moment

- Are you the right person to do this? Does someone else have a better nurse–patient/client relationship?
- Is there an optimum time of the day when the patient's/client's treatment is more effective, i.e. when they are less confused or drowsy, in less pain, experiencing fewer hallucinations, less anxiety, less fear?
- Ensure that the patient's pain has been assessed and pain relief given (see Ch. 23)
- Ensure you have as much privacy as is practically possible
- Let the patient/client know you need to talk to them; give them the subject to be discussed rather than just launching in with no preparation at all
- Ensure you are using the most appropriate level of language
- Check whether the patient/client needs their glasses or a hearing aid.

Difficulty with speech and hearing

People can experience physical difficulties in speech/sign production or understanding speech, such as following a stroke or brain injury. In these situations the trauma has affected the area of the brain that enables the individual to comprehend or produce speech. In these situations it is the role of the nurse and carers to promote all other communication channels by encouraging the patient/client to draw, write, gesture, point or use a more sophisticated communication tool such as speech synthesis, which is the generation of speech sound by computer. Working in collaboration with the SLT can be very beneficial. People who are very breathless find it difficult to speak (see Ch. 17).

Some patients/clients have problems with hearing, which present barriers to communication. Nurses may need to work with patients/clients who lipread or use signing. It may be necessary to work with a sign language interpreter or ensure a referral to an audiologist or SLT in order to achieve effective communication (see Ch. 16 for further information).

Medication

Medication can have a significant effect on communication; in some cases it can cause dry mouth or excess salivation (e.g. clozapine), nausea and indigestion, all of which influence the person's motivation to engage in conversation. If patients/clients are embarrassed or concerned that they will not be able to speak properly or control their mouth, they could be reluctant to speak. In this situation the nurse needs to reassure the patient/client by offering time, a non-judgemental attitude, fluids and oral care to suit their specific needs, and ensure that all steps are taken to reduce the negative effects of the medication.

Cultural factors acting as barriers

It is important for nurses to think about many of the issues already covered and their own experiences when considering cultural differences in communication and how these can challenge health professionals and people who use the services.

REFLECTIVE PRACTICE Box 9.22

Tell me about your culture

- What makes your culture different from others?
- What are the defining values of people from your culture?
- How do other people recognize your cultural identity?
- What dress code do you follow?
- What foods do people from your culture eat?
- How do people from your culture spend their leisure time?
- What religion do people from your culture follow?
- Does this mean you have certain times to pray, or specific holidays?

Student activity

- Answer the questions above.

The questions serve two purposes/points. First, you may recognize them – either you have asked people these questions or questions like them, or people may have asked you. Second, the questions highlight how very difficult these seemingly clear enquiries are to answer and how they encourage the development of generalizations about people from other communities and cultures that may not be helpful (Henley & Schott 1999).

Whenever people discuss difference, there is a tendency to make value judgements regarding those perceived as being different. In this chapter difference, sameness, foreign, British, multilingual, bilingual, unilingual . . . all these notions are of difference but in no way is one difference more or less valued than another. This is not to say that 'everyone is the same really' – people are not; everyone holds different thoughts, beliefs and values, and comes from a multitude of cultures and experiences.

When discussing communication difference it must be noted that some examples used to highlight issues are not positive; however, there are other examples that provide ideas for good practice, which nurses are strongly encouraged to employ.

This text can only offer generalizations about language and communication differences; however, nurses need to develop the skills and knowledge to meet people's individual needs. Never assume that because someone is from a certain country or background, they follow a specific faith, support a particular political party or speak a certain language; to assume anything would be to reduce the nurse's flexibility and ability to meet the need of others.

One of the assumptions that we often make, in a valiant attempt to understand people from other communities, is to ask people about their culture because from our perspective their culture is very different and we expect all parties to recognize this (Box 9.22).

Differences in language and communication rules

Despite sharing a great deal, there are differences in the way language is used to communicate. For example, there are differences in prosody, i.e. tempo, speed, rhythm and pitch of speech.

Intonation

Intonation is the way words are said, the degree of emphasis given and the rise and fall of the pitch in a sentence. The singsong of spoken English or a tonal language such as Chinese shows great variety in the application of intonation. However, the raise in the pitch of voice at the end of a sentence indicates the speaker has asked a question and this is true for many languages.

British English speakers and speakers of other languages in the same family tend to use a narrow range of tone in speech; when these speakers hear the intonation of people who use a wider range of tones they can be interpreted as brash or even aggressive.

People who use tonal languages change the meaning of a word by changing the pitch level. The meaning of the word is dependent on the pitch, either rising–falling, or falling–rising. When people with native tonal languages learn 'tune' languages, it may take some time to learn and develop the singsong skills. As a result they may sound monotone and a little harsh to the ears of a tune language user, resulting in confusion about the emotional content of the statement.

Emphasis

In *British* English emphasizing a word. . . .
In British English emphasizing a word. . .
In British English *emphasizing* a word. . .

In British English emphasizing a *word* changes the meaning of the sentence; in language, meaning is changed by the speed of delivery, the loudness or softness of the word. Again there is plenty of room for confusion. This often leads to anxiety, thereby creating 'noise' which affects the message. Emphasizing important information enables the nurse to help the patient/client/child listen to the message in a more useful way, e.g. 'Please tell me if at any time you want me to stop and I will.'

Loudness

A loudly spoken word or sentence suggests urgency or importance in many languages, but it can also suggest submission to authority, as well as authority over the situation. Softly spoken words also have different meanings that include showing respect for the listener and emphasizing the authority of the speaker; in some languages it suggests professionalism and in others it is used to express anger (Crystal 1999). Nurses who meet someone who is culturally Zulu for the first time may find it odd that they may speak quietly and deferentially to them. This may appear to a British English speaker as if the person is overly polite, shy or may even be hiding something. However, it is the norm to show respect to others in this way using the voice courteously.

Sentence structure

In British English sentences tend to be structured as subject–verb–object, e.g. 'The nurse answered the telephone'. In other languages there is a topic–comment structure, such as: 'The library is open, I will go in an hour.' The way people structure their conversations also differs from language to language. Some people like to map out the situation before getting to the point to give the listener as much background as possible. Some people would find this difficult to follow and at worst find the speaker rude and evasive. Other people will get straight to the point and add the context later, which – while time saving – can also be interpreted as brusque. It is important for nurses to know how to present information; if they are unsure whether to get straight to the point with a patient/client, colleague or carer, they should listen to how the person speaks to them. Gently reflecting their style may improve communication.

Taking turns and guggling

British English speakers lower their voices when they are ready for the listener to speak but in Southern Europe the speaker offers the listener a brief pause in which to speak. British English speakers allow longer pauses in their conversations to give the listener the cue to speak. Clearly people could be confused with the signals and may interpret the long pause or lack of pause as rudeness or poor listening skills.

In some communities it is acceptable to talk at the same time as the speaker on the same subject as a mark of agreement and listening; this sharing of conversation space is also seen in twin, sibling and close friendship conversations. Again it is a mark of involvement, of closeness. However, some linguistic communities would see this as poor manners and shoddy interpersonal skills. British English speakers tend to like clear turn taking.

British and other sign language users also take turns in sequence rather than signing at the same time. Signing at the same time as someone else is considered rude, though not as impolite as holding a person's hands when they are signing in order to stop them making their point, no matter how much the listener may disagree.

Guggles are important in some languages (see p. 235); there are even guggles in sign language. However, in some languages, being still, maintaining a passive facial expression, not making a sound and making little eye contact is a sign from the listener that they are listening and attentive.

It is important that nurses do not assume that there is only one way of encouraging people to speak. The Western model of developing rapport in order to work in partnership with others is not the only way. In order to work within the social, interpersonal and linguistic 'rules' most effectively requires an individual who shares the first and preferred language of the person (Henley & Schott 1999). The services of a qualified interpreter may be needed (see below).

Working with interpreters

When the communication barrier is due to the nurse not speaking the patient's/client's language, a third party who speaks both languages will be needed (Henley & Schott 1999).

A person who can speak two or more languages is not the same as an interpreter. Interpreting is a learned skill, and working with an interpreter is also a skill that has to be learned. Furthermore, interpreters are a professional body of people, most of whom work to exacting codes of ethics and professional standards. Interpreters are skilled in enabling each party to understand the culture of the other, particularly where cultural differences would cause misunderstandings.

Without quality interpreting services, people can be misdiagnosed, mistreated, undiagnosed, uninformed, etc. If the interpreter is untrained these issues are unresolved. Ultimately this means that people's health suffers, carers are unable to support the process effectively and many service users avoid the health service, believing that they will not receive any sort of service.

Summary

- Nurses are encouraged to reflect on their own skills, to develop their awareness and understanding of those with whom they will work.
- This chapter introduces the skills that underpin this area of interpersonal communication and relationship.
- All nurses can enhance their communication skills and relational skills by using the *Essence of Care* benchmarking tools for communication (NHS Modernisation Agency 2003) to focus their development.
- The benchmarks identify good practice in communicating as expected by clients, colleagues and carers.
- Once confident in behaving in ways that produce the outcomes that clients and carers expect, nurses can develop finer communication skills that will truly enhance therapeutic relationships between patients/clients, carers and colleagues and increase the effectiveness of resources.
- Good communication skills are the underpinning foundation on which to base all other nursing interventions.
- Understanding how language is constructed, learned and what part it plays in the development of 'self' in a social world enables the nurse to monitor, evaluate and adapt their communication to meet the needs of the person.
- Recognizing the power of language in developing and sustaining working relationships with others is vital when influencing others ecologically.
- Utilizing reflective exercises, wider reading and focused action plans to develop a lifelong learning portfolio of development will help nurses become skilled communicators in the future.

Self test

1. Describe the stages of a two-way communication process between a nurse and a client.
2. List three factors that could seriously affect the quality of your message.
3. List three functions of play in healthcare settings.
4. Define empathy.
5. Give examples of open and closed questions.
6. List the stages of the therapeutic relationship.
7. List some cultural differences in language and communication.

Key words and phrases for literature searching

Assertiveness
Body language
Communication barriers
Courtesy
Customer care
Emotional intelligence
Empathy
Interpersonal skills
Listening skills
Positive regard
Proxemics
Self-awareness
Therapeutic relationships

Useful websites

Empathy and Listening Skills and Psychological Hugs	www.psychological-hug.com Available July 2006
Language and Culture: An Introduction to Human Communication	http://anthro.palomar.edu/language/default.htm Available July 2006
The Northern School of NLP and Associated Studies	www.nlpand.co.uk Available July 2006

References

Adair J 1998 Effective leadership. Pan Publications, London

Argyle M 1994 The psychology of interpersonal behaviour. 5th edn. Penguin Press, London

Armstrong DF, Stokoe WC, Wilcox SE 1996 Gesture and the nature of language. Cambridge University Press, Cambridge

Binney G, Wilke G, Williams C 2005 Living leadership: a practical guide for ordinary heroes. Financial Times Prentice Hall, London

Boysson-Bardies B 1999 How language comes to children. MIT Press, Cambridge, MA

Buchanan D, Huczynski A 2004 Organisational behaviour: an introductory text. Financial Times Prentice Hall, London

Crystal D 1999 The encyclopaedia of language. Cambridge University Press, Cambridge

Egan G 1998 The skilled helper – a problem management approach to helping. 6th edn. Brooks Cole, Pacific Grove, CA

Fiske J 1993 Introduction to communication studies. 2nd edn. Routledge, London

Fromkin VA, Rodman R 1997 Introduction to language. 6th edn. Harcourt Brace, Sydney

Gibbs G 1988 Learning by doing: a guide to teaching and learning methods. Further Education Unit, Oxford Brookes University, Oxford

Goleman D 1997 Working with emotional intelligence. Bloomsbury Press, London

Guirdham M 2002 Interactive behaviour at work. 3rd edn. Financial Times Prentice Hall, London

Hall M 2000 The source book of magic. Crown House, Carmarthen

Hargie O (ed) 1996 The handbook of communication skills. Routledge, London

Henley A, Schott J 1999 Culture, religion and patient care in a multi-ethnic society. Age Concern, London

Holmes J 2001 Introduction to sociolinguistics. Longman, London

Kurtz S, Silverman J, Draper J 2004 Teaching and learning communication skills in medicine. 2nd edn. Radcliffe Publishing, Oxford

Lewin K, Llippit R, White RK 1939 Patterns of aggressive behaviour in experimentally created social climates. Journal of Social Psychology 10:271–301

Mullins LJ 1995 Management and organisational behaviour. Pitman, London

NHS Modernisation Agency 2003 Essence of care: patient-focused benchmarks for clinical governance. Online: www.modern.nhs.uk/home/key/docs/Essence%20of%20Care.pdf Available September 2006

Nursing and Midwifery Council 2004 code of professional conduct: standards for conduct, performance and ethics. NMC, London

O'Brien LM 2000 Nurse–client relationships: the experience of community psychiatric nurses. Australian and New Zealand Journal of Mental Health Nursing 9:184–194

Pinker S 1994 The language instinct. Penguin, London

Varcarolis EM 1998 Foundations of psychiatric mental health nursing. Saunders, Philadelphia

Wolvin AD, Coakley CG 1985 Listening. WC Brown, Dubuque, IA

Further reading

Bennett M 2001 The empathic healer. Academic Press, San Diego, CA

Glasper AE, Richardson J 2006 A textbook for children's and young people's nursing. Churchill Livingstone, Edinburgh

Holland S, Ward C 1997 Assertiveness: a practical approach. Speechmark Publishing, Oxon

Institute of Leadership and Management (ILM) 2004 Making communication work (ILM Super Series). 4th edn. Pergammon Flexible Learning, Oxford

Tribe R, Raval H 2002 Working with interpreters. Brunner-Routledge, London

Wilson K, Ryan V 2006 Play therapy. Non-directive approach for children and adolescents. 2nd edn. Baillière Tindall, Edinburgh

10

Sleep, rest, relaxation, complementary therapies and alternative therapies

Ah Nya Plant

Glossary terms

Allopathic
Alternative medicine
Biological body 'clock'
Biorhythm
Circadian rhythm
Complementary therapy
Diurnal rhythm
Holistic
Integrated medicine
Jet lag
Melatonin
Rest
Shift work
Sleep
Sleep disorder
Vital force

Learning outcomes

This chapter will help you to:

- Understand why rest and sleep are important to maintain good health
- Describe the physiological control of sleep
- Describe the stages of the sleep cycle
- Outline factors that affect normal sleep patterns
- Outline sleep patterns in different age groups
- Identify factors that disrupt normal sleep patterns
- Describe some common sleep disorders
- Apply simple measures to promote sleep and rest
- Outline the use of complementary therapies in the promotion of sleep, rest and well-being
- Understand the concept of integrated health
- Describe the range of complementary therapies available
- Understand the need to access these therapies in a safe manner.

Introduction

Thy best of rest is sleep.

William Shakespeare (Measure for measure, Act 3, Scene 1).

Maslow's hierarchy of basic human needs comprises five or seven levels. The first level physical/physiological needs, such as food and water, are necessary for life. These physiological needs, which also include sleep and rest, have the greatest priority.

Sleep, relaxation and rest maintain, enhance and restore the person's physiological, psychological and social well-being. Nurses in all care settings are involved in helping and guiding people to attain optimum health and well-being. An important aspect of this is to promote daily routines and lifestyle that enables the individual to enhance the body's normal way of achieving rest by relaxation and sleep. The nurse's role is especially important during illness or following injury when the restorative functions of sleep are most needed for reducing stress and promoting healing. Unfortunately, many patients/clients have problems getting sufficient rest and sleep, particularly so in hospital. Inadequate sleep and rest may, for example, be caused by anxiety, pain, the environment or specific treatments.

The first part of the chapter provides an overview of sleep, including physiological control, the sleep stages and functions. The factors that cause disturbances of sleep, effects of sleep deprivation and some specific sleep disorders are addressed.

The nursing interventions employed to promote rest and sleep throughout the lifespan are discussed in some depth and include the assessment of sleep, sleep hygiene/pre-sleep routines and the sleep environment, and the role of relaxation, orthodox medications and herbal products in promoting sleep. The outline of relaxation (see Ch. 11) and herbal products used in relation to rest and sleep provides a link to the section about complementary and alternative medicine (CAM).

In the last part of the chapter the integration of complementary and alternative therapies with conventional healthcare is discussed. There is information about the use of some therapies and how they can be accessed and utilized safely to promote rest, relaxation and sleep. In addition, some examples of the wider uses of CAM are provided.

Sleep, rest and relaxation

Sleep, rest and relaxation, as already stated, are necessary for well-being and health maintenance. Sleep is an altered state of consciousness, accompanied by a reduction in metabolism and skeletal muscle activity. It occurs naturally in humans and follows a 24-hour biological rhythm (see below).

During sleep, the arterial blood pressure, heart and respiratory rates all decrease and skin blood vessels dilate. It has long been accepted that sleep is important for restoration and repair of cells and tissues. Growth hormone (GH) secretion increases during sleep and cell division in many tissues takes place.

However, there is evidence that, apart from the brain, all other organs undergo just as effective restoration during relaxed wakefulness (Horne & Reyner 1988, 1997). This highlights the importance of relaxation and rest periods during the day, e.g. breaks from work and the need for relaxation and relief from anxiety. Babies and children need a balance between active play, restful relaxed activities such as sitting on a carer's lap to listen to a story and sleep.

Protected time for rest and relaxation is important for patients/clients in hospital and other care settings. People can become exhausted by long visiting hours and the interventions from health professionals that are intended to restore health (Box 10.1).

Sleep is also thought to help revitalize mental activities such as learning, memory, reasoning and emotional

REFLECTIVE PRACTICE Box 10.1

Protected rest times

Periods of rest and relaxation are important for everyone but particularly so during illness.

Student activities

- Find out what happens in your clinical area or local hospital with regard to having protected rest/quiet times for patients/clients.
- Think about how you would feel if you were unwell and admitted to an area where there is activity throughout the day, visitors, nursing care, treatments and visits to other departments for investigations and therapy.

adjustments. Studies of junior doctors working extended shifts indicate that they have concentration lapses and make more serious errors than when their shift length was curtailed to less than 16 hours (Lockley et al 2004).

Biorhythms

Biorhythms are the cyclical patterns of biological functions unique to each individual, e.g. sleep–wake cycles, fluctuations in body temperature, blood pressure, heart rate, mood and some hormone secretion. Biorhythm cycles may follow a 24-hour day–night (circadian) pattern or a longer period such as a woman's menstrual cycle.

The sleep–wake cycle is a good example of a physiological process that follows a circadian (Latin: *circa* [about] and *dies* [day]) or diurnal daily pattern. A 'biological clock' synchronizes the sleep–wake cycle with the 24-hour clock, which people use to determine daily and social activities. It follows a day–night/light–dark rhythm of around 24 hours, thus giving rise to individual sleep patterns and different times for going to bed such as 20.00 hours, midnight or even the early hours of the morning.

Physiology of sleep

The physiological control of sleep involves a functional area in the brain, the reticular formation (RF), sometimes known as the reticular activating system (RAS), other brain structures, neurotransmitters (chemicals) and the hormone melatonin (Fig. 10.1). An outline is provided here and readers requiring more detail should consult Further reading (e.g. Montague et al 2005).

When a person is asleep, the body is relaxed and they are not conscious of external stimuli such as noise or internal stimuli such as hunger. The stimulating mental activity such as thoughts about events of the day or preparatory work for the next day diminishes as the person begins to feel drowsy and falls asleep. However, if these stimuli are very intense and strong the person wakes up and consciously responds to the stimuli. The sensory nerve pathways receive and convey nerve impulses upwards to the cerebral cortex ('conscious brain'). They arise in response to stimuli such as light, noise, pain, temperature and hunger. Likewise, descending messages from the cerebral cortex enable the person to respond accordingly, e.g. getting up to have a snack if hungry or lying awake thinking of a solution to a problem. It appears then, that the balance of impulses to and from the cerebral cortex controls the sleep–wake cycle.

Reticular formation – the reticular activating system

The RF or RAS is a functional system, which comprises diffuse neurones found throughout the brain stem (midbrain, pons and medulla oblongata). It has connections with the cerebral cortex, thalamus, hypothalamus, cerebellum and spinal cord. The RAS is important in the control of motor activity, some autonomic functions and the regulation of sensory inputs en route to the cerebral cortex.

The RAS controls the sleep–wake cycle, the state of cortical awareness and consciousness. Ascending sensory impulses, e.g. sound and light, stimulate the RAS and this increases cortical activity and the person wakes. Consciousness is maintained through the activity of various feedback mechanisms that involve the RAS, cerebral cortex and skeletal muscles. When the RAS is inhibited, RAS activity is low and the person becomes relaxed and falls asleep. Thus a quiet, dark room promotes sleep, whereas increased stimuli to the RAS increases its activity and the high level of excitation prevents the person from relaxing and falling asleep. Stimulating factors, e.g. anxiety, being upset, hunger, thirst, physical discomfort and noise can prevent sleep. RAS functioning is inhibited by drugs, e.g. anaesthetic agents, sedatives, anxiolytic drugs that reduce anxiety, and by alcohol and nervous system problems.

The biological 'body clock'

Normally adults sleep at night and stay awake during the day. This timing of sleep that corresponds with darkness and light is what constitutes a circadian rhythm. It is thought that this is controlled by a group of cells called the suprachiasmatic nucleus (SCN) found in the hypothalamus in the brain (see Fig. 10.1). The SCN, identified as the 'biological clock', is stimulated by visual information from the retina of the eye. This explains why light is the primary controlling stimulus for the biological clock's daily rhythm and why humans go to bed at night.

The SCN is connected to the pineal gland situated in the centre of the brain (see Fig. 10.1). The SCN controls secretion of melatonin, a hormone, from the pineal gland. The secretion of melatonin exhibits a 24-hour cycle and fluctuates in relation to light. It appears that darkness stimulates its secretion and light inhibits it. Thus levels of melatonin are high at night but low during the day. It is thought that melatonin may play an important role in regulating the sleep–wake cycle. It is noted to be higher in children than in adults and may explain why children sleep more than adults (see pp. 256–257). Ongoing research into the effects of melatonin include:

- Looking at its effects of lowering body temperature, hence inducing sleep
- Its role in the treatment of jet lag (see p. 258)
- Its relationship to winter depression and seasonal affective disorder (SAD) (Box 10.2, p. 254)
- Its potential as a natural sleeping pill in treating insomnia (sleeplessness) and its possible role in the reproductive function (Widmaier et al 2005).

Neurotransmitters involved in sleep physiology

There are several neurotransmitters involved in controlling the sleep–wake cycle. These chemicals are produced in the RF and elsewhere in the brain. It is thought that neurotransmitters affect the sleep–wake cycle by influencing the level of activity in the RAS, causing the transition from sleep to arousal to waking and vice versa. Changing levels of neurotransmitters cause the shift from one state to another and give rise to two types of sleep: non-rapid eye movement sleep (NREM) and rapid eye movement sleep (REM) (see p. 254). The neurotransmitters include:

- 5-hydroxytryptamine (serotonin)
- Noradrenaline (norepinephrine)
- Acetylcholine
- Histamine
- Hypocretin
- Dopamine
- Gamma-aminobutyric acid (GABA).

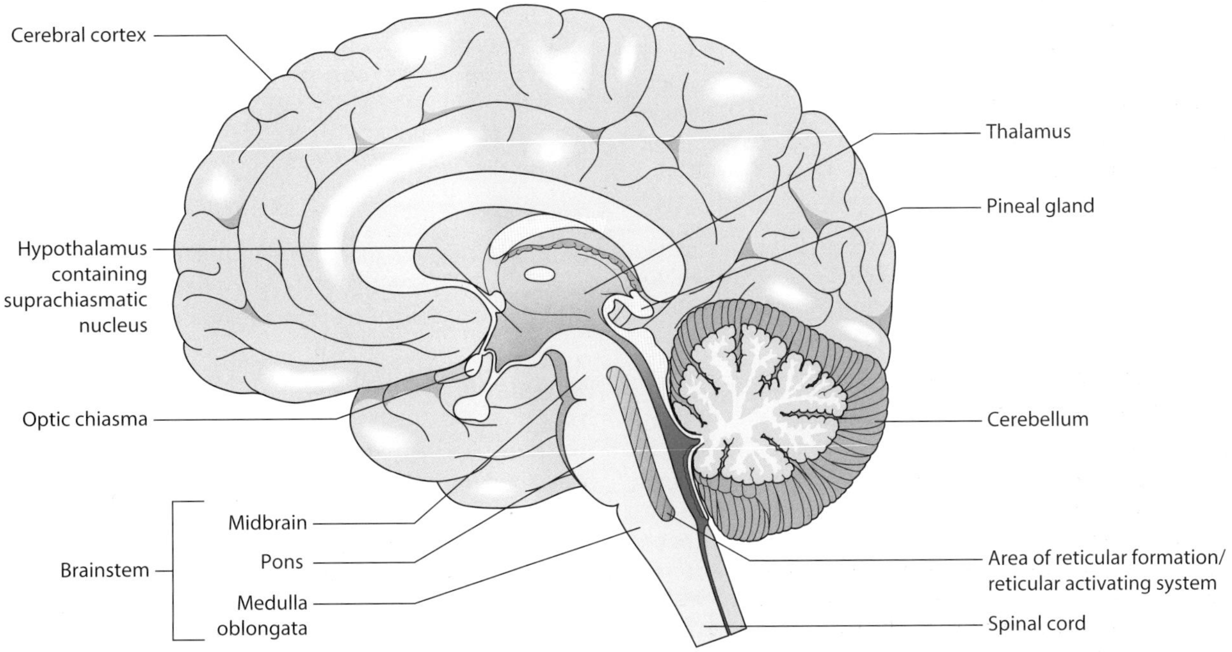

Fig. 10.1 Areas of the brain involved in control of sleep

CRITICAL THINKING Box 10.2

Seasonal affective disorder

The symptoms of SAD include:

- Disturbed sleep, early morning awakening, a desire to oversleep or sleep longer and daytime sleepiness
- Reduced concentration
- Tiredness, lethargy, inability to carry out normal routines
- Low mood and mood swings
- Increased appetite, particularly for carbohydrate and sweet foods
- Reduced libido
- Loss of interest in work, socializing and hobbies.

In severe SAD, symptoms may also include:

- Stress and anxiety and inability to tolerate stress
- Feeling hopeless, depressed and despairing.

Student activities

- Access the NHS Direct website and find out the causes of SAD.
- What types of treatment are available for people with SAD?
- What support is available for sufferers?

[Resources: Lambert K and Kingsley CH 2005 Clinical neuroscience. Worth, New York; NHS Direct. Online: www.nhsdirect.nhs.uk/he.asp?ArticleID=333 Available July 2006]

Box 10.3 **Characteristics of the different stages of the sleep cycle**

Wakefulness – alert, awake, eyes open, relaxed, drowsy, feeling tired, eyelids getting 'heavier', eyes may close, head relaxed, droops, lacks concentration and attention, sleepy but not asleep.
NREM (orthodox) sleep – 50% in neonates, 20% in preschoolers, 70–80% in young adults and variable in older adults:

- Stage 1 – time taken to enter this varies, normally takes about 1–7 minutes, light sleep, lack of awareness continues, muscles relax, heart and respiratory rates are stable. Easily roused by moderate stimuli
- Stage 2 – lack of sensitivity more marked, muscles more relaxed, becoming more difficult to rouse
- Stage 3 – occurs about 20 minutes after the person falls asleep, moderate deep sleep occurs and the person is very relaxed and very difficult to waken. Body temperature and blood pressure drop
- Stage 4 – a progression of stage 3. Deep sleep, only strong stimulation such as shaking will rouse. Sleepwalking, talking, nightmares and tooth grinding (bruxism) may occur in some people.

REM (paradoxical) sleep – about 50% in neonates, 20% in young adults and variable in older adults. This stage normally begins at the end of each sleep cycle. Therefore, REM sleep occurs approximately every 90 minutes, each episode lasting about 10 minutes. The deepest sleep and greatest relaxation occurs and the person is difficult to rouse. Dreaming occurs, rapid eye movements behind closed eyelids, possibly the person is visualizing and following the events of the dream. There is a marked increase in brain oxygen consumption. Blood pressure, pulse and respiratory rates vary more than during NREM sleep.

Stages of sleep

There are two types of sleep, named according to whether or not the eyeballs can be seen to move behind the closed eyelids, i.e. NREM sleep and REM sleep. For young adults, a normal night's sleep of about 8 hours comprises around 70–80% of NREM sleep with the remainder spent in REM sleep. Subjects observed during NREM and REM sleep show distinctive features of brain wave patterns, changes in muscle tone, heart rate and breathing.

NREM sleep

NREM (orthodox) sleep, which occurs first, has four stages. Box 10.3 outlines the characteristics of these stages. Sleep begins with the person relaxed, feeling drowsy and then proceeds from stage 1 to stage 4. This normally takes 40 minutes. The process then reverses, moving back through NREM stages 3 and 2 followed by an episode of REM sleep. If the sleep is uninterrupted, it continues in this cyclical fashion (Fig. 10.2). In adults the cycle repeats four to five times in an average night's sleep, each cycle lasting about 90 minutes. However, the time spent in stages 3 and 4 declines as the night progresses and more time is spent in REM sleep. The amount of REM sleep differs between age groups and during the individual's lifespan. In NREM sleep, there is progressive muscle relaxation and reduced muscle tension. Blood pressure, heart and respiratory rates all decrease. The gonadotrophic hormones, which stimulate the gonads (ovaries and testes), and GH are released during NREM sleep. When awakened during NREM sleep, dreaming is rarely reported.

REM sleep

REM sleep is also known as paradoxical sleep, because the brain wave pattern resembles that of the waking state, but paradoxically the sleeper is difficult to arouse (see Box 10.3). During REM sleep oxygen consumption is high and, when awakened, subjects report that they have been dreaming. REM sleep is associated with an increase in and irregular blood pressure, heart and respiratory rates. There is rapid eye movement. Although twitches of facial muscles may occur, there is loss of skeletal muscle tone throughout the rest of the body.

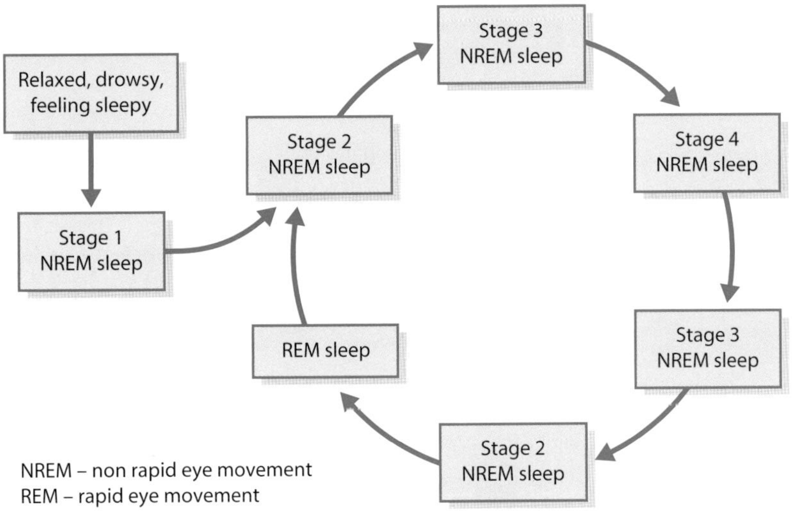

Fig. 10.2 Stages of sleep in adults

Functions of sleep

The functions of sleep are not clearly understood, hence there are several hypotheses regarding this. One of these suggests that during REM sleep, dreaming enhances and facilitates the chemical and structural changes that the brain undergoes during learning and memory. Dreams may also provide the expression of concerns in the 'subconscious'. In one study, soldiers who were woken during dream sleep found extreme difficulty in coping and completing tasks the next day. This demonstrates that dreaming is an important function of sleep, possibly a means of filing away the stimulating experiences of the day (Rottenberg 1992).

Neonates sleep for long periods, probably to recover from the process of birth. During sleep, relaxation of skeletal muscles and a reduction in metabolic processes occurs. This helps to conserve energy and, together with the release of GH, growth and cell/tissue repair such as during wound healing are enhanced (see Ch. 25).

The proper functioning of the immune system is also linked with sleep. For example, interleukin-1 (a signalling protein produced by some white blood cells), which has an important role in the inflammatory response (see Ch. 25), fluctuates in parallel with normal sleep–wake cycles (Widmaier et al 2005).

Effects of sleep deprivation

Most, if not all, nurses can relate to the effects of not enough sleep such as lack of concentration, irritability and poor performance of skilled tasks (Box 10.4). An increase in accidents, e.g. driving home after night duty, and domestic and work-related accidents due to impaired judgement and human errors are all related to sleep deprivation.

Sleep deprivation is associated with reduced function of the immune responses, thereby reducing the individual's resistance to infection. It may also induce mental health problems and even psychotic behaviour if it is accompanied by stress.

REFLECTIVE PRACTICE Box 10.4

Sleep deprivation

Think about times when you have not had enough sleep for whatever reason.

Student activities

- Reflect on tasks that you found more difficult, e.g. programming the video recorder or calculating a drug dose.
- Were you aware of any changes in the way you interacted with other people?
- Do you think that your concentration was affected, perhaps during a lecture or a handover report?

The effects of sleep deprivation vary from person to person and some examples are outlined in Box 10.5. These effects can become problematic and may cause the individual to seek help. If poor sleep habits are not resolved they can develop into a chronic problem such as insomnia (see p. 261). The most effective treatment for sleep deprivation is elimination or correction of factors that disrupt sleep patterns. Nurses should be proactive in helping the person to achieve and retrieve lost sleep.

Factors that affect normal sleep patterns

A person's normal sleep pattern is determined by factors that include:

- Genetics – being a 'morning or evening type'
- Individual needs – sleep patterns show huge individual differences
- Culture (Box 10.6, see p. 256) – such as a 'nap' after lunch, or an afternoon siesta in Mediterranean countries and a late evening meal when it is cooler. In many cultures children stay up late and eat

Box 10.5 **Examples of the cumulative effects of sleep deprivation**

- Loss of appetite
- Headaches
- Feeling cold due to fall in body temperature
- Poor coordination
- Overwhelming desire to sleep
- Tiredness
- Hallucinations
- Irritability
- Mood swings
- Confusion/disorientation
- Increased aggressiveness
- Poor concentration
- Reduced ability to perform skilled tasks
- 'Microsleeps' lasting a few seconds. These may be dangerous, e.g. while driving or operating machinery.

REFLECTIVE PRACTICE Box 10.6

Cultural influences on sleep patterns

Consider the cultural influences on the sleep patterns of an adult patient/client.

Student activities

- How does their sleep pattern differ from a typical pattern of being awake all day and sleeping for 8–9 hours at night?
- To what extent have they had to change their sleep pattern since being in hospital/care home or having care at home?
- Think about how individual sleep patterns can be maintained in a care setting.

with the extended family and this may require adjustments during hospitalization

- Body mass index (see Ch. 19)
- Physical activity
- Age is an important factor and is discussed in more detail below.

Box 10.7 provides an opportunity to consider your own sleep pattern and the factors that influence it.

Sleep patterns during the lifespan

Normal sleep patterns change throughout the lifespan in order to meet the different requirements during growth, development and maturation. The amount of sleep required by a newborn baby is very different from that needed by an older adult. The duration, quality and quantity of sleep are all subject to change, not just the time spent sleeping (Fig. 10.3).

Infancy and childhood

In the first week of life, infants are usually asleep for 16 hours out of the 24 hours, but this is interspersed with waking for frequent feeds. Establishing a sleep pattern is important and a pre-sleep bedtime routine can be introduced as early as 6 weeks. This helps the infant to learn the 'sleep cues' and enhances settling down at bedtime (Box 10.8).

By the age of 3–4 months a pattern of sleep begins to develop and infants sleep around 8–10 hours during

REFLECTIVE PRACTICE Box 10.7

Normal sleep patterns

Consider your typical sleep pattern.

Student activities

- How many hours sleep do you normally have?
- How many hours sleep do you need to feel fresh and alert the next day?
- Think about the factors listed in the text. Which ones have been important in determining your sleep pattern?

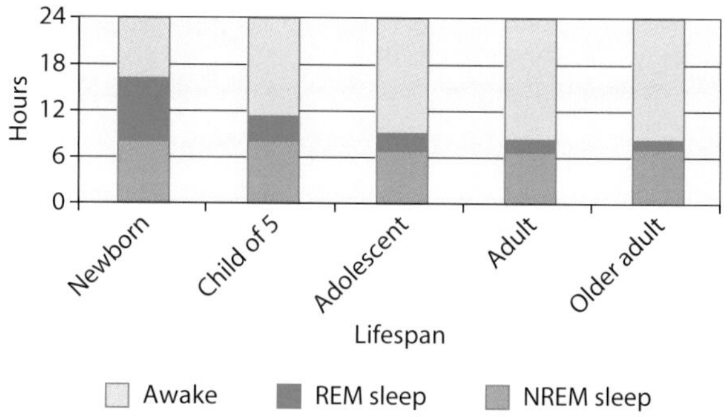

Fig. 10.3 'Typical' sleep pattern changes throughout the lifespan

HEALTH PROMOTION Box 10.8

Helping infants to sleep at night

You are on a community child health placement and many parents/carers have told the health visitor that they cannot get their baby to sleep at night or that the baby seems to cry excessively.

Student activities

- Using the resources below, prepare a summary of the main advice for parents about getting infants to sleep and dealing with crying.
- Find out why some infants have bouts of colic and what can be done to prevent it or relieve its effects.
- Discuss with your mentor the importance of establishing a nighttime sleeping pattern in infants.

[Resources: Cry-sis – www.cry-sis.org.uk/sleepproblems.html; NHS Direct Babies crying – www.nhsdirect.nhs.uk/en.aspx?articleID=645; Parentline New baby and sleep – www.parentlineplus.org.uk/index.php?id=123 All available July 2006]

the night and wake up early in the morning. Normally infants and toddlers have sleeps during the day but the duration reduces and eventually ceases when the toddler reaches the age of 3 years. However, those who are more active will sleep less. Sleep disorders affecting children are outlined later (see pp. 261–262).

Once the child starts school, the amount of daily activity and the overall health of the child will dictate how many hours of sleep are required. Children aged between 4 and 5 years spend, on average, about 10–11 hours sleeping at night.

Adolescents/young adults

Adolescents and young adults need sufficient sleep to cope with the period of rapid growth that occurs. Most young people are engaged in physical and mental activities at school, college or work and socializing in the evenings and at the weekend. Normally by bedtime, they should have no difficulty falling asleep. However, it is normal for those who extend their activities past midnight to sleep on in the mornings, especially at weekends when they may sleep until lunchtime. An average adolescent sleeps 8–9 hours per night but this will vary according to the demands of study, socializing, sport, part-time work, etc.

Adulthood and midlife

During adulthood and midlife sleep requirements vary between individuals. Some people may need 10 hours whereas others need as little as 4 hours of sleep at night. Some women find that their sleep patterns change during the time around the menopause. Sleep may be disrupted by hot flushes and night sweats.

Older adults

In common with other age groups the sleeping patterns and sleep requirements of older adults vary considerably. It is a misconception that older people require less sleep. In fact, the total amount of sleep does not change as age increases. However, the time spent sleeping at night decreases because people wake more often during the night. But the loss of nighttime sleep is offset by an increase in daytime naps and rest time. Also, the quality of sleep deteriorates, as there is a progressive decrease in REM sleep and NREM sleep (stage 4).

The fragmented sleep patterns in older adults may be explained by changes in sleep regulation due to age-related alterations in the circadian rhythm of melatonin secretion. There are changes in both the amount and timing of melatonin rhythm (Skene & Swaab 2003). There may be reduced sensory stimuli and less awareness of time. Patients with dementia are particularly likely to experience changes in sleep patterns and circadian rhythms (Box 10.9).

Chronic illnesses may also interfere with the regulation of sleep and also reduce sleep quality. For example, people who suffer pain due to arthritis may find it difficult to get comfortable or they are woken by pain. Medication may affect sleep patterns, e.g. the person taking diuretic drugs, which increase urine production, may waken several times during the night to pass urine (see Ch. 20).

CRITICAL THINKING — Box 10.9

Sleep patterns in dementia

Frank has dementia and lives with his daughter. She tells you that he does not seem to know whether it is day or night. It is increasingly difficult to get him to go to bed and he wanders about the house at night.

Student activities

- Access the article by McCurry and Ancoli-Israel (2003).
- What changes in Frank's sleep pattern, e.g. increased daytime napping etc., might be observed?
- How can Frank's daughter improve his nighttime sleeping pattern?

[Resource: McCurry SM and Ancoli-Israel S 2003 Sleep dysfunction in Alzheimer's disease and other dementias. Current Treatment Options in Neurology 5(3):261–272]

ETHICAL ISSUES — Box 10.10

Waking a patient/client

Dan, who has severely depressed moods, is an inpatient in an acute mental health unit. He finds it difficult to get to sleep and wakes very early in the morning. Dan went to bed quite early at 22.00 hours and had just fallen asleep when the nurses realize that he has not had his medication.

Student activities

- Consider the choices available to the nurse in charge (see Ch. 7).
- Think about what you would do and discuss this with your mentor.

Factors disrupting normal sleep patterns

Many factors can disrupt normal sleep patterns, both in terms of quality and quantity of sleep. Disruption to normal sleep patterns is usually caused by a combination of several factors. These include lifestyle factors, environment, psychosocial factors, physiological factors, physical and mental health problems and the effects of medication.

Nurses in all care settings can help to eliminate factors which disrupt or prevent sleep and promote those which enhance relaxation, rest and sleep. However, there will be occasions when it might be necessary to disturb a person's sleep in order to perform observations or give care or medication. This is best avoided if possible, and simple measures such as revising medication timing or doing observations without waking the person should be considered (Box 10.10).

Box 10.11 Jet lag

Travelling through time zones causes the biological body clock and circadian rhythms to be desynchronized with the new environmental timing. The effects, which are more marked if travelling east, include:

- Symptoms of loss of sleep, e.g. headache (see also sleep deprivation, p. 255)
- Disrupted sleep pattern, i.e. unable to sleep at night, early waking and daytime sleepiness
- Reduced efficiency
- Low mood.

[Resources: (No author listed) 2004 Clinical facts. What you need to know about . . . jet lag. Nursing Times 100(36):30; Revell VL, Eastman CI 2005 How to trick Mother Nature into letting you fly around or stay up all night. Journal of Biological Rhythms 20(4):352–365

Lifestyle factors

Lifestyle factors and changes in daily routines can disrupt normal sleep patterns. These may include:

- A change in the person's usual pre-sleep routines can prevent sleep. These routines may be disrupted by being in hospital or nursing home
- Eating a heavy meal late at night can cause discomfort
- Inappropriate diet in infants can lead to bouts of colic that disrupt sleep for the infant and prevent parents/carers from getting sufficient sleep (see Box 10.8, p. 256)
- Constipation may be a cause of sleepless nights in all age groups (see Ch. 21)
- Waking due to hunger
- Consumption of high levels of caffeine contained in coffee, tea, cola-type drinks and chocolate can increase the time taken to get to sleep
- Nicotine from tobacco smoking causes problems falling asleep, staying asleep and may cause daytime sleepiness. Interestingly, nicotine patches may cause a reduction in REM sleep and early morning waking
- Drinking alcohol leads to a speedier onset of sleep but disrupts sleep patterns later in the night and affects the quality of sleep
- Longer or different work schedules such as shift changes, working or studying late into the evening. Shift working is discussed further below
- Travel through different time zones leading to 'jet lag' (Box 10.11)
- Overstimulating play or using some computer games near to bedtime can prevent children getting to sleep
- Strenuous exercise or energetic play near bedtime. Although fatigue due to moderate programmed exercise/physical activity can promote relaxation and a good night's sleep, exercise too late in the evening can extend the time it takes to fall asleep (sleep latency)
- Frequent late nights socializing can disrupt sleep patterns.

Shift working

People whose work routines involve rotational night shifts may experience difficulty adjusting to changes in sleep patterns. The work schedule forces the person to sleep against the biological 'body clock' when it perceives it is time to be awake and active. Sometimes it takes several weeks before a person's biological body clock can adjust to the new bedtime hours.

Nurses who are subjected to changing shift work patterns may report feeling rundown, physically exhausted, irritable and have difficulty staying alert when at work. The health of nurses working shifts including nights has consequences for patient safety. Suzuki et al (2004) found there to be significant associations between medical errors, e.g. incorrect patient identification, drug errors, etc., and being mentally in poor health, with night or irregular shift work, and age. A review by Monk (2005) concludes, 'older people have more trouble coping with shift work'. This has important implications for the UK nursing profession, where 28% of registered nurses are over 50 years of age (NMC 2005).

Research studies with night shift and overtime workers indicate that interruptions of sleep patterns can aggravate existing medical conditions and increase the risks of cardiovascular, gastrointestinal and reproductive dysfunctions (Scott 2000).

Environment

External factors including temperature, ventilation, lighting and the level of noise adversely affect the ability to fall asleep and remain so. These factors can be a problem in all care settings including the person's own home. Nurses should be aware that people in health/social care settings might take some time to adjust to sleeping in a strange environment. People discharged home or being nursed at home can also find their sleep disrupted, e.g. by having to have their bed downstairs. Examples of the many external factors that disrupt sleep patterns include:

- Noise levels such as that caused by other patients, staff, equipment or activity in hospital. Paradoxically, a person may find it difficult to sleep if they move to a quieter environment such as a care home in a rural area when they are used to city centre noises
- Lighting – some people need complete darkness to sleep whereas others such as babies and children may need the reassurance of low-intensity lighting
- Temperature – being too hot or too cold. The ward/room temperature may be the problem or the amount of bedding. Infants may sleep better if swaddled in a blanket but overheating has been associated with sudden infant death syndrome (SIDS) (Box 10.12).

HEALTH PROMOTION Box 10.12

Minimizing the risk of sudden infant death syndrome

Sudden infant death syndrome (SIDS) (also known as 'cot death') is the unexpected sudden death of an infant. Overheating, a prone sleeping position, being in an environment where people smoke and respiratory illness and infection have all been highlighted as risk factors.

Advice for parents/carers includes:

- Put babies down to sleep on their backs and at the foot of the cot to prevent them wriggling under bedclothes (Fig. 10.4)
- For the first 6 months have the baby sleep in a cot in your room
- Do not have your baby in bed with you if you or your partner is very tired, have had medicines, alcohol or drugs that can make you drowsy or are a smoker (The Foundation for the Study of Infant Deaths 2005). Be aware that you could suffocate your baby if you fall asleep and roll on it. The baby could also get trapped between the bed and the wall, or fall out of bed
- Do not let your baby get too hot. Overheating can be caused by having too much clothing or bedding, or having the room too hot
- Do not let anyone smoke in the same room
- Always obtain advice from a health professional if your baby appears unwell.

[Resource: The Foundation for the Study of Infant Deaths. Online: www.sids.org.uk/fsid Available July 2006]

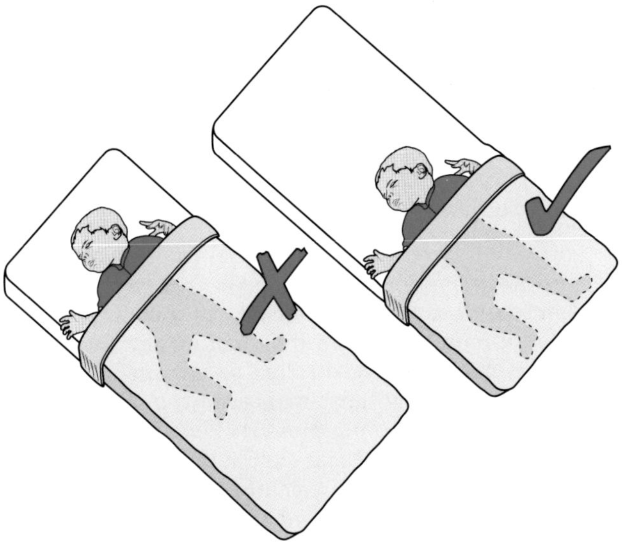

Fig. 10.4 Feet-to-foot sleeping position (reproduced with permission from Fraser & Cooper 2003)

- Poor ventilation – a 'stuffy' ward and odours associated with other people can prevent sleep
- Having to sleep in a room with strangers
- A strange or uncomfortable bed and bedding
- People who usually share a bed with a partner or a pet animal may find it difficult to sleep alone in a single bed
- A change in normal bedtime routine is also a factor.

As discussed earlier, nurses should be aware that patients/clients might become exhausted when they are continually disturbed for observations and nursing care. Some health/care units advocate a rest period after lunch when the ward/floor/unit is closed to visitors and only essential observations or procedures are undertaken during this period (see Box 10.1, p. 252). This ensures that patients/clients are undisturbed and allowed to relax, rest or sleep for a period during the day. In areas such as high dependency or intensive care units an effort should be made to differentiate day from night by, where possible, decreasing noise and the light intensity and keeping interventions to a minimum for a period during the night.

Psychosocial factors

Most people have experienced a sleepless night prior to an interview or an exciting event. It is easy to appreciate that a person who is constantly worrying about finances, work-related issues or having surgery may find difficulty in falling asleep. Emotional problems and anxiety caused by stress and life events throughout the lifespan, e.g. starting school, a new sibling, moving house, children leaving home, retirement or bereavement, can disrupt sleep (see Chs 8, 11). Children may worry about being accepted at school or be affected by relationships with siblings and parents. Adolescents and young adults often have anxieties about relationships, their appearance, exams and employment prospects.

Mental health problems

People with some mental health problems such as anxiety disorders, bipolar disorder (depressed mood or mania), dementia (see p. 257), eating disorders and disordered thought processes may have disrupted sleep patterns. Sleep disruptions can include hyperactivity, difficulties getting to sleep, early waking and excessive sleeping (hypersomnia).

Physical and physiological changes

Changes in physiological parameters, e.g. changes in body temperature and biological rhythms such as hormonal cycles, can disrupt sleep. Some women experience disrupted sleep patterns in the days before menstruation. The hormonal and physical changes of pregnancy may disrupt sleep patterns, e.g. having to pass urine frequently during the early weeks and again towards the end, or difficulties in getting comfortable in bed. Sleep disruption can also be associated with the hot flushes and night sweats experienced by some women as hormone secretion declines during midlife.

Physical health problems

Physical health problems can disrupt normal sleep patterns. Any condition that causes pain or physical discomfort can result in problems with falling asleep or staying asleep. For example, the pain of arthritis, nighttime cramps or restless legs syndrome (RLS) and itching/irritation of skin rashes are among the diverse factors that disrupt sleep.

Most nurses can relate to having a cold and the discomfort of nasal congestion, which prevents or disturbs sleep. People with cardiac or respiratory disorders may be short of breath and may need to sleep sitting up in bed or a chair (see Ch. 17). Those who have episodes of chest pain and irregular heart beats are often afraid to go to sleep because of the fear of a heart attack at night. People with high blood pressure often feel tired and may wake up very early in the morning.

Problems such as indigestion or pain from a peptic ulcer may prevent sleep or wake the person in the night. Changes in weight can contribute to a poor night's sleep. For example, severe weight loss and decreased body mass index (BMI) (see Ch. 19) associated with an eating disorder can disrupt sleep. Although people with a higher BMI tend to sleep better, those who are overweight or obese are at risk of sleep apnoea (see Box 10.15) due to the fat stored around the neck making breathing more difficult.

People who have problems with the urinary system often have to get up during the night to pass urine (nocturia) (see Ch. 20). Nocturia disrupts the sleep cycle and getting back to sleep may be difficult. In older people, nocturia may be caused by heart or kidney disorders, or enlargement of the prostate gland in older men. It is worth noting that this further disrupts sleep in a group who are already sleeping less well at night.

Many problems such as back injuries or joint deformities may force people to sleep in positions to which they are unaccustomed. Assuming an awkward position while attached to monitoring equipment in hospital, or an i.v. infusion, or having a leg in plaster or in traction can interfere with sleep.

People who cannot change their own position in bed, such as those with severe physical disabilities or following a stroke, can suffer discomfort and disrupted sleep. Box 10.13 provides an opportunity for you to consider how a restricted sleep position could affect sleep.

Effects of medication

People who take medication, either prescribed or over-the-counter (OTC), herbal products or illicit drugs may experience sleep disruption. This may be due to side-effects or interactions of the medications with other medication or alcohol, food or beverages. If the medications are required for treatment of chronic illness, e.g. diuretics, it may be necessary to review the dosages and time of administration in order to prevent disruption of sleep. Drug groups that may disrupt sleep include:

- Beta-blockers, e.g. atenolol, may disrupt sleep and cause nightmares
- Diuretics, e.g. furosemide (frusemide), may lead to nocturia
- Some antihistamines, e.g. chlorphenamine (chlorpheniramine), may cause daytime drowsiness
- Antidepressants, e.g. fluoxetine, may cause sleep disturbances – insomnia or drowsiness.

REFLECTIVE PRACTICE — Box 10.13

Sleep positions

Consider a patient/client you have nursed who has had to sleep in a particular position due to their condition.

Student activities

- How has this affected their sleep patterns?
- What nursing interventions were used to overcome the problems?

REFLECTIVE PRACTICE — Box 10.14

Medicines that disrupt sleep patterns

Think about common medications used for the patient/client group in your placement.

Student activities

- Find out if any of the common medications are likely to disrupt sleep patterns or cause daytime drowsiness.
- Are patients/clients routinely informed about side-effects and interactions with other medicines and alcohol?

[Resources: *British National Formulary (BNF)* – www.bnf.org.uk; *BNF for Children* – www.bnfc.org Both available September 2006]

The effects of caffeine, nicotine and alcohol on sleep patterns are outlined above (see p. 258).

Nurses should ensure that people are forewarned about any prescribed or OTC medicines that can affect sleep and advise them to read enclosed information and any warning labels (Box 10.14). Patients should be asked to seek advice if sleep disruption occurs.

Sleep disorders – an outline

Sleep disorders cover a wide range of conditions affecting both adults and children. These include insomnia, snoring, sleep apnoea, narcolepsy, sleepwalking, etc. The commoner sleep disorders are outlined in Box 10.15 but readers requiring more information are directed to Further reading (e.g. World Health Organization 1992, Chokroverty 2000). Fuller coverage of the general interventions to promote sleep is provided below (pp. 262–266).

Sleep disorders will have individual physical effects but they also have a huge psychosocial impact on every area of life. This might include problems with education and study, work and relationships. For example, parents/carers or partners may be prevented from sleeping by snoring, or by anxiety about a loved one who has sleep apnoea or who sleepwalks.

It is important for the nurse to be aware of any limitation of skill in this specialist area. The person/carer/parent who complains of a sleep disorder should be advised to seek specialist help at a sleep clinic and offered

Box 10.15 **Sleep disorders**

Insomnia

This may take several forms – difficulty in falling asleep, difficulty remaining asleep or an inability to go back to sleep after awakening. It may be temporary, lasting a few nights, or may become chronic. Typically the complaint is of insufficient quantity and quality of sleep, but frequently the person obtains more sleep than they realize. Insomnia can affect any age group and causes tiredness/sleepiness, depression, anxiety, lethargy and irritability during the day. A vicious circle develops where worrying about not sleeping prevents the person from getting to sleep.

Management includes interventions to promote sleep, such as good sleep hygiene (rituals to enhance settling and sleep), pre-sleep routines, reducing anxiety, relaxation and improving the sleep environment (see pp. 264–266). If sleep does not occur it is better to get up, read or have a drink and then go back to bed. Sleeping tablets should only be prescribed in the short term such as during hospitalization for surgery. Specialist help may be needed if the problem is not resolved and becomes chronic.

Narcolepsy (excessive somnolence)

This results when sleep–wake regulation mechanisms are not functioning properly. It commonly occurs during the teenage or young adult years. There is excessive daytime sleepiness culminating in a 'sleep attack'. During the 'sleep attack', the person exhibits sudden muscle weakness (sleep paralysis), being unable to move and falling to the ground. REM sleep can occur within minutes. The 'sleep attacks', which happen several times a day, can happen at inappropriate times, e.g. during meals. The person may experience hallucinations and insomnia.

Narcolepsy requires investigation and treatment by a specialist sleep clinic. The person is advised to inform others of the condition. Good sleep hygiene, such as pre-sleep routines and enhancing the sleep environment, is crucial for these patients. Maximum support is needed at home, in the workplace or at school/college.

Sleep apnoea

This is characterized by pauses in breathing – apnoea due to periodic upper airway closure during sleep. This results in a cycle of apnoea–awakening–apnoea throughout the night, disturbing sleep and making it difficult to reach NREM stages 3 and 4.There is also daytime sleeping and risk of accidents. The sudden awakenings are associated with an increase in blood pressure that may eventually lead to an increased risk of strokes and coronary heart disease (see Ch. 17). The condition is more common in men and in people who are overweight or obese (see Ch. 19). Their partners may report very loud snoring and disturbances to their own sleep as a result.

Sleep apnoea requires investigation and treatment by a specialist sleep clinic. Patients should lose weight and avoid alcohol in the evening. If severe, continuous positive airway pressure (CPAP) may be considered (see Ch. 17). Upper airway surgery may be performed.

Sleepwalking (somnambulance)

This occurs during stage 4 NREM sleep and mostly affects children. About 15% of children aged 5–12 years do quiet sleepwalking. After a brief sleep period, they sit up, eyes open, walk purposefully with an unsteady gait and do strange things, e.g. urinating in the wardrobe. Afterwards they may proceed directly to bed again. Adults can also be affected, particularly if anxious or stressed, and may resume sleepwalking as they once did as children. Sleepwalking may be accompanied by violent behaviour.

Management focuses on preventing injury while the person is sleepwalking. It is best to simply watch sleepwalkers to ensure their safety (and that of others), and perhaps guide them gently back to bed, rather than trying to wake them up.

Sleep/night terrors

These commonly occur in stage 4 NREM sleep. The child sits up and screams. They are clearly terrified but are unable to vocalize the source of the fear. They may have some recollection but it is usually very brief and quickly forgotten. However, the arousal is sudden and causes the body to respond physiologically with sweating, an increased heart and respiratory rate and the strong feeling of fear (this also occurs in nightmares). The child may appear to be hallucinating and pushing an imaginary object or person away. Sleep terrors may be accompanied by violent behaviour. Parental attempts to console are not recognized and rejected. Eventually the child falls asleep.

When caring for a patient/client suffering a night terror, it is important to remain calm and reassuring with a quiet, steady voice. It is best to be sure that the person is alert and knows who you are prior to touching or comforting.

Nightmares

These occur predominately during REM sleep. These are dreams that induce a powerful emotional arousal, often causing sudden awakening.

Nurses can provide reassurance by reminding patients/clients where they are and telling them that they are safe, as they may be disorientated when they wake up. Sometimes a drink or a chance to talk helps to calm their fears. An increase in the amount of lighting in the room may help.

(Contd)

(Continued)

Bruxism (teeth grinding)
This usually occurs in stages 1 and 2 of NREM sleep. It may occur in children when the first dentition has erupted. In older children it may be related to anxiety and stress. Bruxism can cause tooth damage and misalignment. Relaxation therapies and talking through anxieties may be helpful (see p. 265 and Ch. 11). Dental and/or orthodontic interventions such as a nighttime mouthguard may be needed to prevent damage to the teeth.

Other sleep disorders
These include jet lag (see p. 258), shift work sleep disturbance (see p. 258), sleep paralysis, nocturnal enuresis (see Ch. 20), those associated with mental health problems (see pp. 257, 259) and neurological conditions such as epilepsy.

Note: Children with Down's syndrome and other learning disabilities may show several sleep disorders, some of which may be due to physical problems, e.g. disordered breathing and sleep apnoea. Sleep deprivation and related daytime behaviour problems are also apparent (Stores et al 1996).

CRITICAL THINKING Box 10.16

Sleep problems and learning disability

7-year-old Molly has a learning disability. She lives at home, attends school and regularly goes into respite care to give her parents a break. Molly has always been difficult to settle at night but now she becomes distressed at bedtime, pulling her hair and screaming. She only sleeps for 2–3 hour periods and wakes her parents every night. Molly's parents are exhausted and feel that they need help to deal with Molly's sleep problem.

Student activities

- Speak to a learning disability nurse and a health visitor and find out what advice and support they would offer Molly's parents. Ask them if they would consider complementary therapies such as aromatherapy (see pp. 271–272).
- Find out if there is a sleep clinic in your area.
- Are there any special services/schemes such as those provided by Sleep Scotland in your area? Sleep Scotland provides help for families with children with special needs whose severe sleep problems can disrupt family life.

[Resources: Gates B (ed) 2002 Learning disabilities. Towards inclusion. 4th edn. Churchill Livingstone, Edinburgh, Chs 10, 20; Sleep Scotland – www.sleepscotland.org Available July 2006]

information about support groups, e.g. The British Snoring and Sleep Apnoea Association (see 'Useful websites', p. 274). Parents/carers should be encouraged to discuss any sleep problems with their health visitor, children's community nurse or learning disability liaison nurse (Box 10.16).

Nursing interventions to promote sleep, rest and relaxation

The nurse plays a key role in helping patients/clients to obtain sufficient sleep and rest. A holistic nursing assessment that includes normal rest and sleep patterns and pre-sleep routines is central to planning interventions that promote rest and sleep. Patients/clients or parents and carers may also be asked to keep sleep diaries where sleep patterns are disrupted. In addition, this part of the chapter will consider sleep hygiene/pre-sleep routines/rituals and the sleep environment and the role of relaxation, orthodox medications and herbal medicines in promoting sleep. In all of these measures, it is vital to involve the patient/client/child, parent or carer in the assessment and decision-making about appropriate interventions and in evaluating their effectiveness.

Nursing assessment of sleep

It is important for the nurse to have an understanding of the patient's/client's normal sleep pattern and habits in order to plan appropriate interventions and detect departures from normal. Most people suffer disruptions to sleep patterns at some time and the nurse should note whether there is difficulty in falling asleep, frequent waking during the sleep cycle, early wakening or oversleeping and the degree to which the quantity, quality and consistency of sleep are affected.

A holistic assessment should include information that includes:

- How culture, beliefs and religious practices influence their sleep pattern
- The person's understanding of the functions and importance of rest and sleep
- Normal pre-sleep routine, e.g. milky drink, warm bath, a child having a bedtime story, reading
- Sleep environment. For example, do they have their own room, whether a child has a light on in their room and any special toys or 'comfort' items, whether the person shares a bed, or sleeps in a chair
- What time they go to bed
- The length of time it takes to fall asleep (sleep latency)
- Usual duration of sleep in hours
- Whether they wake in the night
- The time they wake up in the morning
- Whether they feel refreshed following a night's sleep

- Does the person feel that their sleep pattern is normal?
- What helps the person to fall asleep or sleep better and what prevents sleep?
- Do they dream or have nightmares?
- Any recent changes in sleep patterns – onset and duration of the problem
- The factors known to affect their sleep pattern such as being alone in the house or being away from home, menstrual cycle, time of year
- Measures taken to promote sleep if normal patterns are disrupted, e.g. altering bedtimes, complementary therapies, using OTC sleeping tablets or herbal medicines or prescribed sleeping tablets
- Do they nap during the day?
- What time is their last large meal?
- Do they have a snack before bed or wake in the night to have a snack?
- Do they smoke or consume caffeine or alcohol in the evening?
- Current lifestyle, work and domestic relationships, social activities including play–rest–sleep patterns for children
- Worries, stress and anxieties that may be affecting sleep, e.g. worries about the health of a loved one, debts, exams
- Ongoing emotional problems such as relationship difficulties
- Usual medication, OTC, herbal medicines, prescribed drugs and use of illegal drugs
- Other therapies, e.g. counselling
- History of conditions, e.g. RLS, migraine or joint pain, that might affect sleep
- History of previous sleep problems such as insomnia
- Recent changes in health status
- Changes in behaviour, e.g. a child who is upset at bedtime after the arrival of a sibling, or increasing daytime sleeping in an older adult with dementia
- Change of environment such as moving into a care home
- Changes to routine such as starting school, different work pattern or shift times, travel across time zones or a new baby in the house.

Keeping a sleep diary

When sleep patterns are disrupted or a sleep disorder is suspected, patients/clients, parents or carers are encouraged to keep a diary. Initially, this can be for 1 week. The contents can help to identify the main problems and highlight factors that relieve or exacerbate sleeplessness. The diary can be used as a tool to assess progress and efficacy of interventions used to improve the person's sleep pattern. Initially this can prove tedious to document but once a routine is developed, it becomes easier. In the author's experience, most people who have a severe sleep problem would do anything to resolve it. It is very important to accept the person's interpretation of their sleep pattern/sleep disruption, even if it does not agree with your own analysis.

It is important to explain from the outset what the aims of the diary are and to support and give positive feedback to the person for persisting with the documentation. It is helpful to provide written instructions (prompters of key phrases and questions) for completing the diary (Box 10.17). Involving children in describing their sleep patterns will be enhanced by providing age-appropriate documentation, such as colouring books, cartoons depicting children sleeping/not sleeping, clock faces with movable hands or the use of stickers for hours slept.

After some time people become familiar with the requirements and 'automatic' documentation occurs

Box 10.17 Keeping a sleep diary

- Use an ordinary diary (day per page) with dates, times and space for writing
- Start the diary on the first day of the week (e.g. Monday) and finish the diary on the same day. This is because most people have set routines from the beginning of the week
- It is useful to have the diary by your bed
- Note the activity and type of meal, e.g. watched TV, snack, a glass of wine, a pizza, before bedtime, for that day
- Note the time you get into bed that night (with the intention of going to sleep)
- Note what time you fell asleep, how quickly you fell asleep or how long you took to fall asleep. If you are too drowsy to write all this down, you can document the approximate time in the diary when you awake or ask your partner (if relevant) to note this down for you
- If you waken during the night, note the time you awoke and what woke you
- If you cannot get back to sleep immediately, note the reason why; note any measures taken to help you to fall asleep again
- Note the time you wake up the next morning and what woke you up
- Note how easy it was to get out of bed in the morning and how long it took before you got out of bed
- Note how you felt when you woke up, and after 5–10 minutes, e.g. did you feel refreshed or very tired? Did you feel like going back to sleep or were you ready to get on with the day's work?
- Note the total number of hours you think you have slept
- Then work out from the diary roughly how many hours you have actually slept
- Note if you thought you had any dreams last night
- Note what your activities are for the day, e.g. important meeting or usual routine day
- Note how you felt for the rest of the day, e.g. fresh, tired, irritable, needed a nap.

Note: Include other relevant information, e.g. upset after a row with partner, period started, really worried about the electricity bill, etc.

	Monday 3rd January
	Busy day at work, got home too late to cook. Had a takeaway curry and 2 large glasses of wine at about 21.00.
22.30	Made a drink of hot chocolate and took it to bed. Tried to look through a magazine but too tired.
23.00	Settled down to sleep.
02.30	Woke up to pass urine.
03.00	Still awake. Not sure when sleep resumed - possibly after 15 min but partner said I 'tossed and turned' for half an hour.
07.00	Woken up by alarm clock, dozed for a few minutes.
07.30	Struggled out of bed, did not feel refreshed. Didn't dream but partner said that I mumbled soon after falling asleep the first time, but he couldn't make out any words. Important meeting at work this morning, very stressful. Felt really tired after lunch. Irritable during the afternoon and snapped at colleagues.

Fig. 10.5 Sleep diary entry

without the instruction sheet. Some people may prefer to use special charts with dates, times and prompters instead of a standard diary. The completion of the diary should coincide with follow-up sessions at the clinic to discuss the results with the nurse, doctor or therapist. Figure 10.5 illustrates a typical sleep diary entry.

Improving sleep hygiene and the sleep environment

Simple changes can improve sleep hygiene such as trying to go to bed and get up at about the same time each day. It is also helpful to avoid using the bedroom/bed for other activities such as working or eating. Developing a pre-sleep routine that helps the person to fall asleep and stay asleep is important. This might involve a bedtime story, a milky drink, warm bath, changing into nightclothes, teeth/denture cleaning and passing urine. In hospital or care home, the nurse should try to maintain the person's pre-sleep routine as far as is possible, and offer assistance as required.

People should be given advice about eliminating factors known to disrupt normal sleep patterns (see pp. 257–260). This might include reducing strenuous physical activity in the evening and encouraging quiet play for children. Some people may need to reduce caffeine intake, e.g. by replacing tea or coffee with fruit or herbal teas. Avoiding an excessive fluid intake just before bedtime can minimize nocturia in children and older people. However, they must have sufficient fluids during the day (see Ch. 19). Others may need to eat their main meal earlier in the evening and have a small bedtime snack. A bedtime snack should be available in hospital or care home if necessary. Excessive daytime sleeping or naps may disrupt sleep at night and people may need advice about reducing naps.

REFLECTIVE PRACTICE Box 10.18

Aiming for silence

Sleep can be difficult to achieve if noise levels are too high or if the type of noise changes. Noise will affect sleep in every setting including the person's home.

Student activities

- Stop and listen to the noise one night in your placement. What types of noise are present?
- Reflect on ways to reduce noise, e.g. talking quietly, reducing the loudness of telephone ring tones at night.
- Find out what design/structural features have been used to reduce noise such as double glazing.

Some patients/clients may wish to carry out religious activities such as prayers before sleep, or need their bed in a position that allows them to face the correct way, i.e. towards Mecca. Some people will want to see a local religious leader or read from a particular holy book. These facilities and privacy should be made available.

It is important to promote sleep by ensuring comfort and providing an environment conducive to sleep before medication is considered. The many simple interventions that promote sleep, either at home or in a care setting, include the following:

- Many adults need a dark environment in order to sleep. Making sure that curtains are drawn and are sufficiently thick is important. Where light is still a problem, such as from streetlights, the person may use eyeshades. As already mentioned, some children can only sleep if there is low intensity light in their room or in a corridor. Some care settings for older adults may also provide minimal lighting to reduce confusion on waking and to reduce the risk of falls if the person gets out of bed
- Reducing noise to a minimum (Box 10.18)
- Check the environmental temperature before bedtime to ensure it is neither too hot nor too cold
- Good ventilation. Some people like a window open. Electric fans may be used on hot summer nights
- Provide a relaxing atmosphere – reduce the lighting in the evening, listen to music, read

- Children can engage in a relaxing/soothing activity before sleep, e.g. colouring, a bedtime story
- Complementary therapies (see pp. 266–273) can be used to enhance relaxation. For example, some herbal products are mildly sedating, e.g. chamomile, lavender and lemon balm (see below and pp. 269–270)
- Try to reduce ward activities well before bedtime
- Ensure bedding is adequate and comfortable, and that pillows are arranged for sleep. Some people in long-term care may want to use their own pillows/pillow cases, but always check local policy and safety issues
- Ensure a comfortable sleep position by using, for example, supportive dressings, splints, extra pillows or a firm mattress if preferred by the patient/client. A old mattress that no longer supports the spinal column should be replaced
- For infants and toddlers make sure that they are clean and dry and change nappies as necessary. Many infants will settle more easily if they have physical contact such as cuddling and touch by gently massaging their head or abdomen or back. Others are comforted by wrapping in blanket, but beware overheating (see p. 259). Quiet singing, music or humming may also help to relax the infant/toddler and promote sleep
- Patients/clients who have pain will require analgesics and/or other pain-relieving measures (see Ch. 23)
- Feeling secure is important in promoting sleep. For example, a child needs to know that parents/carer are downstairs. People receiving care at home need the reassurance of knowing when the care team will visit and how to get help. In hospital/care home people feel more secure if they know who is caring for them. Therefore the night staff should walk round to see everyone before bedtime.

Relaxation and sleep

Anyone who is suffering from altered sleep or significant sleep disorders often complains of feeling stressed, anxious and tense and not being able to relax (Box 10.19). Several research studies have highlighted the efficacy of complementary therapies in improving sleep patterns. Most of these therapies are effective in inducing relaxation and so offer an important clinical contribution to stress-related sleep disorders. For further coverage of relaxation techniques and their uses in a variety of situations such as stress and pain, see Chapters 11 and 23.

In a study by Lichstein et al (1999) participants who received relaxation therapy reported additional benefits that included improved sleep efficiency and reduced withdrawal symptoms during a sleep medication withdrawal programme. Massage and relaxation therapy comprising muscle relaxation, mental imagery and music improved sleep in older patients with cardiovascular illness nursed in a critical care unit (Richards 1998). In a study by Chen et al (1999) acupressure and massage therapy improved the quality of sleep in older people. Herbal medicines are considered below and the wider uses of herbal medicine on pages 269–270.

REFLECTIVE PRACTICE Box 10.19

Relaxation and sleep

Think about a patient/client who has difficulties with relaxing and getting to sleep.

Student activities

- What strategies have you seen the registered nurses, family or carers use to help the person relax at bedtime?
- Find out what relaxation therapies, e.g. massage, are available locally.
- Discuss with your mentor how you can promote sleep by helping patients/clients to relax.

Orthodox medications

Medication may be used to aid rest and sleep for patients/clients who cannot sleep despite the non-pharmacological interventions discussed above. The cause of insomnia should be known; for example, 'sleeping tablets' may be prescribed for a patient who is in hospital following surgery and cannot sleep because of noise. The drugs used to aid sleep include hypnotics (drugs that induce sleep), anxiolytics (drugs such as tranquillizers that reduce anxiety) and analgesic drugs (painkillers) (see Ch. 23). In addition, the dose of antidepressant drugs, such as amitriptyline and mirtazapine, can be adjusted and taken at night to improve sleeping in people suffering from depression. However, hypnotic and anxiolytic use has a number of disadvantages, including:

- Changes to the amount of the time spent in different sleep stages
- Daytime sleepiness and a 'hangover effect' with some hypnotics
- Increased risks of falls in older people
- Tolerance develops to hypnotics after continuous administration of a few days and for this reason they should only be prescribed for short periods: one or two doses for transient insomnia and no longer than 3 weeks for short-term insomnia. Ideally they should only be used for a week with some doses omitted (*British National Formulary* 2005)
- Withdrawal symptoms when discontinued
- Rebound insomnia when discontinued
- Vivid dreams when discontinued.

Examples of the medications used to aid sleep are provided in Box 10.20 (see p. 266) but readers requiring more specific information about indications, side-effects, contraindications, etc. should consult the *British National Formulary*.

Herbal medicines

Valerian (*Valeriana officinalis*), hops (*Humulus lupulus*), lemon balm (*Melissa officinalis*), passion flower (*Passiflora incarnata*), chamomile (*Matricaria chamomilla*) and lavender (*Lavandula angustifolia*) have all been traditionally used in herbal medicine for treating restlessness and sleep disturbances.

Box 10.20 Examples of orthodox medication used to aid sleep

- Benzodiazepines, e.g. diazepam, nitrazepam, temazepam
- Clomethiazole
- Antihistamines, e.g. diphenhydramine
- Zaleplon, zolpidem and zopiclone
- Antidepressant drugs, e.g. amitriptyline, mirtazapine.

Note: Barbiturates are very rarely used for insomnia and only for people already prescribed them for severe insomnia which is resistant to treatment. They should not be prescribed for older people. Hypnotics are not generally used for children, but may be prescribed for sleepwalking and night terrors.

[Resource: *British National Formulary* – www.bnf.org.uk Available September 2006]

It is very important to advise people to avoid self-medication with OTC products, especially herbal products, which are advertised to promote sleep. These products may interact with the person's prescribed conventional medications. It is always safer to consult a trained herbal practitioner who can advise the patient and ensure that the most appropriate herbal remedy is available to help promote sleep in that individual. The principles of herbal medicine are covered more fully on page 269–270.

Box 10.21 Perceptions of CAM

- Individualized care
- A combination of treatments tailored to people's specific needs
- CAM therapists were more friendly
- More time is spent with each person/client
- Person/client receives more information on their disease and its treatment and in simple language as CAM practitioners are more likely to use everyday language (see Ch. 9)
- Consultations are more thorough and take longer
- Therapists actively listen to the person/client
- Therapists show more interest in other aspects of person's/client's life, not just their physical symptoms, including personality, life experiences and social network and support
- Focus is on the person/client, not the disease
- Increased person/client involvement and a wider choice of treatments and management
- Increased touch and less technical equipment
- Increased level of hope and optimism
- Social issues are explored, thus helping the person/client to understand their problem/illness in the context of family and work
- A holistic approach may mean that the person/client can make sense and understand more about the illness because it becomes more personally relevant.

[From House of Lords (2000)]

Complementary and alternative medicine

Complementary and alternative medicine (CAM) refers to the health-related therapies, which are not considered to be part of conventional (mainstream) or allopathic medicine. These therapies tend to be health interventions practised by different cultures over thousands of years. Some CAM therapies offered in conjunction with conventional medicine are described as complementary, e.g. aromatherapy (see pp. 271–272), whereas others, such as osteopathy, provide diagnostic information and are offered as an alternative to conventional medicine. CAM therapies are very diverse. The British Medical Association (1993) concluded that there was no common principle linking the therapies and that there was diversity in approach and delivery.

It is clear that most CAM therapies differ from conventional medicine management in their approach and underlying beliefs, principles and philosophies. It should be noted that there is no one single philosophy shared by all CAM disciplines. Some CAM philosophies are linked to religious practices of the country of origin. They have evolved over centuries of use and are incorporated into interpretations of body functions, health and disease. The majority, if not all, of CAM therapists believe that their view of care embraces all dimensions of the person so there is less divide between the body, mind and spirit, hence the term 'holistic' is often used.

The emergence, development and regulation of CAM

In the late 1980s and early 1990s there was an increase in interest and wider use of CAM in the UK by both the general public and health professionals, especially nurses. Several studies suggest that there were approximately 50 000 CAM practitioners and, of these, 10 000 self-registered practitioners offered CAM alongside conventional care. Five million people consulted a CAM practitioner in 1995. People accessed CAM through CAM practitioners, through other health professionals, including doctors, nurses and physiotherapists who offered CAM, or by purchasing OTC products. These data, though limited, suggest that the public are very interested in CAM. This popularity is not confined to the UK; surveys conducted in Australia, the United States and Europe suggest that the public there are equally keen to use CAM. In Europe, however, a slightly different approach exists in that CAM is practised alongside conventional medicine (DH 1996, Budd & Mills 2000). Several surveys reporting on patient/client satisfaction and the popularity of CAM have identified certain themes and characteristics of CAM therapies (Box 10.21).

Box 10.22 Categories of CAM therapies

Group 1 therapies
These include acupuncture, chiropractic, herbal medicine, homeopathy and osteopathy.
Viewed as the 'big five' in CAM, these offer diagnostic skills, appear to be the most organized and already have an established research base for some aspects of practice. There is increasing NHS provision for the therapies in this group.

Group 2 therapies
Aromatherapy, the Alexander technique, massage, counselling, stress therapy, hypnotherapy, reflexology, shiatsu, meditation and healing form this group. They are often used to complement conventional medicine and do not include diagnostic techniques. There is some NHS provision for these therapies, especially in palliative care settings and with people with a learning disability.

Group 3 therapies (groups 3a and 3b)
3a – Ayurvedic medicine and traditional Chinese medicine (TCM).
3b – Crystal therapy, iridology, radionics, dowsing and kinesiology.

[Adapted from House of Lords (2000)]

This widespread use of CAM raised concerns about having in place rigorous structured regulations to protect public safety and interests. There was a need to consider several related issues such as an evidence base for research, adequate training for practitioners, information resources for the public and what prospects there were for NHS provision of these therapies. These concerns prompted a House of Lords Select Committee report (House of Lords 2000) and the government's response the year after (DH 2001). The report noted that there was a wide range of therapies under CAM (Box 10.22). Some therapies had complete systems of assessment and treatment whereas others complement conventional treatment with various supportive techniques. While some were well regulated, others were very fragmented with no consensus about regulation.

Chiropractic and osteopathy are already self-registered and self-regulated which means that their professional activity and education are regulated by Acts of Parliament. Practitioners must be registered with the General Chiropractic Council or General Osteopathic Council, respectively, in order to practise in the UK.

Integrated medicine

Despite the wide diversity of CAM and its popularity, access to CAM via the NHS remains limited. It would seem that CAM could have a potential role in the management of care in the NHS alongside conventional therapies. A steering committee was set up by the Prince of Wales to consider how CAM and orthodox healthcare in the UK could work more closely together.

The Foundation for Integrated Medicine (now known as the Prince of Wales's Foundation for Integrated Medicine) aims to promote the development and integrated delivery of safe, effective and efficient forms of healthcare. The Foundation encourages greater collaboration between practitioners of all forms of healthcare. Operating as a forum, it actively promotes and supports discussion and acts as a centre to facilitate development and action. Its objective is to enable individuals to promote, restore and maintain health and well-being through integrating the approaches of orthodox, complementary and alternative therapies (Foundation for Integrated Medicine 1998). Hence many practitioners now consider the term CAM to be slightly outmoded and that it is more appropriate to use 'integrated medicine' or indeed 'interprofessional health care' instead.

CAM therapies

This part of the chapter outlines the scope and main characteristics of the 'big five' CAM therapies – acupuncture, chiropractic, herbal medicine, homeopathy and osteopathy – and some of the others, e.g. aromatherapy, that have been integrated into conventional healthcare.

It does not lay claims for efficacy. Where treatment and conditions are linked, it serves only to highlight that a particular treatment exists rather than the author's or editor's opinion or recommendation.

The language used to describe elements of a particular therapy such as 'vital force', 'holism' and 'energies' are existing terms related to that therapy.

Readers requiring information about other therapies such as humour therapy, shiatsu, massage, therapeutic touch, etc. are directed to Further reading (e.g. Rankin-Box 2001).

Acupuncture

Acupuncture has been widely practised in China since the first century BC. It involves the insertion of small needles into specific points on the surface of the body. In the 1970s, it gained wide publicity in the West where it is used mainly for pain relief. Currently in the UK, registered medical practitioners and other healthcare professionals practise acupuncture. At the time of writing acupuncture is not subject to statutory regulation. However, the results of a consultation on the statutory regulation of herbal medicine and acupuncture were published in 2005 (DH 2005) and publication of draft legislation, followed by legislation, is planned.

Acupuncture is a heritage of traditional Chinese medicine (TCM), which also includes the use of herbs, diet, massage, acupressure and relaxation through special exercises. The fundamental principles of TCM are based on the belief that a person functions in harmony with the universe. So health, disease and treatment relates to a person's harmony or disharmony with external forces of wind, damp, dryness and cold, and internal anger, excitement, worry, sadness and fear. Elements such as wood, fire, earth, metal and water are used to describe various states of health and illness. Illness is also defined by two complementary, but opposite, forces – yin and yang – and their perfect balance within the body, which is essential for good health. Yin represents cold, damp, darkness, passivity and contraction whereas yang signifies heat, dryness, light, action and expansion. The interaction of yin and yang gives rise to 'qi' (pronounced 'chee'). Qi is an invisible life energy and is a vital force that flows around the body through meridians or energy channels. There are 12 regular meridians, which run down the body in pairs, six on the left and six on the right.

The meridians are mostly named for the main internal organs through which they pass, e.g. the lungs or kidneys. The even circulation of qi around the body is essential for health. Disruption of flow on a meridian can create illness at any point along it, e.g. a disorder in the stomach meridian (passing through the upper gums) could cause toothache. There are about 365 points along the meridians at which qi is concentrated and can enter and leave the body. It is possible to affect the circulation of qi at these points and acupuncturists insert the acupuncture needles to stimulate or suppress its flow. This is thought to influence the health problem by restoring energetic balance and organ function.

During the first consultation, a standard and thorough interview to establish the presenting problem, past medical history and a physical examination is required. Specific questions and examination related to acupuncture would include:

- Inspection of 'trigger points' related to the pain and reflex points on the trunk
- Evaluation of the strengths and weaknesses of the internal organs by examination of the ear, tongue and pulse.

The treatment involves the insertion of tiny needles in the area of the body where the blocked energy to the circulation network is identified (Fig. 10.6). The needle is usually left in place for 5–20 minutes. However, it is important to protect the person/client from energy depletion so a much shorter time is used for a person who is very tired or frail and old.

If additional activation of the acupuncture system is required, the stimulation is achieved by connecting the needles to an electrical device, by moxibustion (heating the needles with burning mugwort – an aromatic herb) or by gentle manual manipulation of the needles.

Weekly treatments are scheduled until a good response to treatment is obtained, after which follow-up treatments can be every 4–6 weeks or further apart.

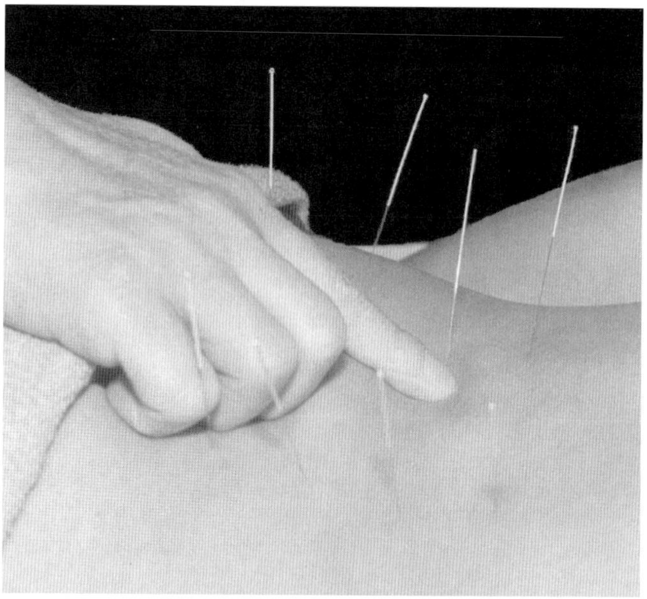

Fig. 10.6 Acupuncture needles in situ (reproduced with permission from Zhu 2005)

> **CRITICAL THINKING** Box 10.23
>
> **Acupuncture in orthodox healthcare**
>
> Orthodox practitioners, e.g. physiotherapists and anaesthetists, use acupuncture to relieve pain and induce sleep. Research by Andrzejowski and Woodward (1996) concluded that sleep patterns in healthy adults improved.
>
> **Student activities**
> - Is acupuncture available in your area of practice?
> - Arrange to talk to a health professional who uses acupuncture to relieve pain and/or promote sleep.
> - What are the contraindications to the use of acupuncture?
>
> [See Further reading, e.g. Rankin-Box (2001)]

Integration of acupuncture into conventional healthcare

The type of acupuncture which is more commonly integrated into orthodox healthcare is 'Western medical acupuncture'. This is acupuncture that has been adapted and is practised by orthodox medical and other health professionals in the West. In some areas of the UK it is available on the NHS. It uses the same needling technique as traditional acupuncture described above but works by affecting nerve impulse transmission and the central nervous system. Acupuncture is effective for anaesthetic and analgesic (see Ch. 23) purposes, especially for musculoskeletal complaints (Box 10.23). Other uses include substance misuse (e.g. smoking cessation), in maternity care, migraine, high blood pressure and digestive disorders. Although traditional acupuncture described above is now a widely accepted Eastern therapy, medical opinion is still divided on its efficacy.

Chiropractic

The term chiropractic comes from the Greek words *cheiro*, meaning 'hands' and *prakticos*, meaning 'doing'. Together this means 'done by hand' or manipulation. Developed in the late 19th century by David Palmer, a Canadian osteopath, chiropractic diagnoses and treats disorders of the spine, joints and muscles. Chiropractics use their hands to manipulate joints and adjust muscles by high velocity, short amplitude thrust and gentle soft tissue massage.

With these techniques the health of the central nervous system and body organs is maintained through realignment of the nerve supply to the affected area. Chiropractic is used to treat musculoskeletal complaints by relieving pain, increasing mobility and improving function.

A chiropractic views the body as a mechanical structure with the key being the spine, which links the brain to the rest of the body. Therefore, any distortion of the spine affects the working of other parts of the body and the reduced 'nerve flow' leads to disease. Chiropractics believe that treatment can ease muscle tension caused by stress or those linked to problems in some internal organs such as the intestine. When the skeletal structure functions smoothly, the body's natural healing processes are free to keep all body systems working in harmony. When body systems are in harmony it is believed that the body has the ability to heal itself from within.

During the initial consultation a detailed case history of the presenting problem, past medical and surgical history as well as lifestyle factors are explored. For example, the person/client is asked about exercise and type of bed used. A full clinical examination of the condition and function of the spinal column will be carried out by asking the person/client to adopt different postures, e.g. lying down, sitting and standing.

Diagnostic procedures include X-rays, neurological tests including reflexes, 'motion palpation' to check the spine and use of a rubber-tipped instrument called an activator. The 'activator' delivers a very small thrust and is used to manipulate the vertebrae. The activator can be used for very frail older people and even babies.

Treatment, usually during the second session, entails using controlled techniques with the hands to adjust and 'unlock' any joint problems. The person/client may hear the joints 'click' during the manoeuvres but these are painless. The first session takes about an hour and subsequent sessions about 20 minutes. The person/client may experience some muscle aches and pains for a few days after the treatment and should be told that this can occur and be reassured that it is normal. Initially the person/client is required to attend two to three times per week with follow-up visits of weekly sessions until the problem is resolved. Chiropractics recommend 'maintenance' visits 6–12 monthly to keep recurring problems at bay. Surgery is never used by the chiropractic and if the problem requires specialist treatment the person/client will be referred to their GP.

Integration of chiropractic into conventional healthcare

A study by Meade et al (1990) reported that chiropractic treatment for low back pain (severe or chronic) was more effective than standard outpatient care. They concluded that consideration be given to introducing chiropractic into the NHS. A follow-up study (Meade et al 1995) confirmed the earlier findings.

Chiropractic can also be used to treat neck and spine problems, muscle, joint and postural problems, sciatica, migraine, sports injuries and gastrointestinal disorders. In the UK, chiropractics are subject to statutory regulation and must register with the General Chiropractic Council in order to practise. Some orthodox practitioners are also trained chiropractics.

Herbal medicine

Over 80% of the world's population use herbs for health maintenance. Herbal medicine, one of the most ancient forms of treatment, is used by every culture to treat disease and promote well-being. It is a system of medicine that uses plants and plant extracts as remedies to treat disorders, promote and maintain good health. There are several subcategories practised in the UK, namely Chinese herbal medicine, Tibetan herbal medicine, Ayurvedic herbal medicine and Western herbal medicine (also called phytotherapy or phytomedicine). Chinese herbal medicine is an integral part of and practised with TCM and acupuncture. This chapter focuses on Western herbal medicine. At the time of writing herbal medicine is not subject to statutory regulation. However, the results of a consultation on the statutory regulation of herbal medicine and acupuncture were published in 2005 (DH 2005) and publication of draft legislation, followed by legislation, is planned.

Conventional medicine uses laboratory-produced drugs which, although derived from plants, are often refined until a single active ingredient has been isolated. Herbal remedies differ from these synthetic drugs in that parts of a whole plant are used as the remedy. Western herbal medicine is a holistic treatment system that seeks to restore the body's self-healing mechanism or 'vital force'. Remedies are prescribed, tailored to the holistic needs of the person, not just the symptoms of the illness. Rather than treating symptoms in isolation, the herbal practitioner looks for the cause of illness such as poor diet, an unhealthy lifestyle or excessive stress, which may have overburdened and imbalanced the body's delicate homeostatic physiological, psychosocial and spiritual domains. Practitioners attribute disease to a disruption in the maintenance of the body's state of harmony or homeostasis. Herbal remedies promote healing by supporting the body's vital force in its efforts to restore homeostasis.

The herbal practitioner's skills lie in knowing the actions of different plant constituents on specific body systems. For example, a plant, or indeed a part of it, may stimulate the circulation or calm the digestive system.

Herbal synergy is a key factor in medical herbalism. According to this theory, parts of whole plants are more effective than the isolated constituents used in synthetic drugs. Herbal practitioners believe that the synergy gives a greater and better therapeutic effect. For example, meadowsweet (*Filipendula ulmaria*), which can be used to treat digestive disorders, contains salicylic acid, the basis of the widely used drug aspirin. However, while aspirin can cause gastrointestinal bleeding, meadowsweet contains tannins and mucilage that protect the stomach lining (Mills et al 2000).

Herbal remedies are extracted from leaves, flowers, fruits, stems, bark, roots, rhizomes, seeds or exudates (e.g. frankincense resin) and other parts of a whole plant which contain a complex mix of active ingredients that produce the plant's medicinal effects. This use of strictly plant products is unlike other herbal traditions (e.g. Chinese herbal medicine) where non-plants (e.g. insects, shells, minerals, animal bone or organs) are also used.

Herbal remedies can be made from combinations of herbs or from a single herb.

Remedies can be given to people/clients in several different ways. These include:

- Infusions of plant parts infused with boiling water (herb teas)
- Tinctures of plant products extracted in alcohol
- Oils
- External applications such as creams.

Every herbal remedy is said to have three effects on the body: to detoxify and eliminate wastes, to strengthen it and help it heal itself and to build up the organs.

The first consultation takes about 1½ hours. A detailed case history of the presenting complaint, past medical history, social history, medications and lifestyle factors are discussed. Diet history is an important aspect of the assessment. If deemed necessary, physical examinations related to the presenting complaint – for example, using a stethoscope to auscultate the lung fields or the heart, or a neurological examination – will be carried out. The management plan is then discussed with the person/client. The relevant remedy could be a tincture or a combination of herbs, teas or creams. The first review is normally at 2 weeks and if the condition is responding well to treatment, follow-up will be at intervals of 4–6 weeks. People's/clients' involvement in their own healing is important and they are advised to actively engage in making lifestyle changes encompassing social context and self-responsibility. Complex cases should be referred to the GP or another appropriate health practitioner and the person/client advised that herbal treatment is not suitable in some cases.

Integration into conventional healthcare

In the UK, some hospitals and GP practices have part-time Western herbal practitioners working within the multidisciplinary setting. However, people/clients who are using herbal treatment are usually self-funding. In Europe, e.g. Germany and France, Western herbal medicine is practised by conventionally trained physicians and integrated into routine medical care. These consultations and treatment, therefore, generally follow the principles of a conventional medical appointment. Herbal medicines can be used to treat a range of diverse conditions including musculoskeletal disorders, menstrual irregularities, anxiety and nervous tension, as well as gastrointestinal upsets. For example, colic in babies may be reduced by the use of dill (*Anethum graveolans*) and fennel (*Foeniculum vulgare*). These may be prescribed as teas for breastfeeding mothers or as tincture drops in juice for older children (Scott & Barlow 2003).

There is a dearth of controlled studies on the efficacy of herbs, especially those used to enhance sleep, and this is an area where nurses can engage in collaborative research with herbal practitioners (Box 10.24).

EVIDENCE-BASED PRACTICE — Box 10.24

Herbal medicine

'As a registered nurse, midwife or specialist community public health nurse you have a responsibility to deliver care based on current evidence, best practice and, where applicable, validated research when it is available.'

Nursing and Midwifery Council (2004, clause 6.5, p. 10)

Student activities

- Consider the extract from The NMC *code of professional conduct* in relation to the use of herbal remedies such as valerian for insomnia.
- Talk to a herbal practitioner about the evidence, to date, for the efficacy of valerian or, if this is not possible, access the articles below and search the literature for further evidence.

[Resources: Coxeter PD, Schluter PJ, Eastwood HL et al 2003 Valerian does not appear to reduce symptoms for patients with chronic insomnia in general practice using a series of randomized n-of-1 trials. Complementary Therapies in Medicine 11(4):215–222; Houghton PJ 1999 The scientific basis for the reputed activity of valerian. Journal of Pharmacy and Pharmacology 51(5):505–512; Leathwood PD, Chauffard F, Heck E, Munoz-Box R 1982 Aqueous extract of valerian root (*Valeriana officinalis*) improves sleep quality in man. Pharmacology, Biochemistry and Behavior 17(1):65–71; [Reference: Nursing and Midwifery Council 2004 The NMC code of professional conduct: standards for conduct, performance and ethics. NMC, London]

Homeopathy

Derived from the Greek words *homoios*, meaning 'like' and *pathos*, meaning 'suffering', homeopathy is a system of medicine that uses remedies prepared from plant, mineral and animal substances. These remedies are taken by mouth in tablet, powder or liquid form or applied as creams.

Hippocrates, in the 4th century BC, proposed that a substance which mimics an illness can be used to cure it. This principle of treating 'like with like' was later developed into homeopathy in the 18th century by a German doctor, Samuel Hahnemann. According to this principle or Law of Similars, 'like cures like', so a substance that produces symptoms similar to the disease can be used to cure the disease. Thus a person's symptom is used as a guide to finding the remedy. For example, being stung by nettles produces a rash, redness and inflammation. The same herb when prepared as a homeopathic remedy can be used to treat allergic reactions producing the same symptoms. Another example is eyebright (*Euphrasia officinalis*), an irritant herb, which can be used to soothe inflamed eyes.

The Law of Potentization in homeopathy relates to the idea that the more a remedy is diluted the more potent it is to heal but at the same time the 'potential' to cause side-effects is reduced. In a typical dilution, one drop of the 'mother tincture' (preparation of the plant material in alcohol) is diluted in 99 drops of alcohol, and then shaken vigorously in a process known as succussion.

Homeopaths view symptoms of illness as a sign that the body is using its natural powers of self-healing to fight back. Accordingly, the body is integrated with a vital force, which maintains it in a state of health. If the body is put under strain, illness can result. Homeopathic treatments stimulate the body's self-healing ability rather than suppress symptoms of the illness.

The first consultation takes about 1½ hours. The person's/client's detailed medical history as well as lifestyle, diet, physical and emotional factors (e.g. mood, likes and dislikes), sleeping patterns, reactions to weather conditions and personality traits are discussed. This exploration of the person's/client's problems and needs is essential so that the best matching remedy can be prescribed. The appropriate remedy may be an animal, plant or mineral preparation, e.g. sepia (cuttlefish ink), aconite (monkshood) and nat mur (sodium chloride) (Phatak 1988). Homeopaths put less emphasis on physical examination and believe that for longstanding problems it is necessary to review the treatment over numerous consultations where the prescription can be altered according to the changes in the symptoms presented.

Integration with conventional medicine

Both medically and non-medically qualified practitioners practise homeopathy. Some GP practices can refer people to a homeopathic hospital.

Osteopathy

The term is derived from the Greek *osteon* 'bone' and *pathos* 'disease'. Dr Andrew Taylor Still, a doctor in the American Civil War in the 19th century, developed this therapy. Osteopaths see the organs of the body as supported and protected by the musculoskeletal system. The bones, joints, muscles, ligaments and other connective tissue provide a framework or scaffolding for the body. If this scaffolding is correctly aligned and working well, the tissues and systems of the body will be healthy.

The initial consultation takes about 1 hour. After diagnosis, massage and manipulation are used to improve mobility of joints and soft tissues. The osteopath will try to look for the reasons behind the fault in the musculoskeletal system. A holistic approach will help to restore the body's ability to heal itself. All aspects of lifestyle, physical, mental and emotional health are seen as important factors influencing physiological health. Poor posture or injury can affect the musculoskeletal system causing pain, strain, impaired local or systemic nerve function and affect the vital organs and body systems. Manipulation of misaligned joints and a focus on soft tissues (muscles, tendons, etc.), treatment to relax muscles and bring back joint mobility will be used. Initially weekly sessions may be necessary until the problem is resolved; follow-up can be 4–6 weekly.

Integration into conventional healthcare

Osteopathy was the first complementary therapy to be subject to statutory regulation (Osteopaths Act 1993). The General Osteopathic Council ensures that practitioners are trained and regulated according to statutory requirements in order to protect public safety and interests. In the UK, osteopaths must be registered with the General Osteopathic Council in order to practise.

The therapy is well supported by many GPs who refer people for NHS-funded osteopathy.

Alexander technique

This is a form of education rather than a therapy where the person is trained to avoid 'bad habits' which give rise to poor posture and then learn to readjust to body alignment. An Australian actor called Frederick Alexander developed the Alexander technique in the late 19th century. The technique is based on the theory that the way a person uses their body affects their general health.

The Alexander technique encourages people to optimize their health by teaching them to stand, sit and move according to the body's natural design and function. This is, in essence, a taught technique and can be taught on a one-to-one basis to any age group.

During the first consultation, the person is asked to go through a series of movements so that their posture and body alignment can be assessed. The first treatment session involves lying down, relaxing the body and light adjustments are made if necessary. Subsequent sessions involve the person sitting or standing while the teacher adjusts posture and re-educates the person to use muscles with minimum effort and maximum efficiency. Further sessions entail different movements involved with standing, moving, sitting, lying down, walking and lifting objects. A session lasts 30–45 minutes, usually twice weekly, and a course may be 15–30 sessions depending on the person's progress.

Integration into conventional healthcare

Although the Alexander technique is not likely to be available on the NHS, most GPs are aware of it and referrals are increasing. It can be used by all age groups and is deemed safe when taught by teachers who have received proper training.

Aromatherapy

Ancient cultures in China, Egypt and India used plant oils combining their medicinal properties with the ancient art of massage. The modern use of plant oils is attributed to a French chemist, Rene Gattefosse, who coined the term 'aromatherapy' in 1937.

Plant material such as flowers, leaves, stems, roots and barks yield oily substances that are refined into 'essential oils'. Distillation (subjecting the plant material to steam till vaporization) is one method of extracting the oils. There are many essential oils, including those extracted from tea tree (*Melaleuca alternifolia*), common lavender (*Lavendula angustifolia*) and frankincense (*Boswellia carterii*). Other oils – known as 'carrier' or 'base' oils – used with essential oils for making massage blends are marigold (*Calendula officinalis*) and grapeseed (*Vitis vinifera*) (Mills et al 2000). A study of lavender essential oil concluded that it reduced restlessness during sleep in a small sample of older people (Hudson 1996). Lewith et al (2005), in a pilot study to evaluate methodology and the efficacy of the aroma of lavender on insomnia, report that women and younger participants improved more than others. In their conclusion the authors indicate that the outcomes favour lavender, and recommend that a larger trial be conducted to draw definitive conclusions.

A few drops of the essential oils diluted in the carrier oil can be absorbed into the body in several ways. These include:

- Through the skin – during massage, a compress or when added to bath water
- Through inhalation – using steam inhalers or a diffuser in a room. Oil molecules enter the nose and reach the central nervous system via the olfactory apparatus and olfactory nerves.

Oils with specific properties can be selected to invigorate or relax the person and induce sleep by influencing mood, emotions and physical well-being (Price & Price 2006). Aromatherapy may be used for simple relaxation but it can be useful in a wide range of conditions that include insomnia, restlessness, stress, anxiety, muscle pain, migraine and other headaches, etc.

The first session involves a holistic history-taking regarding medical history, lifestyle factors and essential oils likes and dislikes. An essential oil blend is selected and used in a full body massage or selected areas of the body appropriate to the client's needs. Advice about home treatments using oils for baths or diffusers may be recommended as appropriate. An initial consultation and massage session may take up to 2 hours. Follow-up sessions usually take about 1 hour if it is for a full body massage. A course of treatment may entail weekly sessions for 4 weeks and fortnightly or monthly thereafter. It is common for clients to have a series of treatment sessions.

Integration into conventional healthcare

Nurses have long promoted the use of aromatherapy as an adjunct to improving patient/client care. Most NHS settings, including hospitals, have set protocols for the practice of aromatherapy by registered practitioners and these must be followed. Aromatherapy can be used for a range of patients/clients in diverse settings. These include people with mental health problems, people with learning disabilities, primary care, intensive care, pain clinics, in wound care and palliative care (Box 10.25).

REFLECTIVE PRACTICE Box 10.25

Aromatherapy in healthcare practice

Think about the patients/clients on your placement.

Student activities

- Reflect on situations where aromatherapy might have been helpful in calming a patient/client so that they could rest or sleep.
- Find out if aromatherapy is available to patients/clients in your area of practice.

Reflexology

In reflexology therapy, pressure is usually applied to the feet, but sometimes to other body parts including the hands or ears to assess the person's health, treat disorders and promote well-being.

Foot massage was practised in China about 5000 years ago and Egyptian tomb paintings depicted men manipulating the feet and hands of others. The basis for reflexology is that there are invisible zones running vertically through the body so that each organ/structure has a corresponding location in the foot, e.g. the urinary tract (Fig. 10.7).

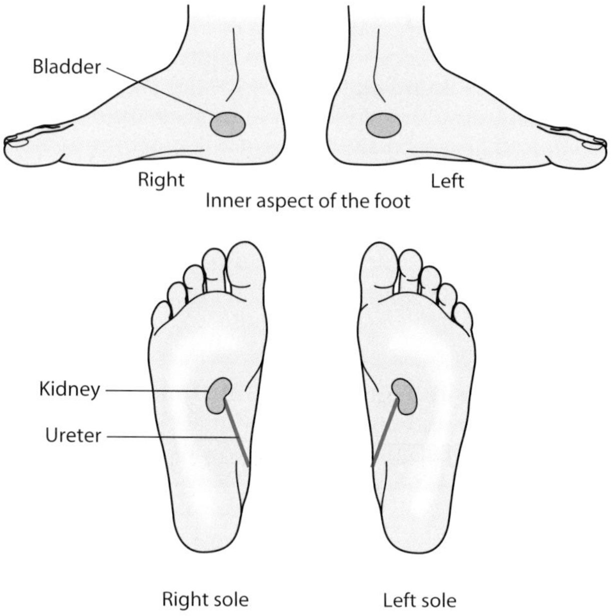

Fig. 10.7 Reflexology pressure points on the feet

To the reflexologist, the feet and hands are a mirror of the body and reference is made to maps of the feet and hands which identify pressure points corresponding to organs and parts of the body (Gillanders 1998). The theory of reflexology suggests that accumulations of waste matter concentrate around reflex points in the form of uric acid and calcium crystals. Treatment of reflex points stimulates natural healing powers and promotes well-being by breaking down the waste material and freeing the flow of energy along the zone.

During the first consultation, which may take an hour or so, the person's past and present health status as well as lifestyle will be recorded. The person will be asked to lie comfortably on a couch and the practitioner will examine the person's bare feet to assess for the presence of existing or potential health problems. The practitioner's hands, fingers and thumbs will stimulate reflex points all over the foot. Talcum powder or any base cream may be used to massage the feet while the practitioner works over the reflex points of the foot. Any discomfort, tenderness or pain is noted, as this may indicate the source of the person's health problem. If necessary, the person will be advised to seek further advice from their own GP.

During a treatment session, a series of movements and techniques involving application and release of pressure are used as the practitioner's hands move from one reflex point to another. A treatment usually lasts approximately 45–60 minutes and several weekly sessions may be necessary until the health problem is resolved. Some people have ticklish or sensitive feet but this is not usually a problem as the practitioner can adjust and maintain the right amount of pressure to suit individual needs.

Integration into conventional healthcare

This therapy can be beneficial in inducing deep relaxation in people, relieving anxiety and improving sleep. Reflexology is used in midwifery practice (Tiran 1996) as well as back pain and gastrointestinal disorders (Botting 1997).

Summary

- The physiological significance of relaxation, rest and sleep impacts on the emotional, cognitive and physical well-being of the individual.
- Insufficient rest and sleep can contribute to impaired judgement and increased risks of adverse effects on the care of patients/clients.
- The nurse has a crucial role in helping the patient/client to identify, manage and resolve factors contributing to sleep disturbances.
- Simple measures to prevent or alleviate sleep disturbances should be employed and medications such as sedatives should be a last resort.
- Patients/clients with serious sleep disturbances should be referred for specialist advice and management.
- Complementary and alternative medicine used by practitioners with recognized qualifications can be used to promote rest and sleep and in the management of sleep disturbances.
- The nurse should be well informed of up-to-date research findings related to relaxation and sleep and, where appropriate, participate in the research

Self test

1. Stage 4 sleep is characterized by being unaware of external stimuli (e.g. noise) or internal stimuli (e.g. hunger). True/false?
2. Light is the primary controlling stimulus for the biological clock's controlling sleep–wake cycles. True/false?
3. Normally the sleep cycle repeats once or twice in an average night's sleep. True/false?
4. During sleep apnoea, the person:
   a. Falls asleep without warning
   b. Stops breathing for short periods during the sleep
   c. Gets up and starts walking about
   d. Talks incessantly in their sleep.
5. How can the nurse improve the sleep environment?
6. Which of the following CAM therapies is subject to statutory regulation?
   a. Alexander technique
   b. Aromatherapy
   c. Homeopathy
   d. Osteopathy.
7. A friend asks you about herbal medications to help with sleep problems. You should:
   a. Say that there are plenty of OTC products available
   b. Advise them to make an appointment for consultation with a trained herbalist
   c. Look up a herbal textbook and advise your friend what to buy
   d. Ask a herbalist and pass on the information to your friend.

Key words and phrases for literature searching

Alternative therapies
Complementary therapies
Insomnia
Integrated medicine
Sleep
Sleep disorders

Useful websites

BBC – *useful information about sleep with many interactive features*	www.bbc.co.uk/science/humanbody/sleep Available July 2006
British Snoring and Sleep Apnoea Association	www.britishsnoring.co.uk Available July 2006
Cry-sis – *provides support for families with excessively crying, sleepless and demanding babies*	www.cry-sis.org.uk Available July 2006
Complementary Therapies in Clinical Practice (*journal*)	http://intl.elsevierhealth.com/journals/ctnm Available July 2006
General Chiropractic Council	www.gcc-uk.org Available July 2006
General Osteopathic Council	www.osteopathy.org.uk Available July 2006
National Sleep Foundation – *US website with useful information about sleep and interactive features*	www.sleepfoundation.org Available July 2006
Narcolepsy Association UK	www.narcolepsy.org.uk Available July 2006
Parentline – *advice about a new baby and sleep*	www.parentlineplus.org Available July 2006
The Prince's Foundation for Integrated Health	www.fihealth.org.uk Available July 2006
The National Center for Complementary and Alternative Medicine (NCCAM) – *part of the US National Institutes of Health*	http://nccam.nih.gov Available July 2006
Wikipedia – *free encyclopaedia; comprehensive information about sleep*	http://en.wikipedia.org/wiki/Sleep Available July 2006

References

Andrzejowski J, Woodward D 1996 Semi-permanent acupuncture needles in the prevention of postoperative nausea and vomiting. Acupuncture in Medicine 14(2):68–70

Botting D 1997 Review of the literature on the effectiveness of reflexology. Complementary Therapies in Nursing and Midwifery 3(5):123–130

British Medical Association 1993 Complementary medicine: new approaches to good practice. Oxford University Press, Oxford

British National Formulary 2005 Online: www.bnf.org.uk Available September 2006

Budd S and Mills S 2000 Professional organisation of complementary and alternative medicine in the United Kingdom. Department of Health, London

Chen ML, Lin LC, Wu SC, Lin JG 1999 Acupressure and insomnia in institutionalized residents. British Journal of Anaesthesia 82(3):387–390

Department of Health 1996 Complementary medicine and the National Health Service. TSO, London

Department of Health 2001 Government response to the House of Lords Select Committee on Science and Technology's report on complementary and alternative medicine. TSO, London

Department of Health 2005 Statutory regulation of herbal medicine and acupuncture: report on consultation. Online: www.dh.gov.uk/Consultations/ResponsesToConsultations/fs/en Available July 2006

Foundation for Integrated Medicine 1998 Integrated healthcare – a way forward for the next five years, a discussion document. The Prince's Foundation for Integrated Health, London

Fraser DM, Cooper MA 2003 Myles textbook for midwives. 14th edn. Churchill Livingstone, Edinburgh

Gillanders A 1998 The essential guide to foot and hand reflexology. Ann Gillanders, Old Harlow

Horne JA, Reyner LA 1988 Why we sleep – the functions of sleep in humans and other mammals. Oxford University Press, Oxford

Horne JA, Reyner LA 1997 Should we be taking more sleep? Sleep 10:901–907

House of Lords 2000 Complementary and alternative medicine: House of Lords Select Committee on Science and Technology 6th report (session 1999–00). TSO, London

Hudson R 1996 The value for lavender for rest and activity in the elderly patient. Complementary Therapies in Medicine 4:52–57

Lewith GT, Godfrey AD, Prescott P 2005 A single-blinded, randomized pilot study evaluating the aroma of *Lavandula angustifolia* as a treatment for mild insomnia. Journal of Alternative and Complementary Medicine 11(4):631–637

Lichstein KL, Peterson BA, Riedel BW et al 1999 Relaxation to assist sleep medication withdrawal. Behavior Modification 23(3):379–402

Lockley SW, Cronin JW, Evans EE et al 2004 Effect of reducing interns' weekly hours on sleep and attentional failures. New England Journal of Medicine 351(18):1829–1837

Meade TW, Dyer S, Browne W, Townsend W, Frank AO 1990 Low back pain of mechanical origin: randomised comparison of chiropractic and hospital outpatient treatment. British Medical Journal 300(6737):1431–1437

Meade TW, Dyer S, Browne W, Frank AO 1995 Randomised comparison of chiropractic and hospital outpatient management for low back pain: results from extended follow up. British Medical Journal 311(7001):349–351

Mills S, Bone K, Corrigan D et al 2000 Principles and practice of phytotherapy. Churchill Livingstone, Edinburgh

Monk TH 2005 Aging human circadian rhythms: conventional wisdom may not always be right. Journal of Biological Rhythms 20(4):366–374

Nursing and Midwifery Council 2005 Statistical analysis of the register. 1st April 2004–31st March 2005. Online. Available www.nmc-uk.org

Phatak SR 1988 Phatak's materia medica of homoeopathic medicines. Foxlee-Vaughan, London

Price L, Price S 2006 Aromatherapy for health professionals. 3rd edn. Churchill Livingstone, Edinburgh

Richards KC 1998 Massage and insomnia. American Journal of Critical Care 7(4):288–299

Rottenberg VS 1992 Sleep and memory, the influence of different sleep stages

on memory [review]. Neuroscience and Biobehavioural Reviews 16:497–502
Scott AJ 2000 Shift work and health. Primary Care 27(4):1057–1079
Scott JP, Barlow T 2003 Herbs in the treatment of children: leading a child to health. Churchill Livingstone, Edinburgh
Skene DJ, Swaab DF 2003 Melatonin rhythmicity: effect of age and Alzheimer's disease. Experimental Gerontology 38 (1–2):199–206
Stores R, Stores G, Buckley SJ 1996 The pattern of sleep problems in children with Downs Syndrome and other learning disabilities. Journal of Applied Research in Intellectual Disabilities 9(2):145–159
Suzuki K, Ohida T, Kaneita Y et al 2004 Mental health status, shift work, and occupational accidents among hospital nurses in Japan. Journal of Occupational Health 46(6):448–454
Tiran D 1996 The use of complementary therapies in midwifery practice: a focus on reflexology. Complementary Therapies in Nursing and Midwifery 2:32–37
Widmaier EP, Raff H, Strang KT 2005 Vander et al's human physiology: the mechanisms of body function. 10th edn. McGraw Hill, New York
Zhu HZ 2005 Running a safe and successful acupuncture clinic. Churchill Livingstone, Edinburgh

Further reading

Barnes J 2002 Herbal medicine: a guide for health care. Rittenhouse, London
Bazil CW 2004 Sleep, sleep apnoea and epilepsy. Current Treatment Options in Neurology 6(4):339–345
Billhult A, Dahlberg K 2001 A meaningful relief from suffering, experiences of massage in cancer care. Cancer Nursing 24(3):180–184
Charman RA 2000 Complementary therapies for physical therapists. Butterworth-Heinemann, Oxford
Chokroverty S 2000 Clinical companion to sleep disorder medicine. Butterworth-Heinemann, Oxford
Ernst E (ed) 2001 The desktop guide to complementary therapies. Mosby, Edinburgh
Mills S, Bone K 2005 The essential guide to herbal safety. Churchill Livingstone, Edinburgh
Montague SE, Watson R, Herbert R 2005 Physiology for nursing practice. 3rd edn. Baillière Tindall, Edinburgh
Payne RA 2005 Relaxation techniques. 3rd edn. Churchill Livingstone, Edinburgh
The Prince's Foundation for Integrated Health 2003 Herbal medicine regulatory working group recommendations on the regulation of herbal practitioners in the UK. The Prince's Foundation for Integrated Health, London
Rankin-Box D (ed) 2001 The nurse's handbook of complementary therapies. 2nd edn. Baillière Tindall, Edinburgh
Reet M 2003 Circadian rhythms and sleep patterns. In: Brooker C, Nicol M (eds) Nursing adults. The practice of caring. Mosby, Edinburgh
Scottish Intercollegiate Guidelines Network (SIGN) 2003 Management of obstructive sleep apnoea/hypopnoea syndrome in adults. Online: www.sign.ac.uk/guidelines/fulltext/73/index.html
Available July 2006
World Health Organization (WHO) 1992 International classification of diseases (ICD-10). 10th edn. WHO, Geneva (last updated 2003). Online: www.who.int/classifications/en
Available July 2006

11

Stress, anxiety and coping

George Hoggarth and Neil Murphy

Glossary terms

Adaptation

Arousal

Burnout

Distress

Eustress

Stress

Stressor

Learning outcomes

This chapter will help you to:

- Discuss the functions of stress and anxiety
- Identify the changes in thinking, feelings, behaviour and physiology that may occur in response to stress or anxiety
- Describe ways in which stress and anxiety can impact on health and behaviours
- Identify common work-related stressors associated with nursing
- Identify strategies to manage own work-related stress
- Identify coping strategies patients/clients/carers may use in response to illness
- Discuss how stress may impact on recovery from illness
- Outline strategies used to reduce the negative effects of stress and anxiety on patients/clients.

Introduction

The word 'stress' was originally used by Selye (1956) to describe the 'pressure' experienced by a person in response to life demands. These demands are referred to as 'stressors' and include a range of life events, physical factors (e.g. cold, hunger, haemorrhage, pain), environmental conditions and personal thoughts.

Stress is a reactive state to demands or potential demands made on the adaptive capacities of the mind and body. It is not necessarily unhealthy, as without stress people would have little motivation to act and could not feel the pleasure of achievement. In many ways stress should be considered a useful and necessary reaction in that, not only does it motivate action, it also prepares the person to take this action. Selye used the term 'eustress' to describe some of the more useful and adaptive forms of stress which enhanced a person's well-being.

However, if people lack the capacity to deal with the demands made upon them, their coping resources may be overwhelmed. In situations in which a person constantly feels under pressure with little respite, or when people experience severe trauma, the adaptive effects of stress can become harmful and may damage health. To describe these types of stressors Selye used the term 'distress'.

The first part of the chapter provides a framework for understanding the causes and effects of stress and anxiety and how these can be used to understand the potential effects on health. These ideas are developed to show how nurses, working in every setting, can apply this knowledge and the associated skills to managing their own stress and to reduce the negative effects of stress on their patients/clients/carers.

Nature of stress

People tend to associate both stress and anxiety with negative effects on health. The media frequently link work stress with health problems, e.g. heart disease, and it is easy for people to make the association between stress and mental illness. Likewise, anxiety is almost always used to refer to an abnormal state rather than a common reactive response. Both stress and anxiety do generate unpleasant feelings and can lead to problem behaviours, but people have feelings for a reason, they have a function. Even when the effects of stress and anxiety seem maladaptive, e.g. difficulty with decision-making, they can usually be explained and understood.

A good place to start in understanding stress is to think about how it may function in shaping and directing our own lives (Box 11.1).

It is important to emphasize how central stress is to life; it is perhaps the main reason people do anything. The feelings associated with stress put pressure on people to act. Taking this idea further, it could also be argued that without successful stress management, there would be less pleasure in living.

Understanding emotion

Stress and anxiety are specific emotional states, with four main elements:

- *Cognition*: The way people understand a situation, how they rate their ability to deal with the situation and considerations of different responses relate to 'thinking' or how people process information. Information processing may involve awareness, although some is involuntary and automatic. The term cognition describes all of these processes
- *Affect*: The way people 'feel' in a situation (good or bad) and how intense these feelings are is referred to as affect
- *Behavioural*: What people do and say
- *Physiological*: The internal changes that take place in order to deal with the situation.

All of these elements interact; changes in one will affect other elements within an integrated system. Emotions provide an ideal example of how the mind and body interact.

REFLECTIVE PRACTICE Box 11.1

A typical day at university

Identify a typical day at the university and recall the things you did during the day. Include getting up, the journey, study periods and break times.

Student activities

- List the things that you liked and disliked during the day and try to identify how they made you feel.
- Did anything really stand out as being particularly exciting or frustrating?
- Can you identify why you did the things you have identified and why some things stand out?

Identifying why you did these things can be difficult; you need to consider your motivation. For example, if you are successful and become a nurse you will be able to earn a living, in a job, which you (hopefully) like and which is valued by others. If you do not attend or study you risk criticism and failure. It is the demands created by the need to succeed and avoid disapproval that motivate people to act, and the anticipation of success can be linked to excitement, pride and pleasure.

Common causes of stress and anxiety

Identifying specific causes of stress is difficult because people, just in the process of living, constantly have to adapt to changes and deal with demands. People always have multiple stressors acting upon them at any one time. A common finding is that the events remembered most clearly are typically those associated with feelings.

Feeling irritated, interested, entertained, anxious and happy can all be considered as potential stressors. The fact that these feelings influence memory and make recall easier is a good example of how affect and cognition interact and influence each other.

In anxiety, a fear-like emotion, it is usually easier to identify specific causes because of the perceived threat. There also seem to be specific types of anxiety responses depending on the nature of the threat (Box 11.2).

Fear is considered to be the basic reactive emotion leading to the typical 'fight or flight' response and is usually initiated by automatic systems. Anxiety, however, almost inevitably involves conscious judgements or appraisals about situations (see Box 11.2).

Box 11.2 **The emotional effects of specific threats**

1. Threats to physical safety/personal existence and integrity, fear of death, pain, mutilation and mental health problems. These are often highly specific situations and are frequently associated with feelings of panic, obvious physical symptoms, e.g. breathlessness, and sensations of impending doom; the person is motivated to escape the threat or, in extreme situations, may freeze – the 'fight or flight' response (see p. 282). Feelings of panic are common; however, individuals who experience them so frequently that they interfere with their lives are said to be suffering from panic disorder.
2. Threats to self-image, fear of social appraisal, disapproval and ridicule are felt in many situations and are associated with more generalized anxiety. Symptoms are typically less intense but more pervasive. The person is uneasy and often feels under scrutiny. This can lead to an overestimation of negative events, motivating them to avoid situations which invite evaluation. Consequently, they may become inappropriately aggressive under pressure to act or comment. Again, these feelings are both common and useful; they help people to learn appropriate social behaviours. When the fears are excessive they inhibit social relationships and lead to generalized anxiety disorder or social anxiety.
3. Threats associated with the loss of something valued or loved (see Ch. 12) can create changes in behaviour similar to depression. The effect of the loss can become overestimated and the affective responses all-consuming. This may lead to withdrawal from social contact and apathy.

Common themes in understanding what causes stress

Despite the difficulties in identifying individual stressors there are some common themes that can be identified as causing most people some stress. People need some stimuli to keep them active and motivated. However, the ability to deal with stress differs between individuals and at a certain point coping resources can fail and performance becomes impaired. There appears to be an optimum level of arousal in which eustress is associated with staying in this optimum range and distress occurs when the stress falls outside the range (Fig. 11.1).

In this model, the arousal (heightened activity including cognitive, affective, physiological and behavioural changes) associated with stress produces the competitive edge; arousal speeds thought processes and quickens reaction. Indeed, when demands are made upon an individual, the increased arousal improves both physical and cognitive abilities in order to meet these demands. However, under- or overarousal is associated with a reduced ability to function effectively.

Change

Change is any event that requires an individual to adapt to an altered situation. Adaptation describes the changes in physiology, cognition and behaviour in response to changes in the environment. Holmes and Rahe (1967) identified a number of life changes and produced a frequently used scale to measure social readjustment. The Social Readjustment Rating Scale (SRRS) allows a person to identify recent life events; a score is allocated to each and totalled to give an overall score (Table 11.1). People who had experienced high-scoring events in the previous year were significantly more likely to become physically ill in the following year than those with low scores. It is

The Yerkes Dodson law argues that a certain level of stress improves performance, but as stress increases there is a gradual deterioration in performance.

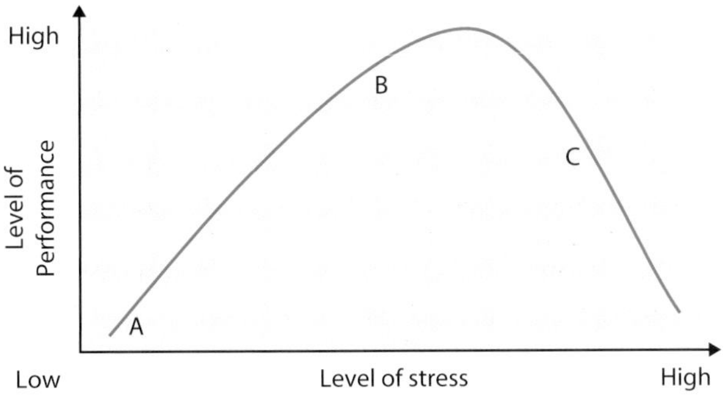

The way that stress affects people is demonstrated at 3 points (A, B and C)

A = no motivation
B = self reward related to speed and accuracy
C = reduced performance and self depreciation

Fig. 11.1 The Yerkes Dodson Law (based on Yerkes & Dodson 1908)

Table 11.1 Social readjustment rating scale (adapted from Holmes & Rahe 1967)

Rank	Life events	Life change unit
1	Death of partner	100
2	Divorce	73
3	Marital separation	65
4	Imprisonment	65
5	Death of close family member	63
6	Illness requiring hospital admission	53
7	Marriage	50
8	Dismissal from work	47
9	Marital reconciliation	45
10	Retirement	45
11	Change in health of close family member	44
12	Pregnancy	40
13	Sexual difficulties	39
14	Gaining a new family member	39
15	Employment changes	39
16	Change in financial state	38
17	Death of a close friend	37
18	Change to a different line of work	36
19	Major arguments with spouse	35
20	Major long-term financial commitment of more than £10000	31
21	Bankruptcy	30
22	Change in responsibility in work	29
23	Son or daughter leaving home	29
24	Major family disagreements	29
25	Outstanding personal achievement	28
26	Spouse begins or stops work	26
27	Moving house	25
28	Change in personal habits	24
29	Trouble with authority figures in work	23
30	Change in work hours or conditions	20
31	Change in school	20
32	Change in recreation	19
33	Change in faith activities	19
34	Change in social activities	18
35	Debts or loan of less than £10000	17
36	Change in sleeping habits	16
37	Change in eating habits	15
38	Holidays	13
39	Christmas	12
40	Minor violation of law (e.g. speeding ticket)	11
TOTAL SCORE		

Note: Scores over 300 in one year indicate an increased risk of stress-related problems and scores less than 150 indicate a low risk.

REFLECTIVE PRACTICE — Box 11.3

Everyday stresses

Think about the ongoing problems of life that cause stress and stress-related health problems. For example, being a long-term carer, reliance on public transport, stressful work, etc.

Student activities

- What everyday problems cause you stress?
- How does this make you feel and behave?
- Reflect on how everyday stresses impact on patients/clients, parents and carers.

CRITICAL THINKING — Box 11.4

Reasons for living

Try to answer the following questions:

- What are the four most important things in your life?
- What makes you feel valued?
- What, if anything, would you risk your personal safety for?

Thinking about these questions can help clarify how important social relationships and shared beliefs are.

important to remember that even events seen as positive still require adaptation and are included as stressors.

Hassles

Lazarus (1981) identified two stress measurements:

- Hassles – events appraised as harmful or threatening
- Uplifts – events appraised as positive.

While people find it easy to identify specific stressful situations, in reality it is ongoing problems of life that are the really significant causes of stress-related health problems (Box 11.3).

Stress can be seen as frustration when things do not turn out as planned; a positive slant is for individuals to view these as 'stumbling blocks'.

People

In social situations people are always aware of others and conscious of the impression they may be making; when there is uncertainty about others' evaluations they feel self-conscious and anxious. In the same way, the availability of social support is an important protector against the negative effects of stress (Box 11.4).

Interpersonal issues are extremely important; the need for acceptance and approval is so powerful it can override even survival needs. People need to feel life has value and meaning. The sense of meaning derives from other people. People appear to devote a great deal of their cognitive resources to dealing with interpersonal issues, which may also be a reflection of, or supported by, some specific inherited elements.

Mediators and the stress response

A number of more general issues also affect the nature and intensity of the stress response. Individual responses to stress and anxiety have both inherited and acquired elements, which interact within the situational context. People clearly differ in a whole range of ways in respect to personality, autonomic reactivity, physical strength, dexterity and intelligence, all of which may affect the stress response. Humans may have certain predispositions that influence stress responses such as learning and remembering. Previous experience is extremely important in moderating a person's reaction to stressors.

In addition, a number of features of the stressful events will influence the responses. These include:

- How important or significant the situation is to the person
- Unpleasant or negative events are more stressful than positive or pleasing events
- Unexpected or unpredictable events tend to cause more difficulty; people cannot plan and are physically unprepared to meet the challenge
- The intensity of a stimulus, e.g. severe pain being more stressful than mild pain
- The duration of the stressful event; stress increases with duration.

The amount of control that a person feels they have over events is also important.

The role of the unconscious

Sigmund Freud (1856–1939) suggested that a person's internal mental world was dominated by primitive, often socially and personally unacceptable, drives. In order to protect self-esteem and mental health these drives were kept out of awareness, in the part of the mind he called the unconscious. However, even though these unacceptable drives were unconscious they did continue to exert 'pressure' to come into conscious awareness and be acted upon.

In a similar way the memories of certain emotionally painful early experiences could also be kept out of awareness to defend the conscious mind from the associated pain. To manage the threat of unacceptable memories or impulses coming into consciousness, Freud suggested that people deploy a range of mental strategies he called defence mechanisms (Box 11.5 and Ch. 8). Defence mechanisms function by distorting a person's view of reality, but even so, Freud considered them to have an important role in protecting a person from psychic pain. While defences can be functional and useful in protecting people from anxiety, Freud also recognized that this protection sometimes came at a very high cost to the individual.

More recent work has emphasized how certain events or experiences, e.g. the experience of illness, activate some of the more primitive unconscious fears that everyone has.

A seminal paper by Menzies-Lyth (1959) also identified a number of ways that organizational and social structures can evolve to support an individual's defences. For nurses, these operate as depersonalization (a way of thinking

Box 11.5 Defence mechanisms

- *Humour*: A very common defence used to manage many of the unpleasant realities of nursing
- *Regression*: The reversion under stress to an earlier or more restricted level of psychological development, e.g. a previously continent child who starts bedwetting when admitted to hospital (see Ch. 20)
- *Suppression*: The dismissal of unpleasant thoughts and distraction are conscious defences everyone uses to manage unpleasant thoughts
- *Repression*: A related mechanism whereby unacceptable emotions, impulses or memories are made unconscious in order to reduce distress
- *Denial* (see repression): A person appears unaware of a stressor that they might reasonably be expected to recognize. For example, a patient/client who professes ignorance about a serious diagnosis despite clear explanation or who appears totally unconcerned about a serious health problem
- *Displacement*: The transfer of emotion away from the correct person, object or experience to a substitute in order to reduce distress. For example, a man may feel guilty following the death of a neglected parent and finding this emotion too distressing to be recognized attempts to displace the guilt about his lack of care onto the nurses by accusing them of neglect
- *Projection*: An individual projects their own unacceptable feelings onto another person in order to render their own feelings more acceptable. A nurse who dislikes a patient but who thinks of themselves as very caring might insist that the patient dislikes them, making their own feelings more acceptable
- *Intellectualization*: An attempt to deal with problems by treating them as an academic or theoretical issue and ignoring the feelings that underpin what the person is saying. This distances the nurse from the painful feelings but is often perceived by the patient as uncaring.

about patients/clients that diminishes their basic humanity and identity). When a nurse relates to a patient/client as an individual the patient's/client's pain and distress can also be very distressing for the nurse to deal with. It is often suggested that nurses should avoid emotional involvement, which in a similar way diminishes or denies the nurse's basic humanity. There is always some level of involvement for the nurse and finding appropriate ways of managing this can enhance the experiences and rewards of being a nurse. However, during periods of high work-related stress there is a tendency to reduce patient-related stress by minimizing the patient's individual distinctiveness, so instead of using names the patient may be referred to by diagnosis or bed/room number.

There can also be a tendency to make moral judgements, that some patients/clients are more deserving of care than others. Patients/clients who engage in behaviours that are disapproved of may be excluded from good healthcare or treated badly. These groups include people who self-injure, smoke or those who do not cooperate with treatment. Because some types of behaviour would be seen as unethical or even abusive, it is only through using defences such as depersonalization, detachment and denial that nurses can continue to act professionally in ways that do not reflect their personal values.

One interesting example of this sort of defence may be found in the use of the obsolete term 'psychosomatic' to describe an illness. The assumption was that psychosomatic conditions were caused by, or aggravated by, stress and anxiety, i.e. 'all in the mind'. Nurses invest a great deal of their self-esteem into their ability to help to treat illness. In addition to helping the patients/clients, this also helps to control the nurse's own anxieties in the face of illness and death. A problem arises when, despite the nurse's best efforts, patients/clients do not get better. This can be seen as a personal failure and a way of dealing with it is to blame the patient/client for the nurse's lack of effectiveness – it is 'all in their mind' and therefore their responsibility.

Identifying stressors

An important function of the development of nursing knowledge is that it allows nurses to predict and manage potential problems that may arise. Nurses need to adopt a holistic approach in an assessment to identify stressors, which includes consideration of the following influences:

- Biological
- Psychological
- Interpersonal/social/environmental
- Spiritual.

Stressors in healthcare rarely affect just the patient/client. They affect relatives, friends and of course nurses involved in their care. The way in which a person behaves in response to the stress will have a significant effect on their future. People often feel angry and irritable when stressed and if this results in aggressive behaviour, they might alienate the people that they rely upon for care and support, thus increasing future stress.

Box 11.6 (see p. 282) considers a range of potential stressors that may impact on specific care situations.

The stress response

The term stress response describes the adaptive physiological changes that take place to enhance a person's ability to deal with demanding or dangerous situations. While the adaptive changes are occurring in response to the stress situation, the internal environment, e.g. blood chemistry, must be maintained within a normal range for optimum cell function. This ability to maintain the internal environment within the normal range is known as homeostasis. Allostatic load refers to the cumulative cost to the body of maintaining homeostasis while responding to stressors; when these resources are overloaded then there is a serious risk to health.

CRITICAL THINKING Box 11.6

Identifying stressors

- Ted is being discharged home 4 days following a heart attack. He works as a bus driver and his wife works shifts in a factory. He smokes but has previously had good health.
- Rhian, who is 12 years old, is attending the day unit for her next chemotherapy treatment. Following the second treatment she suffered unpleasant side-effects. On this occasion her father, who is not known to the staff, accompanies Rhian.
- Pauline has attended the same school for years. Her parents report that she is increasingly withdrawn and uncooperative. She has been told that now she is 18 her care will be transferred to adult services and she will be moving to a day service.
- The police have brought Joseph, aged 19 years, to the unit following what is described as an attempt to burn down the family home while his parents were asleep. He is very distressed, overactive and excitable and feels everyone is trying to harm him.

Student activities

Consider the scenarios above and:

- Identify the significant stressors that may be present and who is most likely to be affected.
- Discuss this with your mentor.

When the potential need for increased mental and physical activity is established, the physiological responses that occur are regulated by two interdependent control systems:

- the autonomic nervous system (ANS), so called because this part of the nervous system is generally outside conscious control
- the endocrine system that uses chemical messaging systems (hormones) (Fig. 11.2).

The ANS is divided into the sympathetic and the parasympathetic divisions, but while periods of stress and anxiety lead to a general stimulation of the nervous system it is the effects of the sympathetic division that predominate.

The sympathetic division is responsible for mobilizing the body's resources in response to stress by releasing the neurotransmitter noradrenaline (norepinephrine) at the effector organs. The adrenal medulla (middle part of the adrenal glands) is also stimulated to release adrenaline (epinephrine) and noradrenaline into the bloodstream. Noradrenaline and adrenaline are related catecholamines, which cause effects that include the 'fight or flight' response of increased heart and respiratory rates, blood pressure, etc.

Releasing factors/hormones from the hypothalamus in the brain stimulate the pituitary gland, which regulates other endocrine structures. Pituitary hormones, e.g. adrenocorticotrophic hormone (ACTH), stimulate the release of corticosteroid hormones from the adrenal cortex (outer part of the adrenal glands). Corticosteroid hormones – known as glucocorticoids, e.g. cortisol – increase the availability of the body's energy resources, alter immune responses and generally prepare the body for action and potential injury. Other corticosteroids – known as mineralocorticoids, e.g. aldosterone – influence sodium and water retention.

Corticosteroids are involved in chronic long-term stress and also influence mood and behaviour. Table 11.2 outlines some examples of the effects of the stress response, their adaptive function and the potential impact on health.

To summarize, the sympathetic nervous system and endocrine system coordinate a response that increases available energy, endurance and pain tolerance and enhances the ability to survive injury. However, as this increased state of arousal is often uncomfortable and is costly in terms of resources, there may be negative health effects associated with both acute short-term stress and chronic long-term stress. In acute states the most significant problems are often due to behavioural changes, whereas the physiological changes occurring in chronic stress appear to increase vulnerability to a range of disorders.

Selye (1956) described the stress response as being triphasic or having three stages: an alarm stage, a resistance stage and an exhaustion stage (Fig. 11.3, p. 285). Selye's model – the General Adaptation Syndrome (GAS) – was the first real attempt to develop a general theory of stress and clarify the role of stress in health and illness. However, the model focused on the underpinning physiology and failed to adequately address psychological and social factors. Despite these problems the model has been highly influential in stress research.

Stress-related health problems

A general view of the effects of both stress and anxiety is that they evolved to influence physiology, cognition, affect and behaviour in order to increase the chances of surviving in difficult and dangerous environments. However, life has changed and the evolved mechanisms are less useful in dealing with the more complex and enduring stress associated with modern life. Stress depletes physical and mental resources while reducing control of behaviour.

Chronic stress in particular is strongly associated with a wide range of health problems because of physiological and psychological 'wear and tear' and inefficient use of energy. This may be associated with behavioural changes that increase other risks and reduce an individual's ability to deal with new challenges.

In someone with a pre-existing vulnerability, exposure to increased stress may be the stimulus to trigger illness; it may then influence recovery and other health-related behaviours. Those with existing conditions may experience a worsening of symptoms, e.g. anginal pain (see Ch. 17) or increased frequency of migraine attacks.

Sociocultural, psychological and biological variables can combine to produce a range of disorders. The interaction between these factors is now widely accepted as the only way to make sense of body functioning. Increasingly, the immune system is becoming the focus for understanding the relationship between stress and illness; this area of study is called psychoneuroimmunology.

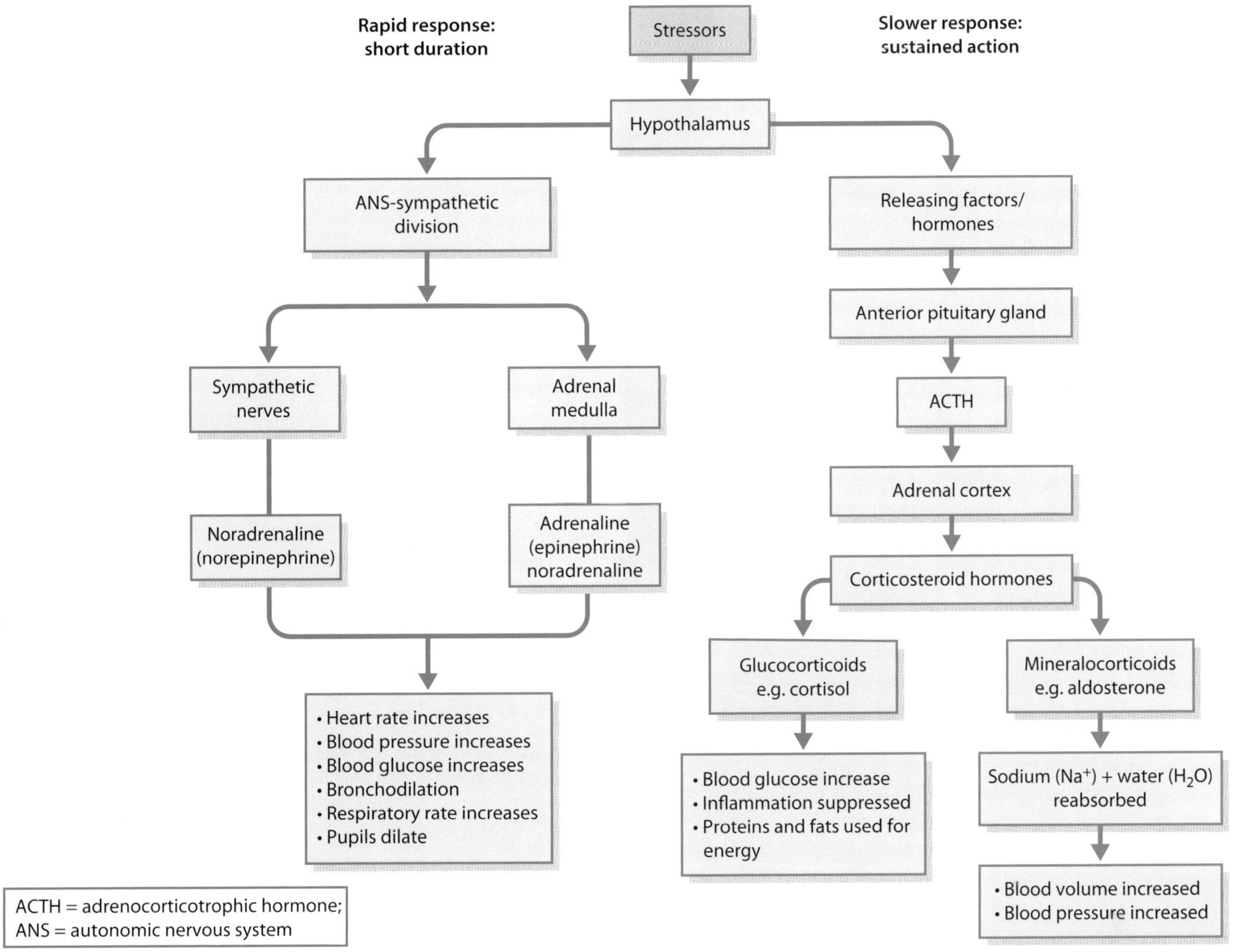

Fig. 11.2 Stress response (simplified)

Table 11.2 Stress response – effects and potential consequences

Effects	Adaptive function	Acute symptoms	Chronic problems
Physical effects			
Increased heart rate and force	Increase in blood supply to tissues	Palpitations	
Increased blood pressure	As above	Headache	Arterial disease: CHD, stroke (see Ch. 17)
Sodium and water retention	Increased plasma volume and blood pressure in preparation for injury		As above
Redistribution of blood supply	Increased blood supply to body core and large skeletal muscles	Skin pallor Gastrointestinal problems	
Increased respiratory rate and volume. Dilatation of bronchi	Increase in oxygenation	Breathlessness	Changes in blood chemistry. Panic
Increased muscle tone	Fast reaction	Trembling	Muscle pain/aches
Immune system stimulation	Migration of leucocytes into tissues	Activation of autoimmune disorders	Slower healing (see Ch. 25)

(Continued)

Table 11.2 (*Continued*)

Effects	Adaptive function	Acute symptoms	Chronic problems
	Body prepares defences in case of injury		Reduced immune surveillance Increased infection (see Ch. 15) and cancer
Increased platelet adhesiveness	Faster haemostasis in case of injury		
Increase in blood glucose and fatty acids	Increased energy		Weight gain Arterial disease. Protein used for energy reduces muscle mass
Increase in basal metabolic rate	Increased energy and endurance	Feeling hot Sweating	Exhaustion Slower healing
Cognitive effects			
Increased alertness	Increased vigilance Avoid danger	Jumpy, overreacts	Sleep disturbance (see Ch. 10)
Focus on potential threat	All mental resources available Increased problem-solving	Cannot concentrate on other things Overarousal reduces efficiency (see p. 279)	Memory disturbance
Sensitized to novel, unexpected, unpredictable, intense, uncontrollable events	Reduces risk, avoids danger	Impulsive/automatic 'fight–flight' behaviours	Avoidance behaviours lead to anxiety states Accident risk increases
Context-specific memories	Potential help in problem-solving, recall previous solutions	Intrusive unpleasant memories Mood links to memories	Negative mood state Past failure affects self-efficacy
Flashbulb memories	Situation labelled as potentially dangerous Reduces exposure to future risk	Memory and mood stay active in consciousness	Non-threatening situations labelled as dangerous Behaviour labelled as unreliable Increases hesitancy and uncertainty
Narrowing of perceptual field	Linked to focusing attention, dealing with threat is the priority	Misses important detail Focuses on irrelevant detail	Memory problems Accident risk increases
Reduced complex problem-solving relates to emotional state	Increased use of rapid automatic responses for danger avoidance	Consequences of behaviour not considered	High levels of arousal significantly impair conscious problem-solving
Rapid associative learning	Rapid identification of potential threats	High potential for association of non-threatening events with danger	Phobias
Emotional effects			
Experienced as a negative affective state	Motivates behaviour to reduce the feelings	Possible aggressive or attack behaviours Inappropriate avoidance/escape behaviours	Feels out of control Relationship or legal problems Use of drugs, alcohol and tobacco
High levels of anxiety; people may freeze	Reduces visibility to potential predators	Unable to function effectively	Reduces self-esteem Other people make judgements of competence
Emotion perceived as evidence for belief	Allows fast responses	People frequently aware that concerns are illogical and feel embarrassed	Maintain self-esteem by defence mechanisms
Managing stressors is associated with self-esteem	Learn to predict potential for effective actions	Self-esteem linked to beliefs about abilities and value	Low self-esteem associated with many mental health problems

Managing stress and anxiety

This part of the chapter outlines the general principles and methods that individuals may use in managing stress and anxiety.

The huge variation in the ways that stress presents and the ways it might affect the person mean that a range of techniques need to be considered. The main reason for this variation is attributable to the fact that, after an

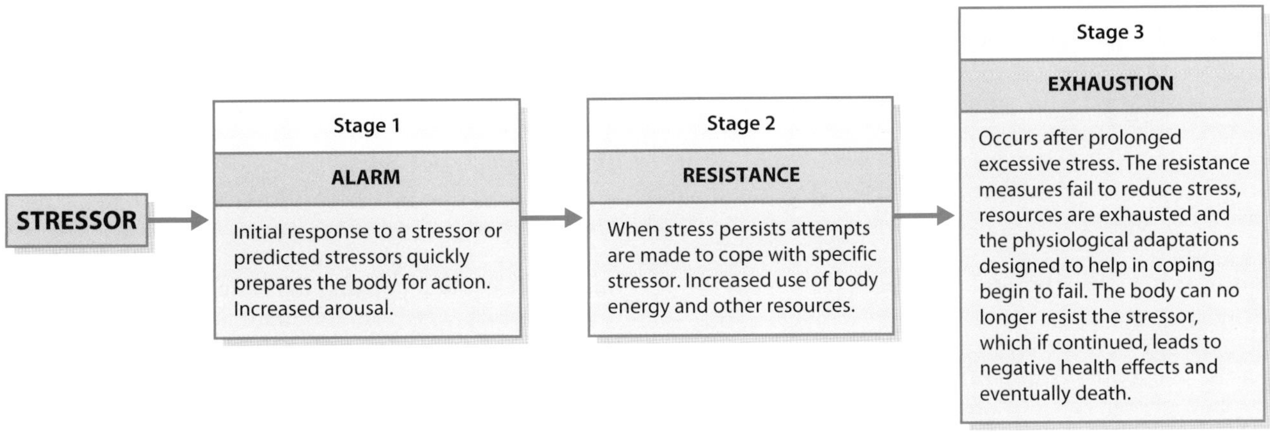

Fig. 11.3 General adaptation syndrome

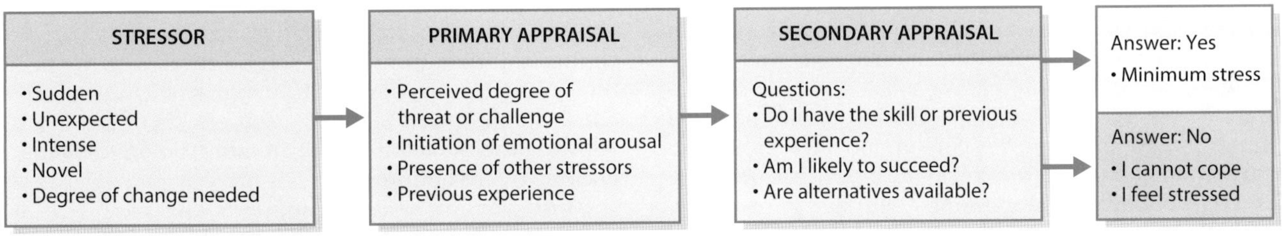

Fig. 11.4 Primary and secondary appraisal of stressors

initial, often automatic reaction to a situation (primary appraisal), people make a series of judgements which will largely control the responses (secondary appraisal).

While recognizing the role of physiology, Lazarus and Folkman (1984) suggested that an individual's previous learning and experience significantly affect the way in which they react to life events; others can look at the same event and come up with differing interpretations. In this view of stress and anxiety it is not the stimulus itself that is problematic, it is the individual's appraisal of the stimulus and their belief about their ability to manage its effect (Fig. 11.4).

This model emphasizes cognition. Judgements are made about the stressor and about the person's ability to change their behaviour or thoughts in such a way as to master or reduce the effects of the stressor. These responses are coping strategies, which may be adaptive (as in managing the event without increasing other problems) or maladaptive (in which the coping strategies might fail or increase stress). This framework is particularly important in understanding many of the principles of stress management.

Everyone uses ways of minimizing stress and improving rest and relaxation (see Ch. 10), such as socializing, reading, listening to music, holidays, etc.

The reaction to stressors/threats and other ongoing actions that people engage in are attempts to manage or modify the stressful situation or the feelings generated by it. While these responses are highly individual they can be categorized into some basic types of coping.

Avoidance

Avoidance commonly involves reducing exposure to stimuli that cause stress or anxiety, attempts to ignore the demands/threats or attempts to suppress the negative feelings. Avoidance is a very common reaction to threat when often the first reaction is to escape, thus avoiding further exposure. To ignore stressors people might engage in distracting tasks, use defence mechanisms (see pp. 280–281) or simply refuse to recognize the importance of the stimulus. People might try to induce positive feelings, e.g. by comfort eating, treating themselves or using stimulant (usually illegal) drugs, sedatives or alcohol.

People frequently resort to sedating drugs and alcohol to help manage the unpleasant feelings associated with stress and anxiety. They might attempt to 'drown out' overwhelming feelings associated with severe trauma, loss or threat by using a sufficiently high dose to induce insensibility.

Anxiolytic drugs, e.g. diazepam, can be used in similar ways during short episodes of intense anxiety or distress but, like alcohol, continued use over long periods is associated with a range of health and interpersonal problems.

Sedation does not address any of the causes or problems faced by people and while they might allow a person to cope with an acute and intense trauma they have no place in long-term management. Continued use is associated with a reduction in effective functioning and an increased risk of dependence.

Currently the role of medical intervention in responding to the normal effects of life events as illnesses to be treated is hotly debated; health staff seem motivated to attempt to remove all types of distress a person might experience. However, chronic stress and anxiety are strongly associated with problems that are considered to be diagnosable illness, depression being very common. Currently the main interventions are based on using antidepressant drugs, e.g. fluoxetine, as improving mood will improve coping.

Dealing with the stressor

The most direct approach to dealing with demands is to take action to meet those demands. This approach is often the most adaptive, particularly for low-level stressors when people can use problem-solving and evaluate the potential consequences of their actions. When the stress experienced is associated with very high levels of arousal, problem-solving is impaired and actions may not be well considered.

Among the most effective and easiest interventions nurses can use to reduce anxiety and stress is to provide useful and understandable information (see Chs 9, 23, 24). Patients/clients should know what to expect in relation to illness, recovery and specific interventions. This is important in allowing the person and their family to prepare themselves and recognize the difference between normal and abnormal sensations – without information every unusual sensation causes anxiety. Nurses may need to adapt information or ways of communicating, and seek help from family and carers when clients find it difficult to understand what is happening to them, e.g. a person with a learning disability or a person with dementia.

To deal successfully with a range of demands people learn and use a series of skills. When demands and expectations are predictable, learning useful skills can be structured and planned (Box 11.7).

When people feel confident in their abilities to control and meet demands, little stress is experienced and successful outcomes become more likely. People often experience positive feelings of achievement when they manage challenging situations and their beliefs about their coping abilities are enhanced. Assertion training by increasing skills in negotiation and relating to others may enhance this perception of control.

Explaining that anxiety is a normal response to many situations is also a useful way of giving people 'permission' to talk about anxieties. Again the nurse must be imaginative in finding ways to help people with learning disabilities or dementia to express/communicate their anxieties.

Imposing structure

In situations that involve multiple and complex stressors the ability to prioritize is important. This could involve making 'to do' lists, prioritizing demands in order of importance and managing the time available to deal with the demands. The principle here is a simple one: for life to be manageable, it needs to be managed (Box 11.8).

Controlling the emotion

Strategies are principally about changing appraisals about the situation. This could involve reassessing the importance of an event and reassessing personal ability to cope with the perceived demands. People may deliberately remind themselves of past successes in managing similar events or make positive statements about their coping abilities. Improving self-awareness helps people recognize the stressors that appear particularly important to them and to recognize the effects of stress early, allowing them to address the situation before the feelings become overwhelming.

Most current research supports the view that it is people's beliefs about the situation and their abilities to cope that control emotional reactions. Changing these beliefs can therefore alter the meaning of the situation and the responses to it. Unfortunately, the underpinning beliefs that inform the way in which people appraise threats or demands lead to habitual and automatic responses based on previous experience. Thus many people are basically unaware of why they feel like they do and as a consequence do not check the accuracy of their beliefs.

The cognitive therapies provide frameworks to help people understand these principles and techniques for re-evaluating belief systems. This involves helping individuals recognize that it is not the event that causes distress, but their beliefs about the event that lead to the

REFLECTIVE PRACTICE — Box 11.7

Dealing with stressors

A student nurse may feel anxious about doing something for the first time, e.g. giving an injection. Preparatory information can reduce anxiety and frequent practice with supervision allows the nurse to feel sufficiently confident that eventually little or no anxiety is experienced.

Student activities

- Think about a nursing intervention that caused you anxiety.
- What helped you to feel confident?

HEALTH PROMOTION — Box 11.8

Time management

Using a diary to note important events, e.g. appointments, submission dates, and keeping track of arrangements is the most effective way of controlling the demands made on time. A diary allows the person to consider the practicalities of accepting extra commitments and to prioritize how much time to devote to each issue. This allows realistic judgements to be made about how many issues can be addressed in the given time.

The diary is only a tool; the person needs to be able to use the information in negotiating their commitments with others and must be prepared to say no when necessary. These ideas help people to deal with stressors in which direct action is appropriate and likely to be useful.

emotional consequences. These beliefs then need to be made explicit and logically examined; examining the evidence for and against beliefs is the basis for disputing their validity. When individuals adopt these methods and use them continuously it is suggested that responses become more grounded in reality, rational and more likely to lead to effective management.

Ellis (1994), who developed a cognitive approach called Rational Emotive Therapy, suggests that people evaluate situations by using simple exclamatory statements about the event. Characteristically, they first make an evaluation of the event, which is sensible and rational, followed by an irrational statement about its meaning. It is the irrational statements which have little or no supporting evidence that cause the emotional reaction. Moreover, people tended to have generalized, irrational beliefs that add to stress interpretations (Box 11.9).

Table 11.3 outlines the sequence of events in creating distress and an example of ways in which people can challenge these beliefs and therefore change the feelings.

People need to identify the beliefs that cause problems and then learn to challenge them. A useful strategy is to note the events/situations which cause stress and then try to identify why they are important. As in the example, this leads to a change from thinking the event controls the feelings to recognition that it is their own beliefs and appraisals that are important. Only then can they start to evaluate their beliefs by examining the evidence on which they are based.

Enhancing coping resources

A wide range of strategies can be used to enhance coping, including:

- Increasing energy reserves by increasing 'wellness' by taking exercise, good nutrition (see Ch. 19) and adequate rest (see Ch. 10), etc.
- Taking responsibility for self-care of chronic disorders increases control and the confidence that enhances

Box 11.9 Common irrational beliefs

- We must be loved by everyone
- Everything we do must be approved of by others
- We must be competent and successful in everything
- Certain things are wrong and the perpetrators should be punished
- When things are not as we like, it is a catastrophe
- I can only be happy when things around me are going well
- It is easier to avoid difficulties and responsibilities than to face them
- Past behaviour will determine our present behaviour
- We are victims of our emotions and have no control over them so cannot help how we feel.

Table 11.3 Example of cognitive sequencing

Stage	Example
A = Activating event – actual or inferred, current or predicted	Student has to present course work to peers and lecturers
B = Beliefs – often in the form of rigid and unqualified demands in the form of 'musts', 'shoulds' and 'oughts' Appraisals are often automatic and habitual – people need to learn how to identify them	Rational appraisal: • People will be evaluating my performance • I will feel and look anxious Irrational appraisal: • My presentation must be perfect or the others will think I am stupid • If they see how nervous I am they will think I'm a useless nurse • If I can't answer questions everyone will know how ignorant I am
C = Consequences – emotional, behavioural and physiological responses to appraisal. Often unpleasant and leads to inappropriate, unhelpful behaviour	Increasing self-focus and anxiety, reducing performance Dry mouth, difficulty speaking, unable to remember points Awareness of each increases anxiety The appraisal becomes a self-fulfilling prophecy and is taken as evidence the beliefs were right
D = Disputing the disturbance-producing appraisals. Subjecting beliefs to rational evaluation. Questioning the evidence for the belief	Are you the only one who is anxious? Isn't it normal? Would you think badly of someone who is anxious? As a student why do you expect to be perfect?
E = Effective – as in the actions chosen. Those based on rational thinking are more likely to be effective in managing stressors	Seeing anxiety as normal and common and accepting that expectations about their own behaviour are unrealistic help to reduce belief Unpleasant feelings reduced with increased likelihood of appropriate behaviours

coping (see Further reading, e.g. NHS Modernisation Agency 2003)
- Learning new skills that will help in dealing with demands or feared situations more effectively
- Learning specific skills that induce feelings of calmness and relaxation, these feelings being incompatible with feeling stressed or anxious (see below).

Relaxation techniques

Over the centuries in a wide range of cultures and under various guises, the ability to relax the body and mind has been seen as an important skill, particularly for those who had to problem-solve and make effective decisions.

If an individual can reduce emotional arousal and focus their thoughts onto problem-solving, then they would be able to more clearly analyse the situations and generate solutions.

The techniques are widely used in healthcare, e.g. pain management (see Ch. 23), insomnia (see Ch. 10), even though the underpinning evidence is inconclusive. However, the feelings induced by effective relaxation techniques are usually perceived by clients as pleasant and restful and there is little evidence of side-effects or safety concerns. Using relaxation becomes more effective with regular practice.

Although there are considerable differences between individual relaxation techniques there does appear to be some common themes. These usually include:

- Control or awareness of the physical body, e.g. position, posture or specific movements
- Control of or an awareness of breathing
- A specific mental focus, e.g. words/phrases (a mantra), visual stimuli, candles, flowers, patterned prayer mats, mental images or fantasy, physical sensations and a gradual shift from external concerns to internal sensations.

Box 11.10 describes one relaxation technique but for more information about other techniques such as imagery, see Further reading suggestions (e.g. Payne 2005). These techniques can be used to help patients/clients or for personal stress management; generally they tend to be most appropriate in situations where direct action or problem-solving is unlikely to be helpful.

Complementary and alternative medicine (CAM) therapies

The role of CAM therapies in healthcare is discussed in more detail in Chapter 10. However, it is important to remember that some of these therapies are linked to particular faiths and will not be acceptable to all groups. There can also be ethical concerns about using methods that do not have an evidence base of research about safety and efficacy.

On the other hand, inducing relaxation is perhaps the one area in which many CAM therapies have shown considerable promise. Meditation, massage, reflexology, yoga and ti chi exercises can all be useful in helping a person manage the effects of stress. Massage techniques are particularly useful in children and in individuals with sensory impairment; the fact that they may reduce pain might also reduce the impact of pain as a stressor.

Box 11.10 A relaxation technique – the parasympathetic flop

- Sit or stand in a comfortable position, and focus your awareness on how your body currently feels, become aware of muscle tension, areas of discomfort and symptoms of stress
- Become aware of your breathing, consider rate and regularity. Take control of your breathing and begin using slow abdominal or diaphragmatic breathing (breathing deeply, push out the abdomen)
- On each breath out, focus on the feelings you get when all of the chest muscles relax and deliberately think about your other muscles relaxing at the same time. Let your body sag, let your shoulders drop and allow your head to lean forward
- Remain in this state, repeating the breathing exercise until you feel more comfortable and then stretch and start moving quite slowly
- Before finishing, return your attention to your body and breathing; you should find that breathing is slower and your body feels more comfortable
- With practice you should be able to relax more quickly and more deeply.

Ability to tolerate stress

Despite the wish for a predictable controllable life, everyone is faced with periods of uncertainty and feelings of helplessness in dealing with the problems of living and indeed dying. There are techniques such as the AWARE technique that people can use to improve stress tolerance. The person is encouraged to:

- **A**ccept the feelings, do not fight or avoid them. Choose to set aside time to think about the things that worry you. Replace rejection, fear or anger of the feelings with recognition and acceptance
- **W**atch it, study the feelings, be a dispassionate observer, learn about them without attempting to change anything. Avoid making judgements of good or bad, watch variations like a bystander
- **A**ct in relation to how you feel; if you want to act anxious then do so, you can also choose to act in different ways. You retain control and choice over behaviour. Slow down if you need to but keep going. The important thing is not to do things simply to avoid the feelings
- **R**epeat the exercise; the more time spent studying your feelings the better, become an expert in your own experiences. The more the feelings become an object of study the less discomfort you will experience

- Expect good outcomes but be realistic; you cannot eradicate anxiety so do not try. During monitoring you will discover variations, notice the good points and pay attention to increasing control.

The role of the nurse

The publication of *Our Healthier Nation* (DH 1998) marked a change in the philosophy of healthcare provided within the NHS. For the first time there was explicit policy direction for a service that previously had focused on treating illness to begin to focus on improving health and preventing illness. The broad and pervasive effects of stress on health, illness and recovery mean that stress management is a key theme in health promotion. Nurses in many diverse settings are often ideally placed to educate patients/clients about the nature and effects of stress. This in itself is a powerful intervention; people commonly misinterpret the effects of stress and anxiety as indicators of serious illness, increasing their anxiety still further.

Nurses can also offer advice or self-help materials to individuals in order to enhance coping skills. Holistic nursing assessment of the healthcare needs of both individuals and of specific groups should include the identification of stressors and current coping strategies used, thus allowing the nurse to offer pragmatic and practical actions that their patients/clients will find useful. The nurse in helping the patient/client to clarify the causes and effects of stress can identify the management strategies most likely to help.

A wide range of health promotion activities can influence stress and coping indirectly – information about health and illness can increase the person's sense of control. In a similar way, interventions designed to promote healthy living such as exercise advice contribute to 'wellness' and increase resistance to the adverse effects of stress.

Stress and people

This part of the chapter describes the more specific aspects of stress that relate to nurses and nursing. This includes work-related stress, which is extremely important in healthcare settings. Stress affecting patients/clients and their carers is addressed with suggested interventions for reducing its adverse effects. In many instances the more general information on causes, effects and interventions can be used to inform the nurse's actions, both in self-care and the care of others.

Stress and nursing

The Health and Safety Executive (2002) estimated that around 500 000 people in the UK were experiencing work-related stress at a level that was making them ill. They also identified that approximately 5 million workers claimed to be stressed or highly stressed in their workplace.

The type of the work that nurses undertake would suggest that it has the potential to be particularly stressful. This is borne out by research that suggests levels of occupational stress to be higher in the NHS than in similar professions. Borrill et al (1996) surveyed over 11 000 NHS staff and found that more than 28% of nurses suffered at least minor mental health problems (typically anxiety and depression) compared to about 18% of the general employed population.

This can be particularly problematic in areas of staff shortages. Harris (2001) observed that 'Health care professionals experiencing high levels of occupational stress can lead to illness, increased absenteeism, high staff turnover, unsafe behaviour and increased accident rates' (see 'Burnout', p. 290).

Employers have a statutory responsibility to provide a working environment in which hazards to health have been identified and actions taken to control exposure to these hazards. Stress has been identified as one such hazard that should be subject to the risk management process (see Ch. 13).

In addition to the increased rate of change, nursing has some features that might account for the high levels of reported stress. One important feature is that nursing is fundamentally an interpersonal activity – nurses deal with people. Many of these encounters are with strangers and in situations that are already emotionally charged where patients/clients and their families are frequently anxious, angry or distressed.

In order to understand the potential for stress it is important to realize that while most nurses would identify angry or aggressive patients/clients as causing stress there are other less obvious issues to consider. These include:

- People who, despite efforts to help them, fail to recover (see p. 281)
- People whose condition affects their verbal and non-verbal communication skills (see Ch. 9)
- People with visible signs of illness, skin lesions or disfigurement
- People who are experts in managing their condition
- People who have been victims of violence or other forms of abuse
- Anxious relatives who complain or become aggressive
- People whose behaviour is bizarre, unpredictable or aggressive
- People whose lifestyles choices may have contributed to their condition, e.g. overeating, smoking, drug or alcohol misuse, high-risk sexual behaviours.

These issues are common to many areas of nursing and often have an emotional impact on the nurses involved in providing care (Box 11.11, p. 290).

There are also significant stressors that arise from the working environment. Those commonly identified by trained nurses include:

- Increasing demands made upon them
- Lack of resources
- Inadequate staffing
- Shift work conflicts with family commitments
- Poor management.

Whereas student nurses frequently have other concerns, some feel that their role is poorly defined, they change work areas frequently and need to balance practice with working on assignments.

REFLECTIVE PRACTICE Box 11.11

Nurses and stress

Identify a patient/client from a clinical placement who caused you to feel uncomfortable or stressed.

Student activities

- Reflect upon the characteristics of this patient/client that caused your discomfort.
- Think about the people, behaviours or conditions frequently seen in your chosen branch of nursing which might generate stress and anxiety for you.
- Consider the importance of attitudes and judgements in dealing with patients/clients.
- Talk to your mentor about some potentially damaging consequences of this type of stress and anxiety for nurses and the care they deliver to patients/clients.

The effects of this stress can manifest in both physical and emotional forms. These forms can be seen in physiological changes and in positive and negative adaptive behaviours.

In the right environment, stress can be highly motivating, with the nurse perceiving the stressors as a challenge, which brings excitement and a sense of achievement and reward. Other less useful ways of coping involve attempts to reduce exposure to further stress by disengaging from emotional aspects of their work; this is commonly seen in the stress-related state of 'burnout'.

Burnout

It is no surprise that some individuals working in high stress environments, particularly if combined with significant external stress and poor levels of support, can begin to feels powerless to contribute effectively at work. This failure of coping resources in the work environment is often referred to as burnout.

Many nurses start training with high hopes and expectations; indeed many people still consider it to be a vocation in which helping others becomes the person's primary goal in life. While humanity should be thankful that such people exist, they often set themselves unrealistically high goals and expectations, dramatically increasing their risk of experiencing burnout.

There is no general definition of burnout but Maslach et al (1996) suggest that it is a syndrome characterized by:

- Emotional exhaustion and excessive tiredness
- Depersonalization (person loses the feeling of their own reality, everything seems dreamlike)
- Reduction in personal accomplishment and the sense of pleasure
- Reduction in morale
- Increased absenteeism
- Changes in interpersonal behaviour and relationship problems
- Increased use of alcohol or drugs
- Reduced concern for, and involvement with, their patients/clients.

ETHICAL ISSUES Box 11.12

Dave

You are on placement with Dave, a fellow first year student. Over the last month he has become snappy with patients/clients, is often late on duty and looks unkempt. He seems harassed and frequently gets personal phone calls that he either asks others to say that he is not there, or takes them on his own.

Student activities

- What do you think might be happening to Dave?
- Identify ways in which you might help Dave. What ethical issues (see Ch. 7) and professional issues should you consider?
- What other actions might you take to reduce the negative effects of this situation?
- Discuss these issues with your mentor.

[Resource: Nursing and Midwifery Council 2004. The NMC code of professional conduct: standards for conduct, performance and ethics. NMC, London (clauses 8.2, 8.3, p. 11)]

Physical symptoms are common and are similar to anxiety:

- Feeling tense all the time
- Muscle pains
- Headaches
- Poor sleep (see Ch. 10)
- Indigestion
- Sweating
- Palpitations.

Experienced over time, the negative effects on performance and relationships can increase the stress and burnout may become associated with more generalized anxiety and depression.

Burnout tends to develop and worsen over time. It commonly starts with feelings that initial expectations are not being met, disillusionment and disappointment. These vague feelings might lead to harder work to attempt to change the situation; if this fails the energy gives way to tiredness and irritability. It is at this point that the symptoms become more pronounced. An important feature of this insidious development is that, as the feelings of helplessness increase, awareness of the problems and their effects diminishes; individuals feel bad but fail to respond to the causes. Burnout can affect the individual, their relationships and the work environment in a range of ways (Box 11.12).

Managing work-related stress

However, while nursing is considered to be a stressful job, several important features of the work counter the negative effects of work-related stress. Nursing can be very rewarding work and if there are good supportive relationships nurses appear to tolerate and cope with potential stressors very well. The ability to discuss work pressures and develop new adaptive skills have been identified as

Table 11.4 Matrix of organizational stress management interventions

	Primary stress reduction	Secondary stress management	Tertiary stress treatment
Individual perspective	Personal stress Time management Assertiveness Communication	Healthy lifestyles Reflection Clinical supervision Mentorship Relaxation Support	Counselling Intervention from Occupational Health Diet Exercise
Group/team perspective	Team building Team role Clarifying boundaries	Group development Diagnosis and intervention Workload analysis Team supervision	Therapeutic teamwork Renegotiate team role
Organization/systems perspective	Job description Clarify roles Individual performance review	Workload management Risk analysis (see Ch. 13) Employee participation	Employee assistance programmes Cultural change

protective so frequently in studies that providing mentorship and clinical supervision opportunities is considered central to good practice. Another important consideration is that an individual who identifies that they are stressed can use the problem-solving process of care planning to meet their own needs.

Schaufeli and Enzmann (1998) developed a matrix that provides a useful summary of the interventions that can be implemented to reduce stress-related problems caused through work (Table 11.4).

Traumatic stress

Some events, particularly if they are sudden, intense and life threatening may so overwhelm a person's coping ability that the capacity to process emotions is impaired. These events include being involved in serious accidents, natural disasters, violent crime or life-threatening illness/injury. In nurses, the sudden unexpected death of a patient, dealing with major incidents/accidents and exposure to threats or violence may generate the same types of response, generally described as an acute stress reaction.

Normal and frequently adaptive responses to extreme stress are shock and denial, both of which 'switch off' the immediate emotional response. Emotional shock is described as feeling stunned, dazed or numb. In health staff dealing with disasters, denial may leave them feeling disconnected from the horror of the situation but more importantly it allows them to function. However, these initial effects are temporary and because they prevent people making sense of the emotions at the time of the event, are typically followed by a number of other effects, which may include the following.

- Feelings are experienced more intensely, often with a sense of threat or danger
- Emotions feel difficult to control
- Vivid memories or 'flashbacks' of the event suddenly and unpredictably come to mind, often associated with intense fear or distress. The 'flashbacks' become a source of anxiety; people might dread them occurring and avoid any potential reminders
- Sleep, eating and interpersonal relationships become disrupted.

For the majority, these symptoms will gradually reduce but how they are experienced and how long they last is highly variable. These variations, as in other stress reactions, are dependent on the person, their interpretation of the situation, other stressors and the availability of support.

Managing traumatic stress

Symptoms persisting longer than 6 months are called post-traumatic stress disorder (PTSD), which may require more specialist help. Therapies are based on cognitive behavioural psychotherapy and some people benefit from antidepressant drugs. Even when the symptoms are severe, many people will recover with appropriate help.

Until very recently the individual was helped to review traumatic experiences in order to make sense of them in a process known as 'critical incident debriefing'. Unfortunately, a critical fact was ignored, which is that the response to serious trauma is adaptive, it protects a person from being overwhelmed. Recent studies on formal debriefing have suggested that not only is there no evidence that it protects people from long-term problems but it also may increase risk (Bisson et al 2000).

The guiding principle in dealing with others who have experienced traumatic stress is to provide a safe, supportive environment with the opportunity to talk if required.

The best interventions appear to be in preparing people to deal with potential trauma. Individuals who understand what reactions can be expected, and how feelings of guilt and responsibility are common but usually inaccurate, are less likely to develop long-term problems. For example, training in the management of aggressive clients should not only address the skills involved, they also need to address the psychological effects of aggression on the nurse.

Stress and patients, clients and carers

Feeling well, being physically fit and well-nourished all contribute to the ability to deal with stressors and contribute to confidence and self-worth.

When an individual's health is compromised they must deal with the added stress associated with their condition, at a time when their coping resources are also reduced. Illness is a poorly defined concept: it may describe the presence of specific disease but the word has much broader connotations. The word can be linked with or used to describe anything that causes evil, harm, pain or trouble, and historically was used to describe things going badly or getting worse. Even when describing specific conditions, the link is with *dis-ease*, i.e. to have no ease.

Many of the common effects of illness present significant physical and psychological challenges that can reduce or exhaust a person's coping resources. These can include:

- Lack of sleep (Ch. 10)
- Malnutrition and fluid deficits (Ch. 19)
- Toxins such as in infections, treatment side-effects, previous substance misuse or the effects of smoking
- Trauma or surgery
- Pain (Ch. 23).

In primary care the interplay between physical and emotional health is well understood; it is estimated that up to 80% of consultations have a significant psychological component. This provides an example of how anxiety can be adaptive: if people were not concerned about their health they might not seek help.

Yet even when the problem is primarily stress-related the person usually presents with physical symptoms, which can make choosing the best interventions very difficult. Healthcare services also often deal with the consequences of social problems, such as poverty or relationship difficulties, which overwhelm coping resources and adversely affect health.

When admission to hospital is required it is likely that this will be accompanied by the sense of threat. This may be intensified for people with learning disabilities and also for carers of people with complex needs. Again the main mediator of the anxiety experienced will be based on the meaning the person attaches to the condition. However, other features appear to significantly increase the potential for stress and anxiety (Box 11.13).

Two related issues, body image and expressing sexuality/sexual identity, can also be highly significant in the person's response to illness (see below).

REFLECTIVE PRACTICE Box 11.13

Stress following admission

- Suddenness and severity of the onset of symptoms
- The danger the person feels, the perceived severity of illness
- Uncertainty about the diagnosis and how long it will last
- The degree of control the person feels they have; this relates to the level of dependence and knowledge of the condition
- Poor previous experiences of hospital and healthcare staff
- The degree of disruption to the person's life
- The potential for full recovery
- The degree of change in function, appearance or body image
- Conditions that affect gender identity
- Embarrassment associated with the condition
- Feelings of guilt/responsibility for their condition, e.g. smokers
- Other significant stressors the person has to manage
- Availability of supportive networks.

Student activities

- Reflect on the patients/clients you have recently nursed. Which of the features above influenced their stress level?
- What was done to minimize the effects?

Body image

Body image is the mental representation people have of their body and physical appearance. The view of physical self is central to the person's sense of identity, social value and self-esteem. Changes in body image, particularly if they involve loss of function, impaired ability to communicate or visible signs of illness and injury can be particularly traumatic. Where the change is likely to be temporary, individuals may simply detach from the situation, putting their life on 'hold' by adopting the sick role and making no attempt to adapt. This avoidance strategy can be highly adaptive in such situations. However, a change that is likely to be permanent often leads to grief-like reactions in which initial shock is followed by profound depression and feelings of anger. In these cases, adaptation can be difficult and delayed.

Expressing sexuality

Expressing sexuality is linked to gender identity, attractiveness, fertility and sexual functioning and gives a person a sense of value and self-esteem. Changes caused by trauma or illness that impact on these areas appear to have emotional effects much more pronounced than would be expected from just functional loss. The presence of visible lesions, stoma formation or loss of body parts, e.g. female breast, or sudden weight changes are all particularly difficult to cope with. Loss of sexual functioning, factors affecting sexual performance, e.g. erectile dysfunction, and infertility may reduce self-efficacy and increase stress and depression.

Coping with illness

Illness can often highlight major differences in the demands made by the situation and the resources a person has available to deal with them. Coping often involves ongoing appraisals and reappraisals of a situation in which individuals may attempt to alter the problem or their emotional responses to the problem.

Attempting to alter the problem is problem-focused coping and depends on the person believing that the problem is controllable or changeable. Ideally, actions should be based on analysis of the situation and planning solutions before the problem is dealt with. However, often actions are based on attempts to confront situations assertively which may involve actions based on anger, thus increasing risk.

Emotion-focused coping strategies that aim to control the emotion are frequently used when the person believes that they cannot change the stressor, either because they believe that they lack the resources/skills or the situation is insoluble, e.g. bereavement (see Ch. 12). Coping can involve attempts to avoid exposure to the stressors or suppressing its effects with alcohol or drugs. Alternatively, a person may seek social support or alter their appraisals of the situation by attempting to reduce its importance.

Social support provides emotional support through empathy, understanding, caring, etc., supporting self-esteem and offering practical help or information. People differ in their needs for social support; for those who like to cope alone, social support can be detrimental.

Helping patients/clients and carers to cope – role of the nurse

The nurse is an important resource which patients/clients and carers often rely upon to reduce the demands made upon them and enhance their coping resources. In serious acute situations where life-saving treatments are required this might be difficult; however, in the longer term, enhancing and supporting the patient's/client's coping skills becomes more relevant.

Although dealing with distressed individuals can be emotionally draining, the nurse needs to maintain an aspect of calm and helpful concern. Nurses can help the patient/client or carer focus on the important issues, provide useful though often limited information, help the person to identify what immediate actions are needed and offer practical help as in acute stress attention and memory may be impaired.

Nurses should anticipate the potential for stress and anxiety in their patients/clients and plan actions to prevent or minimize the more damaging effects. It is important to recognize that many of the anxieties a patient/client may have are realistic and so prevention may be difficult. As there is also the problem that anxiety and stress often interfere with logical thinking and memory, interventions are best made before feelings become too strong, ideally before the stressful event. Patients/clients and their carers, with appropriate and timely help from the nurse, may cope much more effectively.

Patients/clients/carers may also be reluctant to discuss anxieties so as to avoid embarrassment; again the nurse can prevent problems by introducing such subjects into conversation. The effective use of nursing models to inform assessment and interventions should mean that a wide range of issues are specifically addressed, even when they may not appear to be related to the presenting problem. Using a structured approach gives the person 'permission' to talk about difficult subjects.

There are important mediators of stress and anxiety that the nurse must consider in planning care. Cognitively, both stress and anxiety reflect feelings of vulnerability. There is a perception that demands/threats will overwhelm a person's ability to cope.

Stress and vulnerable individuals

Children, some people with learning disabilities and other vulnerable people, who do not understand stressful events and have limited coping resources, will be particularly vulnerable and are more likely to respond differently to life events.

The effects of long-term stress on a child's development have been well documented and have been associated with a wide range of problems in adult life. Gunnar (2004) argues that long-term stress affects emotional areas of the brain. This can alter the child's future ability to deal with stress-related events.

In common with adults, stress in childhood may relate to issues other than illness, such as bullying (see pp. 294–295) or examination pressures. Children's behaviour may change, e.g. becoming withdrawn, tearful, depressed, headaches, etc. Children are affected by stress within the family such as that caused by abusive relationships and domestic violence (see Further reading suggestions, e.g. DH 2000).

Children have limited experience of dealing with demands and limited coping strategies, thus anxiety is a common and frequent experience for children. Young children in particular may also have a very limited ability to communicate their distress to adults. So to understand stress in children it is important to consider the age, the developmental stage and their communication skills.

Children are skilled at judging the emotional state of their parents/carers and can become distressed in response to their parents'/carers' anxiety. This is important for a child who is admitted to hospital, as they have an increased level of stress caused by the reason for the admission and the environment.

Children attempt to make sense of illness and to cope by using much more basic defence strategies, such as regression and repression (see pp. 280–281). Nurses assessing stress and anxiety in children often find that behaviour is a better indicator of a child's distress than their verbal reports (Box 11.14, p. 294). Children commonly become uncooperative. These behaviours may lead to reduced social support or anger in their carers and so can be seen as maladaptive and damaging. Teenagers in particular can be especially difficult by refusing help and by engaging in high-risk behaviours, which include:

- Drug or alcohol misuse
- Smoking
- Crime
- Self-harm.

Table 11.5 (see p. 294) outlines some age-related techniques that nurses, parents or other carers might use to reduce the child's distress.

Children with long-term health problems, e.g. diabetes, when faced with the increased stress associated with the major transition into adolescence, may also start to neglect their condition and increase their health risks.

Box 11.14 Age-related stress behaviours

- *Infant* (birth to 12 months) – sleep problems accompanied by excessive screaming; feeding problems, which may result in weight loss, failure to thrive, etc.
- *Toddler* (1–3 years) – behavioural problems, e.g. difficulties in socializing with other children, may be excessively shy or aggressive (boys are more aggressive than girls)
- *Preschool age* (4–5 years) – social isolation with problems relating to adults and other children
- *Primary school age* – excessive levels of aggression. May exhibit depression. Behavioural problems, e.g. use of violence (learn that violence is a way to resolve conflict)
- *Adolescents* – problems with social interaction and in some cases violent or criminal behaviour.

Table 11.5 Reducing distress in children (Adapted from Huband & Trigg 2000)

Stage	Techniques and aids
Infant	Rocking, patting, holding Use of pacifier (sucking) Use of basic distractions (rattles)
Toddler	Rocking, holding, involvement of parents Distraction: music, bells, rattles, books, party blowers Use of bubbles
Preschool	Touch, stroking Cognitive distraction: counting, imagination games Distraction: favourite games, puppets Story from a favourite book Basic imagery
School age	Stroking hair, back, shoulders Imagery Distraction: music, hand-held games
Adolescents	Massage, imagery, cognitive distraction, relaxation techniques Use of stress ball, music, relaxation and discussion

For nurses working with people with learning disabilities there may be problems in both recognizing and helping to manage stress in their clients. Depending on the nature of the disability the person may have restricted understanding of situations and limited communication skills. In addition, damage to the central nervous system may lead to a reduced tolerance to environmental stimulation, overwhelming their ability to cope. Alternatively, they may become insensitive to stressors, leading to disinhibition and risk taking.

For those with reduced tolerance to environmental stimuli one approach to reducing distress is the use of Snoezelen. This multisensory stimulation technique utilizes lights, tactile surfaces, music and sometimes essential oils (see Ch. 10) to provide an environment that is soothing and relaxing (Box 11.15). Moreover, the client's

EVIDENCE-BASED PRACTICE Box 11.15

Snoezelen use for people with learning disability or dementia

Advocates for Snoezelen argue that it can reduce challenging behaviour and enhance mood and concentration, although reliable evidence is lacking. In a review of the literature, Hogg et al (2001) found that some studies demonstrated a wide range of positive outcomes whereas several studies reported entirely negative outcomes.

Student activities

- Is there a Snoezelen environment in your area?
- Access the article by Hogg et al (2001) and read what they say about research design when studying Snoezelen.
- Locate one study with positive outcomes and one with entirely negative outcomes and discuss their findings with your mentor.

[Reference: Hogg J, Cavet J, Lambe L, Smeddle M 2001. The use of 'Snoezelen' as multisensory stimulation with people with intellectual disabilities: a review of the research. Research in Developmental Disabilities 22(5):353–372]

family can be involved in sessions in order to increase their understanding of the client's feelings, abilities, etc. and enhance family relationships.

Many older people with learning disabilities evaluate their sense of value and their abilities by comparison with people of their own age. This can lead to problems with self-concept and an acute sensitivity to perceived criticism. For some clients the frustrations associated with these social comparisons and their perceived lack of ability may be expressed in low self-esteem, dependency, self-destructive behaviours or difficult behaviours towards their carers. All of these features are associated with reduced ability to deal with potential stressors; the behaviours used in coping often increase stress in both carers and client.

There is still considerable stigma associated with learning disabilities, which can lead to exclusion, rejection and prejudice. Even when prejudice is not present there can be a general insensitivity to the needs of people with a learning disability, which can add considerably to the stress they experience.

Bullying is a stressor commonly identified in children, people with a learning disability and in other vulnerable adults who are considered different in some way (physically, culturally, intellectually), especially if they are seen as less able or weak (Box 11.16).

Coping with serious illness, chronic problems and disability

There are real differences in the way individuals deal with acute illness and the demands of having to adapt to chronic illness, disability and terminal illness (see Ch. 12). Rather than anticipating recovery, the patient/client

Box 11.16 **Bullying**

Bullying can take many forms. Young people have described bullying in the following ways:

- Name calling
- Teasing
- Being pushed or pulled about
- Being hit or attacked
- Your bag/other possessions taken and thrown around
- Rumours spread about you
- Being ignored and left out
- Forced to hand over money/possessions
- Attacked because of religion or skin colour (ChildLine 2005).

Bullying, particularly if it is prolonged, can lead to behavioural problems, which might develop into lifelong problems. Some commonly identified effects include:

- Reduced self-esteem
- Anxiety
- Depression
- Loneliness
- Possible suicidal thoughts (Salmon et al 1998).

These effects can lead to worsening academic grades and school attendance and to a great deal of unhappiness to the point of depression. Unfortunately, bullied individuals are also more likely to be neglected or even rejected by their peers (Shuster 1999), which also reduces potential support.

Individuals who behave differently, either due to learning disabilities or mental illness, often evoke anxiety in other people. Nurses are frequently in situations in which they need to identify those at risk and be able to refer the problem to appropriate agencies.

and family have to learn instead to live with the continued physical, social and emotional effects of their condition.

Having to deal with a serious or life-threatening condition can generate a great deal of anxiety in both the patient and the people to whom they are closest. Following a period of shock or detachment, those involved try to give the situation a meaning; they try to make some sense of the value of their life in the face of death.

Taylor (1983) investigated coping and adaptation in women diagnosed with breast cancer. She suggested that adaptation often involved the patient addressing three main issues:

- *Search for meaning*: This usually involved the woman in trying to identify a reason why she had cancer. Interestingly, 41% of the participants in the study believed that stress played a role. The cancer may be seen as a punishment; self-blame and guilt are experienced and the woman feels helpless. Others see cancer as a challenge, typically undertaking a fundamental review of their lives and re-evaluating how they live.
- *Sense of mastery*: Women held varying beliefs about the degree of control they had over the cancer. Women who believed that they had a significant degree of control were much more likely to try alternative therapies and actively engage in treatment decisions. Even in those who felt little personal control, 50% believed that the doctor did.
- *Self-esteem*: The individual's general belief in her capacity to deal with demands effectively. Even when this belief is not based in reality it still offers significant protection against stressors; in fact Taylor advocates helping the woman to form and maintain a set of positive illusions.

Taylor found more positive outcomes in those women who sought a sense of meaning, who believed they had some control and who had high self-esteem than others in their situation. Why these elements have a direct impact on disease-free survival is not clear, though improved immune function due to effective control of stress may be the most likely explanation.

Improved prognosis has also been seen in patients with good emotional support providing a buffer against stress (Spiegel et al 1989). However, an alternative view is that in avoiding high levels of anxiety individuals are more likely to engage in effective health-promoting behaviours and less likely to become depressed. Depression is associated with just giving up, self-care is neglected and treatments may be ignored. Depression worsens outcomes in a wide range of health problems.

Chronic illness and disability

An acquired disability often means that the client's social roles change and the pressures placed upon the family and carers increase. Throughout there is a need to adapt to many new situations that affect not only health and functioning but also roles and self-concept. Initially, adaptation is resisted but at some point the patient/client must learn to accept the changes and work towards the best outcomes. Patients/clients who fail to make these mental changes often become depressed and possibly self-destructive.

Assessment requires a measure/tool that is inclusive, identifies normal functioning and establishes a baseline from which to evaluate the effect of care at a later date. The assessment also needs to address the needs of the patient's family, as providing long-term care can have profound effects on family and carers. Long-term interventions include many specialist services and collaborative multiprofessional working (see Ch. 3). However it is good practice for a specifically named person to act as care coordinator and to engage the patient and family in all aspects of care.

Rehabilitation

A full discussion of rehabilitation is beyond the scope of this book and readers are directed to Further reading (e.g. Davis 2006). Rehabilitation involves learning ways of coping with chronic (long-term) illnesses or injury. This may involve maximizing physical abilities, learning new skills, problem-solving and changing appraisals about the condition and its consequences. Many conditions may run a prolonged and chronic course, requiring considerable adaptation by the patient/client and those around them. Conditions may be present from birth, requiring life-long help, or they may be acquired after birth as in psychosis, multiple sclerosis or spinal injuries. Many common conditions such as chronic respiratory disease (see Ch. 17), chronic heart failure and arthritis occur in older adults. Unfortunately, the effects of the increased stress, associated particularly with the acquired conditions, may also be instrumental in maintaining or worsening the condition.

Nurses involved in long-term care should adopt an honest and trusting position, which engages the patient/client and maintains motivation to remain as involved in self-care as is practical (see Further reading, NHS Modernisation Agency 2003). This is important, whether recovery is possible or not: patients/clients who maintain a sense of control are generally less distressed and feel less isolated. Honest and accurate information should never be given in a way that removes all hope.

Models in rehabilitation

It is particularly important in long-term care that the guiding model is person-centred, holistic and allows for multiagency collaboration with patients/clients and their carers. The underpinning processes involved in care planning are outlined in Box 11.17 (see Ch. 14).

An example of using a structured approach is in the development of a Wellness Recovery Action Plan (WRAP). The WRAP was developed by Copeland (1997) as a structured system that enables the active monitoring of distressing symptoms in people with long-term mental health problems. However, many of the principles are applicable to most care situations. The development of a WRAP culminates in a plan that aims to modify or eliminate the most distressing symptoms the patient/client identifies. There are five pivotal principles that need consideration when developing a WRAP:

- *Hope*: People must have a reason to make the effort to manage their condition
- *Personal responsibility*: People must recognize that they are not passive recipients of care but actively involved, a partner in care
- *Education*: Learning about the illness allows people to make good decisions
- *Self-advocacy*: Aids self-belief, knowing personal rights and seeing that they are respected; setting goals and working to make them happen
- *Support*: Effective support from family, friends and professionals aids in symptom relief.

The development of a WRAP is dependent on framing what is wanted and needed by the patient/client. Patients/clients, although frequently anxious, do know what they can and cannot do and in developing the plan the patient/client can begin to recognize the collaborative nature of the nurse–patient relationship. In time, and with help from the nurse, the patient/client becomes the expert in their illness or disability.

Box 11.17 Planning long-term care

1. Holistic assessment:
   - Get to know the individuals and their unique problems
   - Establish their expectations
   - Identify the knowledge they have of the condition
   - Identify current coping strategies
   - Identify social support systems
2. Develop a plan on patient/client goals and those of others involved
3. Identify the strategies for goal attainment and equipment/adaptations needed:
   - Identify potential problems and barriers to achievement
4. Identify a named individual to implement the strategy
5. Work within a timeframe for goal completion
6. Set a flexible review date
7. Provide contact details for the key people involved
8. Ensure that the plan is clear and unambiguous
9. Review outcomes with the client and their carers.

Summary

- All nurses need a good understanding of stress and anxiety including stress management.
- Stress and anxiety are complex psychological and physiological responses an individual has in response to environmental demands or perceived threats.
- While people experience stress and anxiety as unpleasant, it serves a useful and adaptive function in motivating behaviour to reduce the demands or potential risk.
- Although stress and anxiety are normal and necessary features of living, there are links between stress and health breakdown. This is particularly evident in long-term stress.
- People always have to deal with multiple stressors and a limited capacity to deal effectively with them. Very high levels of stress almost invariably interfere with a person's ability to function effectively.
- Responses to stress depend very much upon people's beliefs about a situation and their ability to cope. Developing new skills, coping strategies and modifying beliefs are the most effective ways to reduce the negative effects of stress.
- Nursing is fundamentally an interpersonal activity in which nurses are frequently in contact with people who are distressed and need help.
- Nurses experiencing high levels of stress are more likely to engage in behaviour which can be damaging to the health of both patients and the nurses themselves. This chapter has identified work-related stress and self-care as important considerations in the healthcare of other people.
- A range of strategies may be used in the management of stress in both patients/clients and in self-care. Coping styles and strategies will vary from individual to individual and matching the intervention to the individual is an important function of effective nursing assessment.
- All nurses should be able to recognize indicators that might suggest that stress and anxiety are overwhelming a client's resources and more specialized help may be needed.

Self test

1. What is stress?
2. Which four factors aid the understanding of emotional states?
3. In what ways can stress affect performance?
4. What are the stages of the general adaptation syndrome?
5. Eustress is:
   a. Intense stress
   b. Useful adaptive stress
   c. Chronic long-term stress
   d. Stress associated with illness.
6. Which three factors are important in coping with serious long-term illness?
7. What are the five principles for WRAP development?

Useful websites

BBC – *useful information about stress and coping*	www.bbc.co.uk/health/conditions/mental_health Available July 2006
Canadian Mental Health Association	www.cmha.ca/english/coping_with_stress/links.htm Available July 2006
The American Institute of Stress	www.stress.org Available July 2006
The Nursefriendly Stress Resources for Nurses (North American)	www.nursefriendly.com/nursing/stress.htm Available July 2006
Useful resources website	www.teachhealth.com Available July 2006

Key words and phrases for literature searching

Adaptation
Coping strategies
Rehabilitation
Stress
Stress at work
Stress in nursing
Stress management
Theories of stress

References

Bisson JI, McFarlane AC, Rose S 2000 Psychological debriefing. In: Foa EB, Keane TM, Friedman MJ (eds) Effective treatments for PTSD. Guilford Press, New York

Borrill CS, Wall TD, West MA et al 1996 Mental health of the workforce of NHS Trusts – Phase 1, Final report. University of Sheffield and University of Leeds

ChildLine 2005 Stress. Online: www.childline.org.uk Available July 2006

Copeland ME 1997 Wellness recovery action plan. Peach Press, Dummerston, VT

Department of Health 1998 Our healthier nation. TSO, London

Ellis A 1994 Reason and emotion in psychotherapy. 2nd edn. Carol Publishing, New York

Gunnar M 2004 Gunnar Lab. Online: http://education.umn.edu/icd/GunnarLab Available September 2006

Harris N 2001 Management of work-related stress in nursing. Nursing Standard 16(10):47–52

Health and Safety Executive 2002 Work-related stress. Online: www.hse.gov.uk/stress/links.htm Available July 2006

Holmes TH, Rahe RH 1967 The social readjustment and rating scale. Journal of Psychosomatic Research 11:213–218

Huband S, Trigg E 2000 Practices in children's nursing: guidelines for hospital and community. Churchill Livingstone, Edinburgh

Lazarus AA 1981 The practice of multi-modal therapy. McGraw-Hill, New York

Lazarus R, Folkman S 1984 Stress appraisal and coping. Springer Verlag, New York

Maslach C, Jackson S, Leiter MP 1996 Maslach burnout inventory manual. 3rd edn. Consulting Psychologists Press, Palo Alto, CA

Menzies-Lyth I 1959 The functions of social systems as a defence against anxiety: a report on a study of the nursing service of a general hospital. Human Relations 13:95–121

Salmon G, Jones A, Smith DM 1998 Bullying in school: self-reported anxiety and self-esteem in secondary school children. British Medical Journal 317(7163): 924–925

Schaufeli WB, Enzmann D 1998 The burnout companion to study and practice: a critical analysis. Taylor and Francis, Philadelphia

Selye H 1956 (revised 1975) The stress of life. McGraw-Hill, New York

Shuster B 1999 Outsiders at school: the prevalence of bullying and its relation with social status. Group Processes and Intergroup Relations 2:175–190

Spiegel D, Bloom JR, Kraemar HC 1989 Effect of psychosocial treatment on survival of patients with metastatic breast cancer. Lancet 2:888–891

Taylor SE 1983 Adjustment of threatening events: a theory of cognitive adaptation. American Psychologist 38:1161–1173

Yerkes RM, Dodson JD 1908 The relation of strength of stimulus to rapidity of habit-formation. Journal of Comparative Neurology and Psychology 18:459–482

Further reading

Davis S 2006 Rehabilitation. The use of theories and models in practice. Churchill Livingstone, Edinburgh

Department of Health 2000 Domestic violence: a resource manual for health care professionals. Online: www.dh.gov.uk/assetRoot/04/06/53/79/04065379.pdf Available July 2006

NHS Modernisation Agency 2003 Essence of care: patient-focused benchmarks for clinical governance. Online: www.modern.nhs.uk/home/key/docs/Essence%20of%20Care.pdf Available July 2006

Payne RA 2005 Relaxation techniques. 3rd edn. Churchill Livingstone, Edinburgh

Loss and bereavement

12

Catriona Kennedy and Karen Lockhart

Glossary terms

Adjuvant

Bereavement

Cachexia

Chemotherapy

End-of-life care

Grief

Hospice

Nurse specialist

Palliative care

Radiotherapy

Symptom management

Terminal care

Learning outcomes

This chapter will help you to:

- Identify the types of loss individuals experience throughout life
- Identify the stages in the bereavement process and discuss the care of bereaved people
- Discuss the palliative care approach to care, including team working and symptom management
- Identify the services available for people who require palliative care
- Identify the aims of nursing care around death and dying
- Describe the cultural impact of death and dying
- Discuss the main causes of death in the United Kingdom
- Outline the physiology of death and dying
- Identify ethical concerns at the end of life.

Introduction

The death of a significant person is the most difficult loss most people will face and nurses have an important role to play in supporting people who are dying and their families. The first part of this chapter explores issues of loss and bereavement, including death, and the impact of different types of loss on people. Consideration is given to bereavement, including understanding grief responses and planning care.

The middle section focuses on the palliative care approach to care, which encompasses care of people with life-limiting conditions such as cancer, chronic heart disease and some degenerative neurological illnesses. Caring for people at the end of life is a challenging part of the nursing role. Several members of the multidisciplinary team (MDT) are likely to be involved in the care and support of patients/clients with advanced disease and their families. However, nurses are generally the health professionals who have most contact. Nurses therefore have a significant role in supporting individuals through illness, at the end stages of life and families who are bereaved. The skills and knowledge of nurses caring for those with advanced, non-curable illness are crucial to the delivery of high quality care. Strategies for communication and the management of distressing symptoms are discussed. Helping nurses to understand the philosophy of the palliative care approach and the services available is the focus of this section.

The last section is about the care of people facing death – both the person who will die and those who are close to them. A framework for providing care around death is suggested. Finally, ethical concerns at the end of life are identified and the role of the nurse in the last act of care and in the provision of palliative care is identified.

Loss including death

This section considers factors relating to loss and bereavement. Death of a significant other is recognized as a difficult loss to cope with. Nurses are important in helping people to deal with losses which result from injury, illness and death. Therefore it is important to consider how experiences of loss – expected, planned or unexpected – throughout life prepare individuals to cope with significant losses.

Types of loss

Loss and change are part of everyday life and everyone will experience both of these during their lifetime. Loss is experienced in the absence of a person, miscarriage/stillbirth, own impending death, an object, body part, a function (e.g. walking), change related to age/milestones, loss of status, loss/change of job/retirement, a move into a care home, or from institutional to community care, or emotion, which was formerly present. There are several types of loss, the most traumatic of which include:

- Significant person through death
- Separation
- Divorce
- Distance
- Changes in a relationship.

Other losses include:

- Material goods, e.g. due to burglary
- Pet animals
- Objects with sentimental value.

These losses may be thought of as rather less traumatic than that of a significant person. However, responses to loss are individual and linked to a range of other personality and lifestyle factors (Box 12.1). For example, non-animal lovers may find it hard to understand why a person is devastated at the loss of a much-loved pet. As a person's pet may have been their constant companion, the loss is significant and its impact should never be underestimated.

Loss is an inherent part of any change, even where people have decided to make changes such as getting married or having a child. The losses associated with significant life events are expected and normally occur as the person matures from one stage of life to another and makes decisions about how they want life to develop (see Chs 8, 11). If progress through life's normal milestones is not achieved, then feelings of loss may result. For example, parents whose children do not achieve normal life milestones due to disabilities or illness often find it hard to cope. Similarly, if a couple find they cannot have children, apart from dealing with their own feelings, they may feel pressurized by others who expect them to have children. Therefore, response to loss is shaped by context and culture.

Throughout life people form attachments and the stronger the attachment, the greater the loss experienced when that attachment is broken. When an attachment is broken, people cope by revising and reconstructing their life, thereby adapting to loss and subsequent change, often with support from family and friends. Professional intervention may be required if an individual cannot cope with significant loss such as a major change in body image or death. For most people, loss associated with life events they have not 'chosen' is the most difficult to cope with.

REFLECTIVE PRACTICE Box 12.1

Reactions to loss

Identify an object you have recently lost, e.g. keys, handbag, or breakage of a favourite item, etc.

Student activities

- How did you feel?
- Reflect on a situation when you might have underestimated the impact on a person of what you considered to be a 'trivial' loss.

It is likely that many of the feelings you experienced are similar to those associated with loss through bereavement (see this page and p. 301). Therefore, even apparently trivial loss can result in a range of distressing feelings. It is important that nurses do not assume how people feel about loss, as insignificant loss to one person may be catastrophic to another.

Bereavement

In most healthcare settings, nurses will encounter patients/clients and/or carers who are experiencing loss or have suffered bereavement (the loss of somebody or something of value, especially through death). It is often the nurse who assumes the role of helping the patient/client or carer. Bereaved individuals need open acknowledgement of the death and opportunities to display expressions of grief and mourning in order to help them come to terms with the loss. To do this effectively the nurse requires knowledge of what loss is and how people react to and cope with loss. There is also considerable evidence to suggest that professionals working with people who are dying find this enormously stressful (Smith 1992, Phillips 1996, Lockhart-Wood 2001). This type of stress has been referred to as the 'emotional labour' of nursing (James 1989). Through understanding the theories relating to the process of dying and grieving, the nurse is better equipped to support patients and carers in their journey.

For the purpose of this chapter the following definitions (Stroebe et al 2002) will guide understanding:

- Bereavement – describes the situation when a person has died
- Grief – describes the emotional reaction to loss or death
- Mourning – the expression of the emotion which characterizes grief.

Models that describe dying and bereavement demonstrate that these processes usually involve a series of stages and that individuals take varying lengths of time in each stage and may move from one to the other and back again. Thus it is important to remember that each individual's reaction to loss is unique and there is no right or wrong way to grieve.

To date, Elisabeth Kubler-Ross' (1969) 'preparing to die' model of dying has been the most influential. This seminal work was one of the first attempts to explain the process of dying in relation to the emotional and psychological adaptations which accompany the process.

Box 12.2 **Preparing to die**

Denial
This suggests that when given the knowledge that they have an incurable disease the patient will go into denial by refusing to believe that it is true. Denial is now recognized as a protective stage that allows for psychological adjustment to the news. This contradicts the earlier belief that people should be helped out of denial and made to face up to reality. Emerging theory suggests that forcing a person out of denial when they are not ready may be psychologically damaging.

Anger
Families and the patient when coming to terms with a diagnosis of serious illness often feel anger. Anger is often directed towards healthcare staff, especially doctors involved in the diagnosis. It may be perceived that the symptoms were missed or diagnosis took longer and therefore the illness progressed beyond a cure in that time.

Bargaining
Patients and families may seek to 'make deals'; often this is done in private through prayer. It is an attempt to postpone the reality of loss and its presentation may be similar to denial.

Depression
This occurs when the reality of loss is felt and can no longer be denied. It is often accompanied with overwhelming sadness, feelings of loneliness and withdrawal from social activities.

Acceptance
The person has come to terms with the reality of their life now being limited. This is the final and desirable stage of this model. However, it is criticized, as acceptance may not always be achieved and there is a danger of healthcare professionals and other carers trying to push the person through the stages in order to reach this desired state.

[From Kubler-Ross (1969)]

This theory made the previously taboo subject of death and dying one that could be openly discussed. For the first time healthcare professionals were able to relate to a theoretical model which made sense of their patients' behaviours and actions.

The five stages of this model are:

- Denial
- Anger
- Bargaining
- Depression
- Acceptance (Box 12.2).

Anticipatory grief

While Kubler-Ross' model focuses on dying, it has close similarities with the concept of anticipatory grief. Anticipatory grief is grief occurring before death. It differs from post-death grief in its nature and course. Lindemann (1944) was the first to recognize this phenomenon and identified five characteristics of anticipatory grief:

- Guilt – for unresolved issues such as old quarrels
- Somatic (body) distress – physical manifestation of grief, often characterized as feelings of anxiety, sleeplessness, poor appetite, nausea
- Anger (see Kubler-Ross' model)
- Loss of patterns of conduct – inability to carry out daily activities such as getting dressed, work and household chores
- Fixation with the image of the dying person – coping with the changing physical appearance and social standing of the person.

Kubler-Ross noted that common behaviours include denial, reassurance seeking, secrecy about the diagnosis, anger and guilt. There are conflicting views of how helpful anticipatory grief is to the bereavement process, with some authors suggesting that it makes little difference. However, the predominant view is that it is helpful as it helps people to cope and reduces the length of time someone has to adjust to the news of impending death of a loved one. Parkes and Weiss (1983) found that those who have more than 2 weeks to adjust to loss had less difficulty in their adjustment than those who had less than 2 weeks. An alternative argument, however, could be that sudden deaths are more traumatic for the person and invoke a much stronger grief reaction.

One problem, however, is when the dying person appears to live longer than expected; the psychological preparation that goes with anticipatory grief and the state of 'readiness' may be achieved prior to the actual death.

Grief and mourning

Grief and mourning are terms used to describe the emotional reaction to loss or death and the expression of the emotion in relation to this event. Several theories have been proposed to aid understanding of the grieving process. Of these, Worden (1991) and Parkes (1998) are two of the most influential. These two theories complement each other (see Box 12.3, p. 302): Parkes' theory describes the feelings and emotions the person affected by the loss is experiencing during different stages; Worden's theory illuminates the process of adjustment that is necessary to regain equilibrium.

REFLECTIVE PRACTICE Box 12.3

Understanding the grief process

Reflect upon the theories of grieving and their relevance to clinical practice in your branch. You may wish to consider a patient/client and their family you have cared for. Although it is difficult to neatly package the actual experience into stages, you may have recognized some of the characteristics that would indicate the stage of grief.

Student activities

- Discuss your reflection with a mentor or colleague.
- How might knowledge of the theories help you support patients/clients and families?

Parkes (1998) describes four components of grief:

- *Numbness*: This relates to the initial reaction to the news of a loss or that a person has died. This component may last for a period of a few hours to a number of days. Following this is the 'pining' component where feelings of grief are evident.
- *Pining*: The person has intense feelings of pining, often described as 'pangs of grief' The person continues to function with day-to-day essential chores but may seem listless and distant. This component can also have physical manifestations, which include reduced appetite and weight loss, poor concentration and short-term memory impairment. Insomnia may also be a problem resulting in irritability (see Ch. 10).
- *Disorganization and despair*: This component is characterized by continual ruminations over events leading up to the death. For many this will lead to a feeling of the need to apportion blame and anger, which is often directed at the healthcare system. If there were any areas for concern these may become magnified during the grieving process. During this phase the bereaved person may report hallucinations in the form of hearing or seeing the dead person nearby, especially when they are relaxed or drowsy. Usually these hallucinations dissipate when the person becomes more awake.
- *Reorganization*: Finally, reorganization occurs when the feelings described in the preceding components are resolved and the bereaved person has learned to accept and adapt to life with the loss or without the person who has died. It has been suggested that this component may take a long time to achieve, with some people who have lost someone very close such as a spouse or child not really recovering until well into the second year following the death (Parkes 1998).

Parkes suggests that the components of grief must be worked through to enable the individual to 'let go' of the person they have lost and to be able to move on with their lives. He likens this process to the loss reaction and period of adjustment that people display when they have become disabled through the loss of a body part.

While each of these components is seen to be of equal significance, it is important to remember that people often do not clearly signal when one component is complete and they have moved into the next component. Indeed the boundaries are often blurred and people may oscillate between components before moving on. Parkes stresses the importance of allowing people to express their emotions and states that repression of grief is harmful and may result in delayed reactions and complicated grieving. Equally, obsessive grieving is harmful and may lead to chronic grief and depression.

Parkes' theory describes the feelings relating to different stages of the grieving process. This is complemented by Worden's theory of 'grief work' which focuses on the tasks that need to be completed to achieve resolution of these feelings. People sometimes talk about someone who has been recently bereaved as being in a 'state of mourning'; however, Worden (1991) suggests that mourning is an active process which has to be 'worked' at. In his seminal work, Worden (1991) asserts that there are four 'tasks' of mourning that must be worked through in order for the person affected by the loss to be able to come to terms with their loss. They are:

- *Task 1 – To accept the reality of the loss*: Even when death is expected, once it has occurred it is often accompanied by a sense of unreality. The first task of mourning therefore is to come to terms with the reality that the person has died. Part of this is also to accept that reunion is not possible and separation is permanent.
- *Task 2 – To work through the pain of grief*: It is necessary to work through the pain of the grief or it will manifest itself through physical or psychological symptoms or aberrant behaviour such as anxiety or anger outbursts. One of the aims of grief counselling is to help the client work through the pain of the grief and to allow the expression of emotions and feelings to permit resolution so that grief is not carried with them throughout their life.
- *Task 3 – To adjust to an environment in which the person is missing*: Realization that life is different without the dead person occurs from 3 months following the loss. This may involve the gradual coming to terms with living alone and/or raising children alone. It may be that the bereaved individual relied upon the person to do many of the manual tasks around the home or to take care of the finances. Adjustment through learning how to accomplish these tasks alone is an example of what is seen as part achievement of this task of mourning.
- *Task 4 – To emotionally relocate the deceased and move on with life*: This task describes the work of finding an appropriate place for the dead person in the bereaved individual's emotional life, enabling them to move on and live effectively again. Incompletion of this task may be characterized by a holding on to the past and making a pact with oneself never to love again.

> **CRITICAL THINKING** Box 12.4
>
> ### Bereavement in children and young people
>
> Sue is dying and she and her partner have talked about how they can best prepare their children (Colin aged 15 and Kate aged 9) for Sue's death and life without their mother.
>
> **Student activities**
>
> - Access the Winston's Wish website and look at the services they offer and the activities and suggestions they have to help children and adolescents who are facing the death of a loved one or who are bereaved.
> - Discuss with your mentor how these resources could be used in your branch of nursing.
>
> [Resource: Winston's Wish – www.winstonswish.org.uk Available July 2006]

Factors affecting grief

Many factors influence how people respond to loss and bereavement. Whether the death was expected or sudden has an impact on the bereavement process (see pp. 310–311). However, age, cognitive impairment (e.g. dementia or learning disabilities) and cultural differences are all factors that may influence the process of grieving.

Bereavement in children

Bereaved adults caring for a child are often left to support the child. Many are ill equipped to do so and this often results in a protective instinct to shield the child from the pain of the loss. However, with some support, even very young children are able to grasp the concept of death. Furthermore, studies have demonstrated that children who have suffered bereavement and not been able to express their grief are more susceptible to depression (Weller et al 1991). Thus helping and supporting the child to grieve is important.

In order to help children accept and come to terms with death there are a number of interventions that can be carried out to aid this process (Box 12.4). These include:

- Preparing the child for bereavement
- Supporting parents and carers of the child
- Explaining and talking openly about death with the child
- Encouraging the child's participation in mourning, e.g. attending the funeral
- Resumption of normal activities
- Visiting the grave/special place
- Memory boxes/books

(Black 1996, Winston's Wish 2005).

Bereavement in people with learning disabilities

It is widely accepted that the pattern of bereavement in people with learning disabilities is the same as everyone else, as is the case with people who have dementia. However, in some cases the grief reaction is delayed and is first manifest by a sudden change in behaviour such as violent outbursts and withdrawal. Due to the delay in response, it is often handled inappropriately using medication or behavioural therapy (Hollins & Esterhuyzen 1997). In her study of the provision of education for carers of people with learning disabilities, Bennett (2003) found that many felt inadequately prepared to provide bereavement support to their clients. This may indicate why people with learning disabilities are sometimes inappropriately managed with medications and behavioural therapies.

People with learning disabilities generally do better if they are adequately prepared for the loss and are supported through the bereavement. Crick (1988) identified areas of need in people with learning disabilities who had been bereaved. These include:

- A full understanding of death
- Anticipation of bereavement
- Help and support to express feelings of grief
- An empathic confidante.

Complicated grief

While it is acknowledged that each person's course of mourning will be unique, uncomplicated grief is characterized by the patterns and feelings described above. When grief becomes complicated it can lead to unusual patterns of behaviour. Several types of complicated grief are recognized. These are:

- Chronic grief – mourning is of an excessive duration with the person unable to resume the normal levels of functioning
- Delayed grief – normal mourning is inhibited or postponed, only to return at a later date with great intensity
- Exaggerated grief – the person is overwhelmed by grief and may develop severe depression or rely on maladaptive coping strategies such as alcohol or drug misuse, prescribed or illicit (Kindlen et al 1999).

Palliative care

This part of the chapter explores what palliative care is and how palliative care services are organized within the UK. Nurses have an integral role to play in providing patients and families with high quality palliative care. The term palliative care is derived from the Latin word *pallium*, meaning 'to cloak'. Thus palliative care focuses on symptom relief without curing the illness which is causing the symptoms.

Palliative care has been known by many terms over the years. These include terminal care, hospice care, care of the dying, end-of-life care and supportive care (Payne 2004). Problems have arisen with the terminology used previously. For example, Doyle et al (1998) argue that the term 'terminal care' is confusing because it implies there is little that can be done for the patient. This is in stark contrast to the active and sometimes interventionist nature of palliative care, which may include chemotherapy (anti-cancer [cytotoxic] drugs to destroy cancer cells) and radiotherapy (the use of high energy X-rays to destroy cancer cells). Similarly the term 'hospice care' is misleading as it gives the impression that the approach is limited to those in the care of hospice professionals rather than indicating an approach to care that can be used in any setting and at every stage of the illness journey. This term, however, was first used to denote the hospice movement, which advocated a move away from acute hospital care for patients who were dying of incurable illnesses such as cancer. 'End-of-life' care similarly falls short of what encompasses palliative care as it implies that care is only given when the patient is at a certain stage of their illness. End-of-life care certainly falls within the remit of palliative care but palliative care is much broader, with many authors arguing that it should begin at the time of diagnosis. Palliative care then is essentially care of patients and their families whose illness is no longer curable and should begin when this is known.

What is palliative care?

The World Health Organization (WHO 2004) has provided a useful definition:

> Palliative care improves the quality of life of patients and families who face life-threatening illness, by providing pain and symptom relief, spiritual and psychosocial support from diagnosis to the end of life and bereavement.

In this definition the holistic nature of palliative care is evident as it encompasses the multidimensional approach. The WHO outlines the principles that underpin the approach to palliative care, as follows:

> Palliative care provides relief from pain and other distressing symptoms. It:
>
> - Affirms life and regards dying as a normal process
> - Intends neither to hasten nor postpone death
> - Integrates the psychological and spiritual aspects of patient care
> - Offers a support system to help patients live as actively as possible until death
> - Offers a support system to help the family cope during the patient's illness and in their own bereavement
> - Uses a team approach to address the needs of patients and their families, including bereavement counselling, if indicated
> - Will enhance quality of life and may also positively influence the course of illness
> - Is applicable early in the course of illness, in conjunction with other therapies that are intended to prolong life, such as chemotherapy or radiation therapy, and includes those investigations needed to better understand and manage distressing clinical complications
>
> (WHO 2004).

The WHO definition and the principles of palliative care illustrate the complexity of palliative care. For this reason it is unlikely that any one healthcare professional will be able to deliver palliative care in isolation, rather it has to be a MDT approach. Members of the MDT may vary in their level of input over the course of the patient's illness but examples of people involved are:

- General nurses
- Hospital-based medical staff
- District nurses
- Learning disability liaison nurses
- General practitioners
- Specialist palliative care nurses and doctors
- Physiotherapists
- Occupational therapists
- Dietitians
- Psychologists
- Social workers
- Religious figures
- Complementary therapists
- Volunteers.

Furthermore, it is unlikely that palliative care will be delivered in a single place. Thus health and social care professionals working in hospitals, community, hospices and voluntary sectors must understand the palliative care approach (Box 12.5).

The MDT should have a shared idea of common roles and accepted objectives; in order to achieve these, traditional professional roles may have to be adjusted. There is great value in including family and carers within the team, as many patients express a wish to be cared for in their own homes. Families and carers must be well informed and supported in order for this to happen.

The provision of high quality palliative care is a multidisciplinary endeavour. However, nurses usually work very closely with patients and their families during the course of their illness and in bereavement, and therefore have a central role in providing information, care and support.

REFLECTIVE PRACTICE Box 12.5

Teamwork in palliative care

Think back to a placement where you cared for a patient who had a terminal illness.

Student activities

- Which members of the MDT were involved in their care?
- What distinct roles did each professional have and which roles did they share?
- Discuss teamwork and the MDT with your mentor.

Palliative care for children

The WHO (2004) states that palliative care for children is closely related to adult palliative care and provides principles for care of children with chronic non-curative illness. Palliative care for children:

- Is the active care of the child's body, mind and spirit, and also involves giving support to the family

- Begins when illness is diagnosed, and continues regardless of whether or not a child receives treatment directed at the disease
- Requires health providers to evaluate and alleviate a child's physical, psychological and social distress
- Requires a multidisciplinary approach that includes the family and makes use of available community resources
- Can be provided in tertiary care facilities, in community health centres and in children's homes

(WHO 2004).

Overview of palliative care services

Founding of the UK palliative care movement is widely attributed to Dame Cicely Saunders who pioneered the palliative care approach with the opening of St Christopher's Hospice in 1967. However, it took a further two decades for palliative medicine to be recognized as a medical speciality.

The palliative care approach was developed in St Christopher's Hospice with the aim of providing care that was informed by research and was sensitive to the needs of individual patients. Since then it has proliferated throughout the UK and it is now delivered in a variety of settings:

- Home
- Hospital
- Hospice.

Palliative care has been subdivided into general and specialist palliative care.

General palliative care

This is based on the principles of palliative care and should be a core skill of every clinician. It is widely referred to as 'the palliative care approach'. The aims are to promote both physical and psychosocial well-being and are a vital part of all clinical practice whatever the person's illness or its stage. It includes holistic consideration of the family and domestic carers rather than purely medical/physical aspects.

Specialist palliative care

Specialists in palliative care provide specialist palliative care. According to Finlay and Jones (1995) it:

- Is multidisciplinary
- Is available in both general and hospital practice
- Provides advice and support that bridges the divide between home and hospital
- Provides hospice care
- Provides research, education and support for other professionals using a palliative care approach.

Palliative care in hospitals

Despite evidence that the majority of terminally ill patients wish to die at home, most people die in an NHS hospital. Reasons for this include:

- The need for continuous nursing care for people requiring considerable physical help
- Increasing numbers of older people who live alone
- Requirement for complex symptom control.

Patients may be under the care of general physicians or surgeons and be nursed in general wards. The palliative care approach should be adopted in such cases and there are established hospital palliative care teams in the majority of UK hospitals.

Hospital palliative care teams are ideally multidisciplinary; however, some specialist nurses still work alone. The role of the MDT is to provide specialist advice and support for patients with complex palliative care needs and support and advice for general staff caring for the patient.

While many palliative care team members will have a background in cancer care, their remit extends to other diseases, e.g. heart failure. They provide advice on issues such as pain and symptom management, emotional support for the patient and family, advice and support to hospital staff and the primary care team, liaison with other palliative care services and bereavement care.

Hospice care

Hospice care developed largely from the work of charitable organizations such as Marie Curie Cancer Care, Sue Ryder and Macmillan Cancer Support. The services provided include:

- Hospice inpatient units
- Hospice beds within hospitals and nursing homes
- Hospice at home
- Daycare
- Community palliative care team.

Although hospice inpatient units were initially set up to deal with the needs of patients suffering from terminal cancer, hospice services are increasingly being sought from patients with other terminal illnesses such as motor neurone disease. On the other hand, children's hospices have developed for the needs of a much broader range of diseases as children usually die of degenerative disease (Katz 2004).

Patients are admitted to inpatient hospice care for a variety of reasons, including assessment, rehabilitation, pain and symptom management, short respite stays to help relieve carers and terminal care. The environment is more homely than hospitals, and centres on the individual patient's needs. Families are encouraged to be involved in care where appropriate and visiting tends to be open. Staff normally have access to specialized training and education in palliative care.

The main aim of hospice daycare is to enhance the quality of life of the patient, as well as providing respite for relatives caring for the patient at home. The focus of care is on providing support and advice on pain and other distressing symptoms, as well as providing emotional support and rehabilitation, all of which may enable the patient to remain at home. Most daycare units run as multidisciplinary community services where the patient remains under the care of the GP. The role of healthcare professionals in the daycare unit therefore necessitates close liaison with the patient's GP and other members of the primary care team (see Ch. 3).

Hospice at home provides extra care and support to terminally ill patients in their own homes and offers support to relatives and carers. It supplements the services normally provided by district nurses. 'Hands-on' care and support are provided by a team of qualified nurses and auxiliary staff who provide most, if not all, of the nursing care that would be available in an inpatient hospice. This makes it possible for people to spend the last weeks or months of their illness in familiar surroundings, with their family and friends around them.

Marie Curie nurses care for almost 50% of all people with cancer who die in their own homes (Marie Curie Cancer Care 2005). They provide free expert nursing care and emotional support to families affected by cancer. They are available for periods during the day and night, which helps to reduce patient stress and anxiety (see Ch. 11) and gives carers the opportunity to rest or sleep.

Community palliative care team

A community palliative care team may consist of specialist palliative care nurses who visit patients and families in their own home, or they may be part of a bigger team such as those in a hospice. Increasingly, hospital and community are becoming more closely integrated and working across the boundaries.

Similar to the other palliative care services described above, the role of the community palliative care team includes providing support and advice on pain and other distressing symptoms, providing emotional support for the patient and their carers and also providing bereavement support. Charities such as Marie Curie Cancer Care and Macmillan Cancer Support have led the way in providing community-based support by providing nursing services.

Communicating with patients and families

Communication is central to high quality palliative care. Communication skills are often regarded as 'something nurses can do' (see Ch. 9). However, in palliative care effective communication requires considerable knowledge and skill. Studies exploring the perceptions of patients and families indicate that considerable scope exists to improve meeting their information and communication needs (Wilkinson 1991). Kinghorn (2001, p. 167) states that 'effective and sensitive communication is the heart of comforting, assessment of need, expression of psychological/social/spiritual distress as planning for what may be perceived to be an undesirable and premature end to life'.

Speaking to dying patients and their families is difficult and uncomfortable and is usually led by experienced clinicians. Studies have identified that health professionals often 'block' patients when they seek information (Wilkinson 1991, Heaven & Maguire 1996). It is important to acknowledge that awkwardness when dealing with advanced illness and death is universal and nurses should not view inabilities as personal failings. However, it is the responsibility of nurses and other healthcare professionals to develop, refine and advance their communication skills. While it is necessary to understand theories of communication, reflecting upon clinical practice to reach new understandings is critical (Box 12.6).

REFLECTIVE PRACTICE Box 12.6

Communication skills in palliative care

You may wish to arrange to observe an experienced colleague when they are talking with a dying patient and their relatives or you may already have had this experience.

Student activities

- What was positive and negative about the way the situation was handled?
- What skills and attributes of the clinician were important?

Box 12.7 **WHO three-step analgesic ladder**

Step 1 – Mild pain
Paracetamol or non-steroidal anti-inflammatory drugs (NSAIDs), e.g. diclofenac sodium ± adjuvant. Drugs that are not analgesics act as adjuvants to relieve pain. For example, dexamethasone (a corticosteroid) is used to relieve pain resulting from raised intracranial (within the cranium) pressure, as it reduces swelling of the brain. Other adjuvants include anticonvulsants, e.g. carbamazepine and sodium valproate, or antidepressants, e.g. amitriptyline, for nerve pain. These drugs are used not for their primary action but for the actions that relieve the sensation of pain for the patient.

Step 2 – Mild to moderate pain
Weak opioid, e.g. codeine or dihydrocodeine + paracetamol, or NSAIDs ± adjuvant.

Step 3 – Moderate to severe pain
Opioid, e.g. morphine sulphate + paracetamol, or NSAIDs ± adjuvant.

[From WHO (2005)]

Care and symptom control

There are a variety of symptoms associated with terminal illness, e.g. pain. These are discussed below.

Managing pain in palliative care

Cancer is not synonymous with pain; however, 75% of patients with cancer may experience pain (Twycross 1997). The WHO suggests that up to 80% of patients with

Table 12.1 Reversible causes of breathlessness

Cause	Management
Infection	Antibiotics if appropriate
Anaemia	Iron supplementation or blood transfusion
Pleural effusion (presence of fluid in the pleural cavity)	Drainage of effusion
Bronchospasm (spasm of the smooth muscle of the bronchi leading to bronchoconstriction and narrowing)	Nebulized bronchodilators, e.g. salbutamol
Pulmonary embolism (clot in the blood supply to the lungs)	Anticoagulant therapy
Hypoxia (reduced levels of oxygen in the tissues) may result from any of the above causes. Oxygen therapy is used for hypoxia.	

pain may have their pain adequately controlled by following a simple three-step approach to pain management:

- By the mouth – the oral route of administration should be used whenever possible
- By the clock – patients should be prescribed regular analgesia
- By the ladder – a three-step approach has been suggested by the WHO for managing cancer pain (Box 12.7). If a drug fails to relieve pain, then a drug from the next step up the ladder should be used (see Fig. 23.10, p. 672).

The principles of pain management in adults outlined above are equally applicable to children. Assessment of pain is crucial to effective management. Pain assessment self-report scales have been developed specifically for children such as the 'faces scale' (see Ch. 23).

The WHO pain ladder (see Ch. 23) can be used for managing pain in children. However, calculation of drug dosages is complex and should be calculated according to the weight of the child (Goldman 1998).

Breathlessness (see Ch. 17)

Breathlessness (dyspnoea) is an unpleasant and often frightening sensation of being unable to breathe easily. It is a very common symptom in patients with all types of terminal illness.

Some causes of breathlessness may be reversible and therefore accurate assessment of the cause is vital (Table 12.1).

Care of the breathless patient should be individualized and a multidisciplinary approach is essential. Advice from the physiotherapist is often particularly helpful on positioning patients in a bed or chair, control of breathing rate and relaxation methods (Davis 1997) (see Chs 10, 17). Breathlessness has both physical and psychological elements. Not being able to breathe easily can cause intense fear, which causes the patient and family to become anxious, and the physical symptom worsens. This cyclical pattern requires sensitive support and careful management. Reassurance and support can help reduce anxiety, along with relaxation techniques (see Chs 10, 11) and anxiolytic drugs, e.g. lorazepam.

Excess respiratory secretions

Excess respiratory secretions often become problematic within the last days or hours of life. The build-up of secretions in the airways is due to the patient's inability to cough up or swallow them. This presents as a noisy gurgle during breathing, often referred to as the 'death rattle' as it is associated with the terminal phase. The patient is usually in a state of altered consciousness at this stage and is not aware of the problem; however, it is particularly distressing for the family.

Careful positioning of the patient on their side may assist in relieving the problem for a short time. The registered nurse may carry out regular oral suctioning. Drugs such as hyoscine butylbromide may also be prescribed to reduce the secretions and hence the distressing sounds. These drugs, which also cause sedation, may be given by subcutaneous injection or via a syringe driver (see Chs 22, 23).

Fatigue

Fatigue is the most common symptom experienced by patients with advanced cancer. It is defined as 'a total body feeling ranging from tiredness to exhaustion, creating an unrelenting overall condition which interferes with an individual's ability to function to their normal capacity' (Ream & Richardson 1996, p. 527). Fatigue is a difficult symptom to manage, as it is not merely corrected by rest. There are a number of physical and psychosocial causes of fatigue, some of which can be alleviated. They include:

- Physical factors:
  - anaemia
  - cancer treatments such as radiotherapy, chemotherapy
  - cachexia (emaciation resulting from rapid weight loss, often seen in patients with gastrointestinal or lung cancers as a result of complex metabolic changes)

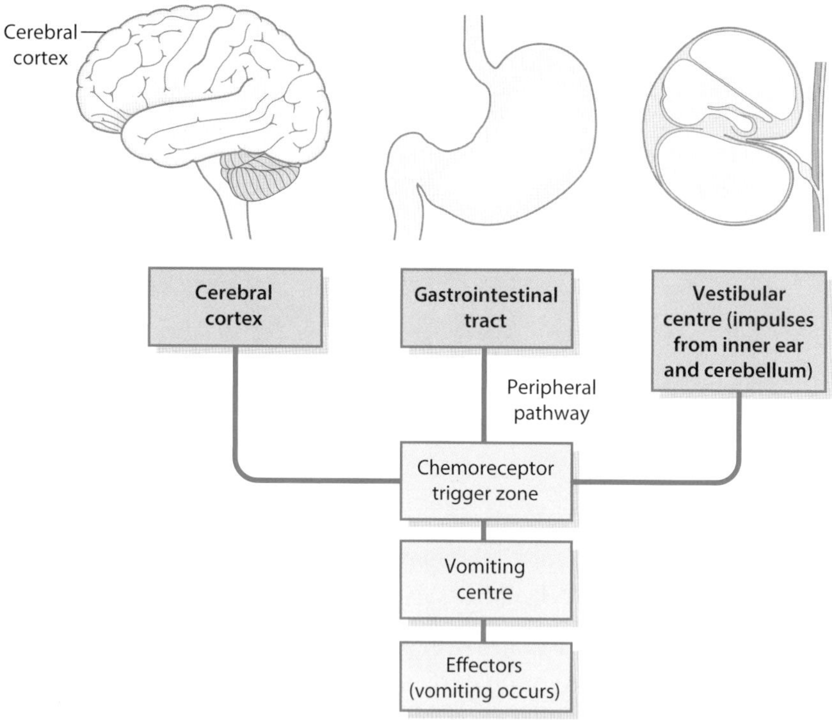

Fig. 12.1 The vomiting reflex (reproduced with permission from Bruce & Finlay 1997)

  - toxic breakdown products from cancer cells
  - coughing
  - breathlessness.
- Psychosocial factors:
  - inactivity
  - insomnia (see Ch. 10)
  - anxiety (see Ch. 11)
  - depression.

Management of cancer-related fatigue is difficult and needs to be tailored to the needs of individual patients. Little research has been done in this area to support management strategies; however, reversible causes such as anaemia should be corrected. Some clinicians report an improvement in fatigue when patients are encouraged to do gentle exercise. It would appear that a balance between periods of rest and activity is the optimum for promoting well-being.

Nausea and vomiting

Patients may feel nauseated and retch for many hours before they vomit or they may not vomit but still suffer the unpleasant sensation of nausea. Nursing care such as ensuring easy access to vomit bowls, tissues and mouthwash, as well as ensuring privacy, can promote the patient's comfort (see Ch. 19). Avoidance of strong odours and food smells can also help to reduce nausea. There are many causes of nausea and vomiting in patients with advanced illness (Lothian NHS Board 2001), including.

- Drugs, e.g. opioids and chemotherapy
- Toxins
- Radiotherapy
- Constipation (see Ch. 21)
- Pain
- Hypercalcaemia (abnormally high level of calcium in the blood)
- Cough
- Anxiety
- Gastric (stomach) irritation or dilatation.

Some of the causes are reversible and treatment of nausea and vomiting depends very much on the cause. Reversible causes must be identified and treated appropriately through accurate assessment.

Vomiting is initiated and synchronized by two centres in the brain: the vomiting centre, which has overall control, and the chemoreceptor trigger zone (CTZ). Both centres respond to various stimuli (Fig. 12.1). The vomiting centre and CTZ contain receptors able to respond to different stimuli arriving from the cerebral cortex, the vestibular centre (impulses from inner ear and cerebellum) and the gastrointestinal tract depending on the cause of vomiting. The receptors include histamine receptors (H_1), acetylcholine receptors (ACh_m), dopamine receptors (D_2) and those for 5-hydroxytryptamine receptors (5-HT_3).

Nurses need to know about the receptors because each type of antiemetic (against vomiting) drug acts at a different type of receptor (Box 12.8). Therefore it is essential to use the appropriate antiemetic drug for the cause of the vomiting. They should always be prescribed and given when nausea and vomiting is anticipated, such as with some chemotherapy drugs. Nausea can be treated with oral drugs; however, alternative routes of administration must be used if the patient is vomiting, e.g. rectal, subcutaneous or intramuscular (see Ch. 22). It is important that the patient with nausea receives regular antiemetic drugs before vomiting occurs. Further reading suggestions (e.g. Prodigy guidance 2004) provide more information.

Box 12.8 Controlling nausea and vomiting – antiemetics and other drugs

- Antihistamines, e.g. cyclizine, are histamine receptor (H_1) antagonists. Used for vomiting following radiotherapy to the head or neck and for motion sickness
- Acetylcholine (muscarinic) receptor antagonists (ACh_m), e.g. hyoscine hydrobromide, are used for motion sickness. They also dry secretions, so may reduce nausea and retching where respiratory secretions are excessive (see p. 307)
- Phenothiazines, e.g. prochlorperazine, are dopamine (D_2) receptor antagonists and also act centrally to block the CTZ. They are used for vomiting associated with radiotherapy, opioids and chemotherapy drugs and widespread cancer
- Metoclopramide acts in a similar way to the phenothiazines but also acts on the gastrointestinal tract. Useful for gastritis, gastric stasis and nausea and vomiting associated with radiotherapy, toxins and opioids
- Domperidone acts centrally to block the CTZ and is used for gastrointestinal problems and nausea and vomiting associated with radiotherapy, toxins and opioids
- Dolasetron and ondansetron act by blocking 5-hydroxytryptamine ($5\text{-}HT_3$) receptors in the gastrointestinal tract. Useful in the management of nausea and vomiting induced by chemotherapy and radiotherapy
- Synthetic cannabinoids, e.g. nabilone, are used where other antiemetics fail to control chemotherapy-induced vomiting
- Aprepitant (a neurokinin-1 receptor antagonist) is used with a $5\text{-}HT_3$ antagonist and dexamethasone for vomiting associated with cisplatin-based chemotherapy
- Benzodiazepines, e.g. diazepam, are used to aid relaxation when vomiting is associated with anxiety
- Dexamethasone (a corticosteroid) may be used alone or with other antiemetics for vomiting associated with chemotherapy.

[Resources: *British National Formulary* (BNF) – www.bnf.org.uk; *BNF for Children* – http://www.bnfc.org/bnfc Available July 2006]

Oral problems

Oral hygiene is very important for patients with terminal illnesses, especially when there is difficulty taking food and fluids or dehydration (see Chs 16, 19). The most common problems encountered are dry or sore mouth, oral thrush (candidiasis) and ulceration.

Constipation

Constipation is a significant problem for patients requiring palliative care and is a particularly distressing symptom. Constipation may also be the cause of other problems such as nausea and vomiting, abdominal pain and cramps, bloating, and faecal soiling and diarrhoea from faecal overflow.

Constipation may have a number of causes, e.g. opioid analgesics. This should be anticipated and a prophylactic laxative prescribed and administered. Immobility, inadequate food and fluid intake, as well as the patient's illness, may all be causes of constipation. As with all symptoms, accurate assessment is crucial to determine the cause of the constipation. The patient's normal bowel habit is recorded in order to assess how this has changed.

Simple measures may help, such as ensuring privacy and acting promptly to requests for a commode or help to get to the lavatory. Interventions that prevent or alleviate constipation are discussed in Chapter 21. Ensuring adequate fibre and fluid intake where appropriate may help; however, with some patients this will not be possible if their illness is advanced.

Terminal agitation

Terminal agitation or restlessness is common in patients in the terminal phase of the illness. At this time the patient may become confused, agitated and may also be hallucinating (a perception of the presence of something which is not there). Care should be taken to identify any treatable causes such as unrelieved pain and constipation. Similarly, if the patient is clear in their thought processes, time should be spent trying to identify if the patient has unresolved issues, as fear and anxiety may exacerbate this symptom.

A quiet, calming environment with familiar surroundings or people known to the patient may help; however, it may be necessary to use sedation to resolve agitation and calm the patient. Opioids can have a sedative effect although their use in this instance is not appropriate as they may induce further confusion and/or hallucinations. Sedative drugs such as haloperidol and/or midazolam can be administered either as subcutaneous injection or via a syringe driver in order to sedate and calm the patient.

Terminal agitation can be very distressing for relatives to watch; however, a simple and clear explanation as to the reasons for the confusion and the strategies used to try to alleviate it may be helpful in reducing their distress.

Death and dying

It has been identified that the palliative care approach is applicable in the early stages of chronic, non-curative illness. However, at the end of life this is particularly appropriate as it promotes quality of life and comfort regardless of the stage of the illness. In this section issues relating to death and dying are considered.

Death may result from trauma, or sudden or progressive illness, and nurses have a role in supporting patients and their family and friends during this time. Personal experiences of death vary and the cause, circumstances and support available influence how individuals experience death and dying. The nurse's actions at the time of death can profoundly affect bereavement, grief and adaptation to the loss. The circumstances surrounding death are unique to each individual and family; however, there are likely to be physical, psychosocial and spiritual needs and the requirement for open and honest information.

Sudden death

When a person dies suddenly this is due to cerebral ischaemia (lack of blood flow to the brain). This can be caused by a stroke, heart attack, cardiac arrest or haemorrhage due to trauma.

Sudden death may result from an acute illness or trauma, accidents or suicide. When death is unexpected, the family and those closest to the deceased are likely to experience profound shock, numbness, disbelief and feelings of chaos and disorder. Sudden death due to accidents, suicide or other trauma is the main cause of death in young adults, particularly males, so meeting the needs of those closest to these patients is challenging (Box 12.9).

Wright (2002) suggests that in grounding sudden death in reality, an individual needs to reach a level of resolution and adaptation with which they can cope. There are three important factors in this process: perception of the event, external resources and inner resources.

Perception of the event

People search for information to help attribute cause and seek an explanation for what has happened. Some people may be unable to cope with information immediately following the bereavement so information giving should be tailored to meet individual needs (see 'Breaking bad news', Ch. 9). Nurses should also consider where people get support and information once their contact with healthcare professionals has ceased.

External resources

It is important to establish what support is available for the bereaved person. Initially support is likely to be provided by family and friends. It is therefore important that nurses identify who can be called upon to provide support, e.g. with transport home from the hospital if a close relative has died suddenly. Careful consideration must be given to what information should be given over the phone by the registered nurse who does not know the person and how they are likely to respond, especially if a relative is being asked to come in to an emergency department. Dealing with sudden death is demanding and requires sophisticated communication skills (see Ch. 9). Knowing what to say and when is important and nurses need to discern what information to give the bereaved person who may be so shocked they cannot think what to ask.

For hospital-based staff, contact with people who experience the sudden death of a loved one may be extremely limited. For many bereaved people the full impact of their loss may not be apparent for some time following the death. Untimely, unexpected and traumatic deaths may cause severe and prolonged grieving. It is therefore important for nurses to be aware of local resources and types of help available and to give this information to bereaved relatives, including information relevant to different faiths. One such source of support is Cruse Bereavement Care, which exists to promote the well-being of bereaved people and help them to understand their grief and cope with their loss (see 'Useful websites', p. 317).

Inner resources

Very individual coping strategies will be used by bereaved people in order to deal with the crisis of sudden death and its aftermath. When a sudden, unexpected death occurs there is usually no opportunity to be present at the time of death. This is thought to complicate the grieving process and how people cope with the bereavement. One of the most important issues in helping people to accept the reality of the death is knowledge of what happened at the end and nurses can help (Box 12.10). Relatives may ask

CRITICAL THINKING Box 12.9

Sudden death due to suicide

Ben, who was 25 years old, suffered from severe depression. He committed suicide while a voluntary patient in a mental health unit.

Discuss with your mentor the potential impact of Ben's death on his family and friends and the staff.

Student activities

Visit the Office for National Statistics website (www.statistics.gov.uk) and find out:

- How many people commit suicide per 100 000 of the UK population.
- How suicide rates vary by age, gender and geographical location.
- Which day of the week is the commonest for suicide.

CRITICAL THINKING Box 12.10

Death of a child

Louisa, the eldest of three children, has recently been killed in a road traffic accident. Her parents are devastated and her mother cannot accept that Louisa is really dead. They have visited the mortuary many times to see Louisa and spend long periods of time there. They are increasingly distressed following each visit.

Student activities

- Consider why Louisa's mother needs to visit the mortuary repeatedly.
- Discuss with your mentor how staff could help Louisa's parents and younger siblings.

if the person suffered or what their last words were and registered nurses should not avoid giving this information or indeed any information they have. Rather than traumatizing relatives, as is often thought to be the case, it is likely that providing information will help them cope with the reality of the situation.

Viewing the body is also important in achieving understanding of the loss. Generally, even in traumatic death, relatives who view the dead person, especially if they were not present at the time of death, find this helpful (Wright 2002). Preparation of the bereaved for viewing a loved one is an important nursing role that can help to lessen the impact of seeing significant changes in body colour or trauma (see pp. 312–313).

Expected death and palliative care

Gradual expected death occurs when there is failure of one or more organs and/or systems that maintain the internal environment of the cells (homeostasis). As the internal environment deteriorates, an increasing number of cells and tissues malfunction, leading to system failure. For example, when the respiratory system fails, hypoxia (reduction of oxygen in the tissues) and hypercapnia (increased carbon dioxide in arterial blood) will result in the failure of other organs including the heart and brain (see Ch. 17).

When death is anticipated and expected, patients and families experience profound and individual physical and emotional consequences. Dealing with these experiences is crucial to the process of accepting and responding to the situation. Whatever stage of acceptance and resolution individuals have reached as the end of life approaches, appropriate care around the time of death is arguably one of the most challenging and responsible aspects of the nursing role.

The palliative care approach is applicable throughout the illness trajectory and, in the later stages of life, represents the best of care by combining the clinical, holistic and human dimensions of care. Uncontrolled physical symptoms in the last stages of life increase levels of distress for both the patient and family members (see pp. 306–309). Furthermore, the intense emotional impact for family members following death increases their risks of morbidity and mortality during the bereavement phase (Parkes 1998).

Recognizing that death is approaching

Knowing when a patient is likely to die is usually very important for family members, some of whom will normally wish to be present at the time of death. For people of many faiths it is especially important for the patient to have the next of kin present as religious rituals must be performed to ensure the dying person passes on to the next life (see pp. 314–315). Families may ask if they should take a break from sitting at the bedside or when they should contact other family members who live at a distance. An important role of the nurse at the end of life is ensuring that family members are alerted to the imminence of death and have privacy to say their goodbyes and grieve. While it is not possible to predict exactly the last stages of life, there are recognized signs that death is imminent (adapted from National Council for Hospice and Specialist Palliative Care Services 1997). They include:

- Profound weakness – usually bed-bound requiring assistance with all care
- Gaunt physical appearance
- Drowsy or reduced cognition – may be disorientated, restless, have difficulty in concentrating and scarcely able to cooperate with carers
- Diminished intake of food and fluids
- Difficulty swallowing medications
- Breathing changes/excess secretions
- Incontinence
- Decreased urine output
- Cold extremities
- Cyanosis.

Causes of death and the need for palliative care

People die in their own home, in a hospital, hospice or a residential/nursing home. Increased life expectancy and the shift from infectious diseases to degenerative diseases such as cancer, heart disease or stroke as causes of death have meant that deaths are concentrated in old age. Many people facing death live alone and lack informal support.

Addington-Hall (1996) surveyed the symptoms experienced in the last year of life in three groups of patients: those with cancer, heart disease and stroke. Symptoms including pain, nausea and vomiting, etc. were prevalent in advanced cancer. People with heart disease had breathlessness and people dying from strokes experienced mental confusion and incontinence. Significantly, this survey revealed that while people with cancer experienced more symptoms, the duration was shorter than for the other two groups. Palliative care is frequently associated with cancer; however, there is increasing recognition that all patients with advanced, non-curable illness require palliative care.

Main causes of death in the UK

The 2001 census of the population of the UK identified that, for the first time, people over 60 years of age form a larger part of the population (21%) than children aged less than 16 years (20%) (National Statistics 2003a). Furthermore, people aged 85 and over have increased to 1.9% of the population. These population trends correspond with life expectancy (the expectation of number of years of life at birth), which continues to improve. In addition, 'the infant mortality rate has fallen dramatically throughout the 20th century' (National Statistics 2003b, p. 7) (Fig. 12.2, p. 312).

In the year 2000, around 80% of deaths were of people over 65 years of age compared with 20% in 1901. However, improvement in life expectancy is accompanied by significant rises in the so-called degenerative diseases which can be linked to lifestyle factors such as cancers and cardiovascular diseases. Therefore the correlation between life expectancy and healthy life expectancy is important, as evidence to date suggests that while life expectancy is

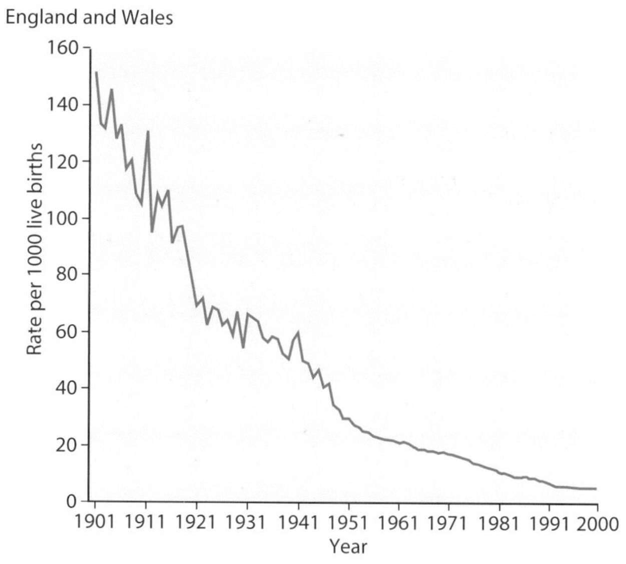

Fig. 12.2 Infant mortality rate 1901–2000 in England and Wales (reproduced from National Statistics, Health Statistics Quarterly (18) Summer 2003, with permission of HMSO Licensing)

CRITICAL THINKING Box 12.11

Causes of death

Select a cause of death relevant to your chosen branch, e.g. suicide/injury undetermined deaths, sudden infant death syndrome, child deaths due to accidents or deaths from heart disease.

Student activities

- Compare numbers of deaths at different ages, gender and regions for the UK.
- Investigate local data for the same cause of death by searching strategic health authority, primary care trust and health board statistics/reports. Are there differences between UK, national and local data?

[Resources: National Statistics 2005 Annual update 2003 mortality statistics: cause (England and Wales). Health Statistics Quarterly (25) Spring 2005. Online: www.statistics.gov.uk/downloads/theme_health/HSQ25.pdf; Northern Ireland Statistics and Research Agency – www.nisra.gov.uk/publications/default.asp?cmsid=20_22_37&cms=demography_Vital%20statistics_Deaths+by+cause&release=future; Scottish Executive – www.scotland.gov.uk/Topics/Statistics/17861/10369 All available July 2006]

increasing, healthy life expectancy is not, and the 'burden of disability' towards the end of life is increasing. Cardiovascular diseases and cancer are significant causes of death of adults in the UK and most European countries. These trends are predicted to continue due to increasingly sedentary lifestyles, smoking and diets high in saturated fats (National Statistics 2003a).

It is important for nurses to understand population trends and causes of morbidity (incidence of a disease) and mortality (numbers of deaths) as they are involved in meeting the health needs of populations and caring for patients and families around the time of death (Box 12.11).

Death states and the physiology of dying

In order to help nurses cope with patients, relatives and their own feelings around the time of death, it is useful to understand what is happening when people die. Death may be sudden due to accident or illness, or be 'expected', for example when a patient has an advanced non-curable illness such as chronic respiratory disease, cardiovascular disease or cancer.

Death as a process begins with the failure of a body system, which then affects other systems (see p. 311). Medical interventions, which can keep people alive even when vital functions have been lost, have created difficulties in deciding when a person can be declared 'dead'. This is particularly so when brain function is lost and a person's body may continue to function or be supported on a ventilator/respirator. Distinctions are normally made between three states:

- *Permanent vegetative state (PVS)*: The cerebral cortex is irreversibly damaged but the vital centres in the brain stem remain intact so breathing occurs spontaneously, the heart beats and blood circulates. The person's eyes may open and reflexes remain intact, which can make it difficult for relatives to accept that recovery is impossible. Brain cells are extremely sensitive to hypoxia and irreversible damage occurs if the blood supply is interrupted for 2–4 minutes.
- *Brain stem death*: If the brain stem is irreversibly damaged the patient will be deeply comatosed and breathing will cease unless artificial ventilation is used to maintain life. Brain stem death is confirmed by a series of tests performed on more than one occasion. Further information about brain stem death can be found at www.surgical-tutor.org.uk/core/trauma/head_brain.htm.
- *Certified death*: Once circulatory and respiratory function have permanently ceased, a person can be legally certified as dead (see p. 315).

The physiological and physical events occurring at death include:

- Pupils become fixed and dilated
- Immediate loss of muscle tone including sphincter relaxation (the bladder and bowel may empty at the time of death)
- Once circulation has ceased, the internal environment of the body deteriorates rapidly
- Rigor mortis (stiffening of the body) commences a few hours after death as muscle cells are depleted of energy (adenosine triphosphate [ATP]) and calcium levels in the cells rise, leading to binding together of the muscle proteins (actin and myosin)

Box 12.12 **A framework for palliative care, dying and death**

Communication
- The patient (if able) and carers should participate in decision-making about care
- Time and opportunities should be given for patients and relatives to seek and be given information
- Instructions should be written down and contact numbers given/obtained.

Coordination
- Effective care requires a collaborative approach using palliative care specialists as required, for example:
  - clinical nurse specialists
  - Marie Curie nurses
  - palliative medicine consultants
  - hospice/hospital palliative care teams
  - community physiotherapists and occupational therapists
  - social workers and counsellors
  - spiritual advisors
- A primary nurse in a hospice/hospital or a lead district nurse if the patient is at home should coordinate nursing care and collaborate with other team members involved.

Control of symptoms (see pp. 306–309)
- Each patient should have their symptoms, problems and concerns (physical, psychological, social, practical and spiritual) assessed, recorded, discussed and acted upon in accordance with their agenda
- In the last days/hours of life, only medications that control or prevent distressing symptoms should be given. Generally the only drugs needed in the final stages of life are:
  - analgesics (usually subcutaneous via a syringe driver; see Chs 15, 23)
  - anticonvulsants
  - hyoscine for 'rattle'
  - tranquillizers.

Continuity
- Regardless of where the patient is located, care should be seamless and healthcare professionals should ensure information is transferred, e.g. to out-of-hours service or hospice.

Continued learning
- All healthcare professionals must be committed to continued learning to ensure optimum care for patients and carers and know how to access and appraise evidence on which to base practice.

Carer support
- Emotional support – carers need support, to be listened to and kept informed. They should be encouraged to participate in care as appropriate and in accordance with the wishes of the patient
- Practical support – if the patient is at home, practical support such as night sitters, respite care and equipment, e.g. commodes, should be provided
- Bereavement information about sources of support/counselling should be provided
- Staff support – professional carers need support as caring for dying patients is challenging and emotionally draining. Reflection and clinical supervision are some of the methods by which nurses may receive support (see Ch. 11).

Care of the dying
- Caring for patients in the last days or hours of life requires particular interventions:
  - stopping non-essential interventions, e.g. wound dressings and drugs, if this would cause considerable discomfort
  - considering comfort measures
  - psychological and religious/spiritual support
  - bereavement planning
  - communication
  - care after death.

[Adapted from National Council for Hospice and Specialist Palliative Care Services (1997) and Thomas (2004)]

- The face will normally stiffen before the hands and feet, and maximum rigor will develop between 12 and 48 hours after death depending on environmental conditions
- Rigor mortis wears off when the tissues begin to decompose as enzymes digest cell proteins
- Some cells may survive within the tissues for some time but as cells die the enzymes begin the process of digestion
- Tissues soften and liquefy and bacterial contamination accelerates the digestive process. Iron sulphide is produced which stains the tissues green and black.

Care around the time of death

Whether a patient dies suddenly or the death is expected, the actions of those involved in caring for the patient and family are of utmost importance. Care that meets the needs of individuals around the time of death has been shown to impact on how well they cope following bereavement. Providing care when a patient reaches the last stages of life is an important nursing role. Regardless of the clinical area, nurses are likely to care for people who are dying. All nurses therefore require appropriate knowledge to inform care planning.

The Macmillan Gold Standards Framework (GSF) is designed to offer guidance to primary healthcare teams to improve the planning of palliative care so they can meet the needs of patients and carers. Evaluation of the GSF has shown that its implementation has improved care (Thomas 2004). While designed for primary care, the seven principles of the GSF provide guidance for nurses involved in caring for dying patients regardless of the clinical setting. Box 12.12 (see p. 313) outlines a framework for care.

Integrated care pathways (ICPs), a multidisciplinary care tool designed to enhance communication and continuity of care (see Chs 3, 14), are increasingly being used and evaluated in palliative care. Information about ICPs in palliative care is provided in Further reading (e.g. Ellershaw & Wilkinson 2003).

Providing support and information around the time of death is important, particularly where a patient may be classified as being either brain stem dead or in a PVS. Tactful handling is required at a time when nurses may be struggling with their own feelings (Box 12.13). Many relatives may not have seen a dead person before so preparation and gentle explanation are necessary.

Cultural aspects of dying and death

If nurses are to provide appropriate care at the end of life they must understand and meet the spiritual and cultural needs of individuals. Different cultures and societies approach death and grieving differently and nurses need to communicate with patients and families to establish what their needs and wishes are and ensure particular requests are communicated among the MDT. Nurses should establish if patients have any religious beliefs, as some patients may not have a belief or faith. They may, however, have requests for care around the time of death, e.g. humanists who neither believe in God nor an afterlife but celebrate the life that has been (British Humanist Association 2005). Table 12.2 provides an

REFLECTIVE PRACTICE Box 12.13

Personal experience of death

If you have experienced the death of someone close to you, reflect on the things others said or did, both helpful and unhelpful. If you have not experienced the death of someone close, think what might be helpful.

Student activities

Discuss the helpful things with your mentor or another experienced nurse.

Table 12.2 Religious practices around the time of death (adapted from Open University 1992)

Faith	As death approaches	When death is imminent	Immediately after death
Buddhism	Dying person needs opportunities to meditate A monk or religious teacher should visit the dying person to talk and chant passages of scripture	The ideal is to die in a fully conscious and calm state A monk or fellow Buddhist may chant to encourage a peaceful state of mind	No special requirements relating to care of the body Buddhists from different countries will have different traditions
Christianity	Some Christians may want prayers or anointing with oil by a minister or priest	As appropriate a priest or minister should be notified Some Christians will wish to receive communion or the last rites	No special requirements
Islam	Other Muslims, normally family members, join the dying person in prayer and recite verses from the Quran Dying person may wish to face Mecca (south-east in the UK)	The declaration of faith (Shahada) is said	Non-Muslim health workers should ask permission to touch the body and use disposable gloves The body must be kept covered Soon after death there is a ritual of washing the body by same sex Muslims Post mortems are disliked
Judaism	A rabbi may be called to join the dying Jew in prayer and facilitate confession	The dying person should not be left alone Jews present will recite psalms and, when death occurs, the Declaration of Faith (Shema)	Health workers should handle the body as little as possible and cover with a white sheet The Jewish burial society will collect the body and perform a ritual wash before burial Post mortems are disliked

(Continued)

Table 12.2 *(Continued)*

Faith	As death approaches	When death is imminent	Immediately after death
Hinduism	Hindus may receive comfort from hymns and readings from the Hindu holy books Some patients may wish to lie on the floor The family should be present	A Hindu priest may be called to perform holy rites A dying Hindu should be given Ganges water and the sacred Tulsi leaf placed in the mouth by the relatives A person should die with the name of God being recited Hindus often wish to die at home	The family will normally wash the body themselves If no family member is available health workers should wear gloves, close the eyes and straighten the limbs Jewellery and religious objects should not be removed
Sikhism	A dying Sikh may receive comfort from reciting hymns A relative or any practising Sikh may do so instead	A Sikh person should die in the name of God, Waheguru being recited Some may want to have holy water (Amrit) in the mouth	Health workers should not trim hair or beards and the body should be covered with a plain white cloth The five symbols of faith should not be removed from the body: • Kesh – uncut hair • Kangha – a comb which keeps the hair bun or jura in place • Kara – steel bangle worn on the left wrist • Kirpan – symbolic dagger worn under clothes • Kaccha – special underpants or shorts

overview of religious practices around the time of death (see also the BBC website in 'Useful websites', p. 317).

Caring for people who are dying or bereaved requires knowledge of specific cultural and religious rituals in order to provide culturally aware care. Nurses need to know who to contact and when from the person's own culture or religion to ensure traditional practices are followed and the patient's wishes are met. The best way to ensure appropriate end-of-life care is to take sufficient time to explore and assess the wishes and needs of the patient and family. Integration of cultural issues into care assessments and care planning is crucial as is the communication between team members (see Ch. 9). If the patient's needs are carefully assessed, documented and communicated amongst team members, the experience of dying will significantly improve for those involved (Box 12.14).

Care after death

Certification of death is a legal requirement normally carried out by a doctor. After death, the patient is referred to as 'the body'. The body should receive care – known as 'laying out or last offices or last act of care'– as soon as possible to minimize tissue damage or disfigurement. If the patient has died at home, the undertaker/funeral director or family is likely to attend to the laying out of the body.

It is important to check with the family as some cultures and faiths have important rituals about how the body is treated after death (see Table 12.2). The family should be asked if they wish to be involved as many people find it helpful to accept the reality of the death if they are involved in a final act of care (Box 12.15, see p. 316).

REFLECTIVE PRACTICE — Box 12.14

Meeting cultural and spiritual needs

In your current/next clinical placement find out how cultural issues are addressed.

Student activities

Find out if:

- There is access to information about death and dying practices for different groups.
- There are established links with local religious/spiritual leaders.
- Cultural issues and wishes are ascertained, recorded and communicated within the healthcare team.
- Patients/families are able to adhere to cultural/spiritual practices, e.g. fasting times.

[Resource: Neuberger J 2004 Caring for dying people of different faiths. 3rd edn. Radcliffe Medical Press, Oxon]

End-of-life ethical issues

Ethical issues at the end of life are complex and require careful consideration. Although students are not responsible for making care decisions at the end of life, they will be exposed to ethical issues and may contribute to debating issues and the plan of care. Decision-making in palliative care is governed by the ethical principles of respect of autonomy, beneficence, non-maleficence and justice (see Ch. 7).

NURSING SKILLS Box 12.15

The final act of care/last offices

- Wear appropriate protective clothing for the control of infection (see Ch. 15). In some circumstances, such as patients with HIV/AIDS, full last offices are not carried out in the ward area. The body is usually labelled, e.g. 'danger of infection', and transported to the mortuary sealed in a protective body bag. The mortuary and undertakers are always informed about the presence of infections. Check local protocols regarding the use of infection labels and body bags
- Insert the person's dentures and use a rolled up towel under the chin to keep the mouth shut prior to the onset of rigor mortis (this should be removed before the family visit)
- Wash the body as necessary and ensure the body is labelled with the patient's details according to local guidelines
- Remove all intravenous infusions, urinary catheters (drain urine prior to removal), drains, etc. unless the death is associated with a serious accident or suspicious circumstances and is to be reported to the Procurator Fiscal or Coroner. In these instances all drains etc. are left in place
- Dress the body in a clean gown or pyjamas – consult the family about this. When a child dies they may have chosen a favourite outfit to be worn
- Brush and comb the hair and shave the face if required (if this was their normal preference)
- Ensure removal, recording and safekeeping of jewellery according to local guidelines (checking this is in accordance with the wishes and beliefs of the patient and/or family)
- Cover the body to the shoulders with a clean sheet
- Tidy the area around the bed, removing unnecessary equipment and charts
- Organize chairs around the bed for family members
- Allow the family as much time as they need to say their goodbyes
- Stay with the family to offer support as needed although you should establish if they want time alone
- Discuss with the family the arrangements for collecting belongings and official documents
- Provide information about local undertakers or other services families may find useful, e.g. Cruse Bereavement Care (see 'Useful websites')
- If a post mortem is required, this must be explained carefully and sensitively to the family by a registered nurse or a doctor
- Provide information for relatives about registering the death
- Provide the booklet *What to do after a Death* (Box 12.16).
- Aftercare for family/friends – identify follow-up care and support
- Care of health professionals and other carers. Support systems should be identified and used.

CRITICAL THINKING Box 12.16

What to do after a death

Think about the type and presentation of information needed by family or friends after a death.

Student activities

- Access the '*What to do after a death*' (available as pdfs for England and Wales and for Scotland) information from the website below.
- Find some information provided by an organization such as Cruse (see 'Useful websites').
- Find out what information is used locally.
- Discuss the different forms of information with your mentor. Think how these may need adaptation if the bereaved person has a learning disability.

[Resource: Rights and responsibilities: death and bereavement – www.direct.gov.uk/RightsAndResponsibilities/Death/fs/en]

ETHICAL ISSUES Box 12.17

Hydration at the end of life

The provision of nutrition and hydration is a part of the nursing role and failing to meet these needs may be seen as failing to work within the Nursing and Midwifery Council *code of professional conduct: standards for conduct, performance and ethics* (NMC 2004). However, in palliative care the beneficial effects of hydration are inconclusive and hydration may not be essential for comfort in the last stages and may even cause discomfort by increasing respiratory secretions and urinary output.

The psychological and emotional aspects of hydration must be considered alongside the physiological effects when active hydration is considered as part of care. Deciding whether it is acting in the patient's best interests is complex and requires regular review of the evidence to support clinical decisions, the patient's condition, prognosis and wishes of the patient and the family.

Student activities

- Consider the perspectives of the patient, family and professional staff.
- Discuss with your mentor the issues relating to hydration at the end of life.

At the end of life there are numerous issues that present ethical dilemmas for those involved. These include:

- Active nutrition and hydration (Box 12.17; see also Ch. 19)
- Decisions about whether to resuscitate or not (see Ch. 6)
- Extraordinary versus futile treatments
- Withholding and withdrawing treatments (Box 12.17; see also Ch. 6)
- Hastening death.

Summary

- Holistic care at the end of life is multidimensional and multiprofessional in focus and embraces the needs of patients and those closest to them.
- Palliative care as an approach is applicable at all stages of the illness journey.
- Nursing care is aimed at managing physical and psychological needs and difficult symptoms, and involves helping the person and family adapt to, and cope with, the resulting role and lifestyle changes.
- Patients requiring palliative care are cared for in most healthcare settings so all healthcare professionals involved need knowledge of the palliative care approach.
- Caring for individuals who are dying and their families is a challenging, but rewarding, aspect of nursing care.
- Nursing care of the bereaved person is aimed at moving towards accepting the reality and adapting to life.
- Effective communication is central to high quality palliative care.
- Perhaps the most important nursing role is that of 'being alongside' or 'being a companion' to those who are dying and providing comfort for their family.

Self test

1. Define the following:
   a. Bereavement
   b. Grief.
2. Explain the palliative care approach to care.
3. List six members of the MDT providing palliative care.
4. Describe the emotions that a bereaved person may experience.
5. What are the causes of fatigue in advanced illness?
6. List the responsibilities of the nurse in providing the last act of care.

Key words and phrases for literature searching

Bereavement	Pain management
Death	Palliative care
Dying	Quality of life
Loss	Symptom management

Useful websites

BBC	www.bbc.co.uk/worldservice/people/features/world_religions/index.shtml Available July 2006
Cancer Research UK	www.cancerresearchuk.org Available July 2006
CancerBACUP	www.cancerbackup.org.uk Available July 2006
Cruse Bereavement Care	www.crusebereavementcare.org.uk Available July 2006
Hospice Information Service	www.hospiceinformation.info Available July 2006
Macmillan Cancer Support	www.macmillan.org.uk Available July 2006
Marie Curie Cancer Care	www.mariecurie.org.uk Available July 2006
National Council for Palliative Care (NCPC) (*many useful publications*)	www.ncpc.org.uk Available July 2006
PRODIGY (*guidance available for many palliative care issues, e.g. cough, dyspnoea, respiratory secretions*)	www.prodigy.nhs.uk/guidance Available July 2006
Scottish Partnership for Palliative Care	www.palliativecarescotland.org.uk Available July 2006

References

Addington-Hall J 1996 Heart disease and stroke: lessons from cancer care. In: Ford G, Lewin I (eds) Managing terminal illness. Royal College of Physicians, London

Bennett D 2003 Death and people with learning disabilities: empowering carers. British Journal of Learning Disabilities 31(3):118–122

Black D 1996 Childhood bereavement: distress and long-term sequelae can be lessened by early intervention. British Medical Journal 312(7045):1496

British Humanist Association 2005 Online: www.humanism.org.uk/site/cms Available July 2006

Bruce L, Finlay T (eds) 1997 Nursing in gastroenterology. Churchill Livingstone, Edinburgh

Crick L 1988 Facing grief. Nursing Times 84(28):61–63

Davis CL 1997 ABC of palliative care: breathlessness, cough, and other respiratory problems. British Medical Journal 315:931–934

Doyle D, Hanks G, MacDonald N (eds) 1998 Oxford textbook of palliative medicine. 2nd edn. Oxford University Press, Oxford

Finlay I, Jones R 1995 Definitions in palliative care. British Medical Journal 311:754

Goldman A 1998 ABC of palliative care: special problems of children. British Medical Journal 316:49–52

Heaven K, Maguire P 1996 Training hospice nurses to elicit patient concerns. Journal of Advanced Nursing 23:280–286

Hollins S, Esterhuyzen A 1997 Bereavement and grief in adults with learning disabilities. British Journal of Psychiatry 170:497–501

James N 1989 Emotional labour: skill and work in the social regulation of feelings. The Sociological Review 37(1):15–42

Katz JS 2004 Overview. In: Payne S, Seymour J, Ingleton C (eds) Palliative care nursing: principles and evidence for practice. Open University Press, Buckingham

Kindlen M, Smith V, Smith M 1999 Loss, grief and bereavement. In: Lugton J, Kindlen M (eds) Palliative care: the nursing role. Churchill Livingstone, Edinburgh

Kinghorn S 2001 Communication in advanced illness: challenges and opportunities. In: Kinghorn S, Gamlin R (eds) Palliative nursing. Bringing comfort and hope. Baillière Tindall, Edinburgh

Kubler-Ross E 1969 On death and dying. Macmillan, New York

Lindemann E 1944 Symptomatology and management of acute grief. American Journal of Psychiatry 101:141–148

Lockhart-Wood K 2001 Nurse–doctor collaboration in cancer pain management. International Journal of Palliative Nursing 7(1):6–16

Lothian NHS Board 2001 Lothian Palliative Care Guidelines. Lothian NHS Board, Edinburgh

Marie Curie Cancer Care 2005 Online: www.mariecurie.org.uk Available September 2006

National Council for Hospice and Specialist Palliative Care Services [now The National Council for Palliative Care (NCPC)] 1997 Changing gear – guidelines for managing the last days of life in cancer. NCPC, London

National Statistics 2003a Census 2001 – National Report. Online: www.statistics.gov.uk/census2001/census2001.asp Available July 2006

National Statistics 2003b Twentieth century mortality trends in England and Wales. Health Statistics Quarterly (18) Summer 2003. Online: www.statistics.gov.uk/downloads/theme_health/HSQ18_revised_21Aug03.pdf Available July 2006

Nursing and Midwifery Council 2004 code of professional conduct: standards for conduct, performance and ethics. NMC, London

Open University 1992 Religious practices wall chart. The Open University, Department of Health and Social Welfare, Milton Keynes

Parkes CM 1998 Coping with loss: bereavement in adult life. British Medical Journal 316(7134):856–859

Parkes CM, Weiss RS 1983 Recovery from bereavement. Basic Books, New York

Payne S 2004 Overview. In: Payne S, Seymour J, Ingleton C (eds) Palliative care nursing: principles and evidence for practice. Open University Press, Buckingham

Phillips S 1996 Labouring the emotions: expanding the remit of nursing work. Journal of Advanced Nursing 24(1):139–143

Ream E, Richardson A 1996 Fatigue: a concept analysis. International Journal of Nursing Studies 33(5):519–529

Smith P 1992 The emotional labour of nursing. Macmillan, London

Stroebe MS, Hansson RO, Stroebe W, Schut H 2002 Handbook of bereavement research: consequences, coping and care. American Psychological Association, Washington, DC

Thomas K 2004 Caring for the dying at home. Radcliffe Medical Press, Oxon

Twycross R 1997 Symptom management in advanced cancer. 2nd edn. Radcliffe Medical Press, Oxon

Weller RA, Weller EB, Fristad MA, Bowes JM 1991 Depression in recently bereaved prepubertal children. American Journal Psychiatry 148:1536–1540

Wilkinson S 1991 Factors which influence how nurses communicate with cancer patients. Journal of Advanced Nursing 16:677–688

Winston's Wish 2005 For grieving children and their families. Online. Available: www.winstonswish.org.uk

Worden JW 1991 Grief counselling and grief therapy. Tavistock/Routledge, London

World Health Organization 2004 WHO definition of palliative care. Online: www.who.int/cancer/palliative/definition/en Available July 2006

World Health Organization 2005 WHO's pain ladder. Online: www.who.int/cancer/palliative/painladder/en Available July 2006

Wright B 2002 Death, grief and loss. In: Walsh M (ed) Watson's clinical nursing and related sciences. 6th edn. Baillière Tindall, Edinburgh

Further reading

Department of Health 2006 NHS Help is at hand. A resource for people bereaved by suicide and other sudden, traumatic death. Online: www.dh.gov.uk/assetRoot/04/13/90/07/04139007.pdf Available September 2006

Diamond J 1998 Because cowards get cancer too. . . Vermillion, London

Dickenson D, Johnson M, Katz JS 2000 Death, dying and bereavement. Open University Press, London

Ellershaw J, Wilkinson S 2003 Care of the dying. A pathway to excellence. Oxford University Press, Oxford

Faull C, Carter Y, Daniels L 2005 Handbook of palliative care. 2nd edn. Blackwell, Oxford

Gordon T 2001 A need for living. Wild Goose Publications, Glasgow

Holland K, Hogg C 2001 Cultural awareness in nursing and health care. Arnold, London

Kennedy C 2003 Death and dying. In: Kindlen S (ed) Physiology for health care and nursing. 2nd edn. Churchill Livingstone, Edinburgh

Lugton J, McIntyre R 2006 Palliative care: the nursing role. 2nd edn. Churchill Livingstone, Edinburgh

Picardie R 1998 Before I say goodbye. Penguin, London

Prodigy guidance (2004, minor update 2005) Palliative care – nausea/vomiting/malignant bowel obstruction. Online: www.prodigy.nhs.uk/palliative_care_nausea_vomiting_malignant_bowel_obstruction Available July 2006

SECTION 4

Developing nursing skills

Safety in nursing practice

13

Emma Briggs

Glossary terms

First aid

Harm reduction

Moving and handling

Risk assessment

Risk management

Standard precautions

Violence and aggression

Learning outcomes

This chapter will help you:

- Discuss the importance of health and safety for practitioners and individuals receiving care
- Describe the role of risk assessment in harm reduction and identify common potential or actual risks in a clinical area
- Outline the legislation in place to maintain safety and prevent accidents
- Identify the main nursing considerations in relation to standard precautions (for detail see Ch. 15), managing aggression, fire safety and moving and handling (for detail see Ch. 18)
- Describe the principles of first aid and the action required for burns and poisoning.

Introduction

The International Council of Nurses (2004) describes the nursing role as promoting health, preventing illness or caring for ill, disabled or dying people along with acting as an advocate and promoting a safe environment. An individual's health and their safety are very closely linked, and a fundamental part of nursing care is to identify factors that influence a person's safety. This may include actual factors, e.g. being unable to drink that has led to dehydration and confusion in an older adult, or potential hazards, e.g. if a toddler is given a very small toy they are at risk of choking.

Healthcare practitioners have a responsibility to look after their own safety and that of the people they work with. Many issues have the potential to affect everyone in a care setting, e.g. poor handling techniques could result in an injury to the patient/client, yourself and a colleague. Therefore, the overwhelming emphasis in this chapter is on promoting the health of everyone concerned through prevention, identifying the risks and eliminating or minimizing them through safe practice. This is achieved by exploring:

- The process of risk assessment
- The legislation in place to maintain safety
- The principles of moving and handling
- Standard precautions
- First aid
- Preventing and managing violence and aggression
- Fire safety.

Subsequent chapters address harm reduction further, e.g. infection control (Ch. 15), safe administration of medicines (Ch. 22), patient assessment (Ch. 14) and nursing care. These are all elements of safe practice and require further reading to aid your development and understanding. Additionally, a safe practitioner is able to identify and minimize hazards for patients/clients, a fundamental part of the Nursing and Midwifery Council's (NMC 2004) *Code of Professional Conduct*. This requires being able to demonstrate a number of other qualities and skills, as outlined below. These skills are used throughout this chapter while addressing diverse safety topics and will help you to develop into a safe practitioner.

A critical or questioning approach

This means that you will ask if something is unclear, or tactfully challenge practice. It is important to develop the confidence to speak up if you do not understand or you think safety may be compromised. It is possible to discuss such concerns with mentors, senior clinical staff or university teaching staff, depending on the situation.

Recognize limitations of knowledge and skills, and seek support

Self-awareness is an essential skill for all nurses and knowing the limitations of your knowledge and clinical skills means that you are less likely to try something beyond your capabilities (which may go wrong). Where you are

REFLECTIVE PRACTICE Box 13.1

Relationships between nursing, health and safety

Student activity

Take a piece of paper and on the left-hand side write down the main activities nurses do in everyday practice. On the right hand side write down how this helps the person's health and reduces harm (and is therefore concerned with their safety). The examples below should help you to start:

Nursing activity	How this improves health and maintains safety
Helping someone to eat and drink	Provides energy and nutrients for daily life and recovery Prevents malnutrition and health deteriorating Able to go home more quickly, maintains independence
Pressure area care	Prevents pressure ulcers developing
Helping people with their medication	

unsure, always seek support from mentors, read around the topic and speak to teaching staff if necessary.

Use of evidence-based practice

Nursing practice should be based on interventions that are known to be safe, effective and informed by research findings (see Ch. 5), clinical expertise and the patient's/client's own wishes.

Use of reflection during and after practice situations

Reflection (Ch. 4) is a valuable learning tool and helps to make sense of situations, apply the theory behind a topic, highlight the positive points and identify areas for future action.

Before moving on, complete the exercise in Box 13.1 to explore the relationships between nursing, health and safety.

Risk assessment

Risks are taken in our everyday lives: some result in positive gains such as winning a lottery; others have negative outcomes, e.g. taking part in a contact sport can result in injury. Risks are also managed regularly to reduce the likelihood of negative outcomes occurring, e.g. wearing seatbelts and having airbags decrease the risk of injury in the event of a car accident.

In clinical practice the word 'risk' tends to be associated with negative outcomes (Jacobs 2000) and there are many potential and actual hazards that can cause harm to patients/clients and staff. Nurses need to identify hazards and reduce the likelihood of harm occurring to any party. This may be as simple as mopping up water on the floor to stop people slipping or more complex such as using an electric hoist to help clients who cannot stand to transfer from their bed to a chair safely. Much of nursing practice focuses on helping people to remain safe and this section explores the way in which risks are identified and reduced to minimize potential harm. The principles of risk assessment are discussed here, illustrating common issues across all nursing specialties. However, people receiving care may have unique health issues and require an individual assessment, and this is explored on page 324.

Risk assessment principles

A hazard has been defined by the Health and Safety Executive (2003a, p. 3) as 'anything that can cause harm, e.g. chemicals, electricity, working from ladders' and a risk as 'the chance, high or low, that somebody will be harmed by the hazard'. It is important to understand the relationship between hazards and risks. A lightning strike presents a serious hazard that can result in death but the risk, or likelihood, of it happening to an individual in their lifetime is very small. Even when you know what the hazards and risks are, other factors can increase or decrease a risk. Going out into wide, open spaces during a thunderstorm may increase the risk of being struck by lightning. Clinical practice can also illustrate this. When drawing up or giving injections, needles are never resheathed because of the potential hazard of a needlestick injury and transmission of blood-borne viruses, e.g. hepatitis B, human immunodeficiency virus (HIV) (see Ch. 15). The risk of a needlestick injury is greatly reduced if nurses adhere to the guidance, but lack of knowledge or understanding about the importance of this increases the risk of an injury occurring to the nurse. Before reading the rest of this section, complete the activity in Box 13.2.

It may not be possible to eliminate risks completely but by identifying the hazard, risk and associated factors the chances of harm occurring can be minimized. This process is called risk management and the first stage is known as risk assessment. There are several reasons why risk assessments are undertaken, including patient/client welfare and ethical and professional responsibilities, including a duty of care to protect vulnerable people (Ch. 7). The *NMC Code of professional conduct* (NMC 2004, p. 10) emphasizes nurses' responsibilities in one of the key standards: 'You must act to identify and minimize risk to patients and clients.' Risk assessment is also an integral part of health and safety legislation (see p. 327).

The process of risk assessment may sound complicated, but it is essentially an examination of the factors that could cause harm to people in a care environment so that precautions can be taken to prevent injuries (HSE

CRITICAL THINKING Box 13.2

Hazards that can cause accidents

Student activities

Examine a kitchen or bathroom in your placement, or your own home if this is not possible. Identify:

- What accidents could happen in the area.
- Potential causes of accidents (hazards) and who could be harmed.
- Any information displayed warning staff of hazards.
- Measures in place to reduce the likelihood of accidents, e.g. temperature controls on hot water taps of baths or equipment available if an accident occurs, e.g. fire blankets.

2003a). The activity in Box 13.2 is the start of a risk assessment. There are usually five stages to risk assessment:

- Step one: Look for the hazard
- Step two: Decide who may be harmed and how
- Step three: Evaluate the risks and decide whether existing precautions are adequate or more should be done
- Step four: Record the findings
- Step five: Review the assessment regularly and revise if necessary.

These stages are explored in a series of text boxes using a moving and handling example from each nursing specialty. The scenarios focus on hazards for staff and patients/clients and follow one of the basic principles, i.e. looking after your joints and your back (not stooping, twisting, reaching or lifting people).

Step one: Look for the hazard

This involves walking round a clinical area to identify what sort of things could cause harm to people, talking to the staff to find out what problems they experience and examining accident and sickness records to identify any particular patterns (HSE 2003a). Examples of this are provided in Box 13.3.

Step two: Decide who may be harmed and how

This essentially refers to the staff and patients/clients involved, but must also include visitors and employees who may be in the clinical area temporarily, e.g. cleaners, contractors, etc. (HSE 2003a). Now read Box 13.4, which builds on the moving and handling scenarios above.

Step three: Evaluate the risks and decide what should be done

This stage of the risk assessment involves looking at the likelihood of harm occurring (remember the being struck by lightning scenario?) and deciding whether the risk is high, medium or low. Then the risk has to be made as small as possible by taking precautions (HSE 2003a). This could include using equipment and educating staff so that they are aware of the risks and can take precautions themselves. Box 13.5 gives two examples of how this may be done.

Box 13.3

Risk assessment in nursing settings – Step 1: Look for the hazard

- Ward B2 is a surgical ward with 28 beds, three bathrooms, a shower room and four single cubicle toilets. Recently two patients have fallen in the toilet area and a risk assessment was requested to try to identify factors contributing to the falls. It was noted that one toilet cubicle was small, the toilet seat low and there were no grab rails for patients to use. The floor was also slippery when wet. This represents a hazard for both patients and staff.
- Sunshine Hospice cares for a range of children and young adults with life-limiting conditions and their families, providing respite, palliative or terminal care. The risk assessment examined three rooms built for toddlers and their families. The cots are at a fixed height (do not move up and down for taller and shorter carers) and on one, the cot side is broken. This is a hazard to any child and all cots pose a risk for parents and staff who have to lean over them to care for children.
- The Richard Smith Education Centre is a school for children and young adults (4–17 years) with learning disabilities and the pupils have a range of abilities and needs in terms of health and social care. The risk assessment is taking place in the new multisensory relaxation room – a room with fibreoptic lights, music and soft furnishings, a technique also known as Snoezelen (see Ch. 10). Children with severe learning disabilities will be regularly transferred from their wheelchairs to the floor to engage in activities. There is currently no equipment to help carers transfer the children who may therefore be tempted to lift them.
- Rosehill House is a residential facility for older adults experiencing mental health problems including dementia. The largest bathroom on the first floor is the most frequently used by staff helping clients to bathe because of the space available. The bath is fitted to the back wall and floor on the left-hand side, and clients have to climb into and out of the bath themselves. Staff have expressed concerns about clients getting into and out of the bath safely, particularly if there is an emergency and they need to get the client out quickly. There is currently no equipment available.

Step four: Record the findings

With each scenario above, the results of the risk assessment must be recorded. Healthcare organizations usually have specific documentation for this process. Written

CRITICAL THINKING Box 13.4

Risk assessment – Step 2: Decide who may be harmed and how

Student activities

For each setting in Box 13.3 identify:

- Who may be harmed? Think about the physical and emotional effects.
- How may this occur? What has caused the accident?

The example from Sunshine Hospice is given below to start you off.

Who is at risk of being harmed?

- Any child is at risk of physical injury if placed in the broken cot. This would cause severe distress and pain to the child, the parents and staff
- Fixed height cots mean that staff and parents are at risk injuring themselves

How may they be harmed?

- A child in the broken cot may fall out, trapping their fingers or limbs or sustain a major injury that could be fatal
- Staff and parents may injure their backs leaning over fixed height cots and may then be unable to care for the child or continue to work.

Box 13.5

Risk assessment – Step 3: Reducing the risks

Ward B2

There have already been two accidents with patients using toilets on B2 so the risk of further injury is high. Installing non-slip flooring, grab rails and a raised toilet seat can minimize the risk. Each patient must be assessed for using the toilet; they need to be independent as the area is too small for staff to assist safely. Reviewing staff knowledge of how to deal with a fallen patient would also be a useful exercise.

Richard Smith Education Centre

Staff and pupils are at high risk of injury if pupils are moved to and from their wheelchairs without equipment. Installing a hoist to transfer children safely should reduce this risk. Staff will also need education on use of the hoist.

records also demonstrate that employers have abided by the law (HSE 2003a) and can complete the final stage.

Step five: Review the assessment and revise if necessary

Risk assessments need to be reviewed regularly and when there are any significant changes. A date is often set to remind people when to review the assessment.

REFLECTIVE PRACTICE Box 13.6

Risk assessments in practice

Generic risk assessments should be available in each placement.

Student activities

1. Locate some of the risk assessments and policies in your placement, for example:
   - Moving and handling
   - Infection control
   - Drug policy and safe storage of medications.
2. Find out what hazards have been identified in your placement and how they have been reduced.

The risk assessments described here could be applied to a number of patients/clients or staff and the focus is the specific task, e.g. transferring people from a wheelchair to the floor. This is often referred to as a generic assessment and comes under health and safety law. Therefore it is the responsibility of the employer to carry this out although senior management may delegate the assessment to a specific individual trained in risk assessment and who regularly works in that clinical area (Box 13.6). Nurses have a duty of care (see Ch. 6) to follow the procedures that reduce the risk, such as using equipment provided and to report situations where safety is compromised.

Individual risk assessments

A person's health and social care needs are unique and nursing assessment (Ch. 14) includes identifying actual or potential hazards that can affect their health. A wide range of assessment tools have been developed to help nurses and other healthcare professionals identify whether people are at risk of specific factors such as mal nutrition or pressure ulcers (see Fig. 14.3, p. 357). Box 13.7 lists some of these tools and sources of further information. Most assessment tools offer a checklist and a scoring system, with the overall result giving an indication of the degree of risk, e.g. high, medium or low risk of developing pressure ulcers. The assessing nurse can then decide how to minimize those risks.

Assessment tools are designed to help nurses in practice identify particular risks but they do not replace clinical judgement. For example, a nutritional assessment tool might indicate that a patient admitted for surgery is currently at a low risk of malnutrition (see Ch. 19). However, the patient will spend at least 4 hours fasting prior to surgery (Ch. 24) and thereafter may not be able to eat or drink for several hours or experience nausea and vomiting. They will therefore be at higher risk of developing malnutrition and this indicates the importance of regular reassessment.

Box 13.7 **Examples of specific risk assessment tools**

Area of risk assessment	Further information
Falls risk assessment	Cooper G 2003 Developing an evidence based approach to falls – risk assessment. Professional Nurse 19(1):19–23
Moving and handling	Raine E 2001 Testing a risk assessment tool for manual handling. Professional Nurse 16(9):1344–1348
Nutritional intake	Arrowsmith H 2000 A critical evaluation of the use of nutritional screening tools by nurses. British Journal of Nursing 8(22):1483–1490 BAPEN, Malnutrition Advisory Group 2003 The Malnutrition Universal Screening Tool (MUST). Online. www.bapen.org.uk Available July 2006
Pressure ulcer development	Waterlow J 1998 History and use of the Waterlow card. Nursing Times 94(7):63–67
Suicide risk assessment	Frierson RL, Melikian M, Wadman PC 2002 Principles of suicide risk assessment. Postgraduate Medicine 112(3): 65–66, 69–71

The discussion on generic risk assessments above highlighted a common issue across all nursing specialties, namely moving and handling. For individual assessments a number of branch-specific issues arise. Risks are taken as part of growing up and everyday life as we develop and learn. This may occur on many different levels, e.g. crossing a busy road, smoking cigarettes or drinking alcohol, starting a new relationship or embarking on a career, and these can often be a case of trial and error. Risk taking is a natural part of life and if people who have learning disabilities or mental health conditions are overprotected, this can lead to social exclusion and infringement of their rights and dignity (Alaszewski & Alaszewski 2000).

To promote social inclusion, people need to be allowed to take reasonable risks to aid their development by promoting independent living and social activities. The regulatory body that preceded the NMC, the United Kingdom Central Council for Nursing, Midwifery and Health Visiting, published guidance on risk management for people with learning disabilities and mental health problems (UKCC 1998). The guidelines suggested that risk assessment should consider client care, the care system and the local environment. Risks still need to be reduced to a minimum and agreed by the multidisciplinary team and client but the value of risk-taking should be recognized. Box 13.8 presents a case study and an opportunity for reflection on a number of issues discussed here.

CRITICAL THINKING Box 13.8

Promoting independent living and social activities

You are on a 4-week placement at a busy day centre for young adults with mild to moderate learning disabilities. Tom is 17 years old and you have been working closely with him for the past week. When he first arrives he confides in you saying he had a fight with his mum before he left home. After discussing this further, you find out that he had asked for three things for his 18th birthday: a rally car, a mountain bike and to go to the cinema with his girlfriend Cheryl who also attends the day centre. His mum had said that he would not be allowed to drive but Tom was more upset about not being able to go to the cinema alone with Cheryl. The cinema is 4 miles from Tom's home and he and his mum usually travel together on the bus. He has never used public transport alone.

Student activities

- Why do you think Tom's mum is concerned about risks and safety?
- Do you think her concerns are realistic?
- How do you think the issue could be resolved so that social inclusion for Tom and Cheryl is promoted?

Health and safety legislation

Legislation plays a major role in promoting safety of individuals and public health in general. This section briefly examines the regulations in place in the UK to prevent accidents and ill health and also the health and safety responsibilities of employers to protect staff and the public.

Maintaining safety and promoting health

Wide-ranging legislation exists to promote public health and safety including:

- Supply of clean water
- Food standards
- Environmental protection
- Sewage treatment
- Fire precautions
- Safety standards for manufacturers
- The provision of a National Health Service.

Governments also publish specific public health strategies such as *Saving Lives: Our Healthier Nation* (DH 1999a) and *Choosing Health: Making Healthy Choices Easier* (DH

2004) which focus on reducing death rates from cancer, coronary heart disease and strokes, mental health illness and accidents (see Ch. 1). Specific documentation and targets have followed in the form of National Service Frameworks, e.g. for children, older people, mental health, coronary heart disease, diabetes, cancer (see www.dh.gov.uk for publications).

One government target is to reduce death and injury rates from accidents in the home by 20%; another is a 40% reduction in road accidents (including a 50% reduction in the number of children seriously injured on roads). The proposals seek to reduce the 10 000 lives lost per year to accidents and focus on the main causes within each age group:

- Accidental injury and pedestrian accidents in children
- Road traffic accidents in young and middle-aged adults
- Falls in people over 65 years.

The preventative measures proposed include an increase in traffic calming measures, design of safe play areas for children, changes in building regulations, the use of safety glass for doors and road safety training for children. The National Institute for Health and Clinical Excellence (NICE 2004) provided guidance on assessment of older adults with the aim of preventing falls and minimizing their recurrence. Falls prevention campaigns have also been launched, aimed at educating older adults. Where accidents do occur, the target is for faster diagnosis and effective treatment to improve health outcomes. By undertaking the activities in Box 13.9 you will find out more about assessment and prevention of falls in older adults.

Nurses across all specialties may have a number of roles to play in accident prevention as they come into contact with people at various stages of their lives for health promotion and treatment measures in various settings including the community, hospitals, clinics, schools and walk-in centres. This may be as part of a local education or screening programme on accident prevention for patients/clients or their families. Nurses are also heavily involved in people's care after accidents have occurred and this provides opportunities for assessment and education to prevent further accidents.

HEALTH PROMOTION Box 13.9

Falls prevention

80% of falls in the home involve an older adult; they may result in fractures, long-term disability and are a major cause of mortality in this age group (DTI 1999). Even minor falls can result in loss of confidence, loss of mobility leading to social isolation and increased dependency and disability. The *National Service Framework for Older People* (DH 2001) sets specific targets for reduction in the number of serious injuries resulting from falls and appropriate rehabilitation of people who have fallen. Many multidisciplinary teams have been established to assess individuals and run falls prevention programmes.

Student activities

1. Read the NICE (2004) guidelines about preventing falls in older people. Consider the extent to which they are implemented in your placement.
2. Identify how the elements of a falls prevention programme listed below may help prevent falls in older people:
   - Exercise classes and keeping active
   - Emphasizing healthy eating
   - Wearing appropriate, well-fitting footwear
   - Being aware of changes in health and eyesight
   - Preventing illness
   - Adjustments in the home, e.g. lighting and grab rails
   - Dealing with the fear and anxiety.

[Resources: Department of Trade and Industry 1999 Avoiding slips, trips and broken hips. DTI, London; Department of Health 2001 National service framework for older people. DH, London; NICE 2004 Falls: the assessment and prevention of falls in older people. Online: www.nice.org.uk/CG021 Available July 2006]

Health and safety in healthcare settings

The Health and Safety at Work Act (1974) is the main piece of UK legislation that places specific responsibilities upon employers to protect the welfare of people at work and the public. Under this Act, many subsequent regulations have been issued which deal with specific topics such as manual handling and the safe use of equipment. Although employers are responsible for providing a safe working environment, employees have responsibilities for:

- Following the regulations
- Taking reasonable care of their own safety and that of others
- Implementing any training and education given
- Reporting unsafe conditions.

Health and safety is essentially everyone's responsibility. This section presents the main legislation that applies to clinical practice (Table 13.1) and summarizes the key points.

The Health and Safety Commission (HSC) and the Health and Safety Executive (HSE) enforce health and safety law in the UK under criminal law, as opposed to civil law, which focuses on personal claims for compensation (see Ch. 6). This means that employers may be heavily fined, or worse, for failing to comply with health and safety regulations. The HSW Act (1974) laid out general duties for employers to:

- Provide a safe working environment
- Identify hazards and reduce them
- Provide information and training for employees
- Arrange safe transportation and handling of articles and substances (HSE 2003b).

Table 13.1 Main health and safety regulations under the Health and Safety at Work Act (1974) (based on HSE 2003b)

Regulation	Date or most recent amendment	Main aim
Management of Health and Safety at Work	1999	Ensures employers carry out risk assessments, implement changes and appoint qualified people to provide information and staff training
Workplace (Health and Safety and Welfare)	1992	Ensures employers cover range of health and safety issues, e.g. ventilation, heating, lighting, seating, welfare facilities
Health and Safety (Display Screen Equipment)	1992	Lays down requirements for people who work with visual display units (computer screens)
Personal Protective Equipment at Work	1992	Ensures that employers provide protective clothing and equipment for employees
Provision and Use of Work Equipment	1998	Ensures that employers provide safe equipment for use at work
Manual Handling Operations	1992, amended 2002	Lays down requirements for the movement of loads by hand or involving bodily force
Reporting of Injuries, Diseases and Dangerous Occurrences	1995	Employers must report work-related accidents, diseases and dangerous occurrences
Control of Substances Hazardous to Health	2002	Ensures that employers identify hazardous substances, assess risks to employees' health and take appropriate action to reduce risks
Noise at Work	1989	Ensures that employers use systems that protect people's hearing in noisy environments
Electricity at Work	1989	Electrical systems are safe and well maintained
Health and Safety (First Aid)	1981	Ensures employers provide adequate first aid equipment and personnel

The Management of Health and Safety at Work Regulations (1999) were more specific and requires employers to carry out:

- Risk assessments
- Risk reduction
- Risk and accident monitoring
- Health surveillance
- Consultation with staff.

These two pieces of legislation provide the background and general principles for health and safety but is useful to look at some of the more specific regulations highlighted in Table 13.1 and their implications for clinical practice.

Control of Substances Hazardous to Health (COSHH)

Chemicals and other substances used at work can be hazardous to people's health and employers must control exposure to prevent harm occurring (HSE 2003c). Hazardous substances include chemicals, gases, dust and biological agents (blood and blood products, micro-organisms) that can cause illnesses ranging from mild allergic reactions to occupational asthma and death. Risk assessments are therefore carried out and precautions put in place, including:

- Educating staff
- Providing personal protective equipment
- Health surveillance
- Formulating policies for dealing with hazardous substances, e.g. disposal, spillages and emergencies.

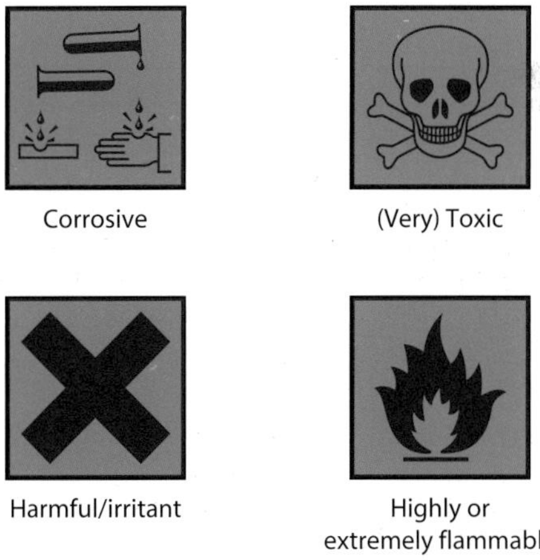

Fig. 13.1 Hazard signs (reproduced with permission from HSE 2002a)

Manufacturers must also supply information and warning labels on hazardous substances, both domestic and industrial (Fig. 13.1). These highlight whether the chemical is an irritant, corrosive, highly toxic or flammable and it is important to be familiar with these (Box 13.10).

Reporting of Incidents, Diseases and Dangerous Occurrences Regulations (RIDDOR)

Accident statistics, covering the period 2001–2004 (HSE 2004a), are shown below:

- 235 people lost their lives at work (2003/4)

HEALTH PROMOTION Box 13.10

Recognizing hazardous chemicals

The hazard signs in Figure 13.1 appear on chemicals and toxic substances used at home and in placements. You should always read the labels on products you are using.

Student activities

- Identify these hazard signs on domestic cleaning products.
- Locate these hazard signs in your placement, e.g. on handwashing products and disinfectants.

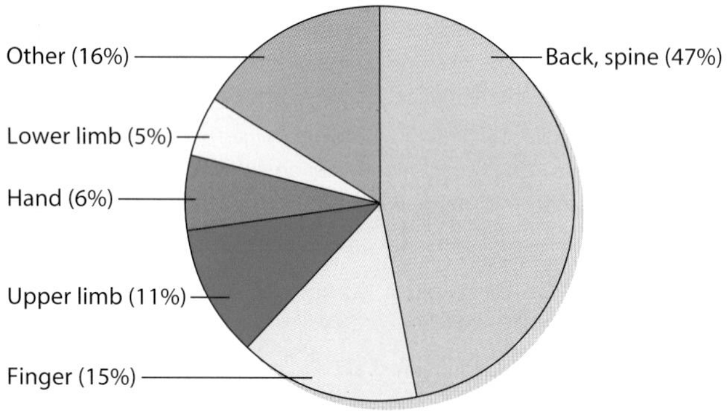

Fig. 13.2 Sites of injuries lasting over 3 days caused by handling accidents (2001/2) (reproduced with permission from HSE 2004b)

- 154 430 people experienced other injuries at work (2002/3)
- 2.3 million people experienced an illness that began or was worsened by their work (2001/2).

In 2002/3 injuries for the health services included:

- Slips and trips – caused 667 serious injuries to staff and patients, and were the most common injuries to nurses
- Moving and handling – caused 53% of staff injuries (HSC 2004).

Figure 13.2 illustrates the areas of the body affected by handling accidents. The government and the HSC have set a target for a 10% reduction in health service accidents between 1999/2000 and 2009/2010.

RIDDOR aims to ensure that accidents and near misses are documented and reported to the HSE so that these can be investigated if necessary and harm reduction measures implemented. Reportable incidents include a patient/client, visitor or member of the public or staff experiencing one of the following:

- A dangerous occurrence that happens in practice, e.g. collapse of equipment or explosion
- An injury that lasts for more than 3 days or a work-related disease, e.g. a severe allergy
- A major injury, e.g. fracture, amputation, or injuries leading to acute illness, unconsciousness or death.

In nursing practice, all accidents and near misses are documented using the local NHS electronic or paper incident forms (Fig. 13.3) which health and safety representatives of the healthcare organization then review and report to the HSE as necessary.

In addition to the general targets for reducing accidents in the health service, the government established the National Patient Safety Agency (NPSA) to reduce the estimated 900 000 patient safety incidents and near misses every year. As well as advising on particular universal issues, e.g. intravenous infusion pumps, the NPSA collect and analyse incident reports from across the country. This information is used to advise on preventative measures and to build a culture of safety and learning within the health services (NPSA 2004) (Box 13.11).

Equipment used at work

Provision and Use of Work Equipment Regulations (PUWER 1998) and Lifting Operations and Lifting Equipment Regulations (LOLER 1998) are designed to cover a range of industries but both ensure that equipment used at work is:

- Suitable for use
- Well maintained
- Regularly inspected
- Only used by trained individuals
- Fitted with essential safety devices and warning labels (HSE 2002).

In addition, LOLER relates to equipment such as electric hoists that should be tested at 6-monthly intervals and have safe working loads (maximum patient/client weight) clearly marked on them (HSE 2000).

Manual Handling Operation Regulations 1992 (amended 2002)

Moving and handling includes lifting, lowering, pushing, pulling, carrying or moving loads such as inanimate objects, and helping people to move. Nursing involves many of these activities on a day-to-day basis and using incorrect techniques or failing to use equipment provided puts practitioners at high risk of injury. Musculoskeletal injuries occur frequently at work in the UK and have considerable economic implications (see Box 13.12). Many of these injuries are preventable and the Manual Handling Operation Regulations lay out the requirements under health and safety law and the responsibilities of employers and staff.

This section introduces the principles of safe practice but moving and handling must not be undertaken without completing a specific course that addresses the theory of safe handling and allows practice of techniques (Box 13.13). Readers should refer to Chapter 18 for further guidance on helping patients and clients to move.

There are five key stages to planning and executing a handling manoeuvre to reduce the risk to the handler and patient/client.

1. *Avoid unnecessary handling*: Is the manoeuvre really necessary? Can the person do it themselves if given enough time, adequate instructions or the right

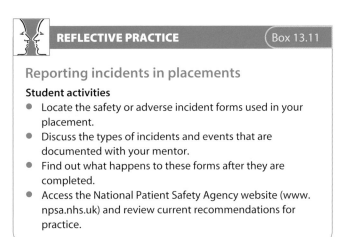

Incident form	**St Stephen's NHS Hospital Trust** **CONFIDENTIAL**
1. Which best describes the incident? Accident ☐ Violence/abuse ☐ Fire incident ☐ Ill health ☐ Formal complaint ☐ Clinical patient incident ☐ Other ☐ **2. Details of the person affected:** Name: Address: Date of birth: Male / female:	**7. Outline the circumstances of the incident:**
3. Did the person receive attention? Yes / No **4. Did the person suffer physical ill health or injury?** Yes / No Body part affected: Nature of the injury: Cause:	**8. Describe any remedial or action taken:**
5. Where and when did the incident occur? Exact location: Department: Date of the incident:	**9. Identify any witnesses:**
6. Details of violence / abuse situation Nature: threat of physical abuse / actual physical violence / verbal abuse / intimidation / racial or sexual harassment / sexual assault Name and details of the assailant:	**10. Date:** **Signature**

Top copy (blue) send to Safety Office. Middle copy (pink) send to Head of Department. Bottom copy (yellow) to be retained.

Fig. 13.3 Incident report form

REFLECTIVE PRACTICE Box 13.11

Reporting incidents in placements

Student activities

- Locate the safety or adverse incident forms used in your placement.
- Discuss the types of incidents and events that are documented with your mentor.
- Find out what happens to these forms after they are completed.
- Access the National Patient Safety Agency website (www.npsa.nhs.uk) and review current recommendations for practice.

Box 13.12

Musculoskeletal injuries in the UK and NHS

- Across all industries in the UK, 1.1 million people suffered musculoskeletal disorders in 2001/2, most commonly back injuries (see Fig. 13.2)
- This accounts for half of all work-related ill health, an estimated 12.3 million lost working days and £5.7 billion in costs to society (HSE 2004b)
- In the NHS, moving and handling injuries are responsible for 40% of all sickness absence, accounting for £400 million a year
- One in four nurses has had time off with a back injury sustained at work.

[From DH 2002]

equipment? Is it necessary to move equipment or boxes?

2. *Assess the risk*: If the task cannot be avoided then assess it using 'Task, Individual, Load and Environment' as a framework (TILE, see p. 330).
3. *Plan the move*: Decide on the most appropriate posture or technique.
4. *Prepare for the move*: Gather the right equipment, number of people required and make sure they are all clear about the technique and the instructions.
5. *Perform the manoeuvre*: Ensure that smooth controlled movements are used and your back is in a natural vertical position (Fig. 13.4).

Box 13.13 **Recommended components of moving and handling training**

- Functions of the spine
- Importance of back care, posture and risk factors contributing to back pain and injuries
- Current legislation and professional guidelines
- Assessment of risks:
  - tasks
  - individual capability (own and that of others)
  - loads (inanimate and human)
  - environment
- Importance of ergonomic approach
- Local policies
- Principles of normal human movement and promotion of client independence
- Safe handling of inanimate loads
- Handling strategies for clients with impaired immobility
- Dealing with unpredictable occurrences
- Use of equipment
- Problem-solving.

[Based on DH 2002]

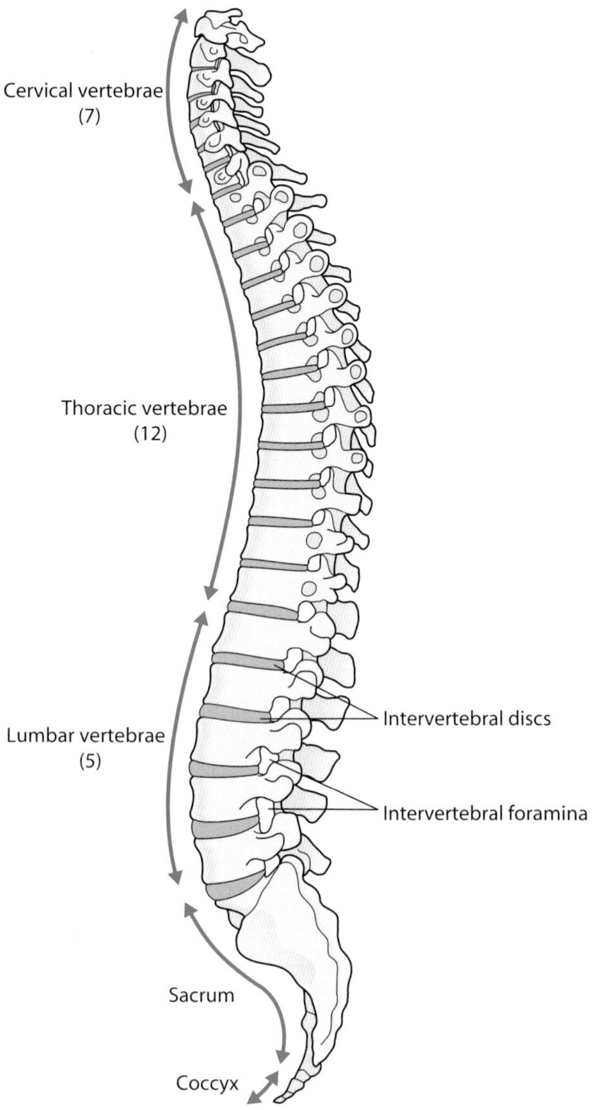

Fig. 13.4 Anatomy of the spine (reproduced with permission from Waugh & Grant 2006)

Moving and handling require an approach similar to other health and safety issues and one of the first stages is a risk assessment. This may be:

- Generic, i.e. referring to a group of people and a particular task, or
- Specific, i.e. relating to a particular patient/client and their individual handling needs.

The TILE framework

This helps to think through the move using biomechanics (the study of human movement) and ergonomics (the science of design and fitting the work environment to the worker). Both of these disciplines contribute to the understanding of how to prevent injuries. TILE is discussed below based on the guidance from the HSE (2004b) and Johnson (2005).

The task (T)

Assessing the task means identifying the factors that may cause injury and eliminating or reducing them. The HSE (2004b) suggest that the following questions be asked:

- Does the task involve holding or manipulating loads at a distance to the trunk?
  Holding an object close to the trunk means that it is easier to control and there is less risk of back injury compared to holding it at a distance or at arms' length.
- Does the task involve twisting, stooping or reaching upwards?
  Stooping, twisting and reaching greatly increase the risk of injury because they place stress on the lower spine. These actions must be avoided in moving and handling tasks by using legs and feet to move rather than twisting at the trunk and by remaining close to the load or patient/client.
- Does the task involve excessive carrying of inanimate objects across a distance or excessive lifting or lowering?
  Carrying objects over long distances or repetitive lifting or lowering can cause fatigue and increase the risk of injury. Equipment, such as a trolley, reduces the risk of injury from carrying. Also, heavier items should be stacked on shelves at waist height so they are not lifted from the floor or high shelves.
- Does the task involve pushing and pulling?
  Pushing and pulling may be a safer technique than lifting but it can still put the handler at risk of injury. For example, pushing a heavy load along an uneven surface or up a slope could be unsafe.

- Can the load suddenly move?
  If the contents of a half full box are not secure they may shift during movement so the load needs to be secure to be safe. If the task involves people, there is always a risk of unexpected movements so the likelihood of this occurring is reduced by making sure the patient/client knows their role and what to expect so they do not become frightened or uncooperative.
- Are there sufficient rest periods for handlers?
  The greater the physical effort, the greater the risk of injury, and inadequate rest periods mean that muscles and joints do not get a chance to recover.
- Is the correct equipment available?
  As part of the risk assessment, the equipment available for the task needs careful consideration. There is a wide range of aids available, from sliding sheets that reduce friction and help people move up in bed, to electric beds and hoists that assist people to sit up, transfer or stand (see Ch. 18). During your moving and handling practical training, you will have the opportunity to practise with a range of equipment used in placements. Equipment must be well maintained and checked before each use. It is important to be aware that all equipment has a safe working load, i.e. an upper weight limit for use, usually marked on larger pieces of equipment such as hoists. This is why it is important to document patients'/clients' weight as part of nursing assessment (Ch. 14). Infection control precautions also need to be considered, e.g. whether equipment can be disinfected with alcohol wipes or if special laundering arrangements are necessary.

Individual capabilities (I)

This refers to the assessment of handlers' abilities. Nursing activities should not require great physical strength but general fitness and regular exercise are important as these reduce the risk of injury. We must also assess our ability to be involved in moving and handling on a daily basis. Classroom trainers or clinical staff must be alerted to any pre-existing or current injuries that could prevent you from being involved in safe moving and handling. People with existing injuries and those who are, or have recently been, pregnant require an occupational health assessment.

Inappropriate clothing can restrict movement during handling manoeuvres or encourage adoption of awkward postures to protect the handler's dignity, and both situations increase the risk of injury. Most uniform policies include trouser suits that allow freedom of movement and footwear that is flat and provides plenty of grip. It is therefore important to follow local uniform policies.

The load (L)

The manual handling guidelines identify a number of factors for consideration regarding the load (if it is an inanimate object) or the patient/client involved. For objects, it is important to have an indication of their weight. This is often printed on boxes or can be judged by gently rocking the item before deciding whether to lift it. The size of the load is considered and whether it is possible to split it in two to make handling easier. Other areas to consider are the type of grip to use and whether the item could be too hot or sharp to handle.

Patients/clients should not be lifted because of the risk of injury to the person and the handlers. Nurses must assess people's capabilities and then determine the best technique or equipment to help them move. One difficulty is that people do not come as a standard size, with handles, or with their height and weight printed on the side. Many people receiving healthcare have the added complication of ill health and attachments such as intravenous infusions and urinary catheters. Therefore specific assessment must be carried out for each patient/client before carrying out manoeuvres. Care settings including NHS Trusts should have their own moving and handling assessment documentation as part of the nursing care plan; some of the key areas that require consideration are outlined in Box 13.14.

> **Box 13.14 Summary of the TILE assessment for moving and handling**
>
> **Task (T)**
> Assess and minimize the risks that cause injury, e.g. holding the load or person away from the trunk, twisting, stooping or reaching, considerable lifting, lowering or carrying distances for objects and pushing or pulling. Assess the need for team handling and think about the range of equipment available including its safe working limits, its condition and last recorded service.
>
> **Individual (I)**
> Assess the capabilities of staff, e.g. their age, gender, height, physical fitness, previous injuries, current or recent pregnancy, training, knowledge or experience, and wearing of restrictive clothing or inappropriate footwear.
>
> **Load (L)**
> - *Objects*: Assess the weight, dimensions, contents (loose, heavy at one end), bulky, harmful (hot or sharp) and whether it is difficult to grasp
> - *People*: Assess their mobility and ability to weight bear, physical health, history of falls or confusion, understanding and concordance, attachments (intravenous infusions, catheters) and risk of moving unexpectedly, e.g. first time out of bed, prone to muscle spasms or seizures.
>
> **Environment (E)**
> Assessment includes adequate lighting, temperature (especially extremes of heat and cold), flooring (for slippery or uneven surfaces, carpet, gradient), obstacles and weather conditions if outdoors.

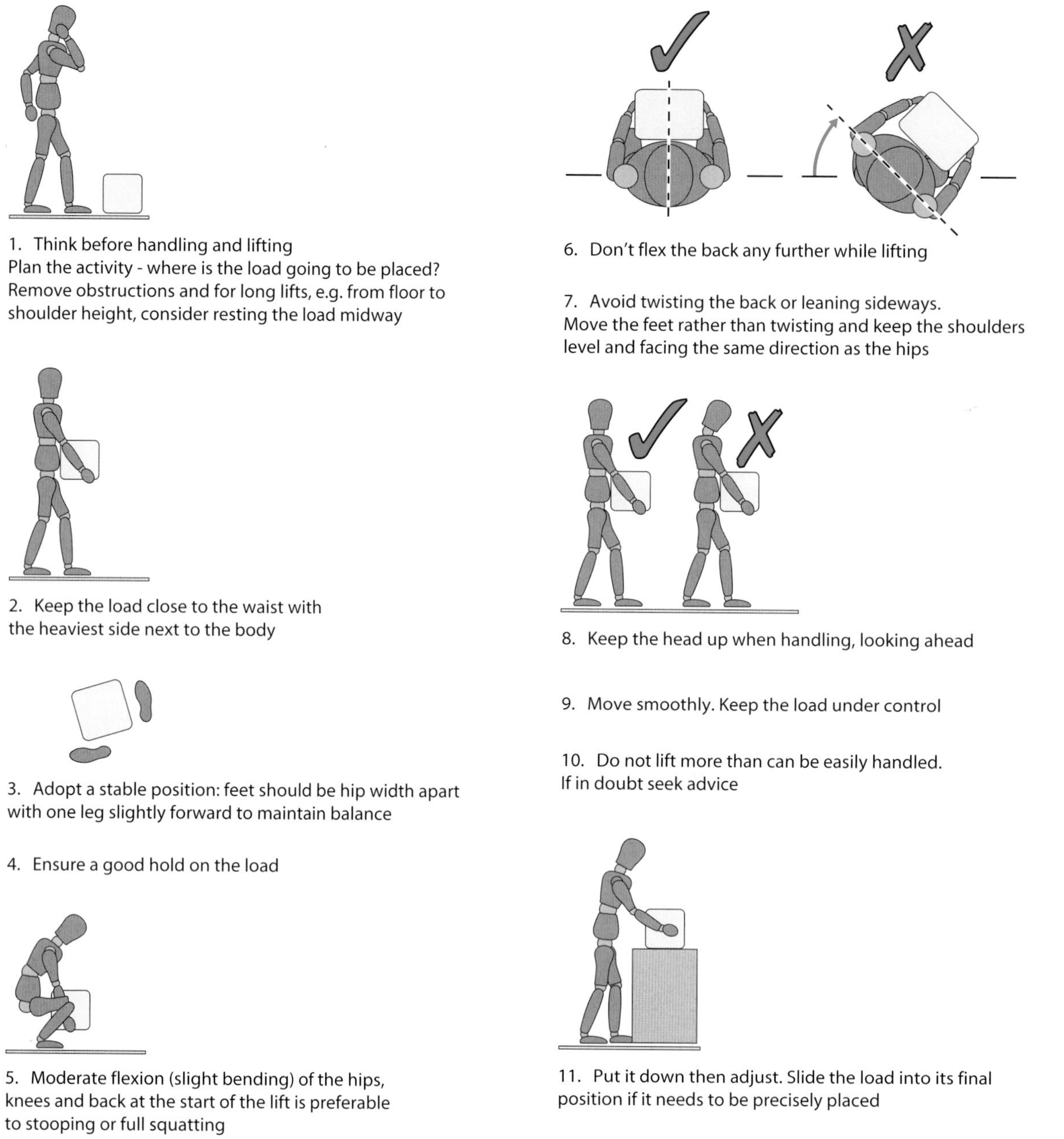
1. Think before handling and lifting
Plan the activity - where is the load going to be placed? Remove obstructions and for long lifts, e.g. from floor to shoulder height, consider resting the load midway
2. Keep the load close to the waist with the heaviest side next to the body
3. Adopt a stable position: feet should be hip width apart with one leg slightly forward to maintain balance
4. Ensure a good hold on the load
5. Moderate flexion (slight bending) of the hips, knees and back at the start of the lift is preferable to stooping or full squatting
6. Don't flex the back any further while lifting
7. Avoid twisting the back or leaning sideways.
Move the feet rather than twisting and keep the shoulders level and facing the same direction as the hips
8. Keep the head up when handling, looking ahead
9. Move smoothly. Keep the load under control
10. Do not lift more than can be easily handled.
If in doubt seek advice
11. Put it down then adjust. Slide the load into its final position if it needs to be precisely placed

Fig. 13.5 Handling technique for inanimate objects (reproduced with permission from HSE 2004b)

The environment (E)

There are many factors in the environment that can increase or decrease the risk of injury to handlers and patients/clients. It is important to assess whether there is adequate lighting; non-slip flooring; a floor gradient or potential obstacles, e.g. doors, furniture, stairs. Extremes of temperature can also alter people's concentration levels and physical abilities. Moving and handling need to be planned to ensure that none of these factors contributes to an injury. There must be sufficient space to avoid awkward postures or techniques and it is important to be alert to hazards that may cause you and the client to slip or trip.

Moving and handling procedures cannot be completely risk-free but the TILE framework allows major hazards to be identified and reduces injuries to staff and patients/clients through using the correct technique and equipment. Figure 13.5 illustrates a good handling technique for lifting an inanimate load and Chapter 18 examines specific techniques for helping people to move.

First aid

This term describes the initial treatment or assistance given to an individual who is injured or unwell before the arrival a qualified healthcare professional, e.g. paramedic or doctor. The aim is to preserve life, prevent worsening of a condition and promote recovery (Mohun et al 2002). This section discusses first aid at work, the general principles of first aid and how to deal with some specific emergencies, i.e. burns and scalds, and suspected poisonings.

All employers must provide first aid facilities, equipment and personnel under the Health and Safety (First-Aid) Regulations 1981 (HSE 2003b), including:

- First aid boxes
- Trained first aiders who have undergone a HSE approved course
- Specialist equipment if there are particular hazards and therefore a higher risk of accidents.

Green posters may also advertise where the nearest first aid box is located and the names of trained first aiders. Some clinical areas may be better equipped to deal with emergencies than others, e.g. comparing a hospital ward and a day centre for older adults. However, all are required to conduct risk assessments and provide appropriate facilities.

Administering first aid outside placements can be very different as equipment is not readily available. Also, not all nurses are trained first aiders although they do have knowledge that is useful in an emergency situation. First aid and emergency skills are part of pre-registration programmes as required by the NMC. The NMC *Code of Professional Conduct* (2004) also describes the duty of care that nurses have outside work in an emergency situation. Often nurses are concerned about expectations of them but any first aid provided is judged in relation to the particular circumstances and against what can reasonably be expected from someone with their level of knowledge, skills and abilities (NMC 2004). This means that expectations of an experienced nurse working in an Emergency Department would be much higher than a student nurse who has only completed a basic life support course.

Some people may be concerned about the legal aspects of first aid provided outside the healthcare environment and being held to account if events do not go as well as anticipated. Similar to the NMC guidance, so long as first aiders have acted in a reasonable manner and this conforms to any training given, they will be in a safe position. The casualty would have to have had experienced further harm as a direct result of first aid given to be in a situation to sue for compensation (Dimond 1993).

This section introduces the basic principles of first aid and subsequent chapters deal with specific situations (Box 13.15). As well as reading the information in these chapters, there are other considerations that can help to develop knowledge and confidence. Some first aid skills are included in nursing programmes and attending a recognized training course to become a qualified first aider may help (see 'Useful websites', p. 347). Remember that first aid should 'do no harm' and that recognizing the limitations of one's knowledge and skills is important; however, you may be the only person present who has attended a basic life support or first aid course and simple measures will often help save someone's life or prevent their condition worsening.

Box 13.15 First aid covered in this book

Chapter	Topics
13	Principles of first aid, dealing with burns, scalds, poisoning
14	Effects of heat and cold: heat exhaustion, heatstroke, hypothermia, frostbite
16	Disorders of consciousness: head injury, seizures
17	Respiratory problems: choking, suffocation, smoke inhalation, asthma Circulatory problems: cardiopulmonary resuscitation, shock and haemorrhage, fainting; myocardial infarction (heart attack), angina (chest pain)
18	Musculoskeletal problems: sprains and strains, dislocations, fractures
25	Wounds: abrasions, lacerations, puncture wounds, bites and stings

FIRST AID Box 13.16

Principles of first aid

1. Assess the situation
2. Check that the area is safe for you and the casualty
3. Make an initial assessment of the casualty
4. Prioritize injuries:
   - Airway (A)
   - Breathing (B)
   - Circulation (C)
5. Call for help
6. Provide first aid.

Student activity

Test your knowledge of first aid by accessing quizzes online, e.g. www.bbc.co.uk/health/first_aid_action/first_for_fun.shtml Available July 2006.

Dealing with emergencies and prioritizing

Emergency situations can be difficult to deal with as people may be distressed, in pain or confused and there may be more than one injury or a number of people involved. However, it is important that you remain calm and apply some simple principles (based on Mohun et al 2002) that will help to organize your thoughts and decisions on the most appropriate action. The principles of first aid are listed in Box 13.16 and described below.

Assess the situation

Make a brief visual assessment of what has happened, looking for evidence of danger or potential hazards for yourself and the casualty. The most important rule of first aid is that you never put yourself in danger otherwise you too may become a casualty. Once you have determined that it is safe, introduce yourself to the casualty or bystanders and ask them to describe what has happened.

Check the area is safe for you and the casualty

Can you safely remove potential dangers such as obstructions or switching off electric sockets? Only remove the casualty from the situation as a last resort and only if there is imminent life-threatening danger.

Make an initial assessment of the casualty and give emergency first aid if necessary

Chapter 16 discusses how to make an initial assessment of a collapsed individual by checking their responsiveness and then:

- Airway (A)
- Breathing (B)
- Circulation (C).

If the casualty has more that one problem, e.g. they are unconscious and their arm is bleeding, deal with problems in the ABC order, i.e. make sure their airway is clear, they are breathing and then attend to the source of the bleeding. If there is more than one casualty you will have to prioritize and decide who requires the most immediate attention. Again, use the ABC assessment. Quiet or unconscious casualties often require the quickest attention. You know that those who are crying or shouting at least have a clear airway, are breathing and also have a pulse. However, they will still need reassurance and assessment of their injuries so encourage bystanders to stay with, and reassure them.

Call for help

In a placement, call for help immediately by shouting and using emergency buzzers where available. You may be asked to put out a 'crash call', a telephone call to the switchboard that will alert the resuscitation team. Clearly state that there has been a cardiac arrest and give the name and location of the area. The National Patient Safety Agency (2004) asked NHS Trusts to standardize their crash call number to '2222' so that the emergency number is always the same. Ensure that you find out the emergency number on the first day of each new placement.

Outside of placements, you will need to telephone 999 (in the UK) to summon emergency services. This phone call is free from public phone boxes and most mobile phones. State the emergency service required (ambulance, police, fire brigade, coastguard) and you will be put through to the appropriate call centre. You will be asked for your name and location and to provide the number of casualties and describe their injuries.

Provide first aid

Provide first aid and stay with the casualty until help arrives. Healthcare professionals will make their own assessment of the situation but your information about the event, your observations and the treatment given are useful to them.

After the event

Dealing with emergencies can be stressful and you may experience a range of emotions afterwards (Ch. 11). It is also quite natural to reflect on the situation, your role, what went well and what you would do differently if the situation occurred again. You might find it helpful to talk to your mentor or your personal tutor at university to help make sense of events or for advice about alternative sources of support.

Being a first aider in a serious incident can affect people weeks or even months later. Reliving the event in some way, avoiding situations that remind people of the event, sleeplessness and experiencing symptoms of stress may suggest that the first aider is experiencing post-traumatic stress disorder (Mohun et al 2002) (see Ch. 11). If this happens it is wise to seek the support of a general practitioner (GP) or counsellor.

Dealing with burns and scalds

Around 100 000 people attend Emergency Departments in England and Wales annually because of burns. Most are caused either by dry heat (e.g. flames) or moist heat (e.g. steam, hot liquids or fat) (DTI 2003), although industrial and domestic chemicals can also cause burns along with high and low voltage electrical sources, radiation (including sunburn, X-rays and radioactive sources) and extreme cold (e.g. frostbite).

The skin is the largest organ in the body and is discussed in more detail in Chapter 16. The epidermis and dermis make up the two main layers of the skin and burns

Box 13.17 Types of burn

Superficial
- Only involves the epidermis and heals well
- Redness, swelling and sometimes blistering
- Painful and sensitive.

Partial thickness
- The epidermis and dermis separate, forming fluid-filled blisters
- Redness and swelling
- Painful and sensitive
- Require medical treatment in children and if more than a minor burn in adults.

Full thickness
- Deep burn involving dermal, subcutaneous and muscle layers
- May appear waxy, charred or leathery
- No pain sensation due to damaged nerve endings
- Need urgent medical attention, specialist burns treatment and skin grafts.

can involve both layers; in severe cases, the underlying subcutaneous fat and muscle layers are also affected.

Burns are classified according to the depth and percentage of the body surface area involved. Box 13.17 illustrates the three depths of burn injury: superficial, partial thickness and full thickness.

The extent of burns may initially be estimated using the 'rule of nines' (Fig. 13.6): the greater the area affected, the greater the risk of shock caused by fluid loss. In adults, medical attention is needed for anything more that a minor superficial burn. A doctor should see children with what appears to be a superficial burn. Medical attention should always be sought for burns affecting the face, groin, hands and feet. When more than 15% burns in adults is present specialist burns care in hospital is necessary. This figure is 10% burns in children where

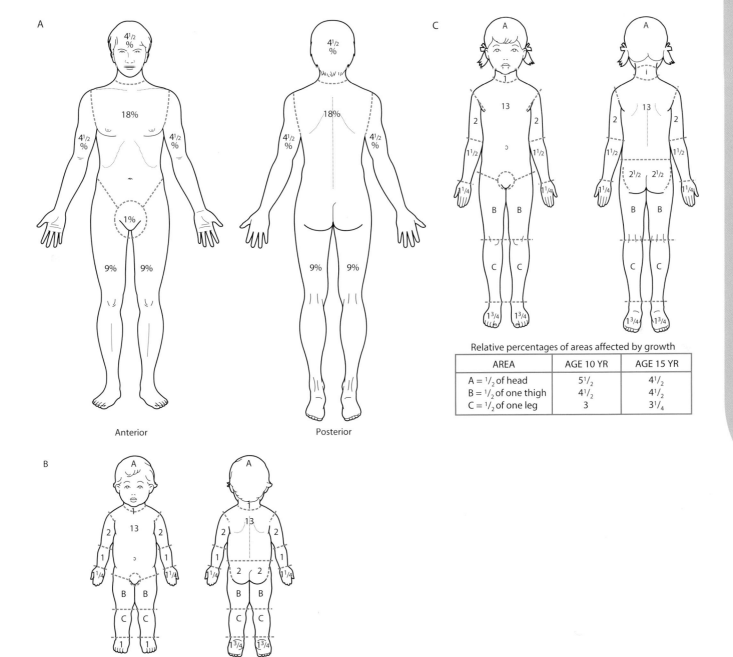

A

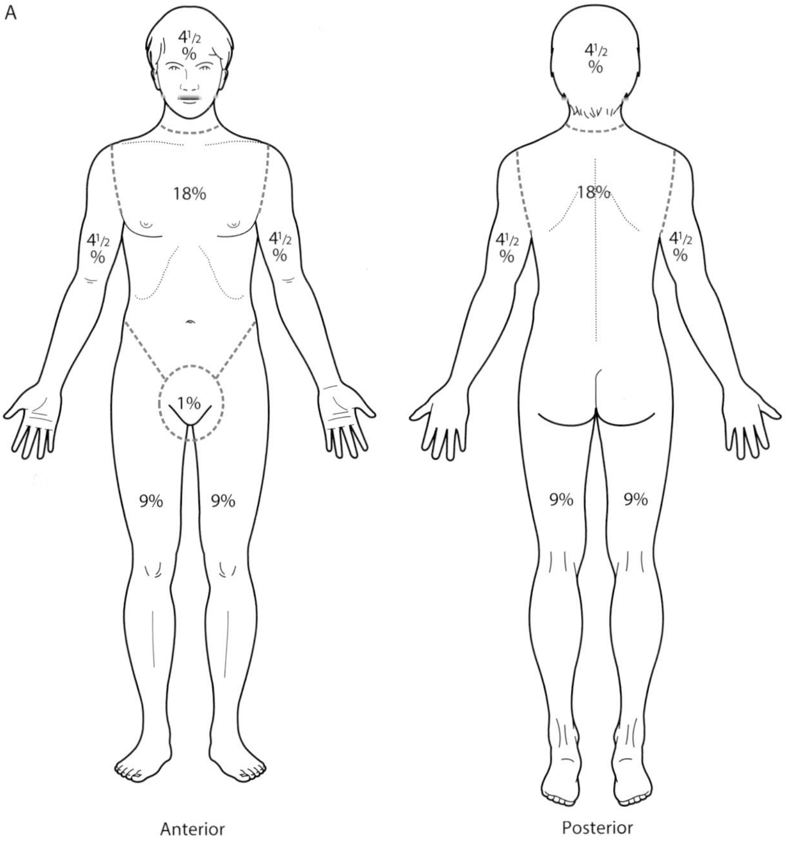

C

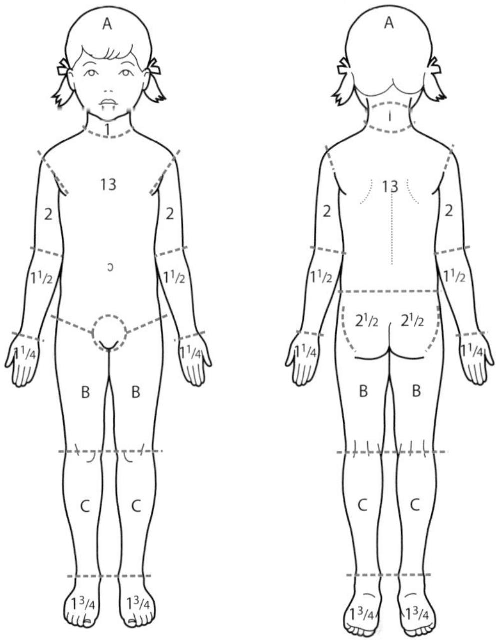

Relative percentages of areas affected by growth

AREA	AGE 10 YR	AGE 15 YR
A = 1/2 of head	5 1/2	4 1/2
B = 1/2 of one thigh	4 1/2	4 1/2
C = 1/2 of one leg	3	3 1/4

B

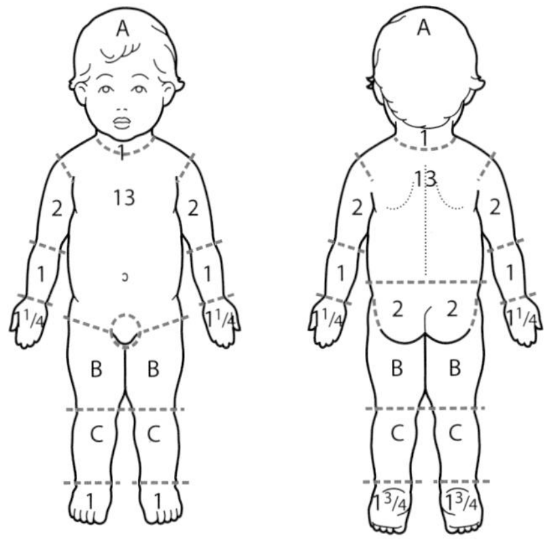

Relative percentages of areas affected by growth

AREA	BIRTH	AGE 1YR	AGE 5YR
A = 1/2 of head	9 1/2	8 1/2	6 1/2
B = 1/2 of one thigh	2 3/4	3 1/4	4
C = 1/2 of one leg	2 1/2	2 1/2	2 3/4

Fig. 13.6 Estimating the extent of burns and scalds in adults and children: **A.** Adults: the rule of nines (reproduced with permission from Waugh & Grant 2006). **B.** Children up to 5 years (reproduced with permission from Hockenberry et al 2003). **C.** Older children (reproduced with permission from Hockenberry et al 2003)

FIRST AID Box 13.18

Burns and scalds

Recognition

Tissue damage as described in Box 13.17.

Aims of treatment

- Establish and maintain airway, breathing and circulation
- Cool the affected area to remove the heat to limit tissue damage and provide temporary pain relief
- Transfer to hospital if appropriate.

Treatment

- Place the burn under cool running water (not ice cold as this will damage the skin) for 10–20 minutes or, if this is not possible, use a jug or container to pour water over the area
- Remove any rings, jewellery and watches that may cause constriction later on due to swelling
- Do not remove any clothing stuck in the wound
- Gels and sprays that cool minor burns are not recommended because of difficulty in controlling the cooling effect once applied (Lawrence 1996)
- For large burns, the casualty is at risk of hypothermia because of the cooling effect of the water. Help to keep the casualty warm by covering unaffected areas
- Superficial burns: cover with a non-adhesive dressing
- Partial or full thickness burns: cover the wound with clean, non-fluffy material (to avoid sticking) to reduce the risk of infection and provide protection while being transported to hospital. Cling film is ideal (although ensure the skin has been cooled and discard the outer layer of film that may be contaminated).

FIRST AID Box 13.19

Poisoning

Recognition

- Casualty may report history of accidental or deliberate poisoning
- Evidence of empty containers, bottles or syringes (if a drug overdose is suspected, watch for used syringes in the area or in pockets that could cause a needlestick injury)
- Drowsiness or loss of consciousness
- Nausea and vomiting when poisons have been ingested.

Aims and treatment

- Maintain or establish airway, breathing and circulation
- Identify poison by asking the casualty, if possible, and looking for clues in the area
- If unconscious, treat as outlined in Box 16.29, p. 454
- Treat any other injuries found
- Call for help to arrange transfer to hospital without delay, even if there are no symptoms.

Ingested poisons

- The casualty is more likely to vomit and protecting their airway becomes a priority
- Vomiting should not be induced because casualties may inhale the vomit blocking their airway
- If mouth-to-mouth resuscitation becomes necessary then protect yourself with a specially designed plastic resuscitation face shield (Fig. 13.7) (Mohun et al 2002).

Inhaled substances

- The danger with inhaled substances, e.g. carbon monoxide gas or smoke, is that the contaminant is still present in the atmosphere
- Work environments where hazardous gases are used have specialist breathing equipment available and trained personnel in case emergencies arise
- If inhalation is suspected, the most appropriate course of action is to summon the emergency services.

a modified chart is used to calculate the extent of burns because of the different sizes of children (Fowler 2003). Box 13.18 describes the management of burns and scalds.

Electrical burns

Extreme caution is required when there are electrical burns to ensure that the casualty is no longer in contact with the source of electricity. It may not be possible to attend to them until it has been confirmed that the current has been turned off (Mohun et al 2002). Anyone who has experienced an electrical burn must seek medical attention because the current may have interfered with the electrical activity of the heart.

Chemical burns

For burns caused by chemicals splashed onto skin or into the eyes, ensure that the water flushing the area runs away from the body so that it does not come into contact with any other region causing further burns. Unlike burns caused by heat, where clothes should be left untouched, it may be necessary to remove contaminated clothing. First aiders must wear protective clothing including heavy-duty rubber gloves and apron to protect themselves. When arranging for the casualty to be transported to hospital, ensure that paramedics are aware that chemicals are involved. Finally, burns caused by cold injuries, e.g. frostbite, require different treatment and should not be cooled (see Ch. 14).

Dealing with poisoning

A poison is any substance that enters the body in sufficient quantities to cause temporary or permanent damage. Poisons may be accidentally or deliberately ingested, inhaled, splashed on the skin or injected. Signs and symptoms vary according to the amount and type

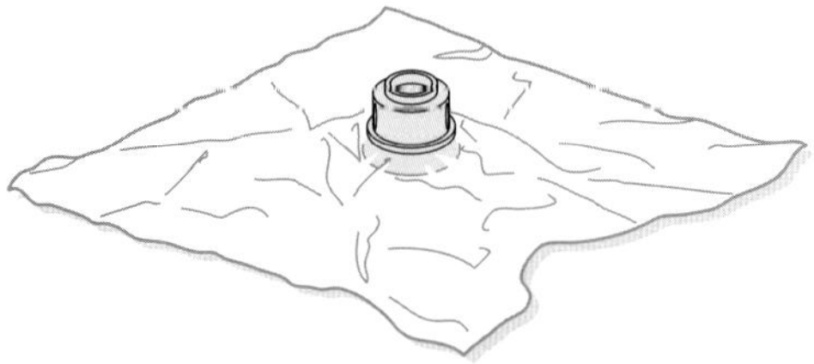

Fig. 13.7 Resuscitation face shield

of poison involved and its route of entry. Box 13.19 shows the principles of dealing with a suspected or known poisoning.

In clinical areas, healthcare practitioners have access to one of six UK centres that comprise the National Poisons Informati on Service (www.npis.org). This service includes a 24-hour emergency helpline and a toxicology database of known poisons and recommended treatments.

Infection control and standard precautions

Preventing the spread of infection is one of the most important nursing roles and is concerned with safety, preventing ill health, and promoting health and well-being in individuals or groups of people. This section briefly introduces key concepts of safe infection control practice and Chapter 15 examines them in more detail.

Standard precautions, previously known as universal precautions, were introduced in North America to reduce the risk of transmitting blood-borne viruses such as HIV and hepatitis B to healthcare workers. Both terms describe infection control guidelines that minimize the risk of coming into contact with body fluids (including blood, urine, faeces and other body secretions and excretions), non-intact skin and mucous membranes. The standard precautions outlined in Box 13.20 are used with every person receiving care, regardless of their infection status, in order to protect healthcare practitioners and prevent the spread of infection.

There are several routes by which bacteria, viruses, fungi and other infectious agents can be transmitted including inhalation, direct contact, ingestion and inoculation. However, effective handwashing has been repeatedly shown be the most important factor in reducing the spread of infection. Knowledge of appropriate handwashing techniques (see Ch. 15) and the necessary frequency is therefore essential (Box 13.21).

Many healthcare procedures are invasive, meaning that they use sharp devices that penetrate the skin or body in some way such as needles or surgery (Horton & Parker 2002). This carries the risk of needlestick injury to practitioners and also transmission of blood-borne viruses after devices have been in contact with patients/clients. Sharps therefore require careful handling and disposal (see Ch. 15). Sharps bins are special containers that conform to British Standard Institute specification

Box 13.20 Standard precautions

- Apply good handwashing technique (p. 401) at appropriate intervals including before and after contact with patients/clients and after gloves are removed (see Box 15.10, p. 405)
- Avoid using sharps whenever possible
- Use safe procedures when handling and disposing of sharps (see Ch. 15)
- Prevent puncture wounds, cuts and abrasions, especially in the presence of blood or bloodstained fluids
- Protect the skin, mucous membranes of eyes, mouth and nose from blood splashes by using appropriate personal protective equipment, i.e. gloves and aprons, when in contact with body fluids, non-intact skin and mucous membranes (see Ch. 15)
- Cover wounds or skin lesions with a waterproof dressing and avoid unnecessary invasive procedures
- Clean up spillages of blood and body fluids promptly using hypochlorite disinfectant
- Follow local policies for sterilization and disinfection of instruments and equipment (see Ch. 15)
- Dispose of contaminated waste safely (see Ch. 15).

[Based on Wilson (2001) and Horton & Parker (2002)]

Box 13.21 When handwashing is carried out

Handwashing is undertaken:

- Before and after:
  - any patient contact
  - handling invasive devices
  - dressing wounds
  - contact with immunocompromised patients
  - handling food or drinks.
- After:
  - contact with body fluid or handling equipment contaminated by body fluid
  - handling clinical waste and used linen
  - removing gloves
  - coughing and sneezing
  - using the lavatory.
- Before leaving the clinical area.

[From Wilson (2001, p. 136)]

REFLECTIVE PRACTICE Box 13.22

Standard precautions in practice

Student activities

1. Locate the sharps container(s) in your placement:
   - What information needs to be documented on the side of the bin, when and by whom?
   - Where are sharps containers placed for collection and disposal?
2. Discuss the measures in place to prevent needlestick injuries with your mentor.
3. Find out the procedure for dealing with and reporting needlestick injuries.
4. How is clinical and non-clinical waste segregated and disposed of?
5. What are the arrangements for segregation and collection of different categories of linen?

which ensures that they are yellow in colour, puncture resistant, leak-proof, clearly marked with three-quarters lines indicating when they should be closed, suitable for incineration and marked with hazard signs.

In the community, some pharmacies and organizations offer needle exchange programmes for intravenous drug users. These harm-reduction programmes aim to help individuals reduce the risk of contracting hepatitis B or HIV by supplying clean needles and safely disposing of used equipment (see www.drugsinfo.org.uk for an example).

Clinical waste must be carefully managed to ensure that toxic or hazardous materials are handled, transported and disposed of safely. There are regulations surrounding clinical waste that needs to be segregated under the Environmental Protection Act (1990). This includes using appropriate bags for household waste such as paper and flowers which can be sent to landfill, yellow clinical waste bags for materials contaminated with blood or body fluids, and sharps containers that need to be incinerated (Wilson 2001). Hospital linen also has a colour coding system which determines how laundry bags are handled (see Ch. 15).

Infection control and standard precautions are an essential part of all healthcare practitioners' everyday practice to ensure the safety of staff, patients/clients and the wider community. Chapter 15 is therefore an important chapter to read. Carrying out the activities in Box 13.22 will help you examine practice and familiarize yourself with infection control procedures and policies for handling, storage and disposal of clinical waste in your placement.

Principles of managing violence and aggression

Developing safe practice involves identifying potential risks and minimizing them, and the issue of violence and aggression is no exception. People are at highest risk of this when engaged in work that involves:

- Dealing with the public
- Providing care and education
- Working with people who are confused, have mental health problems or behavioural challenges
- Working alone
- Handling valuables or medication
- Working with people under stress or those who misuse alcohol or drugs (Royal College of Nursing [RCN] 2003a, HSE 2004c).

Nurses from all branches may be involved in these situations. However, the fear of violence and aggression can be out of proportion to the risks: although verbal aggression is more common and physical harm comparatively rare (Bibby 1995, HSE 2004c), both can have detrimental effects on practitioners. This section is about awareness and prevention. Being aware of the factors that can lead to aggression helps to develop the interpersonal communication skills that prevent incidents where aggression may occur and defuse tense situations.

As the phrase 'violence and aggression' may hold slightly different meanings for different people, it is useful to briefly describe and define the term so that we are able to recognize it when it occurs and deal with incidents appropriately. The RCN (2003a, p. 3) offers the following definition: 'Any incident in which a health professional experiences abuse, threat, fear or the application of force arising out of the course of their work, whether or not they are on duty.'

Some organizations such as the RCN (2003a) and the Department of Health (1999b) simply use the term violence, others use violence and aggression interchangeably and some differentiate between the two. Both terms are used here referring to non-physical (aggressive) and physical (violent) behaviours (Box 13.23).

Minimizing violence and aggression

The reasons why violence and aggression occur are usually complex; for an in-depth discussion, refer to Mason and Chandley (1999) who examine the wider issue of violence in society. For healthcare practitioners there may be a number of additional factors that contribute to an increased risk of witnessing or being involved in an incident. People receiving healthcare may be anxious, tired, in pain, confused, frustrated by waiting times, under the influence of drugs or alcohol, have mental distress or a history of violence – and all of these predispose to unpredictable behaviour. Nursing often takes place in stressful situations and treatment or facilities may be granted, denied or delayed (RCN 2003a).

Over recent years there has been increasing concern in the nursing media and general press about increases in violent incidents towards healthcare staff. However,

Box 13.23 **Types of violence**

Aggression (non-physical violence)

- Verbal abuse including racial and sexual harassment
- Swearing
- Shouting
- Name calling and bullying
- Insults
- Innuendo
- Deliberate silence
- Threatening gestures or postures
- Harassment, in all its forms
- Threatening use of dogs
- Abusive phone calls

Physical violence

- Kicking
- Punching
- Head-butting
- Biting
- Spitting
- Scratching
- Use of weapons
- Assault causing physical injury
- Sexual assault
- Assault causing death
- Deliberate self-harm

[Based on Bibby (1995)]

this is difficult to illustrate because previously there was no clear definition, as well as considerable underreporting (Bibby 1995). The national media also focus heavily on serious incidents and often on individuals with mental health problems; however, it is important to be mindful of the stereotypes that can arise from this. Most people with mental health conditions are at greater risk of harming themselves than other people (Jones & Jackson 2004).

NHS Trusts have explicit strategies for reducing the number of violent incidents towards staff and systems for recording these events. Violence and aggression in the workplace have an immediate impact on individuals involved, their colleagues and also potential long-term consequences. Employers have a duty of care under the HSW Act (1974) (p. 326) to identify risks and take preventative measures. A risk assessment must involve all staff and key stages of the process (see p. 322). NHS Trusts must focus on specific areas including the environment, education provided to staff and methods of communication (DH 1999b).

Environment

The Department of Health (1999b) made a number of recommendations relating to clinical areas. Examining the environment in which care is delivered can identify factors that may trigger or contribute to aggressive or violent incidents (Box 13.24).

Although creating a pleasant but safe patient/client environment is important (Box 13.25), this involves a balance between providing a friendly area and adequate security (National Audit Office 2003). In one department, protective glass screens actually increased tension for staff and clients and were therefore removed and replaced with other preventative measures (HSE 2004c).

Box 13.24 **Improving the healthcare environment to decrease violence**

- Waiting rooms and reception areas need to be clean, hospitable with clear direction signs and notices
- Extremes of temperature and overcrowding may contribute to people's discomfort
- Comfortable seating arrangements should be provided along with measures that relieve boredom, e.g. television or radio (but ensure noise is minimized) and reading materials
- The environment should be laid out to ensure that areas restricted to patients are locked and that there is a clear line of sight between areas wherever possible
- Adequate lighting is also needed and closed circuit television (CCTV) can be a useful deterrent against violent behaviour, especially outside, e.g. in car parks
- Where there is a greater risk of violence, or staff are isolated, a panic button system will alert others to the need for help.

[From DH (1999b), RCN (2003a)]

REFLECTIVE PRACTICE Box 13.25

Providing a safe environment

Student activities

1. Consider your current placement or one you have recently worked in:
   - Are the waiting and reception rooms clean and spacious, and do they have comfortable seating?
   - Are direction signs clear?
   - Are there measures to relieve boredom?
   - Is CCTV used?
2. Discuss your observations with your mentor.

Education

One of the key strategies for reducing violence towards healthcare staff is education to ensure that practitioners are aware of the safety issues and how to prevent or defuse a situation. Violence and aggression training is usually included in nursing programmes and is likely to involve the theory and practice of:

- De-escalation techniques, i.e. methods of preventing and defusing violent behaviour
- Breakaway techniques, i.e. methods of physically escaping from someone's hold.

The training received by clinical staff and student nurses depends on the nature of the areas in which they will be working and the risk assessment results.

Box 13.26 **Verbal and non-verbal cues that suggest that people are agitated**

- Awkward or tense posture
- Facial expressions
- Hand gestures
- Increased restlessness
- Excitability
- Pacing up and down
- Speech patterns such as increased speed, loudness, threatening remarks or refusal to communicate or withdrawal.

[From Mason & Chandley (1999), RCN (2003a)]

In low-risk environments, e.g. operating theatres, staff training may include basic theory and de-escalation techniques. In high-risk areas, e.g. where challenging behaviour is common, or in mental health secure units, training will also usually include breakaway and restraint techniques.

The NHS Security Management Service (NHS SMS; www.cfsms.nhs.uk) was created in April 2003 with the policy and operational responsibility for the management of security within the NHS. NHS SMS has launched a comprehensive strategy to better protect staff and property in the NHS, with a particular emphasis on tackling violence. This replaces work previously undertaken under the NHS Zero Tolerance campaign.

Improving communication and preventing incidents

Safe nursing practice includes promoting effective communication between staff and patients/clients at all times (Ch. 9). Observation and interpersonal skills are often the key to preventing or defusing a situation by firstly looking for verbal and non-verbal cues that suggest that people may be agitated (Box 13.26).

Awareness of factors that can predispose people to violence and aggression (p. 339) is useful. Mason and Chandley (1999) remind readers of the need to be mindful of stereotypes and prejudices that may arise. For example, not everyone with dependence on alcohol or mental distress becomes violent, and external appearances, e.g. tattoos, piercing, do not represent particular attitudes or behaviours.

Interpersonal skills and non-verbal behaviour can help to resolve situations and prevent them from escalating. Key to all situations is the need to maintain respect and dignity for the people involved and to appear calm and confident (Mason & Chandley 1999). Box 13.27 identifies good practices that may help to prevent or de-escalate a situation.

If more critical situations arise, these principles still apply and a confident, calm approach is still needed although it may not be appropriate to intervene. When possible, withdraw from the situation and think about moving other people away from the area too. Being aware of the environment you work in is also important – knowing how to summon help (e.g. other members of staff, security, police) and the general layout of the area along with the exit points. Avoid talking to people in confined spaces or corners if you recognize that a situation may become hostile. It is a good idea to suggest that all concerned move into a more suitable area to discuss the issue. Communication between staff is equally important to ensure everyone's safety. Always inform staff when you are leaving a clinical area, where you will be and when you will return. This is good practice so that if an emergency occurs, e.g. fire or cardiac arrest, colleagues are aware of your location.

Staff working in the community may have specific needs as they usually work individually or as part of a small team. Risk assessments are still carried out, as in other clinical areas, and specific arrangements made for times when practitioners are out on duty. This should include the use of mobile phones to keep in contact, a system of informing other staff where they are and the approximate time they expect to return. The NHS Security

NURSING SKILLS Box 13.27

Preventing and de-escalating potentially violent situations

- Wherever possible, make a good initial contact by introducing yourself, perhaps shaking hands and asking the client their preferred name
- Maintain a relaxed, open posture and ensure that your non-verbal behaviour is not threatening
- Demonstrate that the person has your full attention through your body language, i.e. is directed towards them, and avoid distracting behaviours such as foot tapping, fiddling
- Encourage the conversation by asking open-ended questions and acknowledging their feelings, e.g. 'I can see that you must have been feeling frustrated if you have been waiting' – do not attribute blame
- Try to solve the problem or find someone who can help, but do not make promises you cannot keep. Ask the person what they think could be done to resolve the issue
- Share the problem by using the term 'we', e.g. 'we need to work together on this so that you receive the medication on time in future'
- Avoid behaviours that may escalate the situation, including use of jargon, retaliatory remarks, sarcasm, swearing, ridiculing, trivializing the client's feelings or using phrases such as 'Don't be daft' or 'Calm down'
- If tension continues to escalate it may be helpful to agree to take a break or change venue. Alternatively, if you feel the patient/client is reacting badly towards you, with their agreement, it may be helpful to refer them to someone else.

[Based on Bibby (1995), DH (1999b), Mason & Chandley (1999), RCN (2003a)]

Management Service (2003) introduced a pilot scheme for community staff where they carry identity cards with built-in mobile phone technology. If staff feel threatened they can press a button on the back that covertly records interactions, which can later be used as evidence, and a device that allows their whereabouts to be located in emergencies. Other arrangements may include a 'buddy' system where two members of staff are present during the initial client assessment or it may take place in a local clinic (DH 1999c).

Communication between agencies such as emergency departments, police, GPs and social services is also important. The RCN and NHS Executive (1998) describe a case where a district nurse was requested to visit a patient in their home to re-dress a dog bite wound. The gentleman's GP notes revealed reports from the emergency department recording several attendances there following dog bites from his son's bull terrier and also after being involved in fights. Social services documentation revealed that his grandchildren were also on the Child Protection Register. As a result of the communication between agencies, the district nurse arranged wound care at the health centre rather than visiting him at home and advised the gentleman to return to the emergency department for out-of-hours care if necessary in order to maintain her own safety.

Dealing with and reporting violent incidents

Much of the discussion on violence and aggression has dealt with preventing incidents and defusing or de-escalation. Unfortunately, because of the complex nature of violence it can still occur despite the use of these techniques. The actions required in these incidents focuses on the immediate responses and then detailed follow-up and evaluation (RCN 2003a).

Immediate responses involve dealing with the emotional and physical needs of the practitioner(s) affected. In the case of violent assault, this may mean first aid and people usually experience a range of emotional reactions. This could include a 'crisis' phase where people feel shocked and numb but after the adrenaline has subsided, they feel physically and mentally exhausted (RCN 2003a). People need to feel that they are not alone when incidents have happened and healthcare organizations should have support mechanisms in place for staff who have experienced violence. This may include debriefing sessions for staff and patients/clients involved to make sense of events, long-term counselling and follow-up.

An important part of the evaluation is documenting and reporting aggressive and violent incidents using appropriate documentation so that follow-up action can be taken, hopefully preventing further incidents. However, staff may not want to document incidents for a number of reasons. These were highlighted by the National Audit Office (2003) who found that some staff thought:

- The incident was accepted as part of the job
- The incident may reflect badly on them
- No action would be taken.

A number of campaigns and education programmes aimed to address these concerns have highlighted that violence and aggression are not acceptable and do not reflect upon either the individual concerned or their skills.

Details of incident documentation include:

- The people involved
- Any known trigger factors and causes
- The location
- Any injuries or absence from work as a result (DH 1999b).

It may also be necessary to complete health and safety forms associated with RIDDOR. Given the emotional nature of events, the person completing the form should always receive help from senior staff to recall and document the incident (RCN 2003a). It may also be appropriate to inform the police.

The continued care of someone who has become violent is often not considered. They too may be shocked and upset by their behaviour and may wish to discuss the event from their perspective (RCN 2003a). Agreements can be drawn up between patients/clients and healthcare organizations regarding anti-social behaviour, discussing terms and conditions under which they will receive healthcare. These written agreements may mean that care is withdrawn if violent behaviour continues; however, it must always be made clear that it is the behaviour that is being rejected, not the person (Taylor 2000).

In extreme circumstances, e.g. a client is seriously endangering their own safety or that of others, other methods may be used to protect them and others. In specialist areas such as forensic mental health nursing, 'time out' and seclusion are used for short periods to help divert

REFLECTIVE PRACTICE Box 13.28

Close observation

Lucy McFarland is 22 years old and has been treated for severe depression for 6 years. She has been admitted to an acute mental health unit after a second attempt to take her own life with an overdose of antidepressants. With Lucy's agreement, staff searched her belongings to remove any articles she may use to harm herself and have been maintaining close observation. This means that staff check her activities every 15 minutes and she is not allowed to leave the unit unaccompanied. This duty is shared by several staff who rotate hourly. The ward is often short staffed and regularly employs agency staff which means that Lucy often does not know the nurse observing her.

Student activities

- How do you think Lucy is likely to feel about being under close observation?
- How do you think her privacy, dignity and rights may be affected?
- How can staff make the process of close observation better for her?

aggressive behaviour, reduce sensory stimuli, encourage internal control and disrupt the source of provocation (Mason & Chandley 1999).

However, if more extreme measures are employed, such as observation and restraint, healthcare providers must have clear policies regarding their use and practitioners involved require specialist training. These techniques remain controversial because they prevent a person doing what they want to do, restrict their liberty and, when used inappropriately, can be considered a breach of human rights and abuse (NMC 2002, RCN 2004). Unfortunately, people have also been injured or have died during physical restraint, which has led to a number of investigations and recommendations for practice.

Where techniques such as observing people at regular intervals (see Box 13.28) are used because people have become aggressive or are at risk of suicide, the emphasis is on a therapeutic intervention (rather than a custodial approach) and encouraging positive interactions. A balance needs to be struck between ensuring people's safety and maintaining their privacy, dignity and autonomy (Jones & Jackson 2004).

Restraint

Restraint is a technique that also raises issues of human rights (see Ch. 6) and its use requires careful thought about safety issues. Restraint can include a wide range of explicit and subtle controls such as bedrails (Box 13.29), medication, locked doors, stair gates, arranging furniture to impede movement, controlling language or body language or withdrawal of aids such as walking frames or spectacles (RCN 2004). Most of these practices are unethical and solutions to safety issues must be found that do not affect people's dignity and independence (see Ch. 7). RCN (2004) guidelines contain a range of strategies for nurses working with older adults, including investigating physical causes of behaviour changes, e.g. dehydration, urinary tract infection, hunger and thirst.

The RCN (2003b) also published guidance for nurses regarding the restraint of children and young people, particularly for painful procedures. Chapter 7 discusses the ethical issues surrounding restraint in clinical practice in more depth.

Careful consideration needs to be given to the types of situation where restraint (overt or hidden) or seclusion and observation can be used, assessing the risk to the person and their human rights (Box 13.30).

Fire safety

Fire represents one of the greatest hazards to people's safety with potentially devastating consequences. There need to be three ingredients for a fire to start:

- A source of fuel
- A source of ignition
- Oxygen (Fig. 13.8).

Removing any one of these ingredients means that a fire cannot start and, by lowering the chances of the three coming together, the risk from fires is reduced.

Box 13.29 Risk assessment: safety rails

Safety rails (also known as bed rails or cot sides) are used in hospitals, people's homes and care homes when people, of all ages, are at high risk of falling out of bed. However, they can also be a source of injury and people have climbed over the top and fallen or become trapped between the bars and asphyxiated. Therefore their use needs careful consideration and the following points are based on guidance from the Medical Devices Agency (2001), now merged with the Medicines Control Agency.

Risk assessment

- *Are bed rails actually necessary and is the person at risk of falling out of bed?*
- *Are the safety rails compatible with the bed and the mattress?* The manufacturer's instructions must be followed and electric (profile) and divan beds need rails designed for this specific use
- *Is the safety rail fitted correctly?* Is there a risk of entrapment because of the size of the space between the rails and the bed or headboard?
- *Fitted bed rails*: Some profile beds have fitted bed rails, usually in two sections, with a gap in the middle. Extra care is needed when adjusting the bed, e.g. moving the head end up to help the person sit up, as there may still be a risk of entrapment
- *Using a safety rail bumper*: Quilted or sponge covers are available to go over the top of safety rails and may reduce the risk of entrapment.

Patient/client factors

- *Is their head or body small enough to fit through the bars or the rail and the mattress?* Children need special types of rail because of their smaller size
- *Are they confused or agitated?* This puts them at greater risk of injury
- *Will they need to get out of bed at night?* Consideration needs to be given to how people will alert staff to the need to get out of bed.

Inspection and maintenance

All bed rails must be inspected before use to ensure that they are working properly and regularly maintained so that they remain in good order.

REFLECTIVE PRACTICE Box 13.30

Restraint

Terrance Thornton is an 83-year-old man who has developed dementia and has recently moved into a residential home. He is confused in his new surroundings, especially at night when he has been becoming agitated, shouting at staff and prone to wandering. Care home staff installed safety rails to stop him getting out of bed but as a result he is unable to go to the toilet independently. Staff insist on providing continence pads when helping Mr Thornton to get ready for bed.

Student activities

- How are safety rails being used as an indirect method of restraint?
- What are the consequences of using safety rails and what further problems may occur?

Similar to many other safety issues, legislation (Fire Precautions Act 1971 and Fire Regulations 1992 and 1997) aims to prevent fires by ensuring that employers:

- Carry out a fire risk assessment
- Provide fire detection and warning systems
- Provide an emergency plan and means of escape
- Provide facilities for fighting fire
- Provide fire safety training, normally annual training in healthcare settings.

In addition, all healthcare premises must obtain a Certificate of Firecode Compliance to ensure that they have met all current regulations.

Fire risk assessment

A fire risk assessment must identify all the fire hazards (e.g. sources of fuel, ignition) and the people at significant risk, especially those who have impaired mobility, sight or hearing. This information is used to identify improvements needed and to formulate an emergency evacuation plan (Home Office et al 1999).

Fire detection and warning systems

All large buildings must have fire detection systems that trigger an alarm system or alarms that can be activated at fire points, usually by breaking the safety glass. There may be different fire alarm sounds, e.g. continuous for the immediate area and intermittent for other sections, so it is important to know the local arrangements.

Emergency plans and means of escape

Hospitals are often organized into compartments that provide fire-resistant walls, ceilings and floors for a specified period of time. This reduces damage to buildings and increases survival rates, as initial evacuation is usually horizontal into the next compartment rather than down stairs (Home Office et al 1999). Emergency plans should discuss evacuation of people of differing mobility and availability of equipment such as evacuation chairs and ski sheets for immobile people on mattresses (see Fig. 13.9). Local training enables you to understand the arrangements for specific placements.

Facilities for fighting fire

Healthcare premises must provide facilities for fighting fires such as sprinkler systems and hose reels. In addition, fire extinguishers and fire blankets are located in appropriate areas such as kitchens so that people who have been trained to use them can tackle small fires. Figure 13.10 illustrates the different types of fire extinguisher.

Fire safety training

This section has introduced the basic principles of fire safety but within your nursing programme and throughout your career, fire training should be undertaken annually. This ensures that you are aware of local procedures, any new changes and can rehearse emergency situations. Carrying out the activities in Box 13.31 will highlight your fire safety awareness.

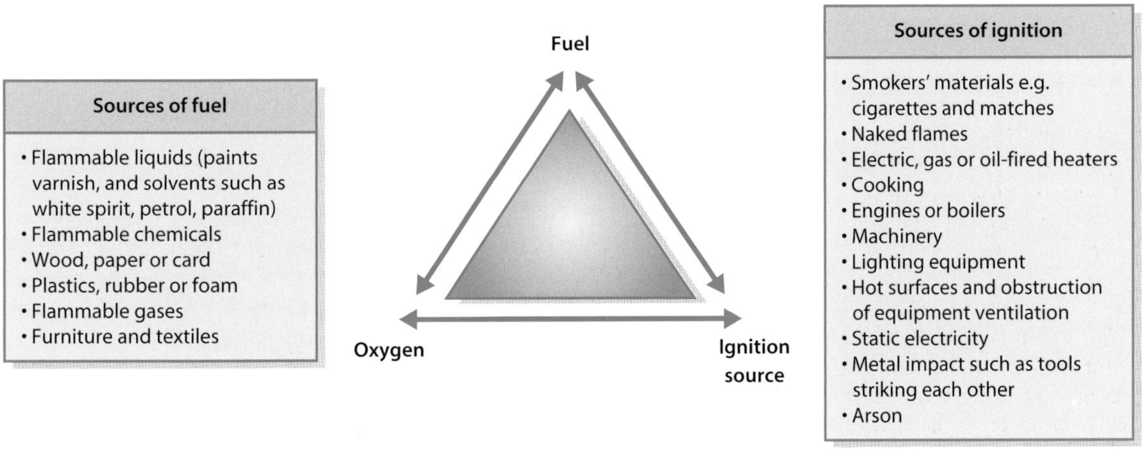
Sources of fuel
• Flammable liquids (paints varnish, and solvents such as white spirit, petrol, paraffin)
• Flammable chemicals
• Wood, paper or card
• Plastics, rubber or foam
• Flammable gases
• Furniture and textiles
Fuel
Oxygen
Ignition source
Sources of ignition
• Smokers' materials e.g. cigarettes and matches
• Naked flames
• Electric, gas or oil-fired heaters
• Cooking
• Engines or boilers
• Machinery
• Lighting equipment
• Hot surfaces and obstruction of equipment ventilation
• Static electricity
• Metal impact such as tools striking each other
• Arson

Fig. 13.8 The fire triangle (reproduced with permission from The Home Office et al 1999)

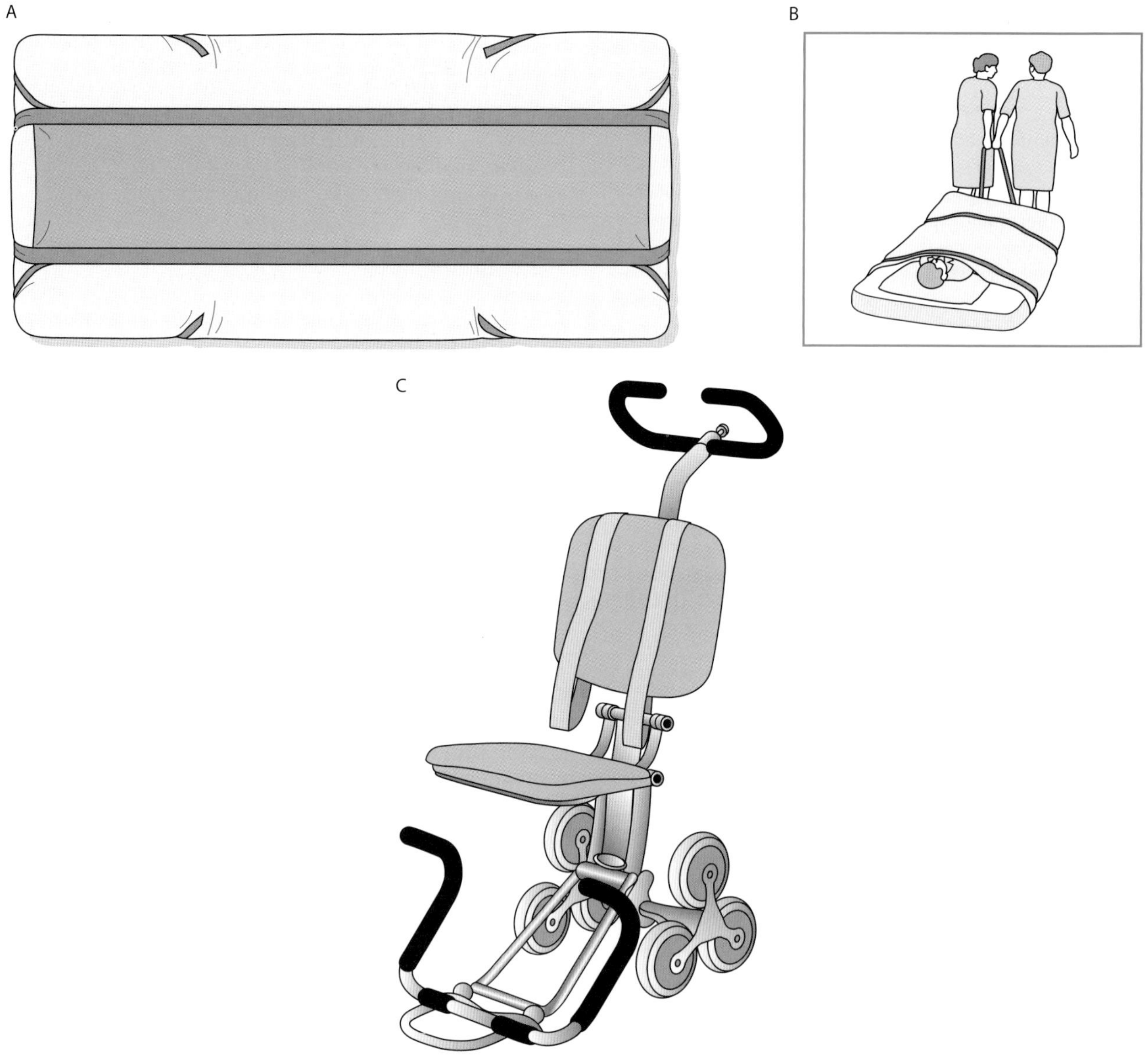

Fig. 13.9 Emergency evacuation equipment: **A.** Ski sheet to be placed under a mattress. **B.** A ski sheet in use. **C.** An evacuation chair that can be used on stairs

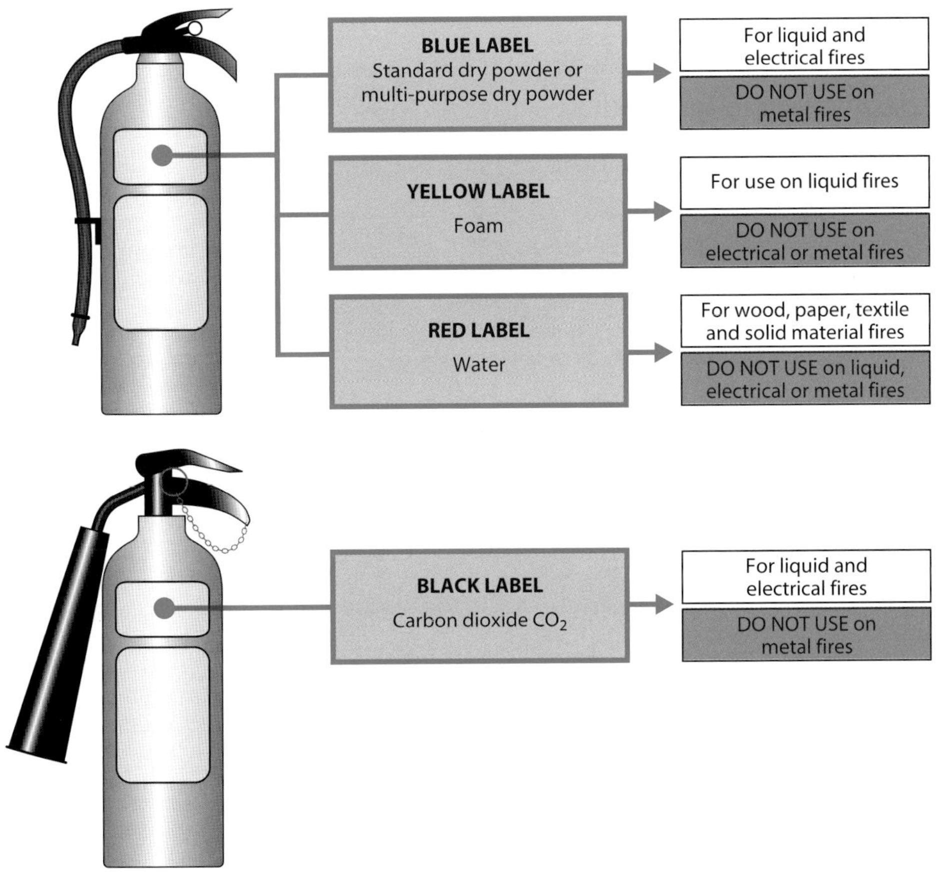

Fig. 13.10 Types of fire extinguisher (based on The Home Office et al 1999)

REFLECTIVE PRACTICE Box 13.31

Fire safety

Student activities

Consider an area of your college or university that you visit regularly and find out:

- Where are the nearest fire exits?
- How they are signposted?
- Where are the nearest points for raising the alarm in case of a fire?
- When are the fire alarms tested?

In each new placement, it is essential to familiarize yourself with the locations of fire points and read the fire action notices that give instructions. You should also:

- Find out how to contact the switchboard or the fire brigade.
- Locate fire extinguishers in the area and correctly identify the types of fire they can be used to tackle.
- Discuss fire evacuation procedures with your mentor.

Summary

- Harm reduction in any area of healthcare begins with risk assessment and includes five stages.
- Risk assessment can be generic (relating to a group of patients/clients, staff or a particular task, e.g. fire hazards, moving and handling) or specific (examining the needs of individuals).
- Health and safety in the workplace is governed by legislation. Nurses need an understanding of this and their responsibilities relating to COSHH, RIDDOR, moving and handling. They must implement training given, follow procedures, use equipment designed to improve safety, take reasonable care of themselves and others, and report any safety concerns.
- Standard precautions and handwashing are essential to prevent the spread of infection.
- Violence and aggression include verbal and physical abuse towards an individual. Many factors can lead to aggressive behaviour and clinical areas conduct risk assessments to identify contributing factors and put in place measures to reduce incidents occurring.
- Core safety skills require theoretical knowledge and rehearsal for practice. These include moving and handling, fire safety, resuscitation and de-escalation techniques. They are part of nursing programmes and annual updates are necessary.
- First aid requires training and practice that builds the confidence needed to deal with emergency situations. This is included in nursing programmes and other organizations also provide training.
- As well as a number of core safety skills, becoming a safe practitioner also means developing a questioning approach, recognizing one's limitations and using evidence-based practice and reflection.

Self test

1. What is the first stage of a risk assessment?

a. Decide who might be harmed and how

b. Look for the hazard

c. Check accident records

d. Ask staff about their experiences of working in the area.

2. What is the principal UK legislation protecting health and safety of employees?

a. Management of Health and Safety at Work Regulations (1999)

b. Workplace (Health and Safety and Welfare) Regulations (1992)

c. Health and Safety at Work Act (1974)

d. Manual Handling Operation Regulations (1992 amended 2002).

3. The acronym TILE can be used to remember the risk assessment areas for moving and handling. What does the 'individual' category relate to?

a. The patient or client

b. The individual staff member working with you

c. Individual capabilities of the handlers

d. The individual load.

4. After your moving and handling training session, you are examining the electric hoist in your clinical area. The information on the hoist tells you that it was serviced 3 months ago. When is it due to be tested and serviced again?

a. 9 months

b. 6 months

c. 3 months

d. Next month.

5. A client you are looking after slips on the way to the bathroom but quickly gets up because he is embarrassed. Do you:

a. Report what you saw to the qualified staff and let them know he has no injuries

b. Investigate whether he has any injuries, respond appropriately and complete an incident form

c. Complete an incident form documenting your account of events

d. Contact your health and safety representative or local Health and Safety Executive office.

6. How long should a burn be placed under cool running water?

a. Up to 5 minutes

b. 5–10 minutes

c. 10–20 minutes

d. 15–25 minutes

7. A gentleman you are looking after is becoming restless and says he is fed up with the care he has received and he feels nothing has gone right. What is your reaction?

a. Ask him to calm down before you sit and speak to him

b. Tell him that it has nothing to do with you

c. Document his concerns and tell him you will let the qualified staff know later

d. Acknowledge his feelings and explore why he is feeling this way.

8. Carbon dioxide fire extinguishers are used for which types of fire?

a. Wood, paper, textiles and solid materials

b. Liquid and electrical fires

c. Liquid fires only

d. None of the above.

Key words and phrases for literature searching

Fire precautions
Health and safety regulations
Moving and handling/patient handling
Risk assessment
First aid
Violence and aggression

Useful websites

BackCare	www.backcare-helpline.org/index2.php Available July 2006
British Red Cross	www.redcrossfirstaidtraining.co.uk Available July 2006
Department of Health Back in Work – *moving and handling in the NHS*	www.nhs.uk/backinwork Available July 2006
Counter Fraud and Security Management Service (CFSMS) – *replaced the Department of Health zero tolerance campaign in 2003*	http://www.cfsms.nhs.uk/ Available July 2006
Health and Safety Executive	www.hse.gov.uk Available July 2006
National Patient Safety Agency	www.npsa.nhs.uk Available July 2006
NPSA Patient Safety e-learning programme	www.npsa.nhs.uk/health/resources/ipsel Available July 2006
Royal Society for the Prevention of Accidents	www.rospa.com Available July 2006
St Andrew's Ambulance Association – *various regional addresses and telephone numbers*	www.firstaid.org.uk Available July 2006
St John Ambulance	www.sja.org.uk Available July 2006

References

Alaszewski A, Alaszewski H 2000 Risk: empowerment and control. In: Alaszewski A, Alaszewski H, Ayer S, Manthorpe J (eds) Managing risk in community practice: nursing, risk and decision-making. Baillière Tindall/RCN, Edinburgh

Bibby P 1995 Personal safety for health care workers. Arena, Aldershot

Department of Health 1999a Saving lives: our healthier nation. TSO, London

Department of Health 1999b Managers' guide – stopping violence against staff working in the NHS. DH, London

Department of Health 1999c Managing violence in the community. DH, London

Department of Health 2002 Back in work campaign. DH, London

Department of Health 2004 Choosing health: making healthy choices easier. DH, London

Department of Trade and Industry 2003 24th (final) annual report of the home and leisure accident surveillance system: 2000–2002 data. DTI, London

Dimond B 1993 Legal aspects of first aid and emergency care: 2. British Journal of Nursing 2(13):692–694

Fowler A 2003 The assessment and classification of non-complex burn injuries. Nursing Times 99(25):46–47

Health and Safety at Work Act 1974 HMSO, London

Health and Safety Commission 2004 Comprehensive injury statistics in support of the revitalizing health and safety programmes: health services. Online: www.hse.gov.uk/statistics/industry/index.htm Available September 2006

Health and Safety Executive 2000 Simple guide to the Lifting Operations and Lifting Equipment Regulations 1998. HSE, Sudbury. Online: www.hse.gov.uk/pubns/index.htm Available July 2006

Health and Safety Executive 2002 Simple guide to the Provision and Use of Work Equipment Regulations 1998. HSE, Sudbury

Health and Safety Executive 2003a Five steps to risk assessment. HSE, Sudbury

Health and Safety Executive 2003b Health and safety regulation: a short guide. HSE, Sudbury

Health and Safety Executive 2003c COSHH: a brief guide to the regulations. HSE, Sudbury

Health and Safety Executive 2004a HSE statistics. Online: www.hse.gov.uk/statistics/index.htm Available July 2006

Health and Safety Executive 2004b Manual handling: guidance on regulations. HSE Books, Norwich

Health and Safety Executive 2004c Violence at work: a guide for employers. HSE, Sudbury

Home Office, Scottish Executive, Department of Environment (Northern Ireland) and Health and Safety Executive 1999 Fire safety: an employer's guide. TSO, London

Horton R, Parker L 2002 Informed infection control practice. 2nd edn. Churchill Livingstone, Edinburgh

International Council of Nurses 2004 The ICN definition of nursing. Online: http://www.icn.ch/definition.htm Available July 2006

Jacobs L 2000 An analysis of the concept of risk. Cancer Nursing 23(1):12–19

Johnson C 2005 manual handling risk assessment – theory and practice. In: Smith J (ed) The guide to the handling of people. 5th edn. BackCare, Teddington

Jones J, Jackson A 2004 Observation. In: Harrison M, Howard D, Mitchell D (eds) Acute mental health nursing: from acute concerns to capable practitioner. Sage, London

Lawrence JC 1996 First-aid measures for the treatment of burns and scalds. Journal of Wound Care 5(7):319–322

Mason T, Chandley M 1999 Managing violence and aggression: a manual for nurses and health care workers. Churchill Livingstone, Edinburgh

Medical Devices Agency 2001 Advice on the safe use of bed rails. MDA, London

Mohun J, John K, Lee T (eds) 2002 First aid manual. 8th edn. Dorling Kindersley, London

National Audit Office 2003 A safer place to work: protecting NHS hospital and ambulance staff from violence and aggression. TSO, London

National Health Service Security Management Service 2003 Using technology to protect staff. Online: www.cfsms.nhs.uk

National Institute for Health and Clinical Excellence 2004 Falls: the assessment and prevention of falls in older people. Online: www.nice.org.uk Available September 2006

National Patient Safety Agency 2004 Alerts and advice. Online: www.npsa.nhs.uk Available July 2006

Nursing and Midwifery Council 2002 Practitioner–client relationships and the prevention of abuse. NMC, London

Nursing and Midwifery Council 2004 The code of professional conduct: standards for conduct, performance and ethics. NMC, London

Royal College of Nursing 2003a Dealing with violence against nursing staff: an RCN guide for nurses and managers. RCN, London

Royal College of Nursing 2003b Restraining, holding still and containing children and young people. RCN, London

Royal College of Nursing 2004 Restraint revisited – rights, risk and responsibility: guidance for nursing staff. RCN, London

Royal College of Nursing and National Health Service Executive 1998 Safer working in the community: a guide for NHS managers and staff in reducing the risks from violence and aggression. RCN, London

Taylor D 2000 Student preparation in managing violence and aggression. Nursing Standard 12(14):39–41

United Kingdom Central Council for Nurses, Midwives and Health Visitors 1998 Guidelines for mental health and learning disabilities nursing. UKCC, London

Wilson J 2001 Infection control in clinical practice. 2nd edn. Baillière Tindall, Edinburgh

Further reading

BackCare 1999 Safer handling of people in the community. BackCare, Teddington

BackCare and Royal College of Nursing 2005 The guide to the handling of people. 5th edn BackCare, Teddington

Health and Safety Executive 1997 Violence and aggression to staff in the health services: guidance on assessment and management. HSE Books, Norwich

Hockenberry MJ, Wilson D, Winkelstein ML et al 2003 Wong's nursing care of infants and children. 7th edn. Mosby, St Louis

Horton R, Parker L 2002 Informed infection control practice. 2nd edn. Churchill Livingstone, Edinburgh

Mason T, Chandley M 1999 Managing violence and aggression: a manual for nurses and health care workers. Churchill Livingstone, Edinburgh

Waugh A, Grant A 2006 Ross and Wilson anatomy and physiology in health and illness. 10th edn. Churchill Livingstone, Edinburgh

14 The nursing process, holistic assessment and baseline observations

Pauline Hamilton and Theresa Price

Glossary terms

Apnoea
Arrhythmia
Assessment tool
Auscultation
Blood pressure
Bradycardia
Discharge planning
Holistic assessment
Hypertension
Hypotension
Hypothermia
Nursing model
Nursing process
Pulse
Pyrexia
Tachycardia
Vital signs

LEARNING OUTCOMES

This chapter will help you:

- Identify the stages of the nursing process and discuss the value of using a problem-solving approach to care
- Discuss how the use of a model of nursing can enhance patient/client care
- Explore the approaches to nursing care used in different settings
- Identify the need for careful documentation as part of nursing practice
- Discuss different nursing assessment strategies
- Explain how body core temperature is assessed using tympanic, oral, axillary and rectal routes, and with different types of thermometer
- Accurately assess adults' and children's temperature, pulse, blood pressure, respirations, height, growth and weight with reference to normal values
- Explain the nursing interventions used to manage pyrexia and hypothermia.

Introduction

This chapter provides an introduction to the nursing process and how it can be applied with different individuals who have varied healthcare needs. It acknowledges the diversity of nursing and provides examples of how the nursing process can be applied in child, mental health, learning disability and adult settings.

The key nursing skills required for holistic assessment are included, with emphasis on the need for effective verbal and written communication skills to promote accurate assessment followed by effective nursing intervention. Tools that assist in the assessment of individuals are explored as well as some models of nursing and approaches to care planning.

Assessment of a person's health status includes the measurement of four vital signs: body temperature, blood pressure, pulse and respirations. In addition, a person's weight, height and, in children, the growth rate may be measured. This chapter explains how each of the vital signs is measured and recorded.

Assessment usually takes place:

- When a person is admitted to a healthcare system
- If there is a change in health status
- To monitor change as a result of treatment, e.g. administration of medication
- Before, during and after surgery.

The nursing process

Nursing and healthcare delivery systems throughout all branches of nursing are diverse. The philosophies that underpin approaches to nursing vary enormously. In the past, the medical model was prevalent in many areas of nursing. Using this approach, nursing care usually followed the medical diagnosis and was focused on the physical condition of the person. In addition, nurses often used intuition to initiate care delivery. Arguably intuition does inform care delivery although it should be used in combination with other measures. The practice of nursing is based on interpersonal relationships (see Ch. 9), with other technical aspects of nursing following.

In recent years there has been a move away from the medical model, recognizing the individuality of patients/clients and the need to address issues that go beyond the scope of physical care and medical diagnosis. However, medical diagnosis not only affects the needs that people may have, but also has an impact on other aspects of life. Thus, there is an attempt to provide holistic care to all groups of people requiring support from nurses and other healthcare professionals (Chin & Kramer 2004). There is also an increasing body of nursing knowledge available to support different nursing strategies and approaches to care, i.e. evidence-based practice (see Ch. 5). This too has an impact on care given. The decision to utilize a particular approach to care should therefore be based upon the unique needs of the person and family, as well as the nursing context (Fawcett 2000, Chin & Kramer 2004).

Yura and Walsh first described the nursing process in 1967 as a means of adopting a problem-solving approach to nursing care. The nursing process provides a systematic way of examining people's problems with a view to providing intervention that would move towards resolving the problems. Their view was that nursing comprises more than intuitive care and that a systematic approach would allow further analysis of the problems that people present with and how they might be resolved. It should be noted that problems identified are problems of the person, not nursing problems. Thus, management of these problems should be person centred (Yura & Walsh 1967).

The nursing process can be applied in all nursing settings although the way in which it is applied depends on the health needs of patients/clients, the skills of the nurses and the care environment. The nursing process is cyclical and has a number of stages:

- Identify with the person what the problems are – *assessment*
- Make plans to address the problems – *planning*
- Take steps to manage the problems – *implementation*
- Reflect on what has happened – *evaluation*.

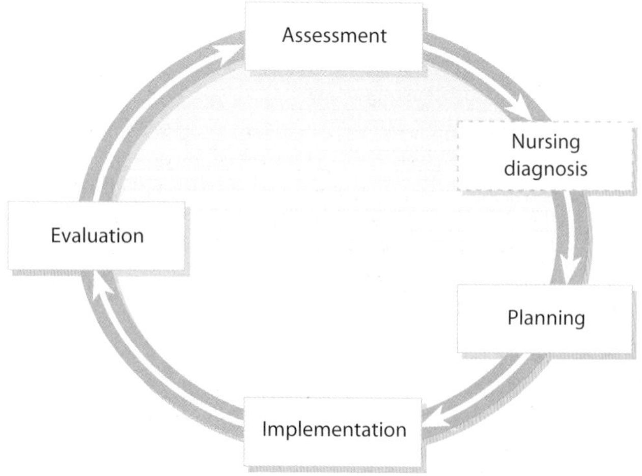

Fig. 14.1 The nursing process (reproduced with permission from Brooker & Nicol 2003)

Sometimes a fifth stage is added to the nursing process – the nursing diagnosis stage – which fits between the stages of assessment and planning (Fig. 14.1). The nursing diagnosis stage has been adopted more in North America than in the UK. The North American Nurses Diagnosis Association (NANDA) has provided standardized nursing diagnoses for many situations (Walsh 1998). Nursing diagnosis explains the effect of the medical diagnosis. For example, the patient may have suffered a heart attack (myocardial infarction) and so one of the nursing diagnoses may be 'central chest pain'. Nursing diagnosis has been used to standardize terminology and assist the process of audit, a mechanism to measure quality of care to determine if standards are being met. The other four stages are discussed below.

The nursing diagnosis stage relates to the diagnosis of nursing issues, which may be based on an underlying medical condition but differs from the medical diagnosis. Medical diagnosis is the identification of disease from examination of symptoms and presenting features, whereas nursing diagnosis is more about gaining understanding of the person's situation, which may have wider implications for the person and also impact on other healthcare professionals (Barker 2001a, NANDA 2001). The approach to planning care influences whether or not the nursing diagnosis stage is included. Patterns of care delivery vary and the UK is moving towards multidisciplinary ways of working with documentation being designed to incorporate multidisciplinary terminology.

As the nursing process is cyclical in nature, evaluation can lead to reassessment if required. If patient/client goals (see p. 358) have been achieved, care can be stopped relative to the goal or the plan of care may be modified if the goal has not been fully achieved.

While the nursing process can be applied in different settings, it is helpful to use a tool that will provide further guidance appropriate to the needs of people and the care setting. This can be achieved by the use of a model of nursing (see p. 359). The stages of the nursing process are explored below.

Assessment

The first stage is assessment of the patient's/client's and family's needs. Assessment involves collecting information (data) about the person and using that information to make decisions about what care, support or intervention is required. Decision-making involves organizing and interpreting the information collected. Professional judgement may also contribute towards the decision-making process. Assessment documentation and techniques vary according to the setting, e.g. outpatient, inpatient, short stay, ambulatory care, rehabilitation, day care, primary care based in the home, clinics or surgeries. Risk assessment is discussed fully in Chapter 13; however, it is an integral part of the assessment process.

As assessment is the cornerstone of establishing what a person's needs are, so the quality of assessment is pivotal to the success of the nursing process. Successful nursing intervention hinges on a complete and thorough assessment being undertaken. Even throughout the other stages of the nursing process, the nurse continues to assess the response to care and success of interventions. Thus assessment is an ongoing process. The aims of assessment are to:

- Determine the needs and potential needs of the person and their family
- Gather information on which a plan of care may be based
- Document information that will provide a basis for reassessment and evaluation
- Act as a mechanism for quality care
- Fulfil statutory obligations
- Aid the structure of nursing knowledge.

Assessment is a complex, time-consuming activity that requires many skills. Assessment of someone's needs should be performed jointly with the person whenever possible. Establishing people's own perspective of their problems helps to create partnership working and assists in providing person-centred care that is holistic in nature. Sometimes this is not possible due to the nature of the person's problems, for example in a high dependency setting when the patient is unconscious, or in a mental health assessment unit when a client is confused and disorientated.

The information required in any given assessment situation will be determined by the nursing context. Confidentiality should be maintained in all settings (Nursing and Midwifery Council [NMC] 2004; see also Ch. 7). Information should be collected systematically to ensure that important issues are not overlooked. A combination of observation, interview and measurement is required to provide a full assessment (NANDA 2001).

Observation is a key nursing skill that informs the overall assessment process. Observing is a form of data collection made by using the senses. Visual observation can relate to all aspects of the person. General characteristics of the person's appearance and physical signs such as skin condition can be observed (see Ch. 16). Touch is also used to assess characteristics such as the temperature of a person's skin, presence or absence of pulses or signs of dehydration such as dry, inelastic skin (Barker 2001a). Smell can be used to assess dimensions of a person in relation to the environment, such as chemicals in the air. In relation to the person, alcohol may be smelt on their breath or smoke on their clothes.

Interactions with other people can be observed, e.g. verbal and non-verbal communication (see Ch. 9). People's behaviour can also be observed, e.g. their reactions to a particular situation, including emotional signs such as crying. Observations should be systematic to ensure the fullest information is gathered.

To complete assessment accurately, practitioners should strive for objectivity. Personal interpretations of observations should be avoided. For instance, when describing a person's physical characteristics, it is desirable to retain objectivity and, where possible, to be specific. For example, blood pressure '180/95' instead of 'blood pressure high', or 'smiles frequently' rather than 'happy'. Essential nursing skills include objective measurement. Equipment such as a thermometer to measure temperature (p. 373) or sphygmomanometer to measure blood pressure is often used (p. 381). Height and weight may be measured with the use of a measuring tape and set of scales (p. 386). Quantifiable information is therefore acquired through the use of equipment as well as direct observation.

Information can be collected in a variety of ways, depending on the situation. The initial assessment of people attending an emergency department will differ greatly from the assessment undertaken by a practice nurse who is immunizing a family going abroad on holiday. The practice nurse makes an assessment of what is required for the safety of the travellers in the longer term, whereas the emergency department nurse makes an initial short-term assessment of the person in relation to their priority for treatment.

Holistic assessment

For assessment to be comprehensive, it should be undertaken in a holistic manner. Thus, the following dimensions of need should be assessed (Fawcett 2000):

- Physical
- Sociocultural
- Spiritual
- Psychological
- Emotional.

While people may present to the nurse with similar medical or social problems, it is only by thorough and systematic assessment that includes the physical, psychological, sociocultural, spiritual and emotional dimensions of their lives that a truly individualized plan of care can be developed. It can, however, be difficult to separate the dimensions, as they are all interrelated and can impact on a person's health in different ways (Box 14.1).

CRITICAL THINKING Box 14.1

Holistic assessment

Anna is a young married woman with small children who is undergoing radiotherapy treatment for cancer. She may experience physical side effects including fatigue. The fatigue may cause anxiety, as Anna may be less able to look after her children and fulfil family obligations. She may consider not completing the course of radiotherapy to allow the fatigue to diminish. It is only by undertaking a holistic assessment that the impact of the treatment on Anna and her family's lives can be ascertained.

Student activities

- Think about the dimensions of holistic care and try to identify more aspects of Anna's life that may be affected.
- Assuming that Anna's children had left home and the other circumstances were unchanged, identify the potential differences that Anna and her children may face.

The nurse's role is to identify and react to a person's response to their own situation. Thus, while a medical condition is acknowledged when assessing a patient or client, it only forms part of the assessment. The aim is to acquire the fullest information necessary without gathering irrelevant information.

Priorities of assessment may differ within the different branches of nursing. In mental health, assessment may concentrate initially on psychological and social dimensions since much of the care of people with mental health problems centres on human responses to illness (see p. 366). With children it is appropriate to use a child and family-centred approach (see p. 367). The benefit of such an approach is that it addresses the needs of the family as well as the child. Learning disability assessment also has unique characteristics, which are discussed later. Nurses working in many settings will meet people with a learning disability as most live in the community and access health services in the usual ways, e.g. though primary care via their GP or practice nurse. What is important is that the principles discussed on page 351 are incorporated into the assessment process.

The nurse will undertake a decision-making process to make sense of the data collected from the assessment and formulate a plan of care. Thus the nurse's assessment of the patient/client will form the nursing history. An example of the types of questions that the nurse may ask is provided in Box 14.2.

Box 14.2 Questions that may be asked during the assessment interview

Breathing

1. Physical:
   - What is the rate and pattern of breathing?
   - Is breathing affected by activities or environmental factors?
2. Psychological:
   - Is there a need for breathing or relaxation exercises?
   - Is there a chance that emotion may affect breathing?
3. Sociocultural:
   - Are there influences on the person's behaviour, e.g. smoking?
   - What are the person's health beliefs (see Ch. 1) about coughing, expectorating or using inhaled medication?
4. Environmental:
   - Are there factors influencing breathing, e.g. medication, position in bed, dampness, irritants?
5. Politicoeconomic:
   - Are there constraints on resources that affect breathing, e.g. housing issues, financial issues?

Eating and drinking

1. Physical:
   - What is the person's weight?
   - Are there barriers to preparing nutritious food?
   - Are there any problems with chewing or swallowing?
2. Psychological:
   - What is the person's understanding of a healthy diet?
   - Are there any issues expressed about body image?
   - Are there any dietary likes/dislikes?
3. Sociocultural:
   - Are there cultural influences regarding eating and drinking?
   - Are there any customs to be observed regarding food preparation, eating and drinking?
4. Environmental:
   - In what sort of environment does the person usually eat and drink?
   - Are there facilities for safe storage and preparation of food?
5. Politicoeconomic:
   - Are there constraints on choice of food due to the person's financial situation or transport?
   - Is there access to information about healthy choices?

Communication

1. Physical:
   - Are there physical barriers to communication, e.g. hearing/speech?
   - Are there any special means of enhancing communication, e.g. sign language?
   - Is there evidence of pain?
2. Psychological:
   - Are there any behavioural, mood or perception issues that affect communication?
   - Is there anxiety about the present situation?
   - What are the person's previous pain experiences?
3. Sociocultural:
   - Are there any language/dialect barriers?
   - Do cultural factors influence communication?
   - What are the person's beliefs about pain?
4. Environmental:
   - Do environmental factors inhibit or support communication?
5. Politicoeconomic:
   - Does the person have access to media resources, e.g. telephone, Internet?
   - Do economic factors inhibit communication?

Controlling body temperature

1. Physical:
   - Is the person's temperature within the normal range?
   - Are there any problems/conditions affecting body temperature?
   - Can the person control their body temperature?

2. Psychological:
   - Can any aspect of the person's behaviour/ mood alter body temperature?
   - Can the person respond to changes in temperature?
3. Sociocultural:
   - Are there social or cultural influences affecting protection from cold/heat?
4. Environmental:
   - Does the person have control over temperature changes, e.g. central heating?
5. Politicoeconomic:
   - Is the person able to respond to temperature changes, e.g. purchasing a fan?

Working and playing

1. Physical:
   - Does the person have an occupation/is the person a carer/is the person a parent?
   - What, if any, are their leisure pursuits?
   - Are occupation/family/leisure commitments affected by the present situation?
   - Is breathing affected by activities or environmental factors?
2. Psychological:
   - What is the person's reaction to the present situation, e.g. anxiety, denial, contentment?
   - Does the person have enough information/ support to deal with the current situation?
3. Sociocultural:
   - How has the person's social role been affected by the present situation?
   - Are there obligations that will not be met due to the person's health status?
4. Environmental:
   - Are there any risks affecting the person, e.g. occupational safety?
   - Have any environmental factors contributed towards the person's current health status?
5. Politicoeconomic:
   - Are there economic concerns due to the present situation?
   - Does the person have access to information and support regarding finances and rights?

Sources of information

Information can be gathered for assessment purposes from:

- The patient/client – the primary source
- Other people or records – secondary sources.

Primary source

The patient or client should be the primary source of information, including children and young people as developmentally appropriate, as it is important to elicit their own perspective of their situation. To successfully interview the patient/client, the nurse needs to be a skilled communicator; questioning, actively listening and eliciting information (see Ch. 9). Often assessment is undertaken in difficult circumstances, e.g. emergency admission to hospital is an anxiety-provoking event for patients and their relatives. Crisis intervention within community mental health nursing is another occasion when assessment is required, usually following a series of difficult events leading up to the need for intervention. The initial impression the nurse may have of the patient/client and their family can influence the ease with which the nurse is able to elicit reliable information. If the nurse gives the impression of being disinterested or hurried, it is unlikely that an accurate assessment will be made. Assessment should form the beginning of a trusting relationship between the nurse and patient/client and provides the person with the opportunity of putting their view of their current situation forward. There may be occasions when the patient/ client is unable to provide information, through illness, confusion, being too young or having difficulty with communication, e.g. learning disability.

Secondary sources

These are used together with the primary source. Biographical data can be confirmed from previous health records. It is important to confirm the currency of this information in case of changes in circumstances such as someone being widowed or having moved house. Social and medical history can often be confirmed from other health records. Other practitioners can also offer information about patients/clients. For example, key workers of individuals living in residential or nursing homes can provide information if a client is hospitalized. Patient-held records or patient passports are also used, when available. Past medical history is also important to assess along with the current health situation. This can reveal information that may impact on the current situation, such as knowledge of allergic reactions to a drug or relevant information about the person's prior experience. Family members and significant others can also be rich sources of information about the patient/client and how their current situation is affecting their ability to cope with daily living.

Discharge planning

Prevention of early readmission may be avoided if discharge planning is robust enough to support the person on discharge. Inadequate planning and coordination can lead to unnecessary suffering and can also have a major impact on the resources needed to support the person. Preparing a patient/client and their family for discharge from hospital is an integral part of nursing care (Scottish Intercollegiate Guidelines Network [SIGN] 2003). In many cases discharge is the most important aspect of a hospital admission for the patient/client and their family. In addition, the way it is managed can influence its success (Department of Health [DH] 2000).

As many hospital admissions are very short, planning for discharge should be incorporated into the initial assessment and even pre-assessment stage. During surgical pre-assessment visits (see Ch. 24), people are given information regarding requirements for going home

Discharge Summary

PATIENT'S NAME .... DISCHARGE DATE ....

DISCHARGE ADDRESS ....

....

....

COMMUNITY CARE ASSESSMENT NO ☐ YES ☐ DATE ....

INFORMATION	✓	DATE	SIGNATURE
Patient aware			
Relative/carer aware			
Mode of transport			
Social worker/services			
Community nurse			
Physiotherapy			
Other			
Specific care instructions			
Aids/prosthesis			
Follow-up appointment			
Medication & education			
Equipment to take home			
Valuables/property			
Medical certificate			
G.P. letter/informed			

COMMUNITY CARE OUTCOME

Fig. 14.2 Discharge schedule

following surgery or other invasive procedures. If a patient lives alone and is unable to have someone stay with them following discharge after day surgery and/or an anaesthetic, an overnight hospital stay may be more appropriate. Thus social, physical, psychological, economic and environmental aspects of assessment are crucial in providing relevant information that will inform a safe discharge. With many people being discharged following hospital admission for acute problems, or longstanding chronic problems, complex management plans and packages of care may be required and therefore a coordinated approach to discharge planning is required. Early supported discharge teams are in place in some specialties such as orthopaedics and care of older adults. Within these services, there is explicit inclusion of discharge criteria in the care planning documentation. The nurse caring for the patient has a responsibility to ensure that a multidisciplinary approach is taken when required. Clinical governance is the provision of first class services to users, achieved by creating a framework within which evidence-based practice can be achieved (Chs 3, 5). This requires that discharge planning is documented and is an integral part of care delivery, emphasizing the need for the nurse to work in partnership with other professional groups and agencies (DH 2000).

The nature of the patient's health needs or presenting problems will inform discharge planning; for hospitalized patients, nurses also need to enquire about the perspectives of carers. Most patients do not exist without a network of significant others who can provide information about them; they must also be consulted about certain aspects of care such as the transition from home to hospital, or hospital to home. Without the support of significant others, it is often not possible to achieve a successful discharge. Within the assessment stage of the nursing process, discharge planning is a vital aspect of providing seamless care across primary and secondary care settings. Therefore family and sociocultural aspects also need to be explored during the assessment stage. Figure 14.2 shows a sample discharge schedule.

The assessment interview

The planned assessment interview that forms the basis of the nursing history can take place in many settings. The health visitor may conduct an assessment of a child's developmental progress at home surrounded by parents and other family members. Alternatively, the assessment might be in a situation of crisis, such as a serious injury following an accident. Whatever the situation, there must be structure to the interview. The focus will be not only on the documentation being used but also on the person being interviewed. It is important to include both. The use of documentation alone will not allow the whole spectrum of issues to be captured. The first interview allows the nurse to gather baseline information about the person. Comparisons against this information will be ongoing. In some settings the interview will be conducted by a doctor and a nurse such as in acute mental health admissions (Barker 2001a). The advantage of this is that the client will not have to repeat similar information to different professionals. There is also the benefit of engaging in multiprofessional working, with all health professionals sharing care of the patient to provide a cohesive service (Barker 2001b).

Privacy

At all times during the assessment process, privacy must be respected. This may be easier to achieve in some settings than in others, e.g. when an interview room is available. In the patient's/client's home or in a busy department where there are many other people, it may be more difficult to achieve and therefore careful consideration is needed. In the home it may mean asking other family members to leave the room, or in the department it may be necessary to speak quietly behind screens. Other barriers to effective communication need to be identified and remedied, e.g. environmental noise affecting concentration could be avoided by moving to a quieter area. Language barriers may be overcome by the use of interpreters from within the family or the health provider organization. Confidentiality should be maintained if interpreters are being used. It should be recognized that factors affecting the quality of the interaction between the nurse and the person may have an adverse effect on the quality of care provided (see Ch. 9 and Box 14.3).

Interpretation of information

The nurse will undertake a decision-making process to make sense of the data collected from the assessment and formulate a plan of care. Nurses need to be aware of their own beliefs, values and attitudes as well as their level of knowledge and competence. Assumptions should not be made about the condition of a patient/client. Not all patient/client observations, such as blood pressure measurements, can be validated. For example, it is difficult to measure the level of anxiety a patient is experiencing (see Ch. 11). As such, nurses need a degree of self-awareness to ensure that value judgements and assumptions are not made regarding the person's situation.

Staging assessment

The use of a step-wise approach to assessment is sometimes appropriate, with some aspects of the assessment process being undertaken immediately while others are undertaken later. For example, an older adult being admitted to a care home may have a full assessment undertaken over a period of 1 week to minimize the effects of relocating on their usual routines and ability to adapt. An unconscious child admitted to an emergency department would need immediate assessment to allow priorities of care to be established.

It is sometimes inappropriate to explore every aspect of assessment at the initial interview. In some mental health and learning disability settings, client assessment may be undertaken incrementally as the therapeutic relationship is established. This is also the case in situations when a person is moving into long-term care, e.g. a nursing home. If this is the case, the nurse assessing must take responsibility for ensuring full assessment is

REFLECTIVE PRACTICE Box 14.3

Sharing personal information

As part of the admission process for entry to your nursing course, you may have had to undergo occupational health screening.

Student activities

- Reflect on the situation where someone you had not previously met has asked you to reveal personal information.
- Consider how you felt about divulging personal information to a stranger.
- How did the approach of the person affect your feelings at the time?

completed. This can be useful if the patient/client needs time to adjust to their new situation before discussing sensitive issues with the nurse.

Documentation

Documentation of the nursing process, at each stage, is an important way to communicate to other members of the healthcare team how the patient/client is progressing and responding to interventions. Documentation must be comprehensive and accurately reflect the health status of the patient/client. Accuracy is achieved by recording information precisely, e.g. 'the patient had 150 mL of tea, toast and scrambled eggs' rather than 'good appetite', as appetite varies from person to person, and also from nurse to nurse, thus making the assessment subjective. It is a professional requirement to record nursing interventions and the information collected to inform the intervention, as nursing documentation is a legal document (NHS Quality Improvement Scotland 2004, NMC 2005).

Assessment documentation takes different formats according to the setting (Box 14.4). Electronic records of care are being implemented gradually throughout the UK as information technology systems are developed to support healthcare delivery (DH 2000). Patient-held records are also used. People who have chronic conditions are being encouraged to be empowered through self-management plans, particularly in community settings. For example, in asthma care when a person attends the practice nurse, the GP and an outpatient department, it is useful for them to have one record that can be used by all professionals to improve continuity of care across primary and secondary care settings. Increasingly, multidisciplinary documentation is being developed with the whole team having access to the records. Confidentiality should be maintained at all times regarding documentation, irrespective of the mechanism being used (NHS Quality Improvement Scotland 2004, NMC 2004).

The Joint Future Report (Scottish Executive 2000) advocates single shared assessment between health and social care agencies. Single shared assessment is intended to simplify the assessment process, be person centred and clarify responsibilities for providing care.

CRITICAL THINKING Box 14.4

Assessment issues

Assessment documentation varies between placements and client groups, and may be paper based or electronic.

Student activities

- Ask your mentor to show you the assessment documentation available in your placement.
- Consider whether the documentation would also be suitable for use with other groups such as children, older adults and people with a learning disability or mental health problems.
- Discuss the limitations of the documentation for each group of people.
- Discuss the benefits of using documentation that is tailored to a particular client group.

Making this process work, however, requires commitment from all healthcare providers as it may mean the erosion of traditional professional barriers and boundaries. It is envisaged that single shared assessment will be most applicable to older adults and people within the community. Increased multidisciplinary and interagency working may enhance shared ways of working towards common goals for people using health services. Person-centred approaches require commitment from personnel in all organizations involved with clients, entailing a more consumer-orientated approach putting the patient/client central to planning of their healthcare. These approaches present challenges to all groups of health professionals, especially those accustomed to a discipline-specific approach to care. The underpinning philosophy of shared assessment is that it is 'needs led' rather than 'service led'. Additional information about shared assessment can be found on the Department of Health website www.dh.gov.uk/NewsHome/YourHealthYourCareYourSay/fs/en.

Assessment tools

As part of the assessment process, it may be necessary to collect further detail about a particular aspect of need. Additional data can add to holistic assessment. Assessment tools, developed by nurses (practitioners and researchers), provide a validated method of eliciting information with a view to minimizing patient/client risk. Assessment tools, as part of risk assessment, form part of the overall assessment process and will be dependent on the unique needs of the patient. Tools devised by other professional groups are also used by nurses, e.g. the Glasgow Coma Scale and Paediatric Glasgow Coma Scale (see Ch. 16). An example of a commonly used assessment tool is the Waterlow scale, a pressure ulcer risk assessment tool (Fig. 14.3; see also Ch. 25). This is used to predict the level of risk of an individual developing pressure ulcers, taking their overall condition into account (Box 14.5). Tools should be appropriate to the client group to optimize their effectiveness. Risk assessment (see Ch. 13) should be performed

A

WATERLOW PRESSURE ULCER PREVENTION/TREATMENT POLICY

RING SCORES IN TABLE, ADD TOTAL. MORE THAN 1 SCORE/CATEGORY CAN BE USED

BUILD/WEIGHT FOR HEIGHT	◆	SKIN TYPE VISUAL RISK AREAS	◆	SEX AGE	◆
AVERAGE BMI = 20-24.9	0	HEALTHY	0	MALE	1
ABOVE AVERAGE BMI = 25-29.9	1	TISSUE PAPER	1	FEMALE	2
OBESE BMI > 30	2	DRY	1	14 - 49	1
BELOW AVERAGE BMI < 20	3	OEDEMATOUS	1	50 - 64	2
BMI=Wt(Kg)/Ht (m)^2		CLAMMY,PYREXIA	1	65 - 74	3
		DISCOLOURED GRADE 1	2	75 - 80	4
		BROKEN/SPOTS GRADE 2-4	3	81 +	5

MALNUTRITION SCREENING TOOL (MST) (Nutrition Vol. 15, No. 6 1999 - Australia)	
A - HAS PATIENT LOST WEIGHT RECENTLY YES - GO TO B NO - GO TO C UNSURE - GO TO C AND SCORE 2	B - WEIGHT LOSS SCORE 0.5 - 5kg = 1 5 - 10kg = 2 10 - 15kg = 3 > 15kg = 4 unsure = 2
C - PATIENT EATING POORLY OR LACK OF APPETITE 'NO' = 0; 'YES' SCORE = 1	NUTRITION SCORE If > 2 refer for nutrition assessment/Intervention

CONTINENCE	◆	MOBILITY	◆
COMPLETE/ CATHETERISED	0	FULLY	0
URINE INCONT.	1	RESTLESS/FIDGETY	1
FAECAL INCONT.	2	APATHETIC	2
URINARY + FAECAL INCONTINENCE	3	RESTRICTED	3
		BEDBOUND e.g. TRACTION	4
		CHAIRBOUND e.g. WHEELCHAIR	5

SCORE
10+ AT RISK
15+ HIGH RISK
20+ VERY HIGH RISK

SPECIAL RISKS

TISSUE MALNUTRITION	◆	NEUROLOGICAL DEFICIT	◆
TERMINAL CACHEXIA	8	DIABETES, MS, CVA	4-6
MULTIPLE ORGAN FAILURE	8	MOTOR/SENSORY	4-6
SINGLE ORGAN FAILURE (RESP, RENAL, CARDIAC,)	5	PARAPLEGIA (MAX OF 6)	4-6
PERIPHERAL VASCULAR DISEASE	5	**MAJOR SURGERY or TRAUMA**	
ANAEMIA (Hb < 8)	2	ORTHOPAEDIC/SPINAL	5
SMOKING	1	ON TABLE > 2HR#	5
		ON TABLE > 6 HR#	8

MEDICATION - CYTOTOXICS, LONG TERM/HIGH DOSE STEROIDS, ANTI-INFLAMMATORY MAX OF 4

#Scores can be discounted after 48 hours provided patient is recovered normally

B

REMEMBER TISSUE DAMAGE MAY START PRIOR TO ADMISSION, IN CASUALTY. A SEATED PATIENT IS AT RISK

ASSESSMENT (See Over) IF THE PATIENT FALLS INTO ANY OF THE RISK CATEGORIES, THEN PREVENTATIVE NURSING IS REQUIRED A COMBINATION OF GOOD NURSING TECHNIQUES AND PREVENTATIVE AIDS WILL BE NECESSARY

ALL ACTIONS MUST BE DOCUMENTED

PREVENTION

PRESSURE REDUCING AIDS	
Special Mattress/beds:	10+ Overlays or specialist foam mattresses. 15+ Alternating pressure overlays, mattresses and bed systems 20+ Bed systems: Fluidised bead, low air loss and alternating pressure mattresses Note: Preventative aids cover a wide spectrum of specialist features. Efficacy should be judged, if possible, on the basis of independent evidence.
Cushions:	No person should sit in a wheelchair without some form of cushioning. If nothing else is available - use the person's own pillow. (Consider infection risk) 10+ 100mm foam cushion 15+ Specialist Gell and/or foam cushion 20+ Specialised cushion, adjustable to individual person.
Bed clothing:	Avoid plastic draw sheets, inco pads and tightly tucked in sheet/sheet covers, especially when using specialist bed and mattress overlay systems Use duvet - plus vapour permeable membrane.

NURSING CARE

General	HAND WASHING, frequent changes of position, lying, sitting. Use of pillows
Pain	Appropriate pain control
Nutrition	High protein, vitamins and minerals
Patient Handling	Correct lifting technique - hoists - monkey poles Transfer devices
Patient Comfort Aids	Real Sheepskin - bed cradle
Operating Table Theatre/A&E Trolley	100mm(4in) cover plus adequate protection

Skin Care	General hygeine, NO rubbing, cover with an appropriate dressing

WOUND GUIDELINES

Assessment	odour, exudate, measure/potograph position

WOUND CLASSIFICATION - EPUAP

GRADE 1	Discolouration of intact skin not affected by light finger pressure (non-blanching erythema) This may be difficult to identify in darkly pigmented skin
GRADE 2	Partial thickness skin loss or damage involving epidermis and/or dermis The pressure ulcer is superficial and presents clinically as an abrasion, blister or shallow crater
GRADE 3	Full thickness skin loss involving damage of subcutaneous tissue but not extending to the underlying fascia The pressure ulcer presents clinically as a deep crater with or without undermining of adjacent tissue
GRADE 4	Full thickness skin loss with extensive destruction and necrosis extending to underlying tissue.
Dressing Guide	Use Local dressings formulary and/or www.worldwidewounds

IF TREATMENT IS REQUIRED, FIRST REMOVE PRESSURE

Fig. 14.3 The Waterlow scale (reproduced with permission from Judy Waterlow © 2005)

CRITICAL THINKING Box 14.5

Using assessment tools

- Two-year-old Jane has been admitted to a children's ward with suspected meningitis. She has a generalized rash and moving is painful.
- Isa Oliver (84) has been admitted to an orthopaedic ward through the emergency department after a fall at home. She has previously been in good health and independent at home. She has a fractured hip and is scheduled for surgery today.
- Imad Jumaa (68) lives in a nursing home. He has dementia and poor mobility due to arthritis. He is doubly incontinent and is unable to attend to his own hygiene needs. Imad has difficulty with communication.
- Fred Maxwell is 28 years old and has a learning disability. He lives in a house with four other service users who are supported by carers. He also has physical disabilities and mobilizes with a wheelchair. Fred is underweight and his appetite is poor; he needs help with personal hygiene and feeding, and is incontinent of urine.

Student activity

Using the Waterlow scale (see Fig. 14.3), assess the level of risk the people above may have of developing pressure ulcers (see Ch. 25 for further information, including other pressure ulcer risk assessment tools).

at appropriate times, e.g. when there is a change in the health status of a patient/client. It is important that all staff using an assessment tool are familiar with its use.

Planning

This stage of the nursing process involves identifying the person's problems or needs and what nursing care, intervention or support is required. The care plan should be written down and contain clear statements about how the person's goals will be achieved (see below). The patient/client should also be involved in this stage if possible. The format of the care plan depends on the particular setting. As well as establishing the person's existing problems, any potential problems are also identified. Learning disability nurses may also concentrate on a client's strengths as well as weaknesses.

Prioritizing care

Planning also incorporates prioritizing care according to the needs of the individual and seriousness of the problems. Life-threatening situations such as airway obstruction must be considered and acted upon before wider health needs such as the desire to stop smoking. Determining priorities is achieved through an understanding of the theory and concepts underpinning nursing (Chin & Kramer 2004). Involvement of the person in this stage of the nursing process also assists in prioritizing care according to their wishes if there are no life-threatening issues. Through communication, mutually agreed goals can be set, based on the person's perception of their situation.

Box 14.6 **Actual and potential problems**

59-year-old Rashid was admitted to hospital with a left-sided weakness and investigations show that he has had a stroke. Rashid is left handed. One of his actual problems is that he is unable to move his left side, which might affect his mobility, skin integrity and independence.

Actual problem

- Unable to move left side.

Potential problems

- Negative impact on self-esteem
- Help required with eating and drinking
- Reduced mobility (see Ch. 18)
- Pressure ulcers (see Ch. 25)
- Deep vein thrombosis (see Ch. 23)
- Muscle weakness
- Limb contractures
- Inability to attend to personal hygiene
- Loss of independence.

Actual and potential problems

The aims of planning are to:

- Solve actual problems (or meet health needs)
- Minimize the risk of potential problems
- Reduce recurring problems
- Assist in the development of coping strategies for problematical health issues
- Build on strengths.

Consequently, nurses need to be able to 'see beyond' the present situation and use their knowledge and expertise to avoid complications and potential problems occurring (Box 14.6). It can be seen from Rashid's situation that the impact of one problem can potentially create many other problems for him that transcend different dimensions of need (p. 351).

Goal setting as part of care planning

Goals are set to enable measurement of the success, or otherwise, of the nursing interventions planned to meet them. Different types of nursing action are often required to meet the goals. For example, different members of the healthcare team may deliver different aspects of the care required. Which member of the team delivers the care to an individual depends on the complexity of their care and on the skills of the members. Competent healthcare assistants may perform some nursing interventions, e.g. they may be able to assist people to maintain personal hygiene. However, for some therapeutic interventions, the registered nurse (RN) would be required to monitor some parameters such as central venous pressure.

Goals can be either short or long term. They should be person centred and achievable. To assist in this,

Box 14.7 Short- and long-term goals

Eddie has been admitted to the ward with breathlessness. In relation to this the following goals may be appropriate.

A short-term goal may be:
- To reduce Eddie's respiratory rate to less than 20 breaths per minute within 2 hours.

The goal may be achieved by:
- Careful positioning in bed; sitting upright well supported with pillows or leaning on a bed table (see Ch. 17)
- Administration of prescribed medication (see Ch. 22)
- Administration of prescribed oxygen therapy (see Ch. 17).

A long-term goal may be:
- To cope with mild breathlessness prior to discharge.

The goal may be achieved by:
- Education regarding breathing exercises prior to discharge
- Teaching Eddie to reduce activity that provokes breathlessness
- Referral to the physiotherapist.

goals should be SMART and incorporate the following characteristics:

- **S**pecific – state clearly what is to be achieved
- **M**easurable – be made quantifiable
- **A**chievable – must be able to be achieved by the patient/client
- **R**ealistic – possible for the patient/client to achieve
- **T**ime orientated – have a time limit by which the goal can be achieved and evaluation undertaken.

A goal could be 'the patient should drink 2.5L of fluid within the next 24 hours'. Within this goal, it would have been assessed that the patient is capable of taking fluids orally, making it achievable and realistic. It is specific because it states the amount of fluid to be taken, is measurable as fluid intake and is time orientated as there is a timeframe allocated to its achievement. Box 14.7 provides an example of short- and long-term goals. If goals are unrealistic and unachievable, this can lead to disappointment of both the patient/client and the nurse. As a consequence, the therapeutic relationship may be adversely affected.

Implementation

Putting the care plan into action forms the implementation stage of the nursing process. Implementation should incorporate current evidence-based practice (Ch. 5). The care plan may encompass physical, psychological, social, emotional and environmental interventions. Implementation may also include activities that are outwith nurses' expertise, e.g. it may be appropriate to refer the patient/client to another healthcare professional such as an occupational therapist for assessment of dressing ability. This referral is the nurse's responsibility and is recorded in the care plan. Such multidisciplinary working and collaboration should assist in providing holistic care.

Evaluation

Evaluation determines if the planned intervention has been effective in achieving the goals set. The goals are reviewed to determine whether or not the patient has met them or is moving towards meeting them. At this stage the goals can be modified or changed according to the patient's/client's response to the interventions. If a goal has been achieved, this is documented. If a goal has not been achieved, the nurse should question why this is the case, and reassess the patient. Perhaps the goals did not encompass the SMART characteristics or the patient's/client's condition may have changed, making the goals unrealistic. Health needs are dynamic and thus require periodic reassessment. Evaluation is an ongoing action that forms part of the cyclical nursing process. However, evaluation is only possible if clear criteria have been applied to the goals. Evaluation of care can be used as part of nursing audit (see Ch. 5).

Nursing models

A nursing model, also known as a 'conceptual model', is a tool used to guide nurses as they engage in the nursing process and can be viewed as a practical way of putting the nursing process into action. There are many different nursing models, as nursing takes place in very diverse situations, with the needs of people varying enormously, and some of these are explored in this section. As nursing models have different philosophical assumptions underpinning them, each presents a unique perspective of nursing knowledge and nursing practice.

Most nursing models are based upon four concepts, which are said to form the essential structure of nursing. The relationship that emerges between the nurse and patient/client will depend on these four concepts:

- The person – the nature of the patient/client having a dimension of 'wholeness' or holism
- Nursing – a helping process with interpersonal relationships at its core
- Health – the goal of nursing is to assist people to achieve an optimum state of health, whether or not they are 'ill' (see Ch. 1)
- The environment – the physical constructions of the world and society within it (Chin & Kramer 2004).

Each model adapts the nursing process according to its own relationship between the four concepts and the particular nursing approach. Emphasis on the four concepts varies according to the theoretical underpinning of the model. Thus, each model represents a unique view of nursing and its relationship to practice (Fawcett 2000). Within the four branches of nursing, therefore, different

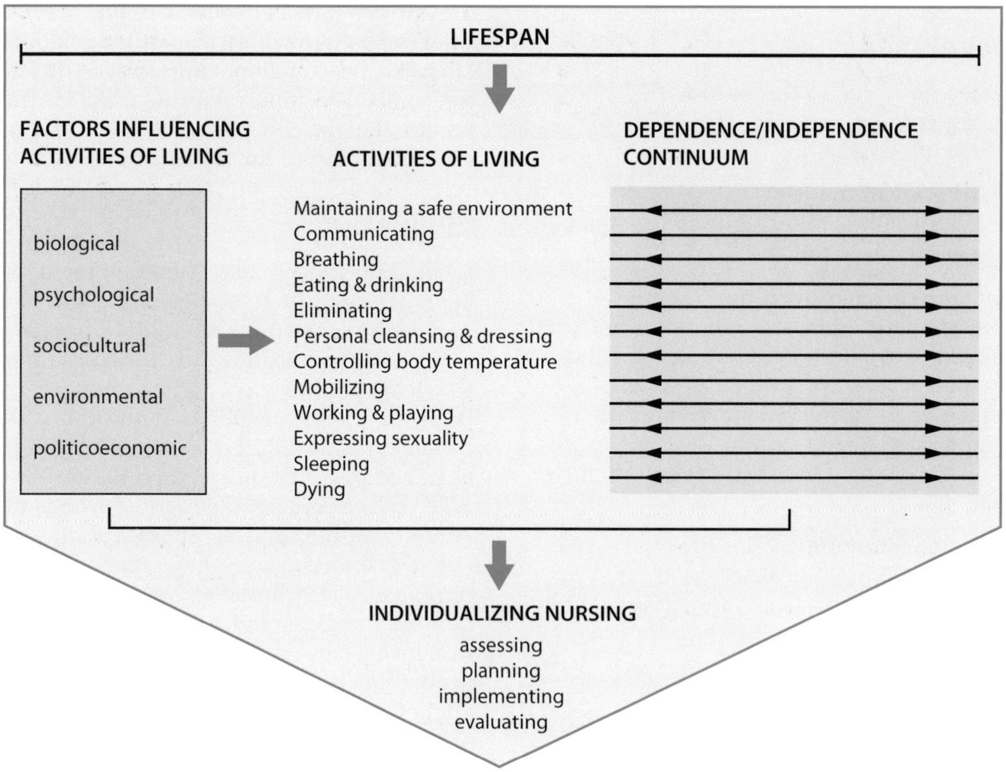

Fig. 14.4 The model of nursing (reproduced with permission from Roper et al 1996)

models are used. Models also vary within primary and secondary care settings, highlighting the diversity of nursing practice. Central to the use of any nursing model is the need for nurses to have excellent communication skills (see Ch. 9).

The Roper, Logan and Tierney model for nursing

The Activities of Living Model was developed in the UK by Roper, Logan and Tierney who first published the *Elements of Nursing* in 1980. Their work developed some of the central components of Virginia Henderson's earlier definition of nursing (see Ch. 2). There are two parts to this model: the model of living and the model for nursing (Fig. 14.4). Over the years it has been refined, indicating that nursing is a dynamic profession, constantly developing in response to external influences.

According to Roper et al (2000), five interrelated components form the core of the model of living:

- The individual
- Activities of living (ALs)
- Lifespan
- Dependence/independence
- Factors influencing the ALs.

The individual

According to Roper et al (2000), individuality in living acknowledges that each person has a unique way of performing the ALs according to where they are on the lifespan, the degree of dependence/independence they have and the influences of biological, psychological, sociocultural, environmental and politicoeconomic factors. Individuality in living is concerned with how an individual experiences and performs ALs according to their preferences, abilities and attitudes.

Activities of living

Roper et al (2000) suggested that 12 activities are essential for survival:

- Maintaining a safe environment (Ch. 13 + others)
- Communicating (Ch. 9)
- Breathing (Ch. 17)
- Eating and drinking (Ch. 20)
- Eliminating (Chs 20, 21)
- Personal cleansing and dressing (Ch. 16)
- Controlling body temperature (see p. 368)
- Mobilizing (Ch. 18)
- Working and playing (Ch. 8 + others)
- Expressing sexuality (Ch. 8 + others)
- Sleeping (Ch. 10)
- Dying (Ch. 12).

It is evident that the activities cannot be viewed as mutually exclusive as they are dimensions that interlink with each other (Box 14.8). For example, it is not possible to consider elimination without considering eating and drinking. The care planning questions in Box 14.2 (see p. 352) can be used to consider planning the care that may be needed to meet dependence in ALs.

CRITICAL THINKING Box 14.8

The relationship between factors influencing ALs and the interdependence of ALs

Jane is 17 years old and lives with her mother and 11-year-old sister. Jane's parents are divorced and her father is not in contact with them. Her mother has chronic arthritis and is physically dependent on Jane to support her with running the house. Jane helps her mother to get into the shower in the evenings and collects her prescriptions. She also does the shopping, cleaning, ironing and supervises her younger sister with homework and getting ready for school. Jane is at college full time and on Friday evenings her friends often go the student union then on to a nightclub. Jane is usually too tired to join them.

Student activities

- Think about how Jane may experience social isolation from her peers (working and playing).
- Consider the psychological impact that home circumstances may have on Jane (sleeping).
- Identify ways in which Jane could get additional support to ease her situation (maintaining a safe environment).

Lifespan

The lifespan is considered to be a continuum with changes occurring along it from birth to death. Throughout this time, every aspect of living is influenced by biological, psychological, sociocultural, environmental and politicoeconomic factors.

The five stages of life identified by Roper et al (2000) are:

- Infancy
- Childhood
- Adolescence
- Adulthood
- Old age.

Throughout these periods, levels of dependence and independence vary. An infant is vulnerable and dependent on others for survival and love. Childhood and adolescence are affected by cultural issues, sociocultural norms and subcultures (see Ch. 8) and are dominated by the family. In adulthood, work and family affect lifestyle. In old age, individuals may have an illness that affects their level of independence, e.g. arthritis which can impair mobility.

Factors influencing the ALs

There are five main factors that can influence daily living (Roper et al 2000), as outlined below.

Biological factors

In the context of the model of living, biological factors relate to physical and physiological performance. While there are predetermined genetic influences affecting physical characteristics such as skin colour, hair colour, height or genetically determined diseases such as haemophilia, other factors can also affect physical characteristics and function. In wartime, if a child is deprived of food, growth may be affected, resulting in slower rates of growth and development. Thus, environmental and politicoeconomic issues may also affect physical factors. Biological factors associated with ageing may affect a person's ability to work, thereby impacting on their sociocultural status.

Psychological factors

Mental and intellectual activity begins in childhood and continues through adolescence, adulthood and into older age (see Ch. 8). The stimuli within these lifespan phases vary. In childhood, development begins through sensory stimuli that can be influenced by family issues such as having siblings who may spend time playing with the toddler. In adolescence, development can be affected by the place of the child in the family and the expectations placed upon them. Thus environmental factors may also influence psychological development. Development across the lifespan is discussed in Chapter 8.

Sociocultural factors

Ideas, values, knowledge and beliefs are embedded within cultural norms of groups within society (see Ch. 8). Thus, many variations exist among the population from which patients and clients will come. Culture is unique to groups of people and can affect the behaviour of individuals. It is important to remember that cultural beliefs may have a profound impact on lifestyle and the responses of people who need to access health services. Dietary practices can have an impact on biological factors; for example, vegetarians may have a low iron intake leading to low blood haemoglobin levels and anaemia. Religion may affect how individuals respond to treatment options, e.g. Jehovah's Witnesses may reject blood transfusion as a treatment option compatible with their beliefs. Therefore sociocultural aspects may impact on biological and psychological factors.

Environmental factors

Environmental factors include housing, the atmosphere, noise and sound. Any of these elements can influence the other factors. Atmospheric pollutants such as carbon monoxide can aggravate respiratory conditions such as asthma, thereby having an impact on biological and psychological factors. Noise pollution can cause anxiety that may impact on psychological and biological functioning, e.g. by causing insomnia and anxiety.

Politicoeconomic factors

The economy, law and the state comprise the politicoeconomic factors that impact on individuals. People are governed by fiscal measures such as the need to pay council tax. Local and national economies also affect people and consequently their behaviour. For example, people on low incomes have limited choices on which to spend their money. Asylum seekers who are given vouchers as part of their financial support may have few choices about where they can exchange them. This may lead to lack of choice

CRITICAL THINKING Box 14.9

Factors influencing activities of living

For groups such as asylum seekers, people with a learning disability or people with chronic illness, consider the extent to which they may have control over the factors that influence ALs.

Student activities

- Work through the ways in which the five factors that influence activities of living affect your patients/clients by reflecting on the scenario above. Draw on any experiences you have had in practice. If you have not encountered such situations, make use of the information you have read.
- Think of an occasion when one of the five factors that influence ALs has affected your own well-being and how that occasion affected other aspects of your life.

and being unable to follow dietary customs, thus impacting on biological and psychological factors.

It can be seen that the main themes of the model are inextricably linked and the activities in Box 14.9 highlight this.

Roy's adaptation model

Sister Callista Roy developed this model in the USA in the 1960s. It has been refined over the years to make it suitable for nursing in the 21st century (Roy & Andrews 1999). The basis of Roy's model is that individuals must adapt to a constantly changing environment. The health of the individual is a reflection of that adaptive process. It is a behaviourist model as it is concerned with the way in which individuals behave in response to changing circumstances. Behaviourism is the study and observation of how individuals behave (see Ch. 4).

Roy's behaviourist model is based on the following two philosophical assumptions:

- That veritivity (true values and meaning of humankind, the purposefulness of human existence) is the principle of human nature, i.e. individuals exist with a common purpose of humankind
- That humanism is central to the individual, i.e. that human experiences are central to knowing and valuing.

The model is based on the following two scientific assumptions:

- That there are interdependent parts of an individual, working in unity. Control mechanisms are involved in the functioning of the system, and for every stimulus there will be a range of behaviours.
- The capacity and ability of the individual to respond to the stimuli, from both the internal and external environment, relates to the adaptation level.

Within the model, there are three types of stimuli (systems). These are:

- Physiological
- Psychological
- Social.

Roy and Andrews (1999) state that there is an interrelationship between these three systems, with all of them working together to maintain a balance within the individual. For example, if a person is physically unable to drink fluids due to a swallowing problem they may become dehydrated, and thus the internal body environment may be affected. Equally, if someone is trekking across the desert with no water to drink, their social system is affecting their physiological status as they are unable to access fluid to prevent dehydration. Thus the systems are interrelated and interdependent, interacting with each other at all times.

According to Roy, if an individual adapts to these stimuli, it could be said that they are healthy. Most people cope effectively with constant changes to their internal and external environments. During a heat wave, for example, an individual may drink more fluids, slow down their level of activity and increase the ventilation of their home. An individual who is unable to make these changes, such as a toddler, may be considered to have an ineffective response to the stimulus of heat. If the individual has not adapted to the stimuli then the role of the nurse is to assist the person to adapt to it. Thus the focus for the nurse is to identify the stimuli to facilitate adaptation in the individual patient/client. Roy acknowledges the individuality of people and so there will be no complete state of balance applicable to everyone. Therefore the nurse must recognize the needs of individuals.

Roy discusses the adaptation level of individuals as forming an adaptive range. Behavioural responses to stimuli can be effective, adaptive stimuli, or maladaptive. The factors that cause problems of maladaptation are called stimuli and there are three types:

- *Focal stimuli* – the internal or external stimulus immediately affecting the person
- *Contextual stimuli* – any environmental factors contributing to the focal stimuli
- *Residual stimuli* – previous experience or attitudes or beliefs (Roy & Andrews 1999) (Box 14.10).

Adaptive modes

There are four adaptive modes within Roy's model that serve as a framework for assessment. It is believed that a person's response to stimuli can be observed in these adaptive modes:

- *Physiological adaptive mode* – physiological balance, i.e. homeostasis
- *Self-concept adaptive mode* – psychological integrity, moral, spiritual
- *Role function mode* – social integrity, managing social interaction
- *Interdependency mode* – emotional and affective (moods or emotions) behaviour.

CRITICAL THINKING Box 14.10

Thinking about Roy's model

The activities below will help you consider how Roy's approach could affect you as a student nurse.

Student activities

- Imagine you are driving through busy traffic to an appointment with your tutor and you are late. You are approaching traffic lights and they turn red. Think about the effect that focal, contextual and residual stimuli may have on your judgement.
- Your second clinical placement is far away and the shift patterns there will cause travelling problems. Consider how the focal, contextual and residual stimuli may affect your adaptation to the situation.
- Suggest two behavioural responses to undertaking an assignment. (For example, an adaptive response may be the creation of a mind map to assist your planning, while an ineffective response would be doing nothing.)

Roy states that these four modes contribute towards the promotion of adaptive goals leading to integration and wholeness. Nursing intervention would be required if there is a need deficit.

Assessment

With Roy's model, assessment is advocated using three stages.

- Stage 1 – examine the adaptive modes; identify if coping is adequate
- Stage 2 – detailed assessment; identify focal, contextual and residual stimuli
- Stage 3 – make a nursing diagnosis based on adaptation status; plan the nursing intervention based on the nursing diagnosis.

Planning

Planning should identify SMART patient-centred goals (see p. 359) that should incorporate the following:

- *Ineffective behaviour to be changed*: For example, if a patient is pyrexial (see p. 369) the goal may be to 'assist patient to regain normal temperature range by providing cool drinks, administering antipyretic medication and monitoring temperature 4-hourly'.
- *Adaptive behaviours to be reinforced*: For example, if a patient has stopped smoking since admission to hospital, the goal may be to 'provide positive reinforcement and assist distraction from smoking through a range of activities such as listening to the radio, reading health education literature and providing access to smoking cessation helpline'.

Evaluation

This involves exploring whether the goals have been met, thus determining if the adaptation response has

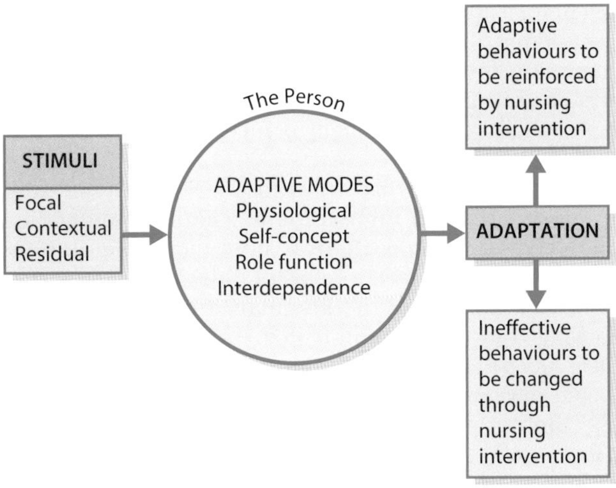

Fig. 14.5 Roy's adaptation model

been achieved effectively or ineffectively. Reassessment occurs at this stage.

Figure 14.5 shows the nursing process as it relates to Roy's adaptation model.

Integrated care pathways

As an alternative to nursing care plans, integrated care pathways (ICPs) may be used. ICPs are sometimes called integrated care plans, care protocols or care maps. The ICP is a single document in which all members of the multidisciplinary team (MDT) record their care. The ICP details expected problems, interventions and outcomes for a specific disorder or group of people. These are devised with explicit agreement by local groups of multidisciplinary and multiagency staff. The aim is to provide a comprehensive service to a group of service users or patients with a specific condition. The introduction of ICPs has been driven by government strategy, which aims to provide improvements in quality of care (DH 2001a). Care pathways are devised on the basis of current evidence for best practice. Much of the evidence on which care is based is informed by the National Institute for Health and Clinical Excellence (NICE) and SIGN, part of NHS Quality Improvement Scotland.

The MDT agrees on the format of the record that will be used by all professionals, not just one group, e.g. nurses. The pathway anticipates the expected requirements for care and the outcomes for the patient within a specified timeframe. SMART goals (see p. 359) are incorporated into the care pathway. It is still important to have the patient at the centre of the care pathway to ensure that the required standard of care is met (Yura & Walsh 1967). Individual assessment is still undertaken, often based on the assessment process associated with a nursing model. It is important that the philosophy of the assessment meets the needs of the patient/client group. For example, a patient undergoing surgery that may impact on their self-image, such as limb amputation, needs to be assessed psychologically and emotionally to determine their ability to adapt. Thus the assessment may be based on Roy's adaptation model. So, although the ICP is multidisciplinary, within its development it is vital that the nursing approach is robust enough to incorporate holistic care (Box 14.11).

While the initial pathways focused mainly on surgical procedures and interventions where the outcome is relatively predictable, there is now increasing development of pathways in the fields of older people and mental health, indicating the acceptance of increased team working and accountability for providing quality care (DH 2001b). However, for problems that require prolonged periods of intervention, ICPs are still considered less appropriate. Development and implementation of ICPs is challenging to professional groups. The benefits of using ICPs include:

- Enabling monitoring of standards of care
- Transparency of documentation
- Enhanced understanding of other professional roles
- Improved team working.

Variance

There are often reasons why a patient will not follow the expected path of recovery or response such as the presence of other health issues from any aspect of their life, i.e. physical, psychological, emotional, spiritual, sociocultural or environmental. This does not necessarily mean that the pathway is unsuitable for the patient, but rather it may highlight the unique features of any individual who requires care. If a patient varies from the expected pathway, this is documented on the care pathway, including whether the variance was avoidable or not. For example, other diseases impacting on patient progress is unavoidable whereas a delay in having a test performed is avoidable.

CRITICAL THINKING — Box 14.11

Integrated care pathways

Having a single document can help to provide an integrated approach to care, with shared working between professionals encouraging greater understanding of others' roles and responsibilities.

Student activities

Find an ICP used in your placement and then consider the following:

- Which nursing model does it incorporate?
- Who you think should be responsible for overseeing the ICP record?
- What benefits there are for the relationships within the MDT when ICPs are used?
- How might the nature of the relationships of MDT members impact on the standard and quality of care given to patients/clients?
- What benefit might there be to patients/clients when ICPs are in use?

Planning care for people with learning disability

The focus on the needs of people with learning disability is embedded in national strategies published in the government's White Paper *Valuing People* (DH 2001b). The Scottish Executive (2002) published *Promoting Health, Supporting Inclusion*, a strategy document to guide practice and the Welsh Assembly Government (2002) has an equivalent, *Inclusion, Partnership and Innovation*. These strategies, along with societal changes, have provided frameworks for the move towards social inclusion for those with learning disability. The underlying key principles of these documents are:

- Rights
- Independence
- Choice
- Inclusion.

Therefore, in order to care for people with learning disability, these key principles need to be included in the planning process. Individuals with learning disability often have complex health needs. While specialist learning disability nurses are in a strong position to begin to assess and meet these needs, generalist nurses may also assess the person's needs if the four key principles above are encompassed in their care. It is desirable for people with learning disability to achieve citizenship within the communities in which they live. In order to facilitate citizenship, nurses in all settings need to be able to assist people with learning disabilities to make informed decisions about their health and health issues.

When planning care for individuals with learning disability, traditional ways of care planning may not always fully encompass these key principles. Many learning disability nurses consider that nursing models are too focused on the medical model. An alternative to using the traditional nursing models was advocated by O'Brien (1987) who focused on the concept of 'normalization'. This approach advocated a way to improve the quality of life of clients although the focus was on services rather than individuals. Nonetheless, this approach has been used successfully to plan and deliver care packages. The development of the term 'social role valorization', referring to the support of valued social roles for those who are at risk of being devalued within society (Gates 2002), has largely superseded normalization.

As the spectrum of learning disability is very wide, ranging from mild to profound and complex, the only way to plan and provide supportive care is by placing the individual at the centre of the planning process.

Person-centred planning

Person-centred planning is a way of working in partnership with people and their families to achieve personal autonomy, which is pivotal to realizing the policy aims for people with learning disability (Scottish Executive 2004). As people with learning disability often have unmet health needs, another aim in caring for these people is to help the person have more control over their health (Gates 2002). For people who have difficulty in articulating their views, an advocate may assist in eliciting their views and thoughts. An advocate may be a paid care worker or a family member or friend.

Person-centred planning aims to assist people to choose the lifestyle they want. Acknowledgement of the person's disability is made, with acceptance of their need for support on their own terms. The focus is on capacity and capacity building, which means working towards maximizing ability.

Person-centred planning can be achieved by sharing of power between the person, family and professional (O'Brien & O'Brien 1998). Any significant person involved with the client may be involved, e.g. paid support workers or those who act as advocates for the person such as family members. Support workers may be part of the MDT such as learning disability nurses, resource workers, physiotherapists, speech and language therapists, occupational therapists and psychologists. Learning about the person is crucial to developing an understanding of their needs. Careful listening (see Ch. 9) and consultation are essential to fully assess the individual. Person-centred planning is a process that takes time and usually starts with a planning meeting. The key features of person-centred planning are shown in Box 14.12 and some are described in more detail below.

REFLECTIVE PRACTICE — Box 14.12

Person-centred planning

- The person is at the centre of the planning process
- Family members and friends are partners in planning
- The plan reflects what is important to the person, the capacities of the person and the support that is required
- The plan leads to actions that are about life, reflecting what is possible and not just about services that are available
- The plan results in ongoing listening, learning about the person and further action (Sanderson 2002).

Student activities

- A useful way to think about person-centred planning is to work through *Our Plan for Planning* (see below) which describes what people want during and after planning meetings and specifically highlights what support people do and do not want from care staff.
- Reflect on the extent of person-centred planning you have seen used with people with a learning disability and discuss this with your mentor.

[Resources: Sanderson H 2002 Person centred planning. In: Gates B (ed) Learning disabilities, toward inclusion. 4th edn. Churchill Livingstone, Edinburgh; People First Manchester and Liverpool 1997 Our plan for planning. People First, Manchester]

Consulting the person throughout the planning process

If the person with learning disabilities has been involved with planning before, it is sensible to talk to them about how they would like to plan, e.g. whether they want a meeting and, if so, what kind of meeting and how they want to be involved. If they are new to planning, it is important to spend time explaining the purpose of planning and looking at different options. Box 14.13 summarizes how this process may work for an individual.

HEALTH PROMOTION — Box 14.13

Craig's story

Craig, who is 32 years old, lives at home assisted by his family and a group of part-time support workers. He has learning disabilities, is unable to speak and moves his hands and eyes to communicate. Craig attends a day centre three times a week. While at the day centre Craig sleeps a lot. His family and support workers describe him as witty and lively, but staff at the day centre find him disinterested and uncommunicative.

It was decided to make a plan for the future. Craig's family asked him who he would like to be involved in the planning. Craig invited staff from the day centre. He asked for the two members of staff he felt most comfortable with. They were happy to come as they thought that Craig might not be getting the most from his time in the day centre. The meeting was held in Craig's home and took up most of an evening.

During the planning meeting, Craig communicated to the group that he was interested in learning to play a musical instrument, finding a girlfriend and making changes that would allow him to make new friends. It was the first time that anyone had realized Craig had these ambitions and no one thought it was impossible to achieve them. Staff from the day centre then recognized that the reason Craig was different at the day centre was probably because he felt he did not know the staff too well and they did not know fully how to communicate with him.

The people who attended the meeting then worked together to change things. Craig now attends a weekly music class with a support worker. One of the staff from the day centre has spent time in Craig's home to get a better understanding of his needs. The next stage of the plan is to find other activities that interest Craig and, like the music class, he will attend these with a support worker. In time, it is planned that he will reduce the time he spends at the day centre as other activities increase. Things are slowly changing for the better and Craig is now involved in every decision that is made.

Student activity

Visit the Scottish Consortium for Learning Disability website (www.scld.org.uk) and find out how one agency is trying to achieve the goals of the government strategies for people with learning disability.

The person chooses who to involve

Unlike traditional planning, it is for the person with learning disabilities to decide who they want to include in the planning process and how. This is easy to say but, with existing services, this is very different from the way meetings are typically organized. If the people around those with learning disabilities cannot find a way to help them make and communicate that decision for themselves, then they must decide in good faith who they think the person would want to involve. A good starting point is thinking about 'people who know and care about the person' which may well yield a different answer from 'people who provide a service to this person'.

The person chooses the setting and timing of meetings

If a meeting takes place it should be at a time convenient to the person with learning disabilities, with the people they wish to invite and be in a place where they feel 'at home'. The planning should be carried out in a way that is accessible to the person with learning disabilities. Graphics, tapes, videos or photos are often used.

Approaches in mental health nursing

In common with learning disability nursing, mental health nursing has also been driven by policy development to become user focused. The trend towards community-based care continues with many services provided by mental health nurses. There is emphasis on caring for people who have enduring mental illness such as schizophrenia. The shift away from institutional care has led to examination and scrutiny of approaches to planning and implementation of care. The following key principles underpin care planning in mental health settings:

- Advocacy
- Consent
- Autonomy
- Relationships
- Communication
- User involvement.

In mental health nursing the approach used is also person centred (Barker 2001b). A person-centred approach builds on the seminal work of Peplau (1952) who espoused the strengths of the therapeutic relationship between the nurse and the person. Building on the work of Peplau is the notion of the professional relationships the nurse has with other professionals as well as the need for a person-centred nurse/person relationship that is not driven by the power of the nurse (Barker 2001b).

The Tidal model

The Tidal model (Barker 2001b) was developed from a study into the need for mental health nursing. It is a multidimensional approach to the provision of mental health care. The philosophy is that people can recover from the experience of mental health problems and that nurses can assist clients to return to their daily life. Therefore the philosophy is about helping people to cope with their problems and find solutions through their own experiences. As it is not about 'fixing them', this model has an empowering approach.

The Tidal model represents the unique contribution that nurses make to the care of people with mental health problems, though it also acknowledges the close relationships with other health and social care practitioners. One of its features is that a care continuum exists. The care continuum straddles the primary and secondary care settings with the premise that the needs of the person should be the focus of care and not the setting. The assumption is that the need for nursing lies wherever the person is, rather than within the 'compartments' of primary or secondary care. Other features of the model are:

- Active collaboration with the person and family, if appropriate, to plan and deliver care
- Empowerment of the person though the narrative of illness and health
- Integration of nursing with the services provided by other members of the MDT
- Resolution of problems of living and promotion of mental health through narrative-based interventions in individual and group sessions.

The role of the nurse is twofold:

- To form a therapeutic relationship with the person and, where appropriate, the family
- To cultivate professional relationships with other workers and professionals who may be involved in the care of the individual.

Barker (1996, p. 236) illustrates the core basis of the Tidal model:

> Life is a journey undertaken on an ocean of experience. All human development, including the experience of illness and health, involves discoveries made on the journey across that ocean of experience.
>
> At critical points in the life journey the person experiences storms or even piracy (crisis). At other times the ship may begin to take in water and the person may face the prospect of drowning or shipwreck (breakdown). The person may need to be guided to a safe haven to undertake repairs, or to recover from the trauma (rehabilitation). Once the ship is made intact or the person has regained the necessary sea legs, the ship may set sail again, aiming to put the person back on the life course (recovery).

Barker (1996) asserts that there are three dimensions within the model:

- *World* – the need to be understood, including having the personal meaning of illness and distress validated by others
- *Self* – emotional and physical security
- *Others* – medical, psychological and social interventions, e.g. housing, finance, occupation, leisure.

The aim of assessment and planning within the three dimensions is to allow the person to verbalize their own experience to determine how their needs can be met.

The narrative basis of the model suggests that the 'self' of the person-as-the-expert can be explored through careful inquiry by the nurse. Therefore, the therapeutic relationship between the nurse and person is crucial to allow construction of the person's experience through narratives. The care plan should document the needs of the person expressed in their own words rather than in professional language or in the third person. Thus the lived experience of the person can be documented.

The aim of the Tidal model, using a person-centred approach, dovetails with best practice statements regarding engagement with the person to work towards person-centred care (Barker 2001b, NHS Quality Improvement Scotland 2004).

Further information about approaches to mental health nursing can be found in the Useful Websites list on page 388.

Approaches to planning care for children

Partnership in care is advocated as the desired approach to caring for children recommended in the National Service Framework (DH 2003). *Every Child Matters*, the government strategy that followed The Children Act (2004), provides further aspirations and policies about the integrated partnership approach to caring for children across society (see Chs 3, 6). The services that children require change as they develop and encounter illness or vulnerability. The key to providing excellent care is in the relationships that develop between the nurse, the child and the family as well as those that the nurse has with other professional agencies and services. Respecting parents and the family means recognizing that:

- Parents are usually the expert on the child
- Parents may have other children to care for and may need to balance the needs of the other children and the child requiring care
- Parents may have to take time off work to attend outpatient or primary care appointments, or during hospital admission
- Parents may have health issues themselves which may influence their ability to be fully involved with the child
- Healthcare and hospitalization can impose financial hardship on the family (DH 2003).

The Nottingham model (Smith 1995) and Casey's partnership model (Casey 1988) are prominent in children's nursing. Both models are based on respect for the wishes of the family and negotiation of care needs. The main differences between them are that the Nottingham model includes the child and the family as 'the client', whereas Casey views the child as 'the client'. However, a partnership approach is central to them both.

The Nottingham model

While the philosophy of this model includes the family as partners, it is still important to include the child in the decision-making process where possible. By doing this, dignity and respect for the child are maintained. As the model uses a holistic approach, taking account of the wider influences that can affect a child's health, the family's perception of health in relation to the child should be assessed when the history is being taken during admission.

Hospital admission can be very disruptive, not only to the child but also to the wider family. The child may have alteration in normal functioning that spans the physical, psychological, social, emotional and/or environmental dimensions of life (DH 2003). To minimize the trauma associated with hospital admission, a welcoming environment is necessary to enable the process of negotiated care to be established. A routine that allows a child's normal activities to be undertaken in relation to activities of living is encouraged, particularly in respect of education and recreation. Play is an important element of the nursing care provided (see Chs 8, 9) and forms an important aspect of pain management (see Ch. 23). The family or main caregivers should be considered the experts on young children. Their knowledge of the child's behaviour and level of independence can be communicated to the nurse and the plan of care is developed jointly. Assisting the family to retain some control over their lives, while meeting the needs of their child, is desirable. This often means that the family will be involved in direct care giving. To provide this type of family-centred care, the family must have clear guidelines about what to expect from the nurse. Therefore, nurses caring for children need to be excellent communicators. Older children and young people are often the experts about their own conditions and associated care (DH 2000).

If hospital admissions are planned (elective), some of the fear associated with hospital admission can be allayed. Receiving written and verbal information prior to admission may help reduce anxiety for the child and their family. It may also reduce recovery times. Pre-admission schemes can also reduce some of the fears and anxiety by providing an opportunity to visit the environment and meet with some of the staff (Smith et al 2002). The Nottingham model follows the steps of the nursing process from assessment, planning, implementing and evaluating care.

Negotiated care

Negotiated care refers to a two-way process between the nurse and the child and their family. The relationship between these people should be based on mutual trust and respect. With each person's contribution being equally valued, an agreed plan of care can be made. The process of negotiation begins at the assessment stage. The level of family involvement should be frequently reassessed as the situation may change, as can the needs of the family. Thus parental participation in direct care delivery may vary over time.

Building an equal partnership

An equal partnership can be developed through the nurse assisting the family to acquire the additional knowledge and skills of caring needed. Equipping the family with knowledge can empower them. Factors that can build the partnership include:

- A positive attitude of the nurse that includes the family in care delivery if desired
- Willingness of the nurse to share information, knowledge and skills
- The ability of the nurse to educate, teach and support others.

Casey's model

This also incorporates negotiated care and partnership building with the child and family. According to Casey (1998), the key elements of paediatric nursing assessment are:

- The nature of the health problem and the child and family's understanding of it
- The developmental effects the health problem has on the child
- The family's situation, its responses to the problem and the nature of the coping
- The wishes of the family and educational needs
- The usual routines of the child
- The child and family's expectations of care and treatment.

Documentation and record keeping

Documentation and record keeping apply to every aspect of nursing intervention. Accurate record keeping is an essential and integral part of professional practice and personal professional development (NMC 2005; see also Ch. 7). Records may be required for legal purposes (see Ch. 6) and audit (Ch. 5). The quality and accuracy of record keeping can reflect standards of care.

Timely and accurate records may highlight changes in a patient's/client's condition by providing a graphical record of their health status, demonstrating trends and changes over time, e.g. with charts used for baseline observations (see Fig. 14.9, p. 376).

Vital signs

Assessment of a person's health status includes the measurement of vital signs that include temperature, blood pressure, pulse and respiratory rate. This section uses an evidence-based approach to measuring vital signs. A number of factors can influence the information obtained from these measurements, including changes to the environmental temperature or metabolic activity and exercise or eating. Nursing care of people with abnormally high and low body temperature is explained. At the end of this section, measurement of height and weight is described. These measurements indicate general health or underlying illness that may require investigation, monitoring and/or treatment.

Nurses measure, record and interpret vital signs and use the information to plan and implement appropriate nursing interventions as well as to evaluate the effect of care and treatment. Vital signs are usually all measured at the same time.

Body temperature

Core body temperature in health is in the range of 36.4–37.3°C ± 0.2°C. It is measured in degrees (°) Celsius (C), and is relatively constant. Body temperature is an indicator of the balance between the amount of heat being generated by cellular processes and the excess that is lost. Efficient cellular metabolism requires the maintenance of body core temperature and organs that are located within the core, such as the brain, heart and liver, function best around 37°C. This is called the 'set point' and serious problems occur if temperature deviates much from this.

Distribution of body heat

Heat is generated by cellular metabolism; therefore areas of high metabolic activity such as the liver or exercising skeletal muscle have the highest temperatures. The locations that are considered to best reflect the body's inner or 'core' temperature are the heart and brain. Peripheral regions, which are nearer to the environment, are cooler as they are more exposed to the lower ambient temperature outside the body. Temperature sensors placed on the skin surface estimate peripheral or 'shell' body temperature. Body core temperature (BCT) can be measured using a variety of instruments that may be placed in sites such as the ear canal, oral cavity, axilla or rectum. Figure 14.6 shows body temperature at different sites.

Heat balance

Maintaining body temperature within the normal range requires a balance between heat produced by the body and its loss to the environment. Heat balance is achieved through the interplay of mechanisms that conserve heat and others that promote heat loss.

Heat conservation

When sensors in the hypothalamus detect a fall in temperature they trigger a set of responses that promote heat conservation. These include:

- *Vasoconstriction* – peripheral blood vessels constrict, diverting blood away from the extremities, thus limiting heat loss from the body to the environment
- *Piloerection* – body hairs are erected, trapping warm air against the body surface (skin)
- *Shivering* – generates heat
- *Reduced sweating* – facilitates heat conservation.

Behavioural responses include putting on more clothes, exercising or moving towards a source of heat.

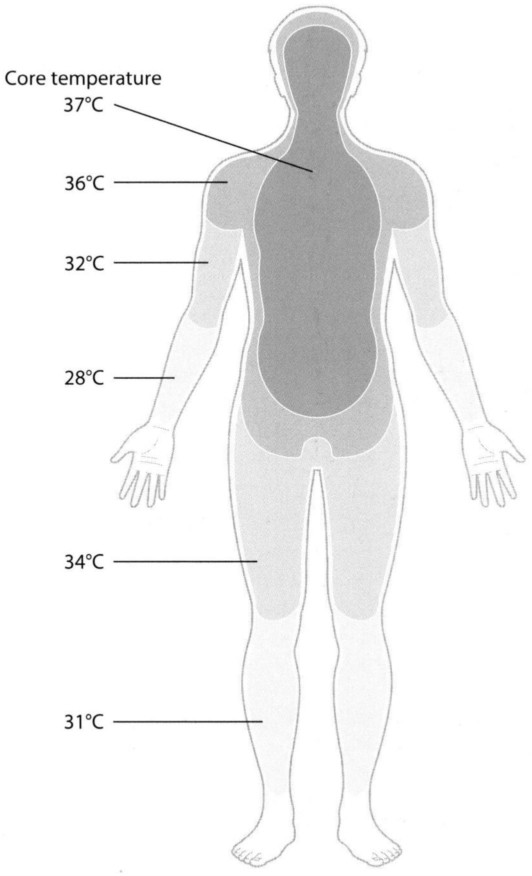

Fig. 14.6 Body temperature at different sites (reproduced with permission from Brooker & Nicol 2003)

Heat loss

If core temperature rises above the set point, the body initiates physiological mechanisms that promote heat transfer. These include:

- *Vasodilatation* – dilatation of peripheral blood vessels, which facilitates heat transfer to the cooler environment of the skin
- *Increased sweating* – facilitates heat loss as sweat evaporates from the skin
- *Increased rate and depth of respirations* – promotes heat loss in expired air
- *Decrease in cellular metabolism* – reduces heat production.

Behavioural mechanisms activated by the brain also promote heat loss. These include taking off clothes or wearing lighter clothes, drinking cold fluids or lifting the arms away from the body.

Physiological influences on body core temperature

There are several factors that influence BCT, as outlined below.

Diurnal cycles

BCT varies throughout the day. Variations are normally within a range of 0.5–1.0°C over 24 hours, with the highest point of 37.2°C at around 6 pm and lowest (36.7°C) around 6 am. People having their temperature measured daily should therefore have this carried out at the same time each day to avoid normal diurnal variations.

Age

In infants, temperature regulation is labile because their physiological heat-regulating mechanisms are immature, and this can continue until puberty. Babies and small children therefore need to be dressed appropriately for the environmental temperatures around them. Heat production is increased in infants and children due to deposits of brown fat around the neck, back and viscera (the organs within the abdominal cavity). The only role of brown fat is to generate heat, and therefore shivering is not usually observed in this age group. Children also have a higher basal metabolic rate than adults, due to increased tissue growth rates. The consequence of a higher metabolic rate is a higher mean BCT.

Older adults may have a lower mean BCT that is also more influenced by ambient temperature. Therefore, should an older person develop an infection, BCT may not rise significantly. Ageing processes tend to reduce muscle mass, which reduces heat production capability in older adults. Additionally, loss of subcutaneous tissue (insulating fat), reduced basal metabolic rate and altered vasoconstriction/vasodilatation mechanisms influence heat loss and production.

Menstrual cycle

Hormones released throughout the menstrual cycle also influence temperature. Increased cellular metabolism occurs at ovulation and body temperature rises by up to 1°C for the remainder of the cycle.

Other factors

Exercise increases heat production. Stress, pain and illness can also increase body temperature, whereas fatigue and headache can decrease it.

Environmental influences on body temperature

Environmental temperature extremes can raise or lower body temperature. The changes depend on the extent of exposure, air humidity and the presence of convection currents.

Smoking cigarettes or cigars can increase oral temperature.

Care of people with temperature abnormalities

Body temperature can deviate from the normal range as a result of excess heat production, minimal heat loss or minimal heat production. It may:

- Rise resulting in pyrexia (fever, BCT above 37.5°C) or hyperthermia (BCT above 40°C) due to failure of heat loss mechanisms (see Further reading: Edwards 2003)
- Fall, resulting in hypothermia (BCT below 35°C).

Table 14.1 Pyrexia: phases and nursing interventions

Condition	BCT	Phase	Signs and symptoms	Cause	Nursing interventions
Pyrexia	37.5–39.9°C	1. Chill	Skin is pale and feels cool and dry Shivering, goose bumps (piloerection) Person complains of feeling cold BCT rises and rigors may occur during this phase	Constriction of peripheral blood vessels Immune response triggers heat generation strategies to kill invading bacteria	Keep person covered in light clothing Add blankets to assist heat conservation
Hyperpyrexia	40.0–42.0°C	2. Plateau	Skin flushed and feels dry Pulse and respiratory rates elevated. BCT remains high Dehydration and dry mouth	Set point elevated Increased cellular metabolism and oxygen consumption	Provide mouthwashes/oral hygiene and fluids or ice chips to suck Provide an easily digestible diet high in energy to meet increased energy needs If temperature above 39°C antipyretics and cooling measures may be prescribed
	42–36.4°C	3. Defervescence	BCT initially elevated but returns to normal Pulse and respiratory rates remain elevated Skin moist, flushed and hot Profuse sweating Dehydration may occur	Vasodilatation of peripheral blood vessels and sweating facilitate heat loss Dehydration and increased cellular metabolism: contribute to raised pulse and respiratory rates	Provide cool dry clothes and bedding Sponging with cool water may promote comfort Continue oral hygiene and fluids as above; a fluid balance chart may be used to monitor hydration status (See Ch. 19) Assess risk of pressure ulcers (see p. 357, Ch. 25) as moist skin increases this risk Continue prescribed antipyretics and cooling measures

Disorders such as heatstroke, hypothermia and frostbite may occur when environmental temperatures are extreme. The first aid for people with heatstroke and frostbite is outlined in this section.

Caring for patients with pyrexia or hyperpyrexia

Pyrexia is present when elevated temperature readings have been recorded at different times throughout the day, rather than a single raised reading. Pyrexia is often caused by an infection and has three stages. The first stage, during which BCT rises, can induce vigorous shivering or 'rigors'. Shivering generates metabolic heat with a subsequent rise in BCT, which the body uses to mount a response against the invading pathogen. The stages and the nursing care required are outlined in Table 14.1. Elevated BCT increases basal metabolic rate and oxygen consumption and, in hyperpyrexia, there is serious disruption of brain and other organ function. Children under the age of 5 years are prone to febrile seizures and the first aid needed is described Box 16.36 (p. 457).

Two major strategies can be used to manage elevated body temperature:

- Antipyretic medication, e.g. paracetamol, ibuprofen, aspirin (not used for children under the age of 16 years because of the potential risk of Reye's syndrome, see Ch. 23) that reduce BCT
- Cooling interventions (see Table 14.2). The evidence to support cooling strategies for children is presented in Box 14.14. However, cooling patients remains an area of nursing practice that is ritualistic and lacking in clear evidence (Price et al 2003).

Aggressive forms of cooling such as the use of cooling mattresses or covering the whole body with ice are sometimes required for patients who develop temperatures above 41°C as this may cause serious and sometimes fatal consequences.

Prolonged exposure to hot sunlight or high environmental temperatures can result in the development of a serious condition known as heatstroke where measured BCT can be as high as 45°C. People at risk include:

- Those exercising or engaging in strenuous activity in high environmental temperatures, especially when combined with high humidity
- Children
- Older adults
- Those with coexisting heart disease or metabolic disturbances, e.g. diabetes or hypothyroidism

Table 14.2 Advantages and disadvantages of cooling interventions

Cooling intervention	Advantages	Disadvantages
Fanning – rotary mobile fans blowing over body surface, using a variety of speeds	Perceived patient comfort Convenient Cheap	Shivering and vasoconstriction Spread of airborne microorganisms No evidence to support use in ill patients
Cool water bathing – sponging with cloths soaked in either ice-cool water or tepid water	No shivering Reduction in BCT	Time consuming Discomfort and vasoconstriction with iced cloths
Ice cooling – ice packs applied to areas where major arteries are near the skin surface, e.g. axillae, groins, neck	Surface cooling on area surrounding pack Rapid cooling	Vasoconstriction, which limits heat transfer from core to the skin causing heat conservation
Cooling blankets/mattresses – can be water filled and placed under patient, or air filled and put over patient Temperature controlled thermostat	Rate of fever reduction faster than traditional methods Control over temperature setting	Expensive to buy or rent Uncomfortable, so generally only used on comatose patients No more effective than traditional methods

EVIDENCE-BASED PRACTICE Box 14.14

Cooling strategies for pyrexial children

Watts et al (2003) undertook a systematic review that considered the use and timing of cooling strategies used in the care of pyrexial children.

Main points

- Reviewed the effectiveness of drugs including paracetamol and ibuprofen in reducing pyrexia
- Considered the use of external cooling strategies
- Fever was defined as 37.5–41°C measured either orally or at the tympanic membrane, 38°C if measured rectally
- Children between 0 and 5 years, with an even distribution of males and females
- Ten randomized controlled trials evaluated
- Effectiveness of intervention determined by a series of outcomes which included effect on body temperature, the presence of febrile convulsions, increased comfort or reduced irritability.

Conclusions

- Antipyretic drugs were effective in reducing fever in seven of the studies
- The combination of antipyretics and sponging with cool water was more effective in reducing temperature
- Four studies indicated that tepid sponging appeared to increase comfort
- Lack of evidence to support the use of antipyretics alone
- Parental education for caring for a febrile child should be encouraged.

Student activities

- Consider the nursing interventions in Table 14.1.
- Find out what cooling strategy is used to manage pyrexial patients/clients in your placement.
- Search the nursing literature for articles that evaluate different cooling strategies.

[Resource: Watts R, Robertson J, Thomas G 2003 The nursing management of fever in children: a systematic review. International Journal of Nursing Practice 9:51–58]

- Those taking recreational drugs such as Ecstasy, alcohol or medications such as diuretics (see Ch. 22) that may impair heat loss mechanisms.

Recognition of heatstroke and the necessary interventions are shown in Box 14.15.

Caring for patients with hypothermia

Hypothermia is present when BCT is below 35°C. It is described as mild, moderate, severe or profound (see Table 14.3). Hypothermia usually occurs accidentally as a result of exposure to low environmental temperatures and people at the extremes of age are the most vulnerable. Awareness of and providing interventions that will minimize the risk factors for hypothermia can often prevent its occurrence. Risk factors in infants, adults and older adults are outlined in Box 14.16.

Hypothermia can also occur in hospital. For example, some anaesthetic drugs lower BCT, as do some interventions, e.g. infusing large volumes of unwarmed fluids or irrigating body cavities with cool fluids in theatre. Postoperatively it is therefore important that temperature is carefully assessed and monitored (see Ch. 24).

FIRST AID — Box 14.15

Heatstroke

Recognition

Usually there is sudden onset of some or all of the following signs and symptoms:

- Hot dry skin
- Flushed skin
- Headache
- Excessive thirst
- Nausea
- Numbness, tingling, muscle cramps
- Dizziness
- Restless
- Mental confusion.

Observations

- Temperature above 40°C
- Tachypnoea (increased respiratory rate)
- Tachycardia (pulse rate >100 bpm in an adult).

Aims of treatment

- To recognize the presence of heatstroke
- To remove the cause
- To reduce body temperature
- To transfer the casualty to hospital.

Treatment

- Remove the source of heat – move casualty into shade or out of the sun
- Lie casualty down and provide reassurance
- Loosen clothing and remove any items of unnecessary clothing if possible
- Sponge with cool water
- Dial 999 for an ambulance
- Check and record respiratory rate, pulse rate and level of response.

Box 14.16 **Risk factors for hypothermia**

Infants

- A large surface area in relation to body weight. As the skin is a heat exchanger, heat loss is relatively high
- Their inability to put on more clothes or turn the heating up when feeling cold.

Adults

- Cold environmental conditions such as when hillwalking or skiing, especially when not wearing appropriate clothing, and water sports accidents, which result in immersion in cold water that leads to very rapid heat loss
- Excessive alcohol consumption and drug misuse that cause both vasodilatation and impair perception of the cold. As a result, people may become inadvertently exposed for prolonged periods.

Older adults

- Impaired ability to control body temperature
- A reduction in temperature sensor (thermoreceptor) effectiveness
- Poor nutrition due to loss of appetite or physical constraints that make it difficult to cook; a low dietary energy intake will reduce heat production
- Loss of the shivering reflex
- Environmental factors such as living in a cold house with little money for heating.

Table 14.3 Effects of hypothermia

Description	Range (°C)	Clinical effects
Mild	32–35	Reduced metabolic rate that reduces oxygen consumption, slows down drug metabolism Severe shivering Pallor BP, pulse and respirations begin to fall Urine output increases due to diminished production of antidiuretic hormone Mental confusion, hearing fades
Moderate	28–31.9	Myocardial irritability; cardiac arrest that may not respond to cardiac resuscitation Unresponsive to environment Loss of shivering response Increased blood viscosity and clot thrombus formation
Severe	20–27	Unable to regulate temperature; loss of brain stem reflexes
Profound	<20	Death

The physiological effects of hypothermia are outlined in Table 14.3 and patients require careful observation for their presence. Severe hypothermia requires treatment in a high dependency area or intensive care unit.

Restoring low BCT to normal requires careful management. The following parameters should be assessed:

- Blood pressure (see p. 380)
- Heart rate (see p. 378)
- Respirations (see p. 384)
- Oxygen saturation (see Ch. 17)
- Temperature – should be measured using a tympanic thermometer (see p. 374) or an internal probe
- Urine output.

Management involves warming, which can be active or passive depending on the severity of hypothermia; however, it is dangerous to rewarm a patient too quickly. In mild hypothermia the aim is to increase BCT by 1–2°C per hour and this can be achieved by:

- Closing windows and doors
- Only removing clothing if the room is warm
- Removing wet or cold clothing
- Making sure the person is dry and wrapping them in blankets
- Wearing a hat to minimize loss through the head, which can be considerable, especially in children
- Active surface warming including blowing warm air over body and surface heaters
- Warming of intravenous fluids – these may be used in moderate and severe hypothermia, when rapid rewarming is required to prevent damage to vital organs.

In frostbite, peripheral blood flow is reduced in tissues that are exposed to freezing temperatures. This is an attempt to conserve heat by limiting heat loss from the skin. Frostbite or cold injury develops as the poor peripheral blood supply causes injury or permanent destruction of the tissue as it becomes deprived of oxygen and ice crystals form in the tissues. If left untreated, gangrene (death of tissues due in an inadequate blood supply) will occur. The parts of the body most at risk of developing frostbite are the facial features such as the ears, nose and cheeks, and extremities such as the hands, fingers, feet and toes.

The following situations or circumstances can lead to the development of frostbite:

- Exposure to sub-zero temperatures that is exacerbated by a high wind chill factor
- The wearing of wet and/or poorly insulated clothes, e.g. walkers, mountain climbers or during water sports
- Some medical conditions, e.g. diabetes, peripheral vascular disease
- Use of recreational drugs and/or alcohol, which cause vasodilatation as well as impairing perception of the cold.

Recognition and first aid management of frostbite are described in Box 14.17.

FIRST AID Box 14.17

Frostbite

Recognition

- Early signs include pins and needles, pale skin and numbness of affected tissue
- Later the tissue becomes hard and mottled blue in colour
- If gangrene occurs the tissue becomes black.

Aims of treatment

- To recognize the development of frostbite
- To remove the casualty from the cause
- To warm the affected area
- To transfer the casualty to hospital.

Treatment

- Move the casualty to a warm area
- Remove any jewellery or clothing from the affected part
- Warm the affected part by using the casualty's own body heat or your own warmth
- Bathing in warm (not hot) water
- Do not rub the affected part as the skin becomes red and hot, and blisters may appear due to warming
- Give paracetamol for pain.

[Adapted from Mohun 2002]

Body temperature assessment tools

Estimation of body core or peripheral temperature can be made at different sites using a variety of instruments. Instruments include tympanic membrane probes, electronic thermometers, disposable chemical dot thermometers and the glass-and-mercury thermometer.

Each device has advantages and limitations (see Table 14.4) and therefore individual needs must be assessed. Should intervention to manage abnormal body temperature be required, it is necessary to select a thermometer that can be used to make frequent or continuous measurements. This must be accurate and reliable at the top and bottom of the scale, and be appropriate for the person's age and individual needs.

Electronic thermometers

The electronic thermometer (Fig. 14.7) usually consists of a battery-operated device that displays a digital readout of the temperature measured during a preset recording time, usually between 20 and 50 seconds. Attached to the device by a cable is a probe, which is most commonly placed in the mouth, axilla or rectum. Protecting rigid probes with a plastic disposable cover and cleaning them between each use prevents cross-infection. Disposable flexible probes may be used for continuous temperature monitoring which has been found to produce reliable information (Henker & Coyne 1995, Giuliano et al 2000).

Table 14.4 Sites and thermometers – a comparison

Thermometer	Site used	Advantages	Limitations
Electronic thermometer probes	Oral cavity, axilla	Easy access Good blood supply	Does not correlate with tympanic or pulmonary artery temperature
	Rectum	Well insulated from external environmental influences on temperature	Not recommended for use with newborns or children
Tympanic membrane thermometer	Auditory canal	Good blood supply Fast measurement (<5 seconds) Easy to use Accurate and reliable	Expensive Ambient temperature may influence temperature within auditory canal Use without specific training may cause unreliability of measurement Poor correlation with oral electronic thermometry auditory Earwax, blood, foreign bodies and other matter in the canal lower the temperature reading so use is precluded in patients who have recently had ear or neurosurgery Hearing aids must be removed before measurement is carried out
Chemical dot thermometers	Oral cavity, axilla, forehead	Ease of access Disposable – reduces cross-infection Low cost	Lacks sensitivity in measuring elevated body temperature Underestimates oral temperature, overestimates axillary temperature Some require 3-minute placement time
Glass-and-mercury thermometer	Oral cavity, axilla, rectum	Inexpensive Reliable Easy access	Requires long placement time (2–3 minutes oral, 3–6 minutes for axilla and rectum) Risk of breakage in people with epilepsy, children and confused or restless adults Cross-infection risks Health and safety risks associated with using mercury in practice, being phased out in practice areas
	Axilla		Unreliable in hypothermia Lacks accuracy and reliability when there is poor skin–thermometer contact or generalized vasoconstriction

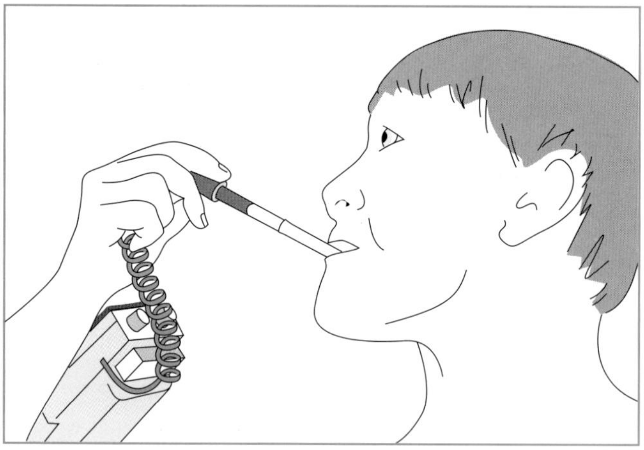

Fig. 14.7 Oral electronic thermometer (reproduced with permission from Nicol et al 2004)

However, the device requires regular calibration, and the site used to measure temperature influences reliability. For example, the axillary placement is affected by environmental temperature and the oral placement depends on its position within the mouth and the cooperation of the patient.

Tympanic thermometers

Tympanic thermometers measure temperature at the tympanic membrane (eardrum). Because the tympanic membrane is in close proximity to the hypothalamus, measurement here accurately reflects the BCT. The tip of the instrument contains a probe, protected by a disposable sheath, which is placed into the ear. Some manufacturers recommend that the pinna is pulled upward and back for an adult and down and back for a child. This action straightens the external ear canal, creates a seal from external air temperature and facilitates correct insertion of the probe (Fig. 14.8).

The probe detects heat emitted from the tympanic membrane in the form of infrared energy. The resulting signal is processed and displayed as a digital readout. Temperature is measured and displayed within 3 seconds of activation and the instrument bleeps on completion. The tympanic thermometer measures body temperature accurately between 25 and 43°C.

Tympanic thermometers are widely used in healthcare settings, probably because they are convenient, easy and quick to use. Although their use relies on accurate technique, a number of studies have confirmed accuracy of measurement (Gilbert et al 2002).

However, there are some limitations to their use (see Table 14.4).

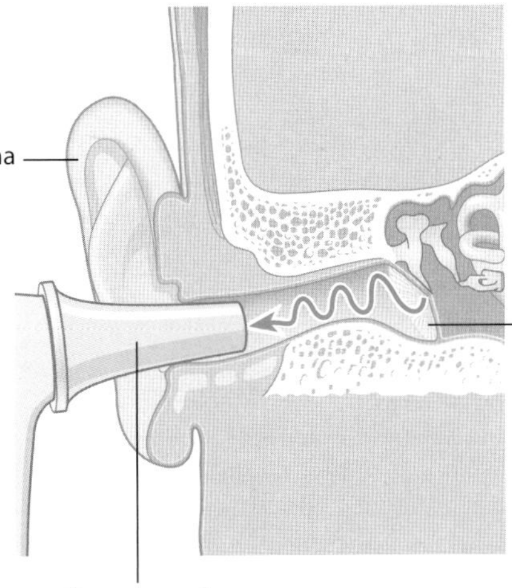

Fig. 14.8 Using a tympanic thermometer (reproduced with permission from Nicol et al 2004)

Single-use thermometers

Single-use thermometers, such as chemical dots, are convenient, easy to use, non-invasive and also disposable. The thermometer consists of a plastic strip, with a series of chemically impregnated paper dots, which is placed in the oral cavity or the axilla. The dots change colour with heat. The final reading can usually be taken in up to 3 minutes depending on the manufacturer's instructions. A study of their use in critically ill patients (Potter et al 2003) suggests that they are useful and reliable. However, the instrument lacks accuracy, as it can over- and underestimate pyrexia. While this thermometer may be useful as a screening tool, it is therefore not appropriate for use in patients who require cooling interventions to manage elevated temperature (Erickson et al 1996, Potter et al 2003).

Glass-and-mercury thermometers

Glass-and-mercury thermometers have been used to measure body temperature in community and hospital settings for many years. The thermometer can be placed in the axilla, the sublingual pocket or rectum, although the last two sites are no longer recommended due to the risk of toxicity if the thermometer breaks. The use of mercury in clinical practice has been subject to review in view of problems relating to mercury toxicity and dealing with mercury spillage. In addition, the use and disposal of mercury in instruments within healthcare settings has been subjected to standards for the Control of Substances Hazardous to Health (COSHH) (see Ch. 13). The associated risks have led many healthcare settings to stop using this type of thermometer altogether.

The glass tube contains mercury located in a bulb at one end. Before use, the thermometer is grasped at the other end from the bulb, and shaken using a flick of the wrist. This returns the mercury back to the bulb. Mercury expands on exposure to heat, and so travels up a column within the tube when placed in contact with the body. The point at which the mercury stops is recorded as the temperature. Graduations of 0.1°C are marked on the glass tube between 35 and 40°C. Temperature is read by holding the thermometer at the opposite end from the bulb and rotating it slowly, at eye level.

Box 14.18 outlines an investigation into the accuracy of different thermometers.

EVIDENCE-BASED PRACTICE Box 14.18

Comparison of thermometers

Within clinical practice a number of different instruments are used to measure body temperature. Dowding et al (2002) conducted an experimental study comparing:

- Tympanic membrane thermometers
- Digital thermometers
- Disposable thermometers.

Measurements were compared to those obtained by the glass-and-mercury thermometer placed in the axilla.

Conclusions

- Temperature readings for the digital thermometers placed in both the oral cavity and axilla were lower than those obtained by glass-and-mercury thermometers.
- The disposable thermometers tested in the oral cavity showed readings that were lower than those obtained using glass-and-mercury thermometers. Conversely, readings taken in the axilla were higher than those obtained using glass-and-mercury thermometers.
- Results for both the digital and disposable thermometers were statistically and clinically significant.
- Tympanic thermometers showed no significant difference in temperature between readings measured by glass-and-mercury thermometers.
- Tympanic readings did not show variability in readings between observers.

These conclusions suggest that tympanic thermometers are reliable indicators of body temperature.

Student activities

1. Find out what types of thermometer are used in your placement.
2. Read the article by Dowding et al (2002) and identify:
   - Limitations and advantages of the thermometers used in your placement
   - Potential problems when using glass-and-mercury thermometers placed in the axilla.

[Resource: Dowding D, Freeman S, Nimmo S et al 2002 An investigation into the accuracy of different types of thermometers. Professional Nurse 18(3):1666–1668]

Thermometer placement sites

Temperature varies widely throughout the body (see Fig. 14.6, p. 369) and it is therefore important to remember

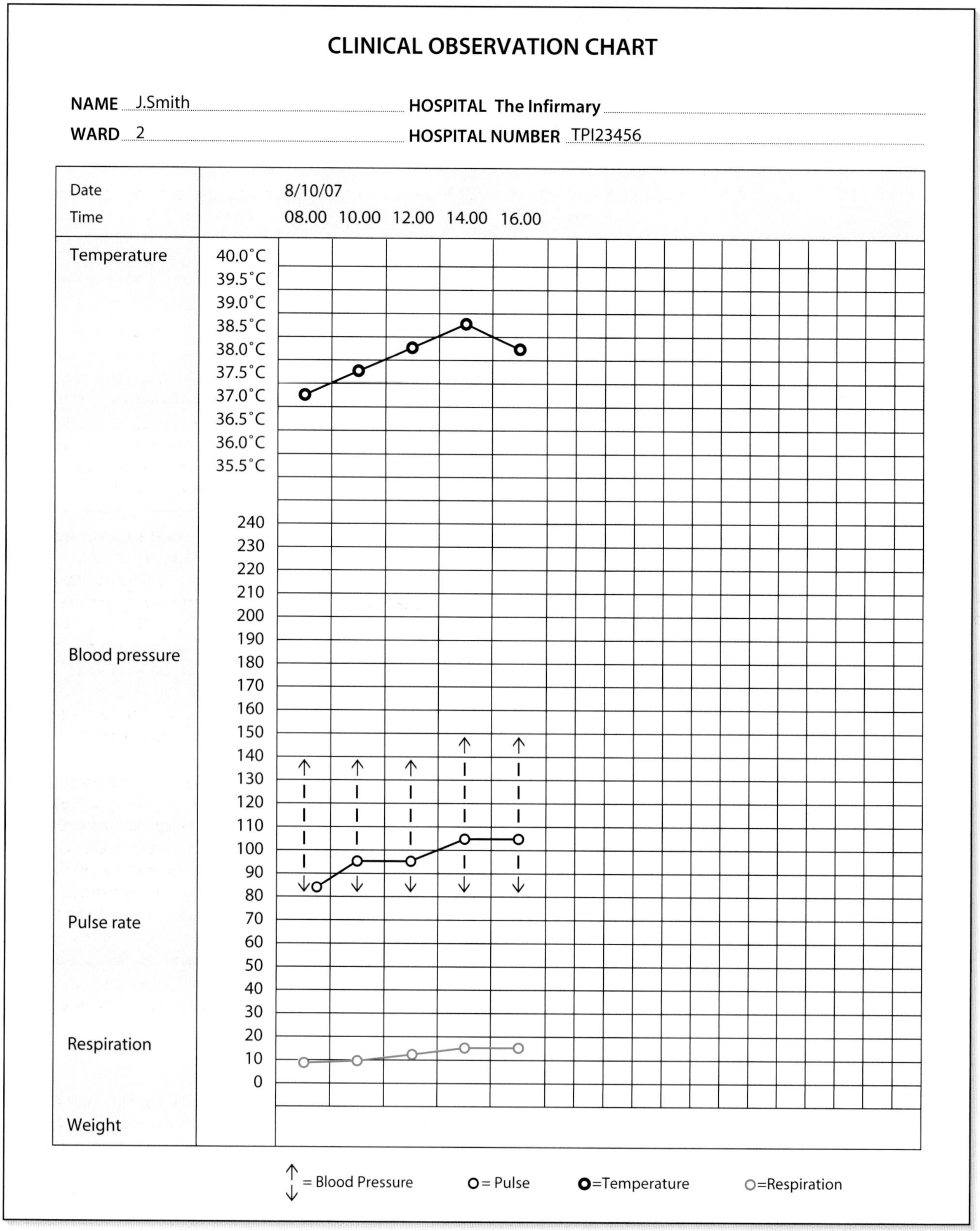

Fig. 14.9 Clinical observation chart

that, if a temperature trend is required, the same site is used for each measurement. As a result of site variation of temperature, it is erroneous to believe that one location is more accurate than another. For example, BCT measured at the pulmonary artery is usually higher than the oral or axillary sites because the mouth and skin are exposed to the cooling influences of ambient temperature. In contrast, BCT will be lower than that found in the rectum due to the heat generated from metabolic activity of microorganisms in the rectum. Commonly used sites for measuring body temperature include the oral cavity, the tympanic membrane, the axilla and the rectum which are discussed below. Measurement of blood temperature within the pulmonary artery is considered to be the most accurate reflection of BCT – the 'gold standard'. This is because blood returning from major organs to the heart reflects the average temperature of the major internal organs. However, measuring pulmonary artery blood temperature is an invasive technique that is confined to critical care areas as are other sites including the pharynx, oesophagus and bladder.

Oral cavity

The thermometer is placed in the sublingual pocket at the junction with the tongue, which is close to the sublingual artery and therefore equates well with BCT. This site may not be suitable for young children who are at risk from biting the probe, especially if they are afraid and/or uncooperative.

Tympanic membrane

The probe is placed in auditory canal and can be used for adults or children (see Fig. 14.8).

Axilla

An electronic, chemical dot or glass-and-mercury thermometer is placed under axilla and the arm holds it in place. This site can be used for adults, infants and children. In children, the arm is held gently against the body to keep the thermometer in place.

Rectum

The rectum can be used for adults although it is not commonly used in children in the UK. It is never used in newborns because of the risk of rectal perforation. If a non-disposable temperature probe is used, a disposable sheath is applied and discarded after use. The thermometer is cleaned according to local policy before and after use.

Skin

A disposable probe attached to the skin surface can be used for adults or children.

Interpreting temperature measurements

The temperature measured should be recorded. In hospitals this is usually on a clinical observation chart (Fig. 14.9). Measuring and recording the temperature on to the chart, either every few hours (1–4 hourly) or daily, will reveal a trend for body temperature. If body temperature is elevated above the normal, then cooling interventions can be initiated (see p. 370). Recording the body temperature every few hours while the patient is being cooled will demonstrate whether the strategy is lowering the temperature back to normal.

Pulse

Nurses frequently perform assessment of the pulse, which is the rhythmic expansion and relaxation of an artery caused by ejection of blood from the left ventricle when it contracts. Knowledge of the rate, volume and rhythm produces information that assists in the assessment and evaluation of health status or response to interventions. This section outlines anatomy and physiology of the pulse and explains how it is assessed.

Principal pulse points

The pressure wave, or 'pulse', of blood travelling along some arteries can be felt using the fingers at points of the body where an artery lies close to a bone (Fig. 14.10). This is the 'peripheral' pulse, and it can be assessed by palpation (gentle compression of an artery using the fingers, against a bone). The most commonly used site is the radial artery at the wrist (see Fig. 14.11).

The carotid arteries are located in the neck at each side of the larynx (see Fig. 14.10). They provide blood to the brain and are easily accessible. This is sometimes referred to as a central pulse. However, only light pressure should be applied to one artery at a time, in case the blood supply to the brain is restricted. During cardiopulmonary resuscitation, the carotid artery is palpated by trained healthcare practitioners to detect the return of a pulse (see Ch. 17).

The femoral artery may be used to assess the pulse, especially when the blood pressure is low, as peripheral pulses in the arm and lower leg can be difficult to palpate. Peripheral vascular disease restricts blood flow to the lower limbs and it may be necessary to establish the presence of pulses in the legs to confirm blood flow to the extremities. The popliteal, posterior tibial and dorsalis pedis (also known as 'pedal') pulse sites are used to assess whether circulation is present in specific parts of the leg and foot. The popliteal pulse can be difficult to palpate and considerable practice may be required to master this.

Normal pulse rate

The rhythmic pulsation of blood in the arterial system is counted and recorded as the pulse rate (see Box 14.19) and normally represents the rate at which the heart beats, i.e. the heart rate. The normal resting rate in adults is between 60 and 100 beats per minute (bpm). In adults, tachycardia is the term given to pulse rates greater than 100 bpm; bradycardia describes a pulse rate below 60 bpm.

Factors that affect heart rate

The pulse rate varies depending on the degree of activity within the autonomic nervous system. Stimulation of the

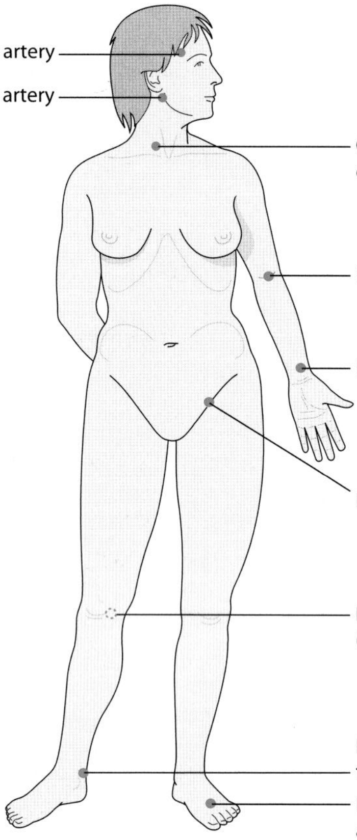

Fig. 14.10 The main pulse points (reproduced with permission from Waugh & Grant 2006)

sympathetic nervous system and the release of adrenaline increase heart rate, whereas parasympathetic activity decreases it. Due to their higher metabolic rate, children have a faster pulse rate than adults (see Table 14.5).

Stressors such as pain, fear and anger increase the pulse rate as they increase sympathetic activity. The rate also increases with exercise and pyrexia, and may alter due to the effects of medications and some diseases such as those involving the heart, lungs or blood (see Ch. 17). Medication such as digoxin is given to patients with heart failure, to improve myocardial contraction and reduce the heart rate. Salbutamol, used to control the symptoms of asthma, can cause tachycardia.

Assessing the pulse

The radial pulse can be found at the inner aspect of the wrist below the base of the thumb and medial to the radius, or wrist bone. It is palpated by placing two fingers, usually the index and third, and applying gentle pressure on the radial artery (Fig. 14.11). Measuring the pulse is described in Box 14.19. The regularity and strength are also assessed (see below). Radial, popliteal and pedal pulses may be difficult to locate in adults who are cold or when the environment is cold and those with:

- Peripheral vascular disease, which impairs peripheral circulation
- Low blood pressure (hypotension, see Ch. 17)

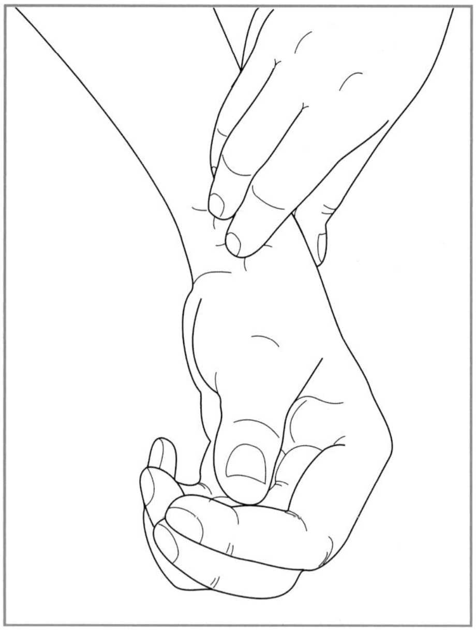

Fig. 14.11 Taking the radial pulse (reproduced with permission from Nicol et al 2004)

NURSING SKILLS Box 14.19

Taking the pulse

Equipment
- Watch with second hand
- Observation chart.

Preparation
- Explain the procedure and seek verbal consent; maintain respect and dignity at all times
- The person should be lying or sitting down. Allow the person to rest for 30 minutes after physical activity, emotional upset or smoking
- Wash hands as per local policy.

Procedure
- Select the pulse site
- Apply pressure gently but firmly with flat fingers until the pulse is palpated
- Count the number of beats for 1 minute using a watch with a second hand. If a regular rhythm is noted, the pulse can be counted for 30 seconds and the number of beats is doubled
- Note further characteristics of the pulse:
  - rhythm (regular or irregular)
  - force or volume
- If the respiratory rate is to be measured, this is usually carried out discreetly while recording the pulse (see Fig. 14.16)
- Handwashing according to local policy
- Record pulse rate on the observation chart (see Fig. 14.9)
- Report and document any changes/abnormalities.

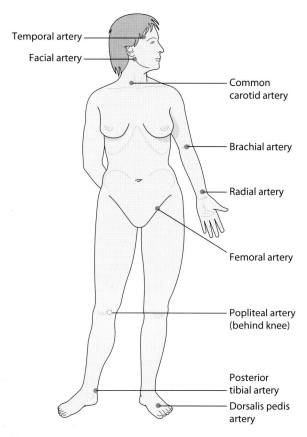

- Cardiac arrhythmias (see Ch. 17)
- Peripheral oedema (see Chs 17, 19).

Regularity
When counting the pulse rate the regularity is also noted, as this reflects the cardiac rhythm. Normally the rhythm is regular as the heart contracts regularly. However, young people may have a rhythm disturbance, known as sinus arrhythmia, which alters with inspiration and expiration. People who have heart disease may have an irregular rhythm due to disordered electrical conduction within the heart, e.g. atrial fibrillation (see Ch. 17). Heart irregularities can be investigated through an electrocardiogram (ECG) (see Ch. 17). An irregular rhythm should always be reported immediately.

Volume
The force of the pulse is also assessed. The terms used to describe force or volume are:

- *Normal* – the pulse is easy to feel
- *Bounding* – pulse feels 'springy' due to an increase in force of cardiac contraction or circulating blood volume; usually found in the presence of infection
- *Thready* – pulse feels weak, difficult to palpate and difficult to count, which may be due to dehydration or haemorrhage
- *Absent* – indicates a blockage of the palpated artery or, together with other observations such as skin colour, cardiac arrest.

Factors that influence the force include the circulating blood volume and the action of hormones on blood vessel walls causing vasoconstriction or vasodilatation.

Features of the pulse in newborns, infants and children

Pulse rates in children vary with age; normal ranges are shown in Table 14.5. There are other specific factors about the pulse and its measurement children that are outlined below.

Apical pulse
The apical pulse is a central measurement, which is the most accurate recording of heart rate in children under 6 years and also in adults who may have heart disease with rhythm disturbances. The apical (apex) beat is located at the apex of the heart. Measurement of the apex/radial pulse in adults is explained in Chapter 17.

The apical pulse is detected using a stethoscope and listening to heart sounds at the apex of the heart (the pointed end of the ventricle). In children, placement of the stethoscope is dependent on age. The stethoscope is placed:

- At the 4th intercostal space and slightly lateral to the left midclavicular line in children under 7 years of age
- At the 5th intercostal space on the left midclavicular line for children over 7 years old (Wong et al 2001).

Table 14.5 Pulse rates for children

Age (years)	Pulse rate (beats per minute)
0–1	110–160
1–2	100–150
2–5	95–140
5–12	80–120
Over 12	60–100

Reproduced with permission from Mackway-Jones et al (2005)

Special considerations include:

- The apical pulse is used to measure the heart rate under the age of 2 years
- Heart rate should be assessed while a baby or child is asleep or at rest, as crying, eating or sucking increase heart rate
- Peripheral pulses in the arms and legs are difficult to palpate.

Blood pressure

This section outlines what blood pressure is and the factors that affect it in health; for more detail you should consult your physiology textbook. The equipment needed and how to measure blood pressure are explained. It is important to be familiar with the early material in this section before attempting to practise blood pressure measurement.

Blood pressure (BP) corresponds to the pressure exerted on arterial walls as blood moves through them. BP measurements provide information about cardiovascular status, which can assist in the diagnosis of disease or evaluation of treatment. Two measurements are made and usually recorded in millimetres of mercury (mmHg):

- *Systolic pressure*, which represents the greatest pressure in the main arteries following contraction of the left ventricle
- *Diastolic pressure*, which is the lowest pressure in the main arteries and occurs at the end of ventricular relaxation while the heart is at rest, before the next cardiac contraction.

The convention for writing blood pressure is to put the systolic pressure first and then the diastolic, e.g. 120/70 mmHg.

Factors that determine blood pressure

BP is determined by several factors including the cardiac output, venous return, blood volume, peripheral vascular resistance (the resistance within arteries and arterioles) and elasticity of large arteries. BP is dynamic, and so varies over the course of the day depending on body demands.

Cardiac output
This is the amount of blood ejected by the heart per minute and is approximately 5.25 litres/minute in adults.

This is determined by the stroke volume (SV) and heart rate (HR), meaning that:

$$\text{cardiac output} = \text{stroke volume} \times \text{heart rate}.$$

In the resting adult, approximately 70 mL of blood is ejected from each ventricle every time the heart contracts. This is called the stroke volume. If the heart muscle is weakened by disease, then stroke volume may be reduced, lowering BP.

The factors affecting heart rate are outlined above and changes in heart rate directly affect the cardiac output.

Venous return

This is the volume of blood that is returned from the veins to the right atrium. In health, the heart pumps this volume out again, meaning that cardiac output is the same as venous return. Skeletal muscle contraction, the respiratory pump and the effects of gravity influence venous return. During exercise, increased skeletal muscle contraction increases venous return, which in turn increases blood pressure. The treatment for fainting (see Box 17.14) involves raising the legs, which increases venous return, overcoming the effects of gravity.

Blood volume

If the blood volume falls, e.g. due to haemorrhage or dehydration, then BP will also fall (see baroreceptor reflex below).

Peripheral vascular resistance

Resistance to blood flow is increased by arterial and arteriolar constriction, which increases BP. Arterial and arteriolar dilatation reduces peripheral vascular resistance and lowers BP. The diameter of these vessel walls is controlled by the baroreceptor reflex (see below).

Elasticity of large arteries

The elasticity of the large arteries, which is their ability to distend and recoil, also contributes to resistance. Elasticity tends to decrease with age and disease, thus increasing resistance, and so BP generally rises with age.

Control of blood pressure

Although BP varies depending on the factors mentioned above, it must always be sufficient to maintain blood flow to the vital organs, otherwise serious problems arise. Control is:

- Short term (see baroreceptor reflex below)
- Long term through regulation of blood volume by the kidneys, which produce the hormone renin that triggers the production of angiotensin and aldosterone. These substances increase BP by causing vasoconstriction and increasing retention of sodium and water (see Ch. 20).

Baroreceptor reflex

Baroreceptors are nerve endings, sensitive to stretch, that are found within the arch of the aorta and the carotid sinuses (located in the area where the common carotid arteries divide into their internal and external branches). When rising BP stretches them, the baroreceptors send impulses to the cardiovascular centre (CVC) in the brain stem. The CVC responds to increases in BP by sending impulses to the heart, which reduces the heart rate, and to blood vessels, which results in vasodilatation. Both of these responses lower BP and are reflex changes mediated by the autonomic nervous system. A fall in BP results in the reverse actions, namely increasing the heart rate and vasoconstriction, that both increase BP to maintain adequate perfusion to the vital organs.

Postural hypotension is a fall in BP that occurs when standing up from a lying or sitting position that is fairly common in older adults and people receiving antihypertensive medication, e.g. atenolol. It occurs because there is a delay in the baroreceptors responding to changes in posture and results in dizziness or fainting. If postural hypotension is observed, or the person is taking certain antihypertensive drugs, then BP should be measured in both the lying and standing positions.

Chemoreceptors

These nerve ending are sensitive to circulating chemicals, especially blood carbon dioxide levels. They are involved not only in the control of respiration, but also send inputs to the CVC. If BP falls significantly and/or if there is severe disruption of respiratory function, the CVC responds to chemoreceptor stimulation by increasing the heart rate and stroke volume, and causing vasoconstriction in an attempt to increase BP.

Blood hormone levels

Adrenaline (epinephrine) and noradrenaline (norepinephrine) act on:

- The heart muscle, increasing the heart rate and strength of contraction
- Blood vessels, causing vasoconstriction.

Other hormones and chemicals also influence BP and you should consult your physiology textbook for more detail.

Figure 14.12 summarizes the mechanisms involved in the control of BP.

Blood pressure values

Adult BP is normally in the range of 100–130 mmHg systolic and 60–90 mmHg diastolic. The British Hypertension Society recommends that optimal BP should be $<120/<80$ (Williams et al 2004). Table 14.6 shows normal BP values for children.

Hypertension (high blood pressure) is defined as systolic blood pressure greater than 140 mmHg or diastolic blood pressure greater than 90 mmHg (Williams et al 2004). Hypotension describes BP lower than the normal range of 100 mmHg systolic and/or 60 mmHg diastolic. Hypertension and hypotension are explored further in Chapter 17.

Equipment used for BP measurement

BP is usually measured by non-invasive means using either the auscultatory or electronic method. The equipment required includes a sphygmomanometer, which

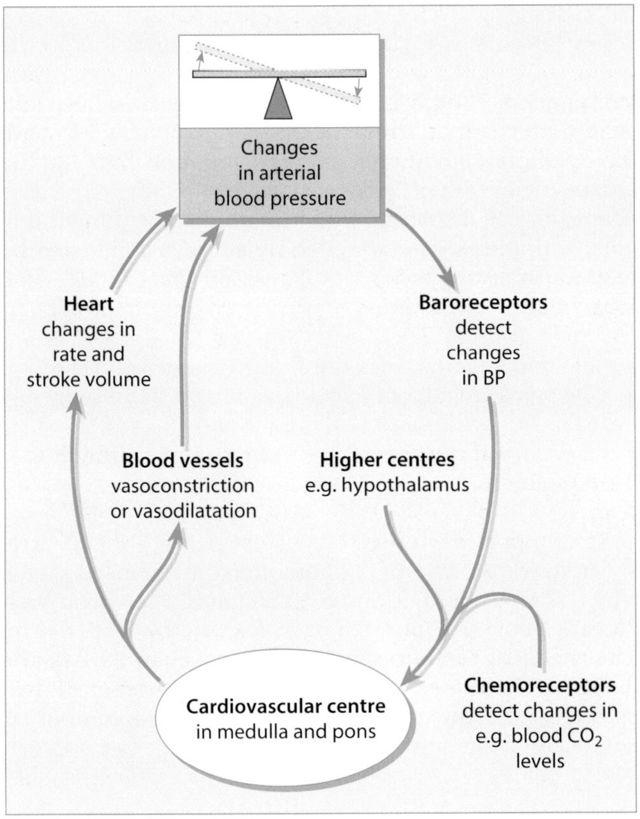

Fig. 14.12 Summary of the main mechanisms in blood pressure control (reproduced with permission from Waugh & Grant 2006)

Table 14.6 Normal BP values for children

Age (years)	Blood Pressure (mmHg)	
	Systolic	Diastolic
0–2	95	55
3–6	100	65
7–10	105	70
11–15	115	70

Reproduced with permission from Hull & Johnston (1999).

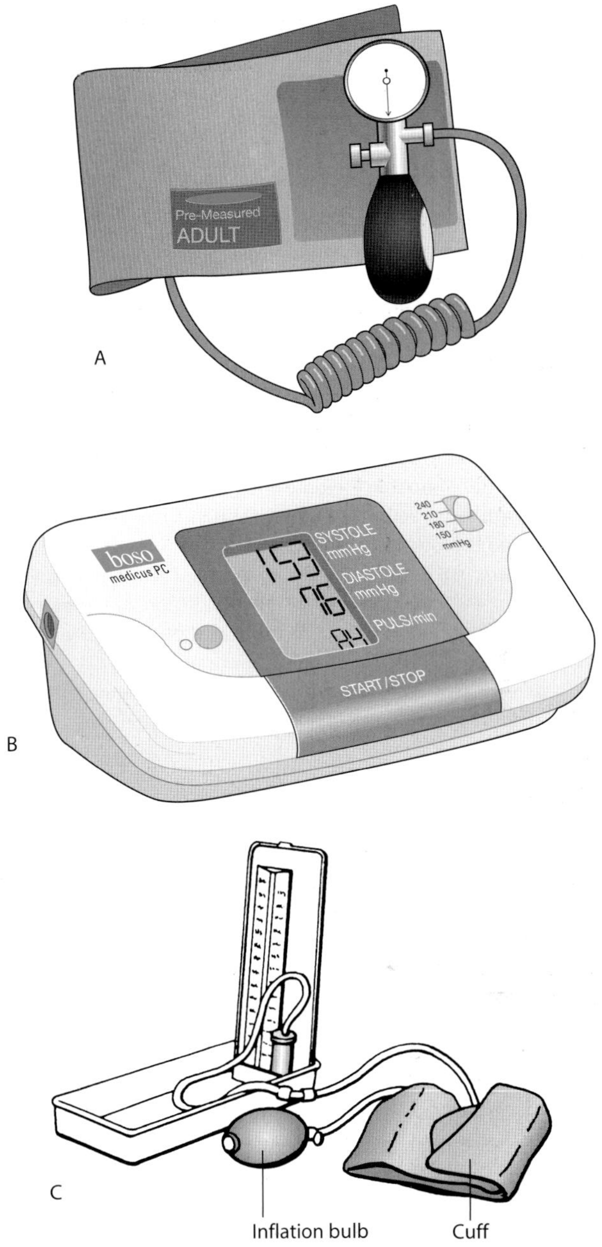

Fig. 14.13 Sphygmomanometers. **A.** Aneroid. **B.** Electronic. **C.** Mercury (reproduced with permission from Jamieson et al 2002)

may be aneroid, electronic or mercury, and an appropriately sized cuff (see Table 14.7). BP is sometimes continuously monitored through the invasive method using a catheter inserted into an artery, a technique beyond the scope of this book as it is confined to the care of critically ill people.

Sphygmomanometers (Fig. 14.13)
The mercury sphygmomanometer has been used for many years; however, health and safety concerns regarding the use and disposal of mercury in the workplace have emerged and therefore these may no longer be in use in your placements. Alternative methods of BP measurement are aneroid or electronic sphygmomanometers, which are being increasingly used.

The aneroid sphygmomanometer is less bulky and more portable than the other types. It does not use mercury and is widely viewed as a safe alternative that has quickly gained acceptance. However, the aneroid monitor has been found to be less reliable as it often underestimates BP. It is not recommended for use in hospitals because it rapidly deteriorates due to high usage and also needs frequent calibration (O'Brien et al 2003, Williams et al 2004). Aneroid sphygmomanometers require regular calibration with a mercury sphygmomanometer to ensure their accuracy.

The electronic sphygmomanometer includes a pressure sensor within the cuff that registers the systolic

CRITICAL THINKING — Box 14.20

How reliable is non-invasive BP measurement?

BP is often recorded on a single occasion and one-off readings do not necessarily reveal trends of a person's BP.

- *Variability over the day*: BP varies over the course of a day in order to meet different requirements such as exercise and other activities, e.g. eating, sleeping, smoking.
- *White coat syndrome*: This is an increase in BP ascribed to anxiety or anticipation of BP measurement by healthcare professionals.
- *Postural hypotension*: See page 380.
- *Arrhythmias*: Irregular heart rhythms may result in variations in the sounds heard from beat to beat as well as differences in the time between each beat. As a consequence, recordings made using the auscultatory method can be inaccurate.
- *Pregnancy*: BP is monitored closely as conditions arising during pregnancy may result in hypertension. In addition, BP can fall when lying supine if the fetus obstructs the inferior vena cava, reducing venous return.
- *Observer error*: The wrong technique or faulty equipment can lead to inaccurate readings.

Student activities

1. Read the article by Thomson et al (2002) and identify some of the factors that contribute towards a loss of accuracy when measuring BP.
2. BP equipment is frequently used in many placements and needs regular checks to ensure that measurements will be accurate. In your placement:
   - Identify the types of sphygmomanometer used.
   - Find out how often they are calibrated and how this is carried out.
   - Identify the different sizes of BP cuffs available and whether they are suitable for use with all the patients/clients there (see Table 14.7).
   - Find out when and how they are cleaned.
   - Examine the cuffs for signs of wear and tear. If they are in need of repair, discuss the further actions required with your mentor.

[Resource: Thomson J, Gillespie A, Curzio J (2002) Changes in equipment for blood pressure measurement. Professional Nurse 17(6):350–353]

and diastolic pressures, which are then displayed digitally. The advantages of these machines are that they require little instruction, eliminate observer bias, and can also display heart rate, mean BP, and the time and date, simultaneously. However, they are often very sensitive to movement and can still be inaccurate in patients with irregular heart rhythms such as atrial fibrillation. No stethoscope is needed and therefore this is not an auscultatory method of BP measurement.

All forms of non-invasive BP monitoring have a number of limitations (Box 14.20).

BP cuffs

Some BP cuffs are supplied in two separate parts: the cover (or sheath) and an inner inflatable bladder. Both components should be inspected before use. The cuff should be clean and intact. The tubing attached to both the sphygmomanometer and the inflation bulb should also be intact with no leaks or signs of perishing. Concerns about the use of mercury and aneroid sphygmomanometer equipment were revealed by surveys conducted by Markandu et al (2000) and Thomson et al (2002) who found that:

- The cuff sheaths were often dirty and split
- The rubber bladders had perished and the tubing leaked
- The balloon release valves were leaky or difficult to manoeuvre.

It is important to use the correct size of BP cuff, irrespective of the type of sphygmomanometer used (Table 14.7). The bladder within the cuff should encircle at least 75–80%, but not more than 100%, of the upper arm. The width of the cuff should be more than 50% of the length of the upper arm. An underestimation of BP will be recorded if the cuff is too large; overestimation of BP will occur if the cuff is too small.

Measuring BP

The important points are explained here and the entire process of BP measurement is outlined in Box 14.21. BP in both arms should be measured and recorded on the first visit.

Measuring BP in newborns, infants and children

Although BP may be measured less frequently in children than in adults, further consideration must be given to the following:

- It may be necessary to palpate BP as auscultation of the brachial artery is difficult in babies and small children.
- The lower edge of cuff should be closer to the antecubital fossa.
- The thigh is used to estimate BP in children under 1 year old.
- BP should be recorded when a baby is asleep or resting. Crying, sucking and eating increase BP.
- Allay any anxiety before measurement. Young children may feel more secure if BP is taken while sitting in a parent's lap.

Further information can be found in Trigg and Mohammed (2006).

Inflating the cuff

Inflation of the cuff compresses the brachial artery (see Fig. 14.14). The cuff is inflated automatically when using an electronic sphygmomanometer. When a mercury or aneroid sphygmomanometer is used, the bladder inside the BP cuff is attached to an inflation bulb with a release valve, which allows the cuff to be inflated manually.

Table 14.7 Estimated BP cuff sizes

Indication	Width (cm)	Length (cm)	BHS guidelines Bladder width and length (cm)	Arm circumference (cm)
Small adult/child	10–12	18–24	12 × 18	<23
Standard adult	12–13	23–35	12 × 26	<33
Large adult	12–16	35–40	12 × 40	<50
Adult thigh cuff	20	42		<53

Reproduced with permission from British Hypertension Society (2004).

NURSING SKILLS Box 14.21

Measurement of BP

Equipment
- A sphygmomanometer (see p. 381)
- An appropriately sized cuff (see Table 14.7)
- A stethoscope for auscultatory methods
- An observation chart (see Fig. 14.9) or medical/nursing notes.

Preparation
- Wash hands as per local policy
- BP measurement should be explained, including the feeling of 'tightness' in the arm, and verbal consent obtained; maintain respect and dignity at all times
- The person should be seated, lying supine for at least 5 minutes, or standing for 1 minute before the procedure begins. They should be relaxed and not moving or speaking
- The arm is supported at the level of the heart (mid sternum) and held straight but relaxed, ensuring that no tight clothing constricts the arm
- The cuff (see p. 382) is applied:
  - with the centre of the bladder marked on the cuff over the brachial artery (see Fig. 14.14)
  - with the lower edge of cuff 2–3 cm above pulsation of the brachial artery
  - in mercury and aneroid sphygmomanometers so that the tubing emerges 'up the arm' as movement of the tubing across the antecubital fossa can create artefactual sounds
- If a mercury sphygmomanometer is used, the column of mercury should be vertical and at the observer's eye level. The mercury level must be at zero before measurement and in a position so that it can be easily read by the observer.

Measurement using a mercury or aneroid sphygmomanometer
- Estimate the systolic pressure beforehand by:
  - palpating the brachial artery
  - inflating the cuff using the bulb until pulsation disappears
  - deflating cuff until pulsation is felt; the point at which pulsation appears is an estimate of the systolic pressure
- Then inflate the cuff to 30 mmHg above the systolic level, estimated earlier; at this point the brachial pulse will no longer be felt
- Place the diaphragm of the stethoscope over the brachial artery and slowly deflate the cuff at a rate of 2–3 mm/s until you hear regular tapping sounds – this is phase 1, the systolic pressure (see Fig. 14.15)
- Systolic pressure and diastolic pressure are recorded to the nearest 2 mmHg
- Measure diastolic pressure – phase 4 (see Fig. 14.15): abrupt muffling sounds become soft and blowing in quality just before the sounds disappear (phase 5) – this point is recorded as the diastolic pressure
- Completely deflate and remove the cuff to prevent any further compression of the limb
- It may be necessary to repeat the procedure for both lying and standing positions
- Clean the diaphragm of the stethoscope according to local policy
- Wash hands according to local policy
- Record the pressures heard as soon as possible after assessment, noting the position of the patient/client (lying, standing or sitting down) and the arm used. This may be on an observation chart (see Fig. 14.9) or in the notes
- Report and document any changes/abnormalities.

Note: NICE (2004) recommends that pressures in both arms should be recorded on the first visit and that the arm with the highest BP should be used in future.

[Resources: British Hypertension Society 2004 How to measure blood pressure. Online. Available: www.bhsoc.org; NICE 2004 Hypertension – management of hypertension in adults in primary care. Clinical Guideline 18. Online. Available: www.nice.org.uk/pdf/CG018quickrefguide.pdf Both available July 2006]

Korotkoff sounds

The auscultatory method relies on the detection of a series of sounds. If the mercury or aneroid sphygmomanometer is used, a high-quality stethoscope with clean, well-fitting earpieces is used. Earpieces are placed in the ears pointing towards the nose. The diaphragm is placed on the brachial artery in the antecubital fossa (Fig. 14.14) to listen to sounds in the brachial artery. These are known as Korotkoff sounds, which are divided into five phases (Fig. 14.15). The first phase can be heard as a clear

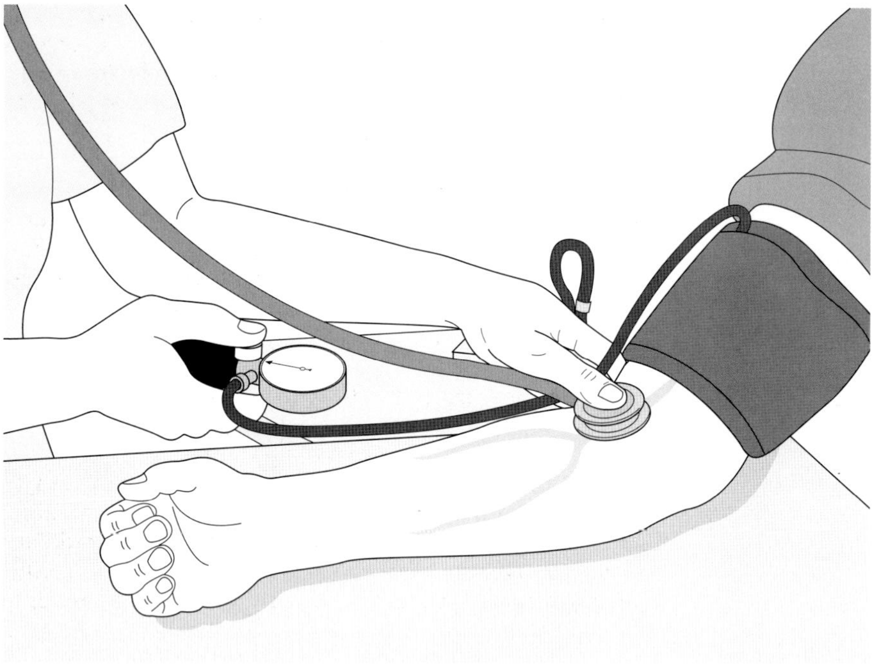

Fig. 14.14 Stethoscope over the brachial artery (adapted with permission from Nicol et al 2004)

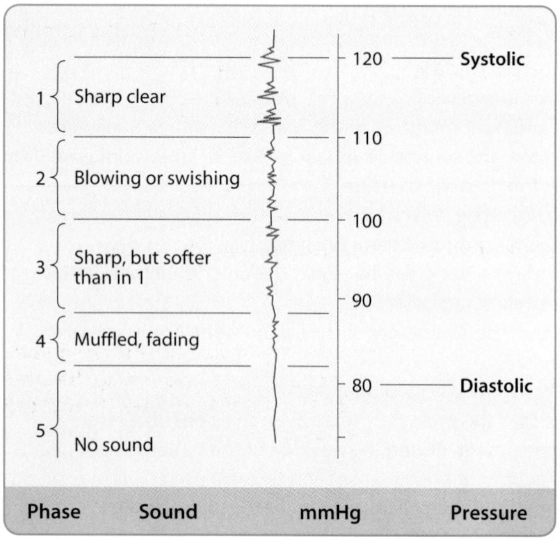

Fig. 14.15 Korotkoff sounds (reproduced with permission from Hinchliffe et al 1996)

tapping noise via the stethoscope as the cuff is deflated. This is the systolic blood pressure and represents phase 1. Muffled whooshing noises are usually heard during phases 2 and 3. The sound becomes much more muffled and softer during phase 4 before it disappears at phase 5. The diastolic pressure is normally recorded at the end of phase 4. However, if the sounds continue until 0 mmHg, then the point at which the sounds change at phase 4 is recorded.

Assessing respirations

The accuracy and frequency of recording of respirations is of vital importance. Respiratory rate recording has been shown to be a crucial indicator of serious deteriorations in health status. Decreases in the respiratory rate (less than 8 breaths per minute) and depth have been noted in the hours preceding cardiopulmonary arrest. It has also been suggested that assessment of respiratory rate is not performed as accurately or as frequently as it should be (Kenward et al 2001). Additionally, there appears to be an overreliance on the use of peripheral oxygen saturation monitors to determine respiratory function (Garrard & Young 1998, McQuillan et al 1998). Analysing and assessing respiratory status requires the observation of several different factors, which are outlined below.

At rest, breathing should be regular, effortless and quiet. However, exercise or breathing difficulties may cause alterations to the rate, depth, rhythm and sound of breathing. Rate and depth of respirations may also change as a result of pain, pyrexia, emotional states and body position, as well as breathing difficulties such as 'shortness of breath' (dyspnoea). They are also influenced by the use of drugs such as nicotine in cigarettes, and opioids, e.g. morphine (see Ch. 23), as well as cocaine and amfetamines. Assessment of respirations is described in Box 14.22.

Respiratory rate

Breathing occurs in cycles. The first phase is inspiration, which is followed by a short pause before expiration (see Ch. 17). The rate and depth of breathing are controlled by the respiratory centre located in the medulla oblongata. Blood levels of carbon dioxide and oxygen, as well as pH (acidity), are the main influences on respiratory rate. Chemoreceptors located in the brain stem, carotid arteries and the aortic arch monitor and respond to changes in the blood levels of carbon dioxide, oxygen and pH. An increase in blood carbon dioxide levels ($PaCO_2$) and a fall in blood pH (increased acidity) activate the chemoreceptors that respond by increasing the respiratory rate,

NURSING SKILLS Box 14.22

Assessing respirations

- The patient should be comfortable and relaxed
- Unusually, the patient is not informed that their respirations are going to be counted
- Accuracy and reliability of measurements are increased by counting for a full minute
- Respiratory rate is recorded over 1 minute by observing the rise and fall of the chest wall. If breathing is shallow, it may be easier to count movements using a hand placed lightly on the chest or abdominal wall although the patient may be aware of this
- Each cycle is counted discreetly (Fig. 14.16), usually after taking the pulse
- Other factors also assessed at this time include:
  - respiratory rhythm (see p. 386)
  - depth of breathing (see p. 386)
  - effort of breathing, e.g. use of accessory muscles (see p. 386)
  - noises associated with breathing (see p. 386)
  - patient's colour, e.g. presence of cyanosis (see Ch. 17)
  - presence of cough or production of sputum (see Ch. 17)
- The respiratory rate is recorded on the observation chart (see Fig. 14.9) or patient/client notes
- Any abnormal findings are reported and recorded in the notes.

which increases the elimination of CO_2 and raises blood pH. Breathing can also be influenced by external factors such as pain, emotion or voluntary control. For more information about breathing and its control, you should consult your physiology textbook.

Counting respiratory rate in adults

Respiratory rate is the number of respirations per minute and is recorded as RR. In adults, the normal adult respiratory rate is 12–18 respirations per minute. Tachypnoea is the term used to describe a respiratory rate that exceeds 20 per minute; absence of breathing is known as apnoea.

Counting respiratory rate in infants and small children

In babies under 12 months old, it is recommended that a stethoscope is used to listen to air movement in the lungs to count the breaths per minute. Average respiratory rates for children are shown in Table 14.8. The child should be relaxed and quiet before measurement is made by lightly placing a hand on their abdomen to count the breaths.

Table 14.8 Children's average respiratory rates

Age (years)	Respirations per minute
Under 1	25–35
1–5	20–30
5–12	20–25
Over 12	15–25

Reproduced with permission from Hull & Johnston (1999).

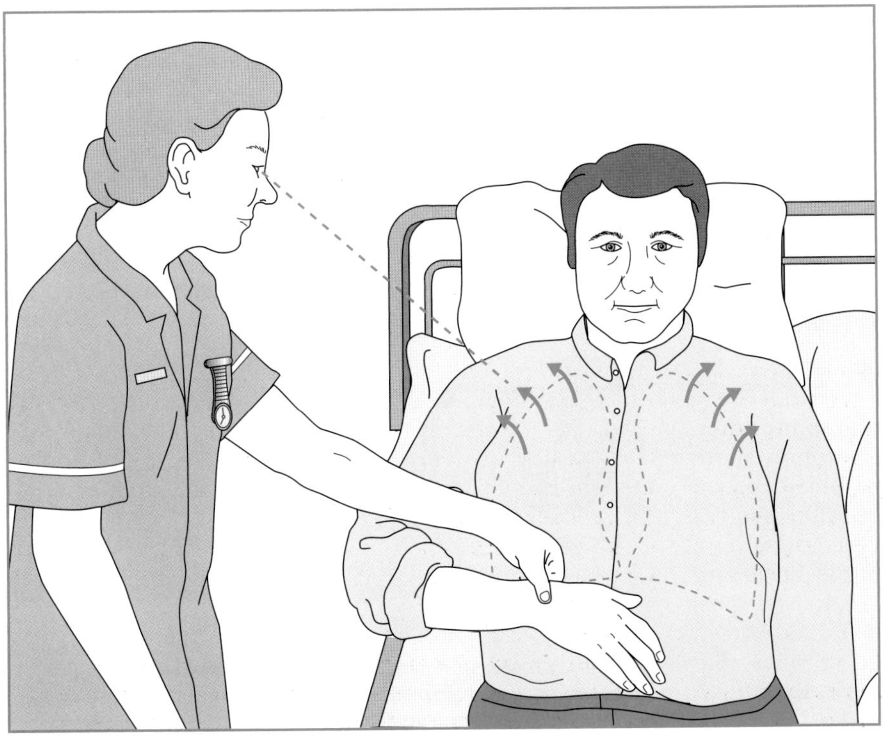

Fig. 14.16 Monitoring the respiration rate while apparently counting the pulse (reproduced with permission from Nicol et al 2004)

If this is not possible, it may be necessary to observe breathing while the child is quietly interacting with a parent or playing.

Respiratory rhythm

Breathing is usually regular in healthy adults. It may be described as regular or irregular and can be influenced, for example, by emotions such as fear or crying and during breath-holding or panic attacks. Babies often have a less regular rhythm, possibly due to incomplete development of the normal respiratory control systems (see Ch. 17).

Abnormal respiratory rhythms

Alterations in rhythm can also be observed in patients with neurological dysfunction that has impaired the respiratory centre within the brain stem.

Damage or poor blood supply to the brain stem can result in an irregular rhythm and rate called Cheyne–Stokes breathing. In this condition breathing patterns change between shallow and slow and deep and rapid, with varying periods of apnoea in between. This type of breathing is often present in the end stages of terminal illness and precedes death.

Depth of breathing

The depth of a breath is determined by the volume of air inhaled. In healthy adults, during relaxed breathing, this is about 500 mL and is called the tidal volume. This and other indicators of respiratory status may also be measured by nurses, especially in people with chronic respiratory conditions such as chronic bronchitis and asthma (see Ch. 17).

The depth of breathing is described as normal, shallow or deep and is observed by watching the rise and fall of the chest wall. These are, however, subjective observations and so open to interpretation. Expansion of both sides of the chest should be the same, i.e. 'equal'.

The term hypoventilation is used to describe shallow slow breathing, which implies limited chest movement. Hyperventilation is used to describe fast and deep breathing, and considerable movement of chest wall may be seen.

Deep, regular breaths may be 'Kussmaul' respirations, caused by an increase in blood acidity (low blood pH). This can arise as a result of uncontrolled diabetes.

Effort of breathing

Normally, at rest, breathing is regular, effortless and quiet. During exercise, the breathing pattern becomes more active as body oxygen demand rises and blood carbon dioxide levels increase (hypercapnia). Exercise involves the movement of more air into and out of the lungs, more quickly and forcibly, and also employs the accessory muscles of respiration, i.e. the internal intercostal muscles and the muscles in the neck and shoulders. Forced expiration is facilitated by the abdominal muscles contracting and pushing the diaphragm upwards. Expiration is no longer passive, but becomes forced.

Noises associated with breathing

Although breathing is normally quiet, alterations to breathing patterns can also include changes to the sound of breathing. Whistling noises called wheezing due to constriction of the airways can be heard on expiration in people with chronic lung disease such as bronchitis or asthma. Obstruction of the larynx results in high-pitched noises during inspiration, which are termed stridor.

Children experiencing breathing difficulties can also develop associated vocal noises such as grunting, wheezing and stridor. In addition, they may hold themselves rigidly, have a retracted neck and nasal flaring (Trigg & Mohammed 2006).

Height and weight

Height and weight parameters are neither vital signs nor physiological indicators of immediate health status although extremes of weight should alert healthcare professionals to associated health risks. Measurement of these parameters should be made on admission to hospital or as part of a community assessment. Body mass index is a useful guide to whether an adult's body weight is appropriate for their height (see Ch. 19). Knowledge of a person's height and weight is needed to calculate drug doses, including anaesthetics, and fluid and nutritional requirements, especially in children. Children may also be regularly weighed and measured to monitor rates of growth and weight gain, which are important in monitoring their health status and development.

The height and weight reference tool used for monitoring children in the UK is the UK90. This tool was devised following a survey of height and weight distribution in children between 1978 and 1990 (Cole et al 2000). A child's height and weight can be compared with normal values from the age of 22 months to the age of 18 or 21 years. The tool also includes normal criteria for head circumference and stage of puberty.

Measuring weight and height

Measuring body weight requires the use of accurate, calibrated scales and is recorded in kilograms (kg). Shoes

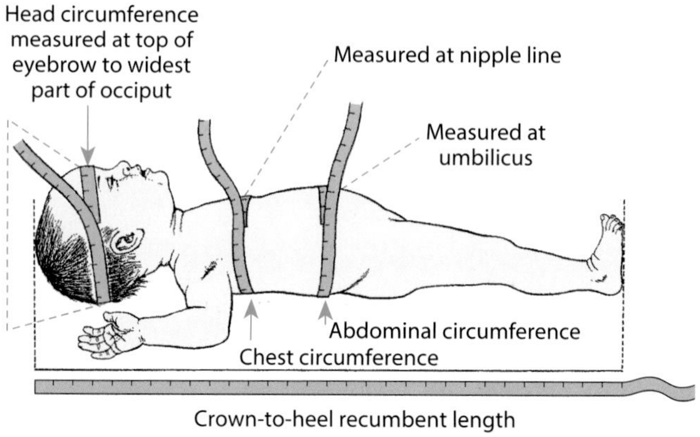

Fig. 14.17 Measurement of head, chest, abdominal circumference and crown to heel length (reproduced with permission from Wong et al 2001)

and excess clothing should be removed and the person is asked to remain still while on the scales until a reading is obtained. Chair or bed scales can be used to estimate weight in people who cannot stand up unaided. If serial measurements are made, this should be at the same time each day or week and in similar clothing. Daily weight may be recorded to assess, for example, fluid loss in response to diuretic drugs. When weight loss is a longer-term goal (e.g. in obesity), it may be monitored weekly.

Height is measured in metres (m), using a fixed measure. Adults and children over the age of 2 years should stand with their back against a wall or scale. The head should be in the midline and the heels, buttocks and backs of shoulders should touch the wall. A moveable rod is placed on the top of the head, parallel to the floor, to assist in reading the measurement. For children under 24 months, their length is measured instead of the height. The child is placed on their back and their head is gently held in the midline. The knees should be held and pushed down until the legs are flat on the table and the child's body is extended (Fig. 14.17). Length, in centimetres (cm), is measured using a measuring tape. In children the circumference of the head, chest and abdomen may also be measured.

Summary

- The nursing process provides a framework for assessing, planning, implementing and evaluating care.
- Assessment is pivotal to the provision of effective nursing care.
- Assessment is a complex activity that requires various nursing skills including observation, measurement, communicating, documenting, interpreting and decision-making.
- Nursing care must be evidence based to meet the aims of clinical governance.
- Approaches to care must be tailored to the needs of groups of people or individuals.
- Assessment of body temperature is required to detect ill health or evaluate patients' progress.
- Methods of thermometry include tympanic, electronic probes and chemical dots. Instruments can be placed in sites such as the ear canal, axilla and mouth, and on skin.
- Assessment of the pulse and BP provides information about general health and cardiovascular status.
- Assessment of respiratory function requires measuring the rate and depth, as well as noting other factors such as effort and noise of breathing.
- Weight and height are not vital signs but are assessed, especially in children, to determine fluid, nutritional or drug requirements.

Self test

1. The first stage of the nursing process is:
   a. Diagnosis
   b. Assessment
   c. Implementation
   d. Planning.

2. The key approach to planning care in mental health and learning disability nursing is:
   a. Family centred
   b. People first
   c. Person centred
   d. Population centred.

3. A tympanic thermometer should not be used in the following situations:
   a. Deafness
   b. Presence of a chest infection
   c. Blood, wax or other material in the auditory canal
   d. Low blood pressure.

4. Cooling strategies such as cool water sponging or fanning can be used to:
   a. Reduce temperature in a person who has warm moist skin
   b. Reduce temperature in a person with cool dry skin

c. Reduce temperature in a person who is having febrile seizures

d. Reduce temperature in a person who has a temperature of 37°C.

5. In health, the normal core temperature range is:

a. 35°–36°C ± 0.2°C

b. 36°–38.5°C ± 0.2°C

c. 37°–38.5°C ± 0.2°C

d. 36.4°–37.3°C ± 0.2°C.

6. You are asked to measure a person's BP. The reading you obtain is 165/98 mmHg. What term should be used to describe this result?:

a. Hypotensive

b. Hypertensive

c. Within the normal range

d. Tachycardia.

7. The same patient appears to be very agitated. He had found it difficult to park his car and was consequently late for his appointment. You measure his radial pulse and find it is 110 beats per minute. What term is used to describe the pulse rate?

a. Bradycardia

b. Apnoea

c. Tachycardia

d. Within the normal range.

8. In a healthy adult what is the normal respiratory rate (in breaths per minute)?:

a. 20–30

b. 25–30

c. 35–40

d. 12–18.

Key words and phrases for literature searching

Assessment tool
Blood pressure
Body core temperature
Holistic assessment
Hypothermia
Nursing history
Nursing model
Nursing process
Person-centred care
Pulse
Pyrexia
Respiratory rate
Sphygmomanometer
Tachycardia
Thermometry
Vital signs

Useful websites

British Hypertension Society	www.bhsoc.org Available July 2006
Person-centred planning	www.nwtdt.com Available July 2006
Tidal model	www.tidal-model.co.uk Available July 2006
Waterlow scale	www.judy-waterlow.co.uk Available July 2006

References

Barker P 1996 Chaos and the way of Zen: psychiatric nursing and the 'uncertainty principle'. Journal of Psychiatric and Mental Health Nursing 3:235–243

Barker P J 2001a Assessment in psychiatric and mental health nursing: in search of the whole person. Nelson Thornes, Cheltenham

Barker P 2001b The tidal model: developing an empowering, person centred approach to recovery within psychiatric and mental health nursing Journal of Psychiatric and Mental Health Nursing 8:233–240

British Hypertension Society 2004 How to measure blood pressure. Online: www.bhsoc.org Available July 2006

Brooker C, Nicol M 2003 Nursing adults: the practice of caring. Mosby, Edinburgh

Casey A 1988 A partnership with child and family. Senior Nurse 8(4):8–9

Chin PL, Kramer MK (eds) 2004 Integrated knowledge development in nursing. 6th edn. Mosby, St Louis

Cole TJ, Bellizzi MC, Flegal KM et al 2000 Establishing a standard definition for child overweight and obesity worldwide: international survey. British Medical Journal 320(7244):1240–1243

Department of Health 2000 The NHS plan: a plan for investment, a plan for reform. TSO, London

Department of Health 2001a Shifting the balance of power. TSO, London

Department of Health 2001b Valuing people: a new strategy for learning disabilities for the 21st century. TSO, London

Department of Health 2003 Getting the right start: National Service Framework for children. TSO, London

Erickson R, Meyer L, Woo TM 1996 Accuracy of chemical dot thermometers in critically ill adults and young children. Journal of Nursing Scholarship 28(1):23–28

Fawcett J 2000 Analysis and evaluation of contemporary nursing knowledge: nursing models and theories. Davies, Philadelphia

Garrard C, Young C 1998 Suboptimal care of patients before admission to intensive care. British Medical Journal 316(7148): 1841–1842

Gates B (ed) 2002 Learning disabilities, toward inclusion. 4th edn. Churchill Livingstone, Edinburgh

Gilbert M, Barton AJ, Counsell CM 2002 Comparison of oral and tympanic temperature in adult surgical patients. Applied Nursing Research 15(1):42–47

Giuliano KK, Giuliano AJ, Scott SS et al 2000 Temperature measurement in critically ill adults: a comparison of tympanic and oral methods. American Journal of Critical Care 9(4):254–261

Henker R, Coyne C 1995 Comparison of peripheral temperature measurements with core temperature. AACN Clinical Issues 6(1):21–30

Hinchliffe SM, Montague SE, Watson R 1996 Physiology for nursing practice. 2nd edn. Baillière Tindall, London
Hull D, Johnston DI 1999 Essential paediatrics. 4th edn. Churchill Livingstone, Edinburgh
Jamieson EM, McCall JM, Whyte LA 2002 Clinical nursing practices, 4th edn. Churchill Livingstone, Edinburgh
Kenward G, Hodgetts T, Castle N 2001 Time to put the R back into TPR. Nursing Times 97(40):32–33
Mackway-Jones K, Molyneux E, Phillips B et al (eds) 2005 Paediatric life support: the practical approach. 4th edn. BMJ Books/Blackwell, Oxford
Markandu ND, Whitcher F, Arnold A et al 2000 The mercury sphygmomanometer should be abandoned before it is proscribed. Journal of Hypertension 14:31–36
McQuillan P, Pilkington S, Alan A et al 1998 Confidential enquiry into quality of care before admission to intensive care. British Medical Journal 316(7148): 1853–1858
Mohun J 2002 First aid manual: the authorised manual of St John Ambulance, St Andrews Ambulance Association and British Red Cross. 8th edn. Dorling Kindersley, London
Nicol M, Bavin C, Bedford-Turner S et al 2004 Essential nursing skills, 2nd edn. Mosby, Edinburgh
NANDA 2001 Nursing diagnosis: definitions and classification 2001–2002. NANDA, Philadelphia
NHS Quality Improvement Scotland 2004 Best practice statement: admissions to adult mental health in-patient services. NHS QIS, Edinburgh
Nursing and Midwifery Council 2004 Code of professional conduct: standards for conduct, performance and ethics. NMC, London
Nursing and Midwifery Council 2005 Guidelines for records and record keeping. NMC, London
O'Brien E, Asmar R, Beilin L et al 2003 European Society of Hypertension recommendations for conventional ambulatory and home blood pressure measurement. Journal of Hypertension 21:821–848
O'Brien J 1987 A guide to personal futures planning. In: Bellamy G, Willcox B (eds) A comprehensive guide to the activities catalogue: an alternative curriculum for youth and adults with severe disabilities. Paul H Brookes, Baltimore
O'Brien J, O'Brien CL (eds) 1998 A little book about person-centred planning. Inclusion Press, Toronto
Peplau HE 1952 Interpersonal relations in nursing. Putnam, New York
Potter P, Schallom M, Davis S et al 2003 Evaluation of chemical dot thermometers for measuring body temperature of orally intubated patients. American Journal of Critical Care 12(5):403–408
Price T, McGloin S, Izzard J et al 2003 Cooling strategies for patients with severe cerebral insult in ICU (Part 2). Nursing in Critical Care 8(1):37–45
Roper N, Logan W, Tierney A 1996 The elements of nursing: a model of nursing based on a model of living. 4th edn. Churchill Livingstone, Edinburgh
Roper N, Logan W, Tierney A 2000 The Roper, Logan and Tierney model of nursing. 5th edn. Churchill Livingstone, Edinburgh
Roy C, Andrews HA 1999 The Roy adaptation model. 2nd edn. Appleton and Lange, Stamford, CT
Scottish Executive 2000 Community care: a joint future. Report of the joint future group. Scottish Executive, Edinburgh
Scottish Executive 2002 Promoting health, supporting inclusion. Scottish Executive, Edinburgh
Scottish Executive 2004 People with learning disabilities in Scotland: health needs assessment report. Scottish Executive, Edinburgh
Scottish Intercollegiate Guidelines Network 2003 The immediate discharge document. SIGN Edinburgh
Smith F 1995 Children's nursing in practice: the Nottingham model. Blackwell, Oxford
Smith L, Coleman V, Bradshaw M (eds) 2002 Family centred care. Palgrave, Basingstoke
Thomson J, Gillespie A, Curzio J 2002 Changes in equipment for blood pressure measurement. Professional Nurse 17(6):350–353
Trigg E, Mohammed T (eds) 2006 Practices in children's nursing: guidelines for hospital and community. 2nd edn. Churchill Livingstone, Edinburgh
Walsh M 1998 Models and critical pathways in nursing: conceptual frameworks for care planning. 2nd edn. Baillière Tindall, London
Waugh A, Grant A 2006 Ross and Wilson's anatomy and physiology in health and illness, 10th edn. Churchill Livingstone, Edinburgh
Welsh Assembly Government 2002 Inclusion, partnership and innovation: a framework for realising the potential of learning disability nursing in Wales. Briefing paper 3. Welsh Assembly, Cardiff
Williams B, Poulter NR, Brown MJ et al 2004 Guidelines for management of hypertension: report of the fourth working party of the British Hypertension Society – BHS IV. Journal of Human Hypertension 18:139–185
Wong DL, Hockenberry-Eaton M, Wilson D et al 2001 Wong's essentials of pediatric nursing. 6th edn. Mosby, St Louis
Yura H, Walsh M 1967 The nursing process. Appleton Century Crofts, Norwalk, CT

Further reading

Brooker C, Nicol M 2003 Nursing adults: the practice of caring. Mosby, Edinburgh
Cook K, Montgomery H 2006 Assessment. In: Trigg E, Mohammed T (eds) Practices in children's nursing: guidelines for hospital and community. 2nd edn. Churchill Livingstone, Edinburgh, Chapter 3
Edwards S 2003 Temperature regulation. In: Brooker C, Nicol M (eds) Nursing adults: the practice of caring. Mosby, Edinburgh, pp. 75–92
Holland K, Jenkins J, Solomon J, Whittam S (eds) 2003 Applying the Roper, Logan and Tierney model in practice. Churchill Livingstone, Edinburgh
Jamieson EM, McCall JM, Whyte LA 2002 Clinical nursing practices. 4th edn. Churchill Livingstone, Edinburgh
Middleton S, Roberts A 2000 Integrated care pathways: a practical approach to implementation. Butterworth-Heinemann, Oxford
Nicol M, Brooker C, Meyer J 2003 Adult nursing: setting the scene. In: Brooker C, Nicol M (eds) Nursing adults: the practice of caring. Mosby, Edinburgh
Nicol M, Bavin C, Bedford-Turner S et al 2004 Essential nursing skills. 2nd edn. Mosby, Edinburgh
Waugh A, Grant A 2006 Ross and Wilson anatomy and physiology in health and illness. 10th edn. Churchill Livingstone, Edinburgh

Preventing the spread of infection

15

Kate Rennie-Meyer

Glossary terms

Aseptic technique
Colonization
Commensal
Disinfection
Fomite
Healthcare-associated infection
Normal flora
Nosocomial infection
Opportunistic infection
Resident flora
Sterilization
Transient flora

Learning outcomes

This chapter will help you:

- Explain the relationship between microorganisms and infectious diseases
- Distinguish nosocomial, community-acquired and iatrogenic infections
- Describe the components of the chain of infection and give examples of factors involved at each stage
- Define common terminology related to infectious diseases
- Identify the key elements of standard infection control precautions and additional precautions
- Explain how and when standard precautions are used in nursing practice
- Describe the purpose of the different types of isolation precautions
- Explain the principles of aseptic technique
- Outline the nurse's role in specimen collection

Introduction

Infections acquired as a result of healthcare have a major impact on patients/clients and healthcare providers. For patients/clients an infection causes anxiety and discomfort, delays recovery and may result in long-term morbidity (ill health) or even death. Quality healthcare is a basic expectation; the public and government reasonably expect that people will not acquire disease because of their treatment or care. Control of infection is a responsibility shared by all healthcare personnel; however, nurses stand in the front line because of their close 'hands on' contact with patients/clients. Therefore, nurses in all areas of clinical practice including hospitals, residential homes, health centres and people's homes provide care for those who are at risk of infection or those who already have an infection. The Nursing and Midwifery Council *Code of professional conduct: standards for conduct, performance and ethics* (NMC 2004) requires nurses to ensure that no action they undertake is detrimental to the safety and well-being of those in their care. Nurses must therefore understand why infections occur, how they are transmitted, and the precautions and methods necessary to prevent the development and spread of infection.

This chapter provides an overview of microorganisms and outlines the incidence of some infectious diseases. It considers the sequence of events that spread infectious diseases and the key features of disease development. The body's defence mechanisms are briefly considered. The next section focuses on the practices required to prevent and control the spread of infection, exploring standard infection control precautions and then additional precautions, including isolation precautions and aseptic technique. Finally, it examines the nurse's role in the collection of microbiology specimens for the laboratory.

Overview of microbiology

Microorganisms are tiny living organisms only visible under a microscope, apart from some fungi. Categories of microorganisms include algae, fungi, protozoa, bacteria, mycoplasma, rickettsia, chlamydia, viruses and prions. Microorganisms are found in:

- Soil
- Water
- Air

- Vegetable matter
- Animals and humans.

For microorganisms to survive in any environment, they must have suitable physical and chemical conditions, nutrients and freedom from hostile competitors. The human body is populated by an extraordinary number of microorganisms, an estimated 1×10^{14} bacteria compared to 1×10^{13} body cells (Tortora et al 2003). These microorganisms (referred to as normal flora or commensals) can benefit the host by providing nutrients, aiding in food digestion and preventing the establishment of more dangerous microorganisms. Normal flora do not populate the entire human body but are located in certain regions, e.g. the skin, mucous membranes and the intestinal tract. Some areas of the body are completely devoid of microbial populations, e.g. the urinary tract, blood and the lungs.

Epidemiology of infectious diseases

Infectious diseases are caused by microorganisms and those that cause infectious disease are known as pathogens. An infectious disease that is transmissible from one person to another is called a communicable disease. Communicable diseases range from relatively mild illnesses such as the common cold to debilitating and lethal conditions such as human immunodeficiency virus/acquired immune deficiency syndrome (HIV/AIDS), tuberculosis and malaria which together accounted for 5.7 million deaths in 2001 (World Health Organization [WHO] 2002). Communicable diseases are categorized according to their frequency and distribution:

- *Endemic*: Always present within a population of a particular geographic region. The number of cases may fluctuate over time, but the disease never dies out completely. Examples include tuberculosis, sexually transmitted infections, chickenpox and mumps.
- *Epidemic*: The sudden outbreak of an infectious disease that spreads rapidly through a population, affecting a large number of people at the same time, e.g. influenza. In hospitals, an epidemic does not necessarily involve large numbers and is recognized when two or more patients in the same ward/unit are infected by the same organism (The Scottish Office 1999).
- *Pandemic*: A disease of epidemic proportions that occurs in many countries simultaneously. HIV is pandemic in that an estimated 34–46 million people worldwide are infected (WHO 2002).

Healthcare-associated infections

Infectious diseases (infections) can be divided into two categories:

- Healthcare-associated infections, also known as nosocomial infections – those acquired within hospitals or other care facilities
- Community-acquired infections – those acquired outside healthcare facilities.

A hospitalized patient may have either type. Community-acquired infections are those that are present or incubating at the time of hospital admission whereas a healthcare-associated infection manifests itself 72 hours or more after admission, and includes infections not apparent until after discharge (Scottish Executive 2002).

Incidence of healthcare-associated infections

In England, healthcare-associated infections account for 5000 deaths per year and are also a significant contributing factor in a further 15000 deaths annually (DH 2003). Approximately 9% of patients entering Scottish hospitals will develop one or more infections during their hospitalization. This is equivalent to over 33000 infections a year (NHS Quality Improvement Scotland 2003). The growing resistance of many microorganisms to antibiotic drugs has exacerbated this situation, making treatment of infections increasingly difficult.

Types and incidence of healthcare-associated infections

Infections resulting from surgical or medical treatment are called iatrogenic infections. In hospitalized patients, iatrogenic infections are frequently attributed to invasive procedures and indwelling medical devices which bypass the body's first line of defence (Fig. 15.1).

Chain of infection

The spread of infectious diseases follows a well-known sequence of events that can be compared to a chain with six links, frequently referred to as the 'chain of infection' (see Fig. 15.2). If all links remain intact and in the correct sequence, then the infection will be transmitted. An infection will not result if the sequence is interrupted. Understanding the characteristics of each link of the chain provides the fundamental knowledge necessary to prevent and control infection.

Infectious agent (pathogen)

The relationship between humans and microorganisms is usually one of balanced conflicts between the host's ability to resist infection and the ability of the microorganism to cause disease. Some microbial species are very adept at avoiding or surviving the body's defence mechanisms. For example, some possess surface structures that attach and anchor them to host cells. Others produce toxins (poisons) that target specific body cells and tissues. A few species manufacture enzymes that dissolve the host's tissues, e.g. necrotizing fasciitis – 'flesh-eating bacteria'.

Reservoirs

The place(s) where pathogens are provided with nutrients and suitable environmental conditions for their survival and multiplication is called the reservoir. Reservoirs may be human, animal or non-living (see Fig. 15.2). However, the principal reservoirs for most infectious diseases are human carriers. A carrier is a person who is, or has been, colonized with a particular pathogen and can transmit it

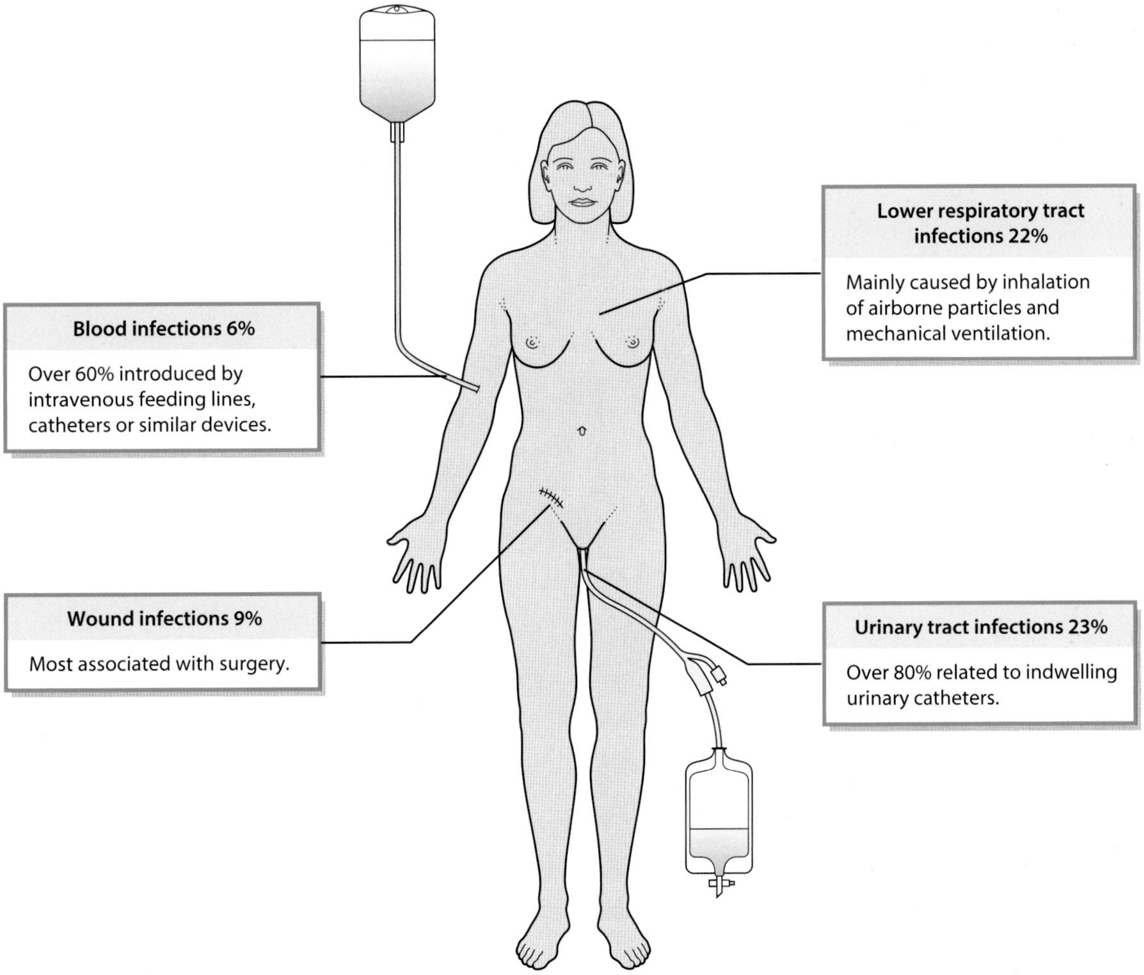
Lower respiratory tract infections 22%
Mainly caused by inhalation of airborne particles and mechanical ventilation.
Blood infections 6%
Over 60% introduced by intravenous feeding lines, catheters or similar devices.
Wound infections 9%
Most associated with surgery.
Urinary tract infections 23%
Over 80% related to indwelling urinary catheters.

Fig. 15.1 Types and incidence of healthcare-associated infections

to others who may then become ill. Various carrier states exist:

- *Temporary*: Usually occurs during the incubation period of infectious diseases, e.g. a person exposed to mumps begins to shed infectious viruses about 48 hours before the first symptoms appear. Those with clinical signs and symptoms of an infectious disease are obvious reservoirs who can transmit the pathogen to others. Pathogens may continue to be shed during the convalescent period that follows the disappearance of symptoms.
- *Asymptomatic*: These carriers shed infectious microorganisms but have never shown any clinical signs and symptoms of the disease. In these cases the carrier seeks no medical attention and takes no precautions against transmission. For example, a third of women infected with gonorrhoea remain asymptomatic (Gould & Brooker 2000) and, unaware that they have the disease, remain untreated and therefore continue to infect other people.
- *Active*: Individuals who have completely recovered from a disease but continue to harbour the pathogen. Active carriers may shed organisms for long periods of time, e.g. carriers of *Salmonella typhi* (that causes typhoid fever) may shed the bacterium for their entire lives. Carriers of hepatitis B maintain the virus in their bloodstream and can transmit the disease to others by items contaminated with their blood or body fluids.

Humans can also become infected with microorganisms that are part of their own normal flora. This is referred to as an endogenous infection and occurs when the normal flora that inhabit one site are transferred to another, e.g. when microorganisms from the colon gain access to the normally sterile urinary tract and cause a urinary tract infection.

Portals of exit and entry

The portal of exit is the route by which a pathogen leaves its reservoir. Some pathogens may leave the host using more than one exit route, e.g. the chickenpox virus exits via respiratory droplets and secretions from skin lesions. Portal of entry refers to the path by which an infectious agent invades a new host. The portal of entry is usually the same as the portal of exit (see Fig. 15.2).

Transmission of infection

To cause disease, a pathogen must be able to survive transfer from its reservoir to a susceptible host. Transmission of pathogens can occur by five main routes (see Fig. 15.2).

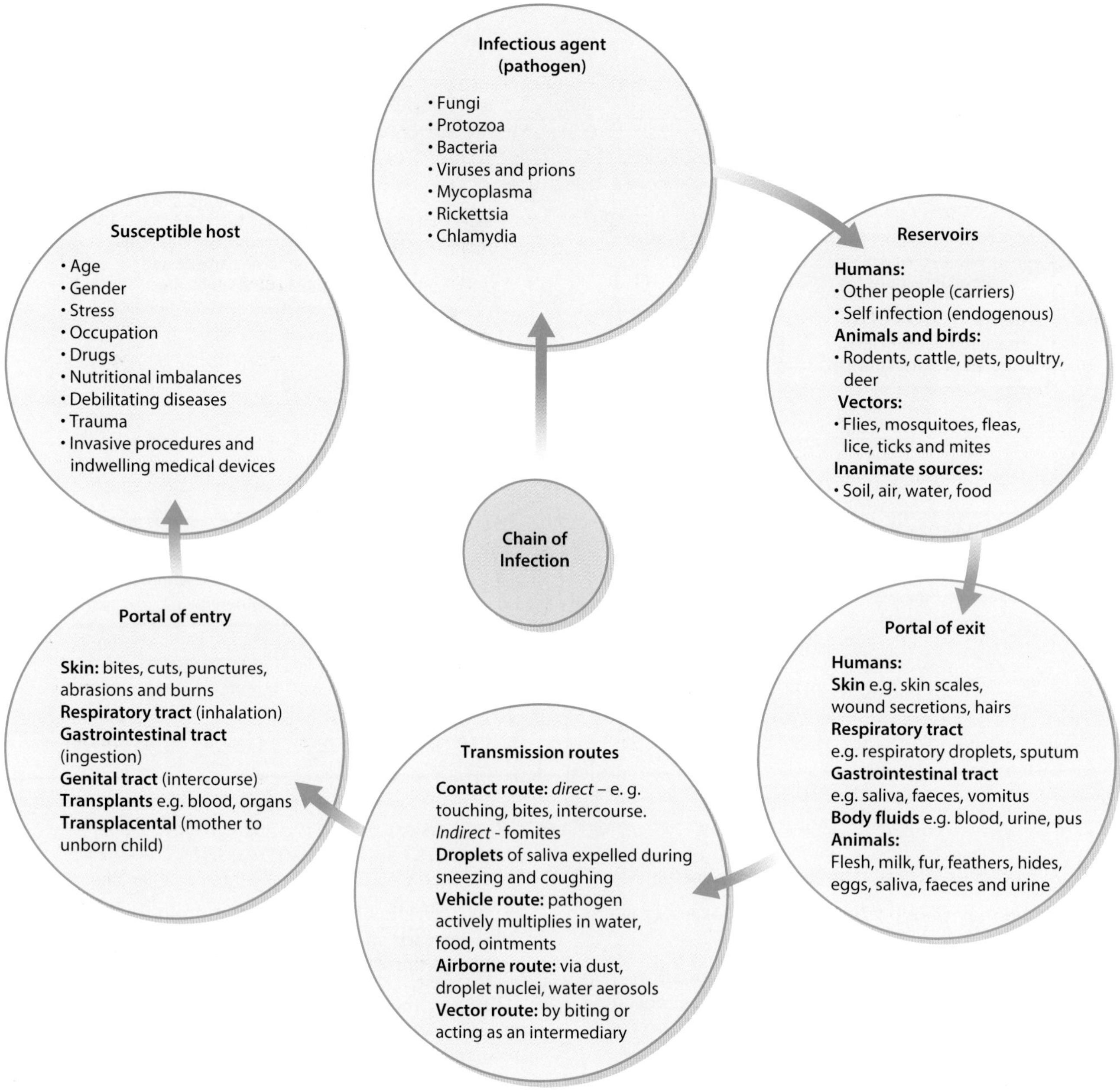

Fig. 15.2 Chain of infection

In healthcare-associated infections the following routes are frequently implicated.

Contact transmission

This is direct, when pathogens are transferred by bodily contact between an infected and uninfected person, e.g. to nurses during bathing or when turning people. Contact transmission may also be indirect, when fomites (inanimate objects) act as an intermediary in the transfer of pathogens, e.g. contaminated instruments or needles. Contaminated hands of healthcare personnel may also transmit infection indirectly and proper handwashing and changing of gloves between patient contacts are essential to prevent transmission of infection by this route.

Droplet transmission

This occurs when an infected person (the reservoir) releases contaminated respiratory secretions into the air when coughing, sneezing and talking, or is subjected to procedures such as suctioning and bronchoscopy. Infected respiratory droplets are propelled short distances (usually a metre or less) and can enter the nasal passages, mouth and conjunctiva of another person, or they can settle on inanimate objects in close proximity to the infected person.

Airborne transmission

This route involves the dissemination of tiny dried particles (usually 5 μm or less) of evaporated respiratory

Box 15.1 **Susceptible hosts**

Age
Congenital infections develop during gestation, while neonatal infections occur in the first 28 days of life. The source of the microorganisms may be the mother's vaginal flora, other infected neonates in a baby unit or the hands of hospital staff. As children grow up, they encounter an increasing variety of social environments and may consequently develop common childhood infections. At the other end of the age spectrum, older adults are prone to infections, mainly due failing immune responses and chronic or debilitating diseases.

Gender
Anatomical differences between males and females explain why urinary tract infections are more common in females than males because the shorter female urethra provides microorganisms with easier access to the bladder (see Ch. 20).

Stress
Prolonged physical or emotional stress alters the body's hormonal balance and reduces resistance to disease. Stress increases the output of cortisol from the adrenal cortex, which suppresses both inflammatory and immune processes. Stress-compromised people often suffer outbreaks of oral or genital herpes lesions or become susceptible to more severe diseases (see Ch. 11).

Occupation
Infectious disease is a persistent hazard of certain occupations, usually when there is increased exposure to pathogens rather than diminished host resistance. Healthcare professionals are frequently exposed to patients/clients shedding virulent human pathogens, veterinary surgeons, agricultural workers and those working in meat processing industries are likely to have a higher incidence of diseases spread by animals and sex industry workers are prone to infections transmitted by sexual intercourse.

Drugs
Both recreational and prescribed drugs can increase susceptibility to infection:

- *Smoking* predisposes to respiratory infections by damaging the epithelium
- *Alcohol*, in excess, increases susceptibility
- *Corticosteroid drugs* suppress inflammatory and immune responses
- *Antibiotic drugs* destroy the normal body flora, encouraging superinfection by extraneous microorganisms
- *Immunosuppressant drugs* lessen the risk of organ rejection following transplantation; however, they suppress the immune response, leaving the person susceptible to opportunistic infections.

Nutritional imbalance
Infections may also be linked to vitamin and protein deficiencies, and this might partly explain why many infectious diseases are higher in parts of the world where undernutrition is widespread.

Debilitating diseases or trauma
Normal defences can be delayed or suppressed by debilitating diseases, e.g. leukaemia, diabetes, kidney and liver diseases, and AIDS. The risk of infection may be increased by some therapies, e.g. radiotherapy and chemotherapy, which can severely depress white blood cell counts. Trauma, e.g. burns, damages the body's surface defences, predisposing to invasion by microorganisms.

secretions (called droplet nuclei). In contrast to droplet transmission in which the particles travel only short distances, in airborne transmission the particles may remain suspended in the air for long periods and can be widely dispersed on air currents. When inhaled by susceptible people, their small size allows them to penetrate the lungs from where they can initiate infection. In hospitals, special air handling and ventilation systems are required to contain infections transmitted by this route.

Susceptible host

The human body has numerous defence mechanisms for resisting the entry and multiplication of pathogens (see Fig. 15.4, p. 398). These mechanisms normally prevent infection unless the pathogen is particularly virulent (liable to cause disease). Lack of resistance to infectious diseases is known as susceptibility. A number of factors reduce an individual's resistance to infectious diseases (Box 15.1). Hospitalized patients are especially susceptible to contracting infections because of their underlying disease, drugs that they may be receiving such as antimicrobial or immunosuppressive agents and procedures that breach the skin and mucous membranes, e.g. surgery, the insertion of indwelling urinary catheters or intravenous catheters (see Box 15.2).

Infectious disease process and associated terminology

There are several possible outcomes when an individual encounters pathogenic microorganisms:

- The pathogen may be eliminated by the body's defence mechanisms
- It may reside in the body without causing any symptoms of disease (colonization)

CRITICAL THINKING Box 15.2

Salmonella food poisoning

Salmonella food poisoning can cause outbreaks of infection in the community and in healthcare premises such as hospitals. The illness is usually self-limiting and short lived but in a proportion of people (usually at the extremes of life) the illness can be life threatening.

In 1984 an outbreak of salmonella food poisoning occurred at a psychiatric hospital in Wakefield, affecting 355 patients and 109 staff. Many of the patients were elderly and 19 died. The investigation that followed traced the source to cold roast beef. The meat had been removed from the kitchen refrigerator in the morning, sliced and then left out for 10 hours before being served.

Between December 2001 and January 2002 an outbreak of salmonella infection occurred in a ward at a busy general hospital in Glasgow, affecting eight patients and two members of staff. Three of the elderly patients consequently died. An investigation into the outbreak (Scottish Executive Health Department 2002) identified that the source of the infection was likely to have been a patient who had the infection on admission. The infection was likely to have then been transmitted to the other patients by one or more of the following routes:

- Patient-to-patient or staff-to-patient contact
- Through inadequately decontaminated equipment and environment
- By contamination of food at ward level and subsequent storage at unsatisfactory temperatures.

Student activities

- Explain why older adults are more susceptible to infection.
- What was the main entry route for this infection?
- How would the pathogen exit the host?
- What measures should have been implemented to prevent the spread of this infection?

- If the pathogen successfully invades and multiplies it will cause an infectious disease.

Infectious diseases are often classified according to their severity, duration and the extent by which they spread throughout the body:

- *Local infection*: Occurs when pathogens are limited to a single body site or system. The signs and symptoms vary depending on the system affected (Box 15.3).
- *Systemic infection*: Pathogens spread from the site of entry via the blood or lymphatic vessels to other tissues and organs. In diseases such as measles and chickenpox, the viruses initially invade the upper respiratory tract and then spread to the skin causing a rash and skin vesicles, respectively.
- *Opportunistic infection*: Arises from microorganisms which are not normally pathogenic in healthy people. However, in those whose immune system has been compromised by illness, treatments or invasive procedures, the normally harmless microorganisms may become pathogenic. Hospitalized patients are especially susceptible to these infections and may need to be nursed in a protected environment (see 'Protective isolation', p. 418).
- *Acute infectious disease*: Develops quickly but lasts for a relatively short period of time, e.g. influenza. Usually follows a set pattern comprising four stages: incubation, prodromal, illness and convalescence (Box 15.4).
- *Chronic infectious disease*: Progresses slowly and has a long and often indeterminate duration, e.g. tuberculosis, hepatitis C, syphilis.
- *Latent infectious disease*: Arises from microorganisms that remain dormant in the body for long periods, but then become active (usually when the person is experiencing physical or psychological stress), e.g. the herpes virus which causes cold sores and the chickenpox virus that may re-emerge later in life causing shingles.

Sometimes it is difficult to detect an infection, for example, in the very young, older adults, those with communication problems and people with mental health problems or a learning disability. The expected signs of infection may not always be obvious and therefore nurses need to be alert to subtle changes in behaviour that may indicate presence of an infection (Box 15.5).

Box 15.3 **Characteristics of local infections**

System affected	Signs and symptoms
Skin	Inflammation: redness, pain, swelling and heat
Respiratory tract	Increased respiratory tract secretions Cough Sore throat Difficulty in breathing (dyspnoea)
Urinary tract	Pain on passing urine (dysuria) Frequency Urgency Urine appears cloudy, possibly 'bloody' and may have a 'fishy' smell
Gastrointestinal tract	Abdominal pain Nausea Vomiting Diarrhoea Poor appetite
Central nervous system	Confusion Drowsiness Stiff neck Headache Intolerance of light (photophobia)

Box 15.4

The four phases of an acute infectious disease

1. *Incubation*: The incubation period is the interval between contact with the pathogen and the development of the symptoms and signs of disease. In some diseases the incubation period is always the same whereas, in others, it is variable, e.g. the common cold: 1–2 days; influenza: 1–3 days; tetanus: ranges from 2 to 21 days. During this period there are no signs or symptoms.
2. *Prodromal*: During this time the person feels 'out of sorts' but is not yet experiencing actual symptoms of the disease. Early signs and symptoms are present but are vague, e.g. fatigue or malaise, mild fever, and some may feel that they are 'coming down with something'.
3. *Illness*: The illness period, or acute phase, is when signs and symptoms of the disease are present, e.g. fever, muscle pains, photophobia, sore throat.
4. *Convalescence*: As the patient's immune response and other defence mechanisms overcome the pathogen, the person gradually regains strength and health is usually restored. Sometimes the convalescent period can be lengthy and, although the individual may recover from the illness itself, permanent damage can be caused by destruction of tissues in the affected area, e.g. deafness may follow middle ear infections.

REFLECTIVE PRACTICE Box 15.5

Changes in behaviour indicative of an infectious disease

Student activity

Consider the changes in behaviour that may be exhibited by the following clients during the prodromal stage of an acute infectious disease:

- A 4-year-old boy
- An adult with a moderate learning disability.

Host defence mechanisms

If microorganisms never encountered resistance from the host, then people would be constantly ill and die from infectious diseases, and eventually the human race would become extinct. In most cases, however, host defence mechanisms are very effective at keeping microbial invaders out. They can be thought of as an army consisting of three lines of defence. If the enemy (the pathogen) breaks through the first line of defence, it will encounter and hopefully be stopped by the second line of defence. If the pathogen manages to escape the first two lines of defence, there is a third line ready to attack it.

The first two lines of defence are referred to as non-specific resistance and are ways in which the body attempts to protect itself against injury and all substances that are harmful to it including pathogenic microorganisms. These comprise external defences and the inflammatory process (see below). The third line of defence is specific to particular microorganisms (called specific resistance) and involves white blood cells (B- and T-lymphocytes) and the production of antibodies that protect the host from one particular foreign substance (see Fig. 15.3).

External defences

The integrity of body surfaces forms an effective barrier to the initial lodgement or penetration by microorganisms. This first line of defence to microbial invasion depends on mechanical, chemical and microbial barriers that combat any attack (see Fig. 15.4).

Inflammation

Inflammation is the second line of defence and is triggered when injury or infection damages tissues. The cardinal signs of inflammation are:

- Redness
- Swelling
- Heat
- Pain.

Loss of function can also occur as a consequence of swelling and pain. In apparent contradiction to the signs and symptoms observed, the inflammatory response is beneficial because it attempts to initially destroy the pathogen and then, if possible, remove it and its by-products from the body. Inflammation limits spread in the body by confining the agent to one specific area. Finally, the process repairs and replaces damaged tissues.

Specific resistance

The third line of defence is the body's immune response, which is triggered when antigens enter the body. An antigen is any material that the body recognizes as foreign, including pathogenic microorganisms, pollen, dust, food components, drugs, insect venom and transplanted tissues. Two processes work together to combat and destroy a specific antigen: cell-mediated immunity and humoral immunity.

This type of immunity results in the production of antibodies and usually confers lifelong resistance to the antigen. For further discussion of these processes, readers should consult their anatomy and physiology textbook.

Development of immunity

The formation of antibodies is the basis of immunization against disease and can be either active or passive.

Active immunity

This provides long-term protection against specific microorganisms. It occurs following an infectious disease when

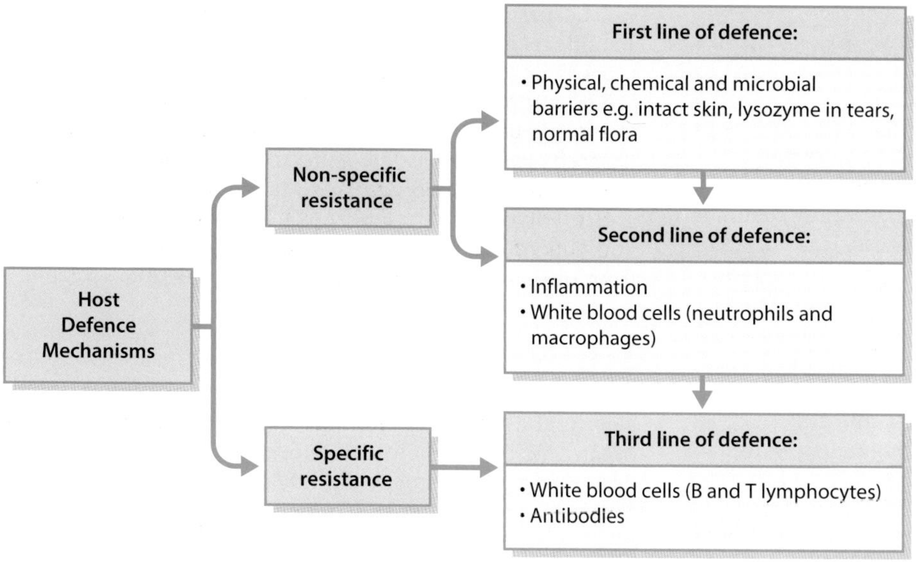

Fig. 15.3 Overview of the defence mechanisms

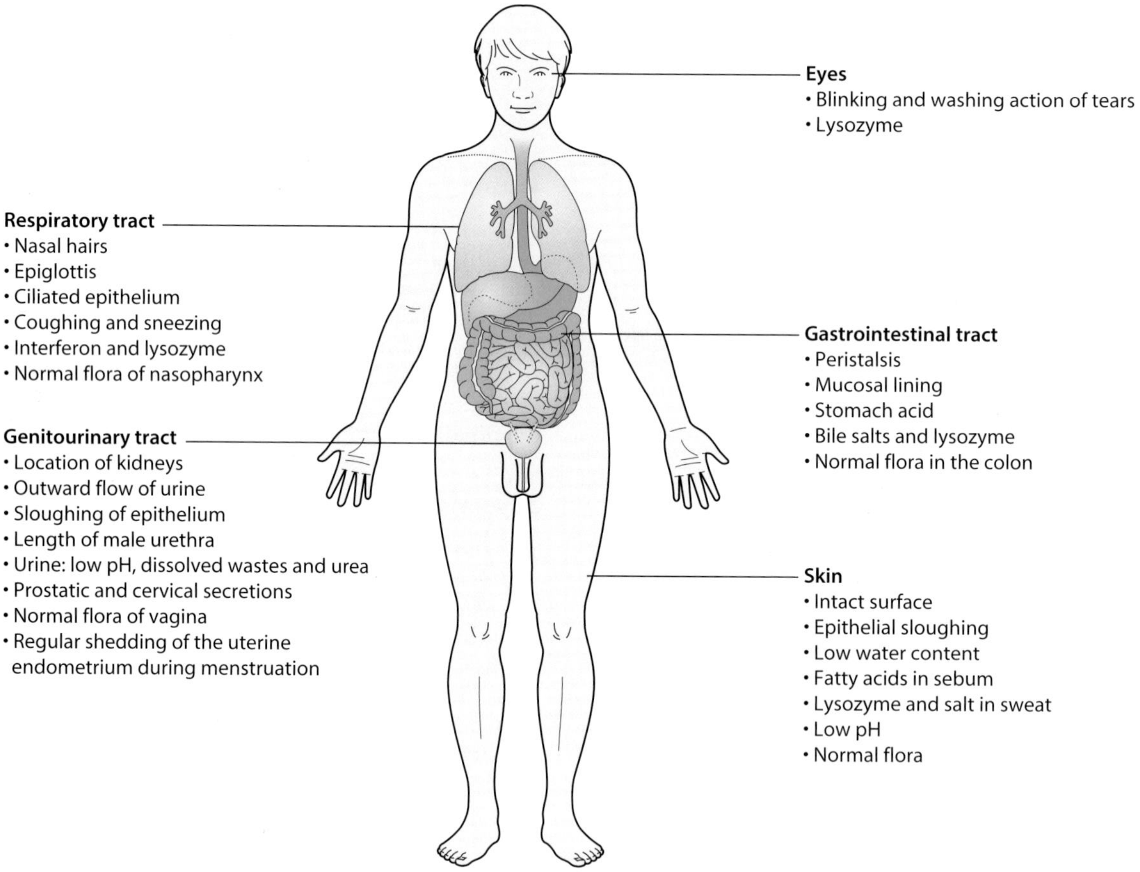

Fig. 15.4 First lines of defence against infection

antibodies are produced within the body (called natural active immunity) or when the person receives a vaccine which stimulates the immune system to produce specific antibodies against a particular agent (called artificial active immunity) (Box 15.6).

Passive immunity

This provides temporary protection against micro-organisms. *Natural passive immunity* is acquired by the developing fetus when it receives maternal antibodies in utero, or by baby when it receives maternal antibodies

> **CRITICAL THINKING** Box 15.6
>
> **Childhood immunization**
>
> After reading adverse publicity about the measles, mumps and rubella (MMR) vaccine, a mother is concerned about having her child vaccinated.
>
> **Student activities**
>
> - Identify accurate sources of information about this topic.
> - At what age is the vaccine given?
> - Consider how you would deal with this situation.

contained in colostrum and breast milk. *Artificial passive immunity* is acquired when a person receives antibodies contained in anti-sera or gamma globulin, e.g. hepatitis B immune globulin is given to protect those who have been exposed to the hepatitis B virus.

Infection control

Infection control refers to the numerous measures that are taken to prevent infections from occurring in healthcare facilities and aims to destroy or remove sources of pathogenic microorganisms by:

- Interrupting the transmission of pathogens
- Protecting people from becoming infected.

These measures break links in the chain of infection. Two tiers of infection control measures are in operation:

- Standard precautions are used for the care of all hospitalized patients at all times, regardless of their diagnosis or presumed infection status (infection is not always detected) and are sometimes referred to as 'universal infection control precautions', 'standard infection control precautions' or 'standard principles'. They reduce the risk of transmission of pathogens present in blood, body fluids, secretions and excretions, non-intact skin and mucous membranes.
- Additional precautions are necessary during clinically invasive procedures (referred to as aseptic technique), e.g. surgery or insertion of an intravenous cannula or urinary catheter. They are also required to prevent the spread of communicable diseases that are transmitted by airborne, droplet or contact routes. These are referred to as 'isolation precautions' and are always used in conjunction with standard precautions. An overview of the principles of infection control is shown in Figure 15.5.

Standard precautions

This section explores standard precautions, which provide guidelines on:

- Hand hygiene
- Personal protective equipment, e.g. gloves, aprons, masks
- Safe use and disposal of sharps
- Safe management of waste and linen
- Decontamination of patient-care equipment (i.e. cleaning, sterilizing, disinfecting).

Hand hygiene

Many infections are spread by contact and the hands are the major vehicles in transfer of potential pathogens in healthcare settings from:

- One patient/client to another
- A contaminated object to a patient/client
- Healthcare personnel to a patient/client or vice versa.

In the mid-19th century, studies by both Ignaz Semmelweis and Oliver Wendell Holmes identified handwashing as the most important feature in preventing transmission of infection in healthcare facilities. Infection control guidelines from national and international organizations have repeatedly acknowledged and supported the view that handwashing remains the most effective measure in reducing the incidence of healthcare-associated infections.

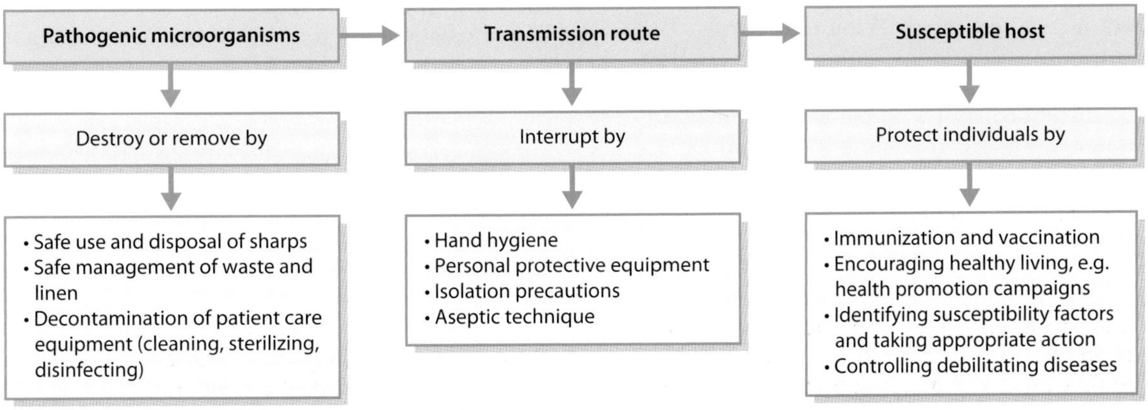

Fig. 15.5 Principles of infection control

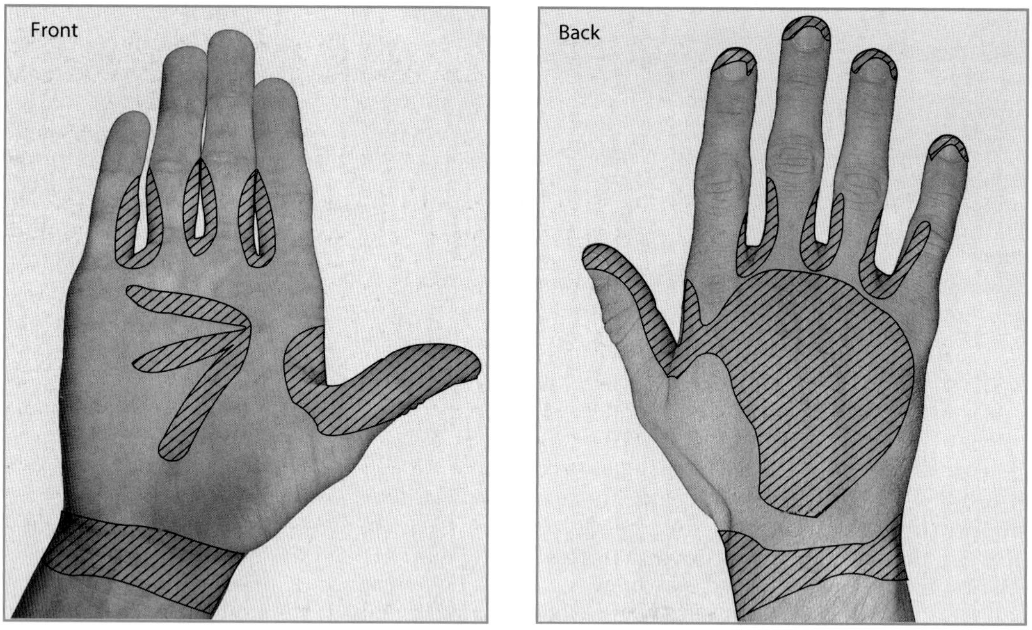

Fig. 15.6 Areas of hands prone to harbouring microorganisms (reproduced with permission from Inglis 2003)

REFLECTIVE PRACTICE Box 15.7

When is handwashing necessary?

Student activities

- Make a list of the times when you wash your hands while on placement.
- Check your answers by consulting Box 13.21 (p. 337).
- Identify any times when your current practice of handwashing requires adjustment.

The purpose of handwashing is to remove potentially pathogenic microorganisms from the skin, of which there are two categories:

- Resident microorganisms (normal flora) that are difficult to remove as they reside in the deep layers of the skin, hair follicles and sebaceous glands (see Ch. 16)
- Transient microorganisms, which represent recent contamination of the hands. They usually colonize the superficial layers of the skin and are acquired during contact with patients/clients and contaminated objects. Transient microorganisms found on the hands of healthcare personnel are frequently implicated as the source of healthcare-associated infections. Fortunately, they are easily removed by routine handwashing (Centers for Disease Control and Prevention [CDC] 2002).

Indications for handwashing

Hands must be washed whenever there is a chance that they may have become contaminated and any time when there is a risk of transmitting infection to others.

Figure 15.6 shows the areas of hands prone to harbouring microorganisms. It is important to be aware that handwashing is one of the most important infection prevention practices and, if not washed at appropriate times, the hands can put patients, residents and clients at risk (Box 15.7). Furthermore, contaminated hands can be a danger not only to the practitioner but also to their colleagues, friends and family members.

Types of handwashing and preparations used

There are three types of hand hygiene used in clinical settings, each of which uses different preparations and is appropriate in different situations.

Handwashing with plain soap and running water (social handwashing)

Plain soap has detergent properties and effectively removes dirt, most organic substances and transient flora from the skin. Handwashing with plain soap and water for 10–15 seconds and rinsing in running water is used routinely in clinical areas (Box 15.8). If the hands are heavily soiled with dirt, blood or other organic material, e.g. when gloves have been torn, handwashing for several minutes may be necessary. It important to recognize that some bacteria grow on soap bars, especially if they are allowed to remain wet (Hateley 2003). Soap bars must therefore be kept dry or liquid soap from a dispenser used instead.

Handwashing with antiseptic preparations and running water (aseptic handwashing)

Antiseptic preparations, e.g. chlorhexidine, povidone-iodine and triclosan, have the same action as plain soap with the additional benefit of killing or inhibiting the growth of resident microorganisms. Some antiseptics continue to perform these actions for several hours after

NURSING SKILLS Box 15.8

Handwashing

Prerequisites to handwashing

- Remove wrist and hand jewellery prior to handwashing because it harbours dirt and the skin underneath is more heavily colonized with bacteria
- Keep nails short as skin below the fingernails harbours high concentrations of bacteria
- Avoid wearing artificial nails, extensions or chipped nail polish, all of which have been shown to increase bacterial counts and impede visualization of dirt under the nails (CDC 2002, NICE 2003).

Handwashing with soap and water

Hands are rubbed together vigorously for a minimum of 10–15 seconds, paying particular attention to the tips of the fingers, thumbs and areas between the fingers (see below).

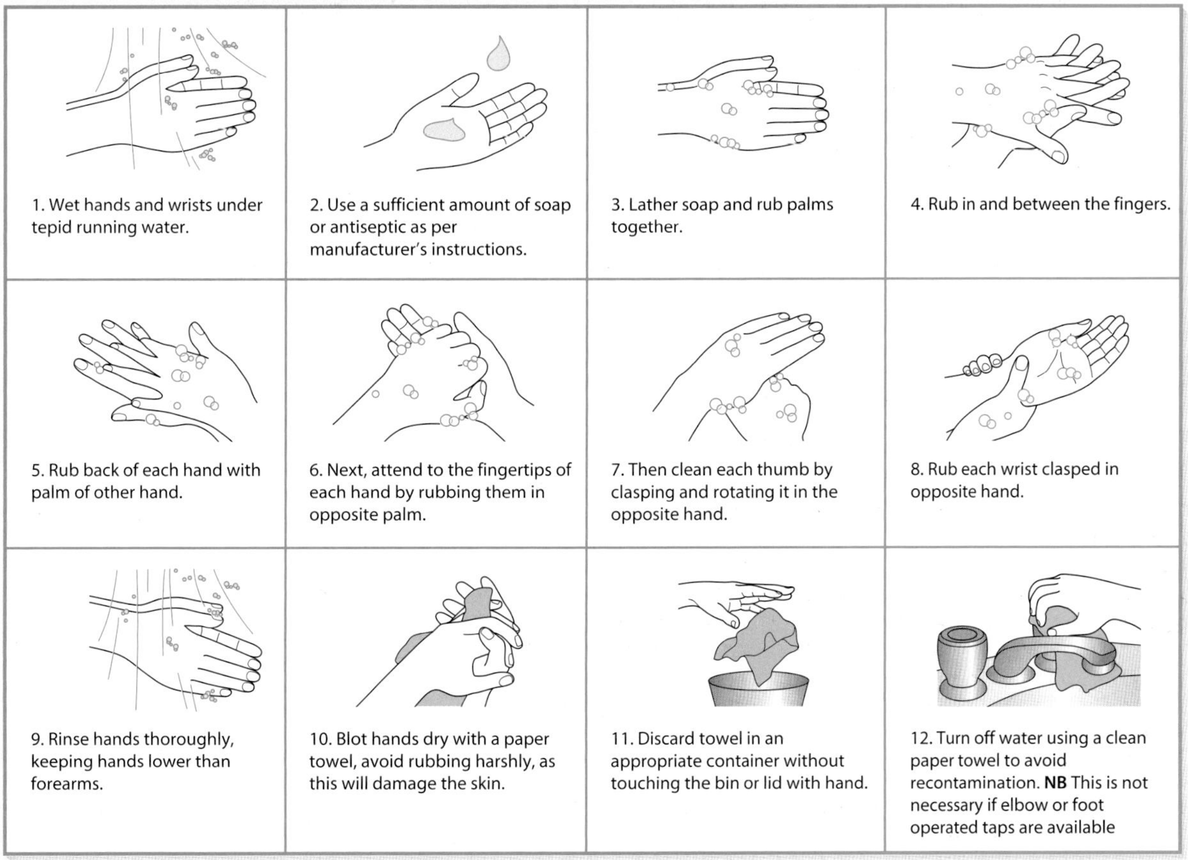
1. Wet hands and wrists under tepid running water.
2. Use a sufficient amount of soap or antiseptic as per manufacturer's instructions.
3. Lather soap and rub palms together.
4. Rub in and between the fingers.
5. Rub back of each hand with palm of other hand.
6. Next, attend to the fingertips of each hand by rubbing them in opposite palm.
7. Then clean each thumb by clasping and rotating it in the opposite hand.
8. Rub each wrist clasped in opposite hand.
9. Rinse hands thoroughly, keeping hands lower than forearms.
10. Blot hands dry with a paper towel, avoid rubbing harshly, as this will damage the skin.
11. Discard towel in an appropriate container without touching the bin or lid with hand.
12. Turn off water using a clean paper towel to avoid recontamination. NB This is not necessary if elbow or foot operated taps are available

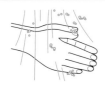

Handwashing (reproduced with permission from the Government of Ontario, Canada)

Skin care

Regular hand decontamination can cause skin dryness. The regular use of moisturizing hand cream increases skin hydration and replaces depleted skin fats. If a particular soap, antiseptic preparation or alcohol product causes skin irritation, the occupational health team should be consulted (DH 2001, CDC 2002).

the hands are washed. Washing the hands with an antiseptic preparation is appropriate in high-risk situations, i.e. before invasive procedures or contact with clients who have compromised immunity and are therefore highly susceptible to infection (see Box 15.8).

Alcohol-based hand rubs

These contain 70% alcohol and emollients (moisturizing agents to counteract the drying effect of the alcohol) and some contain an antiseptic (Hateley 2003). They act rapidly and kill or inhibit the growth of both transient and resident microorganisms. Their use can offer a practical and acceptable alternative to handwashing in certain clinical situations, e.g. between surgical cases in high-volume settings (Fig. 15.7). However, they are ineffective if hands are visibly soiled with dirt, blood or other matter (DH 2001). It is important to remember that alcohol is flammable and toxic if swallowed.

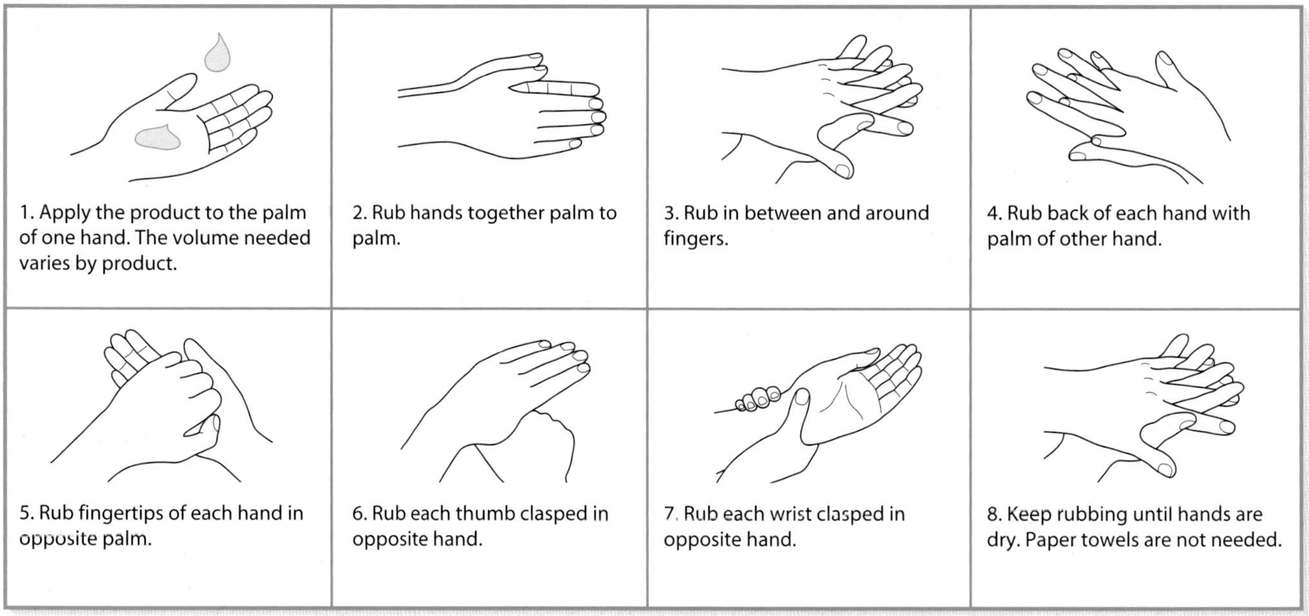
1. Apply the product to the palm of one hand. The volume needed varies by product.
2. Rub hands together palm to palm.
3. Rub in between and around fingers.
4. Rub back of each hand with palm of other hand.
5. Rub fingertips of each hand in opposite palm.
6. Rub each thumb clasped in opposite hand.
7. Rub each wrist clasped in opposite hand.
8. Keep rubbing until hands are dry. Paper towels are not needed.

Fig. 15.7 Decontaminating hands with an alcohol hand rub (reproduced with permission from the Government of Ontario, Canada)

Table 15.1 Handwashing preparations and their indications (from Wilson 2001)

	Hand washing preparations		
Indication for use	**Soap**	**Antiseptic preparation**	**Alcohol rub**
Removes transient microorganisms	✓	✓	✓
Removes resident microorganisms		✓	✓
Effective on physically soiled hands	✓	✓	
For routine use in clinical areas	✓		✓
Suitable for preoperative hand preparation		✓	✓
Hand preparation before invasive procedures		✓	✓

Types of handwashing preparation and their indications

Handwashing preparations and indications for their use are summarized in Table 15.1.

Personal protective equipment

Personal protective equipment (PPE) includes disposable gloves, gowns, aprons, eye protection and masks. They are worn to protect staff and patients from pathogenic microorganisms in both healthcare and community settings. The decision to use or wear PPE is based on a risk assessment (see Ch. 13) associated with a specific patient care activity or intervention (NICE 2003) (Fig. 15.8).

Disposable gloves

The purpose of wearing gloves is to:

- Reduce the risk of healthcare personnel acquiring infections from patients/clients
- Prevent flora from healthcare personnel being transmitted to patients/clients

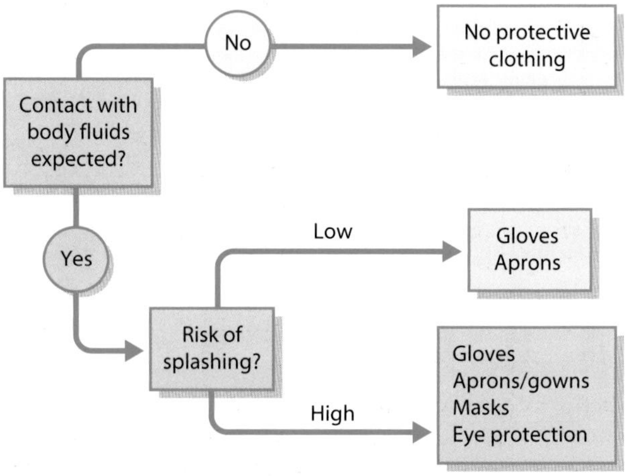

Fig. 15.8 Protective clothing risk assessment and selection

- Reduce transient contamination of the hands of healthcare personnel by flora that can be transmitted from one patient/client to another.

Gloves are worn for:

- All activities that carry a risk of exposure to blood, body fluids, secretions or excretions, e.g. when giving

injections, emptying catheter bags or disposing of bedpans, performing mouth care (NICE 2003)
- Contact with sterile sites, e.g. catheterization, broken skin and mucous membranes, e.g. wound care
- Invasive procedures, e.g. surgery.

Types of gloves and their uses
Gloves are available in a variety of materials including natural rubber latex (NRL), synthetic latex and vinyl. The appropriate type of glove is determined by the activity to be undertaken:

- Latex gloves are used for procedures requiring a high degree of dexterity such as catheterization
- Vinyl gloves, which are looser fitting, are appropriate to wear when giving injections or cleaning up spillage.

Polythene gloves should not be used because of their permeability and tendency to damage easily, exposing both the patient and healthcare practitioner to microbial contamination (Pratt et al 2000, Clark et al 2002).

Gloves can be either sterile or non-sterile and choice is based on the type of activity to be undertaken. Sterile gloves must be worn for any invasive procedure and the technique for putting them on is outlined in Box 15.9. Non-sterile gloves are suitable for activities involving contact with body fluids, e.g. handling urine, wiping up spillage and some 'clean techniques' such as administering injections.

Removal of gloves
Gloves are changed and discarded as follows:

- After contact with each patient
- When performing separate procedures on the same patient if there is a risk of cross-contamination, e.g. mouth care followed by a dressing change
- As soon as they are damaged, e.g. torn or punctured
- On completion of any task not involving patients but requiring the use of gloves
- Before touching any other items, e.g. worktops, pens, telephones, notes.

It is important that gloves are always treated as single-use items and discarded following removal. Wearing gloves does not replace the need for handwashing because gloves may have small defects, may be torn during use or the hands may have become contaminated during removal. Therefore, hand hygiene is essential before their use and after their removal. The technique for removing gloves is outlined in Box 15.10 (p. 405).

Health risks associated with glove use
Pratt et al (2000) and Clark et al (2002) advise that gloves should not be worn unnecessarily as their prolonged and indiscriminate use may lead to skin sensitivity and adverse reactions. Guidelines for reducing latex allergy are shown in Box 15.11.

Many products, in both the home and healthcare facilities, contain natural rubber latex (Table 15.2). Patients/clients may also have allergies and sensitivity to latex and admission to a healthcare facility may put them at risk (Box 15.12). NICE (2003) advise that any sensitivity to natural latex rubber in patients, carers or healthcare personnel must be documented and alternatives gloves made available.

Gowns and aprons

The purpose of wearing water-repellent protection is to:

- Prevent the user's clothing or skin from becoming contaminated with microorganisms which may subsequently be transferred to others
- Prevent the user's clothing or uniform becoming soiled or stained
- Prevent direct transfer or dissemination of microorganisms from the user to others.

When to wear gowns and aprons
Water-repellent gowns are used for procedures where there is a risk of extensive splashing of blood, body fluids, secretions or excretions onto the skin or clothing, e.g. in the operating theatre, dealing with trauma cases in the Emergency Department or during childbirth.

Disposable plastic aprons are worn to protect the front of the uniform from soiling, wetting or contamination that may occur during procedures involving close/direct contact with patients/clients such as:

- Bed making
- Bathing
- Wound care
- Dealing with spillages
- Preparation and serving of food.

In many healthcare facilities, different coloured aprons are used for different activities. Plastic aprons must be worn as single-use items, i.e. for one procedure or episode of patient care (NICE 2003). Care should be taken when removing aprons (see Fig. 15.9, p. 407).

Masks and eye protection

The purpose of masks and eye protection is to protect the wearer where there is a danger of pathogens in blood or other body substances splashing, splattering and spraying onto the mouth, nose and eyes, e.g. dental and operating theatre procedures, airway suctioning, obstetrical procedures.

Eye protection equipment, such as face shields, goggles and spectacles, must be optically clear (scratch- and mark-free), anti-fog and distortion-free, close-fitting and shielded at the sides. They are identified either as reusable after cleaning or for single-use only.

The use and efficacy of masks have been debated for many years. It used to be common practice to wear masks for many procedures, e.g. wound dressings; however, it is now recognized that their use contributes little to patient/client or staff safety. Unless the mask fits closely around the mouth and nose, microorganisms can escape around its edges (Wilson 2001). The movements of the wearer, length of facial hair and level of the voice when speaking, all affect the mask's close fit (Leonas & Jones 2003). Furthermore, if worn for long periods, its filtering efficiency is impaired because moisture collects in the fabric and interrupts the passage of air through the mask (Belkin 1997).

NURSING SKILLS Box 15.9

Technique for putting on sterile gloves

- Sterile gloves are double wrapped. The outside wrapping is not sterile, only the inner wrapping and its contents are
- Check the integrity of the outer wrapping and if you detect holes, rips, or the package is damp or wet, then discard it as the gloves cannot be considered sterile
- Check the expiry date and do not use if this has elapsed
- When putting on sterile gloves, remember that the first glove is picked up by the cuff only. The second glove is then touched only by the other sterile glove (see below).

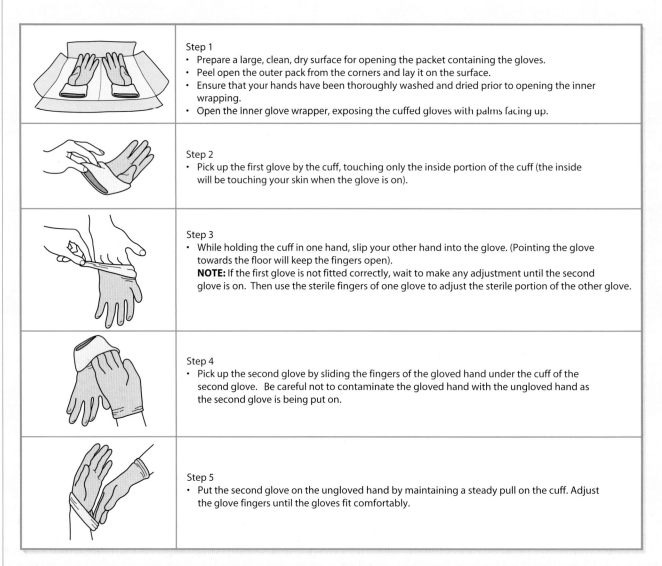

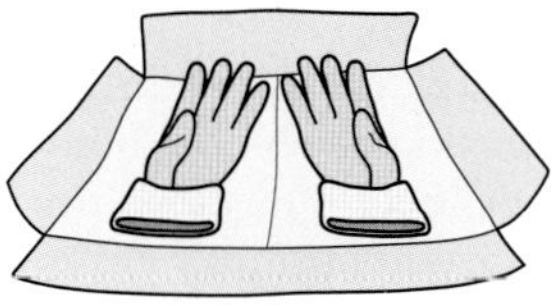	Step 1 • Prepare a large, clean, dry surface for opening the packet containing the gloves. • Peel open the outer pack from the corners and lay it on the surface. • Ensure that your hands have been thoroughly washed and dried prior to opening the inner wrapping. • Open the inner glove wrapper, exposing the cuffed gloves with palms facing up.
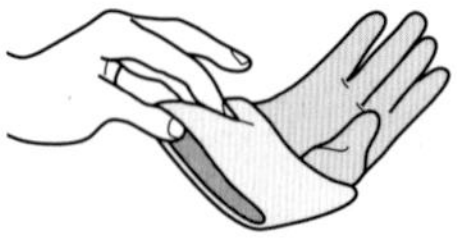	Step 2 • Pick up the first glove by the cuff, touching only the inside portion of the cuff (the inside will be touching your skin when the glove is on).
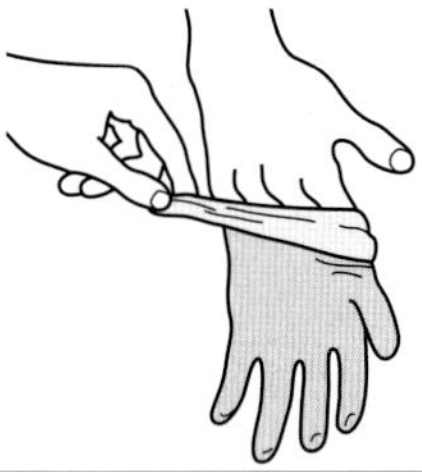	Step 3 • While holding the cuff in one hand, slip your other hand into the glove. (Pointing the glove towards the floor will keep the fingers open). **NOTE:** If the first glove is not fitted correctly, wait to make any adjustment until the second glove is on. Then use the sterile fingers of one glove to adjust the sterile portion of the other glove.
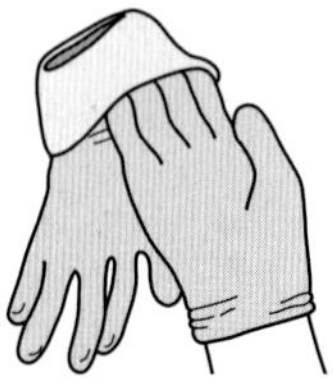	Step 4 • Pick up the second glove by sliding the fingers of the gloved hand under the cuff of the second glove. Be careful not to contaminate the gloved hand with the ungloved hand as the second glove is being put on.
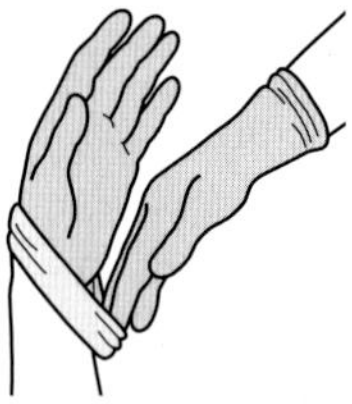	Step 5 • Put the second glove on the ungloved hand by maintaining a steady pull on the cuff. Adjust the glove fingers until the gloves fit comfortably.

Technique for putting on sterile gloves (reproduced with permission from EngenderHealth)

REMEMBER: Sterile gloves can become contaminated:

- If you touch the outside of a sterile glove with an ungloved hand
- If you touch anything that is not sterile including anything outside the sterile area, including your face, clothing, etc.
- If your glove is torn or punctured
- If your gloved hands drop below waist level.

REMEMBER: If your gloves become contaminated:

- Stop whatever you are doing
- Step away from the sterile area
- Remove the contaminated gloves
- If your hands are soiled with blood or other matter, rewash your hands and put on new gloves.

NURSING SKILLS — Box 15.10

Glove removal

- The key to removing both sterile and non-sterile gloves is 'dirty to dirty – clean to clean', i.e. contaminated surfaces only touch other contaminated surfaces: your bare hand, which is clean, touches only the clean areas inside the other glove.
- Avoid letting the gloves snap, as this may cause contaminants to splash into your eyes, mouth or skin, or other people in the area (see below).

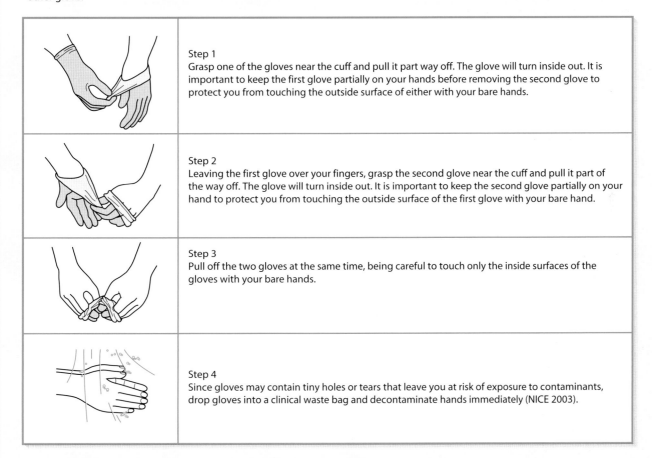

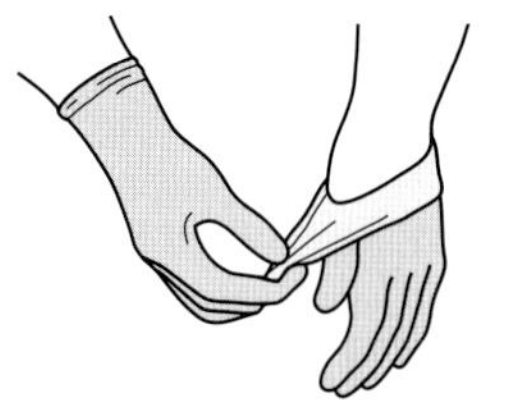	Step 1 Grasp one of the gloves near the cuff and pull it part way off. The glove will turn inside out. It is important to keep the first glove partially on your hands before removing the second glove to protect you from touching the outside surface of either with your bare hands.
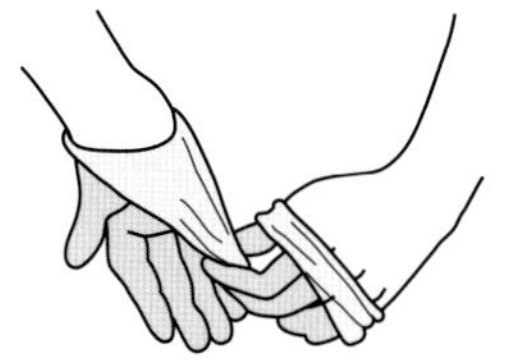	Step 2 Leaving the first glove over your fingers, grasp the second glove near the cuff and pull it part of the way off. The glove will turn inside out. It is important to keep the second glove partially on your hand to protect you from touching the outside surface of the first glove with your bare hand.
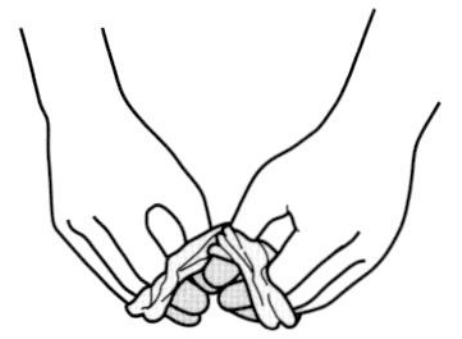	Step 3 Pull off the two gloves at the same time, being careful to touch only the inside surfaces of the gloves with your bare hands.
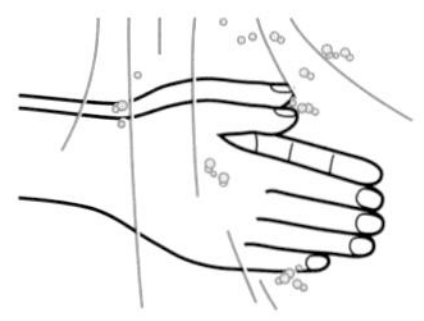	Step 4 Since gloves may contain tiny holes or tears that leave you at risk of exposure to contaminants, drop gloves into a clinical waste bag and decontaminate hands immediately (NICE 2003).

Glove removal (reproduced with permission from EngenderHealth and the Government of Ontario, Canada)

Masks are worn to protect healthcare practitioners when there is a danger of blood-borne pathogens or other body substances splashing or spraying into the practitioner's mouth and nose. Their use is also indicated when caring for susceptible clients, e.g. people with compromised immunity (DH 2001) or in situations when micro-organisms may be transmitted from patients via the airborne route, e.g. meningococcal meningitis (Hateley 2003) (Box 15.13, p. 407). It is recommended that if healthcare workers are likely to be exposed to either tuberculosis or severe acute respiratory syndrome (SARS) a particulate filter personal respiratory protection device (close-fitting masks capable of filtering 0.3 μm particles) should be used. If they are not available then it is better to wear a face-mask than no protection (Health Protection Agency 2004, Occupational Safety and Health Administration 2004).

Safe use and disposal of sharps

In healthcare settings, injuries from needles or other sharp instruments pose a serious danger in transmitting blood-borne viruses such as HIV and hepatitis B and C to healthcare personnel. These infections can be potentially life threatening but are preventable.

What are sharps?

The term 'sharps' refers to any sharp instrument or object used in the delivery of care including:

- Hypodermic needles
- Suture needles
- Scalpel blades
- Lancets
- Sharp instruments, e.g. stitch cutters

Box 15.11 **Latex allergy**

Latex allergy is a reaction to certain proteins in natural rubber latex. The amount of latex exposure needed to produce sensitization or an allergic reaction is unknown although increasing exposure to latex proteins increases the risk of developing allergic symptoms.

Symptoms occurring in sensitized people are variable and usually begin within minutes of exposure but they sometimes develop hours later. Mild reactions involve skin redness, urticaria (rashes) and itching. More severe reactions may involve respiratory symptoms, e.g. nasal congestion, sneezing, itchy watery eyes, sore throat and asthma. Rarely, anaphylactic shock may occur; however, this life-threatening reaction is seldom the first sign of latex allergy.

The National Institute for Occupational Safety and Health (1997) recommend:

- Use of non-latex gloves, e.g. synthetic latex or vinyl, for activities that are not likely to involve contact with infectious materials, e.g. food preparation, routine patient care activities, housekeeping
- Use of appropriate work practices to reduce the chance of reactions to latex:
  - when wearing latex gloves, do not use oil-based hand creams or lotions which can cause glove deterioration
  - after removing latex gloves, wash the hands with mild soap and dry thoroughly
  - practise good housekeeping: clean areas and equipment contaminated with latex-containing dust frequently
- Learning to recognize the symptoms of latex allergy (see above)
- Avoiding direct contact with latex gloves and other latex-containing products if symptoms of latex allergy appear until the Occupational Health Department or a medical practitioner have been consulted
- If you have latex allergy, informing your mentor and taking the precautions advised by your medical practitioner.

Table 15.2 Products containing latex

Household objects	Medical devices
Adhesive tape and bandages	Ambu bags
Balloons	Blood pressure cuffs (bladder and tubing)
Camera eyepieces	Condom urinary collection devices
Carpet backing	Elastic bandages
Computer mouse pads	Electrode pads
Condoms and diaphragms	Enema tubing
Dummies and baby bottle teats	Gloves
Elastic	Goggles
Erasers	Haemodialysis equipment
Handgrips, e.g. kitchen utensils, bicycles	Injection ports on intravenous infusion tubing and fluid bags
Hot-water bottles	Stretcher canvasses
Household rubber gloves	Protective sheets and pillow covers
Paint	Stethoscope tubing
Racquet handles	Sticking plasters
Raincoats	Tourniquets
Rubber bands	Trolley wheels
Rubber toys	Urinary catheters
Shoe soles and waterproof footwear	Vial stoppers
Shower curtains and bathmats	Wound drains and tubes
Swimming fins and goggles	
Tyres	

- Intravenous cannulae
- Contaminated broken glass
- Razor blades.

Most reported sharps injuries involve nursing staff; however, other healthcare personnel including doctors, laboratory, domestic and portering staff may also be involved (Exposure Prevention Information Network [EPINet] 2004) (see Box 15.14).

How injuries occur

Many injuries occur when staff are using and disposing of sharps, for example when:

- Recapping hypodermic needles after use. This is one of the major causes of sharp object injuries (EPINet 2004)
- Manipulating used sharps (bending, breaking or cutting hypodermic needles) which can cause

CRITICAL THINKING — Box 15.12

Contact with latex in the healthcare environment

You are caring for Mary who states that she is allergic to natural rubber latex.

Student activities

- Identify items in your placement that contain natural rubber latex.
- Consider nursing interventions and treatments where contact with natural rubber latex is likely.
- Find out how a latex allergy is diagnosed.

NURSING SKILLS — Box 15.13

Correct use of masks

- The mask should fit snugly over the face, the coloured side facing out and the metal strip at the top
- Position the strings to keep the mask firmly in place over the nose, mouth and chin
- Mould the metallic strip to the bridge of the nose
- Do not touch the mask again until it is removed
- Remove the mask by its ties
- Discard as clinical waste according to local policy
- If the mask is damaged or soiled, replace it immediately.

[Adapted from Health Protection Agency (2004)]

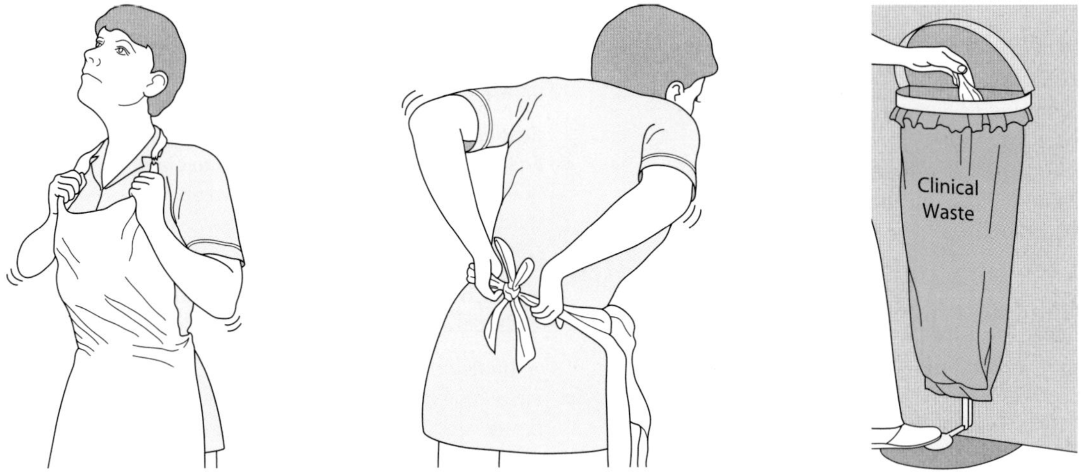

Step 1.
Grasp apron by neck band and tear

Step 2.
Break waist tie

Step 3.
Carefully dispose into clinical waste bin and wash hands

Fig. 15.9 Removing a disposable apron

Box 15.14 — **Incidence and effects of needlestick injuries to healthcare workers**

In the UK, an estimated 100 000 needlestick accidents occur annually to healthcare workers (NHS Scotland 2005). The majority of reported needlestick injuries are as follows:

- 48% involve nursing staff
- 7% involve medical and dental staff
- 20% involve ancillary staff and others including porters, domestic and grounds/estate staff.

Although needlestick injuries may result in local trauma, the principal associated health risk is transmission of blood-borne viral diseases, in particular hepatitis B and C and HIV. The incidence of infection following a needlestick injury varies depending on the virus (DH 2001):

- Hepatitis B: 33.3% (1 in 3)
- Hepatitis C: 3.3% (1 in 30)
- HIV: 0.31% (1 in 319).

The emotional impact of a needlestick injury can be severe and long lasting, even when infection is not transmitted. Not knowing the infection status of the source patient can accentuate the healthcare worker's stress (Bandolier 2003) and this impact can be particularly severe when the injury involves exposure to HIV. In one study of 20 healthcare workers with HIV exposure, 11 reported severe distress, 7 had persistent moderate distress and 2 resigned from their posts as a result of the exposure (Henry et al 1990).

blood inside to splatter or may cause an accidental injury
- One staff member accidentally sticks another staff member when carrying unprotected sharps
- Sharp items are found in areas where they are unexpected, e.g. on surgical drapes or bed linen
- Handling or disposing of waste that contains used needles or other sharps
- Sudden movement by a client at the time of an injection causes a healthcare practitioner to be accidentally stuck.

Preventing sharps injuries

The assessment and management of risks associated with the use of sharps is paramount in health and safety promotion as well as in infection control. Injuries from sharps can be avoided by handling and disposing of them safely (Box 15.15).

HEALTH PROMOTION Box 15.15

Safe handling and disposal of sharps

National and international guidelines are consistent in their recommendations for the safe use and disposal of sharp instruments and needles.

Handling sharps
- Avoid passing sharps from hand to hand
- Minimize handling of sharps
- Do not carry used sharps by hand or pass them to another person.

Sharps containers
- Used sharps must be discarded into a sharps-disposal container that conforms to national standards
- Sharps containers should be located in all areas where sharp objects are used, e.g. treatment rooms, operating theatres, labour and delivery rooms, laboratories
- Containers are located in a safe position – not on floors where they could be kicked over – and out of reach of members of the public, in particular small children. To avoid damage by heat, sharps containers should not be placed near radiators or in direct sunlight (Health Services Advisory Committee 1999).

Disposing of sharps into sharps containers
- Do not remove needles from syringes by hand, or resheath, bend or break them before disposal
- Do not dismantle needles from syringes or other devices, but discard as a single unit
- Dispose of needles and syringes immediately after use
- Place sharps point downwards into sharps container
- Ensure containers are securely closed when three-quarters full
- Ensure containers are disposed of in accordance with local policy
- Needle safety devices must be used where there are clear indications that they will provide safer systems of working for healthcare personnel (NICE 2003).

Managing injuries and exposure to body fluids

Exposure to blood from a sharps injury, bite or splashing into the eyes, mouth or broken skin must always be followed up because of the risk of infection from bloodborne viruses (Box 15.16).

Management of waste

Management of healthcare waste is a crucial aspect of infection control. It is a statutory requirement for healthcare facilities to comply with international, national and local legislation and regulations that relate to the segregation, handling, transportation and final disposal of waste.

FIRST AID Box 15.16

Managing needlestick injuries and exposure to body fluids

Healthcare facilities have protocols to follow if a sharp injury or exposure to body fluids occurs.

First aid
Following any accidental exposure to blood or other body fluids by needlestick, another sharp object or a splash of fluid then:

- Wash the needlestick or cut with soap and water
- Flush splashes to the nose, mouth or skin with water
- Irrigate splashes to the eyes with clean water or saline.

There is no evidence to show that using antiseptics or encouraging the wound to bleed reduces the risk of a bloodborne infection (CDC 2003a). However, many organizations and healthcare facilities within the UK suggest that this should carried out as a first aid measure and this is supported by the WHO (2003).

Management
- Inform the charge nurse immediately
- Attend the Occupational Health Department, Emergency Department or other designated treatment facility. Prompt reporting is essential as post-exposure treatment is sometimes recommended and it should be started as soon as possible.

Whether post-exposure treatment is indicated following exposure to blood or other body fluids depends on a number of factors including:

- The infection status of the person whose blood or body fluids are involved
- The type of exposure, e.g. a splash to the skin versus a deep puncture wound
- Whether or not the casualty has been vaccinated against hepatitis B
- Time elapsed since exposure
- The availability of needed drugs or other therapy.

Documentation
- Complete the relevant documentation for reporting accidents (see Ch. 13).

Classification of waste

Waste generated from healthcare facilities is classified as clinical or non-clinical waste.

Clinical (hazardous) waste

This is generated from many sources including healthcare, veterinary and pharmaceutical establishments. Because of its toxic, infectious or dangerous content it may be hazardous to healthcare personnel, members of the public and the environment. Consequently, special precautions are required to treat and dispose of it safely (Health Services Advisory Committee [HSAC] 1999).

Domestic waste

A considerable proportion of the waste generated in clinical areas is not hazardous to those who come into contact with it and can be safely disposed of as household waste. It is important that this waste is not sent for incineration in order to minimize both disposal costs and damage to the environment (Table 15.3).

Safe handling of clinical waste in healthcare facilities

Disposing of waste safely and economically depends on correct segregation of different types of waste at the point of generation. Waste is bagged, packaged or containerized and must clearly indicate the contents (see Box 15.17).

Safe handling of clinical waste in people's homes

The amount of clinical waste generated by patients/clients in their own homes is much smaller and can usually be disposed of as normal household waste. Used needles, e.g. those used by people with insulin-dependent diabetes, must not be discarded as household waste. Instead, arrangements with local hospitals, clinics, pharmacies or local authorities need to be made regarding their disposal (HSAC 1999). Healthcare personnel, e.g. community nurses and dialysis technicians, who generate clinical waste while treating patients in their homes are obliged by the Health and Safety at Work Act (1992) to transport and dispose of the waste safely (see Box 15.18).

Table 15.3 Categories, containment, treatment and disposal of waste from clinical areas (from HSAC 1999)

Clinical (hazardous) waste	Container colour and disposal
Items soiled by blood or other body fluids: Include wound dressings, swabs, disposable gloves and aprons, materials used to clean up spillages; contaminated waste from patients with transmissible infectious diseases, e.g. tuberculosis and salmonella; disposable nappies from babies, infants, toddlers and others with infectious diarrhoeal diseases	Yellow or orange bag Incineration or heat disinfection followed by landfill
Sharps: Include discarded needles and syringes, cartridges, contaminated broken glass and other disposable sharp instruments including scalpels, razors, lancets, sharp tips of intravenous administration sets, stitch cutters	Yellow sharps container Incineration
Pharmaceutical products and chemical wastes: Include expired and unwanted medicines, cartridges from drug infusion devices, cytotoxic drugs	Collected by ward/community pharmacist who makes arrangements for disposal
Body waste products: Include urine, faeces, body secretions and excretions, plus disposables used for their collection, e.g. bedpans, bedpan liners, vomit bowls	Discharged into sewerage system via sluice, lavatory or macerator
Sanpro (sanitary products) waste: Includes disposable nappies, incontinence pads, stoma bags, urine containers	Yellow bag with black stripes May be incinerated or sent direct to landfill
Domestic (non-hazardous) waste	**Container and destination**
General waste: Includes dead flowers, used hand towels, food (small quantities only), paper wrappings from packs, magazines and newspapers	Black bag at source although some facilities may use clear, green, buff or white bags Sent direct to landfill[AU1]
Cardboard boxes	Folded flat for collection, then direct to recycling unit or landfill
Confidential waste: Paperwork containing sensitive information relating to patients or staff If shredded then recycling unit or landfill	Green/brown bag at source Shredded or incinerated
Glass bottles and jars	When empty, place in a strong box (mark box 'Glass with Care'); put into designated container Recycling unit or landfill
Aerosols, pressurized containers, batteries: May pose a safety and/or environmental risk, i.e. may contain CFCs, prescription medicines, flammable liquids or be explosive in nature	Placed in separately identified containers

NURSING SKILLS Box 15.17

Safe handling of clinical waste

Dealing with clinical waste bags

- All infectious waste (other than contaminated sharps, glassware or sharp-edged waste) must be disposed of into leak-resistant clinical waste bags
- Gloves and aprons should be worn when handling clinical waste bags and containers
- Clinical waste bags must be suspended in an appropriate container, e.g. a foot-operated lidded bin, and the containers positioned at the point of generation
- Bags must not be filled more than three-quarters full and loose contents should never be transferred from bag to bag or compacted by hand. This will avoid injuries from concealed sharps that may have inadvertently been discarded with clinical waste
- All bags must indicate their origin and be labelled with the name of the facility, e.g. hospital ward or department, and the date
- Bags must be sealed at the point of production with a plastic tie, closure or heat sealer. Staples should not be used as they result in puncture holes
- Waste must not be allowed to accumulate in corridors or other undesignated areas because it could cause harm to others.

Dealing with spillages

- Appropriate protective clothing, e.g. non-sterile vinyl gloves and plastic apron, must be worn
- Any spilled fluid must be mopped up with absorbent material, e.g. paper towels
- Carefully place contaminated material in a new clinical waste bag, together with all other spilled clinical waste matter
- Seal and label the bag, and dispose of in line with local policy
- Disinfect the spillage area according to local policy, e.g. hypochlorite
- Remove protective clothing and wash hands.

[From HSAC (1999)]

REFLECTIVE PRACTICE Box 15.18

Management of clinical waste

Student activities

- Identify how clinical waste is managed within your placement from the point of generation to disposal.
- Review practices in relation to clinical waste within your placement.
- Discuss your observations with your mentor.

Management of linen

Used linen, e.g. clothing, towels, sheets, pillowslips, should be laundered:

- Between patient use
- When visibly soiled
- At least weekly (Ayliffe et al 1999).

In healthcare facilities, linen that is soiled with blood, excreta or other body fluids, or contaminated with microorganisms from infectious patients, needs to be handled carefully in order to prevent:

- Contamination of the skin and clothing of healthcare personnel
- Transfer of microorganisms to other patients/clients and environments.

The laundering process should remove evidence of previous use and significantly reduce microbial counts so that the risk of infection to subsequent users is negligible.

Categories of hospital linen

The NHS Executive guidelines (1995) for hospital laundering recommend that laundry should be sorted into three categories (Table 15.4). These recommendations are uncertain for the following reasons:

- There is no evidence that infected linen has higher microbial contamination than other used hospital linen or that double bagging is necessary (McDonald & Pugliese 1996)
- The use of water-soluble bags combined with thermal disinfection for infected linen may cause stains to set. Furthermore, water-soluble bags offer no benefit from an infection control perspective and add to costs (Health Canada 1998)
- Interpretations of the NHS Executive guidelines vary between UK healthcare facilities (Box 15.19).

Safe handling of linen

To prevent the risk of cross-infection it is important that linen in healthcare facilities is handled in the same way for all patients/clients. PPE should be used when handling linen, as follows:

- Plastic aprons when making or changing beds to prevent contamination of uniform/clothing by potential pathogens, and discarded afterwards
- Gloves when handling linen or clothing that is soiled with blood, body fluids, secretions and excretions to prevent contamination of the hands. Following their removal, gloves are disposed of and the hands washed.

Safe handling of soiled linen

Linen is handled with minimal agitation and shaking to avoid the dispersal of microorganisms into the air and onto people or objects in the vicinity.

- Heavily soiled linen is rolled or folded to contain the heaviest soil in the centre of the bundle. Large amounts of solid soil, e.g. faeces, are removed with

Table 15.4 Laundering of hospital linen (from NHS Executive 1995)

Category	Description	Bag type and colour	Laundering process
Used	Normal usage or visibly soiled by blood, body fluids, secretions and excretions	White linen or clear plastic	Sorted before disinfection by washing at 65°C for 10 minutes or 71°C for 3 minutes
Infected	Linen used by patients with certain infectious diseases or as advised by the infection control team Also includes reusable nappies from babies, infants, and others	Red outer bag, containing an inner water-soluble bag	Not sorted prior to washing Water-soluble bag placed unopened in the washing machine and dissolves during the washing process Disinfected by washing at 65°C for 10 minutes or 71°C for 3 minutes
Heat-labile	Fabric likely to be damaged by thermal disinfection, e.g. wool, silk	White bag with a prominent orange stripe or orange plastic bag	Washed at 40°C with hypochlorite added to the penultimate rinse

REFLECTIVE PRACTICE Box 15.19

Dealing with used linen

Healthcare facilities use different terminology when categorizing, segregating and treating linen.

Student activities

Think about your current placement and:

- Compare the categorizing system used with that in Table 15.4.
- Identify the colour of bag used for each category of linen.
- Consider the extent to which handling linen within your placement area corresponds to that outlined in Table 15.4.
- Discuss your observations with your mentor.

a gloved hand and toilet tissue and discarded into a bedpan or lavatory for flushing.

- Containment of linen is achieved by placing it immediately into a collection bag at the site of generation. It should not be temporarily placed anywhere else, e.g. on floors, bed tables, lockers or chairs. The collection bag should be of sufficient quality to contain the wet/soiled linen and prevent leakage during handling and transportation. Bags should not be overfilled, as this may prevent closure or increase the likelihood of the bag splitting during transit to the laundry.
- Rinsing or soaking of linen is never carried out due to the risk of splashing body fluids onto the skin or mucous membranes.
- Ensuring that sharps and other objects are not inadvertently discarded into linen bags minimizes the risk of injury to portering and laundry staff. Some healthcare facilities have a tracking system that requires collection bags to be tagged with the name of the ward/department. This establishes a system whereby extraneous objects found in linen can be returned to the sender.

By careful handling of used linen the nurse can break the chain of infection, thereby protecting patients from healthcare-associated infections (see Box 15.20).

Decontamination of patient-care equipment

Patient-care equipment can act as an intermediary (fomite) in transferring infectious microorganisms from one person to another. It is therefore important that shared or reusable patient-care equipment is decontaminated, i.e. made safe by removing, inhibiting or destroying microorganisms, after use. The term 'decontamination' includes sterilization, disinfection and cleaning. These methods confer different levels of microbial safety on items processed.

Levels of decontamination

The appropriate level of decontamination depends on the risk that the equipment may present in transmitting infection. The following factors are critical to that interrelationship:

- The presence of microorganisms, i.e. their numbers and virulence
- The type of procedure to be performed, i.e. invasive or non-invasive
- The body site where the instrument or equipment will be used, e.g. penetrating tissue or used on intact skin.

The risk of transmission can be categorized as high, medium, low or minimal (see Table 15.5).

Cleaning

This is a physical process that involves decontaminating an item or surface with a detergent solution followed by thorough drying. Cleaning contributes to infection control because it physically removes organic materials, e.g. blood, other body fluids, soil or dust, in which microorganisms can survive. Although cleaning does not necessarily destroy microorganisms, it significantly reduces their numbers and is suitable for low and minimal risk items.

Unless cleaning is carried out competently, infectious microorganisms may be redistributed to other sources and sites (see Box 15.21). Cleaning is also essential prior to disinfection and sterilization, otherwise microorganisms trapped in organic material may survive further processing (see WHO 2003).

HEALTH PROMOTION — Box 15.20

Breaking the chain of infection using standard precautions

Staff Nurse Jones was assigned to care for Mr Green, a patient who had an open draining wound on his left lower leg. When a sample of pus was sent to the laboratory for analysis, the microorganism meticillin (methicillin)-resistant *Staphylococcus aureus* (MRSA) was isolated. Prior to making Mr Green's bed, Staff Nurse Jones washed his hands. Clean linen and a collection bag for linen were placed at the patient's bed. To remove the soiled linen from the bed, Staff Nurse Jones took the following actions:

- Washed his hands
- Wore non-sterile gloves and a disposable plastic apron
- Handled the sheets by the outermost edges so that the soiled area was folded into the centre of the bundle
- Held soiled linen away from his uniform and placed it directly into the linen collection bag
- Removed the gloves and discarded them directly into a waste receptacle
- Washed his hands.

Staff Nurse Jones applied principles of infection control to contain the infectious microorganisms at many points in the chain of infection as shown below.

Link in the chain	Nursing action to break the chain
Infectious agent: MRSA microorganism	
Reservoir: Mr Green's infected wound	Staff Nurse Jones knew the infected wound contained microorganisms that could easily be transmitted to other patients by indirect contact
Portal of exit: Exudate draining from the open wound	Staff Nurse Jones used proper handwashing techniques, wore protective gloves and handled the linen correctly
Mode of transmission: Healthcare workers' hands frequently transfer MRSA by indirect contact	Proper handwashing, gloving and careful handling of used linen
Portal of entry	Microorganisms isolated using standard infection control principles
Susceptible host	None, due to Staff Nurse Jones' adherence to infection control measures

Table 15.5 Categories of decontamination related to risk (adapted from Ayliffe et al 1999, WHO 2003)

Risk	Examples	Level of decontamination required
High: Entry or penetration into the vascular system, body cavities or tissues	Surgical and invasive procedures Intravenous cannulation Urinary catheterization Injections	Sterilization
Medium: In contact with mucous membranes, body fluids or other potentially infectious material	Thermometers Body fluid spills Reusable bedpans and urine bottles Crockery, feeding bottles Vaginal specula	Disinfection: chemical or thermal
Low: Items in contact with intact skin	Sinks and washbowls Lavatory seats Blood pressure cuffs Mattresses Hoists	Cleaning – clean with detergent, rinse and dry Disinfection – for people with known infections
Minimal: Not in direct contact with patients	Furniture Floors Walls Ceilings	Cleaning – including damp dusting, wet mopping, dust-attractant mopping, vacuum cleaning

Sterilization

Sterilization is the complete destruction of all living microorganisms including bacterial spores (spores are a resistant casing produced by several species of bacteria that enables them to survive in adverse conditions, e.g. heat, cold, drying, and most chemicals). When something is sterile, it is devoid of microbial life.

Creutzfeldt–Jakob disease (CJD) and variant CJD present a serious cross-infection risk as the microorganisms resist normal decontamination methods. It is

EVIDENCE-BASED PRACTICE Box 15.21

Good cleaning practices

Although environmental cleaning in most healthcare facilities is the duty of cleaning staff, nursing staff have ultimate responsibility to ensure that the standard of cleaning adheres to national guidelines. As nurses are often required to clean patient-care equipment (e.g. blood pressure equipment, washbowls) and blood and body fluid spillages, it is important that they understand fundamental cleaning principles. Correct handling of cleaning solutions, use of cleaning cloths and ensuring that items are dried after cleaning is paramount. PPE, i.e. gloves and aprons, are worn for cleaning and once the task is completed, the hands are washed before carrying out other duties.

Cleaning solutions

When detergent is dissolved in water, it breaks up and dissolves or suspends grease, oil and other foreign matter, thus facilitating its removal. Detergents are available in various forms, e.g. powders, liquids, sprays, gels and wipes.

Cleaning solutions:

- Must always be freshly prepared and accurately diluted (Gould & Brooker 2000)
- Become contaminated almost immediately during cleaning and their continued use transfers increasing numbers of microorganisms to each subsequent surface cleaned (CDC 2003b)
- Are used instead of hand soap for patient-care equipment, because fatty acids contained in the soap react with the minerals in water, leaving a residue or scum that is difficult to remove (WHO 2003)
- Are disposed of into a sluice or sink in the dirty utility area. They must not be discarded into washbasins (Ayliffe et al 1999).

Cleaning cloths

- Cleaning cloths and mop heads can be another source of contamination, especially if left soaking in used solutions. Washing after use and allowing them to dry before re-use minimizes the degree of contamination (CDC 2003b)
- The same cloth must never be used to clean different areas, e.g. toilets and kitchens
- Disposable, colour-coded cloths are used in many healthcare facilities for use in different areas (WHO 2003).

Drying after cleaning

This is essential because bacteria thrive in moisture. Greaves (1985) showed that washing bowls are still contaminated by bacteria when stored wet and may present an infection risk to the next user.

Cleaning the hospital environment

This is carried out routinely to ensure a clean, dust-free hospital environment. Visible dirt contains microorganisms and cleaning helps to eliminate them. The main methods of removing organic materials are:

- *Dry cleaning*, e.g. sweeping, dusting, which is not recommended because it increases airborne bacterial counts
- *Wet cleaning* using detergent and hot water, which is more effective.

The frequency with which wet cleaning should be carried out depends on the situation, for example:

- Areas visibly contaminated with blood or body fluids must be cleaned immediately
- Isolation rooms and other areas that have patients with known transmissible infections should be cleaned with a detergent/disinfectant solution at least daily
- All horizontal surfaces and toilet areas should be cleaned daily (WHO 2003).

Student activities

Think about your current placement and consider if the following standards apply:

- Bed and cot frames are clean and free from dust
- Floors, including edges and corners, are free from dust
- Patient call bells (if applicable) are clean and free from debris
- Mop heads are laundered daily or are disposable
- Shelves, bench tops and cupboards are clean and free of dust, stains and litter
- Cleaning equipment is colour coded
- Baths, sinks and toilets are clean
- Shower curtains, bathmats, wall tiles and wall fixtures, e.g. soap dispensers and towel holders, are clean, dry and free from mould
- Products for cleaning comply with policy and are used at the correct dilution
- Personal protective clothing is available and appropriately used.

Discuss your findings with your mentor.

important to refer to local policy regarding decontamination processes.

Sterilization is necessary for all high-risk procedures using the methods shown in Box 15.22 (p. 414). Sterilized items need to be stored correctly and checked prior to opening (see Box 15.23).

Disinfection

Disinfection is the destruction or removal of microorganisms to a level that is unlikely to cause infection. It does not guarantee complete removal of all microorganisms because bacterial spores can still survive, i.e. some forms of microbial life may still be present after disinfection.

Box 15.22 Sterilization methods

- *Steam under pressure*: Moist heat sterilization is effective for equipment that can withstand heat and moisture, e.g. metal instruments, surgical gowns, drapes, swabs. Steam under pressure sterilizers were previously called autoclaves (WHO 2003)
- *Dry heat sterilization*: Hot air ovens are used for items sensitive to moisture but capable of withstanding high temperatures, e.g. glass, metal instruments, powders
- *Ethylene oxide gas*: Suitable for heat-sensitive items and devices that contain electronic components, e.g. bronchoscopes. It is extremely toxic and is therefore used according to strict guidelines to ensure staff safety
- *Automated chemical (low temperature) systems*: Sealed chambers containing chemicals, e.g. hydrogen peroxide or peracetic acid, which are used to chemically sterilize immersible instruments including endoscopes and arthroscopes
- *Irradiation*: Gamma radiation is a commercial process used for heat-sensitive items, e.g. plastic syringes, needles, surgical gloves, suturing materials, catheters. Many of these products are single-use items.

REFLECTIVE PRACTICE Box 15.23

Storing and checking sterile items

Student activities

Identify a range of sterile items in your placement:

- How are sterile items wrapped?
- Where are sterile items stored?
- What checks must be made before opening a sterile item?
- Why should sterile items be used immediately and, if they are not, discarded?

Disinfection is necessary for all medium-risk procedures and for equipment used for those with transmissible infections (see Table 15.5). Disinfection can be achieved by thermal and chemical methods (see Box 15.24).

Numerous chemical disinfectants are available to decontaminate equipment and the environment. However, in healthcare facilities the number available is strictly limited (Table 15.6). Furthermore, the use of chemical disinfectants is regulated by the Control of Substances Hazardous to Health (COSHH) Regulations (1999) which are designed to protect against risks to health from hazardous substances in the workplace (see Ch. 13). Each healthcare facility has an infection control policy/manual that gives information about procedures for decontamination (Box 15.25).

Box 15.24 Disinfection

Thermal disinfection

Suitable for items that can withstand heat and moisture but do not need to be sterile. Examples of thermal disinfection equipment used in clinical settings include bedpan washers, dishwashers and laundry machines. Although not frequently used in hospitals, boiling is sometimes used to disinfect medium-risk equipment, e.g. feeding bottles, vaginal specula, ear syringes.

Chemical disinfection

The performance of chemical disinfectants depends on several factors including temperature, contact time, concentration, pH, presence of organic or inorganic matter and the numbers and resistance of the microorganisms. Thermal disinfection is more reliable and should be used in preference to chemicals wherever possible (Wilson 2001). Although chemical disinfectants are widely used and perceived to be safe, there are many drawbacks as identified in the list below:

- Active against a limited range of microorganisms
- Bacterial spores are not easily destroyed
- Their ability to destroy viruses is variable
- Some support the growth of microorganisms
- Poor penetration of organic material, e.g. blood, pus, faeces, milk
- May be inactivated by organic material, e.g. detergents, soaps, rubber, plastics
- Often corrosive, toxic or irritant
- Effectiveness deteriorates with age
- Need to be carefully reconstituted to the manufacturer's specifications
- They are expensive.

Additional precautions

These are used in addition to the standard precautions discussed above; aseptic technique and isolation precautions are explained in this section.

Aseptic technique

Patients in healthcare facilities often acquire infections as a result of invasive clinical procedures which breach the body's normal defence mechanisms, making the tissues vulnerable to invasion by microorganisms. For example:

- Blood infections (septicaemia) after the insertion of an intravenous catheter
- Wound infections following surgery
- Urinary tract infections related to the insertion of an indwelling urinary catheter
- Lower respiratory tract infections, e.g. pneumonia, postoperatively.

Table 15.6 Chemical disinfectants used in healthcare facilities

Group	Uses	Precautions
Alcohol (60–90%), e.g. isopropyl alcohol, methylated spirit	Clean equipment, e.g. trolleys, tabletops, glass mercury thermometers, external surfaces of stethoscopes	Flammable: use in well-ventilated areas, keep away from heat sources, electrical equipment, flames, hot surfaces Toxic: avoid inhalation
Peracetic acid, e.g. Nu-cidex®, Steris-system®	Delicate instruments, e.g. flexible endoscopes, anaesthesia and respiratory equipment, items damaged by heat	Strong smell and should be used in well-ventilated areas May damage rubber and brass after prolonged immersion
Hypochlorite (bleach), e.g. Domestos®, Chloros®, Milton®, Presept®, Haz-tabs®	Environment Non-metallic equipment Disinfection of material contaminated with blood and body fluids	Corrosive to metals Must not be mixed with acids as they may release chlorine gas Can be irritating to the skin, eyes, and respiratory tract
Phenolic (carbolic acid), e.g. Clearsol®, Stericol®, Hycolin®	Environment	Absorbed by rubber and plastics Can cause severe burning of the skin or mucous membranes

NURSING SKILLS Box 15.25

Principles of chemical disinfection

- Check the infection control policy/manual to ensure disinfection is necessary and the recommended product to use
- Wear PPE as indicated
- Clean equipment thoroughly with detergent and water to remove organic materials
- Check the expiry date of the chemical disinfectant – if out of date, do not use
- Dilute the solution as recommended
- Completely immerse equipment for the recommended time
- Discard chemical disinfectant after use (according to local policy), clean container and store dry
- Remove PPE and wash hands.

Student activities

In your current placement:

- Locate COSHH guidelines and the infection control policy/manual.
- Select two chemical disinfectants used in the placement and, from the COSHH guidelines, identify their uses, associated hazards and first-aid treatment recommended in the case of accidental ingestion or inhalation.

Aseptic technique is often referred to as 'sterile technique' or 'no-touch technique'. It includes practices used to render and keep objects and areas sterile, i.e. free of all microorganisms including bacterial spores. Aseptic technique is routinely carried out in a wide range of hospital and community settings.

Indications for aseptic technique

Aseptic technique is carried out during any invasive clinical procedure that enters or penetrates a vulnerable body site such as the vascular system, a sterile body cavity or tissue. Examples of invasive clinical procedures include:

- Wound care
- Insertion of an intravenous cannula or urinary catheter
- Vaginal examinations during labour
- Medical procedures, e.g. lumbar puncture, endoscopy
- Surgical operations and suturing wounds.

Components of aseptic technique

The components of aseptic technique include all the key elements of standard precautions and also focus on:

- Careful preparation of the patient, environment and equipment
- Using an antiseptic solution to decontaminate the hands and the patient's skin (Box 15.26)
- Using only sterile equipment and supplies, e.g. drapes, swabs, instruments, sutures, fluids, catheters
- Creating a sterile working area known as the 'sterile field' where everything within the defined radius is sterile
- Maintaining a sterile working area by safe working practices that prevent contamination of the equipment and supplies.

The principles of aseptic technique are shown in Box 15.27.

Clean technique

Clean technique is a version of aseptic technique. The goal of clean technique is to exclude pathogens from a susceptible site, whereas that of aseptic technique is to exclude all microorganisms (Burton & Engelkirk 2004). When used in conjunction with a 'no-touch' technique

EVIDENCE-BASED PRACTICE — Box 15.26

Antiseptic agents

Antiseptic agents (antiseptics) are chemical solutions that reduce or destroy microorganisms on the skin or mucous membranes without causing damage or irritation. They are used to clean the skin before invasive procedures and also as hand cleansing agents for healthcare workers.

- Antiseptics are used in accordance with the manufacturer's directions, which are designed to ensure that, when used as directed, the antiseptic agent meets its stated efficacy. Like chemical disinfectants, the use of antiseptics is regulated by COSHH Regulations (1999)
- Antiseptics must be discarded after the designated 'use by' date indicated on the label
- Liquid soap dispensers should never be 'topped up', as they are a potential source of contamination because bacteria can multiply within many products. They should be completely replaced, including the dispensing nozzle (Wilson 2001)
- As antiseptics do not have the same destructive powers as chemicals used for disinfection of inanimate objects, they should *never* be used to disinfect equipment or environmental surfaces (WHO 2003).

Student activities

- Identify three different types of skin cleansing preparation used in your placement.
- Find out how they are used and any associated problems indicated in the COSHH Regulations.

NURSING SKILLS — Box 15.27

Principles of aseptic technique

Aseptic technique may vary slightly but the basic principles are similar.

Preparation

- *Environment*: Preferably use a treatment room for the procedure; if not available, the procedure may be performed at the patient's bedside. Ensure that the door or screens are closed to reduce the likelihood of cross-infection by deterring others from walking in and out of the area and to provide privacy
- *Trolleys*: Those used for aseptic procedures must not be used for any other purpose. They should be cleaned daily with detergent and water and dried with paper towels and wiped with 70% isopropyl alcohol solution before use (WHO 2003)
- *Supplies*: Collect the requisite dressing pack, supplementary packs, lotions and any other items required, checking their expiry dates and for damage and sterility (see Box 15.23). Place all supplies on the bottom of the clean trolley
- *Patient*: Explain the procedure to the patient to obtain their consent and cooperation. Position the patient appropriately and comfortably so that the procedure can be performed easily.

Opening sterile packs and supplies and organizing the work surface

- Wash hands or disinfect clean hands with an alcohol-based hand rub
- Place the pack to be opened on the centre of the trolley top. The outside wrapping is not sterile and therefore it is important that the pack is opened correctly to prevent contamination of its contents. Open the inner wrapping, handling the corners only: the opened area forms the 'sterile field'. Henceforth only sterile items can come in contact with this area. The open 'sterile field' must lie flat on the trolley top and never be flattened with the fingers
- Gently slide supplementary packs onto the sterile field ensuring that the outside wrappers do not touch the sterile field. If they do, consider the area contaminated
- Sterile lotions are poured slowly and directly into a gallipot. When pouring liquids the bottle must be positioned clear of the sterile field
- Before organizing the work surface, decontaminate hands again and wear sterile gloves (or use sterile forceps) throughout the procedure.

Maintaining a sterile working area during the procedure

- The area around the procedure site should be surrounded with sterile drapes
- Ensure that only sterile items come into contact with the susceptible site
- Do not allow sterile items to touch non-sterile objects; if in doubt about the sterility of an item or area, consider it contaminated.

Discarding supplies

- After completing the procedure, discard any used sharps immediately into a sharps container and then all waste into a clinical waste bag
- Discard protective clothing into the appropriate waste receptacle
- Wash hands to prevent cross-infection to others.

(not touching the susceptible body area with non-sterile items) clean technique is used for:

- Injecting medications
- Removal of sutures and drains (see Ch. 24)
- Endotracheal suctioning
- Venepuncture and intravenous cannulation.

Clean technique includes all the key elements of standard precautions including:

- Thorough handwashing before and after the procedure
- Wearing suitable PPE, i.e. non-sterile, disposable gloves and apron
- Using and disposing of sharps safely
- Appropriate cleaning, disinfection and sterilization practices
- Correct disposal of waste.

Isolation precautions

Microorganisms cause a wide variety of infections and, for most, standard precautions are adequate to prevent their transmission to healthcare personnel and other patients. However, for patients known to have, or are suspected to have, highly transmissible infections or are colonized by dangerous pathogens, additional precautions are needed. In the past, these were referred to as 'barrier nursing', but are now known as isolation precautions. Some healthcare facilities use the term 'source isolation' to indicate that the patient is the source of the infection and to distinguish them from 'protective isolation', the precautions which may be required for patients who are highly vulnerable to infection.

Principles of isolation nursing

The theory and practice of isolation nursing focus on interrupting the transmission route of microorganisms. Consideration is given to the following elements.

Patient accommodation

A key component of isolation is the appropriate placement of the patient. Some healthcare facilities have infectious disease or isolation units where patients are nursed in single rooms with en-suite facilities, controlled airflow systems and cared for by a team of specialist infection control practitioners. In the UK there are several high-security units for treating patients with highly communicable infections, e.g. Lassa fever and Ebola fever.

In other healthcare facilities, patients are isolated in single rooms within a ward. These settings are less secure than isolation units due to the close proximity of other patients and the frequent contact that healthcare practitioners have with both infected and non-infected patients. Furthermore, the availability of single rooms with en-suite facilities may be limited and, for most patients, rooms and bathrooms must often be shared. When a single room is unavailable, patients with the same microorganism may share a room, a practice referred to as 'cohorting'.

Patient movement

A practice that impinges on isolation measures is moving isolation patients/clients between wards or other healthcare facilities. Glynn et al (1997) identified that five to seven moves were not uncommon in some hospitals. This practice interferes with measures to prevent, control and contain infection and should be avoided. If a patient has to be moved, then it is important that the receiving unit/ward is notified of their impending arrival and the infection control measures required.

Psychological effects of isolation

Society protects itself from those who would do it harm by isolating people: those who have committed serious crimes are isolated in prison; infectious patients are isolated in hospital. In prisons, the degree of isolation varies from high-security confinement to an open approach; however, in hospitals, whatever the degree of isolation it can be a disturbing experience for the patient. In response to their isolation, some patients may become demanding, fussy or irritable. Many patients express feelings of loneliness, abandonment, inferiority and boredom when isolated (Wilson 2001). Isolated patients have significantly higher levels of anxiety and depression, and lower self-esteem and sense of control. In order to promote patients' wellbeing they need to be informed about their condition, its symptoms and treatment, the control measures and their rationale, together with advice about their responsibilities (Lewis et al 1999) (Box 15.28).

It is important to consider the ethical issues relating to confidentiality when caring for people with infectious diseases. Maintaining patient confidentiality is another important concern in isolation nursing (Box 15.29).

Categories of isolation

The three categories of isolation (transmission-based precautions) are:

- Airborne precautions
- Droplet precautions
- Contact precautions.

REFLECTIVE PRACTICE Box 15.28

The impact of isolation

Susan is 20 years old and has a mild learning disability. She is admitted to hospital for investigations. Three days later she develops a fever and a vesicular skin rash. Suspecting that she may have contracted chickenpox and to prevent the transmission of the virus to others, Susan is isolated in one of the ward's single rooms. Isolation in a separate room can be a frightening and anxious time for patients, their relatives and visitors.

Student activities

- Think about how Susan may feel.
- Consider how you would explain the reason for isolation nursing and the precautions needed to Susan.
- Think about how you could minimize the psychological effects of isolation for her.

> **ETHICAL ISSUES** Box 15.29
>
> ## Maintaining confidentiality
>
> Isolation procedures are necessary to reduce the risk of infection to healthcare personnel and other patients. However, by their very nature, they may indicate the type of infection, resulting in a breach of patients' confidentiality.
>
> **Student activities**
>
> Read the NMC *Code of Professional Conduct* (2004, clause 5) and Chapter 7. Then think about the questions below.
>
> - Who has the right to know why a patient is in isolation?
> - Is the patient's right to confidentiality more important than the right of others to protect themselves?

These precautions may be combined for diseases that have multiple routes of transmission, e.g. chickenpox which can be transmitted both by the airborne route and by direct contact with vesicle fluid or respiratory secretions.

Whether used alone or in combination, transmission-based precautions are always used in addition to standard precautions, i.e. by wearing clean non-sterile gloves when touching blood, body fluids, secretions, excretions and contaminated items, and handwashing after removal of gloves. If splashing of blood or body fluids is anticipated then eye protection, masks and plastic aprons are worn. Extra care is taken when handling equipment, sharp items, linen and waste.

Airborne precautions

Airborne precautions are necessary for infections transmitted by the inhalation of droplet nuclei, e.g. tuberculosis, measles and chickenpox.

Isolation (transmission-based) precautions are as follows:

- The patient is nursed in a single room that has a negative atmospheric pressure, i.e. the air flowing into the room is extracted to the outside of the building, not into other patient areas. The door must be kept closed for the air extraction system to operate effectively
- If a single room is not available, the patient may share a room with another patient who has the same infection
- People entering the room must wear masks unless they are known to be immune to the pathogen
- Movement of the patient from the room is limited to essential purposes only. On leaving the room the patient must wear a mask in order to protect others
- The patient is reminded to cover their mouth and nose when coughing or sneezing
- Gloves and plastic aprons are used when handling respiratory secretions
- Hands are washed before entering and after leaving the room.

Droplet precautions

Infections are transmitted by contact with respiratory secretions and large droplets expelled during coughing and sneezing, e.g. mumps, diphtheria and whooping cough. These infections are also spread by direct contact with contaminated items in the patient's immediate environment.

Isolation (transmission-based) precautions are as follows:

- Special air handling and ventilation are not required to prevent droplet transmission
- Patients are nursed in a single room (or in a room with another similarly infected patient)
- Masks are worn when working within 1–2 metres of the patient and used by patients if transportation is necessary (WHO 2003)
- Gloves and plastic aprons are used for contact with infective material
- Hands are washed before entering and after leaving the room.

Contact precautions

Infections are transmitted by direct contact with patients or by indirect contact with surfaces or equipment, e.g. MRSA; some enteric, skin and respiratory infections.

Isolation (transmission-based) precautions are as follows:

- A single room is preferable and essential when the source patient contaminates the environment, or cannot assist in maintaining infection control precautions to limit the transmission of the infection, e.g. infants, children and some people with a learning disability or dementia
- Gloves and plastic aprons are worn for contact with infective material from the patient or their immediate environment
- Hands are washed on leaving the room (Box 15.30).

Protective isolation

This type of isolation is also known as 'reverse barrier nursing' or 'neutropenic isolation'. Certain patients are at increased risk of microbial infections from both endogenous and exogenous sources. This is due to compromised defences such as in severe burns, leukaemia, organ transplants, immunosuppressed states and radiation treatment. Premature infants are also highly susceptible to infection.

Isolation (transmission-based) precautions are as follows:

- These patients are nursed in a total protected environment (TPE)
- TPE includes a private room (with shower and lavatory) where vented air entering the room is passed through high-efficiency particulate air (HEPA) filters. The room is under positive pressure to prevent corridor air from entering when the door is opened

HEALTH PROMOTION

Box 15.30

Breaking the chain of infection using transmission-based precautions

Two young children in a paediatric unit start vomiting and have profuse diarrhoea. Suspecting that the condition may be infectious, both children are moved into a double room and contact isolation precautions initiated. The room has its own toilet facilities and supplies of hand soap, disposable gloves, paper towels, plastic aprons, yellow waste bags, a laundry bag and patient-care equipment. One nurse is assigned to care for both children and wears gloves and a disposable plastic apron when in contact with faeces and vomit, e.g. when changing soiled bed linen, assisting the children with personal hygiene measures. Following each care activity, the nurse removes her gloves and discards them directly into the waste receptacle and thoroughly washes her hands. The nurse applied principles of infection control to contain the infectious organism at many points in the chain of infection as shown in the box below.

Link in the chain	**Nursing action to break the chain**
Infectious agent: Presently unknown. Could be *Salmonella, Shigella*, etc. Awaiting confirmation from the laboratory	Interrupted the microorganisms' transmission route by implementing contact isolation precautions Cohorted the two children with a similar infection in the same room with its own en-suite facilities Assignment of one nurse to care for the two children to reduce the risk of transmitting the infection to others in the unit
Reservoir: Gastrointestinal tract	The nurse was aware that the microorganisms could easily spread to other children by direct/indirect contact
Portal of exit: Diarrhoea	Faeces and vomit were discarded directly into the en-suite lavatory
Mode of transmission: Direct contact, especially via the hands of the children and healthcare personnel. Indirect contact with contaminated surfaces/equipment	The nurse wore gloves and disposable apron for all contact with body excretions and used proper handwashing techniques following removal of gloves and apron Linen was handled carefully and placed directly into the laundry bag; waste was discarded into a yellow waste bag Visitors were instructed to wash their hands before leaving the room All patient-care equipment was decontaminated before it was removed from the room
Portal of entry: Mouth	The nurse ensured that both children carefully washed and dried their hands following each episode of diarrhoea The nurse encouraged the children to refrain from putting fingers and objects into their mouths.
Susceptible host	The infection was not transmitted to other children in the unit due to adherence to infection control measures

- The room must be thoroughly cleaned and disinfected before the patient is admitted
- All items coming into contact with the patient are disinfected or sterilized beforehand
- People entering the room must wear appropriate PPE determined by local policies
- Although standard precautions, e.g. hand hygiene and PPE, are necessary before patient contact, masks are rarely required
- No special precautions are required for the disposal of waste and linen.

Specimen collection

Many different specimens are collected from patients and used to diagnose or follow the progress of infectious diseases. The most common clinical specimens that nurses take for sending to the microbiology laboratory are listed in Box 15.31.

Box 15.31 **Specimens taken by nurses**

These commonly include:

- Cervical and vaginal swabs
- Conjunctival swabs
- Faeces and rectal swabs
- Nasal swabs
- Pus from a wound or abscess
- Sputum (see Ch. 17)
- Throat swabs
- Urine (see Ch. 20).

It is important that the specimen is of the highest quality and collected safely:

- Whenever possible, specimens should be obtained before antimicrobial therapy has started. If this is not possible, the laboratory is informed of the antimicrobial agent(s) prescribed

- The most appropriate time to collect a specimen is during the acute stage of a disease, i.e. when the patient is experiencing symptoms. Some viruses, however, are more easily isolated during the prodromal stage, or onset, of the disease (see Box 15.4, p. 397)
- Timing of the specimen is very important, e.g. urine specimens should reach the laboratory within 2 hours of collection (Wilson 2001). Sputum specimens need to be obtained before a patient uses an antiseptic mouthwash, which can adversely affect the results
- The specimen obtained must be representative of the infection, e.g. a patient with pneumonia must provide a specimen of sputum and not saliva
- Specimen collection should always be performed with care and tact to avoid harming the patient or causing discomfort or embarrassment
- If patients are to collect specimens themselves, e.g. sputum or urine, they need to be given clear and detailed collection instructions.

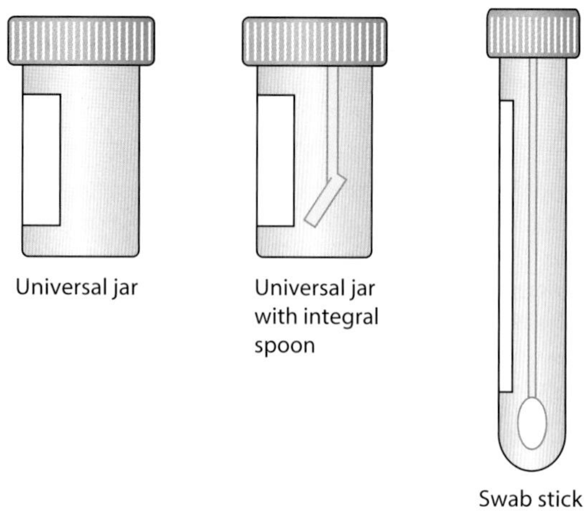

Fig. 15.10 Examples of specimen containers

Collection of clinical specimens

When collecting a clinical specimen for microbiology it must be collected in a manner that will prevent its contamination with either the patient's/client's or healthcare professional's microorganisms. It is important therefore, that standard precautions are implemented:

- Handwashing before and after the procedure
- Wearing PPE, i.e. gloves and aprons.

Sterile containers are always used for the collection of specimens (Fig. 15.10). Care needs to be taken to avoid contaminating the inside of the container or its lid when collecting the specimen, and to ensure that the outside of the container is not contaminated by the contents. The container's lid should be closed tightly to prevent leakage during transportation to the laboratory.

A sufficient quantity of material must be obtained to provide enough material for all the diagnostic tests required. The specimen container is labelled and accompanied by a request form. As a minimum, labels should contain the patient's name, hospital identification number, ward number/name or the requesting doctor's name, the specimen type and the date and time of collection. The specimen container is placed in a double self-sealing bag with one compartment containing the request form and the other the specimen.

When specimens are regarded as infection hazards, e.g. from people with hepatitis B or C, or HIV, they may present an infection risk to portering and laboratory staff; in such cases the specimen container and request form are labelled with biohazard labels.

Transport of specimens

Specimens should be delivered to the laboratory promptly so that the results accurately represent the number and types of organisms present at the time of collection. If delivery to the laboratory is delayed, the pathogens may die or any indigenous flora (non-pathogens) may overgrow, inhibit or kill the pathogens. If the specimen cannot be transported to the laboratory immediately then it may be refrigerated at 4°C (Hateley 2003). However, the refrigerator must be used for specimens only – it must not contain foods or medicines. Blood cultures are never refrigerated but stored at body temperature, in an incubator if necessary.

Summary

- The range of infectious diseases changes rapidly and in recent years new diseases have appeared and some, presumed extinct, have re-emerged.
- Microorganisms can only survive when their growth conditions are favourable.
- Inappropriate use of antibacterial drugs has caused increasing resistance of microorganisms.
- Healthcare-associated infections are preventable but widespread.

- Handwashing is the single most important feature of infection control in healthcare settings.
- Standard infection control precautions are used when caring for patients/clients regardless of whether they have an infection or not.
- Education and training of all healthcare staff are important in preventing the spread of infections and treating those who are affected.
- The mandatory training scheme in infection control for all healthcare staff introduced by NHS Scotland is one way forward, which will hopefully reduce the current incidence of hospital-acquired infections.
- Nurses must keep abreast of current literature regarding infection control; however, learning is only the beginning and what has been learned must then be applied to nursing practice.

Self test

1. The following is a list of a student nurse's daily activities. Indicate the times when nurses wash their hands to reduce the spread of infection:

Activity	Must wash hands	Not necessary
a. Before leaving home		
b. When arriving in the clinical practice area		
c. After bed-making		
d. After handling urine samples		
e. Before using the lavatory		
f. After removing gloves		
g. Before leaving the clinical practice area		

2. Identify the statements that correctly relate to the resident microbial flora of skin:

a. Can be acquired when taking a patient's pulse
b. Survive and multiply in the deep crevices of the skin
c. Are easily removed by handwashing with plain soap
d. Are effectively removed by antiseptic and alcohol-based hand cleansing preparations.

3. Which statement relating to the use of gloves is correct?

a. Hands must be washed following the removal of gloves
b. Polythene gloves are recommended for use in healthcare settings
c. Gloves may be washed and reused
d. Upon removal, gloves should be discarded into a black refuse bag.

4. Identify the correct statements associated with chemical disinfectants:

a. They are general poisons
b. Their effectiveness is impaired by dirt
c. They are inactive against some microorganisms
d. Their use is regulated by the COSHH Regulations (1999).

5. Which is the most common healthcare-associated infection?

a. Urinary tract infection
b. Blood infection
c. Wound infection
d. Lower respiratory tract infection.

6. For each of the practices described below, indicate the situations when a healthcare practitioner may become injured by sharps:

Practice	Is at risk	Is not at risk
a. Bending or breaking a hypodermic needle before disposal		
b. Not recapping a needle and disposing of it directly into a sharps container		
c. Warning a client you are going to give them an injection		
d. Disposing of used sharps into a container less than ¾ full		
e. Detaching a needle from a syringe prior to disposing into a used sharps container		

Key words and phrases for literature searching

Asepsis
Cross-infection
Decontamination
Drug resistance
Handwashing
Infection control
Needlestick injuries
Patient isolation
Respiratory tract infections
Sterilization
Urinary tract infections
Workplace infection risks

Useful websites

Centers for Disease Control and Prevention	www.cdc.gov Available July 2006
EngenderHealth	www.engenderhealth.org/ip/index.html Available July 2006
Eurosurveillance	www.eurosurveillance.org/search/search-02.asp Available July 2006
Evidence Based Practice in Infection Control (EPIC)	www.epic.tvu.ac.uk Available July 2006
Health Protection Agency	www.hpa.org.uk/infections Available July 2006
Health Protection Scotland	www.hps.scot.nhs.uk Available July 2006
Hospital eTool	www.osha.gov/SLTC/etools/hospital/index.html Available July 2006
Infection Control Nurses Association	www.icna.co.uk/ Available July 2006
Medline Plus	www.nlm.nih.gov/medlineplus/infectioncontrol.html Available July 2006
National Institute for Health and Clinical Excellence (NICE)	www.nice.org.uk/page.aspx?o=CG002 Available July 2006
Infection Control	
NHS Plus	www.nhsplus.nhs.uk/nhsstaff/infection.asp Available July 2006
Practical guidelines for infection control in health care facilities (WHO)	www.wpro.who.int/sars/docs/practicalguidelines/practical_guidelines.pdf Available July 2006

References

Ayliffe GJA, Babb JR, Taylor LJ 1999 Hospital-acquired infection. 3rd edn. Butterworth-Heinemann, Oxford

Bandolier 2003 Evidence-based healthcare: needlestick injuries. Online: www.jr2.ox.ac.uk/bandolier/Extraforbando/needle.pdf Available July 2006

Belkin NL 1997 The evolution of the surgical mask: filtering efficiency versus effectiveness. Journal of Infection Control and Hospital Epidemiology 18(1):49–56

Burton RW, Engelkirk PG 2004 Microbiology for the health sciences. 7th edn. Lippincott, Williams & Wilkins, Philadelphia

Centers for Disease Control and Prevention 2002 Guideline for hand hygiene in healthcare settings: MMWR Recommendations and Reports. Online: www.cdc.gov/handhygiene Available July 2006

Centers for Disease Control and Prevention 2003a Exposure to blood: what healthcare personnel need to know. Online: www.cdc.gov/ncidod/dhqp/pdf/bbp/Exp_to_Blood.pdf Available July 2006

Centers for Disease Control and Prevention 2003b Guidelines for environmental infection control in health-care facilities. Online: www.cdc.gov/ncidod/dhqp/gl_environinfection.html Available July 2006

Clark L, Smith W, Young L 2002 Protective clothing: principles and guidance. Infection Control Nurses Association, London

Department of Health 2001 Standard principles for preventing hospital-acquired infections. Journal of Hospital Infection 47(Suppl):S21–S37

Department of Health 2003 Winning ways: working together to reduce healthcare associated infection in England. DH, London. Online: www.dh.gov.uk/assetRoot/04/06/46/89/04064689.pdf Available July 2006

EngenderHealth www.engenderhealth.org/ip/index.html

Exposure Prevention Information Network (EPINet) 2004. Online: www.needlestickforum.net/3epinet/latestresults.htm Available July 2006

Glynn A, Ward V, Wilson J 1997 Hospital-acquired infection. Surveillance policies and practice. Public Health Laboratory Service, London

Gould D, Brooker C 2000 Applied microbiology for nurses. Palgrave Macmillan, Basingstoke

Government of Ontario, Canada

Greaves A 1985 We'll just freshen you up my dear. Nursing Times 6(Suppl):3–8

Hateley P 2003 Infection control. In: Brooker C, Nicol M (eds) Nursing adults: the practice of caring. Mosby, Edinburgh, pp. 253–270

Health Canada 1998 Infection control guidelines (supplement). Canadian Medical Association, Ottawa. Online: www.phac-aspc.gc.ca/publicat/ccdr-rmtc/99vol25/25s4/index.html Available July 2006

Health Protection Agency 2004 Information on face masks and respirators. Online: www.hpa.org.uk/infections/topics_az/SARS/maskFAQs.htm Available July 2006

Health Services Advisory Committee 1999 Safe disposal of clinical waste. 2nd edn. TSO, Norwich

Henry K, Campbell S, Jackson B et al 1990 Long-term follow-up of health care workers with work-site exposure to human immunodeficiency virus [letter to the editor]. Journal of the American Medical Association 263(13):1765–1766

Inglis TJJ 2003 Microbiology and infection, 2nd edn. Churchill Livingstone, Edinburgh

Leonas KK, Jones CR 2003 The relationship of fabric properties and bacterial filtering efficiency for selected surgical masks.

Journal of Textile and Apparel, Technology and Management 3(2)
Lewis AM, Gammon J, Hosein I 1999 The pros and cons of isolation and containment. Journal of Hospital Infection 43:19–23
McDonald LL, Pugliese G 1996 Laundry service. In: Mayhall CG (ed) Hospital Epidemiology and Infection Control. Williams and Wilkins, Baltimore
National Institute for Occupational Safety and Health 1997 Preventing allergic reactions to natural rubber latex in the workplace. NIOSH Publication No. 97–135 (June 1997) Online: www.cdc.gov/niosh/topics/latex Available July 2006
National Institute for Health and Clinical Excellence 2003 Infection control: prevention of healthcare-associated infections in primary and community care. NICE, London. Online: www.nice.org.uk/pdf/Infection_control_fullguideline.pdf Available July 2006
NHS Executive 1995 Hospital laundry arrangements for used and infected linen. HSG(95)18. HMSO, London
NHS Quality Improvement Scotland 2003 Improving clinical care in Scotland: healthcare associated infection (HAI) infection control. NHS QIS, Edinburgh
NHS Scotland 2005 Needlestick injuries: sharpen your awareness. Scottish Executive, Edinburgh. Online. Available: www.show.scot.nhs.uk/sehd/publications/nisa/nisa-00.htm Available July 2006
Nursing and Midwifery Council 2004 Code of professional conduct: standards for conduct, performance and ethics. NMC, London. Online: www.nmc-uk.org/aFramedisplay.aspx?documentID=201 Available July 2006
Occupational Safety and Health Administration 2004 Tuberculosis. HealthCare Wide Hazards Module. Online: www.osha.gov/SLTC/etools/hospital/hazards/tb/tb.html Available July 2006
Pratt RJ, Pellowe C, Loveday HP et al 2000 Epic phase 1: the development of national evidence-based guidelines for preventing hospital-acquired infections in England. Standard Principles: Technical Report. London: Thames Valley University. Online: www.epic.tvu.ac.uk Available July 2006
Scottish Executive 2002 Preventing infections acquired while receiving healthcare, 2002–2005. Online: www.scotland.gov.uk/library5/health/preventinfect.pdf Available July 2006
Scottish Executive Health Department 2002 The Watt Group Report. A review of the outbreak of salmonella at the Victoria Infirmary. Online: www.scotland.gov.uk/library5/health/twgr.pdf Available July 2006
The Scottish Office 1999 Hospital acquired infection: a framework for a national surveillance for the NHS in Scotland. Online: www.scotland.gov.uk/library2/doc15/hai-00.asp Available July 2006
Tortora GJ, Funke BR, Case CL 2003 Microbiology: an introduction. 8th edn. Benjamin Cummings, San Francisco
Wilson J 2001 Infection control in clinical practice. 2nd edn. Baillière Tindall, Edinburgh
World Health Organization 2002 Scaling up the response to infectious diseases: report on infectious diseases 2002. WHO, Geneva. Online: www.who.int/infectious-disease-report/2002/introduction.html Available July 2006
World Health Organization 2003 Practical guidelines for infection control in health care facilities. WHO, Geneva. Online: www.wpro.who.int/sars/docs/practicalguidelines/practical_guidelines.pdf Available July 2006

Further reading

Burton RW, Engelkirk PG 2004 Microbiology for the health sciences. 7th edn. Lippincott Williams and Wilkins, Philadelphia
Gould D, Brooker C 2000 Applied microbiology for nurses. Palgrave Macmillan, Basingstoke
Inglis TJJ 2003 Microbiology and infection. 2nd edn. Churchill Livingstone, Edinburgh
Kowalak JP, Hughes SA, Mills JE 2002 Best practices: a guide to excellent nursing care. Lippincott Williams and Wilkins, Philadelphia
Tortora GJ, Funke BR, Case CL 2003 Microbiology: an introduction. 8th edn. Benjamin Cummings, San Francisco
Wilson J 2001 Infection control in clinical practice. 2nd edn. Baillière Tindall, Edinburgh

16

Caring for the person with physical needs, sensory impairment and unconsciousness

Anne Waugh

Glossary terms

Emollient

Glasgow Coma Scale (GCS)

Infestation

Intertrigo

Maceration

Neurological

Plaque

Prosthesis

Skin flora

Learning outcomes

This chapter will help you:

- Discuss the factors that may influence a person's appearance and personal hygiene
- Describe health-promoting activities that relate to aspects of personal hygiene
- Outline the contribution of the *Essence of Care* (DH 2001) in helping people maintain their personal and oral hygiene
- Explain the nursing interventions that may be needed to assist a person with their personal hygiene activities
- Explain the nursing interventions that will assist communication with people with hearing and/or sight impairment
- State the first aid priorities for assessing a collapsed or unconscious casualty
- Describe the nursing interventions used in caring for an unconscious patient
- Identify relevant sources of information for providing client education on topics included in this chapter.

Introduction

The first section of this chapter explores a range of activities involved in maintaining personal hygiene and appearance, and the factors that may affect them. These activities include many fundamental aspects of care, some of which are highlighted in the *Essence of Care* (DH 2001), emphasizing that a working knowledge of these aspects of care is an important nursing role and also one in which a nurse can 'make a difference'. Sometimes the responsible nurse, who remains accountable for the care that clients or patients receive, may delegate these activities to others in the team. In other cases they may form part of a community care package provided to meet social needs or are carried out informally by carers for a relative. Appropriate nursing interventions are discussed to enable holistic assessment and planning when people need help to maintain their personal hygiene and appearance. In each part of this chapter underpinning anatomy and physiology are briefly reviewed to provide the basis for assessing people's health status and recognizing the presence of abnormalities.

In the middle section, the senses of vision and hearing are reviewed and nursing interventions that will help people with sight and hearing impairment in community and hospital settings are explained.

The final section considers unconsciousness and the related first aid interventions. The nursing care required by an unconscious person is then outlined with the following aims:

- To introduce the idea that assessment and planning of integrated care for a person with substantial physical needs occurs by making links between the fundamental nursing skills explained in this and other chapters of the book
- To show how a holistic approach to care is largely based on combining fundamental nursing interventions appropriately to meet individual needs.

Personal hygiene and appearance

In this section, factors that affect people's personal hygiene and appearance are considered and health promotion activities involving nurses are explored. When assistance is needed, nursing interventions are discussed using the evidence base (see Ch. 5), where available. A range of student activities to promote inquiry is included.

For most people, maintaining their appearance and personal hygiene is an important aspect of their daily routines that, once learned, is often taken for granted to a greater or lesser extent. Many different activities are involved, including:

- Showering, bathing and washing
- Care of the hands, feet and nails
- Care of the eyes, ears and nose
- Hair care
- Facial hair care and shaving
- Dressing
- Maintaining dental health and oral hygiene.

Personal grooming extends to choosing the clothes worn, hair styling and the application of cosmetics and jewellery. The way in which a person chooses to present themselves to others is an integral part of their sexuality.

Children and some adults may need temporary or ongoing assistance with some or all of the activities listed above. Personal hygiene is important for both health and social acceptability and, in most cultures, it is expected that people should be clean and odour free.

Recent attempts to improve fundamental aspects of care in all settings saw the development of best practice statements in the *Essence of Care* (DH 2001). Those relevant to nursing interventions discussed in this chapter include:

- Personal and oral hygiene
- Principles of self-care
- Privacy and dignity.

The best practice statements, or benchmarks, come with a resource pack to help nurses and others rate their current practice against them. By identifying and then improving aspects of current practice nurses can work towards meeting these benchmarks. The best practice statements that relate to personal hygiene are shown in Box 16.1.

Box 16.1 Best practice statements: personal hygiene

- All patients/clients are assessed to identify the advice and/or care required to maintain and promote their individual personal hygiene
- Planned care is negotiated with patients/clients and/or their carers and is based on assessment of their individual needs
- Patients/clients have access to an environment that is safe and acceptable to the individual
- Patients/clients are expected to supply their own toiletries but single-use toiletries are provided until they can supply their own
- Patients/clients have access to the level of assistance that they require to meet their individual personal hygiene needs
- Patients/clients and/or carers are provided with information/education to meet their individual personal hygiene needs
- Patients'/clients' care is continuously evaluated, reassessed and the care plan renegotiated.

[From DH (2001)]

Structure and functions of the skin

The skin completely covers the body, providing a waterproof barrier between the external environment and underlying internal structures. It is self-renewing and self-repairing and consists of three layers (Fig. 16.1):

- The *epidermis* is constantly renewed as the deeper cells divide, migrate upwards and are shed as flat, keratinized cells from the skin surface. Through this process, the epidermis is renewed every 50–70 days, providing for 'wear and tear' of the skin.
- The *dermis* lies underneath the epidermis and consists of connective tissue. It contains collagen and elastic fibres and specialized cells including fibroblasts and macrophages. Structures found in the dermis include blood and lymph vessels, nerve endings, sweat and sebaceous glands and hairs.
- The *subcutaneous layer* consists mainly of adipose tissue (fat) and also varies in thickness. It provides insulation, cushions the underlying structures and acts as a long-term energy source.

Normal skin flora

Following birth the skin surface becomes colonized by commensal bacteria (organisms living in association with another organism, without benefiting it and normally without harming it) and they form the normal skin flora (see Ch. 15). They do not normally cause harm unless they gain entry to a part of the body normally protected by the non-specific defence mechanisms or a person is particularly susceptible to infection, for example when the immune system in compromised following cancer chemotherapy. In hospital, normal flora (commensal bacteria) are replaced by hospital strains that are more likely to be pathogenic (causing illness) and resistant to many antibiotics. This predisposes people to the development of hospital-acquired infection (see Ch. 15).

Appendages of the skin

These include hair and hair follicles, different types of glands and the nails. Hair grows from the bulb at the base of hair follicles (see Fig. 16.1). The arrector pili are small involuntary muscles associated with hair follicles and contraction pulls the hairs erect, causing 'goose pimples' on the skin.

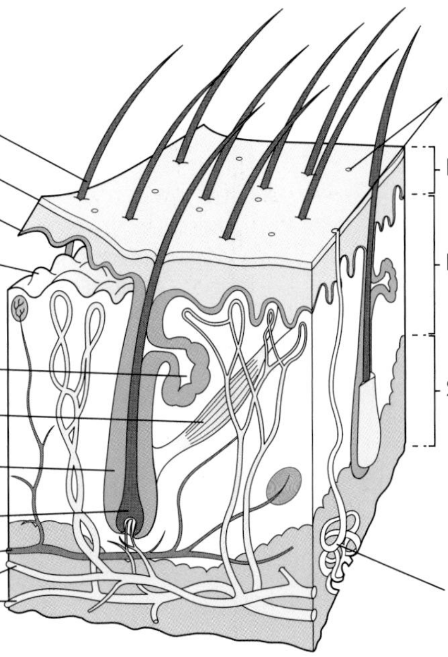

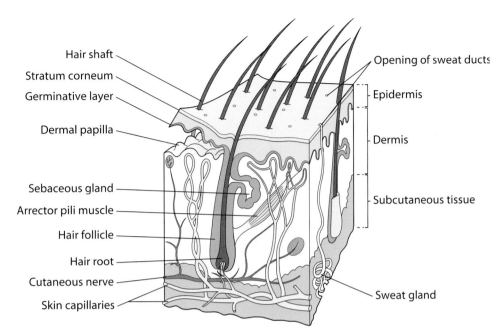

Fig. 16.1 The structure of the skin showing its appendages (reproduced with permission from Waugh & Grant 2006)

Sebaceous glands are present on most parts of the body and become active at puberty. They secrete an oily substance, called sebum, which keeps the hair soft and pliable and the skin supple. It also provides waterproofing and acts as an antibacterial agent, preventing the invasion of microbes.

Sweat glands are also widely distributed throughout the skin and they secrete sweat that consists mainly of water and sodium chloride (salt). Secretion of sweat is increased when either environmental or body temperature is high and by sympathetic nerve stimulation. Excessive sweating leads to dehydration (see Ch. 19). Specialized sweat glands that become active at puberty are found in the axillae and anogenital region. They secrete sweat together with other substances as an odourless milky fluid. When normal flora on the skin act on this, the result is a bad smell, sometimes referred to as 'body odour'.

Functions of the skin

Intact skin acts as a non-specific defence mechanism by providing a waterproof physical barrier plus chemical (acid mantle) and biological barriers that together protect against microorganisms, chemicals and physical trauma.

Control of body temperature is an important function of the skin, with heat loss determined by the amount of blood circulating through its vast capillary network (see Ch. 14).

The skin is also a sensory organ with specialized receptors for touch, pain and temperature. Sensation is mediated by the nervous system (Fig. 16.2, Box 16.2, see p. 428) and provides important information about the environment. It protects people from potentially dangerous situations, e.g. burns from very hot objects. The automatic response to touching something very hot is immediate withdrawal from the hot item. Children learn a great deal about keeping safe through cutaneous sensation. When something causes pain, they quickly learn not to repeat the behaviour. Abnormal sensation puts people at risk from environmental hazards, e.g. stepping into a very hot bath causes scalds.

Limited absorption and excretion of certain substances takes place through the skin. Many drugs are absorbed through the skin, e.g. those contained in transdermal patches (see Ch. 22).

Assessment of the skin

A person's skin condition contributes to their body image and the media encourages people to see healthy skin as an attractive attribute. A major threat to healthy skin is from overexposure to the sun either through occupational or leisure activities (Box 16.3, p. 428). People who have skin conditions often consider themselves unattractive to others and suffer from low self-esteem.

Careful observation of the skin can provide clues about body temperature, hydration and general health of an individual. This can be undertaken informally while speaking to a person when the observant nurse will look at exposed body parts, e.g. the face and extremities, or while recording vital signs. More information can be gained when clothes are removed, e.g. when assistance is needed with activities of living. Formal assessment is needed in some situations, for example, to assess the risk of pressure ulcers (see Ch. 25) and when a person's primary problem is a skin disorder. The characteristics of normal skin are:

- Colour is normal for racial group
- Warm to touch
- Dry surface
- Intact surface.

Knowing the normal characteristics will alert the nurse to the need to report any abnormalities, (e.g. redness, clammy skin, rashes, signs of scratching) that may be present. Signs of scratching may indicate a parasitic infestation.

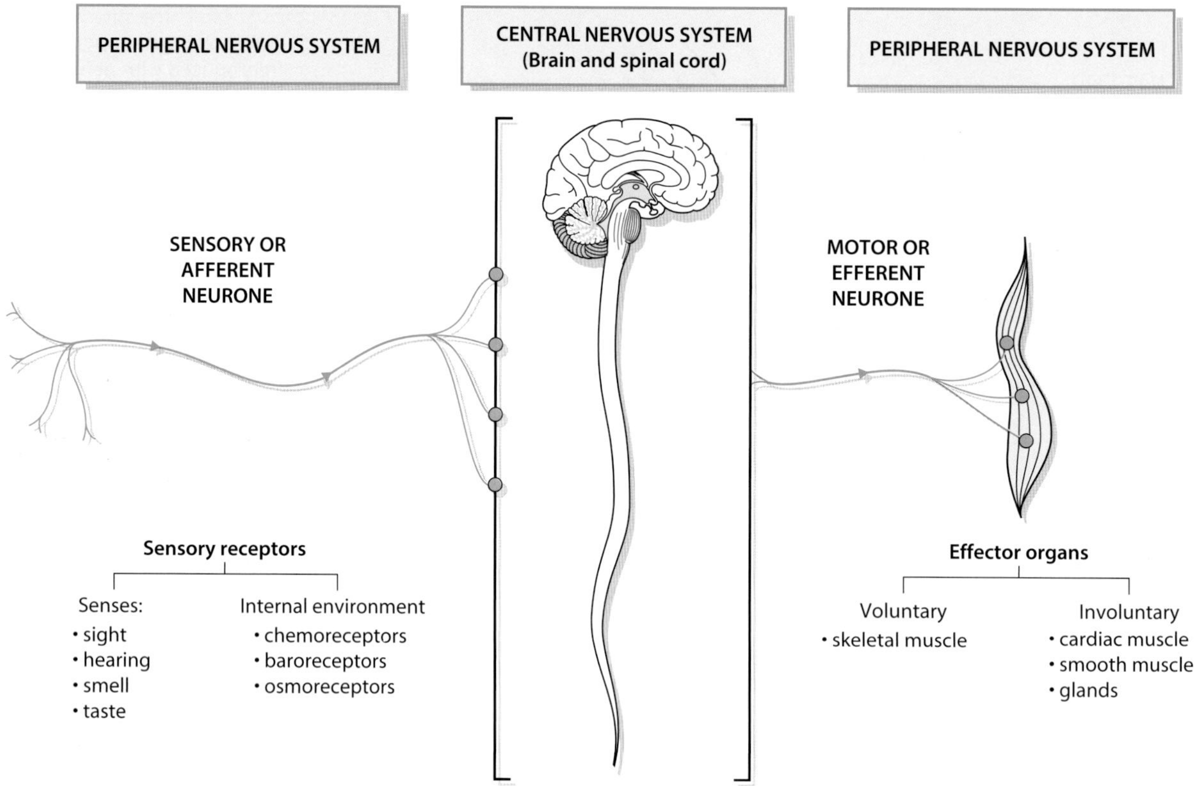

Fig. 16.2 The functional components of the nervous system (reproduced with permission from Waugh & Grant 2006)

Box 16.2

The nervous system

The nervous system consists of two parts:

- the central nervous system comprising the brain and spinal cord
- the peripheral nervous system that includes all other nerves (see Fig. 16.2).

The nervous system controls and integrates body functions. Put very simply, sensory receptors in the peripheral nervous system respond to stimuli either inside the body or in the external environment. This results in generation of nerve impulses that travel to the central nervous system via sensory nerves. After processing in the central nervous system, responses – again in the form of nerve impulses – are conducted through motor nerves to effector organs in the peripheral nervous system, i.e. muscles and glands. Responses may be either voluntary or involuntary.

For a detailed explanation of the components and functions of the nervous system you should refer to your anatomy and physiology textbook.

HEALTH PROMOTION Box 16.3

Preventing skin cancer

Skin cancer is usually the result of too much exposure to the sun. In the UK, rates are increasing and many people do not take the required precautions.

Risk factors

- Skin characteristics: burns easily, fair, freckled, more than 50 moles
- Previous skin cancer: oneself or a family member
- History of severe sunburn.

The SunSmart campaign (Cancer Research UK 2004) advises the following actions to reduce the risks:

Stay in the shade between 11.00 and 15.00 hours
Make sure you do not burn
Always cover up
Remember to take extra care with children
Then use sunscreen – factor 15 or above

Infestation

This is invasion by a parasite that lives on a host, e.g. head lice (see pp. 438–439) and scabies (Box 16.4). Other infestations include body lice that are rare in developed countries but are sometimes found in rough sleepers who lack the facilities for personal hygiene and washing clothes, and pubic lice, also known as 'crabs', that are spread by close contact such as sexual activity and can be recognized by their two large hind claws.

Box 16.4 Scabies

Scabies is caused by infestation of a small parasitic itch mite (*Sarcoptes scabei*) and is acquired from another person during close physical contact. The female burrows along the epidermal layer of the skin, laying eggs and leaving faeces behind. Areas where the skin is thin, including the finger webs and ankles, are commonly affected. As adult mites develop, they feed and burrow, eventually through most areas of the skin, and chemicals in their excreta cause intense itching. The burrows can often be seen on the skin.

Treatment

- Application of pesticide lotions after bathing
- Laundering of clothes and bedding in a domestic washing machine.

Itching can continue for 2–3 weeks until the outer layer of the skin is replaced although the mites will have been eradicated.

Factors influencing appearance and personal hygiene

Many factors that affect people's preferences and routines are considered below. Knowledge of these helps the nurse assess a person's needs so that holistic interventions can be planned and carried out when independence is not possible.

Physical

Many physical factors influence a person's independence in these activities, leaving them with limited ability to undertake some aspects of self-care through to complete dependence on others to meet their needs. These include frailty, impaired movement or inability to use a limb, unconsciousness, difficulty balancing for any length of time and sight impairment.

Consideration of general mobility will indicate whether assistance to get to the bathroom or the use of a hoist or other equipment is necessary (see Ch. 18). In a care setting, equipment such as an intravenous (i.v.) infusion will reduce a person's independence in carrying out activities related to maintaining appearance and personal hygiene.

Breathless and debilitated people may be able to carry out some of the activities required but find trying to complete the whole process themselves exhausting.

If a person is in pain, this will affect both their motivation and ability to undertake or tolerate these interventions. When this is the case, it is important to assess their pain and provide analgesia beforehand.

Psychological factors

Most people feel clean and refreshed after a bath or shower. Someone who is depressed, debilitated or lethargic may not have the interest or energy to engage in maintaining their own appearance and hygiene. This may affect dressing and wearing clean, presentable clothes or extend to complete neglect of personal hygiene. The nurse may need to gently encourage these people to attend to their grooming (Box 16.5). This is also important in people with low self-esteem, low mood or altered body image.

NURSING SKILLS — Box 16.5

Strategies for encouraging personal hygiene

- Provide encouragement by ensuring warmth and privacy for showering or bathing
- Encourage participation by providing opportunity and choice in both buying and use of own toiletries, cosmetics and clothes
- Provide motivation by giving praise for improvements in appearance
- Act as a good role model by ensuring your own standards are appropriate
- Remember that if a person refuses to undertake personal hygiene activities, their wishes must be respected (NMC 2004).

REFLECTIVE PRACTICE — Box 16.6

Caught unaware

It is common to feel uneasy when seen inappropriately dressed by other people.

Student activities

- Recall an incident when you were unexpectedly seen when partially, or wholly, undressed.
- Note down how you felt and provide the reasons for this.
- Identify those people who would not make you feel uncomfortable seeing you in this state.

Social, cultural and religious factors

Cultural and religious norms often influence individual practice. Religious requirements include personal hygiene activities, e.g. Hindus and Muslims require their hygiene needs to be met by nurses of the same sex. In Western cultures communal bathing or showering practices vary although in the UK separate facilities for men and women are usually provided, e.g. swimming pools. In many cultures nudity is considered offensive (Box 16.6). The answers you provided for Box 16.6 may have identified more of these factors.

Environmental factors

In Western countries, living accommodation normally includes an indoor lavatory and a fitted bath or shower. Access to and using the bath, shower and toilet may require the installation of adaptations (see p. 433).

Economic factors

When personal income is low, people may be unable to afford adequate heating for the bathroom or hot water for showering. Similarly, there may be little money to spend on basic hygiene requisites including soap, shampoo, toothbrush and toothpaste.

Lifespan factors

At particular stages of the lifespan there are characteristics affecting both independence in carrying out personal hygiene activities and the actual hygiene activities required.

Infancy

In infancy a parent usually carries out bathing routines and personal hygiene. Infants do not produce sebum (p. **427**) and therefore their skin is susceptible to maceration (softening of the skin caused by continual exposure to moisture) and this predisposes to nappy rash (Box 16.7).

EVIDENCE-BASED PRACTICE — Box 16.7

Nappy rash

Nappy rash is inflammation of those parts of the skin normally covered by a nappy and is minimized by keeping the skin clean and dry. Neonates (newborn babies up to 4 weeks old) pass urine around 20 times per day – this reduces to about 7 times daily by 1 year. Nappy rash does not occur in developing countries where nappies are not used.

Predisposing factors

Contact with faeces is the most important skin irritant and worsens when diarrhoea occurs. Other contributing factors may include:

- Contact with urine
- Maceration or increased hydration of the area
- Chemicals, e.g. from creams and other products applied to the skin
- Trauma if there is friction between a nappy and the skin.

Prevention

This is encouraged by:

- Keeping the skin free from the irritant effects of urine and faeces by regular changing of nappies, ideally each time they are wet or soiled
- Using disposable absorbent nappies – they contain absorbent substances that hold much more urine than conventional nappies
- Using disposable wipes that do not contain alcohol.

Treatment

- Change nappies more frequently
- Use a barrier cream liberally, e.g. zinc and castor oil
- Allow periods without using a nappy
- Use of prescribed preparations.

An information leaflet is available from Prodigy (2004a).
[Adapted from Prodigy (2004b)]

Childhood

During childhood, independence in toileting, washing and dressing is usually established using significant others as role models, not only but also due to physiological development and maturation of the body systems. Through socialization, children learn that personal hygiene is undertaken in privacy or only in the presence of close family members. However, not everyone achieves independence in these activities. For example, children with severe physical or learning disabilities may always be dependent, to some extent, on others.

Puberty

Puberty occurs during adolescence and is accompanied by physical and emotional changes that focus attention on personal grooming and hygiene. Increasing under-arm perspiration develops, necessitating the use of a deodorant. Girls start to menstruate and in boys there is growth of facial hair.

McKinlay et al (1996) carried out a study on clients with severe learning disabilities and found that many were unable to manage menstruation independently (Box 16.8). Interestingly, the suggestions provided by the clients' mothers in the study reflect the information needed by any girl before the onset of menstruation.

At this time there is often experimenting with clothing, hairstyles, cosmetics and jewellery while striving to develop an individual personality and sexual identity. Standards of hygiene may change as development influences the young person's body image and perceptions of self (see Box 16.5, p. 429).

Older adults

In older adults the physical changes of the normal ageing process influence appearance and personal hygiene

HEALTH PROMOTION — Box 16.8

Managing menstruation

McKinlay et al (1996) identified difficulties in about 50% of clients with severe learning disabilities that included:

- Refusing to wear sanitary protection
- Inappropriate disposal of used pads.

Only 20% of clients' mothers had received advice on this topic and provided the researchers with information that they would have found useful prior to their own experiences.

1. Prepare your daughter by:
   - Explaining what will happen and emphasizing this is a normal occurrence
   - Encouraging personal hygiene
   - Telling her to expect blood
   - Showing her a sanitary pad and providing the opportunity to practise using one occasionally.
2. A mothers' discussion group would have been a useful source of advice and support, especially when problems arise.

routines. Age-related changes affecting the skin may impact on nursing interventions and include:

- Dryness
- Thinning, making it more easily traumatized
- Wrinkling
- Longer regeneration time.

To a greater or lesser extent, hair turns white as the colour pigment melanin is replaced by air. An older person may find they can no longer reach their toenails and may require help to cut them. Toenails become thicker and often grow abnormally. Gum disease, which frequently originates in childhood, can result in loss of teeth and the need to wear dentures (p. 442). Physical frailty can make getting into a bath both difficult and unsafe. When this is the case, or there is visual impairment or reduced dexterity, home adaptations and/or aids may be required (pp. 433, 440).

Assisting with bathing, washing and showering

Nursing assessment identifies a person's usual routines and preferences in order to understand their habits (see Ch. 14). This includes the frequency, time of day and what the individual can do independently so that holistic and individualized care can be given as required.

When helping people with bathing and washing, it is important to recognize common nursing practices that may not be conducive to maintaining healthy skin, e.g. use of soap (see p. 432).

Assisting a person with their personal hygiene provides a good opportunity to communicate with them. The nurse can identify not only their preferred hygiene practices but also all other aspects of their general wellbeing and progress. For a dependent person, activities related to personal hygiene can be used to preserve personal choice and individuality when this is not possible in many other aspects of their lives. When a person refuses to undertake any activity, including those concerned with personal hygiene, their wishes must be respected even if this causes the nurse frustration (NMC 2004).

Maintaining privacy and dignity

It is important to remember the importance of privacy and dignity when considering any aspect of personal hygiene, whether assistance is needed or not. The best practice statements (DH 2001) are shown in Box 16.9. These extend to client preference, and Oxtoby (2003) highlights simple interventions, e.g. ensuring bedside screens are completely closed and gowns meet at the back when mobilizing, that will improve people's privacy and dignity. When assisting people to carry out activities involved in maintaining personal hygiene they are likely to feel embarrassed and helpless. Clients' feelings may well be similar to those you recalled while completing Box 16.6 (see p. 429).

Washing and drying the skin

The skin is usually cleaned by washing with soap, or soap substitute, then rinsed and gently patted dry, with particular attention to skin folds and crevices, e.g. under the breasts and between the buttocks. If moisture remains in skinfolds, either through sweating or inadequate drying, irritation and breaks in the skin can develop. This is known as intertrigo. Nursing practices need careful thought to ensure they do not worsen dry skin which is a common problem, especially in older people (Box 16.10, p. 432).

Skin conditions can be painful and people with skin disorders may use prescribed preparations for washing. These people may also feel particularly self-consciousness if they need help with washing because skin problems can affect self-esteem and body image (see Chs 8, 11, 12 and 21). Children may experience additional problems with peer acceptance.

Bathing and showering

A shower is more compact than a bath. It requires less water and is therefore more economical and environmentally friendly. Skin debris is rinsed away more easily by showering than bathing and, for this reason, Muslims and Hindus use running water for washing whenever possible.

Sometimes people need the nurse's guidance about how they can have a bath, e.g. covers are available for plaster casts or a limb can be covered in polythene to keep a wound dry while bathing.

Planning is important when assisting patients to ensure:

- All equipment needed is assembled
- Appropriate intervention is provided
- Privacy and dignity are maintained
- Heat loss is minimized
- Safety is maintained.

Bathing, washing and showering is tailored according to individual needs and preferences. When assistance is

Box 16.9 Best practice statements: privacy and dignity

- Patients/clients feel that they matter all of the time
- Patients/clients experience care in an environment that actively encompasses individual values, beliefs and personal relationships
- Patients'/clients' personal space is actively promoted by all staff
- Communication between patients/clients takes place in a manner that respects their individuality
- Patient/client information is shared to enable care, with their consent
- Patients'/clients' care actively promotes their privacy and dignity, and protects their modesty
- Patients/clients/carers can access an area that safely provides privacy.

[From DH (2001)]

EVIDENCE-BASED PRACTICE Box 16.10

Skin care: emollients

The skin:

- Is afforded chemical protection by the acid mantle (p. 427)
- Has a protective lipid barrier that may be impaired by air conditioning and the use of soap products and other irritants (Holden et al 2002)
- Is often dry, especially in older people, and repeated washing worsens this. Following a small study, Hardy (1996) identified interventions that may improve dry skin including the products used to wash the skin, frequency of washing or showering and use of tepid rather than hot water.

The effects of conventional soap include:

- An alkaline pH that neutralizes the effects of the protective acid mantle
- Depletion of natural skin oils (Holden et al 2002, Jamieson et al 2002)
- Irritating constituents that cause allergies in some people. In particular, perfumes and alcohol can irritate the skin and, when these are constituents of wipes and other skincare products, they must be used with caution.

Emollients

These oil-based substances are applied to soften dry skin. They act by reducing water loss through the skin surface and include:

- Soap substitutes that clean the skin but do not have the side-effects of conventional soap outlined above
- Creams or ointments that are applied to the skin in the direction of hair growth to prevent blockage of hair follicles (Burr 1999). Ointments can be more effective than creams but they are more greasy and can stain clothes and bed linen
- Oils added to the bath that float on the surface or disperse as fine droplets; however, they make the bath surface slippery, thus constituting a potential bathroom hazard for those with mobility problems.

Drying the skin

- This should be by patting rather than rubbing because it causes less friction. Jamieson et al (2002) state that patting also reduces the skin flora and skin infection.

Student activity

Reflect on your placements so far and consider the extent to which skin care has been evidence based.

HEALTH PROMOTION Box 16.11

Safety in the bathroom

To prevent scalding:

- Water temperature should not exceed 43°C (Jamieson et al 2002) and is checked before a person is assisted into a bath or shower.

To prevent slips or falls on wet surfaces (involving the physiotherapist and occupational therapist as required):

- Assess the person's ability to get into and out of the bath or shower independently
- Assess the person's ability to bathe or shower independently
- A non-slip mat should be used in the bath or shower
- A clean, absorbent bath mat should be used when stepping out of a bath or shower
- Dry wet floors promptly.

To call for help when required:

- Leave a call button nearby when a person is left alone.

Note: People with a history of seizures must not be left alone in the bath.

NURSING SKILLS Box 16.12

Principles of bathing infants and children

- Ensure the bathroom is warm and draught free
- An infant should be held securely with their head supported on the nurse's arm or hand during bathing (Fig. 16.3) and the free hand used for washing and rinsing
- Infants quickly lose heat and heat loss is minimized by avoiding prolonged exposure during bathing
- Water temperature must be carefully checked, either by dipping your elbow into it or using a lotions thermometer, to prevent scalds
- A non-slip mat should be used in the bath or shower to prevent slips and falls
- Infants and young children must never be left unsupervised in the bathroom to prevent accidental drowning
- Bathtime is usually a 'fun time' to be enjoyed by both children and carers
- School-age children may need encouragement to take a bath or shower
- Children often dislike having their hair washed as they hate having shampoo suds in their eyes. This can be avoided by providing them with a folded flannel to cover their eyes during hairwashing.

needed, timing may require planning to fit in with other scheduled treatment or therapies. Analgesia, if needed, should be given beforehand to minimize discomfort. The person should have their own toiletries and follow their preferred routines where possible (see Box 16.1, p. 426). Before taking someone to the bathroom, the nurse should check it is vacant, clean and warm and provide the opportunity for the person to empty their bowels and bladder. A mechanical hoist or other equipment may be needed to transfer a person to the bathroom or into the bath (see Chs 13, 18). Safety in the bathroom is an important nursing consideration and the measures taken to prevent accidental slips or falls are shown in Box 16.11.

A towel is wrapped round the person on leaving the bath or shower to keep them warm and maintain their dignity. Principles of bathing infants and children are outlined in Box 16.12.

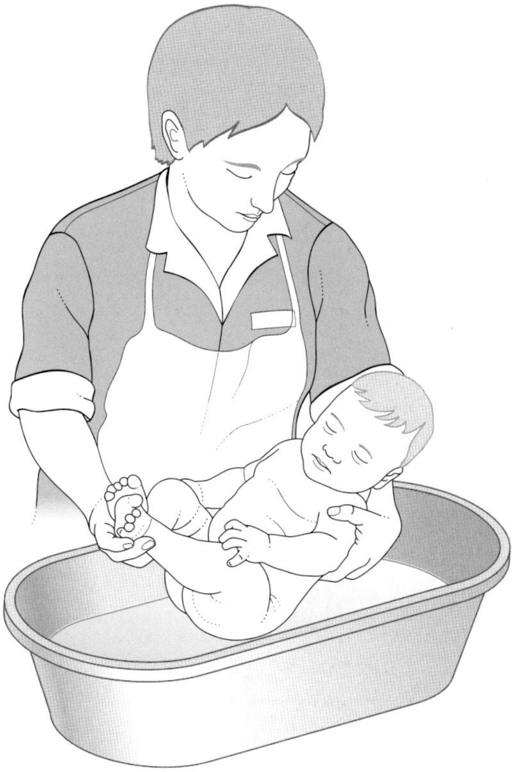

Fig. 16.3 Holding a baby for bathing (reproduced with permission from Trigg & Mohammed 2006)

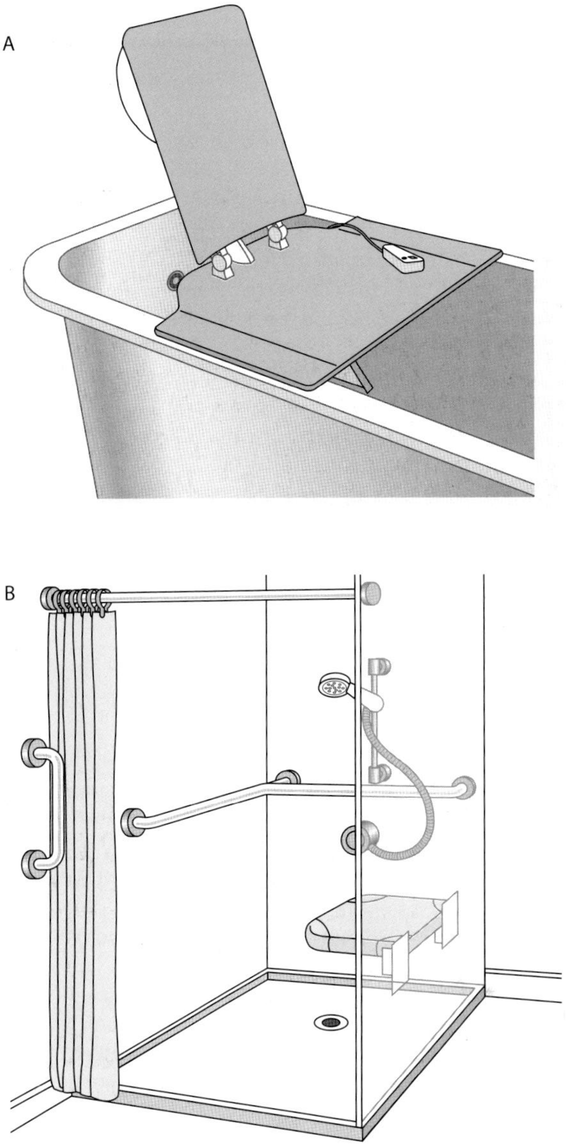

Fig. 16.4 Bathroom adaptations: A. Electric bath lift. B. Accessible shower

After bathing or showering, other aspects of personal care are then carried out, including the use of talc, deodorant and moisturizer; oral hygiene; shaving and styling the hair. Many women apply cosmetics to complete their appearance.

After use, the bath or shower is thoroughly cleaned according to local policy and left tidy for the next person.

Bathing aids

Bathing aids are often used in care settings and home adaptations can also be provided to enable people to remain independent at home (Fig. 16.4). Home assessment is carried out by an occupational therapist and suitable aids identified. Grab rails can be fitted to the walls to assist people getting into and out of the bath and electric bath lifts lower a person into the bath and raise them up again when required. A hoist can be provided at home although assistance from a carer is needed to use this. A shower with a seat can also be installed for people who find standing difficult.

Menstrual hygiene

Menstruation occurs in women between the menarche (first menstruation) occurring during puberty and the menopause (cessation of menstruation). In most women menstrual periods last around a week and take place about every 28 days. During this time there is vaginal blood loss that can heavy to begin with and then reduces. A supply of sanitary pads or tampons is required to absorb menstrual loss. This may need to be provided in care settings, together with hand washing facilities for dependent people. In Western society managing menstruation is a private, personal activity that is generally a taboo subject.

Bedbathing

A bed bath, or blanket bath, is needed to maintain personal hygiene when a person is unable to use the bath or shower or is confined to bed. These people are usually quite dependent and may also be unconscious or confused.

This affords the opportunity for a period of one-to-one communication. The patient should be encouraged to participate as much as their condition allows. Choice of nightclothes and use of a person's own toiletries will enable a person confined to bed to have some involvement in their care. The principles of bedbathing are outlined in Box 16.13 (p. 434).

NURSING SKILLS Box 16.13

Principles of giving a bedbath

- Explain to the person what you are going to do and gain their consent to carry out the bedbath
- Follow local infection control procedures such as handwashing, disposal of laundry, etc.
- Clear the bed area to make space for equipment needed
- Assemble all equipment so the bedbath can be completed without interruption
- Screen the bed space or close the door to provide privacy and avoid embarrassment
- Offer the opportunity to use a bedpan or commode before starting, to promote comfort
- Use the bedbath as an opportunity for communication, to observe the condition of the skin and to assess general progress and well-being
- Assist the person to remove their nightclothes and cover them with a sheet or blanket to preserve their warmth, modesty and dignity
- If two nurses are present, one washes and rinses the skin and the other dries and applies toiletries according to the person's routine and preference
- The face is usually washed first – ask if soap is used for this. Where appropriate, independence can be encouraged by asking the person if they would prefer to do this themselves
- A second facecloth or disposable cloth is used for the rest of the body
- Expose only the part being washed at any time to reduce heat loss
- The further limb is washed first so that the second nurse can dry the limb nearer to them as the second limb is being washed. This also prevents splashing of the clean, dry limb while the second one is being washed. The extremities can be immersed and then washed in the bowl
- The perineal area is washed using a disposable cloth from the front backwards to prevent cross-infection from the anal area (Fig. 16.5). After the area is dried, the water is changed and used cloths discarded
- The back is usually washed last. It is important to remember to part the skin between the buttocks and gently wash the perianal area
- When the person is confined to bed, wet or soiled sheets are changed
- Assist the person into clean bedclothes
- A person confined to bed is then given assistance as required to carry out their other hygiene routines including shaving, cleaning their teeth, hair styling, nail care, etc. These are all much easier when the person is able to sit upright
- Ensure the person is comfortable and has their call bell within reach before leaving the area
- Ensure that all equipment is cleaned or disposed of according to local infection control policy.

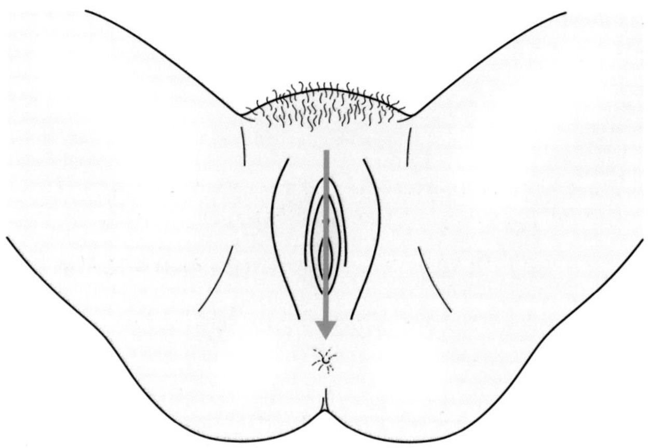

Fig. 16.5 The perineal area: washing from front to back

When the bed bath is complete, other aspects of personal care are carried out, including oral hygiene, shaving and hair styling.

Perineal care

When possible, the patient should be offered the opportunity to carry out personal perineal care themselves (see Box 16.13 and Fig. 16.5). This is often referred to as 'washing between the legs' or 'down there'. Many nurses find carrying out perineal care embarrassing, especially when caring for people of the opposite sex. A dignified and professional attitude will help to put both the nurse and patient at ease.

The nurse must consider cultural needs, e.g. Muslims wash their genitalia in running water after passing urine or faeces. Nurses can provide a jug of water for washing if the person is confined to bed.

Microorganisms normally resident in the bowel are the most common cause infection of the bladder (cystitis). This condition is more common in females whose urethra is shorter and therefore more easily reached by ascending microorganisms (see Ch. 20).

Normally in the male infant the preputial space is incompletely developed, causing the foreskin or prepuce to be adherent to the penis (glans penis). As it is not easily retracted, phimosis (tight foreskin) is normal in early infancy. Through normal development and erections these early adhesions gradually disappear, and the foreskin separates. The foreskin softens and becomes retractable by 2 years of age. Attempts to retract the foreskin for washing etc. before this age must be avoided. However, in uncircumcised men and older male children, the foreskin is carefully retracted and the glans gently washed and dried before the foreskin is repositioned.

Care of the feet, hands and nails

Assessment of the feet is important because problems can often be treated if detected early; without treatment, mobility can become severely restricted. Older people should always be asked if they are able to cut their own toenails as many have difficulty reaching them. The effects of the ageing process on the feet include thickening of the nails and development of calluses and hard skin.

HEALTH PROMOTION Box 16.14

Foot care for people with diabetes mellitus

The following care will protect your feet from damage and ensure you identify any problems that occur promptly:

1. Wash and carefully dry your feet every day, paying attention to the areas between the toes.
2. Inspect your feet when drying them, looking for:
   - Cuts or sores
   - Signs of potential problems including swelling, redness, warmth, pain, cracks or bleeding.
3. Report any ulcers, corns, calluses, blisters, ingrowing toenails or other problems to your foot care specialist (podiatrist).
4. Do not cut your toenails with scissors.
5. Visit your podiatrist for regular checks at recommended intervals, usually between 1- and 6-monthly, and when toenails require cutting.
6. Never walk around barefoot to avoid even minor injury.
7. Ensure your shoes are spacious and well fitting to reduce the risk of corns and calluses developing.

Local policies must always be consulted before trimming nails, because some people are always referred to a podiatrist (a health professional responsible for the management of conditions affecting the feet and/or lower limb) for treatment and cutting of their toenails. 'At-risk' people include those with diabetes mellitus (usually known as diabetes) and poor circulation caused by peripheral vascular disease. It is important that people with diabetes are taught how to look after their feet properly to prevent even minor damage that can progress to serious complications (Box 16.14).

Care of the nails is best carried out after a bath or shower; alternatively, the hands or feet can to be soaked in a bowl of warm water for 15 minutes to allow the nails to soften. A nailbrush can be used to remove obvious matter. The area under the nails is carefully cleaned using an orange-stick or nail file before the hands or feet are dried thoroughly. After drying, the cuticle is gently pushed backwards to prevent it growing over the nails.

Toenails are cut straight across with scissors or clipped using nail clippers. If difficulty is encountered because they are tough, the person should be referred to a podiatrist. Fingernails are usually trimmed using scissors and then filed to the shape of the finger with an emery board. Hand cream and nail varnish is then applied if wished.

Care of the eyes

Anatomy and physiology of the eye is reviewed on pages 445–446 but the importance of the accessory structures of the eye is considered here in order to explain eye care. This may also include care of spectacles, contact lenses or an artificial eye.

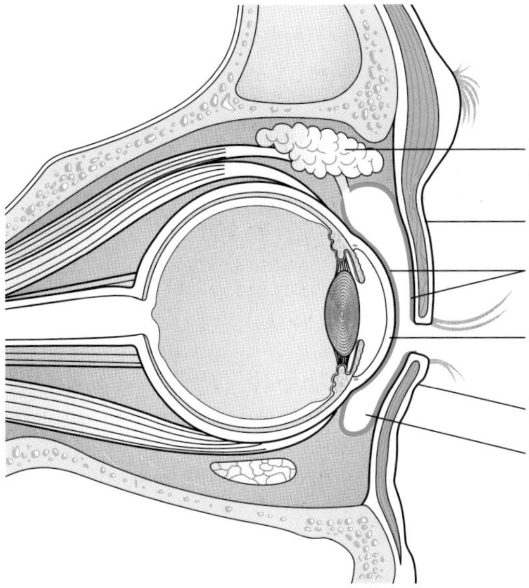

Fig. 16.6 Accessory structures of the eye (reproduced with permission from Waugh & Grant 2006)

Accessory structures of the eye

These include the eyebrows, eyelids and eyelashes (Fig. 16.6). Together they protect the delicate structures at the front of the eye, especially the cornea, from the entry of sweat, dust and other foreign bodies. For example, when a speck of dust enters the eye, copious amounts of tears are produced and the eye waters profusely in an attempt to wash it away. The conjunctiva is a delicate membrane that protects the cornea and also lines the eyelids.

Tears are continually produced by the lacrimal glands and spread across the cornea during blinking, lubricating it and keeping it moist. They contain an antibacterial enzyme, lysozyme, which protects the eye from infection and drains away through a duct into the nose. The inferior fornix is the site for instilling eye medication (see Ch. 22). The areas where the upper and lower eyelids join are called the:

- Medial canthus (inner canthus)
- Lateral canthus (outer canthus).

Eye care

Ensuring the eyes are clean and free from crusting is part of any general hygiene routine and is normally accomplished when washing one's face. Secretion of tears and blinking keep the eyes clean and moist while awake. Unconscious people are at risk from damage to the cornea because the blink reflex is lost and their eyes are therefore kept closed (see p. 458).

Eye care is required is some situations, e.g. presence of discharge. Sometimes it is an aseptic procedure (see Ch. 15) carried out by trained staff for people who have had surgery or trauma to the eye. In other situations, it is a clean procedure (see Ch. 15) (Box 16.15, p. 436).

Spectacles

Spectacle lenses are made from glass or plastic material and both types should be kept clean using the cloth

NURSING SKILLS Box 16.15

Principles of eye care

- Prepare the patient by explaining what you are about to do
- Follow local infection control protocols, e.g. handwashing
- Always use a new sterile eye care pack
- The patient should sit or lie down with their head tilted backwards
- Ask the patient to close their eyes
- If there is an infected eye, clean the non-infected eye first
- Gently swab the lower eyelid with a lint-free swab, lightly moistened with sterile normal saline from the inner canthus outwards
- Take care to ensure the swab does not rise above the lid margin opening the eye as corneal damage may occur
- Use each swab only once
- Repeat swabbing until all the crusting has gone
- Dry away excess saline with a dry swab
- Prescribed medication may then be instilled into the eyes (see Ch. 22)
- Wash your hands.

provided. They can be washed in soapy water and gently dried using a soft cloth to prevent scratching. When not in use, they should be stored in their case (labelled with the person's name in a care setting) to protect them from scratching and to minimize effects of physical damage.

Glass lenses are relatively heavy and can cause soreness on the bridge and sides of the nose. Lighter lenses made from shatterproof material are also safer, especially when people are in situations where an object may hit their eyes. Irrespective of the type of lenses, spectacles should be checked for comfort and fit. This means checking the sides and bridge of the nose and the back of the ears for signs of soreness. A person may have different pairs of glasses for reading and watching TV, and care should be taken to ensure the correct pair is in use.

Contact lenses

Contact lenses are thin transparent discs inserted onto the cornea to correct refractive errors of the eye. They float on a layer of tears and can be hard, soft or gas permeable. The solutions required for the care of the different types of lenses vary and are used according to the manufacturer's instructions. Each lens is kept in a separate labelled container as the two lenses may have different prescriptions.

Handwashing before insertion or removal is essential to minimize the risk of infection or introduction of foreign bodies that will cause inflammation of the conjunctiva (conjunctivitis) or corneal ulcers. Contact lenses are normally removed at night and should not be used when a person is receiving ophthalmic (eye) medication. Use of daily disposable contact lenses eliminates the need for cleaning and storage.

Artificial eyes

An artificial eye, or ocular prosthesis, is required after removal of the eyeball. This may be following trauma, severe infection or removal of a tumour. An artificial eye may be a permanent prosthesis. When it requires care, people usually prefer to carry this out themselves. If assistance is needed, advice from the nurse specialist or ophthalmology department should be sought.

Care of the ears

In order to carry out safe care of the ears it is necessary to be familiar with two important structures: the external auditory canal and the eardrum, or tympanic membrane (see Fig. 16.14, p. 449). Anatomy and physiology of the ear and hearing is outlined on page 449.

It is important to wash the skin covering the external ear as part of bathing or showering. Children often forget to wash behind their ears (Trigg & Mohammed 2006). The ears should be cleaned daily by gentle insertion of the corner of a moist flannel and rotating it into the external auditory canal. Nothing else should ever be inserted into the ear (except a tympanic thermometer or an otoscope). Cotton buds and other objects should not be used to try to remove wax because they can push it further into the external auditory canal and also damage the eardrum (Harkin & Vaz 2003). Hearing impairment may occur when there is build up of wax in the external auditory canal. Excess wax can be removed by irrigation (previously called syringing), a procedure that requires special training. Any discharge from the ear is abnormal and should be reported immediately.

Small children are prone to putting small items into their ears. A foreign body can cause deafness when the external auditory canal is blocked and may also damage the eardrum. Although foreign bodies in the ear are much more common in children they do occur in adults. They also occur in people who unadvisedly use cotton buds or other objects to deal with earwax.

The first aid interventions required should this occur are as follows:

- Do not attempt to remove the foreign body unless it is a live insect. (A live insect can sometimes be removed by gently pouring tepid water into the casualty's ear.)
- Reassure the casualty and stay calm
- Organize transfer to hospital.

Hearing aids

The Royal National Institute for Deaf and hard of hearing people (RNID) (2004a) estimates that two million people in the UK have hearing aids, but a quarter of these people do not use them regularly. A further three million people have a hearing impairment and would benefit from having a hearing aid.

Adapting to using a hearing aid takes time and initially it is worn for short periods that are gradually increased. Hearing aids are described as analogue or digital, depending on the technology they use. Digital hearing aids process sounds better than analogue hearing aids. The NHS

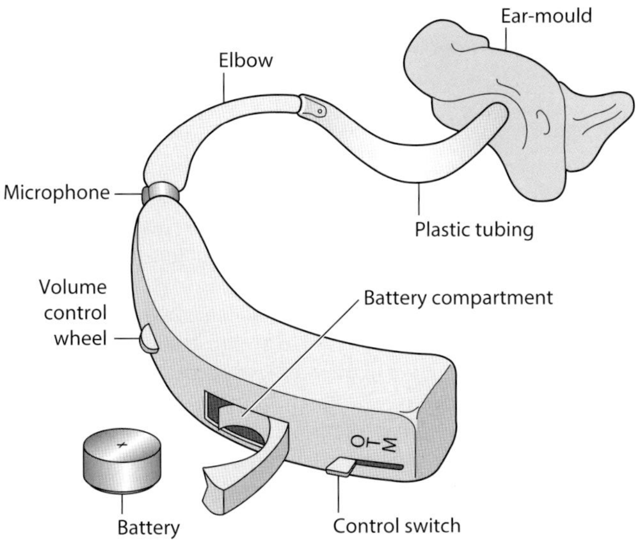

Fig. 16.7 Behind-the-ear hearing aid (reproduced with permission from Gates 2002)

provides, repairs and replaces certain hearing aids free of charge although some people choose to buy their own.

Hearing aids are battery operated and are worn in or around the ear. They amplify sounds but do not restore natural hearing. There are three main designs: body-worn, behind-the-ear and in-the-ear.

Body-worn aids have a small box that can be clipped to clothing. People with severe hearing impairment often use them as they provide the most powerful amplification. They are also widely used by people who also have poor vision and those who find using the controls of behind-the-ear models difficult. In-the-ear aids are not suitable for people with severe hearing loss. The behind-the-ear aid is the most commonly used (Fig. 16.7). They have a small control switch with letters that mean:

- O = aid is turned off
- M = microphone is on and will amplify sound
- T = induction loop, used to pick up radio signals without interference of background noise when an induction loop system is installed (see p. 452).

The microphone detects sound and must be kept clean and dry. The volume control wheel can be adjusted to suit different environments although this requires reasonable manual dexterity. The battery compartment opens, allowing the small battery to be changed. These should be kept out of children's reach as they can swallow them or poke them into their ears or nose. The plastic tubing transmits sound to the ear mould that is specially made for the wearer and should fit snugly. The plastic tubing and ear mould are wiped with a tissue after use. They are disconnected from the elbow and washed in soapy water and dried at least weekly. The plastic tubing needs to be replaced every few months.

Care of the nose

The nose does not normally require special care. Gentle blowing into a handkerchief or tissue removes excess secretions and debris. The use and prompt disposal of tissues is encouraged in care settings to reduce the risks of cross-infection. Harsh blowing should be avoided as it can cause damage to the eardrum and nasal mucosa. When there is a tube situated in the nose, for example a nasogastric tube, there may be accumulation of secretions that can be gently removed using moist swabs or cotton buds.

Children are prone to inserting small objects into their noses causing pain, trauma, blockage and, some days later, infection.

The first aid interventions are:

- Do not try to remove the object as it may be pushed further into the nose, worsening any damage
- Reassure the casualty and stay calm
- Encourage the casualty to breathe normally through the mouth
- Organize transfer to hospital for safe removal of the foreign body.

Hair care

The appearance of a person's hair normally contributes to their self-esteem, personal identity and sexuality. It also provides an indicator of their well-being and is usually clean and shiny. When tangled, dull or unkempt this suggests low self-esteem, low mood or that the person is physically unable to carry out hair care independently.

Most people style their hair using a brush or comb, at least daily. Fine-toothed combs are suitable for short hair; broader toothed ones are better for people with long or curly hair. People with impaired movement of the shoulders or poor handgrip find hairbrushes or combs with large handles easier to use. Brushing keeps the hair clean by removing dead epithelial cells and dust from the scalp and hair.

Haircutting is usually carried out at regular intervals and its style contributes to a person's individual and cultural identity. This aspect of personal hygiene is one of the least private and is normally carried out communally at a hairdressing salon. For people unable to get out and about, arranging for a hairdresser to visit them at home or in a care setting often provides a psychological boost. Hair cutting must never be undertaken without consent of the person involved because some people do not cut their hair for religious or cultural reasons, e.g. Sikhs and Rastafarians. Nurses should be aware of the religious and cultural hair care needs of people in their care. Examples of these are outlined in Box 16.16 (p. 438).

Hairwashing

Hairwashing frequency varies considerably between individuals; younger people commonly wash their hair daily although many other people wash their hair less often. Without washing, the hair becomes greasy as dried sweat and sebum accumulate.

Hairwashing can be carried out as a separate activity or during showering or bathing. Debilitated people often appreciate help with this at a sink in the bathroom. Helping someone style their hair provides a good opportunity for one-to-one communication and improves

Box 16.16 **Hair care – cultural and religious needs**

People of certain faiths keep their hair covered, including:

- Muslim women
- Jewish orthodox women
- Sikh men wear turbans and some Sikh women will also cover their hair.

Moreover, in Sikhism, two of the *Symbols of faith* (the '5 Ks') are to do with the hair:

- *Kesh*: The hair of both sexes is left uncut and worn in a bun (jura)
- *Kangha*: The bun is held in place by a comb known as the kangha. The kangha is of major significance and people will want to wear it or have it with them at all times.

(*Note*: the other *Symbols of faith* for Sikhs are the *kara* (steel bangle), the *kirpan* (symbolic dagger) and the *kaccha* (shorts/underpants).

African-Caribbean people tend to have brittle, crinkly hair and use wide-toothed combs to reduce discomfort and breaking. Pomade is an oil-based product used to enhance shine and smoothness of this type of hair. It is rubbed into the hands and then applied to the hair and scalp. Damp hair may be braided or pleated, but loosely because it tightens as it dries.

NURSING SKILLS Box 16.17

Principles of hairwashing in bed

- Remove the head of the bed and put an empty basin on a chair at the top of the bed
- Position the patient comfortably with their head just over the top of the bed and the neck and shoulders supported with pillows (see Fig. 16.8)
- Place polythene sheeting on the floor and on the pillows
- Cover the pillows with a towel to absorb excess water
- Test the temperature of the water before use to prevent scalding or cooling
- Offer the patient a flannel to cover their eyes to protect them from shampoo lather that can be irritating
- Wet the hair by pouring warm water from a large jug gently through it into the basin – a bed-fast rinser will assist in this process (Baker et al 1999)
- Apply shampoo and massage it gently into the hair
- Rinse off the lather by pouring more warm water through the hair into the basin, repeat and then repeat again with conditioner if the patient wishes
- After the final rinse, towel dry the hair
- Remove all equipment to reduce any hazard from water on the floor
- Ensure that any equipment is cleaned or disposed of according to local infection control policy
- Assist the patient to sit up when possible and, if necessary, help to style their hair using a hairdryer.

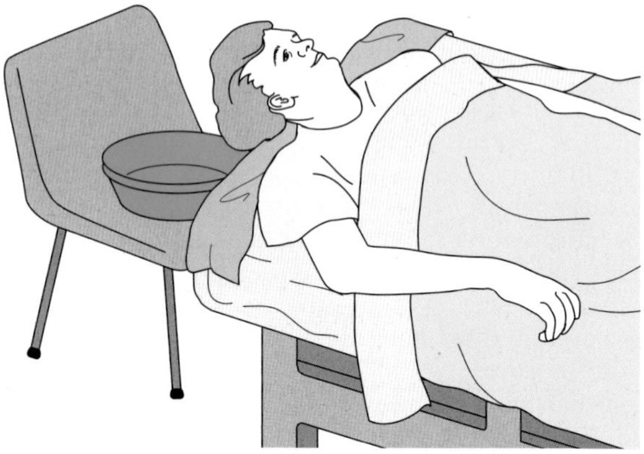

Fig. 16.8 Hairwashing in bed (reproduced with permission from Nicol et al 2004)

their self-esteem. It is important to include the person in decisions about styling when possible to avoid unwanted or inappropriate looks and effects. Chemotherapy and radiotherapy treatment often cause alopecia (hair loss) and people receiving these treatments are given individual advice about hair care. When hairwashing with shampoo and water is not possible or practical, dry shampoo can be used instead. Hairwashing can also be carried out in people confined to bed (Fig. 16.8); the principles for this are shown in Box 16.17.

Head lice

The presence of head lice (*Pediculus capitis*) is also known as pediculosis but, importantly, the presence of nits (the empty cases that remain stuck to the hair after the eggs have hatched) does not indicate current infestation.

Eggs, commonly known as nits, are laid by adult females and firmly cemented to hair shafts near the scalp. The eggs hatch after 7–10 days and adults live for about 1 month. Adult head lice are tiny insects found in the hair with peak prevalence in children between the ages of 4 and 11 years. They are usually found behind the ears and round the hairline. Infestation is often accompanied by intense itching of the scalp and scratching can cause secondary infection.

Fortunately, head lice do not transmit disease to people but there is considerable stigma and social distress associated with their presence. This is compounded by widespread myths and misconceptions about the means of spread and treatment of head lice. They affect people from all socioeconomic groups and show no preference between clean or dirty hair. Head lice can neither jump nor fly. People who have been in close contact with an infested person should be identified and treated if lice are found. They are spread by direct contact with an infested person and cannot survive for long away from the host. There is a lack of evidence to support the commonly held belief that spread occurs through sharing of hair brushes,

EVIDENCE-BASED PRACTICE Box 16.18

Treatment of headlice

Treatment can be chemical or mechanical.

1. Chemical treatment involves the use of pesticides or herbal preparations applied to the hair and scalp. There is widespread resistance to some pesticides, whose use is therefore ineffective, and so treatment options require:
   - Consultation of local policies in healthcare
   - Discussion with a health professional or pharmacist for community settings.

   After chemical treatment, the hair is carefully combed using a fine-toothed comb to remove remaining lice and nits. Two treatments are used 7 days apart.
2. 'Bug busting' is a mechanical treatment using a fine-toothed detection comb to remove headlice from wet hair after conditioner has been liberally applied. This is repeated every 4 days for at least 2 weeks.

Increasing concern about the effects of pesticides, especially on children, is encouraging research into the effectiveness of different treatments. However, there continues to be a lack of consensus about which is best (Prodigy 2004c). A recent study by Burgess et al (2005) suggests that a new chemical may be less irritant to the scalp and less sensitive to resistance than others currently used.

Patient information leaflets are available from Prodigy (2004a)

[Adapted from Prodigy (2004c)]

combs, hair ornaments, hats and scarves (Koch et al 2001, Prodigy 2004c). Treatments are summarized in Box 16.18.

Continued presence of head lice after any treatment may be the result of:

- Non-compliance with treatment
- Incorrect use of the treatment
- Reinfestation.

Care of facial hair

A moustache and beard need daily grooming. Electric trimmers can be used when requested but trimming or removal should never be undertaken without the person's permission as any facial hair may have personal, cultural or religious significance. In frail or debilitated people gentle wiping or washing after meals easily removes any food debris.

Shaving is best carried out after bathing when the skin is softer. It forms part of many men's daily hygiene routines and being unshaven makes many feel unclean. An unkempt appearance can quickly develop, especially in the eyes of their relatives.

Many men use an electric shaver, which is a safe, convenient method that is encouraged in those people who are prone to bleeding because they are taking anticoagulant medication or have a clotting disorder. Electric shavers should never be shared because of the risk of cross-infection.

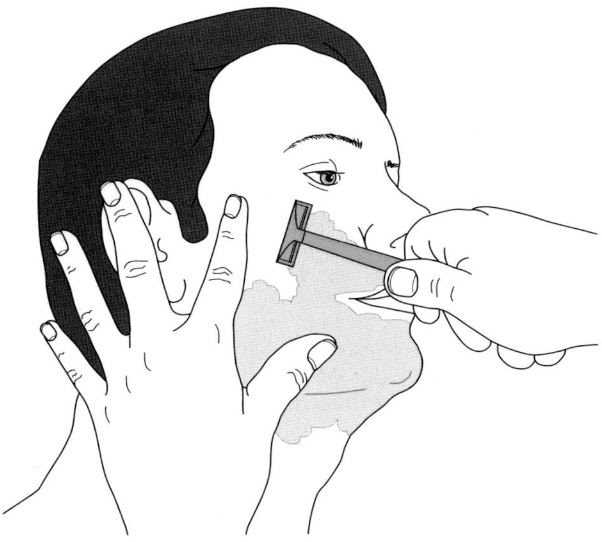

Fig. 16.9 Shaving (reproduced with permission from Nicol et al 2004)

Wet shaving is other men's personal preference. When assistance is required, the person's usual routine should be followed. The face is washed and shaving cream applied and worked gently into the skin until lather is formed. Shaving is carried out using small, firm strokes of the razor in the direction of hair growth over taut skin. The razor is rinsed frequently. People often make facial movements that tighten their skin during shaving to provide a closer shave. The face is usually shaved before the neck. Assistance if needed can be provided by the nurse (Fig. 16.9). Any moles or other lesions should be avoided. When shaving is complete, the face is washed thoroughly. Shaving and the use of aftershave contribute to men's personal identity and sexuality.

Some women normally have more facial hair than others. Excessive facial hair can result from drugs, some endocrine conditions or reduced oestrogen secretion after the menopause. Facial hair in women can be removed either with appropriate depilatory creams or waxing, or disguised using bleaching agents. On no account should it be plucked or shaved unless this is what the woman usually does. Permanent removal, using electrolysis, can be undertaken in certain situations.

Dressing

The clothes people wear normally reflect their traditions and culture. Cultural differences in acceptable modesty exist, especially regarding women who may be expected to wear skirts, cover their legs or cover their faces. Some Muslim women are traditionally clothed from head to foot. Clothes also reflect one's mood and communicate feelings and individuality.

Contemporary clothing is normally made from material that can be easily washed and needs minimal ironing. The type of clothes worn also depends on the context – working clothes often differ from those worn on informal social occasions. Formal social occasions, such as weddings and funerals, often have specific dress codes.

The type and amount of clothes in a person's wardrobe is largely determined by their personal income but also by their hobbies and interest in appearance.

When deciding what to wear, the type of activities that will be undertaken and ambient temperature need to be taken into account. In a cold environment, several thin layers provide more insulation and therefore warmth than one thick layer. This has the additional advantage of allowing the wearer to take off a layer at a time as the temperature increases. In hot environments, thin, pale-coloured clothes made from natural fibres are often preferred because they reflect light and absorb more sweat than synthetic materials. In some situations special clothing is required to maintain health and safety, e.g. UK law requires that a crash helmet be worn when riding a motorcycle.

Everyone should have their own clothes wherever they live. People should be offered choice when selecting clothes to wear although sometimes assistance is needed in making appropriate choices.

Help is sometimes needed with dressing, e.g. if there is a weak limb or side, the affected limb is put into blouses, shirts or trousers first. The same strategy is used when equipment such as i.v. infusion is in use.

Dressing aids

Adaptive devices or aids are available to make dressing easier, especially for people who have difficulty bending or have poor manual dexterity. They can be used to assist with many different items of clothing including socks, stockings, tights and jackets. Fastening clothes can be made easier by using:

- Velcro closures
- Button hooks
- Zip pullers
- Dressing reaches
- Sticks.

The Disabled Living Foundation (2004) demonstrates many of these items. People with visual impairment sometimes use a tactile code such as sewing differently shaped buttons on the inside of garments or sewing tags in different places to tell what colour their clothes are. Those people who have red–green colour blindness may also have a system to distinguish colour, especially of their socks.

Prostheses

Dentures are discussed later in this chapter (p. 442).

People may use a prosthesis or accessories for cosmetic or clinical reasons. For example, a wig can be used as an accessory for a change of appearance but in other situations it is worn to hide alopecia, or hair loss, which may occur naturally or following cancer treatment. People who wear wigs for the latter reasons can be self-conscious, both when wearing them and also if they need to removed for any reason.

REFLECTIVE PRACTICE Box 16.19

Factors that influence personal hygiene and appearance

Manjit Singh Dhillon is a Sikh client you meet during a home visit with the district nurse. He is 85 years old and recently widowed. He is frail and appears rather unkempt. His clothes are also in need of laundering. During your visit Mr Dhillon tells you about the importance of the symbols of Sikhism (the 5 Ks).

Student activities

- Find out about the items that he referred to as the '5 Ks' (see Box 16.16 and Further reading).
- Think about how help with showering or washing will need to be modified, so that Manjit is able to change his shorts (kaccha) in accordance with the teachings of his faith.
- Reflect on the other factors that may be influencing his ability to carry out appropriate personal hygiene and maintain his appearance.

An artificial limb will often affect a person's ability to carry out bathing and showering independently. External breast prostheses are sometimes used following surgical removal of a breast. Many women find them difficult to adapt to because they feel mutilated and unattractive after surgery (see Chs 12, 24).

When it has been established that a person uses a prosthesis the nurse should adopt a tactful approach to identify how and when it is used and any impact it may have on their ability to carry out personal hygiene activities. It is important to consider the person's dignity and ask them prior to removing it for any reason.

Summary – personal hygiene

In summary, assisting someone with personal hygiene and dressing can initially appear simple but tailoring help to meet individual requirements can prove more complex. Box 16.19 provides an opportunity to consider aspects of personal care and the factors that can influence it.

Dental health and oral hygiene

This section reviews anatomy and physiology relevant to the maintenance of oral functioning and health. Effective care required to maintain oral health is considered and the nurse's role in maintaining dental health and oral hygiene discussed.

Oral care is a basic hygiene need in both healthy and sick people. The teeth are essential for biting and chewing a normal healthy diet. For many people, having attractive teeth is an important aspect of their personal appearance and self-esteem.

Anatomy and physiology: the mouth

The mouth, or oral cavity, is the first part of the digestive tract (see Chs 19, 21). The tongue consists of voluntary muscles that enable speech, chewing and swallowing and it is covered with mucous membrane. Taste buds are present in the tongue and the sense of taste relies on the presence of saliva for dissolving chemicals in food to activate the taste receptors. The cheeks and gums are also lined with mucous membrane. The lips are involved in speech and non-verbal communication.

Salivary glands

The three pairs of salivary glands secrete between 1000 and 1500 mL of saliva into the mouth daily. Saliva is essential for a healthy, comfortable mouth and is composed mostly of water. Its effects include:

- Lubrication of the mouth
- Washing away food particles from the teeth
- Minimizing oral infection through the presence of antibacterial enzymes
- Beginning the digestion of dietary carbohydrate.

Teeth

Teeth enable people to eat solid food. At birth there are 20 temporary or deciduous teeth, 10 within each jaw. They erupt between the ages of 6 months and 2½ years (Table 16.1). These are known as the temporary teeth or primary dentition. From around 6 years they are shed and, in time, are replaced by 32 permanent teeth, known as the secondary dentition. There are four different types of teeth (Fig. 16.10A), their shapes being suited to their functions. The incisors and canine teeth are used to bite and tear food; the posterior premolars and molars, with their broader, flat surfaces, are used for chewing and grinding food. The four posterior molars are commonly known as the 'wisdom teeth'.

All types of teeth have the same basic structure (Fig. 16.10B). The crown protrudes through the gum, or gingiva, and the root lies embedded in the jawbone. A hard layer of dentine surrounds the central pulp cavity that contains blood vessels and nerves. The crown has an outer coating of enamel while the root has a layer of cement that holds the tooth firmly in its socket.

Maintaining oral health

Dental health promotion aims to reduce tooth and gum disorders and preserve people's natural teeth. Establishing good oral care and dietary habits therefore begins in childhood (Box 16.20).

Table 16.1 Eruption of the primary dentition (after McDonald & Avery 1994)

Average age of eruption (months) Upper teeth	Teeth	Average age of eruption (months) Lower teeth
10 months	Central incisor	8 months
11 months	Lateral incisor	13 months
19 months	Canine	20 months
16 months	First molar	16 months
29 months	Second molar	27 months

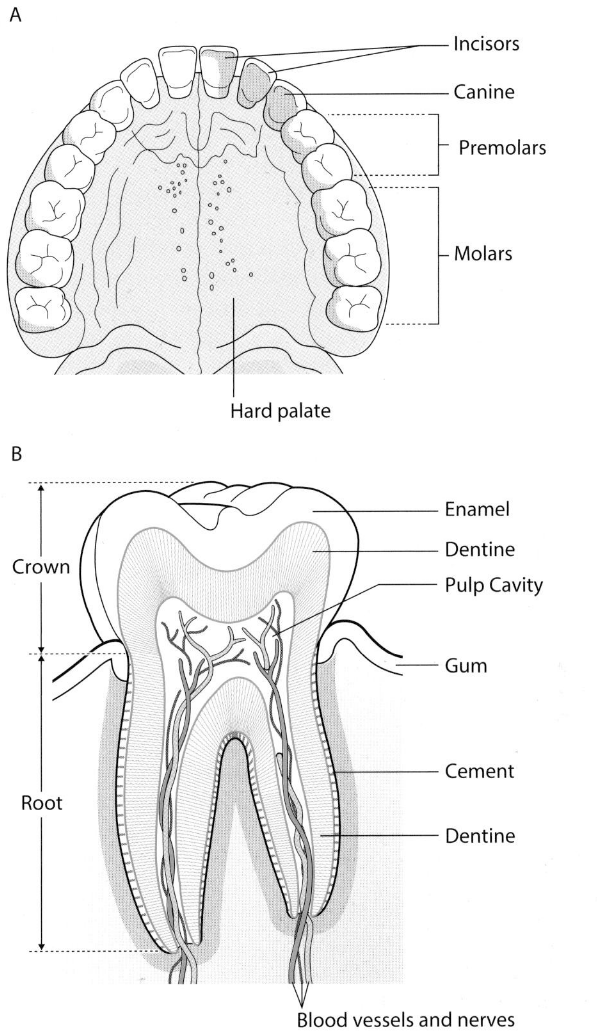

Fig. 16.10 **A.** Types of teeth (second dentition). **B.** Structure of a tooth (reproduced with permission from Waugh & Grant 2006)

HEALTH PROMOTION Box 16.20

Maintaining healthy teeth

- Visit your dentist at least yearly for dental examinations – free NHS treatment is provided for susceptible groups including children, women during and after pregnancy, older adults and unemployed people
- Use fluoride toothpaste; children's toothpaste contains lower levels of fluoride because they are renowned for eating it
- Brush your teeth using fluoride toothpaste at least twice daily and preferably after meals and sugary snacks
- Mouthwashes freshen the breath and can dislodge food debris
- Limit food and drinks containing sugar to mealtimes; using a straw for fizzy drinks delivers fluid to the back of the mouth, avoiding the teeth
- Renew your toothbrush every 2–3 months.

[From British Dental Health Foundation (2004a)]

Teething can be a troublesome time for both infants and their parents. It only occurs during eruption of the primary dentition that begins from around 6 months. Some infants experience drooling and may bite on hard objects while teething, although others can be very irritable.

Regular visits to the dentist from an early age enable discovery of the characteristic smells and sounds of the dental surgery through non-threatening situations. Tooth brushing by parents should begin when the teeth erupt and continuing assistance is needed until manual dexterity is sufficiently developed at around 7 years.

Eating habits should include sugary foods only at mealtimes and non-sugary foods such as cheese or fresh vegetables for snacks between meals. Sugary drinks should never be put in babies' feeding bottles to avoid the risk of dental caries (decay), especially at night. Sugar-free medicines are widely available and encouraged for the same reasons.

During childhood and adolescence falls and trauma can damage the teeth and mouth. Measures to minimize potential hazards and resultant injuries should be considered, including:

- The use of non-slip mats in the bath or shower
- Supervision of children when using play equipment
- Use of mouthguards during contact sports.

The mouth has an extensive blood supply and trauma that causes damage to teeth is likely to be accompanied by profuse bleeding from damaged oral tissues.

Oral care

Effective oral care moistens and cleans the mouth, removes unpleasant tastes and freshens the breath.

Toothbrushing and flossing

Dental health and oral hygiene are maintained by brushing the teeth with toothpaste at least twice daily and ideally also after meals and sugary snacks. This is the most effective way of removing plaque (a sticky film of bacteria that forms on the teeth) and food debris from the teeth and maintaining healthy gums. A small or medium size brush with soft or medium bristles will make it easier to clean the back teeth that can be hard to reach. The toothbrush is held at 45° to brush each surface of each individual tooth. Tooth brushing should take 2 minutes. The amount of toothpaste needed is the size of a pea.

Toothbrushing is followed by daily interdental cleaning with special brushes or by flossing from around 8 years of age. To do this, dental floss is inserted between each tooth in turn and a seesaw action used to pull the floss backwards and forwards between the surfaces. This removes food debris and plaque from the gums and spaces between the teeth that a toothbrush cannot reach. Flossing reduces gingivitis (inflammation of the gums) but should be undertaken with care by people receiving radiotherapy or chemotherapy because their gums are prone to inflammation, bleeding and infection.

People with poor manual dexterity can hold toothbrushes with large handles more easily. Electric toothbrushes tend to have larger handles and also reduce the manual effort needed to brush the teeth.

Care of dentures

Dentures should fit well and provide a good cosmetic appearance. Ill-fitting dentures cause discomfort, difficulty with eating and inflammation, candidiasis (thrush) or ulceration of the gums and oral mucosa.

They can be cleaned using a toothbrush and non-abrasive denture toothpaste although the British Dental Health Foundation (2004b) suggest that a soft nailbrush and ordinary soap are also suitable. Brushing should be carried out over a sink containing water or a soft towel to prevent damage if they are dropped. All surfaces should be carefully cleaned. The person's gums and palate are also brushed and the mouth well rinsed. After brushing, the dentures may be soaked in an effervescent denture cleaner to remove staining and bacteria. Dentures should not be soaked in these solutions overnight (British Dental Health Foundation 2004b). They are more easily inserted when they are wet and therefore do not need to be dried.

Removal of dentures can be embarrassing as people are likely to feel self-conscious without them and may also have difficulty in speaking clearly. Some people sleep with their dentures in situ while others prefer to keep them in a denture pot at the bedside. They should be soaked in water to prevent warping or cracking. Denture pots should be labelled in care settings to avoid mix-ups.

People who wear dentures should still visit the dentist for preventative examinations to ensure they continue to fit well and to detect any oral problems, e.g. oral cancer, at an early stage.

Tooth and gum disorders

Disorders include dental caries, periodontal disease and malocclusion.

Dental caries

Discoloration and then cavities, or caries, develop in the teeth when bacteria present in plaque react with carbohydrates, converting sugars into acids that slowly dissolve tooth enamel. The most susceptible periods are between 4 and 8 years (primary dentition) and between 12 and 18 years (secondary dentition).

If plaque is not removed by brushing the teeth, it hardens forming tartar. Tartar cannot be removed by toothbrushing and accumulation results in gingivitis. The gums are reddened, ulcerated and prone to bleeding when the teeth are brushed. Tartar can only be removed by a dentist or dental hygienist.

Periodontal disease

This results from long-standing gingivitis and becomes increasingly common from the third decade although it often originates in childhood. There is destruction of the gum structures that support the teeth and this accounts for considerable tooth loss in later life. Prevention is by encouraging good dental health from childhood (see Box 16.20, p. 441).

Malocclusion

Malocclusion occurs when the upper and lower teeth do not meet normally because they are uneven, overcrowded or overlapping or when the jaw does not develop normally. Biting and chewing are difficult, there is abnormal wear on the teeth, trauma to oral mucosa and the teeth may also have a poor cosmetic appearance. Orthodontic treatment involving the use of dental 'braces' is usually required in the teenage years to correct this.

Oral assessment and oral hygiene

The mouth has a role in eating and drinking, taste and breathing, and verbal and non-verbal communication, including intimate self-expression (see Ch. 9). If the mouth is causing discomfort this can have a detrimental psychosocial impact in addition to more physical effects including loss of taste, loss of appetite and resultant constipation. Dehydration causes oral dryness and discomfort (see Ch. 19). A dry mouth can also create difficulty with speaking and is exacerbated by mouth breathing and oxygen therapy (see Ch. 17).

Assessment provides a baseline that enables planning and implementation of individualized care and from which oral status can subsequently be evaluated. Best practice statements from the *Essence of Care* (DH 2001) show benchmarks for good oral hygiene practice (Box 16.21).

The oral cavity is carefully inspected using a pen torch and spatula. Signs of a healthy mouth include:

- Oral mucosa, tongue and gums are moist, pink and clean
- Clean, white teeth
- Absence of halitosis ('bad breath')
- Absence of ulcers
- Dentures that, if worn, are well fitting.

Any abnormalities such as redness, dryness, ulceration and a dirty or coated tongue are recorded together with the presence of capped or crowned teeth, fixed braces or dentures. A wide range of factors may cause oral problems (Box 16.22) and if a person in your care has one or more of these, oral assessment requires careful consideration.

Oral assessment tools

Several of these tools have been developed, taking the condition of the oral cavity and a variety of risk factors (see above) into account; however, they have not been sufficiently tested for validity and reliability to recommend them for general use. Roberts (2000a) reviewed some of these tools and then compiled an assessment and intervention tool for older people (Roberts 2001). This is based on a questionnaire and also suggests appropriate nursing interventions. Freer (2000) developed an assessment tool with a scoring scale for use in a neurosciences unit.

Oral hygiene: nursing interventions

When assistance is required with oral hygiene, thoughtful nursing intervention can make a difference; however, Adams (1996) suggests that patient preference is not always taken into account. The aims of nursing interventions are to:

- Maintain or restore comfort of the mouth
- Promote oral health.

When possible, people should be encouraged to carry out their own oral hygiene. For many people, only assistance to get to a sink, where they can stand or sit and brush their own teeth, may be required. A person in bed or sitting in a chair can often also brush their own teeth when provided with a glass of water and a receiver for collecting wastewater.

When nursing intervention is required an evidence-based approach should be used to select an appropriate

Box 16.21 Best practice statements: oral hygiene

- All patients/clients are assessed to identify the advice and/or care required to maintain and promote their individual oral hygiene
- Planned care is negotiated with patients/clients and/or their carers and is based on assessment of their individual needs
- Patients/clients have access to an environment that is safe and acceptable to the individual
- Patients/clients are expected to supply their own toiletries but single-use toiletries are provided until they can supply their own
- Patients/clients have access to the level of assistance that they require to meet their individual oral hygiene needs
- Patients/clients and/or carers are provided with information/education to meet their individual oral hygiene needs
- Patients'/clients' care is continuously evaluated, reassessed and the care plan renegotiated.

[From DH (2001)]

Box 16.22 Factors predisposing to oral problems

- Dehydration
- Inability to eat or drink
- Malnutrition
- Mouth breathing
- Oxygen therapy
- Ill-fitting dentures
- Poor cognitive function and self-neglect
- Antibiotics – alter the normal flora of the mouth and predispose to opportunistic invasion of *Candida albicans* causing oral thrush
- Other medication, e.g. phenytoin (used to control epilepsy)
- Cancer treatment – radiotherapy and chemotherapy damage the rapidly dividing cells of the oral mucosa and also predispose to oral thrush
- Underlying medical conditions, e.g. diabetes mellitus.

technique and solution (Table 16.2). Medication can be prescribed for oral hygiene, e.g. in people undergoing treatment for cancer who have specialized needs (Mallett & Dougherty 2000).

Pieces of fresh pineapple or tinned pineapple chunks contain a protein-digesting enzyme that cleans the tongue (Rattenbury et al 1999). Chewing or sucking them is also refreshing and stimulates salivation.

A technique no longer recommended is the use of a swab wrapped round a pair of forceps because this can damage the oral mucosa (Bowsher et al 1999, Roberts 2000b). Some solutions are also no longer recommended: lemon and glycerine should not be used because the osmotic action of glycerine dehydrates the oral mucosa and the acidity of lemon juice may damage tooth enamel (Bowsher et al 1999); hydrogen peroxide damages granulating tissue and should also be avoided (Roberts 2000b).

There is little evidence to support an optimal frequency for oral hygiene although this is suggested to be between 2 and 6 hourly in ill people. It is often appropriate to moisten the mouth with water, a mouthwash or ice chips more frequently. Chewing gum stimulates salivation and, when sugar-free, does not harm the teeth. A person's fluid status (see Ch. 19) should be reviewed

Table 16.2 Techniques and solutions used for oral hygiene

Technique or solution	Advantages and disadvantages
Technique	
Toothbrush	Gentle use of a soft, small toothbrush followed by rinsing the mouth can be used when there is no inflammation of the oral cavity. This removes plaque and debris from the teeth and gums, and reduces coating of the tongue (Mallett & Dougherty 2000) This technique requires the person to be able to swallow, rinse their mouth and void wastewater safely
Mouthwash	Providing a mouthwash will refresh the mouth when dehydration or nausea is present and after vomiting The effect is short lasting and mouthwash therefore needs to be offered frequently A mouthwash requires the person to be able to swallow, rinse their mouth and void wastewater safely (see Solutions, below)
Moistened foamsticks	These are widely used in oral hygiene to clean and moisten the oral mucosa but they are not effective in removing plaque from the teeth (see Solutions, below) Although there is awareness within the profession that patients may be at risk from biting off and swallowing or inhaling the foam, Roberts (2000b) could not find evidence in support of this concern despite an extensive literature review Foamsticks are suitable for use in people who cannot swallow or rinse their mouths out safely
A swabbed finger	A moist swab round a gloved finger is also effective for cleaning and moistening the oral mucosa; however, it may cause compression of food debris and plaque into the interdental spaces. Plaque is not removed This can be used when a patient is unable to use a mouthwash or swallow safely This technique is not recommended for children or others who may bite the swabbed finger!
Solutions	
Water and normal saline	Both are readily available, convenient and economical solutions to use There is insufficient evidence to recommend saline mouthwashes (Bowsher et al 1999)
Thymol tablets	These are widely used and prepared according to the manufacturer's instructions – normally, one tablet to one glass of water There is no evidence supporting the benefits of their use and some people find the taste unpleasant
Chlorhexidine gluconate	Used as a mouthwash, this solution reduces bacteria and is effective against plaque Long-term use can cause reversible staining of the teeth and tongue
Sodium bicarbonate	Careful dilution (1 level teaspoon in 500 mL; Nicol et al 2004) is required when using sodium bicarbonate because it is strongly alkaline and can damage the oral mucosa. It also has an unpleasant taste There is a paucity of evidence to support its use although it removes mucus and other debris present in the oral cavity It should only be used with care and when other solutions have proved ineffective
Saliva substitutes	For a persistent dry mouth, these sprays are effective for 1–2 hours

when a dry mouth persists as dehydration is not reversed by providing oral hygiene.

Lip salve or soft paraffin may be used to moisturize and prevent cracked lips. It forms an oily film that reduces water loss by evaporation.

Sensory considerations

When planning care, nurses need to consider the effects of sensory impairments on a person's ability to self-care and the implications for effective communication. This section of the chapter introduces some issues related to poor vision and hearing and appropriate nursing interventions.

The eye and vision

The eye is the organ for sight and vision and provides people with important information about their environment and those things in it. It is estimated that around 80% of the sensory information perceived is visual.

Anatomy and physiology of the eye (see p. 435 for accessory structures)

The eyeball consists of three layers (Fig. 16.11A):

- The outer layer includes the transparent cornea at the front of the eye and the sclera, or white of the eye. The posterior part of the sclera provides attachment for the extraocular muscles that move the eyeball in its socket.
- The middle vascular layer comprises the iris, ciliary body and the choroid. The iris is the coloured part of the eyeball and the pupil its central dark space. The pupil constricts in bright light and dilates in dim light. The lens is a transparent body that lies behind the iris.
- The retina forms the delicate inner layer and contains specialized light-sensitive receptors called rods and cones.

The anterior segment of the eye contains aqueous fluid. It is secreted by the ciliary glands and drained away through the scleral venous sinus (see Fig. 16.11A). As

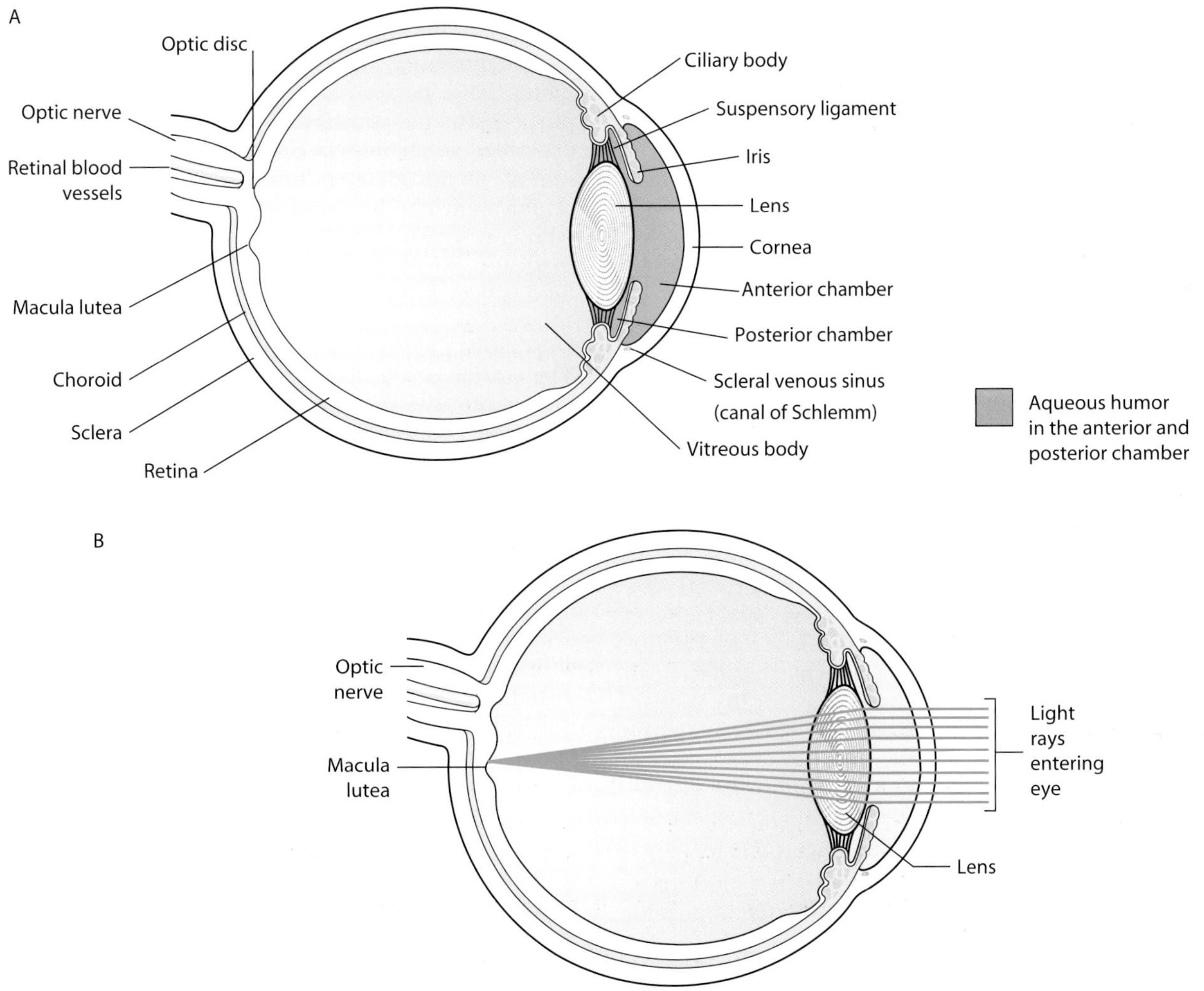

Fig. 16.11 **A.** Structure of the eye. **B.** Focusing of light rays on the retina (reproduced with permission from Waugh & Grant 2006)

production and drainage of aqueous fluid is fairly constant the intraocular pressure in the anterior segment also remains relatively constant.

Light rays entering the eyeball are refracted, or bent, as they pass through the transparent structures at the front of the eye. The lens focuses the light rays towards the retina where a visual image is formed (Fig. 16.11B, p. 445). This stimulates the light-sensitive receptors of the retina, generating nerve impulses that are conducted to the cerebral cortex. Each eye forms an image and both generate impulses that are transmitted to the brain for processing. Binocular vision provides accurate information about the environment, including the speed and distance of objects. If there is only one eye with vision, less detailed information is perceived. This means that even simple visual judgements, such as putting a cup down safely, are more difficult. Visual perception is a complex process and interpretation of visual stimuli seldom occurs alone but takes place alongside that of others, e.g. hearing, taste and smell.

Accommodation of the eye describes the changes that take place to allow focusing on near objects, i.e. those closer than 6 m:

- The shape of the lens changes – it becomes thicker, providing more refraction of the light rays from near objects in order to focus them on the retina. As this requires more effort than distant vision, tiring of the eyes may occur after prolonged close-up activities, e.g. reading
- The pupils constrict
- Both eyes move towards the object being viewed, also known as convergence.

Visual acuity

Eye testing measures visual acuity (VA) to measure visual clarity. The most common method is the 'Snellen type test chart'. The test chart (Fig. 16.12A) is situated in a well-lit area and measurement is carried out 6 m from the chart. This represents 'distant vision' where no accommodation is required. Normal vision is 6/6, meaning that the person can read line 6 at 6 m from the chart. When only the top line can be read, the VA is 6/60. If the top line on the chart cannot be read at this distance, the individual is moved nearer to the chart; if the top line of the chart can be read at 3 m, this is recorded as 3/60. The eyes are tested separately with and without spectacles, if appropriate. For people who cannot speak or read English or those with learning disabilities, alternative charts can be used such as the Snellen 'E' chart (Fig. 16.12B). A chart depicting objects of decreasing size (Fig. 16.12C) can be used in prelingual children.

Sight impairment

Box 16.23 outlines some common types of sight impairment and there are many causes. Diabetes mellitus is a common cause of blindness when the effects of poor blood glucose control damage the retina.

The Royal National Institute of the Blind (RNIB) (2004a) estimated more than 75% of people over the age of 75 have impaired vision, meaning that most older people have some degree of sight impairment. Less than 10% of people with severe or moderate sight impairment are born with impaired vision.

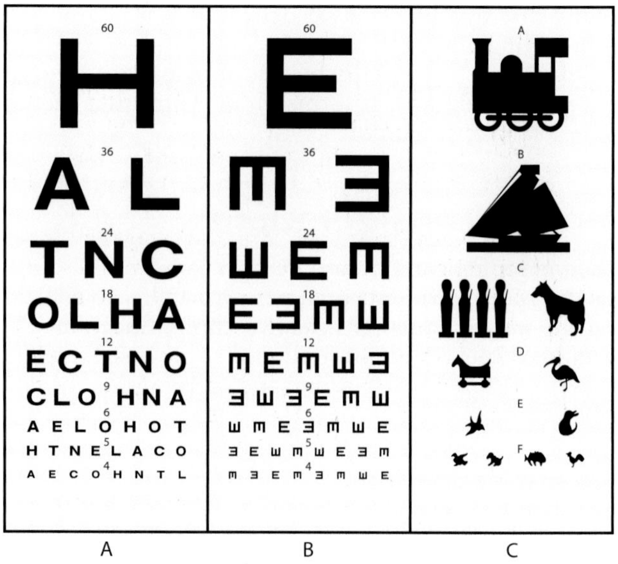

Fig. 16.12 Snellen test type charts: **A**. Snellen letter. **B**. Snellen 'E'. **C**. Recognition of objects (reproduced with permission from Peattie & Walker 1995)

The presence of severe sight impairment does not mean that a person is completely without sight. For the purposes of registration in the UK sight impairment is described as severe when a person can only read the top line of the test chart at 3 m (VA = 3/60). Moderate sight impairment can be registered when VA = 6/60. People who can see further than this in either situation above may also be eligible for registration when their visual field is very limited.

Describing sight impairment

The term 'severely sight impaired' describes those people previously referred to as 'blind'; 'moderately sight impaired' describes those previously known as 'partially sighted'. Some people do not like any of these terms because they feel they are negative and misleading. They may prefer to be described as 'visually impaired' or as having 'impaired vision' or 'visual disability' if they cannot see or are unable to see clearly.

Helping people with sight impairment

Nurses should be aware of the common incidence of visual problems, especially in older people who may not have recognized this themselves. They may observe behaviours that suggest sight impairment that warrant further investigation. These include:

- Holding written material very close to the eyes
- Tendency to explore items by touch
- Appearing startled when someone approaches quietly
- Difficulty in establishing eye contact during speech
- Reluctance to move around, especially in a strange environment
- Avoidance of visual tasks or not noticing things that are nearby

Box 16.23 Types of sight impairment

- *Refractive errors*: In the normal (or emmetropic) eye, light from distant objects is focused on the retina. When this is not the case, corrective lenses can be prescribed to restore normal vision (Fig. 16.13):
  - in *myopia* (shortsightedness) the eyeball is too long and therefore light rays from distant objects are focused in front of the retina. Correction requires a biconcave lens to focus light rays on the retina
  - in *hypermetropia* (longsightedness) the eyeball is too short and near objects are focused behind the retina. A biconvex lens is used to focus the light rays on the retina
  - in *astigmatism* there is abnormal curvature of part of the lens or cornea. Correction is achieved by the use of cylindrical lenses
- *Diplopia*: Means double vision and indicates an underlying problem affecting vision, such as after a stroke
- *Strabismus (squint)*: In this condition, a person cannot align both eyes – one or both of the eyes may turn in, out, up or down, and cannot focus simultaneously on a single point. Children with strabismus may initially have double vision. The cause is unknown and it is present at or shortly after birth
- *Presbyopia*: Becomes widespread after the fourth decade as the elasticity of the lens decreases with age and the ability of the eye to accommodate on near objects deteriorates. It is corrected by use of magnifying spectacles for reading
- *Cataract*: This is opacity of the normally transparent lens. This condition can be congenital or acquired, especially in later life, and is a common cause of blindness worldwide
- *Glaucoma*: Intraocular pressure rises as an abnormality of the production, flow or drainage of aqueous fluid develops. The condition may be congenital or acquired, and acute or insidious in onset. It may result in blindness if untreated
- *Tunnel vision*: Loss of peripheral vision
- *Diabetic retinopathy*: Disease of the retina in people with diabetes mellitus. A leading cause of blindness
- *Age-related macular degeneration (AMD)*: AMD is a leading cause of blindness in people aged over 50. It takes two forms: wet and dry. It affects the macula lutea, an area of the retina which is necessary for seeing fine features and for reading.

- Rubbing the eyes
- Obvious signs of eye problems, e.g. swelling.

It is recommended that people over 60 have their eyes tested annually because eye problems usually develop insidiously and without pain but can have serious consequences including blindness.

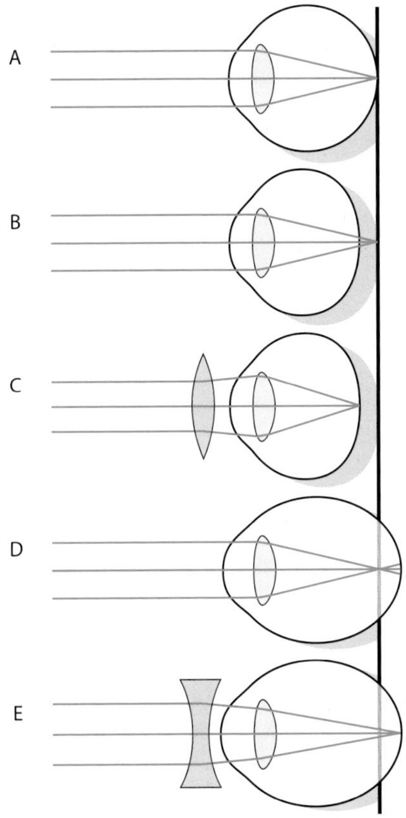

Fig. 16.13 Refractive errors of the eye and corrective lenses. **A.** Normal eye. **B.** Hypermetropia (longsightedness). **C.** Hypermetropia corrected. **D.** Myopia (shortsightedness). **E.** Myopia corrected (reproduced with permission from Waugh & Grant 2006)

The primary aims when caring for people with visual impairment are maximizing independence and maintaining safety. During childhood, specialized help is needed to support the family in achieving this (see Box 16.24, p. 448). Communicating and maintaining a safe environment are therefore the most important activities that the nurse needs to consider.

Communication

Good verbal communication skills are essential and it is important to use normal speech and maintain eye contact when talking to visually impaired people, as the tone and inflexion convey much more than the actual words used (see Ch. 9). People with visual impairment often compensate by increased perception from their other senses. When approaching a visually impaired person this should be from the side of vision, if there is one. Calling their name will alert them to your approach and identifying yourself and others is essential. When leaving, tell them you are going. A call bell should be left at hand in care settings, as the visually impaired person cannot call to a passer-by for help unless they can hear them. The sense of touch is important for people with visual impairment, especially when this occurs together with hearing problems. Sighted people quickly scan their environment for cues about what is happening around them and the nurse must allow more time for visually impaired people to do this. When describing something being 'over there',

HEALTH PROMOTION Box 16.24

Promoting development in children with sight impairment

Aims

1. *To provide support for the child and family*: Information should be provided to enable the family to identify appropriate sources of support and education to meet their needs and to facilitate development of the child into adulthood.
2. *To maximize attachment*: From an early stage, bonding between an infant and its parents is reinforced by mutual eye contact which may be absent. Other cues need to be identified to encourage attachment and to facilitate reinforcement. These can be provided in other ways such as speech, touch or cuddling the child.
3. *To achieve optimum development*:
   - Normal motor development leads to independence and relies heavily on visual stimuli. Non-visual cues and stimuli must be provided instead. Later on the child will need to learn to get around independently outside and a cane or guide dog may be introduced to achieve this
   - Development of play and socialization skills also relies heavily on visual stimuli – imitation being a prime example. More time is required to explain what should and can be done and guidance about other stimuli that encourage development of the other senses, e.g. touch and hearing, provided
   - Education needs to take into account the reliance on non-visual clues. Specialist support will be required to facilitate learning and will usually include learning to read Braille.

[Based on Wong et al (2001)]

a gesture that indicates location often accompanies the words. People with visual impairment may not see these gestures and therefore verbal cues about the location of items can cause confusion. Using more specific language, e.g. the television is beside the window, is helpful.

Written communication can pose challenges for people with sight impairment and simple interventions such as the use of a reading lamp directed towards the material will enhance residual vision, thus assisting reading. Spectacles should always be clean (see pp. 435–436). Many people with sight impairment can read ordinary print but find it is slow and very tiring while others find large print is essential. Books in large print are widely available. Hand-held magnifying glasses can be a useful reading aid. Large writing using a broad, black felt-tipped pen on white paper provides good contrast and is a useful strategy for providing written guidance to people with sight impairment.

Many people with sight impairment enjoy audio material. The RNIB provides a Talking Book Service and audiotapes that can be used in most cassette players are widely available. Headphones may be required to use audio equipment if others nearby are being distracted.

Some people with sight impairment use tactile forms of communication. Braille is a system of raised dots that can be learned by touch and produced using a Braillewriter. Moon is another, simpler form of tactile communication used mainly by older people. Both of these methods are effective but only between those people who can understand them.

An expanding range of technology is being designed to facilitate access to written material through increasing use of computers and the Internet.

Maintaining a safe environment

Many interventions will assist in maintaining a safe environment for everyone, especially for those with sight impairment (RNIB 2004b). Corridors and stairs should always be well lit, well signed and free from moveable and unnecessary items to minimize the occurrence of accidents. This is important at home, in care settings and in public places because many people, especially older people, have some degree of sight impairment although they may not be aware of it.

At home, a sight-impaired person can decide where items are kept and so find them again easily. Orientation to a new environment takes time. Most people will need to be accompanied around a new environment several times before becoming accustomed to new surroundings. Pot-pourri with different fragrances can be used to distinguish areas such as the sleeping area and sitting room. Sight-impaired people should be encouraged to explore parts of their new surroundings by touch. Moving personal belongings should only be carried out after discussion with the person.

Several issues may arise relating to safe use of medication (see Ch. 22). These include difficulty reading small print on labels of the containers, counting of tablets and opening blister packs. Assistance with administration of medication may be needed, especially those instilled into the eye.

People often find bright light and glare uncomfortable, both outdoors and inside on bright sunny days. Wearing ordinary sunglasses may not help because light also reaches the eyes from above and round the sides although a brimmed hat or baseball cap can solve the problem. Clip-on tinted spectacles with side shields that can be worn over normal spectacles are useful because they are quickly removed when going into a dark area.

Services and support

Local authorities maintain registers of blind and partially sighted people to enable planning of services to meet their needs. They provide home adaptations to meet individual needs.

After assessment, mobility aids may be provided to provide navigational independence. These include a white guide cane or, for some people, a guide dog.

The ear and hearing

The ear is a sensory organ that provides important information about the environment. It enables people to hear sounds that are interpreted by the brain. The ear is also the organ that enables people to maintain balance. The anatomy and physiology of hearing is outlined and the

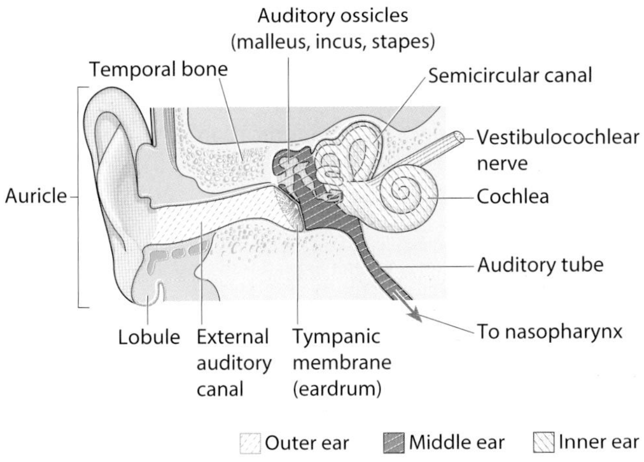

Fig. 16.14 Structure of the ear (reproduced with permission from Waugh & Grant 2006)

nursing interventions that will help a person with hearing impairment are explored.

The RNID (2004a) estimates there are 9 million deaf and hard of hearing people in the UK, with numbers increasing as the population becomes older. The incidence is about 2% in young adults rising to 55% in those over 60 years. Robins and Mangan (1999) highlight common and widespread difficulties faced by hearing-impaired people when communicating with nurses and most other health professionals.

Anatomy and physiology

The ear consists of three parts (Fig. 16.14):

- The outer ear consists of the auricle, or pinna, and the external auditory canal. The external auditory canal extends from the auricle to the tympanic membrane, or eardrum. It is lined with hairs and ceruminous glands that secrete wax.
- The middle ear is an air-filled cavity that transmits sound waves inwards. It contains the auditory ossicles, three tiny bones named according to their shapes: malleus (hammer), incus (anvil) and stapes (stirrup).
- The ossicles extend across the middle ear to the oval window. Air reaches the middle ear from the nasopharynx via the auditory (pharyngotympanic) tube, maintaining atmospheric pressure on both sides of the eardrum. The auditory tube is normally closed but opens during swallowing or yawning.
- The inner ear lies in the temporal bone and consists of the cochlea, vestibule and three semicircular canals, one lying in each plane. The outer bony part encloses the fluid-filled membranous part of the labyrinth. It contains the specialized receptors involved in hearing and balance.

Hearing

Sound waves entering the outer ear are funnelled along the external auditory canal to the eardrum which then vibrates. The vibrations are transmitted and amplified through the middle ear cavity by movement of the ossicles. When the vibrations reach the outer boundary of the inner ear, they generate fluid waves in the membranous cochlea and stimulate specialized receptors located in hair cells of the spiral organ (of Corti). This generates nerve impulses that are transmitted to the temporal lobe of the cerebral cortex where hearing is perceived.

Balance

The vestibule and three semicircular canals have no role in hearing but also contain specialized receptors. These are stimulated by movement of the head generating nerve impulses that are transmitted to the cerebellum providing information about posture and balance.

Assessment and prevention of hearing loss

Nurses play diverse roles is preventing hearing loss and assessment of people's hearing.

Newborn babies have their hearing assessed through the use of sophisticated computer-linked equipment – otoacoustic emission testing (OAE) and/or automated auditory brainstem response test (AABR). Where this equipment is not available, health visitors perform a less reliable distraction test using simple sounds when the infant is between 6 and 8 months of age. Whenever a hearing problem is suspected, children have investigations that include audiometric testing (see below) and careful follow-up. Hearing impairment in children is often accompanied by developmental delay and difficulty with speech. Compliance with childhood immunization programmes is recommended as some infectious childhood diseases can cause deafness, e.g. mumps.

The occupational health nurse is involved in preventing noise-induced hearing loss and hearing tests for those who work in a noisy environment. Under the Health and Safety at Work Act (1974) (see Chs 6, 13) employers must provide their workers with advice about minimizing the risks of noise-induced hearing deficit and provide personal protective equipment, e.g. earmuffs or earplugs, when appropriate. Exposure to regular noise above 100 decibels can lead to noise-induced hearing impairment; this can occur in the work environment or leisure activities, e.g. shooting. Table 16.3 (see p. 450) shows a range of sounds representing various intensities.

Hearing impairment

Interpersonal communication relies heavily on speech and characteristic signs that accompany hearing impairment include:

- Turning one ear towards the speaker
- Apparent lack of attention or poor concentration
- Inappropriate responses
- Often seeming withdrawn or alone
- No response to sounds in the environment
- Asking for information to be repeated
- Speech which is unusually loud or soft
- A person who is easily startled when the speaker initiates conversation.

In adults and older children, hearing loss and deafness are usually measured by audiometry. This investigation

Table 16.3 Hearing impairment – impact on communication

Decibels (dB)	Typical noise	Severity of deafness (RNID 2004)	Impact on communication
150	Severe pain	Profound	BSL may be first or preferred language Use lipreading
140	Jet aeroplane during take off		
130			
120	Thunder, indoor rock concert		
110			
100	Hearing impairment after prolonged exposure		
90	↕ Trains Heavy traffic, workshop	Severe	BSL may be first or preferred language. Use lipreading and hearing aid
80	Loud radio/television		
70	↕ Street noises		
60	Noise in a restaurant	Moderate	Difficulty in following speech without a hearing aid
50			
40	↕ Normal conversation at 1 m		
30		Mild	Difficulty in following speech when there is background noise. Often unaware there is a problem
20	Whisper		
10	Leaves rustling	Normal hearing	None
0	Faintest sounds heard		

identifies the thresholds, or quietest sounds, that can be heard across a range of frequencies, or pitches. Hearing thresholds are measured in decibels (dB). The person being tested is asked to respond by pressing a button when they can hear a tone. The level of the tone is then adjusted until it can just be heard and this level is called the threshold. The greater the threshold level found, the greater the hearing loss.

Hearing impairment varies in severity from mild to profound and can be congenital (present from birth) or acquired (onset after birth). Any hearing impairment is likely to impact on people's ability to communicate (see Table 16.3 and Ch. 9).

Previously unidentified hearing impairment is most commonly encountered when caring for children and older people. The nurse should be aware that many severely or profoundly deaf people also have other disabilities, including learning disabilities. In those under 60, 45% have other disabilities, while in those over 60 years the incidence rises to 77% (RNID 2004a).

There are two types of hearing loss: *conductive*, when sound waves cannot be transmitted though the outer or middle ear to the inner ear, and *sensorineural*, when there is abnormality of the cochlea or auditory nerve that transmits auditory impulses to the brain. Some people have both types of hearing loss.

There are many causes of hearing impairment (Box 16.25). Sometimes people lose their hearing temporarily and it returns when they receive treatment; for others hearing loss is permanent. Accumulation of excess wax in the external auditory canal can cause conductive hearing loss and is a common occurrence in older people. This can be improved, and sometimes cured, by ear irrigation (see p. 436). Deafness occurs most commonly as part of the ageing process known as presbycusis and is common in older people who are often unaware of its presence as the onset is insidious and slowly progressive. Ringing in

Box 16.25 **Common causes of hearing impairment**

- Premature birth
- Infections, e.g. mumps, meningitis; maternal rubella (German measles) during pregnancy
- Accumulation of ear wax
- Older age – known as presbycusis
- Conditions affecting the ear, e.g. repeated middle ear infections (otitis media), Ménière's disease, otosclerosis
- Medication, including aspirin, aminoglycoside antibiotics (e.g. gentamicin)
- Ongoing exposure to loud noise, e.g. at work, night clubs.

Box 16.26 Deafblindness

Around 95% of what people perceive about themselves and their environment comes through the senses of sight and hearing. In 2004, the RNID (2004b) estimated there were about 23 000 deafblind people in the UK, some of whom are completely deaf and completely blind, whereas others have some residual hearing and/or vision.

Facts

- This is also known as dual sensory impairment
- It is sometimes congenital but more often acquired
- Older people are most commonly affected and without appropriate support they can become withdrawn, depressed and isolated. They may lose independence in many areas, including mobility, communication, access to information and enjoying leisure activities
- With appropriate support, deafblind people of all ages can live fulfilling lives at home and in their community. Local authorities may provide guidehelps or communicator guides who help these people take an active part in everyday life
- The organization Sense provides information for people with dual sensory impairment and their carers (see 'Useful websites', p. 461).

the ears, or tinnitus, is a distressing condition that can also be an early sign of hearing impairment.

Describing deafness

It is important to realize that being deaf or hard of hearing can mean different things to different people. People are often comfortable with particular words to describe their own deafness and may feel quite strongly about terms they do not like being used. The RNID (2004b) provides the following guidance:

- Deaf people: generally used term for any degree of deafness
- Hard of hearing people: those with mild to severe hearing loss and also people who have lost their hearing gradually
- Deafened people: those who could hear normally at birth and became severely or profoundly deaf after learning to speak
- Deafblind people: those with very limited hearing and vision (see Box 16.26)
- The Deaf Community: used by many Deaf people whose preferred language is British Sign Language (see p. 452) and who consider themselves part of the Deaf Community ('Deaf', with a capital D, emphasizes their Deaf identity).

Communicating with hearing-impaired people

Deaf and hard of hearing people may communicate in different ways depending on the severity of their hearing impairment. Hearing impairment can be overcome, at least partly, by the use of hearing aids (see pp. 436–437), lipreading, using a computer or sign language. Other strategies used by people with hearing impairment include increased sensitivity to facial expression and other non-verbal behaviours. Some people with mild hearing loss use a hearing aid or lipread. People with moderate hearing loss have difficulty hearing what is said without a hearing aid, especially when there is background noise. People who are more severely deaf may have difficulty following what is being said, even with a hearing aid. Many of these people lipread and some use sign language. Some, but not all, people who are profoundly deaf find that hearing aids are of little benefit and therefore rely on lipreading or sign language (Box 16.27, p. 452). Nurses will usually need the services of an interpreter when communication is through sign language, especially when detailed or complex information is involved.

It is important to be aware that deaf people often find difficulty communicating in group situations, especially when there are rapid changes in speakers and topics. Box 16.28 (p. 452) provides some useful tips that will enhance verbal communication with people who have impaired hearing.

The unconscious patient

In this section consciousness, assessing levels of consciousness and management of the unconscious casualty are explained. Common conditions that affect the nervous system are outlined and neurological investigations and terminology are highlighted. The final part explores the care of the unconscious person as an example of someone who is completely dependent on others for all aspects of nursing care.

The outcome of unconsciousness can be complete recovery, partial recovery or death, often depending on the cause. The timescale is also variable and can last from a few minutes or hours to weeks or longer. There are many different causes, including:

- Trauma
- Poisons, e.g. alcohol, carbon monoxide, drug overdose
- Seizures
- Stroke
- Cardiovascular conditions, e.g. severe blood loss, severe shock, cardiac arrest, myocardial infarction (heart attack)
- Metabolic causes, e.g. severe infection, kidney or liver failure, hypoglycaemia (low blood sugar levels)
- Terminal illness, when recovery will not occur.

Levels of consciousness

When a person is conscious they are awake, aware of their surroundings and interact with it, both consciously and subconsciously. This requires normal functioning of the brain, including the cerebral cortex as well as the brain stem that conducts nerve impulses there for processing. Loss of consciousness is a sign of a serious underlying

Box 16.27 Help for hearing-impaired people

1. Hearing aids – see pages 436–437.
2. Lipreading – only about 40% of the spoken word is understood and less when the speaker has a beard, moustache, a strong accent or exaggerated pronunciation. Comprehension is enhanced by the development of increased sensitivity to non-verbal cues including body language, facial expression and gestures.
3. Sign language and finger spelling (see www.rnid.org.uk):
   - British Sign Language (BSL) is the most widely used UK form. It is a visual–gestural language that uses hand signals, facial expressions and shoulder movements to represent words and ideas. It is widely used by hearing-impaired children and their families
   - Signed English was initially designed to encourage hearing-impaired children with reading, writing and speech, but is also used by people with learning disabilities
   - Finger spelling.
4. Makaton – this is a communication system based on signs, symbols and speech, widely used by both adults and children with communication difficulties including those with learning disabilities. It uses a core vocabulary that focuses on essential daily activities. In the UK, the symbols are based on BSL (see Ferris-Taylor 2003 and www.makaton.org for further information).
5. Other aids for hearing-impaired people:
   - Alerting devices such as lights can be attached to doorbells, alarm clocks and smoke alarms to facilitate communication, enhance independence and promote safety
   - The RNID website and telecommunication companies provide information about equipment for deaf and hard of hearing people
   - The installation of induction loops helps people with a hearing aid or loop listener to hear sounds more clearly by reducing or cutting out background noise. These systems are widely found in public places including theatres, cinemas, banks, shopping centres and train stations (Fig. 16.15). Smaller systems can be installed at home and are useful for listening to the television.
   - Increasingly, specially trained 'hearing' dogs are being used to improve the lives of people with hearing impairments by alerting the person to specific sounds, e.g. smoke alarm, door bell, etc.

Fig. 16.15 Induction loop symbol

NURSING SKILLS Box 16.28

Communication tips for people with hearing impairment

- Gently alert the person to your arrival
- Check the hearing aid, if used, is switched on
- Minimize background noise if appropriate, e.g. television
- Sit or stand at the same level at an appropriate distance from the person – about 1 m if wearing a hearing aid or 1–2 m for lipreading
- Face the person, making sure your face and lips are visible
- If the person lipreads, ensure they are wearing spectacles, if used
- Speak slowly and clearly using your normal tone and inflection
- Use non-verbal communication skills to reinforce your verbal skills, e.g. hands, facial gestures
- Check that the person is following the conversation by asking them to contribute actively at times
- If you are not understood:
  - try using other words to explain yourself
  - raise your voice slightly but use lower tones, never shout
  - use gestures or writing to enhance understanding.

disorder and the nurse must know how to assess an unconscious person and provide appropriate first aid and nursing interventions.

The unconscious casualty

A collapsed casualty is dependent on the actions of others to maintain life, and providing timely and effective first aid interventions is vital (Box 16.29). The principles are always the same although cardiopulmonary resuscitation (CPR) varies depending on age (see Ch. 17).

First aiders should monitor the casualty's response, together with pulse and respiratory rates (see Ch. 14) every 10 minutes, recording them on a piece of paper if available. The condition of a collapsed casualty can change quickly and careful assessment and recording provide important information that will assist in evaluating the casualty's condition, both at the time and later in

FIRST AID Box 16.29

The unconscious casualty

Priorities are established using the framework DR ABC:

Danger – This may be caused by moving traffic, chemicals, etc; ensure the area is safe for both you and the casualty before proceeding
Response – Ask the casualty loudly, 'Can you hear me?' If there is a response, you have established that they are conscious, breathing and a circulation is present. If there is no response, other possibilities are outlined below with the treatment needed

Airway – if there is no response, open the airway (see Ch. 17)
Breathing – assess by looking for the chest rising, listening for signs of breathing and feeling for air movement into or out of the mouth for up to 10 seconds
Circulation – assess by looking at the casualty's colour, feeling for a pulse for up to 10 seconds.

After carrying out the DR ABC assessment you will be able to identify the casualty's response. Treatment depends on whether your observation/assessment of the casualty is that they are:

Conscious and breathing
Treatment:
- Check circulation
- Assess and treat other injuries
- Get help or send someone for help if necessary.

Unconscious and breathing
Treatment:
- Place casualty in the recovery position (see Fig. 16.17A, B)
- Check circulation (see above)
- Assess and treat other injuries
- Send for an ambulance.

Unconscious, not breathing but circulation present
Treatment:
- Give rescue breaths (see Ch. 17)
- Send for an ambulance
- Assess circulation – frequency depends on the casualty's age (see Ch. 17).

Unconscious, not breathing and no circulation
Treatment:
- Taking age into account, commence CPR (see Ch. 17) and send for an ambulance.

(See also 'Basic life support – airway maintenance and cardiopulmonary resuscitation', Ch. 17, pp. 473–478.)

[Adapted from St John Ambulance website: www.sja.org.uk/firstaid/info Available July 2006]

hospital. Level of consciousness is assessed more accurately by using the Glasgow Coma Scale (see below).

Unconscious or partly conscious people must never be given anything orally because they are at risk from choking or inhaling fluid into their lungs and either of these events will have serious consequences.

People with diabetes mellitus may lose consciousness when their condition is not well controlled. This is usually when blood sugar levels fall below normal and is sometimes called a 'hypo' – meaning hypoglycaemia. Many people recognize the onset of a 'hypo' and take a sugary drink or snack to reverse it before they become unconscious. If unconsciousness occurs, the person is treated in the same way as any other unconscious casualty. People with diabetes who have been ill for some time may also lose consciousness through abnormally high blood sugar levels (hyperglycaemia).

There may be evidence of ingestion of drugs or alcohol, e.g. empty bottles or packaging, around an unconscious casualty that will alert the first aider to the possibility of overdose. In either case vomiting can occur and the unconscious casualty is at risk of inhaling vomit unless placed in the recovery position (see Fig. 16.17A, p.460) when vomit will drain from the mouth, keeping the airway open.

The Glasgow Coma Scale (Fig. 16.16, p. 454)

Altered consciousness exists on a spectrum from loss of alertness and drowsiness to coma. These and many other terms used are subjective and therefore unreliable for describing a person's level of consciousness. In order to assess a person's level of consciousness accurately an assessment tool is used, usually the Glasgow Coma Scale (GCS). The scale relies on scores achieved for three independent measurements:

- Best eye response
- Best motor response
- Best verbal response.

Different responses to each of these can be found in people with altered consciousness and these are added together providing a total score at regular intervals. The best score is the maximum of 15 and the lowest is 3. Coma is defined as a score of 8 or less but any value under 15 is significant. Changes in the GCS score are important indicators of altering neurological status. A dot for each response is entered in the appropriate box on the chart.

Assessing the level of consciousness using the GCS is shown in Box 16.30 (p. 454). Sometimes it is not possible to assess best eye opening accurately because neither eye can be opened, e.g. when there is severe swelling, and 'C', meaning 'closed', is entered in the bottom box on the chart. The best verbal response involves the person's ability to speak and understand. When a patient has an endotracheal tube in situ or a tracheostomy that prevents

NURSING SKILLS — Box 16.30

Glasgow Coma Scale (GCS) measurements

Best eye opening (maximum score 4)

- Spontaneous opening (4) – eyes open spontaneously as the observer approaches
- Opening to speech (3) – eyes open when addressed by the observer. It may be necessary to raise the voice slightly or gently shake the shoulder in case the casualty is hard of hearing
- Opening to pain (2) – when there is no response to either of the stimuli above, a painful stimulus is applied. The stimulus must be consistent to detect changes accurately
- No eye opening (1) – even to a painful stimulus.

Best verbal response (maximum score 5)

- Orientated (5) – the person is able state their name and where they are and can also answer simple questions about the year, month and date
- Confused (4) – the person can speak but is not fully orientated to time, place and person
- Inappropriate sounds (3) – the person is unable to engage in meaningful conversation
- Incomprehensible sounds (2) – no recognizable words but may consist of sounds, e.g. moaning and groaning
- No response (1) – no sounds are made in response to either speech or painful stimuli.

Best motor response (maximum score 6)

- Obeys commands (6) – the person can do something that involves movement of muscles above the neck, e.g. to stick their tongue out or tightly close their eyes. This means that even if the person has a spinal injury, they can still be assessed accurately and avoids squeezing of the observer's fingers, which can be a reflex action.
- Localizes pain (5) – when the person cannot respond to commands, applying a painful stimulus may elicit a response. The person attempts to locate or remove the painful stimulus (when this has already been demonstrated for their best verbal response, there is no need to reapply another painful stimulus to assess the motor response)
- Withdrawal from pain (4) – the person responds purposefully by withdrawing a limb from the stimulus but does not attempt to locate or remove it.
- Flexion to pain (3) – there is no purposeful response to the painful stimulus and the limbs flex abnormally in a purposeless way
- Extension to pain (2) – the limbs extend, or straighten in an abnormal way, rather than withdraw or flex in response to a painful stimulus.
- None (1) – there is no limb response to painful stimuli.

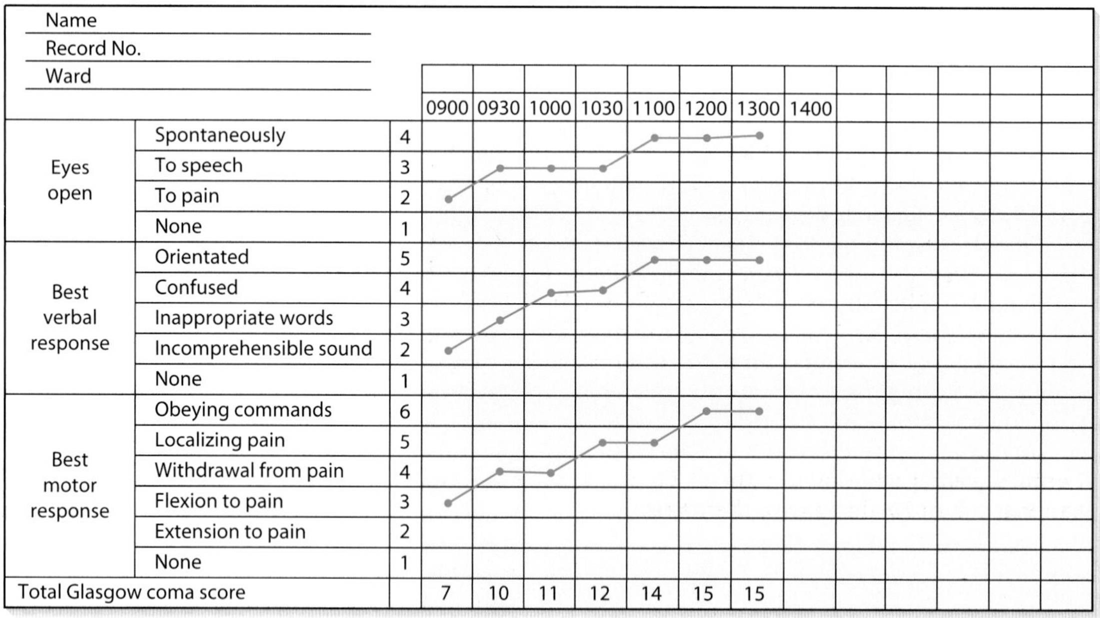

Fig. 16.16 Glasgow Coma Scale

them from speaking, a 'T' is entered in the bottom box on the chart.

Assessment of level of consciousness using the GCS is not reliable for children and modifications are required to take expected developmental milestones into account until their language skills have developed (Box 16.31).

Other situations where GCS findings need careful evaluation include the presence of:

- A learning disability because developmental milestones may not match those expected for the physical size or age

NURSING SKILLS — Box 16.31

Adaptation of Glasgow Coma Scale measurements for children

- Best eye opening – carried out as per Box 16.30
- Best verbal response – the adaptations required are:

Best verbal response		Best grimace response – used for pre-verbal infants
Alert, normal babbling, cooing or words used	5	Spontaneous normal mouth and facial movements
Less than usual babbling, cooing, etc. or spontaneous irritable cry	4	Less than normal spontaneous mouth and facial movements or response to touch
Inappropriate crying	3	Vigorous grimace in response to pain
Occasional whimpering or moaning	2	Mild grimace to pain
No vocal response	1	No response

- Best motor response – carried out as per Box 16.30.

[Adapted from NICE (2003)]

Table 16.4 Outline of common neuro-logical conditions

Cerebrovascular accident (stroke)	Caused by haemorrhage from cerebral blood vessels or a thrombosis, or clot, lodged in a cerebral artery affecting conscious level, sensation, movement, swallowing, speech and/or vision One-sided paralysis (hemiplegia) is often present
Confusion (delirium)	Disorientation to time, place or person It is not an illness but indicates an underlying problem and is common in older people It is usually reversed when the cause is treated
Dementia	Slow, progressive and irreversible memory loss, disorientation and impairment of reasoning that usually affects some older people The most common form is Alzheimer's disease Independence declines in the later stages when there is increasing difficulty with speech and performing routine activities
Epilepsy	Recurrent seizures; affects children and adults (see text)
Meningitis	Inflammation of the meninges, usually caused by bacteria or viruses
Multiple sclerosis (MS)	A common cause of disability in people under 50 years, characterized by an unpredictable series of relapses and remissions Onset may be acute or insidious, and blurring of vision or double vision can be early signs Later, problems with elimination of urine and faeces, speech, vision, fatigue, depression and weakness or paralysis of the limbs are common
Parkinson's disease	Gradual and progressive decline in motor function that results in tremor, rigidity, slowness of movement and difficulty in initiating movement

- Verbal communication problems, e.g. the person cannot speak or English is not their first language.

Neurological observations in hospital

This involves GCS measurement, which assesses level of consciousness, together with several other observations including pulse, blood pressure and respiratory rate; the response of the pupils to light; and limb movements. These are recorded on a single chart, known as a neurological observation chart. A full discussion is beyond the scope of this book but is explained by Bowie and Woodward (2003).

Common conditions affecting the nervous system

In addition to unconsciousness, there are many conditions that affect the normal functioning of the nervous system (Table 16.4). Related associations and groups also provide useful information and some of their websites are included at the end of this chapter. There are also many different investigations used to identify disorders affecting the nervous system (Box 16.32, p. 456). Box 16.33 (p. 456) provides the opportunity to find out what a neuro-logical investigation can involve.

Some of these conditions are very common and you are likely to meet people with them when on placement.

Box 16.32 Common neurological investigations

The following investigations may be used to diagnose or evaluate treatment for disorders of the nervous system:

- X-rays of skull and spine
- Brain scans – computed tomography (CT), magnetic resonance imaging (MRI), positron emission tomography (PET)
- Electroencephalogram (EEG)
- Nerve and muscle function tests, e.g. electromyogram (EMG)
- Lumbar puncture (LP) – cerebrospinal fluid sampling.

A simple explanation of these investigations accessed on the BBC website (BBC 2004) will help you provide patient information; a more detailed nursing explanation can be found in Bowie and Woodward (2003).

REFLECTIVE PRACTICE Box 16.33

Undergoing an MRI scan

Jane is to have an outpatient MRI scan. She has poor short-term memory and becomes confused in new surroundings. Jane keeps asking the staff at the nursing home about what will happen during the test and seems anxious to get more information. She has a moderate hearing impairment and wears a hearing aid.

Student activities

- Find out about MRI scanning.
- Consider how you might feel during this investigation.
- Identify the key information needed by Jane so that she is well prepared for her scan.
- Consider how to provide Jane with information that meets her needs.

There is much terminology used to describe the effects of nervous system conditions and some common terms are defined in Box 16.34.

Box 16.34 Effects of neurological conditions

Amnesia – loss of memory
Aphasia – loss of speech
Ataxia – impaired muscle coordination
Bradykinesia – slow movement
Diplopia – double vision
Dysarthria – difficulty speaking
Dyskinesia – difficulty with voluntary movement
Dysphagia – difficulty swallowing
Dysphasia – difficulty speaking
Hemiparesis – weakness of muscles on one side of the body
Hemiplegia – paralysis of muscles on one side of the body
Paraplegia – paralysis of the lower limbs
Paraesthesia – abnormal sensation, e.g. tingling
Photophobia – intolerance of light
Quadriplegia, tetraplegia – paralysis of all four limbs
Tremor – involuntary muscle movement usually affecting a limb or limbs.

Seizures

These are also known as 'fits' or 'convulsions'. They affect both adults and children and can be frightening to those around when they occur. This can be at home, in a care setting or outdoors and they are relatively common in some people with learning disabilities. One started, a seizure is usually short lived and self-limiting. It cannot be stopped and therefore first aid intervention is based on maintaining a safe environment (see Box 16.35). A seizure may be accompanied by incontinence of urine and/or faeces.

In children under 5 years, seizures are often associated with a high body temperature and are known as febrile seizures (previously called convulsions). First aid interventions (see Box 16.36) therefore aim to reduce the raised body temperature in addition to maintaining safety.

In older children and adults a warning, or 'aura', often occurs before a seizure, meaning that the person is aware that one is about to take place. After a seizure there is often a period of drowsiness and disorientation. When recovery occurs it may be necessary to reorientate the person and explain what has happened.

Nursing the unconscious person

Depending on the cause, nursing care can take place in a variety of settings. These range from a terminally ill person in their own home to trauma casualties in an intensive care unit. In the latter case there will also be many technical interventions; however, the principles of nursing care are the same for any unconscious person. These interventions are explained in different chapters of this book and the art of nursing an unconscious person lies in providing coordinated care tailored to meet their individual needs. Assessing, planning and prioritizing the nursing care for an unconscious person is a complex nursing skill that is carried out by an experienced nurse although providing their care often involves other members of the multidisciplinary team (MDT) including student nurses under the supervision of their mentor. There is no 'standard care plan' for nursing an unconscious person although there are many common nursing problems. Table 16.5 (see p. 458) uses a problem-solving approach to care planning to identify common nursing interventions that may be included in the care of an unconscious person. It is based on the Roper, Logan and Tierney model (see Ch. 14) to enable systematic and holistic assessment of a person's actual and potential nursing problems. There are many references in this table that make it easy to find the full explanation of the relevant intervention. Some aspects of nursing care are discussed in more detail below.

FIRST AID Box 16.35

Seizures in adults

Recognition

Sudden collapse, violent muscle twitching, then muscle relaxation followed by a period of unconsciousness and recovery. *Note*: There are several types of seizure (see Bowie & Woodward 2003).

Aims of treatment

- To maintain a safe environment around the casualty
- To provide care when consciousness returns
- To organize hospital transfer if necessary.

Treatment

- Clear the area of potential hazards
- Ask any onlookers to move away
- Record the time of onset
- Slacken tight clothing, especially around the neck and waist, to assist breathing and place a cushion under the head if possible
- When the seizure is over, observe closely.

If breathing has returned:

- Roll into the recovery position (see Fig. 16.17A, p. 460), check and record breathing, pulse and level of response
- Stay with the casualty until fully recovered
- Record the length of the seizure.

If breathing has not returned:

- Commence resuscitation.

DO NOT:

- Restrain or move the casualty during the seizure
- Attempt to put anything into the mouth.

Transfer to hospital when:

- This is the first seizure
- The seizure lasts for more than 5 minutes
- Unconsciousness lasts longer then 10 minutes.

The care needed is prioritized and always starts with A, B, C:

- Maintain a clear **A**irway
- Monitor **B**reathing
- Monitor **C**irculation.

Several items of equipment are kept at the bedside of unconscious patients. Some items may not be needed if the patient is terminally ill. They are checked each time a new nurse takes over the care to ensure they are still present and in working order in case they are needed in an emergency. They include:

- Suction equipment
- Equipment for administering oxygen
- Oral airway.

Positioning the unconscious patient

In order to maintain a patent airway the recovery position or lateral position is used (Fig. 16.17, p. 460). These prevent the tongue moving backwards and obstructing the airway and promote drainage of any secretions from the mouth and respiratory tract.

Recovery position

The recovery position for adults is mainly used in first aid situations when there are no pillows available to support the casualty (Fig. 16.17A, p. 460). To place someone in this position:

- In a first aid situation, kneel on the ground beside the casualty and remove any large items from their pockets
- Lie them flat on their back with both legs straight
- Position the arm nearest you at right angles to the body then bend the elbow and place the palm facing upwards

FIRST AID Box 16.36

Seizures in children

Recognition

Loss or alteration of consciousness, involuntary muscular twitching, evidence of high fever, not breathing.

Aims of treatment

- To maintain a safe environment around the child
- To provide care when consciousness returns
- To organize transfer to hospital
- To minimize anxiety of the immediate carers
- To cool the child if feverish.

Treatment

- Place pillows around the child to protect from injury
- Record the time of onset
- If feverish:
  - remove clothing down to underwear
  - tepid sponge the child starting at the forehead working downwards.
- When seizure is over, observe closely

If breathing has returned:

- Roll the child into the recovery position
- Check and record breathing, pulse and level of response
- Record the length of the seizure
- Stay with the child until fully recovered
- Remain calm and provide the child and carer with reassurance.

If breathing has not returned:

- Commence resuscitation
- Dial 999 for an ambulance.

DO NOT:

- Restrain or move the child
- Attempt to put anything into the mouth.

Table 16.5 Using a problem-solving approach to plan care for an unconscious patient

Actual/potential problem	Aim	Nursing intervention	Rationale
Maintaining a safe environment			
Emergency situation occurs	To provide rapid and effective intervention	Ensure oral airway and other emergency equipment (p. 457) is at the bedside	Equipment needed is readily available if required
Breathing			
Respiratory or circulatory difficulties	To prevent or detect and report any of the following:		
	• airway obstruction	Nurse in the recovery or lateral position (see Fig. 16.17, p. 460)	Maintains patency of the airway and prevents tongue occluding it
	• inadequate breathing	Observe rate, depth and effort of breathing (see Ch. 14)	Identify changes in respiratory function
	• inadequate tissue oxygenation	Observe skin for pallor or cyanosis	Indicators of decreasing oxygenation
	• circulatory problems	Record pulse and blood pressure (see Ch. 14) as advised	Changes indicate changing condition
	To maintain adequate tissue oxygenation	Administer oxygen therapy as prescribed and maintain safety measures (see Ch. 17)	Increases oxygen available for tissues Prevents fire in the area
Deteriorating neurological condition	To detect and report changes promptly	Carry out GCS and neurological observations (pp. 453–455) as directed	Changes indicate alteration of neurological condition
Communicating			
Unable to communicate verbally Anxiety, fear or disorientation	To provide a safe environment where patient and their relatives understand what is happening	Explain all procedures in simple language before providing interventions	Puts patient at ease and provides a calm, therapeutic environment
		Encourage visitors to speak to the patient	A familiar voice is reassuring
Eating and drinking			
Unable to eat or take oral fluids	To maintain hydration	Administer i.v. fluids as prescribed (see Ch. 19)	Provides optimum fluid requirement
	To maintain nutritional status	Administer nasogastric feeding or parenteral nutrition as prescribed (see Ch. 19)	Meets nutritional requirements which are increased in illness and fever
		Record fluids given on fluid balance chart (see Ch. 19)	Enable accurate evaluation of fluid balance
		Observe for signs of dehydration and fluid overload (see Ch. 19)	Enables early detection and adjustment of fluid therapy
Maintaining body temperature			
Infection	To allow early detection of nosocomial infection (see Ch. 15)	Record temperature as directed (see Ch. 14)	Increased temperature is an early indicator of infection
	To minimize effects of fever	Send specimens for culture and sensitivity (see Ch. 15) as directed	Allows early identification of pathogenic microorganisms
		Provide care for a pyrexial patient (see Ch. 14)	Lowers body temperature and promotes comfort
Personal cleansing and dressing			
Cannot undertake these activities independently	To maintain a high standard of personal hygiene	Give a daily bedbath (pp. 433–434)	Keeps patient comfortable with fresh and clean skin
		Provide oral hygiene (pp. 443–445)	Maintains oral health
		Provide hair care (pp. 437–439)	Keeps hair clean and shiny
		Provide eye care (pp. 435–436) and keep eyes closed with hypoallogenic tape or hydrogel pads	Keeps eyes moist, clean and closed to prevent corneal damage when corneal reflex is absent
Sexuality			
Unable to express sexuality or maintain own privacy	To promote individuality	Close screens when carrying out personal care	Maintain privacy, dignity and individuality
		Use preferred routines and own toiletries	
		Dress in own clothing when possible	

(*Continued*)

Table 16.5 *(Continued)*

Actual/potential problem	Aim	Nursing intervention	Rationale
Mobilizing			
Problems associated with immobility	To prevent development of pressure ulcers	Assess risk using an assessment tool (see Ch. 25)	Identify risk of development of pressure ulcers
		Change position frequently according to risk identified	Prevents prolonged pressure on the skin between firm surface and bony prominences
		Use of pressure-relieving aids (see Ch. 25) as directed	Reduces pressure on skin between bony prominences and a firm surface
	Prevention of deep vein thrombosis (DVT)	Carry out passive exercises as directed (see Ch. 18)	Reduces venous stasis and promotes circulation in the limbs
		Use of other preventive DVT measures (see Ch. 18)	
		Observe for swelling, tenderness or redness of the calves	These are signs of DVT
	To prevent muscle wastage, joint stiffness or contractures	Carry out passive exercises as directed (see Ch. 18)	Exercise of skeletal muscles maintains their tone and reduces muscle wastage. Prevents joint stiffness or contractures
Eliminating			
No control over micturition	To maintain intact skin	Keep skin clean and dry – a penile sheath or catheterization and catheter care may be required (see Ch. 20)	Urinary incontinence predisposes to skin excoriation and breakdown
		Record urine output on fluid balance chart	Enables accurate evaluation of fluid balance
No control over defecation	To maintain intact skin	Wash skin after defecation	Faecal incontinence predisposes to skin breakdown
	To prevent constipation	Record when bowels open in nursing record Increase fibre if possible Administer prescribed laxatives	Low fibre diet, insufficient fluid intake and immobility predispose to constipation
		Observe faecal characteristics (see Ch. 21)	Signs of constipation, diarrhoea or other abnormalities may be evident
Sleeping			
Frequent nursing interventions disrupt circadian rhythm	To promote circadian rhythm (see Ch. 10)	Plan and implement nursing care in an organized manner	Encourages periods of rest and sleep between nursing interventions
Dying			
Terminal illness	To facilitate a peaceful and dignified death	Support the patient and their relatives (see Ch. 12) Encourage relatives to participate in care Understand that some patients will not recover	Provides compassion and understanding in the face of a poor prognosis

- Bend the upper leg and then roll them towards you until the bent leg is across their body. Keeping the upper leg bent will stop them from rolling onto their front
- Place the back of the upper hand under their cheek in a position that keeps their airway clear.

In infants under 1 year the recovery position is achieved by the first aider holding the infant on its side with the head inclined downwards (Fig. 16.17B, p. 460).

Lateral position

Nursing care is more easily carried out in the lateral position (Fig. 16.17C, p. 460), which is normally used in care settings. The patient is positioned as follows:

- Head – supported on one pillow
- Torso – the spine is kept straight and a pillow placed behind the back to provide support
- Arms – the lower arm is brought in front of the patient and placed with the palm upwards. The

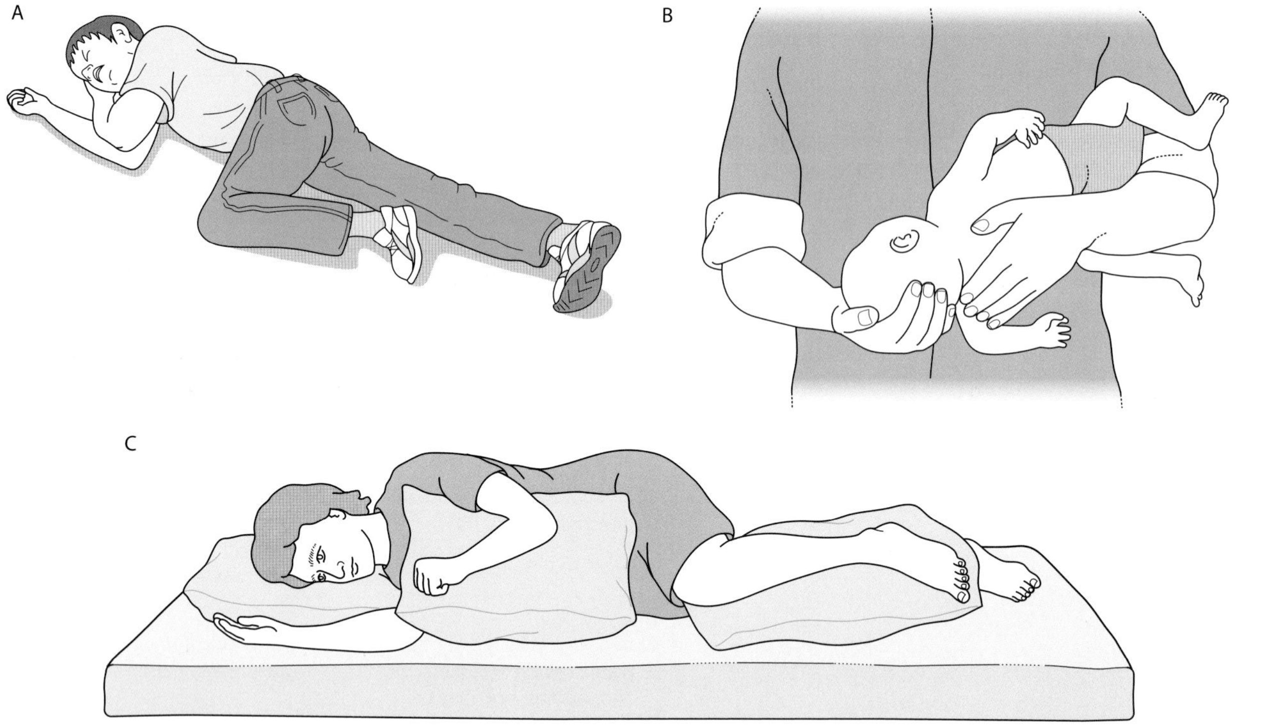

Fig. 16.17 Positioning the unconscious patient: **A.** Recovery position – adults. **B.** Recovery position – infants under 1 year. **C.** Lateral position

upper arm is bent slightly at the elbow and supported on a pillow
- Legs – the lower leg is kept straight and in line with the spine while the upper leg is bent forwards at the knee and supported on pillows.

Communicating with an unconscious person, their relatives and friends

It is important to provide explanations of interventions before they are carried out just as for any other patient. Normal speech is used when communicating with an unconscious patient. As the person is unable to verbalize any fears, concerns or discomfort, the nurse must be especially alert for and report other cues such as restlessness or alterations in vital signs that may indicate pain or changes in the patient's condition. Hearing is the last sense to go and the first to return when consciousness is regained and therefore it is seldom clear to what extent the patient is aware of events around them. In terminal illness, good communication with relatives plays a large part in helping relatives come to terms with not only the current situation but also later on when the patient dies (see Ch. 12).

Visiting someone who is unconscious is stressful and can be a cause of great anxiety, especially when the outcome is unknown or likely to be poor. Anxiety is reduced when visitors are given clear explanations that enable them to understand the treatment and care. At least initially visitors may be limited to close family and significant others to minimize intrusion.

Involvement in the care of their loved one can reduce relatives' feelings of helplessness. Initially relatives can provide information about the person's preferences, lifestyle and hobbies that enables nurses to carry out personal care using preferred routines as far as possible. They are encouraged to speak to the patient and touch them to provide familiar stimuli and may also be asked to provide some favourite tapes or CDs. They may be asked if they want to participate in aspects of personal care and their wishes must be respected whatever decision is reached.

REFLECTIVE PRACTICE — Box 16.37

Care of an unconscious patient

Think about an unconscious patient with whose care you have been involved.

Student activities

- Using Table 16.5, identify which nursing interventions were carried out for your patient.
- Write down the reasons why these were appropriate for that situation.

Planning nursing interventions

Before attending to the patient, consideration is given as to what interventions are required at one time. When the person needs to be turned, this can be followed by oral hygiene, eye care and passive exercises. This will minimize disruption and allow periods of rest, especially important during the night and when seriously ill (Box 16.37).

Summary

- This chapter provides a discussion of fundamental aspects of nursing interventions in relation to personal hygiene activities.
- *Essence of Care* (DH 2001) was designed to improve standards of care and several of the benchmarks have been used here to stimulate learning and reflection on nursing practices you have seen when on placement.
- The high prevalence of sight and hearing impairment, especially in older people, has been highlighted together with some of their effects on people's daily lives. Assessment and nursing interventions for people with these conditions has been considered.
- Care of the unconscious patient has been outlined to show that the nursing interventions for a person with complex physical needs are largely based on coordinating a range of fundamental interventions discussed here and in other chapters.

Self test

1. Define the following terms:
   a. Intertrigo
   b. Skin flora
   c. Plaque
   d. Prosthesis
2. List the priorities when assessing someone who is unconscious or has collapsed.
3. Identify the factors that may influence a person's ability to carry out personal hygiene activities independently.
4. Explain the interventions required to maintain safety in the bathroom.
5. Explain the purpose of best practice benchmarks in *Essence of Care* (DH 2001).
6. Describe the behaviours that may suggest a person has sight impairment.
7. Describe the nursing interventions that would facilitate communicating with someone who lipreads.

Key words and phrases for literature searching

Blindness
Contact lens
Deafness
Eye care
Hearing aids
Mouth care
Oral hygiene
Personal hygiene
Visual impairment

Useful websites

Age Concern (England)	www.ace.org.uk Available July 2006
Alzheimer's Society	www.alzheimers.org.uk Available July 2006
Carers UK	www.carersonline.org.uk Available July 2006
Department of Health	www.dh.gov.uk Available July 2006
Disabled Living Foundation	www.dlf.org.uk Available July 2006
Epilepsy Action (British Epilepsy Association)	www.epilepsy.org.uk Available July 2006
Makaton Vocabulary Development Project	www.makaton.org Available July 2006
Meningitis Research Foundation	www.meningitis.org.uk Available July 2006
Multiple Sclerosis Society	www.mssociety.org.uk Available July 2006
National Institute for Health and Clinical Excellence	www.nice.org.uk Available July 2006
Parkinson's Disease Society	www.parkinsons.org.uk Available July 2006
Prodigy: *practical support for clinical governance*	www.prodigy.nhs.uk Available July 2006
Royal National Institute for Deaf and hard of hearing people (RNID)	www.rnid.org.uk Available July 2006
Royal National Institute of the Blind (RNIB)	www.rnib.org.uk Available July 2006
Sense – *dual sensory impairment*	www.sense.org.uk Available July 2006
Stroke Association	www.stroke.org.uk Available July 2006

References

Adams R 1996 Qualified nurses lack adequate knowledge related to oral health, resulting in inadequate oral care of patients on medical wards. Journal of Advanced Nursing 24(3):552–560

Baker F, Smith L, Stead L 1999 Washing a patient's hair in bed. Nursing Times 95 (5 Suppl):1–2

BBC 2004 Talking to your doctor – medical tests. Online: www.bbc.co.uk/health/talking/tests Available July 2006

Bowie I, Woodward S 2003 Nursing patients with neurological problems. In: Brooker C, Nicol M (eds) Nursing adults: the practice of caring. Mosby, Edinburgh

Bowsher J, Boyle S, Griffiths J 1999 Oral care. Nursing Standard 13(37):31

British Dental Health Foundation 2004a Preventive care and oral hygiene. Online. Available: www.dentalhealth.org.uk

British Dental Health Foundation 2004b Dentures. Online: www.dentalhealth.org.uk Available July 2006

Burgess IF, Brown CM, Lee PN 2005 Treatment of head louse infestation with 4% dimeticone lotion: randomized controlled equivalence trial. British Medical Journal 333(7505):1423

Burr S 1999 Emollients for managing dry skin conditions. Professional Nurse 15(1):43–48

Cancer Research UK 2004 SunSmart – be safe in the sun. Online: www.cancerresearchuk.org Available July 2006

Department of Health 2001 Essence of care – patient focused benchmarking for health care practitioners. Online: www.dh.gov.uk/PublicationsAndStatistics Available July 2006

Disabled Living Foundation 2004 Equipment demonstration centre inventory. Disabled Living Foundation, London. Online: www.dlf.org.uk Available July 2006

Ferris-Taylor R 2003 Communication. In: Gates B (ed) Learning disabilities towards inclusion. 4th edn. Churchill Livingstone, Edinburgh

Freer SK 2000 Use of an oral assessment tool to improve practice. Professional Nurse 15(10):635–637

Gates B (ed) 2002 Learning disabilities towards inclusion, 4th edn. Churchill Livingstone, Edinburgh

Hardy MA 1996 What can you do about your patient's dry skin? Journal of Gerontological Nursing 22(5):11–18

Harkin H, Vaz F 2003 Nursing patients with problems of the ear and hearing. In: Brooker C, Nicol M (eds) Nursing adults: the practice of caring. Mosby, Edinburgh

Holden C, English J, Hoare C et al 2002 Advised best practice for the use of emollients in eczema and other dry skin conditions. Journal of Dermatological Treatment 13(2):103–106

Jamieson EM, McCall J, Whyte LA 2002 Clinical nursing practices. 4th edn Churchill Livingstone, Edinburgh

Koch T, Brown M, Selim P, Isam C 2001 Towards the eradication of head lice: literature review and research agenda. Journal of Clinical Nursing 10(3):364–371

Mallett J, Dougherty L (eds) 2000 Manual of clinical nursing procedures. 5th edn. Blackwell Science, Oxford

McDonald RE, Avery DR 1994 Dentistry for the child and adolescent. 6th edn. Mosby, St Louis

McKinlay I, Ferguson A, Jolly C 1996 Ability and dependency in adolescents with severe learning disability. Developmental Medicine and Child Neurology 38(1): 48–58

National Institute for Clinical Excellence 2003 Clinical guideline 4 – Head injury. Triage, assessment and early management of head injuries in infants, children and adults. Online: www.nice.org.uk Available September 2006

Nicol M, Bavin C, Bedford-Turner S et al 2004 Essential nursing skills. 2nd edn. Mosby, Edinburgh

Nursing and Midwifery Council 2004 Code of professional conduct: standards for conduct, performance and ethics. NMC, London

Oxtoby K 2003 Preserving patients' privacy and dignity. Nursing Times 99(48):18–21

Peattie PI, Walker S (eds) 1995 Understanding nursing care, 4th edn. Churchill Livingstone, Edinburgh

Prodigy 2004a Patient information leaflets. Online: www.prodigy.nhs.uk Available July 2006

Prodigy 2004b Guidance – nappy rash. Online: www.prodigy.nhs.uk Available July 2006

Prodigy 2004c Guidance – headlice. Online: www.prodigy.nhs.uk Available July 2006

Rattenbury N, Mooney G, Bowen J 1999 Oral assessment and care for inpatients. Nursing Times 95(49):52–53

Roberts J 2000a Developing an oral assessment and intervention tool for older people: 3. British Journal of Nursing 9(19):2073–2078

Roberts J 2000b Developing an oral assessment and intervention tool for older people: 2. British Journal of Nursing 9(18):2033–2040

Roberts J 2001 Oral assessment and intervention. Nursing Older People 13(7):14–16

Robins J, Mangan M 1999 Seen and not heard. Nursing Times 95(37):30–32

Royal National Institute for Deaf and hard of hearing people 2004a Facts and figures about deafness and tinnitus. Online: www.rnid.org.uk/information_resources/factsheets/deaf_awareness/factsheets_leaflets/facts_and_figures_on_deafness_and_tinnitus.htm Available July 2006

Royal National Institute for Deaf and hard of hearing people 2004b Deaf and hard of hearing people. Online: www.rnid.org.uk/information_resources/factsheets/deaf_awareness/factsheets_leaflets/deaf_and_hard_of_hearing_people.htm Available July 2006

Royal National Institute of the Blind 2004a Research library statistics on sight problems. Online: www.rnib.org.uk/xpedio/groups/public/documents/PublicWebsite/public_researchstats.hcsp Available July 2006

Royal National Institute of the Blind 2004b How do people with sight problems do everyday things? Online: www.rnib.org.uk/xpedio/groups/public/documents/PublicWebsite/public_everyday.hcsp Available July 2006

Trigg E, Mohammed T (eds) 2006 Practices in children's nursing: guidelines for hospital and the community, 2nd edn. Churchill Livingstone, Edinburgh

Waugh A, Grant A 2006 Ross and Wilson's anatomy and physiology in health and illness, 10th edn. Churchill Livingstone, Edinburgh

Wong DL, Hockenberry-Eaton M, Wilson D et al 2001 Wong's essentials of pediatric nursing. 6th edn. Mosby, St Louis

Further reading

Akhtar SG 2002 Nursing with dignity – Islam. Nursing Times 98(16):40

Brooker C, Nicol M 2003 Nursing adults: the practice of caring. Mosby, Edinburgh

Heath H, Schofield I (eds) 1999 Healthy ageing: nursing older people. Mosby, London

Jootun D 2002 Nursing with dignity – Hinduism. Nursing Times 98(15):38

Kaur Gill B 2002 Nursing with dignity – Sikhism. Nursing Times 98(14):39–41

Mohun J, John K, Lee T (eds) 2002 First aid manual: the authorised manual of St John Ambulance, St Andrews Ambulance Association and the British Red Cross. 8th edn. Dorling Kindersley, London

Redfern SJ, Ross FM 1999 Nursing older people. 3rd edn. Churchill Livingstone, Edinburgh

Breathing and circulation

17

Jillian Riley

Glossary terms

Apnoea
Arrhythmia
Bradycardia
Breathing
Cardiac arrest
Cyanosis
Dyspnoea
Hypertension
Hypervolaemia
Hypotension
Hypovolaemia
Hypoxaemia
Hypoxia
Orthopnoea
Oxygen saturation
Peak expiratory flow rate
Sputum
Tachycardia

Learning outcomes

This chapter will help you:

- Outline the anatomy and physiology of the heart, circulation and blood, and the respiratory tract and breathing
- Describe some common disorders affecting circulation and breathing
- Describe the first aid treatment for common problems with breathing and circulation
- Describe basic life support procedures in adults, children and infants
- Describe the nurse's role in the assessment of circulation and breathing
- Outline some common diagnostic procedures
- Outline the role of health promotion in the reduction of conditions affecting breathing and circulation, and in minimizing the effects of existing conditions
- Describe the nursing interventions for someone with disorders of breathing and circulation
- Understand the principles of rehabilitation for people with disorders of breathing and circulation.

Introduction

The care of people with problems affecting their breathing and/or circulation takes place in diverse settings, from the home to the acute hospital, and includes people of all ages, from the neonate to older adults. Immense change has occurred over the past decade, through technological advances, the development of new drugs and, possibly more importantly, through the shift in focus from the health professional as expert to the concept of the 'expert patient' involved in self-management and decision-making. These have consequently led to change in the care delivered by nurses, some of which is discussed in this chapter.

Assessment of the patient is an important first step in their nursing management and treatment and so, following a brief review of the structure and function of the heart, circulation, blood and respiratory system, the chapter outlines some of the important nursing observations that may be undertaken as part of a holistic assessment. The chapter also outlines some of the more common disorders and investigations used in their diagnosis.

This chapter describes the ways in which the nurse can contribute towards the health of the person with disorders of breathing or circulation, reduce the effects of illness and maximize quality of life for both the patient and their family. Because disorders of breathing and circulation may at times require emergency treatment, some first aid measures are included. The health promoting activities that help to prevent problems with breathing and/or circulation are also explored.

An overview of breathing and circulation

This section provides an outline of the anatomy and physiology of breathing and the circulation. Readers should consult their own anatomy and physiology book for more detail. In addition, an outline of common conditions, basic life support, holistic assessment of the breathing and circulation and investigations are provided.

Life depends on an adequate and continuous supply of oxygen (O_2) and nutrients to the cells and the removal of the waste products of metabolism. Without this, cells will become starved of oxygen and die. The accumulation of waste products such as carbon dioxide (CO_2) also disrupts cell function and eventually contributes to cell death.

Breathing and circulation are therefore fundamental to life and the cardiovascular system (CVS), blood and respiratory system must work together to supply O_2 to the cells and remove waste CO_2. This requires an adequate intake of air and a good blood supply to the lungs in order for gaseous exchange to take place. Oxygenated blood carries O_2 to the cells and deoxygenated blood, containing CO_2, leaves the cells and is transported to the lungs. The CVS is responsible for circulating the blood around the body, and to and from the lungs.

Cardiovascular system – outline of anatomy and physiology

The CVS comprises the heart which pumps blood around the body and to the lungs and the circulatory system of arteries, capillaries and veins through which the blood travels.

The heart

The heart is situated in the thorax, within the mediastinum (the space between the two lungs) with its base inclined to the left (Fig. 17.1). It is protected from injury by the bones forming the thoracic cage, the sternum (breastbone) in front, the ribs and the vertebral column behind.

The wall of the heart has three layers (Fig. 17.2), as follows:

- The outermost layer or pericardium is a double serous membrane which forms the pericardial sac surrounding the heart. It secretes serous fluid between the two layers that provides lubrication and allows the heart to move freely as it relaxes and contracts.
- The middle layer or myocardium comprises specialized cardiac muscle. It contracts (systole) to pump blood around the body and lungs and relaxes (diastole) to fill with blood prior to the next contraction. It requires a plentiful and continuous supply of oxygen, which is supplied by the coronary arteries (see below).
- The innermost layer is the endocardium. This is a smooth layer of cells that enables blood to flow easily through the heart chambers.

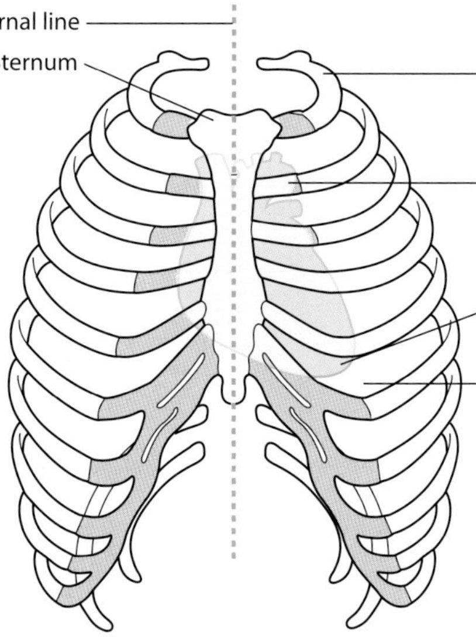

Fig. 17.1 Position of the heart in the thorax (reproduced with permission from Brooker & Nicol 2003)

The heart is divided into four chambers (see Fig. 17.2). The two upper chambers or atria are the receiving chambers that pump blood into the ventricles. The two lower chambers are thick-walled ventricles that pump blood to the lungs (pulmonary circulation) and to the tissues and cells (systemic circulation). The right and left sides of the heart are divided by the septum.

Valves situated at the entrance or exit of the chambers ensure that the blood flows in one direction. The two semilunar valves are the pulmonary valve at the junction of the right ventricle and pulmonary artery and the aortic valve at the junction of the left ventricle and the aorta. The atrioventricular (AV) valves between the atria and ventricles prevent any backflow of blood from the ventricles to the atria as the ventricles contract. The right AV valve (tricuspid valve) lies between the right atrium and ventricle and the left AV valve (bicuspid or mitral valve) lies between the left atrium and ventricle.

Coronary circulation

Three major arteries supply the myocardium with oxygen: the right coronary, the left anterior descending and the circumflex. They branch to form a dense network of arterioles and capillaries that extend throughout the myocardium and ensure that it is supplied with oxygen and metabolic waste products are removed. Once the myocardium has been supplied with oxygen, blood returns to the right atrium via the coronary veins and is transported to the lungs for carbon dioxide removal and reoxygenation. The coronary arteries primarily fill with blood during diastole when the heart muscle is relaxed.

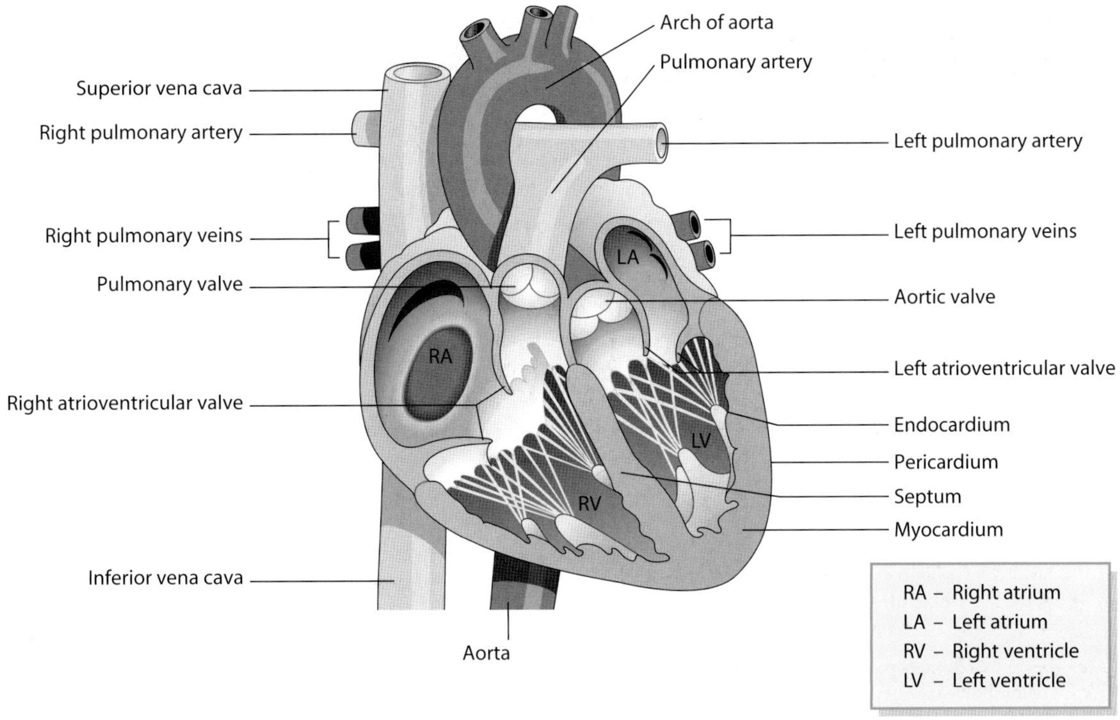

Fig. 17.2 Heart showing the chambers, valves and blood vessels (reproduced with permission from Waugh & Grant 2001)

Conduction

The electrical conduction system of the heart has four main structures (Fig. 17.3):

- Sinus node
- Atrioventricular (AV) node
- AV bundle (bundle of His) and bundle branches
- Purkinje fibres.

The sinus node is known as the 'pacemaker' of the heart because it initiates each heartbeat. It normally fires at a rate between 60 and 100 beats per minute (bpm). From the sinus node, the impulse passes to the AV node causing the atria to contract (atrial systole). From the AV node the impulse passes down the AV bundle in the septum to the right and left bundle branches and the Purkinje fibres. This causes the ventricles to contract (ventricular systole) and eject blood into the aorta and pulmonary artery.

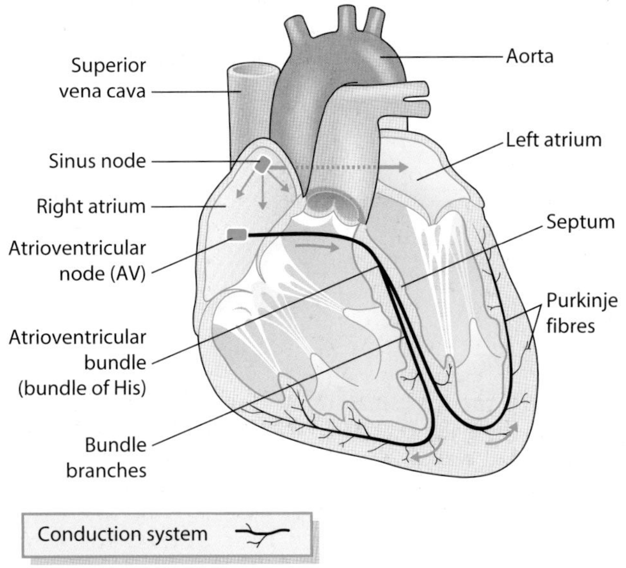

Fig. 17.3 Conduction pathways (reproduced with permission from Brooker & Nicol 2003)

Cardiac cycle

The cardiac cycle is the rhythmic contraction (systole) and relaxation (diastole) of the heart as it fills with blood and pumps it around the body and to the lungs. It comprises a series of stages that occur during a single heartbeat. Normally the whole cycle is completed in less than 1 second. Once one cycle is completed, the next cycle commences to maintain a continuous flow of blood.

The function of the cardiac cycle is to provide an adequate output of blood from the heart. The amount of blood that is ejected with each heartbeat is referred to as the stroke volume (SV), whereas the term cardiac output (CO) refers to the amount of blood ejected from the heart in 1 minute. Hence the equation:

$$\text{Cardiac Output (CO)} = \text{Heart Rate (HR)} \times \text{Stroke Volume (SV)}.$$

Sinus rhythm

Sinus rhythm is the normal rhythm of the heart. It produces a typical waveform comprising five deflections

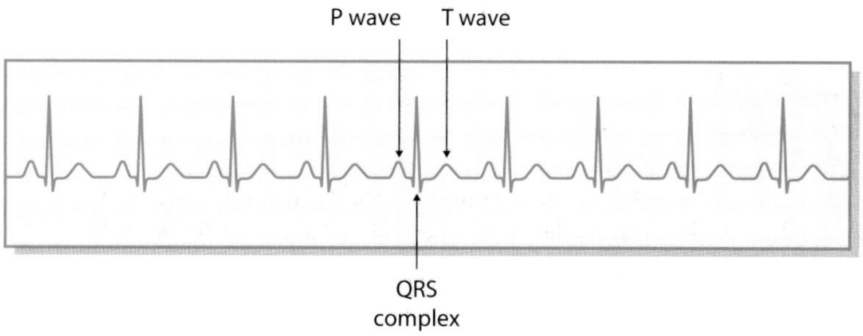

Fig. 17.4 Sinus rhythm (reproduced with permission from Brooker & Nicol 2003)

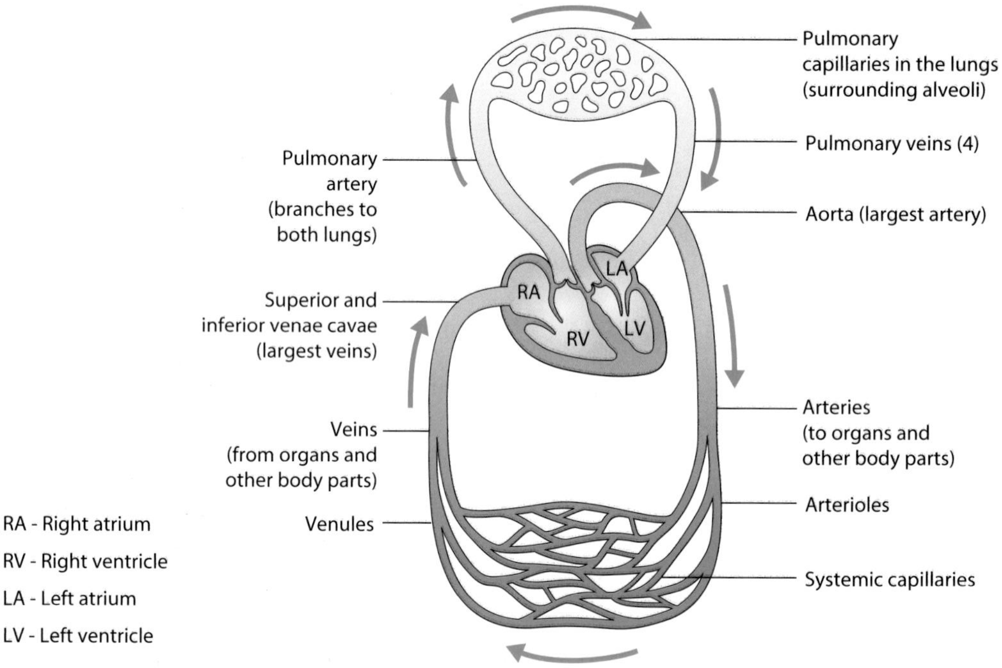

Fig. 17.5 The systemic and pulmonary circulation.

known universally as P-QRS-T (Fig. 17.4). The deflections depicted on an electrocardiogram (ECG) represent the electrical activity in the heart and correspond to the events of conduction and the stages of the cardiac cycle:

- P wave – the first small dome-shaped deflection represents electrical activity through the atria and atrial contraction (atrial systole)
- QRS complex – the larger, narrower deflection represents contraction of the ventricles (ventricular systole)
- ST segment – the period during which the coronary arteries fill with blood
- T wave – the gently rounded deflection represents the resting period of the ventricles when they are relaxed (ventricular diastole).

At rest the adult heart normally beats in response to the sinus node activity at approximately 70 bpm. Sinus rhythm describes any heart rhythm where the complexes described above can be seen and that occurs at a rate between 60 and 100 bpm. In adults, a HR rate <60 bpm is referred to as sinus bradycardia, while a HR >100 bpm is sinus tachycardia.

Systemic and pulmonary circulation

The systemic circulation is the circulation of oxygenated blood from the left ventricle into the aorta, to cells/tissues and deoxygenated blood back to the right atrium of the heart. The pulmonary circulation is the circulation of deoxygenated blood from the right ventricle to the pulmonary artery, to the lungs and oxygenated blood back to the left atrium of the heart.

Thus oxygenated blood returning from the lungs enters the left atrium and passes through the left AV valve into the left ventricle (see Fig. 17.2, p. 465). The left ventricle pumps blood into the systemic circulation through the aorta (large artery) and from there to numerous smaller arteries, arterioles and capillaries, which take blood to the rest of the body (Fig. 17.5). The coronary arteries supplying the myocardium are the first to branch from the aorta. The arterial blood supplies cells with oxygen and nutrients and returns, carrying carbon dioxide and other waste, to the right side of the heart via small veins (venules) and increasingly larger veins. Deoxygenated venous blood returns to the right atrium in two large veins – the superior and inferior venae cavae – and passes through the right AV valve into the right ventricle.

The right ventricle pumps blood into the pulmonary circulation through the pulmonary artery (see Fig. 17.5). The pulmonary artery divides to send a branch to each lung where further subdivisions occur and the blood moves through smaller and smaller arteries and arterioles until they reach the pulmonary capillaries. Gas exchange occurs between the blood in the capillaries and the air in the alveoli of the lungs (see p. 470); carbon dioxide moves from blood to the alveoli and oxygen from the alveoli to the blood.

The oxygenated blood is returned to the left atrium of the heart through venules and larger and larger veins that form four pulmonary veins (two from each lung).

An efficient pulmonary and systemic circulation ensures that the body tissues and organs are perfused with oxygenated blood and waste products are removed.

Blood – outline of anatomy and physiology

Blood is a viscous fluid circulating in the blood vessels. It is a connective tissue and forms the main transport system of the body. The colour depends upon the amount of oxygen it is carrying; well-oxygenated arterial blood is bright red, whereas oxygen-poor (deoxygenated) venous blood is darker in colour.

Blood comprises a fluid part called plasma which forms approximately 55%, and the blood cells which form the remaining 45%. Blood is slightly alkaline with a normal pH range of 7.35–7.45.

Blood volume varies according to body size and age. Adult blood volume forms approximately 7–8% of body weight. An adult male weighing 70 kg has around 5.6 L of blood. Females have a smaller proportion than males; however, during pregnancy, the volume increases by between 20 and 40% in order to maintain blood flow through the enlarged uterus and placenta to supply oxygen and nutrients to the fetus and to remove fetal waste products. Infants and children have a greater proportion, which gradually decreases until adult proportions are reached. At birth the circulating blood volume varies, but is usually around 85 mL/kg. Thus a newborn weighing 4 kg has approximately 340 mL of blood.

The functions of the blood include the following:

- Transports oxygen and nutrients to the cells
- Transports carbon dioxide to the lungs and waste such as urea to the kidneys for excretion
- Helps to maintain fluid, electrolyte and pH balance (see Ch. 19)
- Transports hormones, enzymes and drugs to areas of action
- Distributes heat around the body
- Prevents serious haemorrhage by haemostasis (see p. 468)
- Protects against infection with white blood cells and antibodies.

Plasma

Plasma is the straw-coloured fluid found when blood separates. In the vascular system, plasma provides a medium to carry blood cells. Plasma is between 90 and 92% water and dissolved nutrients, gases, electrolytes, hormones, drugs, waste products and proteins such as albumin, globulins and fibrinogen.

HEALTH PROMOTION Box 17.1

Iron-rich foods

A balanced diet that supplies sufficient iron is needed for the body to produce haemoglobin. Foods rich in iron include:

- Red meat
- Liver
- Dried fruit
- Nuts
- Beans
- Whole grains
- Fortified cereals
- Leafy green vegetables.

Student activities

Access the Food Standards Agency (FSA) website:

- Which vitamin increases iron absorption from food?
- Which beverages can inhibit iron absorption?
- How can a teenage girl who is strictly vegetarian obtain enough iron from her diet?

[Resources Food Standards Agency – http://www.eatwell.gov.uk/healthydiet/nutritionessentials/vitaminsandminerals/iron; www.eatwell.gov.uk/healthydiet/vegaveg Available July 2006]

Blood cells

There are three types of blood cell: erythrocytes (red cells), leucocytes (white cells) and thrombocytes (platelets).

Erythrocytes (red blood cells)

Erythrocytes are the most numerous of the blood cells. They are formed in the red bone marrow and their main function is to carry oxygen. They are biconcave discs that are small enough to pass through small capillaries where the exchange of oxygen, nutrients, carbon dioxide and other waste takes place. Erythrocytes contain haemoglobin (an iron-containing pigment/protein molecule), which is responsible for carrying most of the oxygen transported in the blood. Iron and some B complex vitamins (e.g. folic acid and vitamin B_{12}) are essential for the formation of haemoglobin (Box 17.1).

Leucocytes (white blood cells)

Leucocytes are divided into different groups. These include:

- Granulocytes (polymorphonuclear cells) – neutrophils, basophils and eosinophils
- Lymphocytes
- Monocytes.

All leucocytes have a role in defending the body against microorganisms and other foreign particles. Some leucocytes remove foreign particles such as a bacterium or an abnormal cell by phagocytosis, which involves engulfing and digesting the particle; other leucocytes are part of the immune response through the production of antibodies or destruction of abnormal body cells.

Thrombocytes (platelets)

Platelets are fragments of larger cells found in the bone marrow. They are necessary for blood clotting and haemostasis (control of bleeding from small vessels).

Haemostasis

Normally blood flows freely within the vascular system but when there is significant bleeding from a damaged blood vessel, the process of haemostasis normally prevents major blood loss.

Haemostasis involves four overlapping stages:

- *Vasoconstriction*: The diameter of the blood vessels becomes smaller and blood loss is reduced
- *Platelet plug formation*: Platelets clump together at a site of injury and form a 'platelet plug', which can temporarily stop bleeding until blood coagulation processes are initiated
- *Coagulation/blood clotting* (fibrin clot formation): A complex process with many stages requiring 12 clotting factors, whereby inactive prothrombin (a plasma protein) is converted to active thrombin. In the next stage thrombin converts soluble fibrinogen (plasma protein) to insoluble fibrin and forms a fibrous mesh over the cut vessel. This mesh traps blood cells, a fibrin clot is formed and the damaged vessel is sealed
- *Fibrinolysis*: The final stage where the clot is removed by enzymes once healing is complete.

Blood groups

There are two major blood group classifications: the ABO system and the rhesus system.

The ABO system has four main blood groups – A, B, AB and O – which are defined by the presence of antigens (specific proteins) on the surface of the erythrocyte. People with antigen A are blood group A, those with antigen B are group B. People who have both A and B antigens are blood group AB and those without either antigen are group O.

Someone with blood group A will have anti-B antibodies in their plasma, someone with blood group B will have anti-A antibodies, people with blood group O will have both anti-A and B antibodies while someone with blood group AB will have no antibodies. These antibodies will bind to a foreign antigen and initiate a reaction that destroys the cell such as occurs if incompatible blood is transfused (Bywater & Rawlings 2003) (see p. 498).

It is important to be aware of the different blood groups in order to ensure that when blood is transfused, blood from the correct group is given to the correct person. Table 17.1 outlines the ABO blood group compatibility.

The rhesus group is determined by a further set of antigens on the erythrocyte. People who have the antigens are rhesus positive (Rh[D]-positive) and those without are rhesus negative (Rh[D]-negative). Unlike the ABO system there are no preformed anti-rhesus (anti-D) antibodies. However, if a rhesus negative person receives rhesus positive blood they will develop anti-D. Although this will not cause a transfusion reaction at the time, any future transfusion will initiate a reaction and the donor erythrocytes will be attacked.

During pregnancy a rhesus negative woman who has a rhesus positive fetus may become sensitized and develop anti-D antibodies. During a subsequent pregnancy with a rhesus positive fetus the anti-D antibodies can cross the placenta and cause haemolysis (breakdown) of the fetal erythrocytes. This is a serious condition and can lead to fetal death or the baby may suffer brain damage or die after birth. Women are tested for rhesus group during antenatal care. Anti-D is given to rhesus negative women to prevent the sensitization of the immune system. It is given by injection following events that may lead to sensitization such as bleeding during pregnancy, miscarriage, termination and labour.

Table 17.1 ABO blood group compatibility (reproduced with permission from Brooker & Nicol 2003)

Recipient	Donor			
	A	B	AB	O
A	Yes	No	No	Yes
B	No	Yes	No	Yes
AB	Yes	Yes	Yes	Yes
O	No	No	No	Yes

Respiratory system – outline of anatomy and physiology

The respiratory tract provides oxygen for cellular function and excretes waste carbon dioxide. This is achieved by breathing, where air moves in (inspiration) and out (expiration) of the lungs and by gas exchange in the lungs and at the cells.

Respiratory structures

The respiratory structures (Fig. 17.6) include:

- The nose, pharynx, larynx, trachea and bronchi, which warm, filter and humidify (moisten) air before it reaches the lungs
- The lungs containing smaller bronchi, bronchioles, alveolar ducts and alveoli where gas exchange occurs.

Nose

The first part of the nasal cavity is lined with skin containing hairs that trap large particles from the inspired air. The internal part of the nasal cavity is lined with respiratory mucosa comprising ciliated columnar epithelium containing many mucus-secreting goblet cells. The inspired air is humidified by the moist mucosa and warmed by plentiful blood vessels supplying the respiratory mucosa. The sticky mucus traps dust, bacteria and other foreign particles in the inspired air and the cilia then waft these particles towards the pharynx where they are swallowed and so do not enter the lungs.

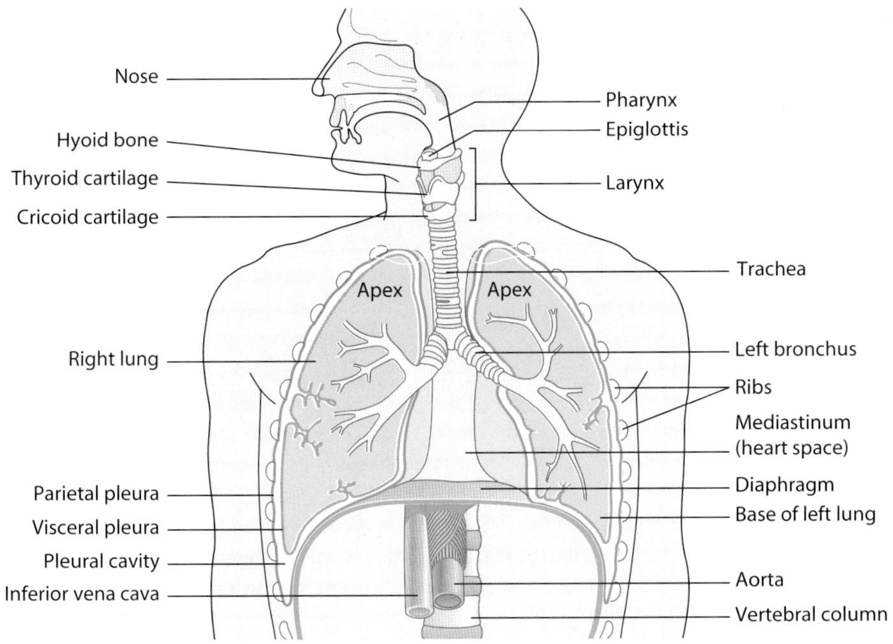

Fig. 17.6 The respiratory structures (reproduced with permission from Brooker and Nicol 2003)

Pharynx

The pharynx is a funnel-shaped passage with three parts: nasopharynx, oropharynx and laryngopharynx. The process of warming, humidifying and filtering inspired air normally continues in the nasopharynx, which is lined with respiratory mucosa (Box 17.2). The nasopharynx is exclusively respiratory, but the oropharynx and laryngopharynx provide a passage for food and fluids in addition to air. The oropharynx and laryngopharynx are lined with tougher stratified squamous epithelium, which is continuous with that of the oesophagus.

The pharynx also contains lymphoid tissue – the nasopharyngeal tonsils in the nasopharynx and the palatine tonsils in the oropharynx – which form part of the body's defences against invading microorganisms.

Larynx

The larynx (voice box) is formed from cartilage, ligaments and membranes. Inspired air moving through the larynx is warmed, humidified and filtered as it passes from the pharynx to the trachea. The vocal cords, which extend from the front to the back of the larynx, are concerned with sound production. Inspired air must pass through the opening between the vocal cords – the glottis – to enter the trachea.

During swallowing, various reflex mechanisms prevent food or fluids from entering the lower respiratory tract. These include:

- Upward movement of the larynx causes the epiglottis (a small flap-like structure attached to the top of the larynx) to close over the opening into the larynx
- Breathing does not normally occur during swallowing
- The soft palate closes off the nasopharynx.

In addition, if food or fluid does enter the larynx, the cough reflex is normally stimulated (see below and p. 484).

Box 17.2 Mouth breathing

Mouth breathing, as may occur in patients with nasal obstruction or dyspnoea (difficult breathing), bypasses the normal processes in the nose and nasopharynx that warm, humidify and filter air and leads to an exacerbation of the breathing problems. The respiratory mucosa will be damaged, the cilia cease to function effectively and mucus secretions become dry, crusty and difficult to expectorate (cough up).

Trachea

The trachea (windpipe) is a continuation of the larynx and is between 12 and 15cm in length in an adult. It divides (bifurcates) to become the right and left main bronchi, with one bronchus going to each lung. The trachea is formed from C-shaped rings of cartilage, which are incomplete at the back. This gives the trachea some flexibility while the cartilage ensures that the airway remains open. The trachea is also lined with respiratory mucosa and continues to warm, humidify and filter air, although warming and humidification is practically complete when air enters the trachea. The mucus continues to trap foreign particles and, in a synchronized process called the mucociliary escalator, the cilia move the mucus with particles upward to the larynx from where it is either expectorated by coughing or swallowed.

Irritation such as that caused by excess mucus or foreign material (food, fluid, etc.) in the larynx, trachea or bronchi stimulates the cough reflex in which a forced expiration expels the mucus and/or foreign material. For further coverage of the cough reflex and the first aid for choking, see pages 484–485.

Bronchi, bronchioles and alveoli

The processes of humidification and warming in the upper respiratory tract are complete, air is saturated with water and warmed to 37°C and most foreign particles have been removed before it enters the bronchi.

Once the right and left main bronchi enter the lungs they divide into smaller and smaller bronchi, bronchioles and finally the tiny alveolar ducts that lead into the alveoli. The larger bronchi are lined with respiratory mucosa and the walls are supported by rings of cartilage and so remain open throughout the respiratory cycle (inspiration and expiration). As the bronchi become smaller they lose the cartilage and the lining gradually changes to non-ciliated epithelium. Further changes occur as the walls become thinner until a single layer of simple epithelium remains in the alveolar ducts and alveoli. This structural adaptation facilitates gaseous exchange.

The alveoli are very small air sacs clustered together and surrounded by a network of pulmonary capillaries. Special cells in the walls of the alveoli secrete surfactant (phospholipid fluid) which ensures a moist membrane needed for gaseous exchange. Surfactant also reduces surface tension and prevents alveolar collapse between breaths. Surfactant starts to be secreted by about 22 weeks' gestation and there is a rapid increase around 35 weeks' gestation (MacGregor 2000). Hence in the preterm infant, surfactant production may be insufficient to maintain patency of the alveoli and lead to respiratory distress (see p. 483).

Oxygen diffuses from the alveolar air, across the very thin layer of cells, the respiratory and capillary membranes into capillary blood (Fig. 17.7). Carbon dioxide leaves the blood and diffuses across the two membranes into the alveoli. The carbon dioxide is excreted during expiration.

For efficient gaseous exchange to occur there must be both adequate ventilation of the lungs and good perfusion with blood. In other words, if the lungs expand and fill with air, this will only lead to effective breathing; there also needs to be good supply of blood to the alveoli for the exchange of oxygen and carbon dioxide.

Lungs

The two lungs are situated within the thoracic cavity, either side of the heart and are protected from injury by the ribs (see Fig. 17.1, p. 464). The right lung is divided into three lobes whereas the left lung is smaller and has only two lobes. Its smaller size is due to the position of the heart in the mediastinum.

A double serous membrane called the pleura lines the thoracic cavity (parietal layer) and covers the outside of each lung (visceral layer). The pleura secretes serous fluid that lubricates the lungs, thus enabling them to move easily as they inflate and deflate. The intact pleura also keeps the lungs inflated.

Breathing (ventilation)

Breathing is the mechanical process by which air moves in and out of the lungs. There are two processes: inspiration, which requires energy and is active, and expiration, which is passive. Expiration is followed by a short pause before the next inspiration. In a normal respiratory cycle (at rest), the amount of air inhaled and exhaled is normally around 500 mL in an adult. This is known as the tidal volume (TV).

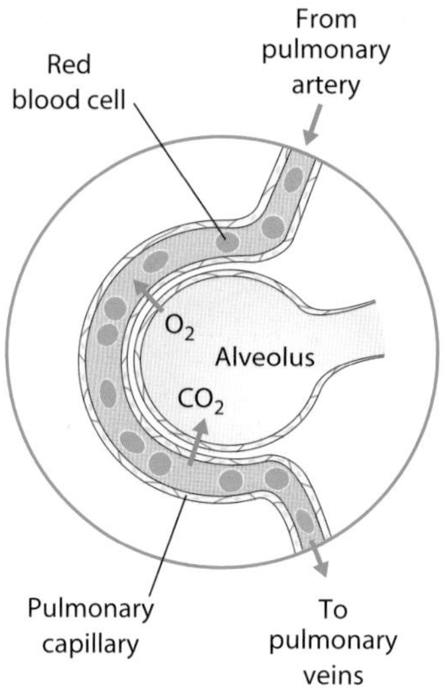

Fig. 17.7 Gas exchange between alveolus and pulmonary capillary (reproduced with permission from Brooker and Nicol 2003)

During inspiration the capacity of the thoracic cavity is increased as the diaphragm (muscle between the thorax and the abdomen) and intercostal muscles (between the ribs) contract. The lungs are stretched, the pressure within the lungs falls and air moves into the lungs in order to equalize the atmospheric and alveolar air pressures.

During expiration, the relaxation of the diaphragm and intercostal muscles leads to an inward and downward movement of the thoracic cage and elastic recoil of the lungs. The pressure in the lungs is greater than atmospheric air and air moves out.

Normal, unlaboured breathing depends on several factors. These include:

- *Compliance*: Healthy lungs distend during inspiration. This distensibility is referred to as lung compliance, which is the effort required to inflate the alveoli. Low compliance increases the effort needed to inflate the lungs and can be caused by lung diseases that reduce elasticity, or situations where surfactant is deficient (see above). Other causative factors include deformities of the thorax that prevent expansion
- *Elasticity*: The natural elasticity of the lungs allows a return to their normal shape following each breath. The loss of elasticity means that expiration must be forced and more effort is needed for inspiration
- *Airflow resistance*: Any narrowing of the airways (bronchoconstriction) such as that occurring in asthma increases the effort needed to inflate the lungs.

Common conditions affecting breathing and circulation

Disorders of the heart and blood vessels, blood and respiratory tract can lead to difficulties with breathing and to circulatory problems. Unfortunately, these are

Table 17.2 Common cardiovascular conditions

Angina pectoris	See Coronary heart disease below
Cardiac arrhythmia	Abnormal heart rhythm. Arrhythmias include: • Atrial fibrillation (AF) (see p. 480) • Supraventricular tachycardia (SVT) • Premature ventricular contraction (PVC) • Ventricular tachycardia (VT) (see p. 474) • Ventricular fibrillation (VF) (see p. 474)
Coronary heart disease (CHD)	Common condition caused by narrowing of the coronary arteries by atherosclerosis. This is atheroma (fatty plaques on the lining layer) accompanied by damage to the lining of the artery, hardening and eventually a partial obstruction to the flow of blood through the vessel Can manifest itself as angina or myocardial infarction and eventually leads to chronic heart failure Atherosclerosis may be caused by a diet high in saturated fats, hypertension and smoking and exacerbated by obesity and lack of physical exercise (see Boxes 17.5, p. 474; 17.7, p. 475)
1. Angina pectoris	Narrowing of the coronary arteries by atheroma is the usual cause of angina but can be due to coronary artery spasm Narrowing leads to a reduction in the blood supply to the myocardium and transient chest pain, which may radiate to the arms (especially the left), abdomen, jaw, neck and throat Pain is often induced by exertion, cold weather and wind, emotional stress and sometimes following a large meal Rest promptly relieves the pain (see Box 17.3, p. 472) Angina affects just under 2 million people in the UK (British Heart Foundation 2005)
2. Myocardial infarction (MI) – 'heart attack'	Occurs when blood flow in the coronary arteries is blocked by atheroma and oxygen does not reach all of the myocardium Usually caused by clot (thrombus) formation where an atheromatous plaque has ruptured – a coronary thrombosis The coronary artery is occluded and unless the artery is reopened, using thrombolytic drugs that dissolve clots or an invasive procedure such angioplasty, the myocardium supplied by that vessel will be damaged (infarcted) MI is a common cause of death in Western countries and, of the 300 000 that occur each year in the UK, about 30% will be fatal (British Heart Foundation 2005) (see Box 17.4, p. 474)
Congenital heart disease	Disorder that develops as the heart is formed and present at birth Common congenital abnormalities include septal defects (hole in the heart) and patent ductus arteriosus (a fetal blood vessel between the left pulmonary artery and the aorta to bypass the lungs) Some may be caused by genetic or chromosomal abnormalities such as septal defects in infants with Down's syndrome Usually treated surgically
Heart failure	The heart fails to pump effectively and is unable to deliver adequate oxygen and nutrients to the cells and tissues It may occur in one side or both right and left Heart failure is usually a chronic condition but it can occur acutely Chronic heart failure is commonly caused by CHD, cardiomyopathy (disease of the myocardium), valvular disease, arrhythmias, hypertension, chronic respiratory disease, etc. (see Box 17.5, p. 474)
Hypertension	Blood pressure that is persistently higher than 140/90 mmHg in adults In children there is no precise definition for hypertension; however, it is generally agreed to be a blood pressure greater than 130/85 mmHg on three consecutive readings In the vast majority of cases, no cause is found and it is termed 'essential hypertension' Secondary hypertension may result from a variety of conditions that include heart and blood vessel disease; kidney disease; endocrine diseases; drugs, e.g. corticosteroids, oral contraceptives, non-steroidal anti-inflammatory drugs (NSAIDs); pre-eclampsia associated with pregnancy (see Box 17.5, p. 474)
Myocardial infarction (MI) – 'heart attack'	See Coronary heart disease above
Rheumatic heart disease	Chronic inflammation and scarring of the myocardium and valve cusps Usually leads to valvular heart disease
Valvular heart disease	Usually affects the mitral or aortic valves but the tricuspid and pulmonary valves can be affected The valve may be either stenosed or regurgitant

common; for example, coronary heart disease (CHD), a disease that affects both breathing and circulation, accounted for 114 000 deaths in 2003 in the UK (British Heart Foundation 2005) and is a major cause of premature death. Disorders of the lungs are also common and appear to be on the increase. In 1999 lung diseases led to 153 000 deaths in the UK (British Thoracic Society 2001).

Diseases that affect breathing and circulation may be acute or chronic and affect all age groups. Some of the more common conditions are outlined in Tables 17.2–17.4.

Table 17.3 Common blood (haematological) conditions

Anaemia	Anaemia occurs when there is a reduced oxygen carrying capacity of the blood and the haemoglobin level falls below 9 g/dL There are several causes including: • Lack of iron and/or vitamin B_{12} or folate (see Box 17.1, p. 467) • Excessive blood loss – acute or chronic • Abnormal haemoglobin – see Haemoglobinopathies (below) • Excessive destruction of erythrocytes – haemolytic anaemia • Bone marrow suppression – aplastic anaemia
Deep vein thrombosis (DVT)	A DVT is a clot that forms in a vein, usually a large vein of the leg or pelvis, but it can occur in the arm Predisposing factors are venous stasis (slow bloodflow), increased blood stickiness and vein damage The risk factors for DVT therefore include prolonged immobility (see Ch. 18), increasing age (>40 years), poor peripheral blood flow, dehydration (see Ch. 19) or clotting disorders Identification of those at risk and prevention is vital (see Ch. 24) See Pulmonary embolus (below)
Haemoglobinopathies	
1. Sickle cell disease	An inherited condition which is due to abnormal haemoglobin, known as HbS Seen in individuals from areas where falciparum malaria is common (equatorial Africa, parts of India and parts of the Eastern Mediterranean) and their descendants in Europe, West Indies and the USA The erythrocytes become sickle-shaped under certain conditions, e.g. hypoxia (reduced oxygen level in the tissues) or dehydration, which leads to reduced oxygen carriage, vessel blockage with pain and infarction and chronic haemolytic anaemia as the abnormal erythrocytes are destroyed in the spleen At-risk populations should be screened for the abnormal HbS
2. Thalassaemia	A group of inherited haemoglobinopathies Thalassaemia can occur in people of all racial groups but is commonly found in people with Mediterranean ancestry The synthesis of globin chains, essential for haemoglobin production, is reduced because of a faulty gene, leading to fragile erythrocytes with impaired oxygen-carrying capacities, which are more rapidly destroyed by the spleen In thalassaemia major (two faulty genes inherited) there is severe anaemia, jaundice and enlarged liver and spleen Those with thalassaemia trait (one faulty gene inherited) may have mild anaemia or be asymptomatic
Leukaemia	A group of malignant diseases affecting the tissues that produce blood cells Leukaemia leads to an overproduction of immature leucocytes in the bone marrow that are released into the blood, suppressing normal production of erythrocytes and platelets, which leads to anaemia and risk of bleeding The lack of mature leucocytes increases the risk of infection There are several types of leukaemia affecting different leucocytes Leukaemia may be either acute or chronic.

FIRST AID — Box 17.3

Angina

Recognition

- Chest pain and pain or tingling in the jaw, throat, arms, back or upper central abdomen
- Pain eases with rest and lasts no more than 15 minutes
- Breathlessness.

Aims of treatment

- Encourage a resting position to reduce the workload of the heart
- Pain relief
- Reduce risk of worsening angina.

Treatment

- Encourage the casualty to sit down in a position that eases the pain and breathlessness
- Most people with known angina will have been prescribed sublingual (under the tongue) glyceryl nitrate (GTN), either as a tablet or an aerosol spray to use when they have anginal pain. The casualty should take this as soon as the angina attack starts
- Call for emergency help (dial 999) if the pain is not relieved after 15 minutes of using the GTN.

Table 17.4 Common respiratory conditions

Asthma	A chronic condition where inflammation causes spasm of the smooth muscle of the bronchi (bronchospasm), leading to bronchoconstriction and narrowing There is paroxysmal dyspnoea with wheezing and difficulty breathing out, a dry cough and tightness in the chest The emphasis is on self-management by patients or carers (see Box 17.6, p. 475) An attack of acute, severe asthma is a life-threatening medical emergency
Bronchiectasis	The bronchi and bronchioles are abnormally dilated and contain copious amounts of foul-smelling purulent (containing pus) sputum It may be localized or more generalized, when it may be associated with cystic fibrosis
Bronchiolitis	Inflammation of the bronchioles, usually caused by a viral infection Occurs mainly during winter months and usually affects infants under 12 months of age
Chronic bronchitis	Inflammation of the bronchi, defined as a cough with sputum for at least 3 consecutive months in 2 consecutive years There is an increase in mucus-secreting goblet cells and loss of cilia caused by tobacco smoke and air pollution A form of chronic obstructive pulmonary disease (see Box 17.7, p. 475).
Chronic obstructive pulmonary disease (COPD)	A group of progressive obstructive lung diseases where airway resistance is increased with reduced airflow, e.g. emphysema, chronic bronchitis or severe asthma (see Box 17.7, p. 475)
Croup	An acute viral infection that causes swelling and/or spasm leading to narrowing of the larynx in children The child will have harsh-sounding (stridulous) 'croupy' breathing Narrowing of the airway gives rise to the typical crowing inspiration
Cystic fibrosis (CF)	A genetic disorder affecting the exocrine glands A screening blood test is available for neonates High levels of sodium in sweat may confirm the diagnosis The affected glands produce viscous mucus, which leads to blocked bronchi or ducts, stasis of secretions, infection and fibrosis The lungs and pancreas are primarily affected, giving rise to repeated chest infections, respiratory problems, digestive problems and heart failure
Emphysema (pulmonary)	Overdistension of the alveoli leading to rupture and a reduction in gas exchange in the lungs Associated with tobacco smoking (see Box 17.7, p. 475) A form of chronic obstructive pulmonary disease (see Box 17.7, p. 475)
Lung cancer	A primary malignant tumour in the lung or bronchi Smoking is the most important factor in its development but exposure to tobacco smoke, asbestos and environmental pollution are also implicated (see Box 17.7, p. 475) Other cancers, e.g. breast, colorectal, often metastasize (spread) to the lung to form secondary cancers
Pneumonia	An acute infection of the lung It may be hospital- or community-acquired, or associated with impaired immune responses
Pulmonary embolism (PE)	A clot that forms in a vein breaks away and travels in the circulation and through the heart to lodge in a pulmonary blood vessel in the lungs (see Deep vein thrombosis, above) Leads to infarction of lung tissue in areas deprived of blood
Tuberculosis (TB)	A notifiable infectious disease caused by the bacterium *Mycobacterium tuberculosis* The BCG (bacillus Calmette–Guérin) vaccine is used to protect those at high risk of contracting TB, e.g. infants born in high-risk areas with 40 cases of TB per 100 000 population or higher

Readers requiring more information should consult the Further reading suggestions (e.g. Brooker & Nicol 2003, Chs 18–20).

Basic life support – airway maintenance and cardiopulmonary resuscitation

Basic life support (BLS) comprises the first aid measures for maintenance of a clear airway, artificial respiration (e.g. rescue breaths) and chest compressions (external heart massage) in people who have suffered a cardiac arrest (also known as cardiopulmonary arrest), or artificial respiration alone if only breathing has stopped. BLS aims to provide an intake of oxygen and maintain the circulation of blood. Cardiac arrest is defined as the sudden cessation of effective output of blood from the heart. The failure of output from the heart means that the circulation is not maintained. There are several forms of cardiac arrest, including:

- *Asystole*: There are no P-QRS-T complexes (see p. 466), the heart is not beating
- *Pulseless electrical activity (PEA)*: An electrical rhythm compatible with a cardiac output, but has the clinical signs of a cardiac arrest

FIRST AID Box 17.4

Myocardial infarction

Recognition

- Sudden crushing chest pain that is not relieved by rest and lasts longer than 30 minutes. Frequently the pain comes on when the casualty is resting and this may distinguish it from stable angina. Severe chest pain may wake them from sleep. The pain is usually central, but may radiate to the lower jaw and the left arm. Pain may also be felt in the right arm, throat, back or upper central abdomen
- Sudden light-headedness, dizziness, giddiness
- Nausea and vomiting
- Grey, ashen skin; cyanosis (blue tinge) of lips and extremities
- Sweating
- Cool extremities
- Anxiety, feeling of impending doom
- Breathlessness – copious frothy secretions that may be white or pink stained if pulmonary oedema occurs (see p. 485)
- Pulse may be rapid, irregular or weak
- Confusion – as insufficient oxygen is supplied to their brain
- Signs of shock, e.g. pallor, light-headed, extremities cool and moist.

May progress to unconsciousness, or the casualty may stop breathing and the heart stop beating (see 'Basic life support', pp. 474–477).

Aims of treatment

- Reduce the workload of the heart
- Obtain medical help as soon as possible.

Treatment

- If the casualty is conscious, put in a half-sitting position with knees bent and with head and shoulders supported. Try to allay anxiety
- If the casualty has a history of heart disease and has medication let them take it
- Summon an emergency ambulance by dialling 999
- An aspirin tablet should chewed but only after checking for allergies or history of bleeding
- Continue to monitor condition. If the casualty becomes unconscious, open their airway and check breathing and place in the recovery position. Be prepared to give basic life support if breathing stops or the heart stops.

Note: Patients should be encouraged to seek help at the earliest possible opportunity. It is important that the public are aware of the symptoms of a myocardial infarction and understand that seeking medical help is vital.

- *Pulseless ventricular tachycardia (VT)*: An arrhythmia with rapid ventricular heart rate but insufficient output to produce a pulse
- *Ventricular fibrillation (VF)*: An arrhythmia with uncoordinated ventricular activity that produces no output of blood.

HEALTH PROMOTION Box 17.5

Salt intake

A diet containing high levels of salt (sodium chloride) is associated with an increase in blood pressure. High blood pressure (hypertension) is a risk factor for coronary heart disease (CHD) and for strokes.

The salt content of unprocessed foods is comparatively low, but added salt is present in many prepared or processed foods, e.g. home cooked meals, cheese, snack foods, ready meals, breakfast cereals, etc. Food products with more than 1.25 g salt/100 g (0.5 g sodium/100 g) are considered high in salt (Mayor 2004).

Adults should be encouraged to keep their salt intake within the recommended daily intake. Parents and carers should be aware that the recommended intake for infants and children is much lower than in adults and depends on age. An even lower salt intake may be advised for people who are hypertensive and for those with chronic heart failure. This is because excess salt intake leads to water retention, which increases the blood pressure and leads to the formation of oedema (swelling due to fluid collecting in the tissues, see p. 479).

Student activities

Use the Food Standards Agency website to answer the following questions:

- What is the recommended salt intake per day for infants, children and adults?
- Find out how to calculate the salt content of a food from the amount of sodium.
- What are the advantages of reducing salt intake?

[Reference: Mayor S 2004 Pass the salt: cutting down on salt to reduce blood pressure. British Journal of Primary Care Nursing 1(4):160–162; Resource: Food Standards Agency – www.salt.gov.uk Available July 2006]

The causes of cardiac arrest include CHD, other heart diseases, hypovolaemia, e.g. severe haemorrhage, electric shock, electrolyte imbalances (see Ch. 19) and severe respiratory problems.

The BLS procedures for cardiopulmonary resuscitation (CPR) outlined below are put in place until the emergency services or hospital cardiac arrest team can start advanced life support (see also Ch. 16). The BLS techniques are different for adults, children and infants. BLS is described using adult procedures and the differences in technique for children and infants are provided in Box 17.8 (p. 478).

Adult basic life support

An adult is defined as a person who has reached puberty for the purpose of providing BLS. If the casualty is outside hospital an emergency ambulance must be summoned by dialling 999 (see below). If the cardiopulmonary arrest has occurred in hospital the nurse should know the internal 'crash call' telephone number for summoning the cardiac

HEALTH PROMOTION Box 17.6

Self-management in asthma

All people with asthma should have a written self-management plan outlining the daily actions they should take to monitor their condition and identify any deterioration. It should suggest alterations to daily management when their condition deteriorates and indicate when professional help is needed.

A personal asthma action plan is available from Asthma UK, which, if used, should be completed by the patient and their doctor or practice nurse.

Any management plan should include the following:

- Record peak expiratory flow rate (PEFR) every morning before medication (see p. 486). If the reading has decreased by 70% of normal then recordings should be taken twice daily. By careful and regular monitoring, it should be possible to recognize when the condition is deteriorating or failing to improve and medical assistance should be sought
- Monitor PEFR recordings twice daily if it deteriorates or there are increased symptoms such as increased wheeze, breathlessness, cough, chest tightness or difficulty sleeping at night
- Use inhalers and other medication as prescribed and use the correct inhaler technique (see p. 491) – the practice nurse should check this on each visit
- Avoid known allergies that trigger an asthma attack, e.g. pets, dust, pollen, etc.
- Smoking cessation
- Avoid contact with people with viral chest infections, as these may trigger an asthma attack.

Student activities

- Access the personal asthma action plan and consider how it helps patients to manage their condition.
- Discuss with your mentor how some degree of self-management of chronic conditions by patients can influence their feelings of control and improve outcomes and hence quality of life. However, total self-management will not be an option for all patients, e.g. those with a learning disability or dementia.

[Resource: Asthma UK Personal asthma action plan – www.asthma.org.uk/all_about_asthma/publications/be_in_control.html Available July 2006]

HEALTH PROMOTION Box 17.7

Smoking cessation

Smoking is a major cause of death and disability. It causes:

- COPD
- Cancer of the lung and other sites such as the mouth, throat and oesophagus
- CHD.

Tobacco was responsible for 6.3 million deaths in the UK between 1950 and 2000 (Cancer Research UK 2005). Smoking is the single most preventable cause of premature death. Helping people to stop smoking and acting to prevent people starting to smoke is a vital role for all nurses.

Student activities

- Access the websites below and consider the smoking cessation advice and help they offer to the public and professionals.
- Find out what smoking cessation facilities are available locally.

[Reference: Cancer Research UK – www.cancerresearch.org.uk
Resources: Action on Smoking and Health (ASH) – www.ash.org.uk; British Heart Foundation – www.bhf.org.uk/smoking; NHS – www.givingupsmoking.co.uk All available July 2006]

arrest team. The National Patient Safety Agency (NPSA) (2004) advised all NHS Trusts in England and Wales to standardize the internal crash call telephone number to 2222. At the time of writing the vast majority of acute Trusts now use 2222 but until all Trusts have converted, individual hospitals may have a different number and all staff should be aware of it.

When initially faced with an adult whom you suspect has experienced a cardiopulmonary arrest, the following procedure should be started immediately:

- Assess for danger. Prior to assessing the casualty or commencing resuscitation it is important to ensure that this would not put you in any danger.
- Assess the casualty's level of consciousness. If they respond to gentle shaking or loud speaking ('Open your eyes', 'Can you hear me') do not move them unless in danger. Check for injuries and get help if necessary. Continue to check condition.
- If they do not respond shout for help and start BLS.
- Open the airway using the head tilt/chin lift method (Fig. 17.8A, p. 476). Place a hand on the forehead and gently tilt the head backwards. Place the fingertips under the casualty's chin and lift the chin. This is used in the adult to bring the tongue forward to prevent it from obstructing the airway. Using this method in an adult requires the neck to be hyperextended and so should not be used when

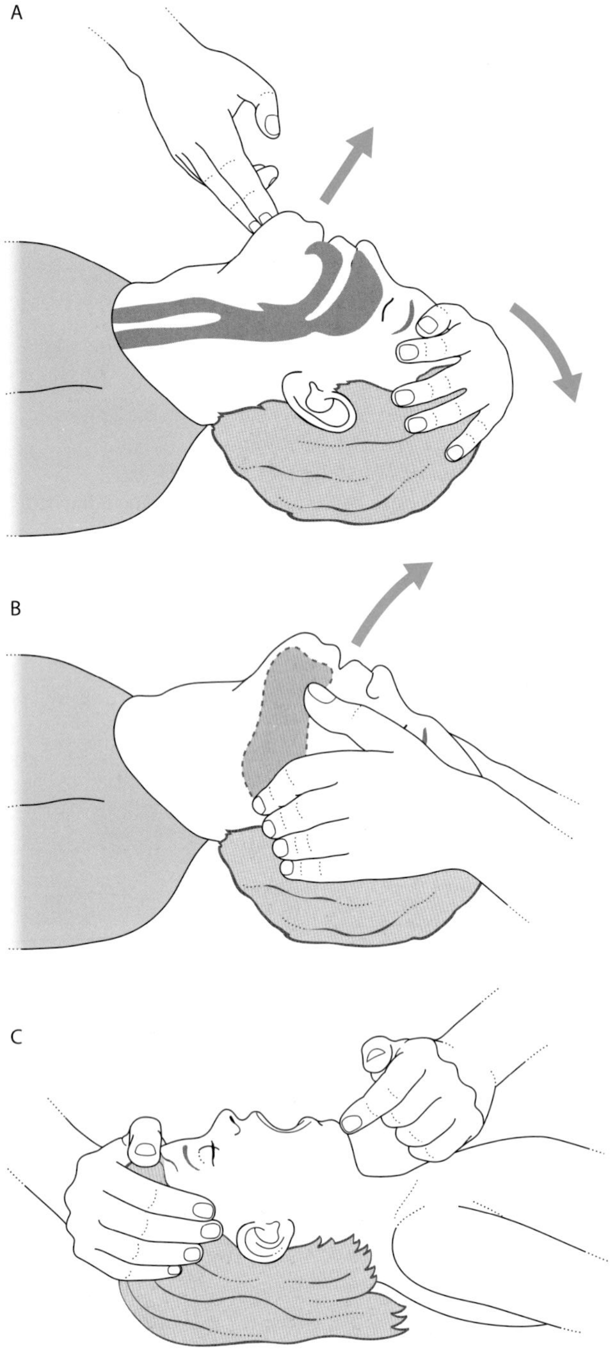

Fig. 17.8 Opening the airway: **A.** Head tilt/chin lift – adult. **B.** Jaw thrust – adult. **C.** Head tilt/chin lift – child (reproduced from Mallik et al 1998 and Huband & Trigg 2000)

a head or neck injury is suspected. If head or neck injury is suspected in an adult, the jaw thrust method is used. For this manoeuvre, the index and middle fingers are placed under the angle of the lower jaw and steady gentle pressure used to move the jaw upwards and forwards (Fig. 17.8B). The mouth should then open slightly.

- The patient should only be moved if it is not possible to open the airway using this action. In this case turn them gently onto their back.
- Remove any visible obstruction or foreign body from the airway. Open the mouth and look into the airway. Only remove obstructions if they are clearly visible and easy to remove. Do not remove well-fitting dentures.
- Check for normal breathing using the 'look, listen and feel' steps. Spend no more than 10 seconds on these steps.
  - look at the chest wall and observe any movement
  - place your ear close to the person's mouth and listen for breath sounds
  - place your cheek close to the person's mouth to feel any movement of air.
- If there is any indication that the person is breathing, turn them into the recovery position (see Fig. 16.17A) and monitor until help arrives.
- If there is no sign of breathing and you are alone – dial 999 immediately. Now start chest compressions (external cardiac massage) immediately. The heel of your hand should be placed in the centre of the chest. The other hand should be placed on top of the first and the fingers interlocked. Firm pressure is then applied with the heels of the hands (Fig. 17.9A). The elbows should be kept straight so that the pressure is exerted downwards. The pressure should be sufficient to depress the sternum by 5–4 cm in an adult to create an effective cardiac output as the heart is compressed between the sternum and the spine and this squeezes blood into the circulation. Pressure any greater than this, however, may cause rib fractures.

  Thirty chest compressions are performed at a rate of approximately 100 per minute followed by two rescue breaths.
- Give the casualty two effective rescue breaths. With the airway open, pinch the soft tissue of the nose with the index finger and thumb and open the casualty's mouth a little. Take a deep breath and place your lips around the casualty's mouth and blow steadily into the mouth over 1 second (Fig. 17.10A). While doing this, you should watch to see whether the chest wall rises. Then take your mouth away from the casualty's mouth and watch the chest wall fall as the air comes out. If you don't see the chest wall rise, check the airway is open and give another breath. Do not attempt more than two breaths before going back to chest compressions.

  Note: In hospital this may be achieved by inserting a plastic airway and using an Ambu bag connected to an oxygen supply to deliver these breaths while waiting for the cardiac arrest team to arrive.
- A lone first aider does 30 chest compressions before two rescue breaths but if two first aiders are present, the 30:2 ratio is used, with one person undertaking chest compression while the other does rescue breaths and maintains the airway. If more than one rescuer is present, another should take over CPR every 2 minutes to avoid fatigue.

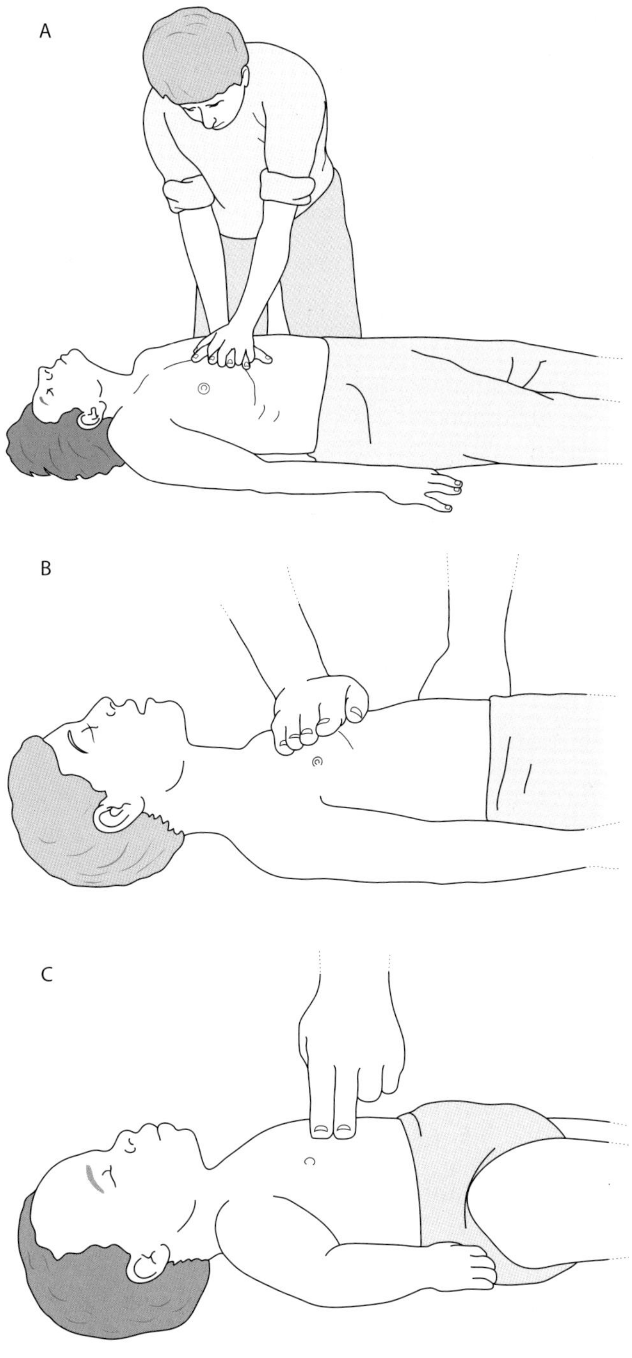

Fig. 17.9 Chest compression: **A.** Adult. **B.** Child. **C.** Infant

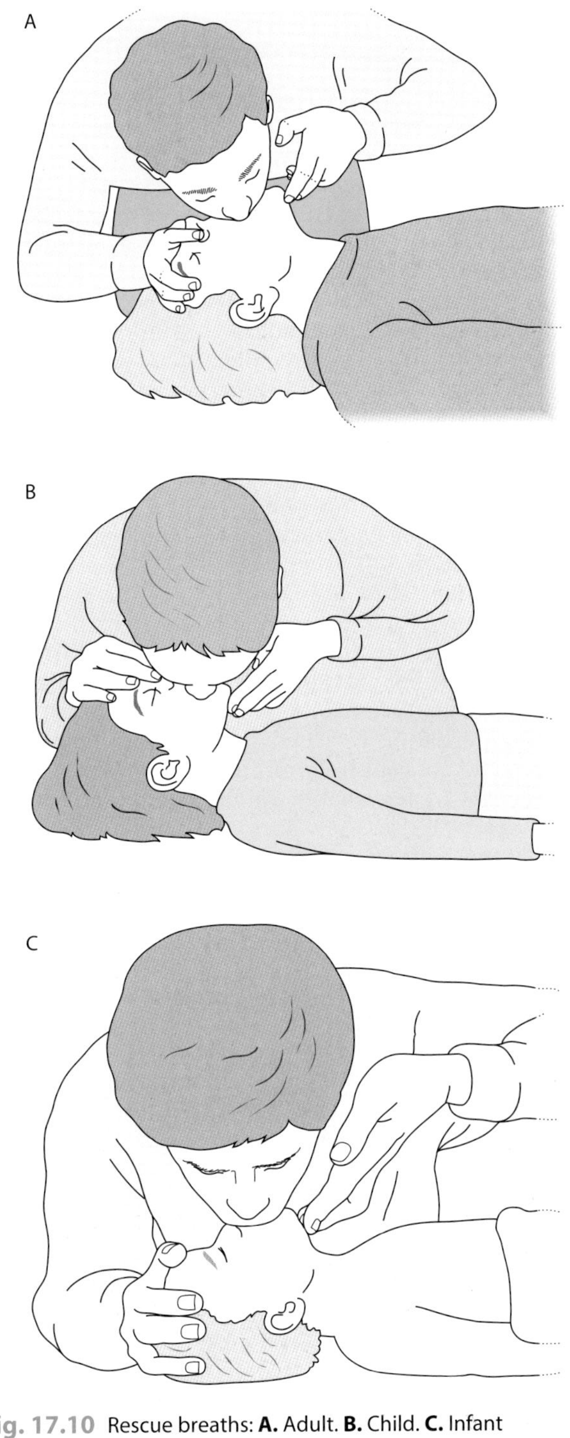

Fig. 17.10 Rescue breaths: **A.** Adult. **B.** Child. **C.** Infant

- Continue CPR until help arrives or the person starts breathing normally

(Resuscitation Council (UK) 2005).

Basic life support for infants and children

A child is defined as a person aged 1 year and up to the age of puberty and an infant as being less than 12 months old for the provision of BLS. The differences between BLS for children and infants and that for adults (see above) are outlined in Box 17.8 (p. 478).

Assessment and observation – circulation and breathing

Assessment and observation form the basis for nursing management and treatment and are therefore key skills to learn. However, observations do not have to be complex, nor require sophisticated equipment. Some of the best skills for assessment and observation are those that involve looking, listening, touching and smelling.

Box 17.8 BLS – differences in techniques for children and infants

- *Assessment of consciousness*: Gently shake the baby or child, speak loudly or call their name if known. They may respond by moving, swallowing, coughing, crying or a verbal response in older children, or breathing (regular breaths more than occasional) may be obvious. If they respond, do not move unless in danger. Check for injuries and get help if necessary. Continue to check condition
- *Opening the airway*: In children and infants the head tilt/chin lift is used but without over-extension because this can cause the airway to close (see Fig. 17.8C, p. 476). Jaw thrust is used if head/neck injury is suspected but this time only the index finger on the lower jaw is used
- *Look in the mouth* and remove any obvious obstruction
- *Check the breathing* as above. If they are breathing, turn them on their side and obtain help. If the child is not breathing, give five rescue breaths. Pinch the nose and place your lips around the child's mouth and blow gently into the lungs (see Fig. 17.10B, p. 477). Only take shallow breaths and do not use all the air in your lungs. While doing this, you should watch to see whether the chest wall rises. As it does so, cease blowing and let the chest fall.

  In infants place your mouth over the infant's mouth and nose and blow gently to give the two rescue breaths (see Fig. 17.10C, p. 477). The amount of air used is that amount that fills your cheeks
- *Check the circulation* by looking for movement, swallowing, etc. If you have been trained, feel for the carotid pulse in children or the brachial pulse (on the inner aspect of the elbow) in infants. If the circulation is present, continue rescue breaths for 1 minute before dialling 999 for an emergency ambulance
- *If circulation is absent* or the pulse is less than 60bpm, chest compressions (external cardiac massage) should be started immediately.

  For children the heel of one hand is placed one fingerbreadth above the junction of the rib margin and sternum (see Fig. 17.9B, p. 477). Pressure is then applied with the heel of the hand with the elbows kept straight. The pressure should be sufficient to depress the chest by about one-third of its depth. Fifteen chest compressions are performed at a rate of approximately 100 per minute followed by two rescue breaths.

  For infants two fingers are used (see Fig. 17.9C, p. 477) or alternatively, the first aider may put their hands around the infant's chest and place one thumb above the other, one fingerbreadth below the internipple line in the centre of the sternum. Again the chest is compressed to around one-third of its depth
- *When CPR is necessary* the 15:2 ratio is continued. CPR continues until help arrives.

[Resources: Resuscitation Council (UK) (2005); St John Ambulance – www.sja.org.uk/firstaid/info]

This section will look at important areas for the assessment of breathing and circulation and include assessment of the skin, the heart rate, blood pressure and respiration.

Although assessment is useful, it only becomes a valuable tool if nurses know what to do with the findings. All data should be recorded in the patient's notes and/or on observation charts (see Ch. 14). Where nurses suspect that the data are abnormal, then the person in charge should be notified as soon as possible.

Skin – general assessment

Assessment of the skin is quick and easy yet provides useful information about both breathing and circulation. Nurses should take every opportunity to assess a person's skin, e.g. while helping them with personal hygiene. More information about skin condition and assessment is provided in Chapters 16 and 25.

In health the skin should be warm, dry, intact and normal colour for racial group. However, with normal ageing the skin becomes drier and loses its natural elasticity. In people with either very pale or dark skin it may be difficult to notice abnormalities such as pallor or a bluish hue (cyanosis). This explains why it is important to also look at the mucosae, e.g. inside the mouth or the conjunctiva inside the lower eyelid, which in health should be pink and moist.

Changes in skin colour

The colour of the skin including the nail beds and the lips and the mucosae can provide valuable information:

- Cyanosis is a bluish hue to skin and mucosae. It is due to hypoxia (reduced oxygen level in the tissues). It may be central cyanosis where the bluish hue affects the lips, the oral mucosa, tongue and conjunctivae, whereas cyanosis affecting the extremities – fingertips, toes, ear lobes or nose – is referred to as peripheral cyanosis
- Extremities that are red in colour are also likely to be warmer to touch. This is more commonly found after exercise or when the patient has a high temperature (pyrexia) and the blood vessels in the skin are dilated (vasodilatation) (see Ch. 14)
- Skin may be very white (blanched) when the blood supply has become so severely reduced that the tissues do not have an oxygen supply. If left untreated the skin will become blackened in colour and gangrene is likely to ensue (see Ch. 25)

- Very pale skin may be associated with anaemia. The lips, oral mucosa and conjunctivae will also be pale because of anaemia (see Table 17.3, p. 472).

Skin turgor and oedema

Assessment of the skin should include turgor and the presence of oedema. Turgor indicates the elasticity of the skin and although this decreases with age, skin turgor may be useful in a holistic assessment of hydration status. Reduced turgor may be an early sign of dehydration (see Ch. 19).

To assess skin turgor, a fold of skin, usually on the back of the hand, is lifted. Once released, it should quickly return to its original position. However, because skin loses its elasticity with age it will not return to its original position so quickly in older people.

Oedema is an abnormal accumulation of tissue fluid between the cells (see Ch. 19). It usually collects in dependent regions such as the legs, ankles/feet or sacral area. For example, if someone spends much of the day sitting in a chair, fluid will collect in the sacral area and ankles. This is partly due to immobility and lack of normal contraction of the calf muscles. Normally muscle contraction squeezes the veins and helps to maintain the return of venous blood to the heart (see Ch. 25). However, dependent oedema is also compounded by gravity, which allows fluid to collect in these areas. Oedema may be seen in people with the following conditions:

- Heart failure
- Venous insufficiency (see Ch. 25)
- Protein deficiency
- Kidney disease
- Liver failure.

However, swollen ankles with some oedema may be found when standing still in hot weather or during pregnancy and are not necessarily a sign of ill health.

The term 'pitting' is used to describe oedema that remains indented or pitted when lightly pressed. This is frequently a sign of more severe oedema.

Oedema is not usually visible until the body has retained at least 4 L of fluid, which is equivalent to approximately 4 kg of weight gain. An accurate way to record fluid balance is through daily weighing and people with heart failure who are prone to fluid retention, for example, are frequently asked to record their weight daily.

Capillary refill time

Capillary refill time is useful for assessing skin perfusion (amount of blood passing through the skin) and cardiac output. Although peripheral areas such as the nail bed may be used, central areas such as the sternum are more useful in people with a poor cardiac output and poor peripheral circulation. To test capillary refill time, two fingers are lightly pressed into the area for a period of 5 seconds. On release, the skin colour should return to normal within 2 seconds. If it takes longer for the skin colour to return, capillary refill time is prolonged and it is likely that the person has a low cardiac output.

Box 17.9 Causes of tachycardia and bradycardia

Tachycardia

A heart rate greater than 100 bpm in an adolescent or adult may normally occur in the following situations:

- During and after exercise
- Anxiety and fear
- Excitement
- Pregnancy
- Excessive alcohol intake
- Pain (see Ch. 23)
- Infection (see Ch. 15)
- Pyrexia (see Ch. 14).

Disorders of breathing and circulation that cause tachycardia include:

- Anaemia
- Hypovolaemia (low blood volume), e.g. following serious haemorrhage
- Breathing problems, e.g. during an asthma attack
- Heart diseases, e.g. heart failure.

Bradycardia

A heart rate of less than 60 bpm in an adolescent or adult may occur in the following situations:

- In a fit and athletic person
- During sleep.

Disorders affecting breathing and circulation that cause bradycardia include:

- Hypothermia
- Heart disease, e.g. after a heart attack (myocardial infarction)
- Some drugs used to treat heart disease, e.g. digoxin or atenolol (a beta-blocker).

Heart/pulse rate

When blood is pumped from the heart there is rhythmic expansion and recoil of the arteries in the vascular system. Wherever an artery is near the skin surface this ejection of blood will cause a pulse, which can be felt when the artery is gently pressed against a bony prominence. In adults and older children this is commonly felt at the wrist where the radial artery crosses the forearm bone, the radius (see Ch. 14). In babies aged less than 6 months HR is determined by using a stethoscope to count the apex beat of the heart (see Ch. 14).

The pulse rate should be easily palpated and is a useful measure of the function of the cardiovascular system. The pulse should reflect the HR and varies with age. It is normally between 60 and 80 bpm in adolescents and adults at rest, although up to 100 bpm is considered normal. In the neonate the HR is faster and is usually between 120 and 160 bpm depending on whether the baby is active, crying, resting or asleep. The HR slows during infancy and childhood to reach adult levels during adolescence (see Ch. 14).

Box 17.9 outlines some situations and disorders in which HR is faster or slower than normal.

A weak and thready pulse is frequently faster than normal and is found in dehydration (see Ch. 19), hypovolaemia or heart failure. A pulse that feels strong and bounding is also frequently fast and may indicate pyrexia, anxiety or hypervolaemia (high blood volume).

When a pulse is noted to be irregular, it should be reported and documented in the nursing notes and on the appropriate charts. Many heart diseases, such as atrial fibrillation (AF), cause an irregular pulse rate and commonly occur in older people. Further investigations should be undertaken an apex–radial pulse should be recorded and an ECG performed.

Apex and radial

Sometimes the radial pulse rate is not the same as the HR (pulse deficit). This can happen if the heart rhythm is abnormal. A disturbance in heart rhythm is called an arrhythmia, e.g. AF where the atria beat very rapidly but only some of the beats lead to a pulse. In these situations the pulse is likely to be irregular and a simultaneous recording of the apex beat and the radial pulse rate is useful (Box 17.10).

Peripheral pulses

Pulses are found wherever a blood vessel lies close to the skin surface. The radial pulse has been described above (see p. 479). Other peripheral pulses (see Fig. 14.10, p. 378) are assessed in a variety of specific situations. Peripheral pulses indicate the flow of blood to the peripheries and how well the heart is functioning. Additionally, they provide information on the state of the individual blood vessels, e.g. checking for the presence of the pedal pulse (dorsalis pedis) in the foot when a person has a suspected blockage in the arteries supplying the leg, or following surgery to clear a blockage (see Ch. 14 for further information).

The electrocardiogram

The ECG waveform depicts the electrical activity of the heart (see p. 466 and Fig. 17.4). It is used to detect arrhythmias and heart diseases such as myocardial infarction. Readers requiring more information about ECG should consult Further reading suggestions.

Blood pressure

Blood pressure (BP) is the pressure exerted upon the wall of the arteries by the circulating blood. It is a useful, non-invasive measurement, widely used in patient assessment (see Ch. 14). BP is usually measured indirectly using a sphygmomanometer (usually aneroid) or an electronic device. Mercury sphygmomanometers are being replaced as a safety measure because of the toxicity of mercury. BP is a routine aspect of health assessment in adults and at prescribed intervals for monitoring condition, e.g. after surgery or for hypertension. BP is less frequently recorded as part of assessment in children; however, in some cases BP can indicate the presence of congenital heart disease or kidney disease.

NURSING SKILLS Box 17.10

Recording apex–radial pulse (adult)

Note: To record an apex–radial pulse, two members of staff are needed.

Equipment
- Stethoscope
- Watch with second hand
- Observation chart.

Preparation
- Explain the observation and seek verbal consent; maintain respect and dignity at all times
- Ensure that the patient is either sitting or lying and allow time for rest following exertion or a situation that could affect heart rate, such as bad news.

Procedure
- Draw the curtains around the bed space to ensure the patient's privacy and dignity
- One nurse places the diaphragm of a stethoscope over the apex of the heart, at the 5th intercostal space and approximately 12 cm to the left of the midline (see Fig. 17.1, p. 464); the other nurse locates the radial pulse
- Using the same watch and commencing at the same time the nurses count the heartbeat for 1 minute
- Help the patient with clothing and replace bedding before opening the curtains
- Clean stethoscope earpieces according to local policy
- Wash hands
- The apex beat and radial pulse recordings are charted in different colours (see local policy)
- Any abnormalities are reported and documented.

If there is a large difference between the two values, it can be concluded that the radial pulse rate does not accurately reflect the heart rate, i.e. there is a pulse deficit. A heart arrhythmia should be suspected and an ECG performed if this is a new sign (Riley 2003).

BP has two measurements and is measured in millimetres of mercury pressure (mmHg). The two measurements reflect different stages of the cardiac cycle (see p. 465): the upper reading, the systolic pressure, when the heart contracts (systole) and the lower reading, the diastolic pressure, when the heart is relaxed (diastole). As the heart contracts, blood is pumped from the left ventricle into the aorta and systemic arteries and this is recorded as the systolic BP. Following ventricular ejection, blood moves along the arteries, and the elastic vessel walls start to recoil. This is then recorded as the diastolic BP (see Ch. 14 for details of measuring BP).

The normal BP range varies with age: in adults the optimum BP is <120 systolic and <80 diastolic, and a normal BP is described as <130/<85 mmHg (Williams et al 2004). In the neonate, BP is normally between 60 and 85 systolic/20 and 60 diastolic mmHg (see Ch. 14).

HEALTH PROMOTION Box 17.11

Lifestyle and hypertension

Several lifestyle factors contribute to hypertension (Williams et al 2004). These include:

- Increase in body weight leading to obesity (see Ch. 19)
- Sedentary lifestyle
- Excessive alcohol intake
- Increased salt (sodium chloride) intake (see Box 17.5, p. 474)
- Environmental stress (see Ch. 11).

Student activities

- Access the NICE information for people with hypertension and consider the guidance regarding lifestyle factors.
- Discuss with your mentor how information about lifestyle changes can help people with hypertension to reduce their blood pressure and the associated risks.

[Resource: National Institute for Health and Clinical Excellence 2004 Hypertension (persistently high blood pressure) in adults. Understanding NICE guidance – a guide for people with hypertension, their families and carers, and the public. Online: www.nice.org.uk/pdf/CG018publicinfo.pdf Available July 2006]

In addition, there are many factors that normally influence BP throughout a 24-hour period (see Ch. 14). These include:

- Posture
- Activity and exercise
- Emotional state such as fear, anxiety
- Presence of pain (see Ch. 23).

A sustained increase in BP is termed hypertension and in adults this is defined as a BP over 140/90 mmHg. For example, Grade 1 (mild) hypertension is systolic pressure between 140 and 159 mmHg and diastolic pressure between 90 and 99 mmHg (Williams et al 2004). BP tends to increase with age in developed countries. Lifestyle factors contributing to hypertension are outlined in Box 17.11.

Hypertension is a serious condition and leads to many problems, e.g. CHD, heart failure, strokes, kidney damage and retinal changes. The BP is recorded on three separate occasions before treatment is commenced for hypertension. This is because there are several factors that may lead to inaccuracies in blood pressure readings in addition to 'white coat' hypertension where the anticipation of having BP recorded causes it to increase. Box 17.12 outlines some interventions to ensure the accuracy of BP measurement and recording.

A low blood pressure that is insufficient to maintain tissue blood flow and oxygenation is termed hypotension. It may be caused by:

- Dehydration
- Hot weather when the arteries dilate (vasodilatation) and dehydration may also be present
- Heart failure

REFLECTIVE PRACTICE Box 17.12

Maximizing the accuracy of blood pressure measurement*

Measures that help to ensure accuracy include the following:

- Ensure the BP device/sphygmomanometer is 'properly validated, maintained and regularly recalibrated according to manufacturer's instructions' (NICE 2004, p. 7)
- Give an explanation about measuring BP to the patient/parent/carer
- Home monitoring may reduce 'white coat' effects. However, NICE do not currently recommend it, as its value has not been established (NICE 2004)
- Provide a relaxed environment
- Do not record BP if the person has been active – allow them to rest first
- Ensure a comfortable temperature – neither too hot nor too cold
- Remove tight clothes that might constrict the blood flow in the brachial artery in the arm
- Position the patient either sitting or lying down, with their arm straight and supported so that the muscles are relaxed
- Use a cuff of the correct size (see Ch. 14)
- Position the device at the correct level
- Record BP in both arms and use the arm with the higher reading on future occasions
- Make a note of the systolic and diastolic readings and record them on the chart and in the nursing notes
- Inform the nurse in charge if the blood pressure has altered by more than 10 mmHg from a previous recording or from the normal BP range for age
- The registered nurse will tell the patient/parent the BP reading, explain any implications and answer their questions.

Student activities

- Think about a recent placement where blood pressure was routinely measured. Which of the measures listed above did you see being used?
- Discuss with your mentor how you might increase the accuracy of blood pressure measurement.

* See also Ch. 14.

[Reference: National Institute for Health and Clinical Excellence 2004 Hypertension (persistently high blood pressure) in adults. Understanding NICE guidance – a guide for people with hypertension, their families and carers, and the public. Online: www.nice.org.uk/pdf/CG018publicinfo.pdf Available July 2006]

- Drugs such as beta-blockers
- Hypovolaemia such as after serious haemorrhage, e.g. from a wound, stomach/duodenal ulcer (peptic ulcer), etc. However, not all bleeding results in hypotension and most people will have to deal with minor bleeding from cuts and grazes. Box 17.13 (p. 482) provides an opportunity to think about the information people need to be able to deal with minor bleeding at home.

HEALTH PROMOTION Box 17.13

Dealing with minor bleeding and cuts and grazes

You and the community nurse are visiting Rodney who lives in sheltered accommodation when the carer mentions that he cut himself the other week. The cut was only small but it bled for a few minutes and no one was sure what they should do. The community nurse asks you to gather some information about dealing with minor cuts and grazes ready for your next visit to the client.

Student activities

- Access the St John Ambulance website and read the advice. You will also find it useful to read the advice about more severe bleeding and shock.
- Consider the information needed by Rodney's carer and think about how you will convey the safety aspects.

[Resources: Mohun et al (2002); St John Ambulance, First aid advice online – www.sja.org.uk/firstaid/info/bleeding.asp Available July 2006]

Hypotension may lead to feelings of dizziness or even fainting (syncope) because insufficient blood and hence oxygen reaches the brain. Fainting can also be caused by other factors. These include:

- Hot weather or a sudden change in environmental temperature
- Sudden change in body position such as standing or getting out of bed too quickly
- Standing still for a prolonged period, causing the blood to pool in the legs
- Emotional upset such as the sight of blood.

The first aid for fainting is outlined in Box 17.14.

FIRST AID Box 17.14

Fainting

Recognition

- Pallor
- Weak pulse
- Light headedness
- Stumble or fall suddenly to the ground.

Aims of treatment

- Restore blood flow to the brain by positioning the person so that gravity assists blood flow
- Deal with the cause.

Treatment

- Check and maintain an open airway (see pp. 475–476, 478) if the person has already fainted
- A person who feels faint should be sat on a chair, leaning forward with their head between their knees, or lie the person down
- Loosen tight clothing at the neck and chest
- Try to ensure fresh air
- Elevate the legs
- Reassure as consciousness returns
- Gradually allow the person to sit up
- Check for injuries if the person fell
- Do not give anything orally until the person is fully recovered, then offer cold non-alcoholic fluids.

Note: If the person does not start to regain consciousness quickly, open their airway and check breathing and circulation (see pp. 475–476, 478). Put the person into the recovery position (see Ch. 16) and call for medical assistance. If necessary, commence BLS (see pp. 473–478).

Central venous pressure

Central venous pressure (CVP) records the pressure in the central venous system or the right atrium of the heart and is a useful measurement to assess fluid status. A catheter is inserted into a large central vein, usually the internal jugular or subclavian vein, and attached to a monitoring device. Frequently a pressure transducer monitors and records the pressure in mm of mercury (mmHg). Occasionally a water column is used, in which case the measurement is recorded in centimetres of water (cmH_2O). Central venous pressure is measured in the acutely ill and as such is frequently seen in intensive care or high dependency units. However, central venous pressures may also be measured in the patient on the general ward and so it is useful to have some idea of the importance of this measurement.

Breathing – general assessment

The assessment of breathing includes respiratory rate, depth and rhythm and assessment of the function of the lungs. Normal breathing at rest is silent, even and regular and is the unconscious active inspiration of air followed by passive expiration. However, both inspiration and expiration may become active with the person forcing air in or out of the lungs. Active breathing usually uses accessory muscles of breathing, the abdominal muscles and the muscles of the neck and shoulders. The use of the accessory muscles occurs in normal deep breathing and is also frequently seen in a person with breathing difficulties (see p. 483).

Respiratory rate

The respiratory rate should be recorded as one of the first observations in all general assessments and is referred to in greater depth in Chapter 14. In addition, the respiratory rate should be recorded as part of ongoing monitoring of vital signs, as 'respiratory rate is a significant predictor of critical illness' (Butler-Williams et al 2005, p. 35). When counting the respiratory rate, breathing should be observed for a 60-second period, with the person at rest. It is also a useful idea to count the respiratory rate without the person being aware and inadvertently altering their breathing rate.

Box 17.15 **Causes of dyspnoea**

- Most respiratory diseases, e.g. foreign body in the airway, asthma, COPD, lung cancer, respiratory tract infection, pneumothorax (air in the pleural cavity causing a lobe of the lung to collapse), pulmonary embolism
- Heart diseases, e.g. arrhythmias such as atrial fibrillation, congenital heart defects, heart failure
- Severe anaemia
- Neurological conditions such as motor neurone disease.

[See Tables 17.2–17.4 (pp. 471–473) for further information about some conditions that affect breathing and circulation.]

The normal respiratory rate varies with age. The normal adult respiratory rate at rest is usually between 12 and 15 breaths per minute, while it is normal for a neonate to breathe at 30–60 breaths per minute (see Ch. 14).

A respiratory rate that is faster than that expected for age (tachypnoea) is normal when caused by:

- Exercise
- Fear
- Anxiety
- Pain
- Fever.

Disorders of breathing and circulation that cause tachypnoea may include:

- Anaemia
- Heart diseases
- Following severe haemorrhage
- Most respiratory illnesses – COPD, chest infection, asthma.

A respiratory rate that is slower then expected for age (bradypnoea) is normal when the person is sleeping; however, it is abnormal when caused by:

- Sedation and opioid analgesics (see Ch. 23)
- Excessive alcohol intake.

Breathing patterns – depth and rhythm

The breathing pattern should be assessed while counting the respiratory rate. When assessing breathing patterns the nurse should observe features that include:

- *Depth of breathing* (deep, normal or shallow): Very deep, sighing breathing (Kussmaul breathing) is a feature of uncontrolled diabetes with associated acidosis (see Ch. 19). Sighing breathing occurs with severe haemorrhage. Shallow breathing occurs if it is painful to breathe deeply such as with rib fractures or following an abdominal or chest operation (see Ch. 24).
- *Difficulty in breathing* (dyspnoea): Difficult or laboured breathing occurs in a variety of conditions (Box 17.15). Orthopnoea describes difficulty breathing when lying flat. A person with dyspnoea may use the accessory muscles of respiration in an effort to move more air in and out of the lungs. In the adult these include the abdominal muscles, the muscles of the neck and shoulders and in extreme situations the person may straighten or arch the back in order to expand the thoracic cage. Accessory muscles of respiration in children include the contraction of anterior chest wall muscles and the nurse should observe for nasal flaring and head bobbing as the child breathes in. Pursed-lip breathing is associated with chronic respiratory diseases.
- *Chest wall movement*: In normal breathing there is symmetrical chest expansion with both sides moving together. Failure of both sides of the chest to expand simultaneously may be a sign of pneumothorax or serious rib fractures (paradoxical breathing). In children asymmetric chest expansion may be a sign of heart failure. Sometimes the chest is sucked inward with each breath (chest recession). The degree of recession gives some indication of the severity of respiratory distress.
- *Regularity of breathing pattern*: The term apnoea is used to denote the absence of breathing for a period of 20 seconds or more. This may occur for short periods and be followed by a period of normal breathing. Apnoea occurring during sleep is more common in people who are obese, those with heart failure or chronic respiratory disease (see Ch. 10).

  In full-term infants an irregular breathing pattern can be normal. There is rapid breathing followed by a short period of apnoea. If the baby's colour and HR do not change then this is normal. However, more prolonged abnormal apnoea occurs in very low birthweight infants, especially in those infants born at or before 32 weeks' gestation (MacGregor 2000).

  Cheyne–Stokes breathing is an abnormal breathing cycle characterized by repeated cycles that begin with slow, shallow breathing, gradually becoming abnormally rapid and deep followed by decreasing depth and rate and a period of apnoea (10–20 seconds). It is usually associated with a poor prognosis and may be seen just prior to death (see Ch. 12).

Abnormal breath sounds

Normal breathing is silent. Any noise that occurs during breathing is therefore abnormal. The noise may occur either during inspiration or expiration. Abnormal sounds include:

- *Stridor*: A high-pitched noise that occurs on inspiration or expiration and indicates a disturbance to the airflow in the upper respiratory tract. Inspiratory stridor is a feature of epiglottitis (inflammation of the epiglottis), which primarily affects children.
- *Stertor*: Snoring sound heard during breathing occurs during sleep and in altered consciousness.
- *Wheeze*: A whistling sound heard on expiration and indicates a resistance to airflow in the lower

FIRST AID Box 17.16

Asthma attack

Recognition
- Great difficulty in breathing
- Wheeze on breathing out
- Anxious, restless and distressed
- Difficulty in speaking
- Cyanosis
- Exhaustion.

Note: Cough is a feature in some people.

Aims of treatment
- Relieve breathlessness where possible
- Alleviate anxiety
- Seek emergency assistance if required.

Treatment
- If the person already has a diagnosis of asthma and has their medication with them, assist them to use their inhalers. Help the casualty to stay calm and relaxed
- If this is the first attack the casualty should be seen by a doctor
- If the attack is severe or prolonged, or is not eased by the medication, summon help by dialling 999
- Stay with the person, reassure and keep them calm until help arrives.

[Resources: BBC – www.bbc.co.uk/health/first_aid_action/action_file_menu.shtml (Select asthma from Breathing difficulties); Interactive test – www.bbc.co.uk/health/first_aid_action/hs_child/hs_asthma.shtml All available July 2006]

respiratory tract such as occurs in bronchospasm (constriction of the bronchi caused by the contraction of the involuntary muscle in their walls). The noise becomes louder as the obstruction to airflow worsens. Wheezing frequently occurs during an asthma attack (see also p. 473). As it occurs when breathing out it is referred to as an expiratory wheeze. First aid for asthma is outlined in Box 17.16.
- *Grunting*: A breath sound heard mainly in neonates. It is a serious sign of worsening respiratory function and professional help should be sought immediately.
- *Rattle*: A rattle is heard both on inspiration and expiration and is associated with secretions in the lower respiratory tract (see p. 490). Sometimes this is associated with end of life when the term 'death rattle' may be used (see Ch. 12).

Cough and sputum

In health, regular deep breathing and ciliary action remove normal secretions and inhaled foreign particles. Secretions are generally swallowed but may be coughed up (expectorated). However, when these mechanisms are ineffective or there is an increase in mucus secretion or foreign particles, the cough becomes essential (Jones & Moffat 2002). A cough is the sudden and rapid expulsion of air from the lungs. Coughing may be voluntary or it may be an involuntary cough reflex. The cough reflex is part of the protective mechanisms that protect the airway from foreign bodies that either irritate or may obstruct the airway. The cough reflex occurs, for example, when food or fluid goes the 'wrong way'.

Choking occurs when there is a partial blockage to the upper airway. The person will be anxious, have difficulty breathing and may start coughing. This may dislodge the foreign body but, if not, urgent treatment may be necessary to prevent asphyxia. This is characterized by severe hypoxia leading to hypoxaemia (reduced oxygen content in arterial blood) and hypercapnia (increased carbon dioxide in arterial blood). Unconsciousness occurs and eventually death without effective treatment. Choking has a number of causes but usually occurs when a foreign body, e.g. food such as peanuts, small toys or pieces of toys, loose tooth, pen top, etc., is inhaled.

The first aid treatment for an adult who is choking is outlined in Box 17.17. The first aid procedures for choking in infants and children differ from those in adults and readers are advised to consult Further reading (e.g. Mohun et al 2002). Obviously it is preferable to prevent choking in the first place by identifying the risks and excluding them whenever possible, such as by choosing toys suitable for a child's age (Box 17.18).

A cough may be described as dry or productive. Coughing may be associated with pain in some chest conditions and following chest or abdominal surgery (see Ch. 24). Prolonged coughing can cause muscle pain and may deter patients from coughing. The nurse should assess levels of pain and ensure that effective pain relief is provided (see Ch. 23).

A dry cough is one that develops without the presence of excess secretions. The cough could result from an irritant in the upper airway such as smoke or cold air and sometimes develops into a 'tickly' cough. Some forms of medication cause a dry cough, e.g. some heart medication such as angiotensin-converting enzyme (ACE) inhibitors. A constant dry cough is frequently a nuisance to the person and may result in them stopping their medication if they think this is the likely cause. For this reason it is important to listen to the patient's complaints and inform the prescriber so that medication can be reviewed.

A productive cough is one where excess mucus or sputum ('phlegm') is present in the respiratory tract. When the airways are inflamed, as occurs during an infection, there is an excessive secretion of mucus, which then accumulates in the airways. The mucus is usually expectorated by coughing. A productive cough may also be found where ciliary action is ineffective. Smoking is known to damage the cilia, and is responsible for the so called 'smokers cough'.

The nurse should observe the colour, consistency, quantity and odour of any sputum produced during coughing and record this information in the nursing notes and charts (Box 17.19). Any changes should be reported to the person in charge.

A specimen of sputum will be sent to the laboratory for microscopy, culture and sensitivity if infection is

FIRST AID Box 17.17

Choking in adults

Recognition
- Struggling for breath
- Difficulty talking
- Pointing to/clutching the throat
- Anxious
- Blueness of the lips and mouth.

Aims of treatment
- Dislodge the foreign body.

Treatment
- Remove debris, dentures and loose teeth from the mouth
- Stand to the side and slightly behind the person, supporting the chest with one hand and lean them well forward
- Use the heel of the hand to give up to five sharp slaps on the back between the shoulder blades (scapulae)
- Check to see if the obstruction is relieved after each back blow
- If the slaps do not relieve the obstruction, attempt the following abdominal thrusts:
  - stand behind the person, with both arms around the upper part of their abdomen
  - ensure the person is leaning forward
  - place your clenched fist between the umbilicus and bottom of the breast bone (sternum) and grasp it with your other hand
  - pull sharply inwards and upwards to dislodge the foreign body
  - repeat this up to five times
- If the person is unconscious it will be necessary to do the abdominal thrusts with the casualty on their back and their airway open (see pp. 475–476):
  - kneel astride the casualty's thighs and use the heel of the hand to press on the abdomen to apply inward and upward thrusts
  - check to see if the obstruction is relieved after each thrust
- If the casualty becomes unconscious the muscles around the larynx relax and some air will pass down to the lungs. BLS (see pp. 473–477) should be started if the casualty is not breathing
- If the casualty is breathing, they should be placed into the recovery position (see Fig. 16.17A,B, p. 460) (Resuscitation Council (UK) 2005)
- If the foreign body is not dislodged and/or the person is unconscious, summon emergency assistance by telephoning 999.

suspected (see Ch. 15). Box 17.20 (p. 486) outlines the safe and effective collection of a sputum specimen. If the patient is unable to expectorate a specimen may be obtained during nasopharyngeal/tracheal suctioning (see pp. 490–491) by using a sputum trap.

HEALTH PROMOTION Box 17.18

Preventing choking in babies and small children

A friend who has a new baby and a toddler aged 18 months tells you that she and her partner are worried about the risk of choking, as they have heard how easily this can happen in babies and small children. She asks you about how they might reduce the risk as much as possible.

Student activity
Visit the websites below and find out how your friend and her partner can minimize the risk of choking in their children.

[Resources: Child Accident Prevention Trust – www.capt.org.uk/FAQ/default.htm; Royal Society for the Prevention of Accidents (RoSPA) – www.rospa.com/homesafety/advice/child/accidents.htm Available July 2006]

Box 17.19

Characteristics of sputum – colour, consistency, quantity and odour

Colour
- White mucoid such as with a severe 'cold'
- Yellow or green sputum containing pus (purulent) in bacterial infections affecting the respiratory tract. Common in COPD and CF
- Red if containing fresh blood or having a 'rusty' appearance if blood is old. Coughing up blood or bloodstained secretions is known as haemoptysis. It may be associated with disease of the lung tissue such as cancer, pneumonia, tuberculosis, trauma; pulmonary emboli causing pulmonary infarction (death of lung tissue); heart diseases such as acute left ventricular failure, mitral valve stenosis; blood clotting disorders, e.g. haemophilia, or anticoagulant drugs. The amount of bloodstaining can vary from blood streaks to a massive haemorrhage. If bloodstained secretions are new, or develop into a frank haemorrhage, the nurse in charge or the medical team must be notified.

Consistency
- Viscous or sticky secretions, which are difficult to expectorate, may occur in dehydration (see Ch. 19)
- Copious watery, frothy secretions are characteristic of pulmonary oedema (fluid in the alveoli), which may be due to heart failure. The secretions are generally white but may have a pink tinge.

Quantity
- Increasing or decreasing amounts of sputum should be documented and reported.

Odour
- Foul-smelling sputum may be a feature of bronchiectasis (see Table 17.4, p. 473) or lung abscess.

NURSING SKILLS Box 17.20

Collection of a sputum specimen

Equipment

- Disposable gloves and apron
- Sterile specimen container and specimen bag
- Request form for microbiology laboratory
- Fresh disposable sputum carton with lid if appropriate
- Tissues
- Mouth wash/teeth cleaning facilities
- Waste bag.

Preparation

- Explain the procedure to the patient to ensure informed consent
- Ensure that the specimen is obtained before the patient uses an antiseptic mouthwash, as this can affect the results (see Ch. 15).

Procedure

- Collect the specimen container, request form and transport bag
- Wash hands and put on plastic apron and non-sterile gloves (Ch. 15) and follow local policy for other protective clothing for specific infections, e.g. tuberculosis
- Ensure privacy to produce a sample
- The physiotherapist may be asked to assist by helping the patient to expectorate
- Ask the patient to cough and expectorate sputum into the sterile container
- Replace the lid on the sterile container and make sure that it is securely closed
- Check that the sample is sputum and not saliva. Observe the sputum and note the characteristics (see above)
- Offer the patient a mouthwash or teeth cleaning facilities, especially if expectorating foul-smelling sputum
- Change disposable sputum carton and observe as required and place in waste bag
- Dispose of used sputum carton/waste bag in the clinical waste bag
- Remove gloves and apron and wash hands
- Label the specimen container with the correct patient information and enclose in a specimen bag with the correctly completed request for investigation form
- Arrange for transfer to the laboratory
- Offer the patient a drink if appropriate
- Record date and time the specimen was collected in the patient's nursing and medical notes.

Peak expiratory flow rate

The peak expiratory flow rate (PEFR) is the greatest rate of airflow out of the lungs and is measured in litres per minute (L/min) during a forced expiration. The normal range for PEFR depends on age, height and gender. It is an important measure of lung function and is frequently used as a guide to monitor the progress of a condition such as asthma or the person's response to their medication. A Wright or mini-Wright peak flow meter is used to measure PEFR (Box 17.21).

NURSING SKILLS Box 17.21

Measuring peak expiratory flow rate (Fig. 17.11)

Equipment

- Peak flow meter and disposable mouthpiece
- Observation chart
- Disposable apron.

Preparation

- Explain the procedure to the patient to ensure informed consent
- Ensure that the reading is taken at the correct time, i.e. before and/or after inhaled medication (see p. 491).

Procedure

- Wash your hands and put on apron
- Attach the disposable mouthpiece and ensure that the meter is set at zero
- Ask or assist the patient to stand or sit upright
- Ask the patient to breathe in as deeply as possible, seal their lips around the mouthpiece and then exhale as forcibly and as quickly as possible
- Make a note of the result and if possible take two more consecutive readings (after resetting the meter to zero) and record the highest. *Note*: It may only be possible to obtain one reading if the patient is distressed by breathlessness, coughing, etc.
- Ensure that any post PEFR medication is given and recorded (see Ch. 22)
- Check that the patient is comfortable
- If the patient retains the disposable mouthpiece for further use, it is stored dry and covered. Otherwise it is disposed of in the clinical waste according to local procedures
- Chart the results and report any changes or difficulties in obtaining three results.

[Further reading: Higgins D 2005 Measuring PEFR. Nursing Times 101(10): 32–33]

Pulse oximetry

Pulse oximetry is used to measure the percentage of saturated haemoglobin in the arterial blood and gives a useful indication of the amount of oxygen in the peripheral blood. Oxygen saturation monitoring is frequently undertaken, either continuously or as a periodic measurement. The normal oxygen saturation range is 94–98%.

The measurement is performed with a non-invasive pulse oximeter, a device comprising a probe connected to a monitor (Fig. 17.12). The probe should be placed where it is in close contact with the blood such as the nail bed or ear lobe. The pulse oximeter measures and displays the peripheral capillary saturation of haemoglobin (SpO_2)

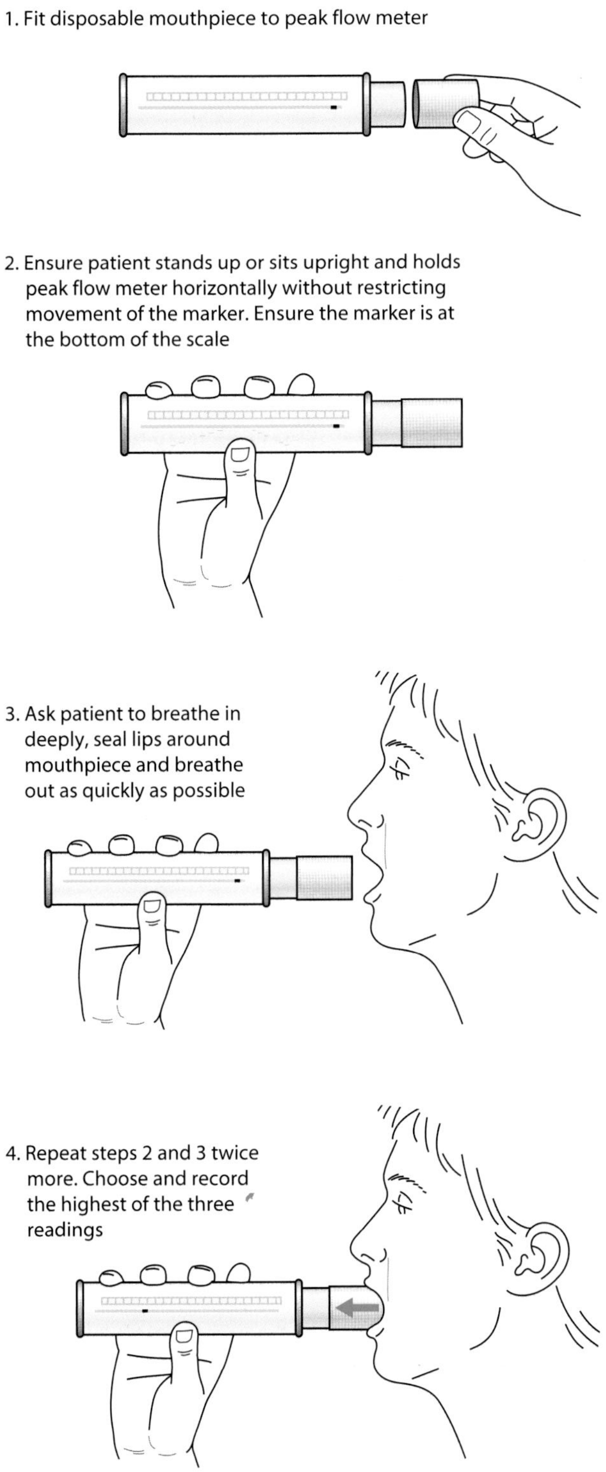
1. Fit disposable mouthpiece to peak flow meter
2. Ensure patient stands up or sits upright and holds peak flow meter horizontally without restricting movement of the marker. Ensure the marker is at the bottom of the scale
3. Ask patient to breathe in deeply, seal lips around mouthpiece and breathe out as quickly as possible
4. Repeat steps 2 and 3 twice more. Choose and record the highest of the three readings

Fig. 17.11 Recording peak expiratory flow rate (reproduced with permission from Brooker & Nicol 2003)

(Allen 2004). Pulse oximetry has limitations and results must be interpreted carefully (Box 17.22).

Arterial blood gas analysis, an invasive procedure, may be used in critically ill people to directly measure the amount of oxygen and carbon dioxide in the blood and other parameters that include blood pH (see Ch. 19).

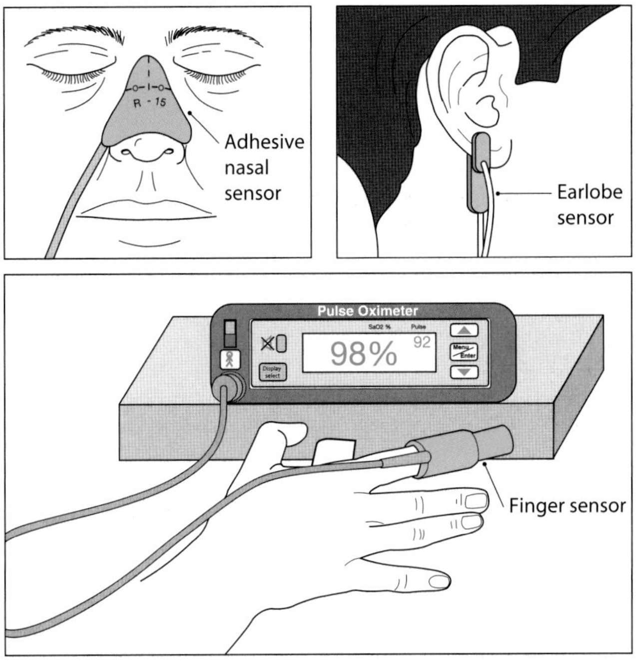

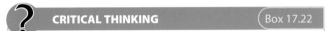

Fig. 17.12 Pulse oximeter and probe (reproduced with permission from Nicol et al 2004)

CRITICAL THINKING Box 17.22

Mr Jones

Mr Jones is to have continuous pulse oximetry monitoring.

Student activities

Read the article by Allen (2004) and answer the following questions:

- Where will you place the oxygen saturation probe?
- What would you do to minimize the risk of inaccurate results?
- What physical signs will the registered nurse take into account when interpreting the readings?

[Further reading: Higgins D 2005 Pulse oximetry. Nursing Times 101(6):34–35]

Pain associated with breathing or circulation problems

Pain is abnormal and, if present, may indicate circulatory or breathing problems. It can be caused by a variety of conditions and may be either cardiac or non-cardiac in origin. As with any pain, it is important for the care team to identify the cause so that appropriate pain relief and management can be planned (see Ch. 23).

The following points should be considered when assessing the person with pain associated with breathing or circulation problems:

- *Precipitating factors*: For example, does the pain become worse with exercise, in cold weather, with deep breathing or movement?

- *Location of pain*: Cardiac (heart) pain is frequently central and may radiate to the back, arms and jaw. Pain caused by circulatory disorders, such as peripheral vascular disease, will occur in the limbs
- *Description of pain*: Cardiac chest pain may be described as a heavy sensation, aching or crushing. If chest pain is described as a sharp pain on inspiration it is likely to be caused by pleurisy (inflammation of the pleura) rather than angina or a myocardial infarction
- *Intensity of pain*: It is useful to use a pain assessment tool and ask the patient to grade their pain. In children, facial expressions can be very useful for the assessment of pain and pain assessment tools used with children often include faces (see Ch. 23)
- *Factors that relieve the pain*: For example, cardiac chest pain may subside on resting or stopping the activity that caused it, or by a change of position, e.g. a person with pericarditis (inflammation of the pericardium) may obtain relief by leaning forward. Chest pain that is muscular in origin may be relieved by a warm or cold compress.

It is important, however, to remember that it is not always easy to ascertain answers to questions about levels and sites of pain. People with a learning difficulty or speech problems can find it difficult to describe pain or its location, while a child's response to pain is linked to their developmental stage (see Ch. 23).

Common investigations – breathing and circulation

There are many different investigations used to identify disorders affecting breathing and circulation and some of these are outlined in Box 17.23. Box 17.24 provides an opportunity to find out what a cardiac investigation can involve.

Box 17.23 Common investigations – breathing and circulation

The following investigations may be used to diagnose or evaluate treatment for disorders affecting breathing and circulation.

- Blood tests – full blood count (FBC), erythrocyte sedimentation rate (ESR), urea and electrolytes, arterial blood gases, blood clotting tests, cardiac enzymes, lipid screening, e.g. cholesterol comprising high-density lipoprotein (HDL) and low-density lipoprotein (LDL)
- Chest X-ray
- Scans – computed tomography (CT), magnetic resonance imaging (MRI), ultrasound/echocardiogram
- Coronary angiogram and cardiac catheterization
- Electrocardiogram (ECG)
- Respiratory function tests – including spirometry, e.g. forced vital capacity (FVC), forced expiratory volume in 1 second (FEV_1), peak expiratory flow rate (PEFR) (see p. 486)
- Sputum specimen for microbiological or cytological examination
- Bronchoscopy.

A simple explanation of some of these investigations accessed on the BBC website will help you provide patients with information; more detailed nursing explanation can be found in Riley (2003).

[Resources: BBC – www.bbc.co.uk/health/talking/tests Available July 2006]

CRITICAL THINKING Box 17.24

Having an echocardiogram

14-year-old Leroy is booked to have echocardiogram. He is anxious about the investigation and that it will show something that will stop him playing football.

Student activities

- Find out what happens during an echocardiogram.
- Consider how you provide Leroy with all the information he needs.

Care of the person with breathing and/or circulation problems

Breathing and circulation problems may affect people of all ages and causes range from respiratory problems such as poor oxygenation, cardiac causes when the heart is unable to pump oxygenated blood around the body or blood disorders when there is insufficient oxygen delivered to the body tissues and organs due to a low haemoglobin level (see Tables 17.2–17.4, pp. 471–473). Problems associated with breathing and circulation such as dyspnoea (see Box 17.15, p. 483) or profound fatigue may impact upon all aspects of life: physical functioning and daily activities, and psychological and social aspects.

This section of the chapter outlines the basic, but essential, aspects of care needed by patients who have breathing and circulation problems, helping with expectoration, inhaled medication, oxygen therapy, respiratory support, blood transfusion and rehabilitation.

Communication and relief of anxiety

Breathlessness is extremely frightening and may increase anxiety, which in turn makes the patient more breathless (Prigmore 2005). Communication is both important yet difficult. Communication is a two-way process and this is difficult for the person who is struggling for breath, has a breathing tube, e.g. tracheostomy (opening in the trachea), requires continuous oxygen therapy or who is too breathless to form words (Box 17.25). The nurse must

REFLECTIVE PRACTICE Box 17.25

Breathlessness

Ron, who has COPD, is very breathless and finds talking increasingly difficult. He feels helpless and anxious.

Student activities

- Reflect on the difficulties that Ron may experience with communicating his physical and emotional needs.
- Consider the impact of severe breathlessness on Ron's ability to interact with his family and friends.

maintain a calm appearance, use gentle touch and appropriate eye contact to provide reassurance. Additionally, alternative communication strategies should be employed such as a pen and pad or a word or picture board. Giving the patient time to express their feelings is clearly important and the nurse should use both verbal and non-verbal cues to ensure that they do not feel rushed. When talking is very difficult, the use of closed questions that do not require long answers may also be useful (see Ch. 9).

Positioning to relieve breathlessness

Patients feeling breathless should be supported by pillows in an upright position, either in bed or in a chair. This will increase their lung expansion, which assists gaseous exchange in the alveoli. Breathing may also be easier if they lean forward slightly on pillows placed on a bedside table (Fig. 17.13).

The breathless person is likely to feel anxious if laid flat. However, if they are comfortable lying down, they should lie with their back straight, again to assist with chest expansion. Opening a window may also help someone who is struggling to breathe.

Personal hygiene and skin care

Patients may need help with personal cleansing and dressing depending on how breathless they are and the degree of fatigue caused by poor oxygenation and the constant struggle to breathe (see Ch. 16). They may need extra time to wash and also the opportunity to rest during personal hygiene. Additionally, if mouth breathing (see Box 17.2, p. 469), they will have a dry mouth and require oral hygiene, mouth washes and ice to suck.

Patients with breathing difficulties are likely to have poor oxygenation and consequently some degree of tissue hypoxia. This, combined with factors such as underlying disease, reduced mobility, sliding down from the upright position and poor nutrition, will make them susceptible to pressure ulcers. It should therefore be assumed that any person with a breathing problem is at risk of developing a pressure ulcer and scoring using a pressure ulcer risk tool should be used so that appropriate measures to prevent their occurrence can be implemented. Regular repositioning, mobilization and the use of pressure-relieving devices should be considered (see Ch. 25).

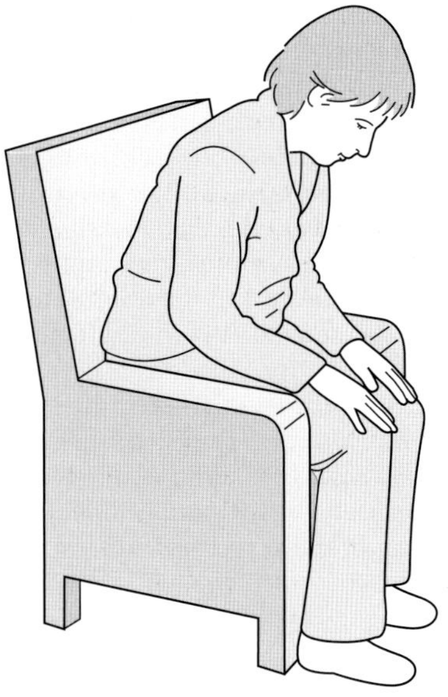

Sitting in chair leaning forward

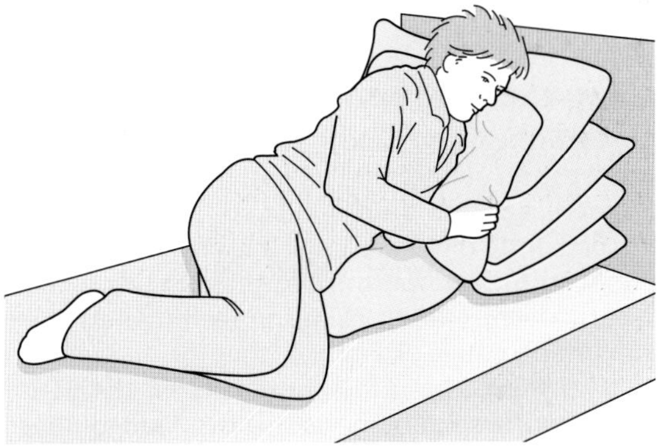

High side lying

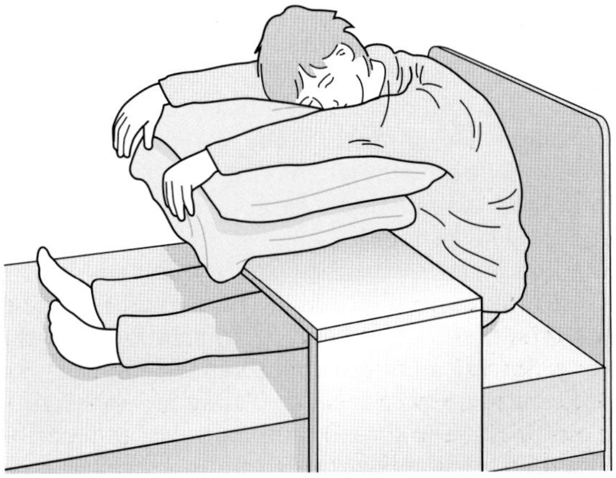

Upright positioning in bed leaning forward onto pillows or bedside table with pillows

Fig. 17.13 Position for relieving breathlessness (reproduced with permission from Brooker & Nicol 2003)

Nutrition and hydration

The breathless patient frequently finds it difficult to eat because of a dry mouth and may also feel nauseated, particularly if they are swallowing secretions. The provision of small, frequent meals helps the breathless person maintain an adequate dietary intake (see Ch. 19). Adequate nutrition to cope with the increased work of breathing is essential in the person with a chronic breathing problem who may also require a high protein diet. The dietitian should be approached for advice.

Mouth breathing makes their mouth dry and uncomfortable. Additionally, the patient may have an increased respiratory rate or pyrexia (see Ch. 14) that will increase fluid loss from the body. Attention to adequate hydration in the breathless patient is essential, not only for their overall fluid balance, but also for their comfort. A dry mouth rapidly leads to cracked lips and discomfort (see Ch. 16) and dehydration (see Ch. 19) and will lead to viscous secretions. Plugging of the airways may result.

Helping the person with expectoration

Increased and/or viscous secretions make breathing more difficult and the nurse should work with the physiotherapist to assist expectoration and maximize breathing effort.

Breathing exercises and coughing

Secretions can be moved and expectorated by deep breathing exercises and coughing. The patient should be encouraged to increase their fluid intake so that they can more easily expectorate the secretions. It is important to provide the patient with clean sputum cartons with lids as required and mouth washes/teeth cleaning facilities after expectoration. A specimen of sputum may be requested (see Box 17.20, p. 486). The nurse should advise the patient to avoid swallowing secretions, as this can lead to nausea.

Patients with chest infections or those who are susceptible to an infection, e.g. postoperatively or with rib fractures, should be encouraged to breathe deeply at intervals. The nurse must ensure that effective analgesics are administered to allow this without pain. Deep breathing with expansion of both lung bases is easiest with the spine straight. This is either in the upright sitting position or with the back straight when lying flat. This will expand the lung bases and facilitate gaseous exchange and clearance of basal secretions.

Breathlessness is extremely frightening and breathing exercises may control and help the person restore their normal breathing pattern during an attack of breathlessness or following a bout of coughing. Usually the patient will find these exercises easier if they are in a half side-lying position. They should be encouraged to breathe out gently while relaxing their shoulders and upper chest. When breathing in, this should also be gentle, and they should feel their lower ribs and upper abdomen expand. They should be encouraged to breathe gently, with minimal effort. Patients prone to panic attacks and attacks of breathlessness should be encouraged to practise this technique.

'Huffing' and coughing are useful techniques to help expectorate secretions. Huffing is thought to be less tiring than coughing and so it is useful to teach this to someone with chronic respiratory disease (Box 17.26).

Box 17.26 **Huffing and coughing**

Huffing
- The patient takes a medium breath in
- They then open their mouth and force the air out. They may find it easier to understand this if it is suggested that they force air out as if they are breathing onto a mirror to clean it
- They should then take a few gentle breaths before repeating this sequence two to three times until secretions are in the upper airway
- One or two coughs should then clear the secretions.

Coughing
- To make an effective cough, patients should breathe in deeply
- Then contract the muscles of the abdomen and chest wall as they forcibly exhale and cough
- When unable to cough effectively, secretions will be retained in the upper airway and suctioning may be necessary.

Postural drainage

Sometimes postural drainage is needed to remove secretions, particularly in patients with chronic respiratory disease. In these circumstances the person lies in bed with the foot of the bed elevated. Gravity then assists the movement of secretions from areas of the lungs. Alternatively, the patient can lie on their side with pillows placed under their waist to gently tip their head down. The physiotherapist will modify the patient's position to drain secretions from particular lobes or lung segments.

In small children with bronchiectasis or cystic fibrosis, a parent or carer may perform postural drainage.

Suctioning

In some circumstances it may be necessary to use suction to remove secretions from the airway. This is more likely when there is an artificial airway such as an endotracheal tube (a plastic tube introduced through the mouth or nose into the trachea to secure or maintain the airway) or tracheostomy tube (Fig. 17.14 and Box 17.27), the person is sedated or unconscious, when there is a poor cough reflex as may occur following a stroke or head injury, or when the patient is too weak to expectorate.

Suctioning should only be undertaken by someone who is competent to do so. The nurse should therefore have been taught how to undertake the procedure and observed in order to confirm competence. Patients and parents can also be taught how to perform suctioning when long-term assistance with clearing of secretions is required, e.g. a child or adult discharged home on home ventilation (see pp. 495–496).

Suctioning should be performed as a clean procedure. The nurse should wash their hands and protect themselves from infection by wearing a clean (not necessarily sterile) glove on both hands, plastic apron and eye protection if necessary.

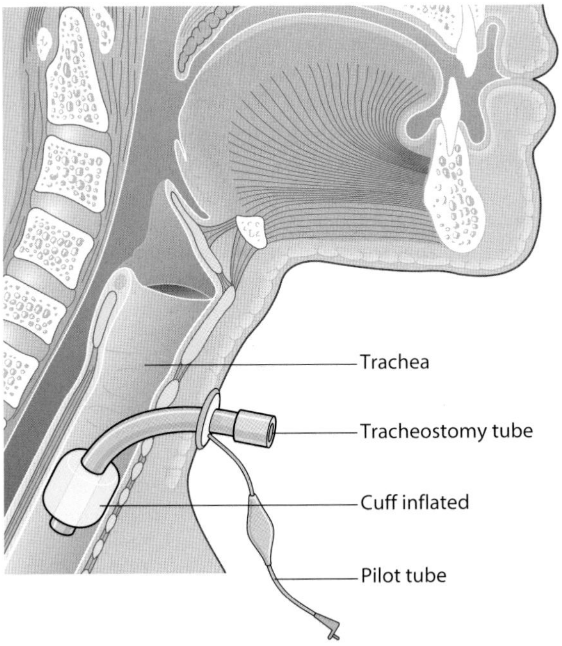

Fig. 17.14 Tracheostomy tube (adapted with permission from Brooker & Nicol 2003)

Box 17.27 Tracheostomy

A tracheostomy is a surgical opening into the trachea through the front of the neck. The tracheostomy is kept open with a tracheostomy tube (see Fig. 17.14). It facilitates breathing, oxygen therapy or clearance of secretions and may be short or long term.

Common reasons for a tracheostomy include:

- Long-term mechanical ventilation (see pp. 495–496)
- Absent laryngeal reflexes, e.g. following a stroke or head injury
- Sputum retention
- Head or neck injury or surgery
- Upper airway obstruction.

[Further reading: Harkin H, Russell C 2001 Tracheostomy patient care. Nursing Times 97(25):34–36; Russell C 2005 Providing the nurse with a guide to tracheostomy care and management. British Journal of Nursing 14(8):428–433]

Readers can find more information about suctioning in Further reading suggestions (e.g. Nicol et al 2004, Higgins 2005).

Inhaled medication

Inhaled medication is frequently used in the management of respiratory diseases such as asthma or COPD because the drug acts more quickly when it is administered directly to the site of action. Drugs administered in this way include bronchodilators (e.g. ipratropium bromide), antibiotics or corticosteroids (see Ch. 22).

There are various ways to administer inhaled medication, including:

- Nebulizers
- Dry powder inhalers
- Metered-dose inhalers.

Nebulizers (Fig. 17.15A, p. 492)

A nebulizer can be used to administer medication or to liquefy secretions with 0.9% saline solution. The drug is inhaled and is rapidly absorbed through the alveolar blood supply. It therefore acts quickly and side-effects associated with oral intake are avoided. Most nebulizers require a flow of gas and will be administered either with compressed air or oxygen. The nebulizer breaks up the solution so that it is inhaled as small droplets suspended in a gas. The use of a nebulizer is outlined in Box 17.28 (p. 492).

Dry powder inhalers

A dry powder inhaler releases medication as the person breathes in. The patient places their mouth around the device and breathes in. The flow generated by their breath releases the medication into particles that can be inhaled. These inhalers are easy to carry around and are therefore convenient to use at work, at home, in the car or at school.

The nurse should ensure that patients are able to use their inhaler effectively. Inhaler technique should always be checked by the practice nurse or general practitioner or before hospital discharge and on a regular basis in clinic.

Metered-dose inhalers (Fig. 17.15B, p. 492)

These are also available for inhaled medication and are frequently used by people with asthma. The inhaler is designed to deliver a dry powder and the medication, which is forced into the lungs.

Before use the inhaler is shaken to distribute the powder evenly within the gas. The cap is removed and the inhaler is held upright. To be effective, the patient should breathe out gently and then place their mouth around the mouthpiece of the inhaler. As they start to breathe in, the canister top should be pressed to release the medication. The breath should be slow and deep, and held for approximately 10 seconds. Usually the prescribed dose is for more than one 'puff' in which case the subsequent doses should be taken after approximately 30 seconds.

Using the inhaler requires a degree of coordination and may therefore not be suitable for children, some people with learning disabilities, some older people or those with poor dexterity (Box 17.29, p. 493). Spacer devices are available which are easier to use (Fig. 17.15C, p. 492). They comprise a large and, usually, cone-shaped device, onto which the inhaler is fitted and are thought to be effective when used with regular breathing.

Oxygen therapy

Oxygen is a drug and should always be prescribed, except in an emergency situation such as cardiopulmonary arrest. The prescription should indicate the oxygen concentration, e.g. 24%, and flow rate in L/min. This includes

NURSING SKILLS Box 17.28

Use of a nebulizer

Equipment

- Nebulizer – mouthpiece or facemask (see Fig. 17.15A)
- Air cylinder if piped supply not available
- Nebulizer/drug solution and prescription sheet.

Preparation

- Explain the procedure to the patient to ensure informed consent
- Ascertain whether PEFR measurements are required before and after drug administration
- Wash your hands and follow local infection control procedures
- Ensure that the patient is in the upright position or on their side with their back straight.

Procedure

- Check the medication and the patient's identity against the prescription sheet
- Place the medication, which is normally diluted with 2–3 mL of 0.9% saline, or the saline alone in the nebulizer base and then reassemble
- Ensure that the mouthpiece or facemask is securely connected to the nebulizer. It is preferable to use a mouthpiece to deliver the solution as there is less wastage
- The gas is adjusted to a flow rate of between 4 and 5 L per minute to ensure the medication is vaporized and a fine spray is seen coming out and a hissing sound heard
- The patient is helped to use the mouthpiece/facemask and encouraged to breathe deeply to ensure the solution reaches both lung bases
- Following use, the nebulizer and mouthpiece/facemask should be washed under running water and left to air dry. The equipment is stored dry in a polythene bag at the patient's bedside. It should be changed every 24 hours to prevent infection
- Ensure that all the solution has been vaporized and assist the patient as necessary, e.g. with expectoration or repositioning
- Record the nebulized drug administration and report any changes in condition.

Note: When more than one medication is prescribed for the nebulizer; they should not be mixed and should be administered one after the other, with the bronchodilator (if prescribed) given first. This will open the airways and facilitate more effective treatment with the second drug. Each nebulizer should be labelled according to the medication use.

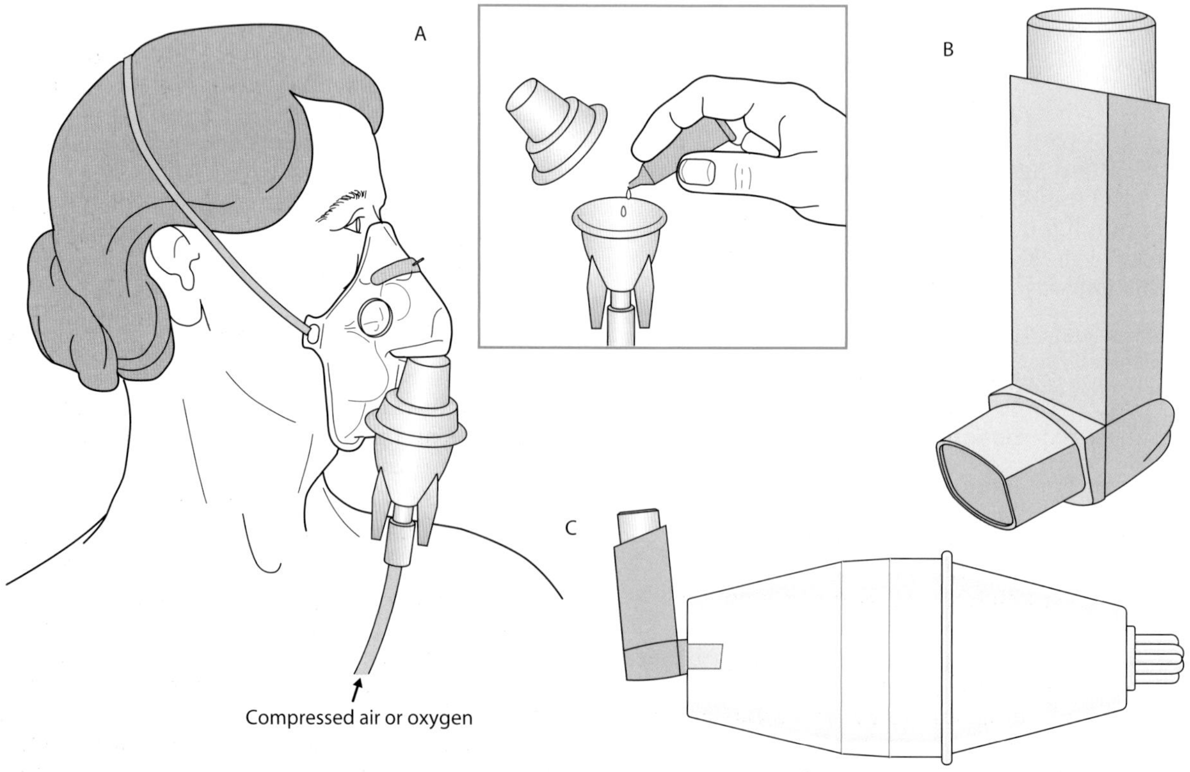

Fig. 17.15 **A.** Nebulizer (reproduced with permission from Nicol et al 2004). **B.** Metered-dose inhaler. **C.** Inhaler with spacer attached

> **CRITICAL THINKING** Box 17.29
>
> **Rosie**
>
> 4-year-old Rosie needs to have inhaled medication to control her asthma symptoms.
>
> **Student activities**
> - Think about how you would explain the use of the inhaler and spacer to Rosie and her parents.
> - How will Rosie's level of understanding and motor skills influence the way you explain how to use the inhaler?
>
> [Further reading: Huband & Trigg, Ch. 16, pp. 144–149 (2000)]

oxygen delivered by any method, e.g. by mask (face or tracheostomy), nasal cannulae or an incubator, etc. Oxygen is given, usually in the short term, to relieve hypoxia while the underlying cause of the problem is urgently sought.

Oxygen is a potentially hazardous substance. It supports combustion and therefore requires certain precautions:

- Electrical devices should be used with caution when oxygen therapy is in use; this includes electrical shavers and children's toys
- Smoking should not be allowed in the vicinity of oxygen
- Oil, grease, alcohol-based solutions and other flammable solvents should be kept away from the vicinity.

Additionally, the administration of high levels of oxygen can be dangerous and may lead to:

- Eye damage in preterm babies – retinopathy of prematurity (previously known as retrolental fibroplasia)
- Lung damage with fibrosis in preterm babies
- The retention of carbon dioxide in people with COPD whose stimulus to breathe is decreased oxygen in their blood (normally the stimulus to breathe is a rising carbon dioxide level in the blood).

Problems associated with oxygen therapy

There are various physical, psychological and social problems associated with oxygen therapy, many of which are similar to those experienced by patients who are breathless (see pp. 488–490) (Box 17.30). The problems include:

- Noise of gas flow
- Drying of airway mucosa – prevented by humidification (see p. 495)
- Dry eyes – ensure that facemask fits well over the nose to minimize leaks
- Dry mouth – provide adequate fluid intake (see Ch. 19) and oral hygiene (see Ch. 16)
- Difficulties with eating and drinking – consider the use of nasal cannulae
- Nausea – give antiemetics drugs as prescribed
- Plastic smell from oxygen mask

> **CRITICAL THINKING** Box 17.30
>
> **Pete**
>
> 15-year-old Pete has required continuous oxygen therapy for the past 2 days. The bridge of his nose is sore and he does not want to wear the facemask any longer. His mouth is dry, he has no appetite and is reluctant to drink. Pete is very quiet and does not want to see visitors.
>
> **Student activities**
> - Why do you think he feels like this and what can the nursing staff do to help?
> - Consider the physical, psychological and social problems associated with Pete's oxygen therapy and write a care plan that will address the specific problems.
> - Consider how these problems could have been foreseen and prevented.

- Soreness caused by facemask or nasal cannulae – the nurse must check regularly for soreness over the nose, the ears or around the nostrils and take steps to prevent skin damage such as adjusting straps to avoid pressure
- Feeling isolated – provide appropriate contact
- Facemask is frightening and may lead to feelings of claustrophobia – minimize by providing information and explanation
- Communication problems (see pp. 488–489)
- Patients removing the facemask – provide information about reasons for oxygen therapy. Consider changing to nasal cannulae
- System disconnection, especially in a confused patient or young child – the nurse should regularly check system integrity.

Oxygen administration systems

Oxygen is supplied via a piped system in hospitals or in standard colour-coded cylinders (black with a white top) in the community and occasionally in hospital (Fig. 17.16, p. 494).

Oxygen can be administered in a variety of ways (Fig. 17.17, p. 494), including:

- Face and tracheostomy masks – the choice of mask depends on the reason for oxygen therapy
- Nasal cannulae/prongs
- Headboxes, oxygen tents and incubators.

The administration method chosen will depend upon age, the reason for administration, whether it is short or long term and where possible the patient's preferences. For example, a young child or baby may not tolerate an oxygen mask and so a headbox or incubator may be used.

Oxygen may be given as a short-term treatment, e.g. postoperatively. However, long-term oxygen therapy (LTOT) may be needed for a patient with COPD, and arrangements must be made for oxygen therapy to be supplied at home (Box 17.31, p. 494).

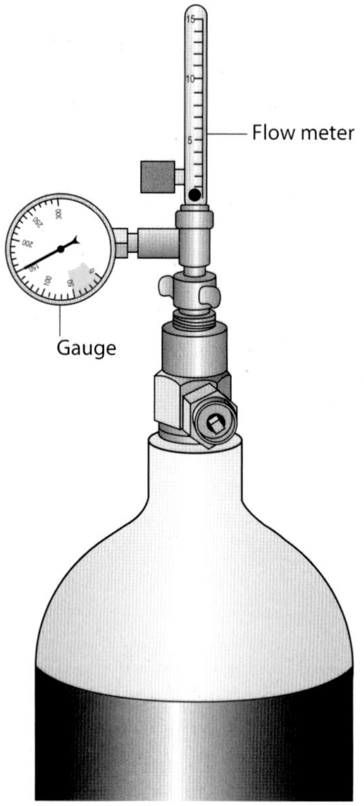

Fig. 17.16 Oxygen cylinder (reproduced with permission from Nicol et al 2004)

Fixed performance Venturi systems (high-flow)

Fixed performance facemasks deliver a high flow of gas achieved by entraining atmospheric air to give a fixed and accurate oxygen concentration (Higgins 2005) (see Fig.17.17A). Masks are available that provide oxygen at various concentrations (24%, 28%, 35%) and the oxygen flow rate is set between 4 and 8 L/min according to the manufacturer's instructions. Specific high-flow masks are

> **Box 17.31 Long-term oxygen therapy**
>
> LTOT is supplied at home for patients with COPD who meet certain criteria; for example, 'Patients should breathe supplemental oxygen for at least 15 hours/day' (NICE 2004, p. 9).
>
> 'Oxygen converters should be used to provide the fixed supply at home for LTOT' (NICE 2004, p. 9). Oxygen converters remove nitrogen from room air to provide a high concentration of oxygen for the patient.
>
> In addition, ambulatory oxygen is supplied to patients having LTOT who want to continue with treatment outside their home.
>
> [Reference: NICE 2004 Chronic obstructive pulmonary disease. Quick reference guide. Online: www.nice.org.uk/pdf/CG012quickrefguide.pdf Available July 2006]

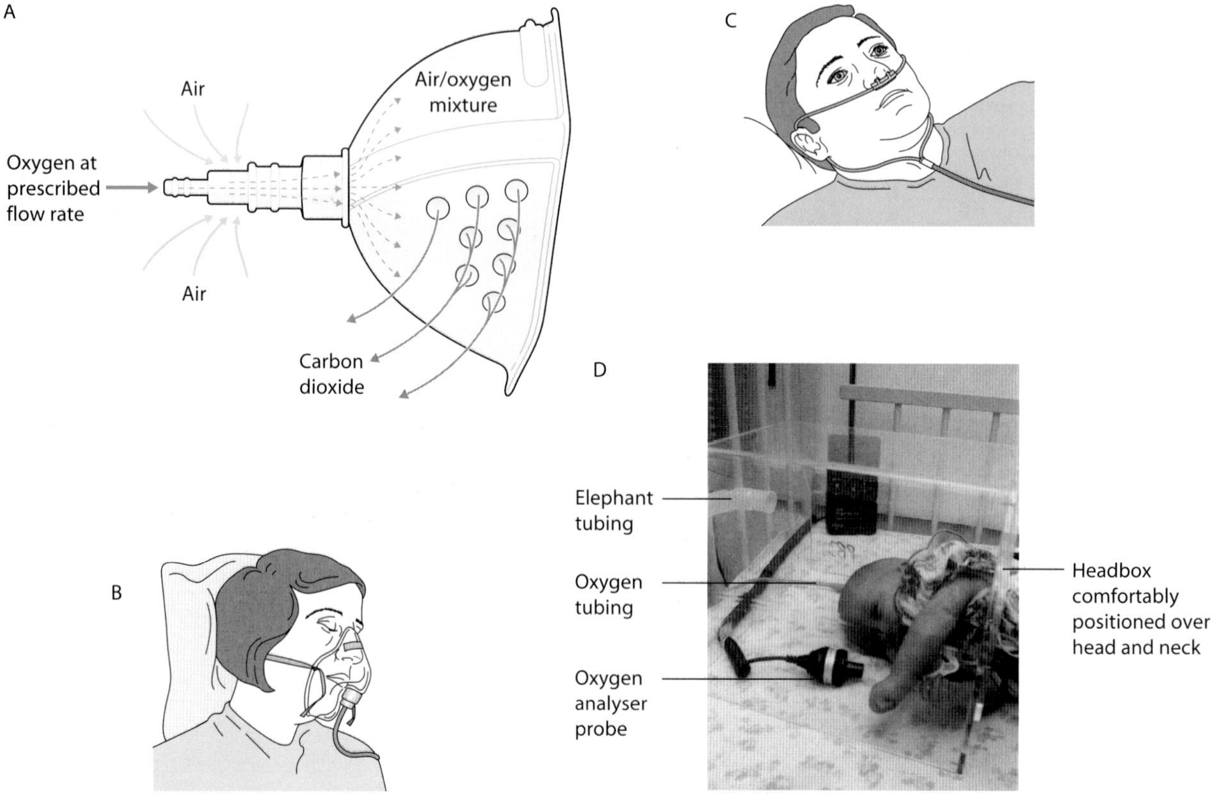

Fig. 17.17 Oxygen delivery systems: **A.** Fixed performance, high-flow Venturi system mask. **B.** Variable flow – Hudson-type mask. **C.** Nasal cannulae/prongs. **D.** Delivery of humidified oxygen via a head box (reproduced with permission from Brooker & Nicol 2003; Nicol et al 2004; Huband & Trigg 2000)

available for use with tracheostomy tubes. Humidification should be used with high-flow masks.

Variable performance systems

These systems use a low-flow mask, e.g. a Hudson mask, and are frequently used either in the emergency situation or for a person recovering from an anaesthetic (see Fig. 17.17B). With an oxygen flow rate of between 6 and 10 L/min, a concentration of up to 60–70% can be given.

Nasal cannulae/nasal prongs

Nasal cannulae/prongs are small plastic tubes, which are inserted into each nostril to administer oxygen (see Fig. 17.17C). The cannulae are secured by tubing over the ears. Oxygen flow rates of approximately 2 L/min are used. Higher flow rates may cause discomfort and drying of the nasal mucosa, which will damage the delicate mucosal lining.

The system enables the patient to also breathe room air and so does not require an elaborate humidification system. Their use also enables the patient requiring oxygen to eat, drink or talk and is therefore useful alongside a standard oxygen facemask for short-term use. Nasal cannulae are available in small sizes for infants and young children.

Headbox, body/trunk box

A headbox is frequently used for infants up to about 8 months of age, requiring oxygen, as it is unlikely that they will tolerate a facemask. Boxes, which are integral to a baby chair, e.g. Manchester chair, are available for older infants (Huband & Trigg 2000). This system allows the infant to be nursed in a more upright position.

The clear plastic headbox is placed around the infant's head and neck. Humidified oxygen is delivered into the box and the infant breathes air with a higher oxygen concentration (see Fig. 17.17D). The oxygen flow rate should be sufficient to prevent the accumulation of carbon dioxide in the head box. An oxygen analyser probe is used within the box to ensure that the infant receives the correct oxygen concentration. The clear nature of the headbox means that the infant can see out while also being observed for signs of deterioration such as increased respiratory rate.

Oxygen tent

Oxygen tents are predominantly used when infants or young children will not tolerate an oxygen mask. The oxygen is supplied to an oxygen tent placed over the bed. The child is free to move in the bed, while still breathing a higher oxygen concentration than room air. However, they are infrequently used today due to their several disadvantages. There is a high concentration of oxygen within the oxygen tent and the risk of fire is increased, observation of the child is limited and oxygen concentration falls every time the tent is opened for monitoring, care or treatment.

Incubator

An incubator is useful for the preterm or sick baby where the percentage of oxygen in inspired air can be easily controlled while also providing a stable temperature. These are frequently used for the very ill or preterm neonate.

Continuous positive airway pressure (CPAP)

CPAP is increasingly used to correct hypoxaemia. A tight-fitting mask is placed around the mouth and nose and positive pressure is applied throughout both inspiration and expiration in a spontaneously breathing patient. CPAP is useful to improve oxygen saturations. Not all patients, however, are able to tolerate CPAP and air swallowing can lead to gastric distension with vomiting and aspiration. Careful monitoring of the patient is important with checks made on respiratory rate and effort, oxygen saturations, blood pressure and heart rate.

Because the mask needs to fit securely the skin condition should also be checked. The bridge of the nose is liable to pressure from the tight-fitting mask. A small piece of DuoDERM® or protective material placed over this area may increase patient comfort. Additionally, it is important to ensure that there is no air leak around the eyes, as the high-flow oxygen can dry and irritate the eyes and cause conjunctivitis.

Humidification

Water vapour is present in atmospheric air to a greater or lesser extent and so when breathing atmospheric air humidification is dependent upon the environmental humidity. Normal air humidity is between 40 and 60% and depends on temperature. Further water vapour is normally added to inspired air as it passes through the upper airways (see pp. 468–469). However, humidification of inspired air is impaired in situations that include:

- Breathing in cold dry air, as with piped oxygen, particularly so with high-flow oxygen therapy
- Mouth breathing (see Box 17.2, p. 469)
- Upper respiratory tract infection
- Dehydration (see Ch. 19)
- When the upper airways are bypassed as occurs with tracheostomy or endotracheal tube.

Various hot- and cold-water devices are available for the humidification of inspired air and one such device is shown in Figure 17.18 (p. 496).

Respiratory support – artificial ventilation

This term refers to the process whereby a mechanical device (a ventilator) ventilates the lungs with gases. It is usually delivered through an endotracheal or tracheostomy tube, which is attached to a ventilator that pushes oxygen into the lungs. They are frequently used in the intensive care unit or operating theatre when the person is unable to breathe adequately. This process is referred to as intermittent positive pressure ventilation (IPPV). Readers requiring more information should consult Further reading (e.g. Woodrow 2000).

Non-invasive intermittent positive pressure ventilation

Artificial ventilation can also be delivered using non-invasive intermittent positive pressure ventilation (NIPPV), also known as non-invasive ventilation (NIV).

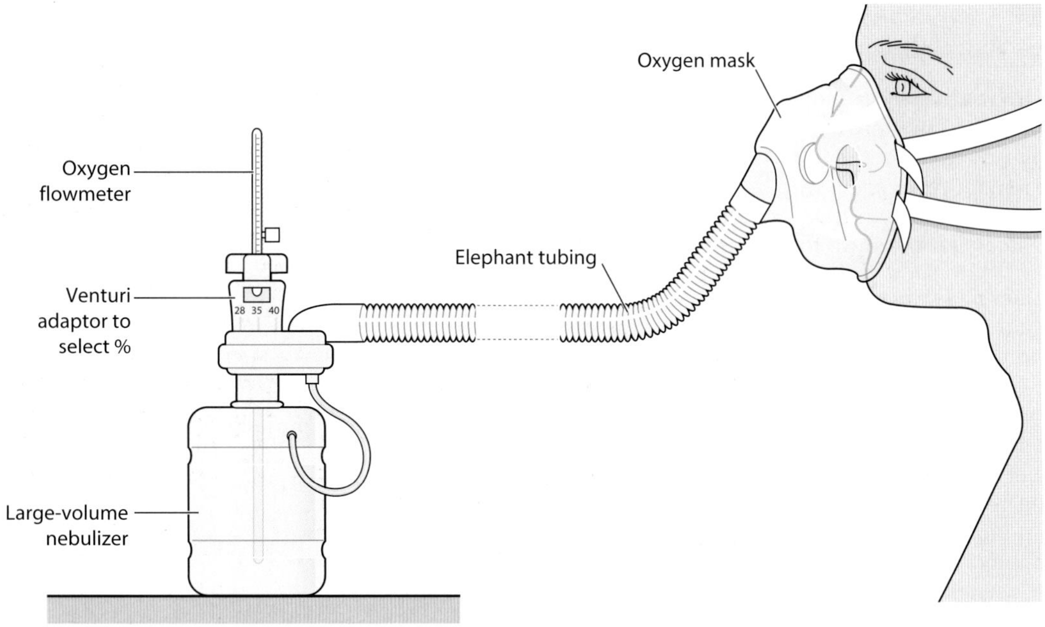

Fig. 17.18 Humidification of oxygen (reproduced with permission from Brooker & Nicol 2003)

A mask is used to avoid the need for an endotracheal tube or tracheostomy.

A mask covers the mouth and/or nose and is attached to a mechanical ventilator that pushes oxygen into the lungs. It is useful in nocturnal hypoventilation, a syndrome related to sleep apnoea (see Ch. 10). It is also used in severe muscle fatigue, neuromuscular weakness, COPD and in severe heart failure. NIPPV may be used almost continuously or on a sporadic basis for someone who only requires support at night. It is therefore increasingly used at home for both adults and children who require longer-term assistance with breathing while living at home. However, if this is to be effective it is essential that not only do the family receive accurate information beforehand, but they also receive adequate support. People on home ventilation understandably worry that they may suffer equipment failure and back-up systems and emergency plans should be decided upon in advance.

Although NIPPV can enable the person to live at home, travel and stay with friends, the device is heavy and awkward to move. It is frequently noisy to use and this may be a significant problem when cohabiting couples share a bed.

Care of patients requiring a blood transfusion

Blood transfusions can be life saving but they are expensive and can be hazardous. The risks associated with a blood transfusion using donor blood include transfusion reactions, fluid overload and also the risk of acquiring variant Creutzfeldt–Jakob disease (vCJD).

A blood transfusion may be required for a variety of reasons, including:

- Anaemia
- Preoperative preparation
- Postoperatively if blood loss is excessive, despite efforts made during surgery to prevent/minimize blood loss
- Haemorrhage causing hypovolaemia, such as after a road traffic accident
- Blood diseases requiring transfusion of clotting factors or platelets.

For the person with anaemia, or awaiting major surgery where blood loss is expected, every attempt should be made to improve haemoglobin levels through measures including oral iron supplements and a diet rich in available iron (see Box 17.1, p. 467).

In the UK, transfused blood is usually obtained from a healthy volunteer donor. Donors are asked a series of health questions and have a check on their haemoglobin level to ensure that the donation will be safe for both donor and patient. All donated blood is screened for hepatitis B and C, human immunodeficiency virus (HIV) and syphilis. In addition, other tests may be performed, e.g. if the donor has recently returned from certain countries. The blood is stored in a blood bank at around 4°C and labelled with the blood group and type.

Whole blood is transfused but various blood components, e.g. platelets, may be used in specific situations (Box 17.32).

Prior to transfusing blood, the recipient's blood should be cross-matched in the laboratory to ensure ABO blood group and rhesus factor compatibility with that of the donor (see Table 17.1, p. 468). This is done to prevent a transfusion reaction where the donor erythrocytes clump together (agglutinate) and block small blood vessels.

Monitoring during blood transfusion

Prior to commencing a blood transfusion it is important to obtain baseline recordings of temperature, pulse rate,

Box 17.32 Blood and blood products

- Whole blood transfusions are given to people who have acute serious haemorrhage, e.g. resulting from trauma, gastrointestinal haemorrhage, surgery, etc.
- Packed cell or plasma-reduced blood transfusions are used when the transfusion is given to raise the haemoglobin level. This ensures that erythrocytes are given without the risk of fluid overload
- Platelet transfusions are given to people with bleeding problems where they lack platelets, e.g. leukaemia
- Fresh frozen plasma (FFP) is used when clotting factors are needed and may be given to the person who is bleeding following surgery. A concentrate of clotting factors known as cryoprecipitate is obtained from FFP
- Other coagulation factors, e.g. factor VIII or IX for patients with haemophilia (inherited bleeding disease where either factor VIII or factor IX is deficient).

blood pressure and respiration rate. These should then be repeated according to local policy during the transfusion, e.g. recorded every 15 minutes for the first hour and thereafter recorded hourly if the person is well and shows no adverse effects until the unit of blood is transfused. However, when more than one unit of blood is given, the observations should be recommenced at 15 minute intervals with each new unit of blood. The early signs of a transfusion reaction, including fever and rigors, should be observed. If a severe reaction occurs, BLS (see pp. 473–478) may be required.

Fluid balance is monitored and recorded and this includes recording the volume of blood transfused. It is generally assumed that a unit of whole blood is 500 mL and a unit of packed red cells is 300 mL. For more accurate recording of fluid volume, the unit of blood should be weighed. Grams of weight approximate to millilitres of volume, i.e. a unit of blood weighing 490 g is recorded as 490 mL.

When monitoring fluid balance (see Ch. 19) it is also important to record urine output. If a transfusion reaction occurs the donor erythrocytes agglutinate and can cause kidney damage. If the patient complains of loin or back pain, a sample of urine should be observed and tested for haematuria (blood in the urine).

Fluid balance is of particular importance in older people, the very young or those with cardiac or respiratory failure, when circulatory overload may lead to hypertension and pulmonary oedema. This is characterized by increasing respiratory rate, dyspnoea and agitation.

Documentation is important. All observations should be clearly recorded. In addition, the start and finish times of each unit of blood should be documented.

Ensuring transfusion safety

Due to the danger associated with the transfusion of incorrect or incompatible blood and other complications, hospitals and community settings have their own strict blood transfusion policy that must be observed. Although blood should be administered at room temperature it should be removed from the blood bank fridge no more than 30 min/1 hour before transfusion, and, preferably, only 15 minutes prior. The local policy regarding the checking procedure on removal from the blood bank and prior to commencing the transfusion, including patient identification, must be undertaken and a qualified nurse should always take responsibility for this procedure.

The safe disposal of equipment is essential. Gloves should be worn when handling blood or intravenous administration sets to protect staff from blood-borne diseases (see Ch. 15).

When completed, the transfused blood packs should be returned to the laboratory if a transfusion reaction is suspected. Otherwise, the disposal of blood bags should be in accordance with the local policy. Due to concerns over vCJD, any blood products or blood waste must be incinerated.

Transfusion complications

Complications associated with blood transfusion include:

- Blood incompatibility (Box 17.33, p. 498)
- Febrile reactions
- Allergic reactions
- Circulatory overload
- Acute bacterial reactions due to contaminated blood
- Delayed complications such as delayed haemolysis (breakdown of erythrocytes), viral infections and iron overload (particularly with regular blood transfusion such as in patients with thalassaemia).

Readers requiring more information about complications should consult Further reading (e.g. Bywater & Rawlings 2003).

Alternatives to donated blood transfusion

Apart from blood conservation through minimizing loss, the alternatives to the transfusion of donor blood include:

- Autologous transfusion – a patient having planned major surgery may donate their blood about 4 weeks prior to surgery. This leaves time for the body to restore the haemoglobin level to normal and will also ensure a ready supply of suitable blood for transfusion when required. By doing this, the risk of incompatibility is eliminated, as is the risk of an acquired disease from donor blood.
- Plasma and volume expanders – albumin, gelatin solutions or modified starch solutions may be used as volume expanders. They add volume to the blood and are useful to treat hypovolaemia. They can be used until suitable blood is available.
- In the future the development of surgical techniques whereby blood is salvaged during surgery and returned to the patient may be used more extensively.

Box 17.33 Blood incompatibility

Transfusion of the wrong or incompatible blood is extremely serious and can lead to life-threatening complications, e.g. kidney failure. It may occur because a mistake has been made with blood samples or the vital bedside checks have not been followed.

Signs and symptoms

- Flushing
- Pain at the cannulation site, abdomen, loin or chest
- Agitation
- Fever
- Shivering
- Hypotension
- Tachycardia
- Nausea and vomiting
- Wheeze
- Headache
- Chest tightness
- Oliguria (reduced urinary output)
- Haematuria.

When a transfusion reaction is suspected the registered nurse should immediately stop the transfusion and obtain urgent medical assistance. The intravenous access should be kept patent with 0.9% saline. The haematologist should be contacted and any remaining blood returned to the laboratory for investigation.

Currently this practice is used for some cardiac surgery.

- Erythropoietin is a normally secreted growth factor for erythrocyte production and so increases haemoglobin. It can be given intravenously as recombinant human erythropoietin and may be a useful adjunct to good nutrition and iron supplements in the person awaiting major surgery (Margereson & Riley 2003).

Rehabilitation for conditions affecting breathing or circulation

Rehabilitation for people with conditions affecting breathing and/or circulation aims to restore someone to as normal a situation as possible (see Ch. 11); for example, for the breathless person, the ability to function in normal activities of daily living such as washing, dressing, cooking and shopping and return to work if possible. This will include issues such as managing their symptoms, advice to prevent worsening of their condition, increasing exercise tolerance and improving psychosocial coping.

Rehabilitation programmes are provided for people after a heart attack and for those with COPD. Programmes should use a holistic approach to focus on the needs of each individual but are likely to involve education, exercise, and counselling and support. For example, a programme for a breathless person will include:

- *Education*: This is an important component for any rehabilitation programme. For the breathless person, this should include information regarding the cause of their breathlessness, strategies to reduce it and lifestyle advice that may prevent the condition worsening, e.g. smoking cessation.
- *Exercise*: This includes teaching breathing exercises and exercises for muscle strength. Respiratory muscle training will reduce the effort required for breathing and hence the fatigue associated with breathlessness. Breathing exercises to reduce anxiety and distress also play an important part as does exercise training to assist with the activities of daily living. The specialist nurse, physiotherapist and occupational therapist should all work together to ensure that the exercises are appropriate for recovery.
- *Counselling and psychosocial support*: For most people with a chronic illness, social support is an important factor in helping them to cope with their condition (see Ch. 11). Positive support can provide emotional, informational and functional support and so help improve self-esteem.

Summary

- Problems with breathing and circulation are common. They reduce quality of life and account for many thousands of premature deaths in the UK.
- Health-promoting activities that include smoking cessation, a balanced diet, weight control and exercise reduce the risk of developing problems with breathing and circulation and minimize the effects of existing conditions.
- All healthcare staff should be familiar with basic life support procedures for infants, children and adults.
- Nurses should be able to respond to an acute situation and provide first aid for disorders affecting breathing and circulation.
- Holistic assessment of breathing and circulation is central to the planning of appropriate nursing interventions.
- Many nursing intervention can alleviate distressing symptoms, such as breathlessness.
- Promoting self-management is key to improving the health of people with breathing and circulation disorders.
- Nurses play a key role in reducing risk and managing chronic disorders of breathing and circulation.
- Rehabilitation programmes for people with conditions affecting breathing and/or circulation aim to restore someone to as normal a situation as possible.

Self test

1. Which arteries supply oxygenated blood to the myocardium?
2. Inspired air is warmed, humidified and filtered in the:
   a. Mouth
   b. Nose
   c. Alveoli
   d. Bronchioles.
3. What is the optimum blood pressure in an adult?
4. How would you instruct a patient to do a PEFR measurement?
5. Which lifestyle factors predispose to atherosclerosis and CHD?
6. In BLS the ratio of chest compressions to rescue breaths in an adult is:
   a. 5:2
   b. 10:2
   c. 30:2
   d. 20:2.
7. How does providing sufficient fluids help patients to expectorate?
8. The administration of high concentration oxygen can cause carbon dioxide retention in patients whose stimulus to breathe is a low blood level of oxygen rather than the normal stimulus of rising carbon dioxide level in the blood. True/false?

Key words and phrases for literature searching

Basic life support
Blood transfusion
Breathlessness
Cardiopulmonary resuscitation
Chronic respiratory diseases
Coronary heart disease
Oxygen therapy
Rehabilitation
Smoking cessation

Useful websites

BBC	www.bbc.co.uk/health Available July 2006
British Committee for Standards in Haematology – *Guidelines*	www.bcshguidelines.com Available July 2006
British Heart Foundation	www.bhf.org.uk Available July 2006
British Thoracic Society	www.brit-thoracic.org.uk Available July 2006

References

Allen K 2004 Principles and limitations of pulse oximetry in patient monitoring. Nursing Times 100(41):34–37

British Heart Foundation 2005 Coronary heart disease statistics. Online: www.heartstats.org
Available July 2006

British Thoracic Society 2001 The burden of lung disease. British Thoracic Society, London

Brooker C, Nicol M 2003 Nursing adults. The practice of caring. Mosby, Edinburgh

Butler-Williams C, Cantrill N, Maton S 2005 Increasing staff awareness of respiratory rate significance. Nursing Times 101(27):35–37

Bywater L, Rawlings E 2003 Nursing patients with blood disorders. In: Brooker C, Nicol M (eds) Nursing adults. The practice of caring. Mosby, Edinburgh

Higgins D 2005 Oxygen therapy. Nursing Times 101(4):30–31

Huband S, Trigg E 2000 Practices in children's nursing. Churchill Livingstone, Edinburgh

Jones M, Moffat F 2002 Cardiopulmonary physiotherapy. BIOS Scientific, Guildford

Mallik M, Hall C, Howard D 1998 Nursing knowledge and practice. Baillière Tindall, London

MacGregor J 2000 Introduction to the anatomy and physiology of children. Routledge, London

Margereson C, Riley J 2003 Cardiothoracic surgical nursing: current trends in adult care. Blackwell Publishing, Oxford

National Patient Safety Agency (NPSA) 2004 Patient safety alert 02. Establishing a standard crash call telephone number in hospitals. Online: www.npsa.nhs.uk
Available July 2006

Nicol M, Bavin C, Bedford-Turner S, Cronin P, Rawlings-Anderson K 2004 Essential nursing skills, 2nd edn. Mosby, Edinburgh

Prigmore S 2005 Assessment and nursing care of the patient with dyspnoea. Nursing Times 101(14):50–53

Resuscitation Council (UK) 2005 Adult basic life support. Online: www.resus.org.uk/pages/bls.pdf
Available July 2006

Riley J 2003 Nursing patients with cardiovascular disorders. In: Brooker C, Nicol M (eds) Nursing adults. The practice of caring. Mosby, Edinburgh.

Waugh A, Grant A 2001 Ross and Wilson's anatomy and physiology, 9th edn. Churchill Livingstone, Edinburgh

Williams B, Poulter NR, Brown MJ et al 2004 British Hypertension Society Guidelines. Guidelines for the management of hypertension: report of the fourth working party of British Hypertension Society, 2004 – BHS IV. Journal of Human Hypertension 18:139–185

Further reading

Brooker C, Nicol M (eds) 2003 Nursing adults. The practice of caring. Mosby, Edinburgh, Chs 18–21

Bywater L, Rawlings E 2003 Nursing patients with blood disorders. In: Brooker C, Nicol M (eds) Nursing adults. The practice of caring. Mosby, Edinburgh

Higgins D 2005 Tracheal suction. Nursing Times 101(8):36–37

Mohun J, John K, Lee T (eds) 2002 First aid manual. Authorized manual of St John Ambulance, St Andrew's Ambulance Association and The British Red Cross. 8th edn. Dorling Kindersley, London

Moore T 2003 Suctioning techniques for the removal of respiratory secretions. Nursing Standard 18(9):47–53, Quiz 54–55. Erratum 2003, Nursing Standard 18(13):31

Moore T, Woodrow P 2004 High dependency nursing care. Routledge, London

Nicol M, Bavin C, Bedford-Turner S, Cronin P, Rawlings-Anderson K 2004 Essential nursing skills. 2nd edn. Mosby, Edinburgh

Sheppard M, Wright M 2006 Principles and practice of high dependency nursing. 2nd edn. Baillière Tindall, Edinburgh

Waugh A, Grant A 2006 Ross and Wilson's anatomy and physiology, 10th edn. Churchill Livingstone, Edinburgh

Woodrow P 2000 Intensive care nursing: a framework for practice. Routledge, London

Mobility and immobility

18

Christine Donnelly

Glossary terms

Active exercises
Dislocation
Flexibility
Fracture
Hazards of immobility
Immobility
Passive exercises
Sprain
Strain

Learning outcomes

This chapter will help you:

- Appreciate the roles that the musculoskeletal system plays in producing movement
- Describe the first aid interventions for fractures, dislocations, strains and sprains
- Understand the principles of safe handling and moving as applied to people
- Discuss the benefits of mobility across the lifespan
- Explain the principles of nursing care that will reduce the hazards of immobility
- Outline the principles of bedmaking
- Describe the roles of nurses, physiotherapists and occupational therapists in assisting people regain mobility.

Introduction

This chapter focuses on human movement and its importance to health. The introductory section provides an overview of the nervous and musculoskeletal systems and their role in movement. The musculoskeletal system comprises the bones, joints and skeletal muscles, each of which is briefly described. First aid for conditions affecting components of the musculoskeletal system is outlined and the principles of nursing care for people with casts, traction and external fixators are explained. The second section explores factors that influence balance, posture and movement. Development of the spinal curves and the importance of maintaining them are described. The next section extends the principles of safe handling and moving that were introduced in Chapter 13 to moving patients/clients, including the use of equipment such as hoists, glide sheets and transfer boards. Helping people to mobilize, including the use of walking aids and wheelchairs, is outlined. In the following section the benefits of mobility and the hazards of immobility are introduced and the problems that people of all ages may experience due to immobility are explained. Active and passive exercises are described. This chapter refers to others that provide more detail about potential hazards of immobility such as pressure ulcers (Ch. 25), deep vein thrombosis (Ch. 24) and constipation (Ch. 21). The principles of bedmaking are outlined. A multidisciplinary approach is normally taken to provide care for people with mobility problems and usually involves at least a physiotherapist and occupational therapist (OT) as well as the nursing team, and their role in promoting mobility is described in the final section.

The nervous and musculoskeletal systems

This section outlines the anatomy and physiology of the musculoskeletal and nervous systems and their roles in mobility. You should refer to your physiology text for more detail of the related anatomy and physiology and to Chapter 16 for a fuller explanation of disorders affecting the nervous system. First aid for fractures, dislocations, sprains and strains is described and the principles of nursing care for people with casts, traction and external fixators are explained. An overview of common disorders of muscles, bones and joints is included.

Nervous system

The nervous system consists of the brain, spinal cord and peripheral nerves that allow rapid communication throughout the body (see Fig. 16.2). Three types of nerve are responsible for conducting impulses:

- *Sensory nerves* from the skin, muscles and other tissues that send impulses to the spinal cord and brain
- *Motor nerves* that carry impulses in the opposite direction and are so-called because they stimulate muscles to contract; some stimulate glandular activity
- *Interneurones* that connect sensory and motor nerves.

Stimulation of motor nerves brings about contraction, or shortening, of the muscle supplied. When motor nerve stimulation stops, the muscle returns to its resting length. Since many motor nerves supply a single muscle, the spinal cord and brain can regulate the strength of a muscle contraction. When only a few muscle fibres (cells) are stimulated, the movement is not very forceful. However, if all the muscle fibres are stimulated at the same time, the contraction is much stronger. For example, moving one's hand gently stimulates fewer muscle fibres than when throwing a stick. Additionally, as different nerves transmit signals to muscle fibres at different speeds, some muscle actions are faster than others.

The musculoskeletal system

The structure and functions of the components of the musculoskeletal system are outlined, together with some common conditions that may affect them. Many of these disorders impair mobility.

Voluntary muscles

Voluntary (skeletal) muscles are those in the body that are attached to two bones with a movable joint between them. One of the bones is usually more stationary at a given moment than the other to allow movement to take place between them. Skeletal muscle has a striped appearance under microscopic examination and muscle tissue has four characteristics:

- *Contractility*, the ability to shorten
- *Extensibility*, the ability to lengthen
- *Excitability*, the ability to respond to nerve stimulation
- *Elasticity*, the ability to stretch and return to its original length.

Muscles come in different shapes and sizes depending on their function, and they usually have a thicker belly and a tendon at each end for attachment to bone (Fig. 18.1). The muscles around the mouth are circular, allowing the mouth to open and close fully during eating, whereas the muscles of the forearm are long and thin, allowing the wrist and fingers to flex while making a fist, and to extend during movements such as waving.

Postural muscles help to keep the upright posture or maintain positions for sustained periods of time and do not tire quickly. Examples include the muscles of the abdominal wall, buttocks and thighs. Active muscles are involved in movements such as typing, running and blinking. They allow muscles to respond appropriately to the tasks they perform but tend to tire quickly (Box 18.1). Muscle

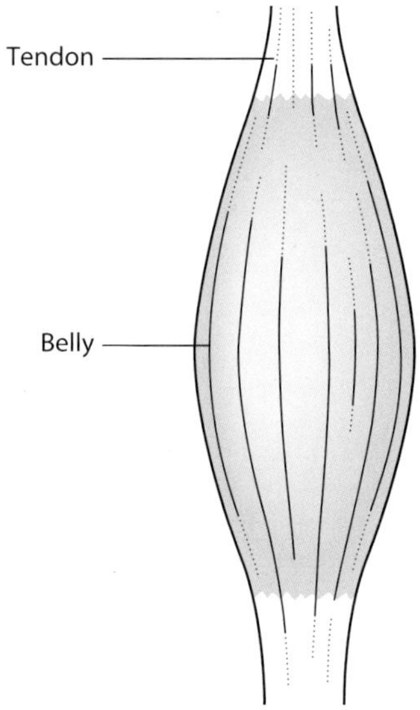

Fig. 18.1 A typical skeletal muscle (reproduced with permission from Greig & Rhind 2002)

REFLECTIVE PRACTICE Box 18.1

Understanding the musculoskeletal system

Student activities

1. Using skeletal muscles:
   - Try clenching your fist and see how quickly you begin to feel discomfort.
   - Now think of how long you can hold a poor sitting position without moving. These differences between muscles are important when exploring patient/client immobility of all ages.
2. Fascia:
   - Try this if you are wearing a jumper or T-shirt. Grasp the hem at one side, gathering a couple of inches of the hem together and pull down on the jumper. Observe how the stress lines from the pulled section spread upwards to the shoulder on the same side and also across to the opposite shoulder as well as along the hem towards to other hip.
3. Effects of postural habits on fascia:
   - Stand in front of a mirror and look at your posture, both front and side views. What do you notice about your posture? You may see that you have one shoulder higher than the other. You may notice that your head tends to lie towards one side or that your shoulders and hips are not aligned. This may be due to the way you carry your rucksack or bag. Do you have a habit of putting your bag on the same shoulder? Does your bag stay more easily on one shoulder than the other? Take a mental note of your own postural habits.
4. Consider the effects on your health of particular postural habits by using what you have learned from activities 1 and 2.

disorders are outlined in Table 18.1 and first aid interventions for strains and sprains, and their subsequent neurovascular checks, in Boxes 18.2 and 18.3, respectively.

Fascia

Fascia is formed from connective tissue, one of the four basic tissues in the body (the others being muscular, nervous and epithelial). Superficial fascia refers to the fatty tissue under the skin and deep fascia refers to the tissue that surrounds muscles, tendons and other organs. The superficial and deep fascias are connected to each other, and the deep fascia that surrounds muscle bellies and tendons is continuous throughout the body. It is incredible to think that the connective tissue surrounding the brain (the meninges) is connected to the fascia in the feet! This is the reason why people with painful knees can be diagnosed

Table 18.1 Disorders of the musculoskeletal system

Disorder	Causes and effects
Muscles	
Cerebral palsy	This condition is primarily neurological but is characterized by neuromuscular abnormalities It can be caused by brain damage due to hypoxia either before or during birth and results in impaired coordination and muscle control Intellect can be unaffected but because clients cannot articulate words easily care must be taken not to assume this is the case although learning disability is sometimes present
Muscular dystrophies	This is a general term used to describe genetically inherited conditions that lead to skeletal muscle wasting without any nerve damage Congenital muscular dystrophy can be present at birth or manifest within the first 6 months of life Signs include generalized muscle weakness and poor head control Duchenne muscular dystrophy is a rapidly progressive condition that only affects boys and is often fatal during adolescence; it is present from birth but may not become evident until around 4 years of age Not all muscular dystrophies are congenital (present from birth)
Strains	Strains occur during overexertion of all or part of a muscle, e.g. the calf muscles during jogging and other keep-fit exercises If a muscle is not warmed up adequately and too much work is demanded of the fibres, it becomes exhausted, and tightens and shortens The signs of muscle strains and the interventions required are shown in Box 18.2
Bones	
Fractures	A fracture is a break in the continuity of a bone, usually caused by excessive force being applied to it In simple fractures the skin remains intact; however, in compound fractures the broken bone protrudes through the skin Figure 18.4 shows different types of fracture: Spiral fractures are common in footballers and skiers because they tend to have the foot fixed in one position, and if the leg and body rotates sharply around it, this causes the bone to fracture (Fig. 18.4B). In comminuted fractures (Fig. 18.4C) there are many bone fragments due to severe damage at the fracture site Fractures are diagnosed by X-ray investigation: it can be difficult to diagnose fractures in children because their bones are softer and are more likely to bend than to break. Fractures of this type are called greenstick fractures (Fig. 18.4D) because the characteristics are similar to bending a green twig. The outer layers of the twig split, while the soft wood underneath only bends Some fractures occur around the epiphyseal plate (see Fig. 18.2). When there is still active bone growth, it is important that these fractures are carefully managed to ensure even growth of bone. Uneven bone growth along the epiphyseal plate will lead to problems with joint alignment, which in turn may cause mobility problems Box 18.5 shows the signs of fractures and the first aid treatment required
Osteoporosis	This condition is characterized by bone fragility, porosity and an increased risk of fractures, especially of the wrist, vertebrae and hip, particularly in women In the UK, one in two women and one in five men over the age of 50 will suffer a fracture due to osteoporosis (National Osteoporosis website, see p. 528) Box 18.4 outlines some of the measures that can be taken to maintain bone density, which will reduce the effects of osteoporosis
Rickets and osteomalacia	These conditions are often referred to as 'sick bones' and result from vitamin D deficiency Both terms refer to the same condition, known as rickets in children and osteomalacia in adults In the UK, people most at risk of vitamin D deficiency are those who get little exposure to sunlight; vulnerable groups include people who cover their limbs for cultural/religious reasons, e.g. Moslems, especially women and children, and older adults who are housebound or resident in nursing homes Lack of vitamin D can lead to generalized bone pain and muscle weakness In children there may be enlarged bone ends, particularly in the wrists, that cause lasting deformity.
Joints	
Arthritis	Inflammation of joints associated with pain, swelling and restricted movement Osteoarthritis: a degenerative disorder usually of weight-bearing synovial joints that commonly accompanies the ageing process, usually due to 'wear and tear' or less often following a previous injury

(Continued)

Table 18.1 *(Continued)*

Disorder	Causes and effects
	Rheumatoid arthritis: this condition also affects most body systems. Initially the affected synovial joints are often the fingers and wrists; later the larger joints, e.g. the hip, also become affected
Dislocations	Dislocations occur when bones are displaced and the joint can no longer function They may be caused when excessive force is placed on a bone, pulling it out of alignment, or excessive pulling on a joint that causes the ligaments to tear A partial dislocation (subluxation) requires the same treatment as a full dislocation (see Box 18.5)
Sprains	Sprains arise when damage to the ligaments that surround a joint occurs (see Fig. 18.7) Damaged ligaments weaken a joint and may leave it prone to further injury or dislocation Damage around the joint may also cause bleeding within it A common cause of sprains to the neck is a whiplash injury commonly sustained in car accidents. This results from a sudden jerking back of the head and neck causing damage to the ligaments, vertebrae and nerves in the neck region Signs of sprains and first aid treatment are shown in Box 18.2
Movement and gait	
Parkinson's disease	This condition is named after Dr James Parkinson (1755–1824) who first identified this progressive neurological disorder, which affects movements such as walking, talking and writing It is typified by tremor, muscle rigidity or stiffness and bradykinesia that typically cause hesitancy in walking, characterized by a shuffling gait and the absence of arm swinging, accelerated walking which can result in falls and difficulty in carrying out fine movements such as buttoning a shirt
Parkinsonism	This describes the symptoms of Parkinson's disease that occur, e.g. following a stroke, or as the result of medication, e.g. chlorpromazine for severe mental distress

FIRST AID Box 18.2

Strains and sprains

Recognition

- Pain
- Reduced function, especially if a joint is affected
- Swelling and bruising.

Treatment (acronym RICE)

- **R**est and support the injured limb in the most comfortable position
- **I**ce is applied to reduce pain and swelling. A pack of frozen vegetables wrapped in a clean tea towel, laid on the affected area for short periods, is very effective
- **C**ompression is applied to reduce swelling. Apply a bandage or compress to the affected limb. The compress can be soaked in Arnica solution, which reduces bruising, made by mixing 10 drops of mother tincture with 250 mL cold water
- **E**levate the affected limb on pillows to reduce swelling
- Check for adequate circulation (see Box 18.3)
- If the casualty is in severe pain or cannot use the affected limb, send to hospital
- Take the casualty to hospital if the pain and swelling do not subside within 24 hours.

with back problems. If the fascia has been damaged in one area, the effects can often be found elsewhere in the body.

Your jumper (see Box 18.1) is a good analogy for the reactions that occur in the fascia when it is shortened

NURSING SKILLS Box 18.3

Neurovascular checks

These are also sometimes referred to as circulation, sensation and movement (CSM) checks, which are carried out to confirm that a cast, bandage or other intervention does not restrict the local circulation. They are carried out as a first aid measure, following discharge with a new cast and in hospital settings.

The frequency is determined by the type of intervention, the extent of damage, any local policy and reduced over time if observations are within expected levels for the particular patient. Any abnormalities (trends or sudden changes) are reported immediately to the charge nurse. The area, often an extremity, distal to the cast is checked for:

- *Temperature*: The area should be warm. Cool or cold fingers are abnormal and may be the result of restricted blood supply to the area.
- *Colour*: The area should be pink. Mottling and white or bluish colour is abnormal and results from impaired blood supply to the affected area.
- *Sensation*: There should be normal feeling in the area. Any tingling, alteration or loss of sensation is abnormal and may be due to compression of nerves due to local swelling.
- *Movement*: The amount of movement of the area. Although this may be restricted, any decrease in previous mobility is abnormal.

or 'knotted' through injury. Have you ever felt knots in your shoulder muscles? Did this affect the arm on that side? The effects of postural change may be distant from the original injury. Understanding that fascia is continuous throughout the body helps to understand some of the problems faced by patients/clients who are immobile or trying to regain mobility following illness or injury. The postural characteristics identified earlier have arisen because the muscles and their surrounding fascia have adapted to your habits and protect the shoulder joint from further injury.

These changes are seldom seen in children because their muscles are more elastic and the fascia returns to a near normal position. They also recover more easily from injuries and awkward movements without obvious lasting effect. Fascia stiffens with age. The longer standing a postural habit, the more the fascia adapts to the preferred, habitual position. Understanding that everyone has habits that affect the underlying muscles and tissues also helps to appreciate mobility difficulties that people may have. This knowledge not only helps nurses to move patients/clients more appropriately but also helps them to understand why someone may complain of hip pain when the problem may originate in their shoulder.

Bones

Bones are dynamic, living structures with nerve and blood supplies. The main functions of bones are to:

- Support soft tissue and provide attachment for muscles
- Protect internal organs from injury
- Allow movement at joints as the muscles attached to them contract.

A typical long bone, such as those of the limbs, has a shaft and two epiphyses (Fig. 18.2). Bone growth takes place at each end of the shaft at the epiphyseal plate. This region consists of cartilage until bone growth is complete when it ossifies. Muscle tendons attach to the outer covering of bone, the periosteum. Hyaline cartilage replaces periosteum at the ends of long bones that form synovial joints.

Before birth the long bones consist mainly of cartilage (Fig. 18.3), which is a tough connective tissue. During pregnancy and early childhood, cartilage is gradually replaced by bone tissue. This process is called ossification and takes place at centres of ossification, initially in the bone shaft and at the epiphyses after birth. Until growth is complete, bones increase in both length and diameter, and a rich blood supply provides the nutrients and energy for the necessary cell division to take place. Several hormones, including growth hormone and thyroid hormones (thyroxine, tri-iodothyronine), are important in growth and development of bones, especially in infancy and childhood, and excessive or impaired secretion results in abnormal bone development. In time, ossification is

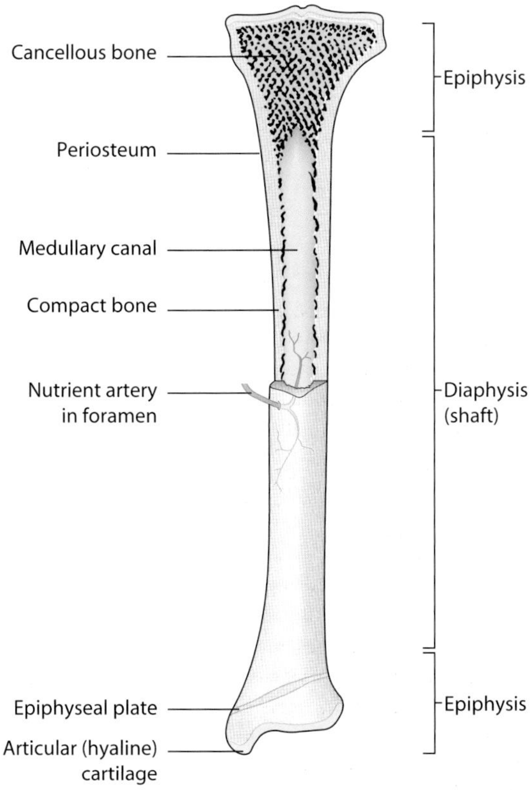

Fig. 18.2 A typical long bone (reproduced with permission from Waugh & Grant 2006)

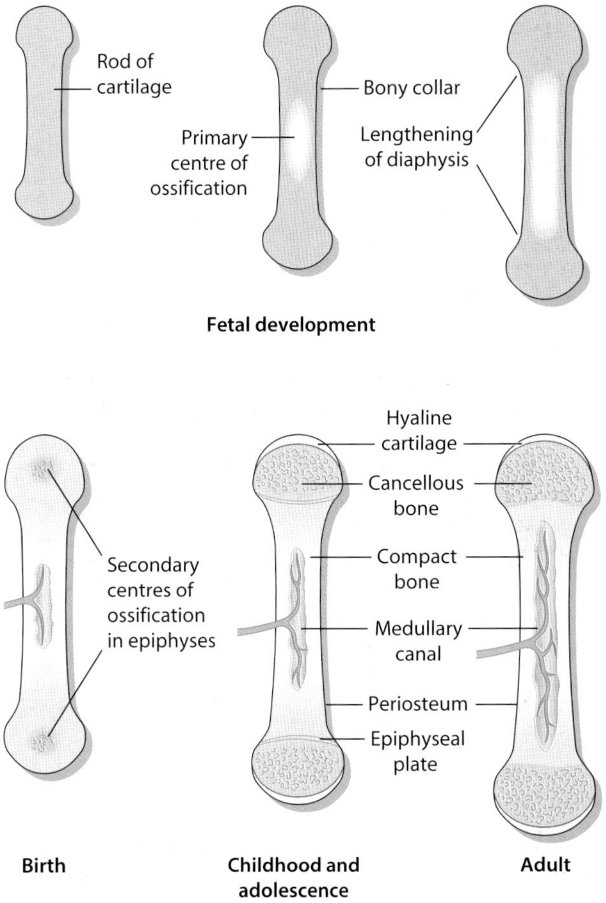

Fig. 18.3 Stages of development of a long bone (reproduced with permission from Waugh & Grant 2006)

sufficient to allow walking to be achieved. Although cartilage offers some protection to the vital organs, it behaves like stiff plastic, having a degree of flexibility, as it does not have the rigid hardness of bone. As a result, children's vital organs are more prone to injury if they fall or are shaken than those of adults and their bones tend to bend, rather than break, causing greenstick fractures (see Fig. 18.4).

At puberty, there is often a sudden increase in bone growth due to the increase in production of the sex hormones testosterone and oestrogen. By the late teenage years, ossification is largely complete. Bones are not fully hardened until their growth stops at about 18 years in females and 25 years in males. Bone mass reaches its peak around 30 years of age. It is important to maintain a lifestyle that maximizes bone density in order to reduce the effects of reduction in later life (Box 18.4). The hardness of adult bone protects vital organs such as the brain, spinal cord, heart and lungs from injury.

Once bone growth is complete, bones continue to replace old bone tissue with new, a process known as remodelling. For example, the lower third of the femur (thigh bone) replaces itself every 4 months in young adults. Following a fracture, new bone tissue is laid down to repair the break. Box 18.5 describes the treatment required for fractures. Bone mass begins to decrease after about 35–40 years of age. In some people the loss of bone mass is excessive and leads to a condition called osteoporosis. Bone disorders are outlined in Table 18.1.

Care of people wearing casts, external fixators or traction

This section introduces the roles of casts, external fixators and traction in immobilizing joints and fractured bones and the principles of nursing care are outlined.

People should be as fully participant in their care as possible, particularly as they will need support and encouragement to adapt to their altered body image, whether it is temporary or permanent and regardless of age. This can be particularly challenging during puberty, which brings about many body changes that can be difficult enough for adolescents to deal with, without the added complication

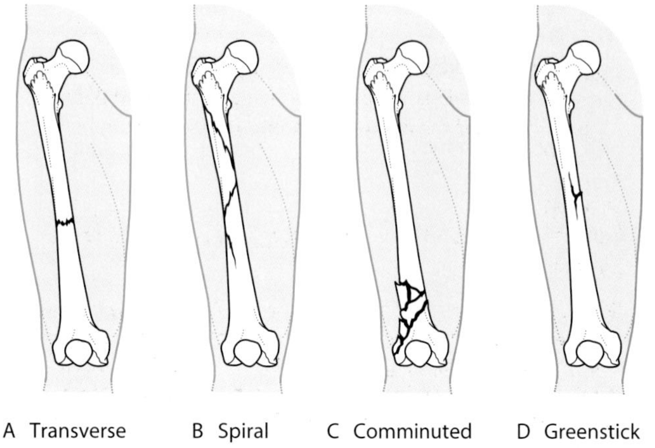

Fig. 18.4 Types of simple fracture

HEALTH PROMOTION Box 18.4

Promoting bone health

To promote bone mass:

- Eat a calcium-rich diet with foods such as milk, cheese and yoghurt (low fat varieties are high in calcium)
- Take regular weight-bearing exercise such as walking, jogging or aerobics for 20 minutes at least three times per week. It is important to be aware that excessive exercise in those with a low body weight and/or eating disorders may result in low oestrogen levels, which means that optimal bone mass is not achieved, predisposing to osteoporosis
- Give up smoking
- Limit alcohol intake to 21 units per week for men and 14 units per week for women
- Avoid consuming excessive amounts of retinol (vitamin A) that is found in fish and dairy products as it is thought to increase the risk of fractures in later life. Vitamin A found in vegetables as carotene is safe.

The National Osteoporosis Society

Student activities

Visit the National Osteoporosis Society website (www.nos.org.uk Available July 2006) and find out:

- How hormone replacement therapy affects bone density.
- Why older adults are advised to increase their intake of calcium and vitamin D.
- The current treatment strategies for people with osteoporosis.

FIRST AID Box 18.5

Fractures and dislocations

Recognition

The cardinal signs of a fracture or dislocation are:

- Pain
- Swelling
- Possible deformity
- Loss of function.

Treatment

This follows the RICE principles outlined in Box 18.2 (p. 504):

- Immobilize the affected limb
- If a bone is protruding through the skin, cover with a clean, wet cloth and place a strand-free dressing round the protruding bone until it is higher than the bone before applying a bandage
- Do not give the casualty anything to eat or drink in case an anaesthetic is required
- Casualties with suspected fractures or dislocations must be sent to hospital.

of being 'different' from their peers because they have to wear a bulky plaster or stay in bed in traction.

- *Care of patients wearing a cast*: Patients who have sustained simple fractures (see Table 18.1 and Fig. 18.4) usually have the fracture immobilized using a lightweight plaster. However, if the plaster needs to be changed after a few days because swelling has reduced, Plaster of Paris (PoP) may be used as it is cheaper and easily removed. It is usually replaced with a harder-wearing, lightweight, waterproof plaster. The principles of care are the same, whichever type of plaster is used (Box 18.6).
- *Care of patients with external fixators* (Fig. 18.5): External fixation is a method of immobilizing fractures that involves insertion of pins above and below the fracture. The pins are secured to external rods. Pin sites are cared for using the principles shown in Box 18.7. After assembly, neurovascular checks (see Box 18.3) are carried out to ensure local circulation is not impaired and that any swelling is not causing nerve compression. The affected limb is raised to minimize swelling and supported using pillows.

NURSING SKILLS Box 18.6

Care of people wearing casts

- Once a plaster has been applied the affected limb is supported on a waterproof pillow, covered by a towel to absorb moisture. The pillow also provides gentle elevation to reduce swelling.
- Fingers or toes are cleaned to remove any debris so that CSM checks (see Box 18.3) can be carried out at regular intervals and any changes or abnormalities reported.
- The person should be encouraged to change their position hourly so that the plaster dries evenly, on all sides.
- When assisting the person to move their affected limb, only the palms of the hands should be used. This avoids causing indentations from thumbs or fingers on the inside of the plaster that could cause pressure on the skin underneath, leading to a pressure ulcer.
- Nothing should ever be inserted inside a plaster to relieve itching, e.g. knitting needles or rulers. These can damage the skin or become lodged in the plaster, causing ulceration, infection or pressure damage.
- The plaster should be kept dry during personal hygiene activities by covering with a plastic bag. This is also important for waterproof plasters, because the lining material is not waterproof.
- Physiotherapists or experienced nurses supply people with appropriate walking aids if a lower limb is in plaster and teach patients how to use them correctly.
- People wearing plasters can usually be discharged early with an outpatient appointment so that progress can be monitored.
- Education plays a vital role in compliance with treatment as the person must be able to care for their own limb and plaster, and identify early warning signs of complications. It is important to involve people in their care and to provide the necessary information both verbally and in writing. Nurses should check that the person understands what is required of them and that emergency contact numbers are prominently displayed on the information sheets.

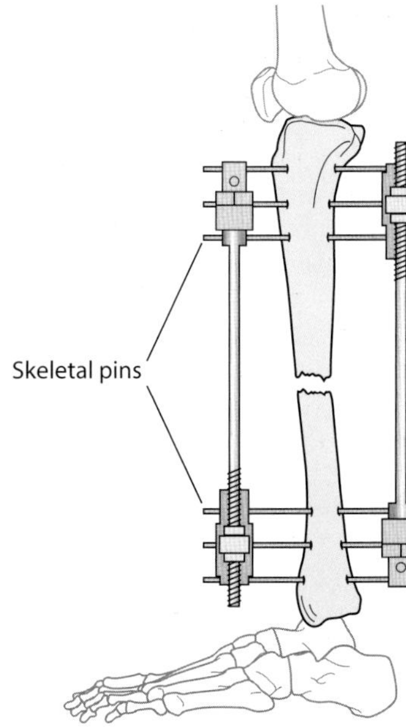

Fig. 18.5 An external fixator (reproduced with permission from Brooker & Nicol 2003)

NURSING SKILLS Box 18.7

Care of pin sites

External fixators and skeletal traction involve the use of stainless steel pins and the insertion sites require specific care because infection of the bone (osteomyelitis) into which they are inserted is a serious complication.

- Frequent observation is carried out as per local policy to detect early signs of inflammation, e.g. redness or swelling, or movement within the bone.
- Cleaning and dressing is performed according to local policy. The evidence for this is largely inconclusive.
- A small non-adhesive dressing is usually applied if there is leakage and the nature and amount are recorded in the nursing notes.

Student activity

Using the resources below, find out more about the care of pin sites.

[Resources: Smith M 2003 Nursing patients with musculoskeletal disorders. In: Brooker C, Nicol M (eds) Nursing adults: the practice of caring. Mosby, Edinburgh, Chapter 27; Temple J, Santy J 2004 Pin site care for preventing infections associated with external bone fixators and pins. Cochrane Database of Systematic Reviews 1:CD004551]

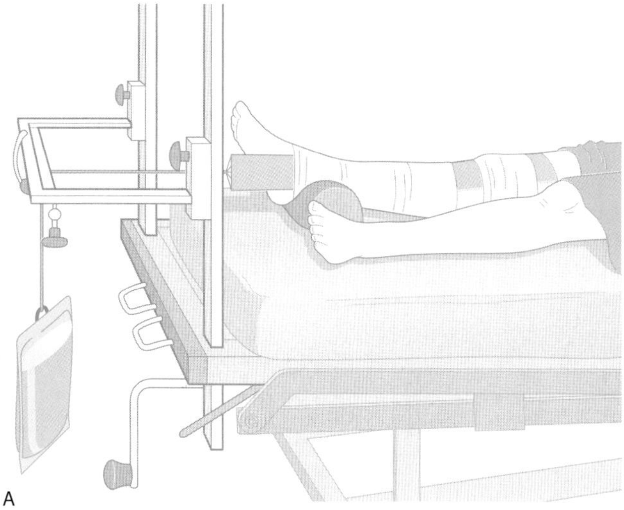

A

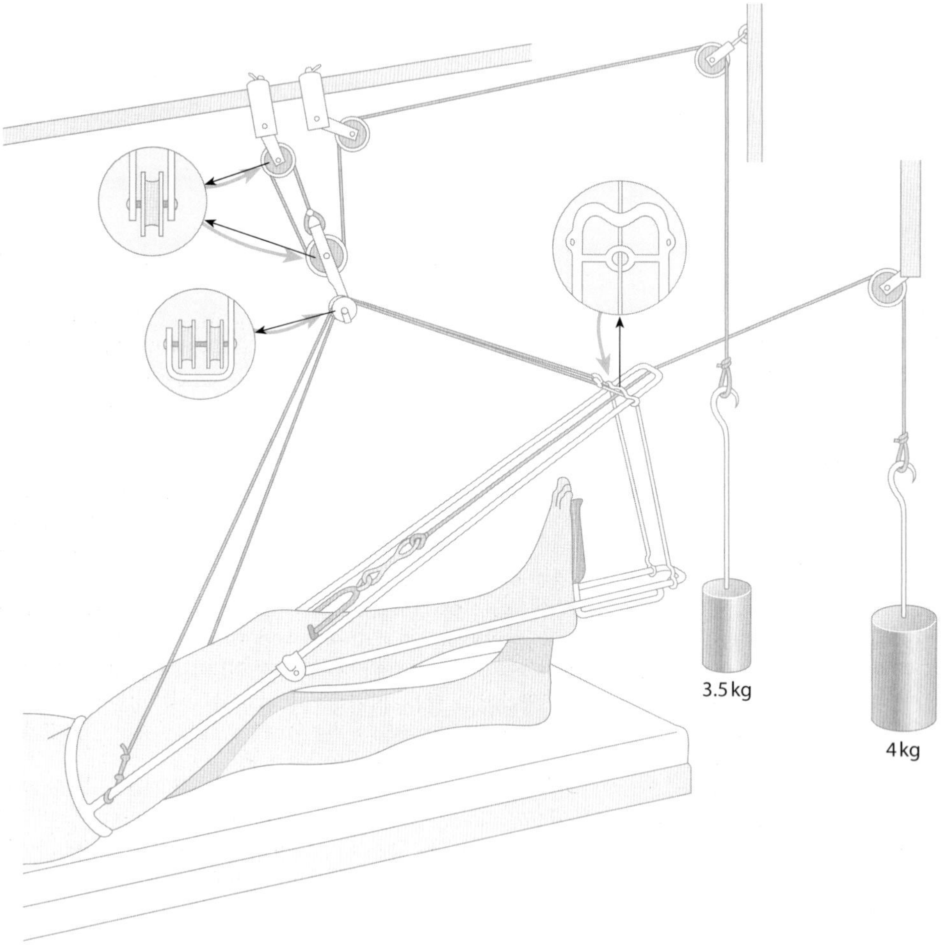

B

Fig. 18.6 Types of traction: **A**. Straight leg skin traction. **B**. Skeletal traction (reproduced with permission from Brooker & Nicol 2003)

- *Principles of care for patients in traction*: Traction is the application of a force (or 'pull') on bones that keeps them and their associated joints in correct alignment. It can be applied to either the skin or skeletal system and both types confine the patient to bed. Figure 18.6 shows different types of traction that can be used to treat fractures or joint injuries. In skin traction the pull is applied via adhesive straps attached to the skin of the legs. In skeletal traction, either pins are inserted through the bone below the fracture or a splint is applied to the lower limb and in both cases a system of pulleys is applied. Pin care is outlined in Box 18.7. The skin under a splint needs extra care to prevent development of pressure ulcers. In traction where weights are applied and hang over the end of the bed, the patient's body provides the

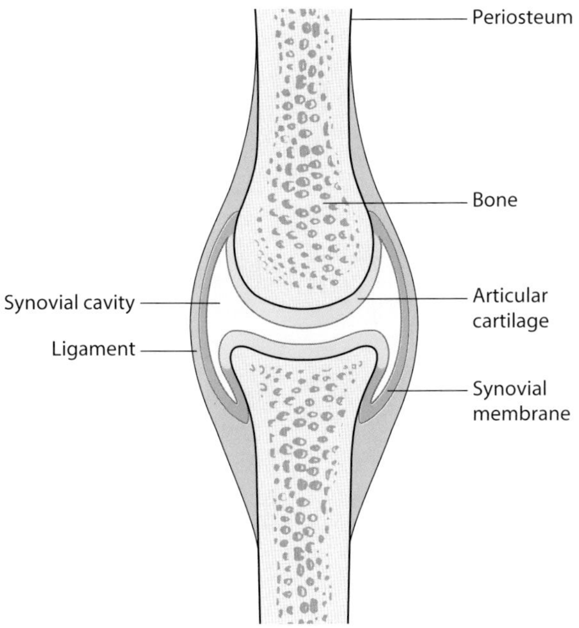

Fig. 18.7 Typical synovial joint (reproduced with permission from Waugh & Grant 2006)

Box 18.8 Movements possible at synovial joints

Movement	Definition
Flexion	Bending, usually forward but occasionally backward, e.g. the knee joint
Extension	Straightening or bending backward
Abduction	Movement away from the midline of the body
Adduction	Movement towards the midline of the body
Circumduction	Movement of a limb or digit so it describes the shape of a cone
Rotation	Movement round the long axis of a bone
Pronation	Turning the palm of the hand down
Supination	Turning the palm of the hand up
Inversion	Turning the sole of the foot inwards
Eversion	Turning the sole of the foot outwards

From Waugh & Grant (2006).

countertraction. It is essential to ensure that traction is maintained by keeping the weights hanging free. It is therefore important to ascertain the nursing care required for the particular type of traction in use and to understand how it is maintained. Enforced immobility conferred by traction increases the risk of hazards of immobility (see Box 18.18, p. 525), e.g. pressure ulcers, and patients are assessed for this risk and appropriate interventions carried out to reduce the effects of pressure (see Ch. 25).

Joints

Joints, or articulations, occur between bones. They hold the bones securely together but may also allow movement. Some joints hold bones together very tightly and do not permit movement, e.g. the sutures of the skull, whereas others, e.g. the hip and shoulder joints, allow a range of movement. This chapter focuses on synovial joints because they are most involved in body movement. It is these movable (synovial) joints that cause most discomfort and pain, and that most often affect mobility if they become diseased or out of alignment.

Figure 18.7 shows a typical synovial joint. The bone ends are covered in hyaline cartilage, which is smooth and shiny. It aids movement between the bones. The joint cavity is lined with synovial membrane and inside is a small amount of synovial fluid, which lubricates the joint. Ligaments consist of white, fibrous tissue and hold the bones together. They are not very elastic and so restrict the amount of movement available and stabilize the joint. Joints are further supported and protected by surrounding muscles, which prevent dislocation (see p. 504) and help to maintain upright posture. Ligaments attach to the periosteum of bones and cross the joint cavity. Twisting a joint, e.g. the ankle, may stretch and tear the ligaments and is known as a sprain.

Muscles work together in antagonistic pairs to allow movements to take place at a joint. Contraction of one of a pair of antagonistic muscles brings about one specific movement and the opposite movement is caused by contraction of the opposing muscle, e.g. the biceps and triceps in the upper arm.

Box 18.8 lists the types of movement available at some joints and Figure 18.8 illustrates some of them. Knowing these movements is important for carrying out passive exercises (movements of joints initiated by an external force, e.g. physiotherapist or nurse, to exercise muscles and joints, see p. 525) or encouraging patients/clients to practise active exercises (movements initiated by an individual that exercise muscles and joints, see p. 525). When caring for people with mobility problems it is important to know the range of movements available at different joints so that they are not moved into positions that could be harmful. This is particularly important when caring for unconscious patients, or following joint replacement surgery. Common joint disorders are outlined in Table 18.1.

Posture, balance and movement

For purposeful movement the body must move in a synchronized manner, with the nervous and musculoskeletal systems working together to ensure that movements are smooth and coordinated, and of the appropriate force for the intended task. To understand why problems with movement occur, it is necessary to know how normal upright posture develops and the principles of human movement and balance. This section explores these areas.

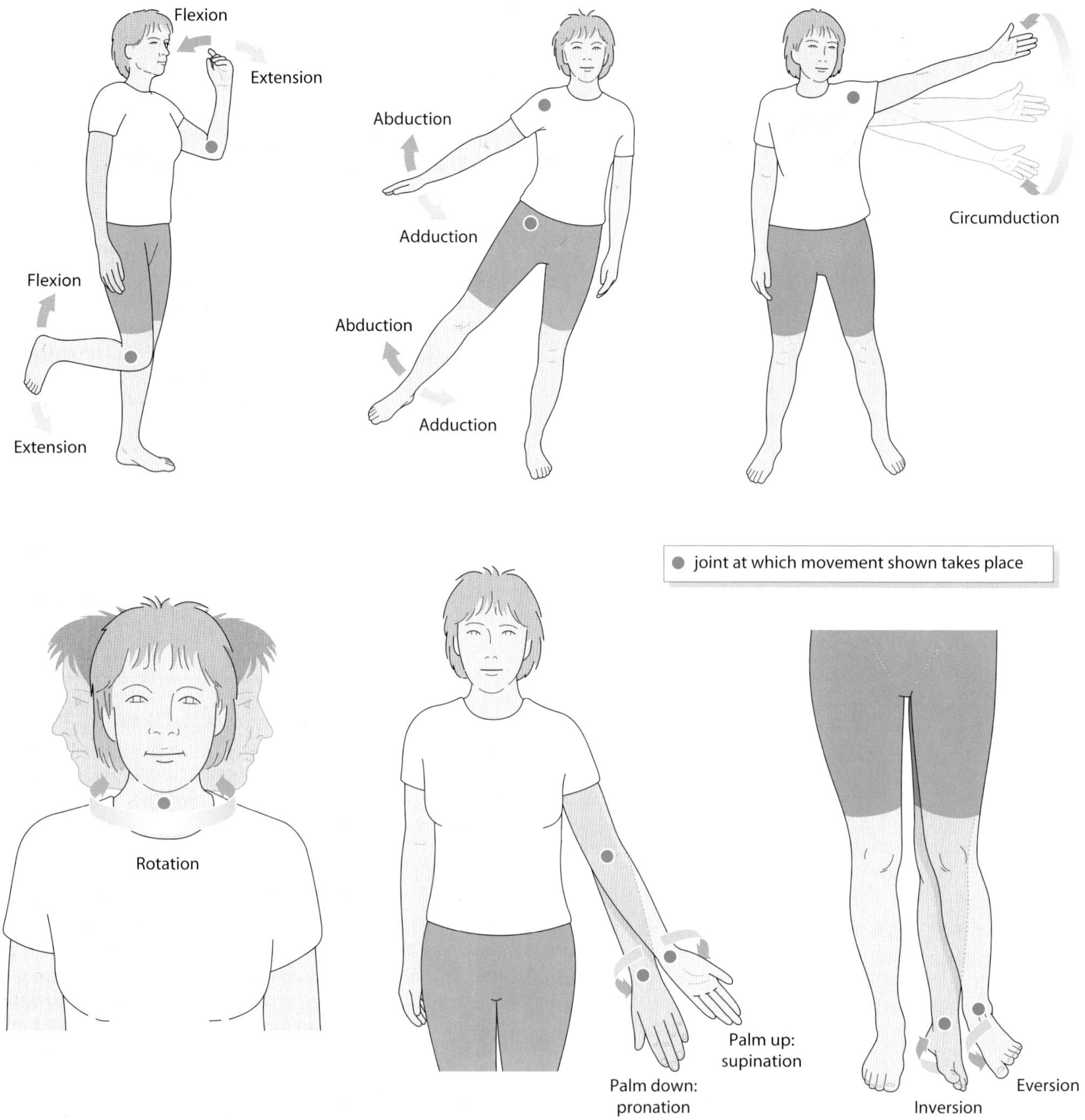

Fig. 18.8 Main movements possible at synovial joints (reproduced with permission from Waugh & Grant 2006)

Development of the spinal curves

Babies are born with one 'C' shaped spinal curve, which is convex posteriorly. They are unable to control movement of the head, arms or legs and depend on natural reflexes to bring about movement, e.g. the rooting reflex where, in response to lightly touching the side of the cheek, a baby turns its head to that side and begins to suck until the reflex disappears, usually at about 3–4 months of age. The head and spine must be well supported when young babies are moved. At about 6 weeks, babies' eyes begin to follow colours and movements. This is accompanied by reflex movements in the back of the neck that strengthen the muscles there. Gradually, the neck muscles become bulkier and stronger, and begin to pull the cervical vertebrae and associated muscles into a secondary concave curve, the cervical curve (Fig. 18.9). This enables the head to move from side to side. As babies learn to turn their heads, the muscles around the neck strengthen further and they begin to hold their heads steady on their shoulders for short periods. This is the first stage in developing head control. Gradually thereafter the shoulder muscles strengthen, enabling the muscles of the upper arm to

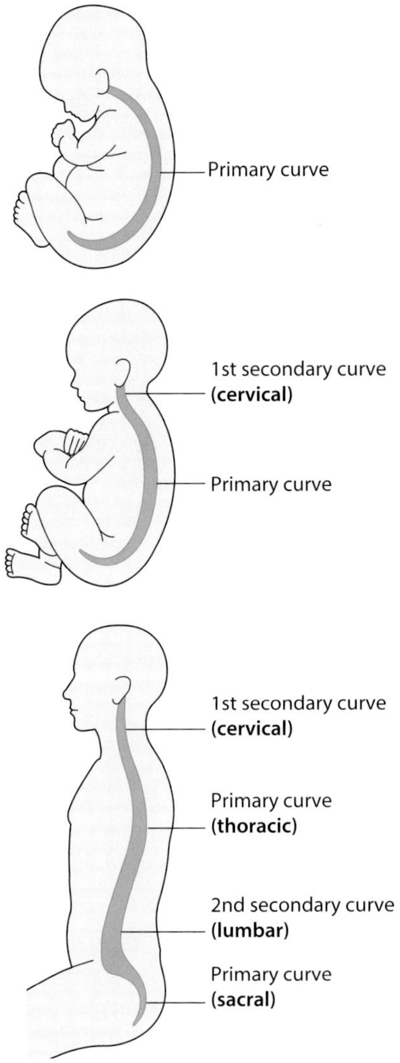

Fig. 18.9 The spinal curves (reproduced with permission from Waugh & Grant 2006)

become stronger, leading to more purposeful movements of the upper limbs.

At about 3–6 months the baby learns to sit up, but the back is still very rounded. At this age the baby begins to roll from side to side (Box 18.9). This rotational movement around the spine develops the muscles of the lower back, leading to the development of the secondary concave lumbar spine (see Fig. 18.9), which in turn allows the pelvic girdle to be suspended in its correct position at the bottom of the spine.

Only when the spine has achieved the lumbar curve can the child begin to walk and graduate to the toddler stage. Eventually the muscles of the upper and lower legs and feet begin to strengthen and the child develops the upright posture. The spinal curves bring the centre of gravity into a straight line (see Fig. 18.9), which allows the body weight to be evenly distributed and helps to maintain balance in all movements.

The thoracic and sacral curves are known as primary curves because they retain the initial convex 'C' shape.

HEALTH PROMOTION Box 18.9

Preventing childhood accidents

From the time that babies can roll over, at 3–6 months of age, they are at risk of rolling off a surface if left unattended. A child's environment needs to be organized to minimize the risk of accidents.

- Children under the age of 5 and people over 65 (particularly those over 75) are most likely to have an accident at home
- 0–4 year olds have the most accidents at home; boys are more likely to have accidents than girls
- Falls are the most common accidents in the home
- Childhood injuries are closely linked with social deprivation and are most common in children from poorer backgrounds (RoSPA).

Student activities

Visit the RoSPA website (www.rospa.org.uk Available July 2006) and find out:

- The reasons why children of different ages are at risk from accidents.
- The precautions that will minimize accidents to children of different ages at home.

The cervical and lumbar curves are known as secondary curves because they develop a concave curvature. A child with severe cerebral palsy, who has poor head control, cannot learn how to make meaningful movements with the rest of their body.

Maintaining the spinal curves

Good posture means that the four spinal curves (cervical, thoracic, lumbar and sacral) are in alignment, with the legs suspended from the pelvis. Strong abdominal and back muscles will help to support the spine in a good position. Weak abdominal muscles allow the pelvis to tilt forwards and the lumbar curve to become exaggerated. Habits that encourage the spine to move out of alignment will affect posture because, over time, the fascia adapts to the repeated, sustained tension in the underlying muscles, leading to discomfort and pain. Therefore, people who usually stand bearing most of their weight through one leg and foot, rather than spreading it equally between both legs and feet, will find their spine moves out of alignment affecting their posture.

Tall children tend to droop their shoulders and keep their heads down, to avoid standing 'head and shoulders' above their classmates. Carrying heavy school bags on one shoulder can also lead to adaptive shortening of fascia and muscle tissue around that shoulder. The incidence of low back, neck and shoulder problems arising in schoolchildren has increased so much that some European countries demand that children are issued with bags that have straps for both shoulders and that they are fitted with wheels so that the bag can be pulled rather than carried if it is heavy. Lockers should also be provided in schools so

HEALTH PROMOTION — Box 18.10

Recommended position for sitting at a computer

These nine steps should be followed when you sit at a computer or workstation:

1. Sit well back in the seat, and adjust the angle and height of the backrest so that your back is well supported.
2. Make sure that the small of your back is well supported.
3. Adjust the height of your chair so that your forearms are approximately horizontal when you use the keyboard.
4. Check that your wrists are in a neutral position.
5. Check that your feet are flat on the floor or use a footrest to take the pressure off the back of your thighs.
6. Make sure the area under your desk is free of clutter so that your feet can move freely.
7. Check that the height and angle of the screen allow you to hold your head in a comfortable position.
8. Use a document holder if you do a lot of copy typing.
9. Make sure that your work area is large enough to accommodate your books and other study materials so that you have enough space to support your arms when you are not using your keyboard.

Working-Well

Student activities

Visit the Working-Well website (www.working-well.org Available July 2006) and work through the exercises there to ensure your workstation is correctly organized.

that pupils only have to carry the books required for one class at any time.

Peer pressure (see Ch. 8) and the need to conform to fit in with a group can have lasting effects on people's posture and mobility. Teenagers tend to slouch, when both standing and sitting, and girls may also slouch because they are embarrassed by development of breasts and comments made by others. It can therefore be difficult to maintain a good posture if it makes an individual stand out from the crowd. However, posture is more than just the ability to stand or sit in a good upright position: it is a balanced action of muscles to maintain all parts of the body in positions that do not involve undue strain, and from which immediate coordinated action of any part of the body is possible.

Normally, babies and toddlers do not have problems with posture unless they are born with an abnormality that predisposes to problems with mobility, such as cerebral palsy, developmental dysplasia of the hip (previously called congenital dislocation of the hip) or a missing limb. However, as children grow older they become more aware of adult habits and often copy them. This is when problems with posture can begin.

Sitting at a computer for long periods also affects the curves of the lower back and neck. Depending on how the head is held while looking at the screen, the other spinal curves alter to try to keep the upper body balanced. For example, in a sitting position, the eyes should be level with the top of the screen so that the head is level. If the head is tilted backwards in order to look upwards, the lumbar spine curvature will be increased, causing both neck and lower back problems. This is why the Health and Safety Executive (see Ch. 13) have regulations about how people should sit when using computers (Box 18.10). The longer people sit at computers in a poor posture, the more likely they are to develop neck, back and other joint problems. It is particularly important for children not to spend too long sitting at a computer because of the damage they can do to their still developing bones and joints. However, the trend for computer games and careers in IT encourages many people to spend long hours at the computer, often without much thought of how this will impinge on their long-term health.

As two-legged upright beings, humans are constantly at the mercy of gravity trying to pull them nearer to the ground. During the course of a day, people lose height as the spine continually counteracts the effects of gravity on their bodies. Water loss from the intervertebral discs (the pads of cartilage between the vertebrae) is another contributing factor. However, after a night's sleep the discs swell again and by the morning, height is regained. Therefore, when measuring a patient's/client's height and weight (see Ch. 14), it is advisable to do this at the same time of day, so that the same conditions prevail. This is particularly important when children are being assessed and/or treated for problems with growth and development.

Effects of ageing on the spinal curves

As part of the normal ageing process, the effects of gravity begin to take their toll on the musculoskeletal system. The 'elderly people crossing' road sign depicts older adults walking with stooped posture and using walking sticks. Although not appropriate for the majority of older adults, this sign clearly demonstrates the combined effects of poor posture and gravity on the musculoskeletal system. There is, however, nothing wrong with stooped posture, as long as the position is not sustained for lengthy periods. Anatomically, the stooped posture is exactly the opposite of upright posture. Muscles work in antagonistic pairs (see p. 509) and when one of the pair is contracting the opposing group relaxes. In the upright posture the muscles classified as extensors (that act to straighten joints) are active, whereas in a stooped posture the flexor muscles (that act to bend joints) are active. Movement between both of these postures is recommended in order to ensure good blood flow to each group of muscles. Regular changes in posture mean that muscle shape also changes between short, fat and tense in the contracted state, to longer, thinner and more pliable in the resting state. This increases blood flow to, through and from the muscles and improves oxygen exchange (see Ch. 17) between the blood and the muscles. At the same time waste products are removed from the muscles. This maintains optimum health of the muscles and their surrounding fascia. Try to move regularly between the upright and slouched postures while reading the rest of this chapter.

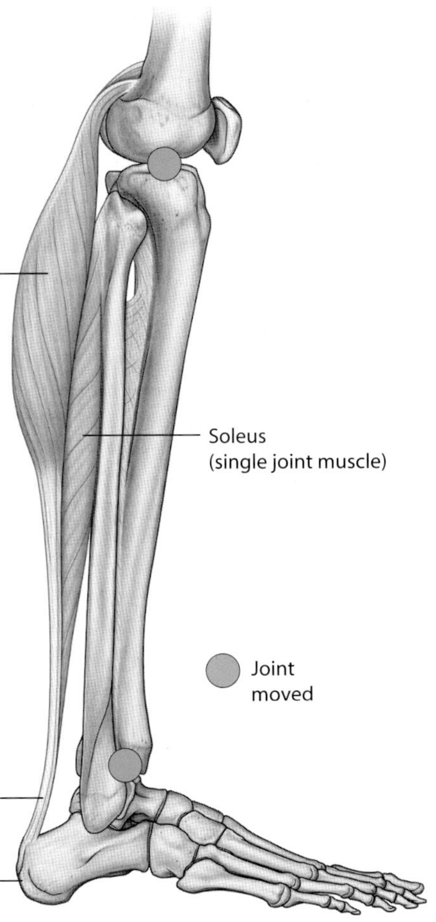

Fig. 18.10 One- and two-joint muscles of the lower leg (reproduced with permission from Drake et al 2005)

Movement

Movement is brought about by the actions of muscles on joints. Some muscles act on more than one joint and these are the most active in producing movements. Single joint muscles are the deeper, postural muscles (e.g. soleus) and two-joint muscles are the more superficial, active muscles (e.g. gastrocnemius) (Fig. 18.10). This arrangement of muscles helps to produce coordinated movement. For a more detailed explanation of the mechanics and physiology of human movement see, for example, Trew and Everett (2001).

Gait

Gait is the term used to describe the manner in which people walk or run. A person's gait can be analysed in a laboratory, which can assist in the diagnosis and treatment of mobility problems such as arthritis. Gait varies depending on:

- People's movement habits
- The ways in which individuals' muscles and fascia have adapted to their habits over time
- Age
- The presence of disease or abnormalities that affect nerves, bones, muscles and/or joints.

Balance is the key to walking. The balance reflexes do not begin to develop until about 6 months of age and, as toddlers begin to walk around 12–13 months (Wong et al 2001), their gait is quite different from that of adults. Children under the age of about 2 years walk with flat feet and their legs more widely apart. About the age of 4 years, children begin to develop the arm swing. As the more balanced adult gait of striking the ground with the heel first and swinging the arms develops, the pace of step and step length increase. This is often lost in Parkinson's disease (see Table 18.1). If someone has a particular way of putting one foot down on the ground, then the other foot has to alter its pattern of movement to accommodate for this.

As posture is about maintaining dynamic balance, whatever happens in one part of the body affects the movement in another part. A Trendelenburg gait is characterized by leaning to the affected side every time the opposite leg swings through to take a step, which is caused by unilateral weakness of hip abductor muscles (gluteals). In older people, the pace of walking and the step length generally decrease. Older adults often suffer from gait disorders that have many causes, one of which may be a fear of falling (Alexander & Goldberg 2005).

Age and disability are the two major factors contributing to changes in gait because both affect posture and balance. Degenerative changes around the hip also tend to reduce stride length. People gradually lose the ability to maintain their balance as they age; therefore, in order to provide a larger base for support to maintain balance, the width of the step also increases slightly.

The joints tend to stiffen with age, which reduces the range of movement. If this happens around the ankle it becomes more difficult to lift the foot free from the ground, leading to dragging of the toes that can predispose to falls. Finally, joint stiffness also affects the spine, leading to loss of rotation and arm swing. Reduction in both of these elements slows the walking speed.

Joint problems that affect gait may be reversible with surgical intervention and include arthritic joints, flat foot (pes planus) and bunions (hallux valgus). Foot drop is another cause that results from compression damage to the peroneal nerve caused by, for example, a prolapsed ('slipped') intervertebral disc. Joint and muscle pain will affect gait. Pain in the hip(s) or knee(s) causes people to spend less time weight-bearing on the affected joint. Fibromyalgia (muscle, tendon and joint pain) and myasthenia gravis (an autoimmune condition) are disorders that both result in weakened and easily fatigued muscles that can impair mobility. Table 18.1 outlines Parkinson's disease, a common condition that affects both movement and gait. Other terms used to describe problems with movement experienced by patients/clients include:

- *Apraxia* – inability to produce coordinated movements
- *Bradykinesia* – unusually slow movement, especially the starting and stopping of movements

- *Dyspraxia* – partial loss of the ability to produce coordinated movements.

Many problems with gait can be attributed to problems with the feet, which is why it is important to refer people with foot conditions, especially older adults, to a podiatrist. These include many easily treatable and reversible conditions such as corns and calluses, nail deformities, verrucae, athlete's foot and other fungal infections.

Efficient handling and moving (EHM)

Many people can be encouraged to move themselves with help, such as verbal encouragement or a hand placed over the muscle groups to be moved, and further intervention is not needed. Good handling and moving skills are paramount to the health and safety of nurses and their patients/clients and are essential to assist people to move safely when they cannot move unaided. Nurses who understand the principles of human movement can apply them not only to care safely for people with mobility problems, but also to protect themselves from injury. Knowing the stages of human development, including ageing, also enables nurses to predict, to some extent, the needs of people of all ages (see Ch. 8).

Details of the current legislation and the principles of safe handling and moving are explained in Chapter 13. This section extends this to include the safe handling and moving of people including:

- Moving people in bed
- Using equipment to assist moving
- Helping people to use walking aids.

Another important text to read is *The Guide to the Handling of People* (Smith 2005). This book details all the moves that can be executed safely (too numerous to mention in this chapter), those that are condemned because they are considered to be a very high risk to nurses and patients/clients, and how equipment can be used to minimize handling and moving injuries. Suggestions are given about the best way of applying the principles of safer moving but it is beyond the scope of this chapter to cover every potential situation that a nurse might come across.

It is important to understand the difference between *efficient* handling and moving, and *effective* handling and moving:

- An efficient movement is one that achieves its goal using the appropriate amount of muscle effort for the demands of the task
- An effective movement usually involves more force than is required to produce the desired action.

Efficient movement is therefore preferable as it is less likely to result in injury to either nurses or patients/clients. Several equally acceptable approaches to EHM are recognized, including:

- *Ergonomic* – involves taking a risk assessment approach (see Ch. 13) to reduce the risks of the procedure to the minimum by redesigning the environment or equipment to enable safer working conditions, e.g. using profiling beds to reduce the amount of patient handling
- *Neuromuscular* – the neuromuscular approach practises specific and patterning conditioning movements to prepare the body to develop a core pattern of movement that is applied to all handling and moving situations (Crozier & Cozens 1997)
- *Biomechanical* – practises bending of the knees and keeping the back straight to maintain the spine in its strongest position.

Principles of safer handling and moving

In order to minimize the risk of injury to either practitioners or patients/clients, it is important always to:

- Apply the approach taught in your university, according to local policy
- Carry out a risk assessment before handling and moving either people or inanimate loads by using the acronym TILE:
  - **T**ask: whether it requires unusual skills or knowledge, can it be mechanized, is it necessary or can it be achieved by other means
  - **I**ndividual: in terms of practitioner experience, knowledge, height and weight
  - **L**oad: in terms of patient/client height, weight, physical and mental capabilities
  - **E**nvironment: assess the space, height of working surfaces and the presence of uneven floor surfaces or carpets; remove unnecessary equipment.

The principles of efficient movement are covered in Chapter 13. Carrying out the exercises in Box 18.11 will remind you of these.

REFLECTIVE PRACTICE Box 18.11

Principles of efficient movement

It is essential that nurses learn to adopt a systematic approach to all interventions that require the handling and moving of people.

Student activities

1. Think back to the first time you had to move a patient/client in bed:
   - Why did you move the patient/client?
   - How did you go about it?
   - Did you plan the move before you started?
   - How successful was the move?
   - Was the patient/client comfortable?
   - Were you comfortable?
2. Now consider how you may have done things differently using the principles of risk assessment and efficient handling and moving.
3. Next time you have to move a person in bed, remember to plan your actions, prepare the area, yourself and the patient/client and reflect on whether or not it made the move easier.

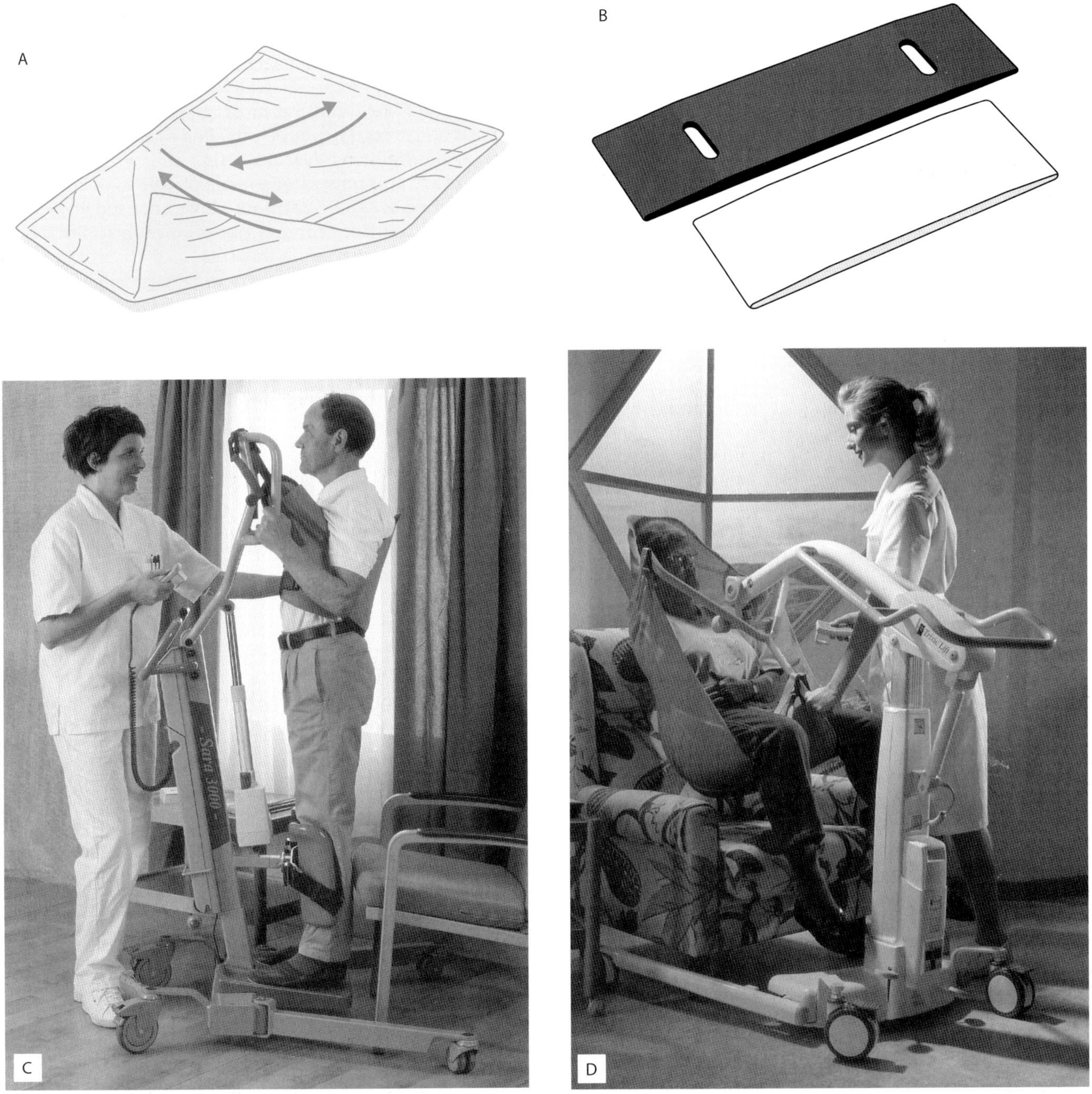

Fig. 18.11 A range of handling and moving equipment: **A**. Glide sheet. **B**. Small transfer boards. **C**. Standing and raising (SARA) hoist. **D**. Trixie hoist (hoists reproduced with permission from ARJO)

Equipment

There are many devices available to assist in moving people (Fig. 18.11). Commonly used equipment and its potential uses are described below. Use of mobility aids such as walking frames, walking sticks and wheelchairs is explained on page 521.

Glide sheets

Glide sheets, also known as slide sheets (see Fig. 18.11A) are often used to help people move in bed or in a chair. There are many different styles, but they all work on the same principle of reducing friction between the skin and the bed or chair surface when they are placed under a surface contact area, e.g. the sacrum, heels, shoulders, head. Some glide sheets enable movement to occur in several directions, i.e. up, down, side-to-side and in a circular movement. These are commonly referred to as multiglide sheets, which are made of thin, low-friction material. Others allow movement in one direction only and are referred to as one-way glide sheets. Typically, a glide sheet looks like a sleeping bag, but is open at both ends and has a slippery inner surface. Once in position, it is possible to move a person using minimal force. Some glide sheets have handles to enable the handlers to take hold of the sheet rather than placing their hands on the individual.

Transfer boards

These are generally fairly solid although some are more flexible than others, and are used to assist in transfers between different pieces of equipment or furniture such as chairs, beds, baths, wheelchairs, trolleys and car seats. They are often referred to as lateral transfer boards since the person being moved usually moves in a sideways direction. Depending on the nature of the transfer, a smaller or larger board may be used. Glide sheets are often used in conjunction with transfer boards as they reduce the handler effort required. Some transfer boards are manufactured with glide sheets attached. These can be useful for bathing. Figure 18.11B shows a small transfer board used for sitting transfers, while larger transfer boards are available for use in bed transfers.

Hoists

Mechanical and electrical hoists are widely used to assist people into and out of bed and chairs. Mechanical hoists usually require more handler effort to operate than electrical hoists. Another benefit of the electrical hoist is that the patient/client can be given the control box and, following instruction and supervised practice, they can operate it themselves. Many people with paraplegia (who have paralysis and therefore functional loss of their trunk and lower limbs) are able to move themselves independently using electrical hoists. There are many different styles and sizes of hoists and it is important to understand how a particular hoist works before using it to move people.

Some hoists are used only to assist people into a standing position for a short period of time, for example to assist with toileting, or while their personal hygiene is being attended to and/or their clothing is being adjusted.

Standing and raising hoist

Figure 18.11C shows a standing and raising appliance (SARA) hoist, which is used only for standing transfers. These standing hoists should only be used when the person being moved can take some of their body weight through their feet. If there is any doubt about this, standing hoists must be avoided and a passive lift hoist that will take the whole body weight used instead. Each hoist clearly displays a safe weight that must not be exceeded.

Passive lifting hoists

Passive lifting hoists are suitable for use in situations where there is any doubt about a person's ability either to move or to comply with instructions. Passive lifting hoists involve the use of slings, made of soft but strong material, that are applied to the patient/client before being attached to the hoist. Disposable slings are sometimes used to minimize cross-infection (see Ch. 15); otherwise the slings should be laundered according to the manufacturer's instructions and local policy. Some slings are also suitable for bathing and toileting. Figure 18.11D shows a Trixie hoist with its slings. Slings are not interchangeable and the correct ones for a specific hoist must be used following the manufacturer's guidelines. Slings are available in a range of sizes and the most appropriate size should be used. A correctly fitted sling adds to the security of a patient/client during the transfer.

There are also hoists that enable people to be raised off the bed while in a lying position. These are used for people with spinal injuries who are not allowed any flexion of the spine and in operating theatres.

Hoists can appear very frightening to people who have never been moved in this way before. Nurses should take time to discuss with patients/clients why they are being moved in this way, describing the benefits to the individual as well as to the nursing staff. Chapter 13 (p. 328) identifies the Health and Safety regulations that must be followed when using equipment such as hoists.

Accessories

Sometimes it is not necessary to use hoists and slides when moving people, and equipment described in this section can be used to assist mobility.

Rope ladders

Rope ladders attached to the end of the bed can be useful for assisting people to move themselves into a more comfortable position independently. Patients/clients need to have good upper limb and head control to be able to pull themselves up into a sitting position.

Turning discs

These consist of two discs that rotate against one another and are designed either for people to sit on or to place under their feet. They are used to assist with turning and can be used independently or with assistance. Generally, it is better to use turning discs with lighter people as the weight of heavier patients/clients can interfere with the turning mechanism.

Using equipment to move people

Nurses must familiarize themselves with any equipment used in people's homes, nursing homes and wards before using it. It is also useful to have experienced being moved using the equipment so that clear explanations can be given to the patient/client. Practical classes at university provide the opportunity to experience being moved in a hoist while under the watchful eye of a trained supervisor and it is a good idea to use these opportunities. They can also be used to discuss with the trainer if a particular piece of equipment is appropriate for a particular care setting. Observing a demonstration using a healthy volunteer who cannot represent your specific patient's/client's needs may not necessarily identify problems with equipment that may be encountered in practice.

Checking equipment

Always check that the equipment is in good working order before using it to move people. Chapter 13 outlines the Lifting Operations and Lifting Equipment Regulations (LOLER) for checking equipment safety on a regular basis. Common faults include:

- Deflated tyres on wheelchairs
- Missing or incorrectly fitting footplates on wheelchairs
- Brakes that are difficult to operate
- Low power or flat batteries on electric hoists
- Tears in slides
- Loose nuts and bolts
- Worn-out slings
- Damaged surfaces on transfer boards.

Risk assessment

Initial assessment of the patient's/client's mobility needs must be carried out by an experienced practitioner and appropriately documented in the nursing notes. Physiotherapists and OTs may be involved in this process, which provides a broad indication of the equipment that may be required to move the patient/client. This part of the patient/client records must be read carefully before any handling and moving activities are carried out. If you are unsure about what is expected, it is essential to seek advice from your mentor. This prevents injury to either patients/clients or nurses by carrying out procedures incorrectly (Box 18.12).

As there is a possibility of litigation when things go wrong, it is always advisable to err on the side of safety. A person in bed is unlikely to suffer harm by waiting a few minutes longer while the appropriate preparations for moving them are made.

Although an initial assessment will have been undertaken, a patient's/client's condition can change at any time. It is therefore important that each time the person is being moved, further assessment of both their needs and the handler's capabilities is carried out.

ETHICAL ISSUES Box 18.12

Condoning unsafe practice

Jootun and MacInnes (2005) examined the extent to which undergraduate students correctly apply taught principles when handling and moving people during placements. They identified many factors that influence practice and can promote the continuance of unsafe practice. In today's society where litigation is increasing and patients/clients are more informed about their care and codes of practice, it is important to carefully consider the ethical dilemmas that may arise each time a patient/client is moved.

Student activities

- Have you ever been asked to carry out a manoeuvre condemned because it carries a high risk of injury?
- Would you make the manoeuvre because it can be easier than refusing, or would you defend your position and refuse to assist?
- Think about the implications for the nurse and a patient/client if harm occurred during a condemned manoeuvre.

Effective communication

Handling and moving people requires effective communication skills (see Ch. 9). Pacing of explanations is important so that too much information is not given at once or causes anxiety or confusion. Children, like anyone else, should not be patronized when equipment is being used; they prefer to be told what is going on and what to expect. For example, telling a child that getting into a hoist is like going on a rocket trip can conjure up an image that may be both frightening and easily misunderstood. People who are frightened do not cooperate easily and inappropriate explanations may lead to breakdown in the nurse–patient/client relationship. Some people are unable to understand explanations about handling and moving equipment, e.g. some clients with dementia or a severe learning disability. In such cases, an empathetic approach and careful handling and moving must be used.

It is good practice to explain what moving a person will involve and to describe any equipment and what it does before bringing it to the bedside. Patients/clients should direct the speed of moving activities. People with poor vision should be encouraged to touch and handle equipment before it is used so they can get a sense of what will be happening to them.

Finding the most suitable equipment

Sometimes it can be difficult to find the ideal piece of equipment to move a patient/client safely, e.g. where there is apraxia or dyspraxia (see p. 513). In these situations physiotherapists must be resourceful in finding and using the right equipment to meet very specific individual needs. Foam wedges, mats and padding are often used to reduce the risk of injury from the equipment itself. These clients can become very agitated and, since they have little or no control over the movements of their limbs, can also be at high risk of injury as can those assisting in the manoeuvre. It is particularly important that only the palms of the hands are used when supporting limbs. Gripping must be avoided as this causes strong contraction of the underlying muscles, making control of the limb even more difficult.

Handling and moving people

This section addresses key issues of moving people with or without equipment. Details about how to carry out specific manoeuvres can be found in the *Guide to the Handling of People* (Smith 2005). Nursing patients/clients in bed usually involves handling and moving them to carry out their care, for example:

- Moving the patient onto and off the bed in a supine position
- Moving the patient up the bed
- Sitting the patient up in bed
- Turning the patient
- Inserting and removing bedpans
- Changing bedding
- Changing dressings
- Dressing and undressing
- Transferring the patient to a commode or wheelchair

- Preparing the patient to stand up
- Putting the patient to bed

(after Holmes 1997).

Helping people to move in bed has been identified as carrying a higher risk of injury than other handling and moving activities (Bertolazzi & Saia 1999). For this reason, it is important that all necessary steps are taken to reduce the risk of injury and to follow the handling and moving guidance given in the nursing care plan.

When moving people in beds or chairs it is important to be aware that the spine is the central axis around which all movement occurs. If a patient/client who has lost power of their arms is required to move one of their hands, the nurse should work from the shoulder girdle. This is because the muscles of the shoulder girdle are postural muscles, built for power, rather than the smaller muscles of the hand, which are built for fine movements. If the hand is moved first, the handlers must bear the load of the whole arm, whereas moving the shoulder first allows the arm and hand to be moved with less effort. Likewise, to move a person's foot, the move is started from the hip.

It is often necessary to support patients'/clients' limbs on pillows while they are being moved in bed. This must be carried out in a manner that both supports and protects the limb, and does not cause pain. Limbs should be supported underneath, either in the palm of the hand or across the forearm, while pillows are being positioned. The limbs should be supported in natural positions (Fig. 18.12) that do not put joints into positions that could result in pain or loss of function. Feet should not be left hanging off the ends of pillows and wrists should be supported in neutral positions.

Turning a person in bed

This technique is used to move patients/clients in bed to minimize the risk of twisting their spines while changing bed linen, placing hoist slings in position or turning them (to minimize the risk of pressure damage, see Ch. 25). Box 18.13 (p. 520) describes the principles of turning a patient/client in bed using a glide sheet.

Regaining balance

When a person has been immobile for a period of time, none of the body systems works to their full potential and a programme of gradual mobilization is required to enable them to regain full independence. After a couple of days in bed with a viral illness, even young people may feel quite wobbly on their legs, dizzy and not up to their usual energy levels, and find carrying out even simple tasks makes them feel tired. The feeling of dizziness experienced after a lengthy period of lying down can be due to postural hypotension. For this reason, people who have been nursed in a supine position (lying flat) are sat up gradually, so that the cardiovascular system can adjust to the new position.

If patients/clients are being nursed on a profiling bed, the head of the bed is gently raised a little at a time. Giving the control box to the patient allows them to raise the head of their bed to a position with which they feel comfortable. They may raise the head of the bed further at a rate they can tolerate, until they are able to sit upright. At this stage they will still need to be supported with pillows and backrests. Thereafter they will need to relearn how to sit up unsupported and regain their sitting balance.

Once sitting balance has been regained, the patient/client can progress to standing and walking. The key points to be aware of are whether or not the patient/client can move from sitting to standing unaided and, once standing, whether or not they will have standing balance. Mobility aids and hoists can be used to assist patients/clients to stand and walk (see p. 520).

Helping a person to sit up in bed

The most efficient equipment to assist a patient to move from the lying to the sitting position is an electric powered, height adjustable, profiling bed. If profiling beds are not available, other equipment can be used on non-profiling beds such as:

- Pillow lifters
- Mattress elevators
- A knee break, which supports the patient's knees in a flexed position in bed
- Passive lifting hoists with slings (see p. 516).

Patients/clients can be encouraged to move themselves in bed using equipment designed for the purpose, e.g. rope ladders or slides, or a combination of these.

As patients recover and become more mobile, the nursing care plan is altered to reflect their improving mobility. Patients should be encouraged to help themselves to sit up by rolling onto their sides, taking their weight through their elbows and pushing themselves up into a sitting position. During any of the aforementioned procedures, the nurse should initially stay beside the patient to offer support if needed and to give advice and encouragement. Once patients have gained confidence in carrying out the move, and the nurse is satisfied that they are capable of moving themselves safely, observation can be carried out from a distance.

Helping a person to get out of bed

Ensure that there is enough space to work safely, taking into account the size of the chair and the amount of space required for turning the patient/client. Box 18.14 explains how to select a suitable chair for a patient/client; however, in reality, choice may be limited. Initially the bed should be level with the upper thigh while the patient/client is being dressed. Once the person is ready to be moved into a sitting position the bed is lowered to allow their feet to touch the floor. Always check that the brakes are securely applied before helping a person to move. Do not lean against the bed when moving a person as the wheels may slip on the floor.

Well-fitting, lightweight slippers should be put on to prevent the person slipping when their feet reach the floor. Shoes should always be worn with socks, to maintain dignity and to prevent chafing of the feet; however, they can add considerably to the weight of the legs, making them more difficult to move.

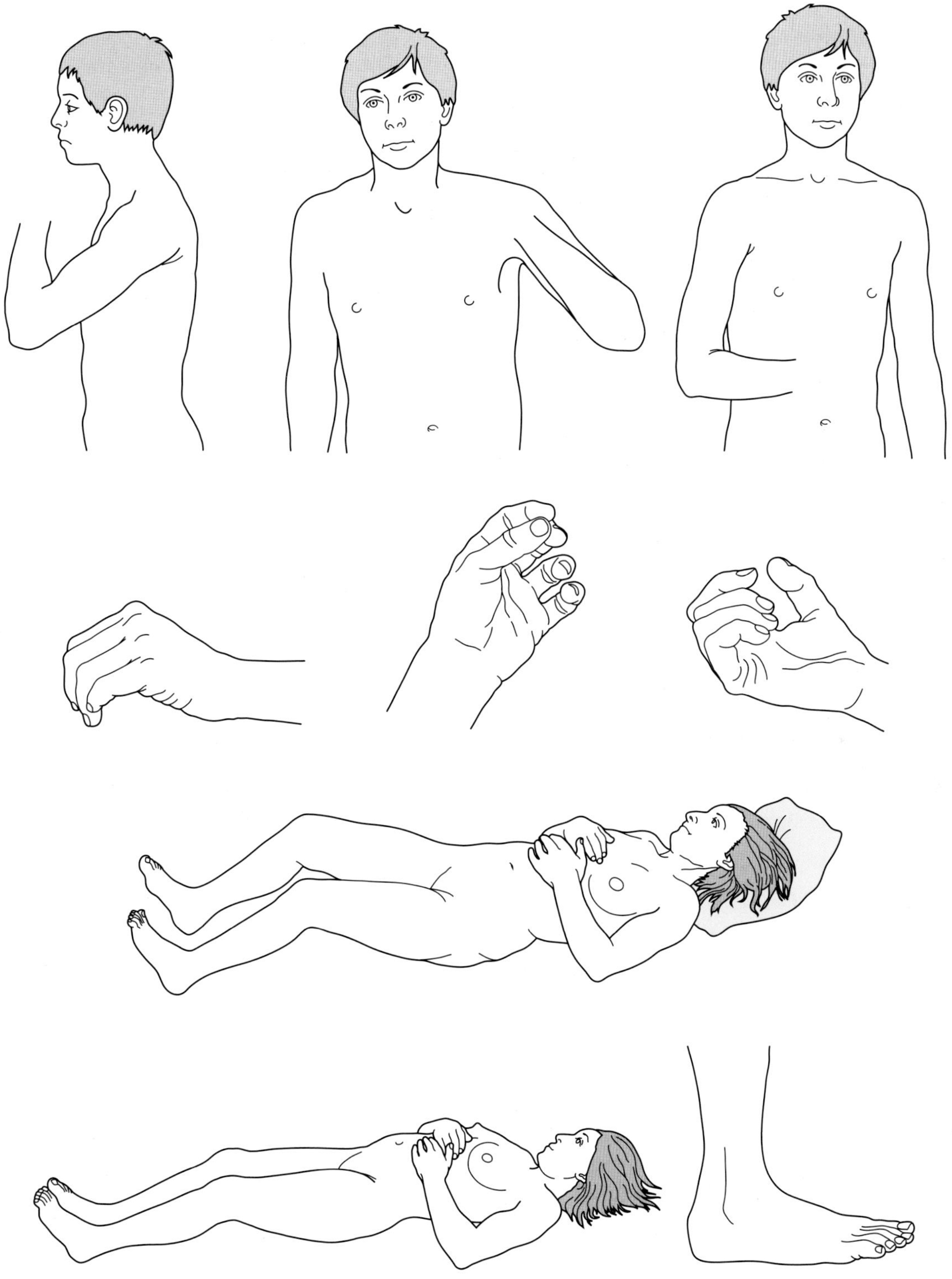

Fig. 18.12 Resting positions of the limbs (reproduced with permission from Peattie & Walker 1996)

The nursing care plan will indicate what equipment to use and how much assistance a patient/client needs to get out of bed and sit in a chair. All equipment requires the assistance of at least one nurse. This includes:

- Passive lifting hoists (see Fig. 18.11D) with slings for people who cannot weight-bear
- Partial weight-bearing hoists and walking harnesses
- SARA hoists (see Fig. 18.11C) for people who have some ability to weight-bear
- Turning discs with frames for people who have good upper body strength and are able to weight-bear. People using these must be able to hold the frame to pull themselves up into a standing position.

NURSING SKILLS Box 18.13

Turning a person in bed using a glide sheet

All handling and moving situations should be risk assessed to identify the number of staff and the equipment required.

- Handwashing according to local policy.
- The procedure is explained and the bed screened.
- When risk assessment requires that two nurses assist, one works at each side of the bed. If only one nurse is assisting, the cot side on the opposite side of the bed should be raised to stop the patient/client falling out of bed.
- With the patient/client on their side, the glide sheet is placed on the bed behind the patient/client, with the open ends towards the ends of the bed.
- Half of the glide sheet is rolled up and placed with the roll behind the patient's/client's back, ensuring that both the hips and shoulders will be lying on the glide sheet when it is unrolled. The rest of the glide sheet is flattened on the bed, as free from wrinkles as possible.
- The patient/client is assisted onto their back.
- The second nurse slides her hands underneath the patient/client and unravels the glide sheet towards her.
- Still on their back, the patient/client is then gently moved on the glide sheet towards one edge of the bed, by one nurse pulling the top layer of the glide sheet towards her.
- The patient/client is then rolled onto their side in the middle of the bed.
- The glide sheet is removed by gently pulling it out from underneath the patient/client.

Some patients/clients require only minimal assistance to stand up from the side of the bed. These people must have good sitting balance and be able to support themselves while sitting at the edge of the bed with their feet flat on the floor. Always allow the patient/client to dictate the speed of the move; it is important that people feel in control and that their needs are respected. A person who has had strong analgesics may not be as quick-thinking as usual and needs to be given short, concise instructions that are easily understood. It is also important to be aware that some drugs may cause postural hypotension, a drop in blood pressure that may cause dizziness or fainting when standing upright.

The physiotherapist can provide specific advice to nurses about positioning themselves to help a particular patient/client.

Helping a person to stand up from a chair

Standing a patient up from a chair is different from standing a patient up from a bed. The main differences are that nurses must accommodate the arms of the chair and the height of the chair is usually fixed. Equipment that may be used includes:

- Riser seats
- Blocks to raise chairs (the chair legs are slotted into raised blocks that increase the height of the chair)
- SARA hoists (see Fig. 18.11C).

Key points to follow when assisting people to stand from chairs are shown in Box 18.15.

NURSING SKILLS Box 18.14

Choosing a suitable chair

Tarling (1997) considers that the following factors should be taken into account:

The seat

- *Height*: Should correspond with the leg length of the seated person, should allow the feet to be flat on the floor with the thighs level and should be firm to help the seated person push up.
- *Depth*: Should correspond to the length from the back of the hips to the front of the knee (a lumbar support will increase this measurement).
- *Angle*: The seated person's hips should be level with their knees. If the hips are higher, a footstool should be used to raise the feet and to reduce pressure on the back of the thighs.

The back

- *Height*: Depends on whether a head support is required. Chair wings impede conversation and encourage slouching to the side, but may reduce draughts.
- *Headrest*: Should be tilted slightly backwards to provide comfortable support. A vertical headrest tends to push the head forward, causing neck pain.
- *Armrests*: If present, these should come well forward so that the person can grasp or push down on them to assist moving to the front of the chair before standing. They should provide support for the elbows without distorting the shoulder position.
- *Chair legs*: Front legs should be vertical and the rear legs angled slightly backwards. There should be a minimum of 13 cm clearance under a chair to accommodate hoists.
- *Style*: Reclining armchairs, supportive chairs, riser and adjustable chairs all promote comfort and independence. Riser chairs have features that assist people to move from a sitting to a standing position with minimal assistance.

Helping people to mobilize

The differences in gait in children, adults and older people (see p. 513) must be taken into account when assisting people to walk. It can be difficult to walk alongside a patient/client who has an altered gait. Helping people with walking carries an increased risk of injuries (Thomas 2005). Allow people with visual impairment to use familiar arm holds for walking, e.g. taking hold of the sighted person's left arm around the elbow and walking slightly behind. Equipment used to assist people with

NURSING SKILLS Box 18.15

Principles for assisting people to stand from chairs

1. Risk assessment using TILE (see p. 514).
2. The nurse stands to the side of the person, with the leading foot pointing in the direction of intended movement, ready to take a step as the person moves.
3. The person's hips are brought close to the edge of the seat.
4. Positioning the person's feet with one foot slightly in front of the other enables a pushing action to assist standing, without the person losing their balance.
5. The person is asked to keep their head in a relaxed upright position, looking forwards.
6. The nurse should be ready to assist the person, if required, by placing their nearest arm across the person's back, towards the furthest away hip, allowing the palm of the hand to make contact with the hip area. The nurse moves their hand into a comfortable position that reduces any overstretching. The nurse's other arm should be moved into a position that allows the palm of the hand to cradle the person's shoulder.
7. Simple instructions are used to direct the movement.
8. The person is encouraged to raise their head to initiate the standing movement and use the armrests to push themselves into a standing position.
9. Simultaneously, the nurse raises their own head and takes a step forward with the leading foot so that on completion of the movement both the nurse and the person are balanced.
10. Before releasing their hold on the person, the nurse checks that the person's weight is equally distributed between both feet and that they have control of their balance.
11. If the person is unable to stand, the nurse's hands will slide off the shoulder and back, leaving the person in a sitting position. The situation should be reassessed and equipment used to move the person from the chair.

walking includes walking sticks, walking frames and crutches. These are all measured and fitted to the person's height by the physiotherapist or registered nurse. Wheeled walkers may be used for children. If a person needs manual assistance with walking, an assessment is carried out and documented in the care plan. This takes account of whether the individual:

- Can control their arms and upper body
- Can maintain balance while standing
- Has an upright or stooped posture
- Can comply with instructions
- Has ever used, or currently uses, walking aids
- Has breathing or respiratory problems that affect their stamina
- Is suffering pain and how this affects their mobility
- Has suitable footwear, e.g. slippers, boots, shoes. Good fitting, supportive shoes are preferable and reduce the potential for falls (see Ch. 13).

The following factors should be also taken into account and assessed prior to mobilizing a person:

- Is the individual expected to walk a long distance?
- What is the reason for walking, e.g. is it to or from the toilet?
- What are the prevailing floor conditions, e.g. linoleum or carpet?
- Does the individual have attachments such as an intravenous infusion or a urinary catheter?

Walking frames

Walking frames are widely used and come in many shapes and sizes according to the function for which they are required. Some walking aids have wheels and are known as rollators. They may have a shopping basket attached so that they can be used to carry light bags. In hospitals, walking frames often have rubber stoppers on the ends of the legs so that the frames do not slip on the floor. Sometimes walking frames are used temporarily as people regain full fitness. For other people, they are a permanent measure to maintain their safety and independence, especially those who:

- Have the ability to weight-bear but may tire easily
- Have a history of falling
- Have painful joints
- Lack confidence.

Walking sticks

Walking sticks or tripods (that have one handle and three feet) provide a similar function to walking frames, but are less bulky. They are often used as a first measure when people become aware that their balance is failing. Many people purchase walking sticks without any advice from a physiotherapist or OT. Most walking sticks are height adjustable and should be set at a comfortable height that allows the elbow to be held in a slightly flexed position. The correct height for the stick is identified by measuring the distance from the person's wrist to the ground while they are wearing their normal outdoor shoes. Normally the stick is used on the side to which the person is most likely to fall, but this is not a hard and fast rule and physiotherapists or OTs can assist in properly assessing the person to advise on individual requirements. Physiotherapists will also measure clients for crutches and tripods so that they are given the correct height of appliance.

Wheelchairs

Wheelchairs offer a degree of independence to some users, but many others are dependent on being pushed around. It is important to understand what a person's expectations are when discussing the use of a wheelchair. The following general principles are useful:

- If a person is completely dependent on others pushing the wheelchair, then it is best to use one with smaller wheels (Fig. 18.13A). This makes it easier for the handler to push the wheelchair outside, because the tyres are not inflatable.
- If the patient/client wishes to move the wheelchair independently it is better to have larger, inflatable

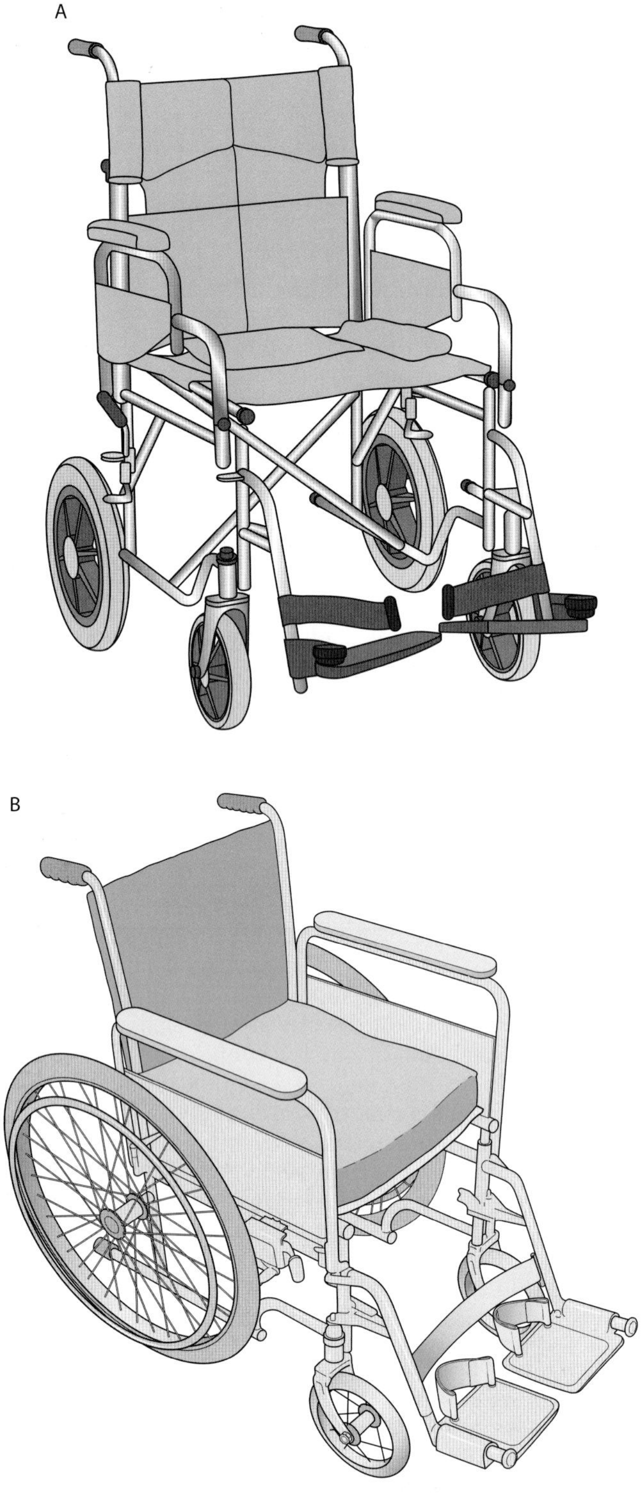

Fig. 18.13 Wheelchairs: **A.** Small wheeled. **B.** Large wheeled

tyres so that the wheels can be turned more easily, causing less damage to the hands (Fig. 18.13B).

Choosing the correct width of wheelchair is important to ensure that the patient/client will not slip out of it. It is also necessary to consider the width of doorways if the wheelchair is for home use. Sometimes it is necessary to remove doors to enable access to rooms. All new buildings must comply with national building regulations, e.g. the Scottish Building Standards Agency (2004), to ensure that they have wheelchair access through at least one door and, thereafter, into at least one toilet and one public room on the ground floor.

Wheelchairs can be designed to suit the specific needs of individual patients/clients. Sometimes the whole seat is moulded around the person's body to accommodate their body shape and offers support in the correct places such as the head, thorax, hips, knees and feet. Back extensions, head extensions, leg extensions and foot plates can all be adapted to meet the individual patient's/client's needs. Many younger people have lightweight frames and wheels on their wheelchairs, particularly if they are likely to be involved in sporting and keep fit activities. Different types of padded seat are available to reduce the effects of pressure (see Ch. 25). Box 18.16 provides information about checking and storage of wheelchairs.

Box 18.16 Wheelchairs

Safety checks

Ensure that:

- All tyres are inflated
- Both footplates are attached and in good condition
- Heel straps are correctly fitted to footplates
- Both brakes are working
- The chair is clean
- Any additional attachments such as padding, head support or leg extensions are securely in place and in good condition.

Storage

- Chairs can be folded for storage.
- Empty chairs are easier to move if they are left unfolded and a wheelbarrow action is used. Take hold of the handles from underneath and raise the back wheels slightly from the floor so that only the front wheels are in contact with the floor.

Falls

Cryer and Patel (2001) identified that, in the community, one-third of people over the age of 65 and 50% of people over the age of 80 will fall at some time. Some of these falls will result in fractures. Dealing with a falling patient is challenging. There are many factors that predispose to falls, including:

- Postural hypotension
- Dizziness
- Alterations in gait
- Stroke
- Fear of falling
- History of previous falls
- Sight and hearing problems
- Poor footwear
- Hazards in the environment

- Poor lighting
- Polypharmacy (Ch. 22)
- Steps and stairs
- Use of alcohol and recreational drugs.

As falls are common, it is very important to be aware of the main predisposing factors in order to prevent or minimize their occurrence. Prevention of falls is explored in Box 13.9 (p. 326). Older adults who are admitted to hospital following a fall are referred to a gerontologist (a physician who specializes in the care of older adults) for further investigation of their physical health and home circumstances. Falling is often the first indication of an underlying problem. It may be the sign of something simple, e.g. a person requires spectacles, or it may be the result of something more serious such as postural hypotension. Gerontologists carry out physical and psychological investigations to identify the cause of falling and the measures required to remedy the situation.

As part of the multidisciplinary team (MDT), gerontologists work in conjunction with nurses, OTs, physiotherapists and social workers to provide the support needed to enable people to return home. By reducing polypharmacy (see Ch. 22), treating previously undiagnosed conditions and putting appropriate mobility aids into the home, many older adults can be enabled to continue to live at home. The benefits of living at home, in familiar surroundings, far outweigh those of living in supported accommodation, e.g. a nursing home. Moving people from their familiar environment can cause confusion and increase the risk of falls. It is also more cost-effective for health authorities to provide support in people's homes than in long-term supported care.

Care of people who have fallen

Normally nurses walk to the side and slightly behind patients/clients when they are escorting them (see p. 520). This means that if a patient/client loses their balance, the nurse can move behind them and begin to control their descent to the ground. However, this should only be undertaken if the following criteria are present:

- There is enough space to enable the nurse and patient to move
- There is no significant height difference between the nurse and the patient
- The patient is not much heavier than the nurse
- The patient is not resisting being handled
- The patient is falling backwards towards the nurse.

Alternatively, the nurse must clear any furniture if possible and allow the patient/client to fall to the ground, particularly if the person is falling away from the nurse.

Once on the ground the patient/client is safe and the situation must then be assessed to find the best means of assisting them to stand up again. It may be necessary to make a patient comfortable on the ground until the requisite help arrives. People should always be assessed for injuries incurred before being moved.

The patient/client may be able to stand up unaided or be able to follow instructions that will help to do this. Some people will have previously been taught how to do this by the physiotherapist. Small children may be lifted manually, but otherwise inflatable cushions or hoists (see p. 516) should be used if patients cannot assist themselves to stand. An incident form is completed according to local policy (see Ch. 13).

The benefits of mobility and hazards of immobility

In order to maintain good health it is important to exercise regularly as there are many benefits of mobility that are often taken for granted (see below). Both weight-bearing exercise (e.g. walking, running, cycling) and non-weight-bearing exercise (e.g. swimming) should be encouraged. Weight-bearing exercises involve overcoming the effects of gravity and are good for maintaining and developing bone mass (see p. 506). Non-weight-bearing exercises, such as swimming, can also be carried out in a hydrotherapy pool (see Box 18.20, p. 527) where the body weight is supported, the effects of gravity are greatly reduced and the joints can be moved more easily.

Sometimes complete immobility is enforced, such as during bedrest or coma, while application of a plaster cast confers immobility of the affected limb. Immobility can be short or long lasting. In these situations it is important to be alert for signs of the many potential hazards of immobility, discussed later in this section. Short-term immobility is less likely to be associated with the potential hazards of immobility. This section explores the benefits of mobility and the potential hazards of immobility across the lifespan.

Benefits of mobility

Keeping mobile is one of the best ways to keep fit. A 20-minute, brisk walk every day will improve the fitness of all body systems, especially the cardiovascular and musculoskeletal systems. Specific health benefits include:

- Maintaining/increasing bone density
- Maintaining/increasing muscle bulk
- Maintaining/increasing the thickness of articular cartilage
- Maintaining/improving joint movement
- Maintaining/improving the circulation and prevention of deep vein thrombosis
- Maintaining/improving respiratory function; deep breathing keeps the lungs free from infection
- Preventing constipation by increasing the transit rate in the intestines
- Assisting in achieving all the activities of living
- Improving mental well-being
- Maintaining independence and social interaction.

The Paralympics clearly show that exercise and fitness can be accessible to everyone and that many people are able to overcome severe disabilities to keep fit although they need to remain vigilant about the hazards of immobility, especially the development of pressure ulcers.

Children

Play normally provides the exercise that children's body systems need to grow and develop in a coordinated manner. Further intervention is unnecessary in children who are able to play actively by participating in, for example, cycling, running, ball games and other weight-bearing activities. However, children who have sedentary hobbies such as playing computer games and watching television will begin to feel the effects of lack of exercise. In addition to becoming overweight, normal muscle bulk does not build up and there may be changes to the normal curvature of the spine. These may have lasting effects on children's health, especially the musculoskeletal system, in later life (see p. 511).

Teenagers

Teenagers also need to exercise and should be encouraged to participate in formal exercise in order to develop their bones and muscles. Weight-bearing activities such as walking, running, dancing, skiing, football and rugby help to increase bone mass during adolescence and delay the loss of bone mass thereafter (see p. 506). During exercise, bones accommodate to the stresses that are applied to them, so that those who exercise regularly have denser bones containing more minerals. Bones alter in shape as extra material is laid down at the points of maximum stress. Swimming is an excellent pastime for health in general but, as it is not a weight-bearing activity, it does not affect bone mass. It is, however, very good for developing muscle tissue and the cardiovascular system.

Aerobic, anaerobic and resistance exercises are all good for promoting general health and well-being. Aerobic exercises involve using large muscle groups, rhythmically, over a period of at least 15–20 minutes, and the muscles have sufficient oxygen to fully utilize fuel molecules and release the energy required for contraction. These exercises are generally low in intensity and long in duration such as walking, cycling, jogging or swimming. Anaerobic exercises require muscles to work very hard in the absence of oxygen and are usually high in intensity and short in duration, e.g. sprinting, squash. The limited duration of this type of exercise is due to the accumulation of lactic acid because fuel molecules cannot be fully utilized without oxygen. Resistance exercise – also called strength training or weight training – increases muscle strength, mass and tone.

Cross-training, i.e. training for different events at the same time, such as cycling, swimming and running, develops all the body muscles at the same rate and people report fewer injuries during exercise. In addition, greater body flexibility is present because one group of muscles is not being built up at the expense of others. Cross-training for any sport prevents people from becoming muscle-bound, which can lead to injury (Stamford 1996). For example, runners who only exercise to build up their stamina for running often find their hard-worked muscles become prone to sprains and tendons prone to inflammation. Their other muscles become weaker in comparison and are therefore more prone to injury. This is seen when Olympic athletes, who have spent years training for a particular event, pull up with a calf or hamstring (the posterior thigh muscles) injury in the most important race of their lives.

HEALTH PROMOTION — Box 18.17

Exercise and older adults

The Department of Health (DH 2004) recognizes the importance of exercising in people of all ages, including older adults, and there are many ways in which communities meet this need:

- Afternoon dances for people who prefer not to go out after dark
- Guided walking/exercises in shopping centres
- Fitness and swimming sessions for older adults.

Student activities

- Visit the websites below and identify the benefits of exercise in older adults.
- Visit the Age Concern website (www.ageconcernscotland.org.uk) and find out what activities help to prevent health issues in older adults.
- In your placement identify people who encourage patients/clients to participate in exercising, e.g. an activity coordinator.
- Find out about activities specifically for older adults in your town.

[Resources: Department of Health 2004 At least five a week: evidence on the impact of physical activity and its relationship to health – www.dh.gov.uk/PublicationsAndStatistics/Publications/PublicationsPolicyAndGuidance/PublicationsPolicyAndGuidance-Article/fs/en?CONTENT_ID=4080994&chk=1Ft1Of; MedlinePlus. Exercise for seniors – www.nlm.nih.gov/medlineplus/exerciseforseniors.html All available July 2006]

Adults and older adults

As people age, the benefits of exercise continue to increase (Box 18.17). The more the muscles and fascia have adapted to postural habits, the less flexible people become (see p. 505).

Hazards of immobility

There are many and diverse hazards of immobility, as listed in Box 18.18. The effects of immobility are the same across the lifespan, but children tend to recover more quickly from a period of immobility.

It is very important for nurses to recognize the potential hazards that patients/clients with limited mobility or who are immobile may face in order to minimize their occurrence. The reasons that people may be at risk from these potential problems are not only physical but also include mental health problems such as depression. In general, the risk of these hazards increases with a person's age, presence of other health problems and the period of immobility. Bedrest, which confines patients

Box 18.18 **Hazards of immobility**

- Poor circulation that may predispose to deep vein thrombosis
- Poor respiratory function that may predispose to chest infections
- Development of pressure ulcers (see Ch. 25)
- Loss of bone density (osteoporosis)
- Joint stiffness
- Muscle wasting
- Constipation
- Potential loss of mental well-being, e.g. depression
- Boredom, isolation
- Impaired social interaction
- Loss of independence that may affect all the activities of living.

to bed, is sometimes prescribed for therapeutic reasons, for example:

- Some medical interventions (e.g. traction) require this
- To prevent the increase in oxygen demand needed during exercise
- To provide rest for seriously ill or debilitated patients.

Following a period of bedrest or restricted mobility, a programme of planned return to full activity may be required. This often involves several members of the MDT, especially the physiotherapist and OT whose roles are described. Falls pose a potential risk in many situations and helping people who have fallen is explained at the end of this section.

Maintaining healthy joints and muscles

When not used, the joints stiffen and the skeletal muscles waste, and both will limit mobility when mobility can be restarted. It is therefore important to maintain the range of movements available at joints and the condition of skeletal muscles when mobilization is not possible. Active and passive exercises can be carried out in bed in these situations. Active exercises are those initiated by people themselves without aid, e.g. flexing and extending the fingers. Passive exercises are those initiated by carers who move a person's joints through the normal range of movements. It is important to know the normal movements at joints so that they are not moved into abnormal and potentially harmful positions. They help to:

- Increase blood flow to, through and from the muscles and fascia
- Encourage blood flow in general, reducing the risk of deep vein thrombosis
- Promote healing and maintain or improve muscle function
- Stimulate the lymphatic system to drain excess tissue fluid and remove potentially harmful microorganisms.

Active exercises

Whenever possible, people are encouraged to actively exercise all their joints. Encouraging patients/clients to meet their own hygiene needs, dress themselves and walk around are all good ways of encouraging active exercises. Safety is always important and it may therefore be appropriate to stay nearby so that patients/clients are not overreaching, e.g. to pick things up, which may affect their balance and result in a fall. When caring for older adults, it is important that they are given enough time to carry out such activities. When nurses intervene too quickly or provide too much assistance, this not only reduces people's capacity for self-care but also increases dependence on others. Sometimes physiotherapists organize classes that promote movement and provide regular exercise.

Patients/clients who are confined to bed can often still carry out active exercises but may need encouragement to move each joint through its full range of movement on a regular basis during waking hours. In addition to keeping the joints and their associated muscles functioning, carrying out active exercises also helps to pass time and gives people some active control over their recovery. Some patients may wish to use weights in order to provide resistance and make the muscles work harder, or they may be taught specific exercises by the physiotherapist. Patients who have undergone mastectomy (removal of breast tissue) or surgery to the elbow should be encouraged to brush their hair using the affected arm to keep the associated shoulder in good condition. Some patients prefer to have the screens drawn round their bed while they are exercising; always check with the patient first.

Passive exercises

Passive exercises are usually carried out by the physiotherapist, nurse or sometimes the patient themselves (see p. 526). When carrying out passive exercises, the joint is supported proximally (towards the centre of the body) and distally (away from the centre of the body) in the palms of the hands and is moved gently within a given range. Over time, the range of movement (ROM) is increased. Often the patient can resume active exercises, but sometimes active movement may never return, e.g. in a person with paraplegia. It is essential that any passive movement applied to a joint and its associated muscles is carried out gently, assessing ('sensing'), through touch, the range of movement available at the joint. As soon as resistance to a movement is felt, or the patient expresses discomfort, the joint is returned to its normal resting position (see Fig. 18.12). It is important that the elbow joint is not passively stretched, as it is easily damaged. You must observe a skilled practitioner performing passive movements before attempting them yourself.

Prevention of deep vein thrombosis

Deep vein thrombosis (DVT) occurs when the flow of blood through the deep veins of the legs and pelvis is slowed and blood clots form within those veins. Damage to blood vessel walls and coagulation problems are also implicated in DVT formation, which sometimes occurs in healthy people on long haul flights, causing 'economy class syndrome'. DVT is dangerous because fragments of the clot may become detached and travel in the veins, through the right side of the heart and lodge in a pulmonary artery in lungs causing pulmonary embolism, which can be fatal. The risk of DVT is reduced by carrying out active or passive exercises (see above) and preventing dehydration (see Ch. 19) during periods of immobility.

Preventing chest infection

When mobility is restricted, the benefits of deep breathing that occur during exercise are lost and deep breathing must be actively encouraged. The aim of deep breathing exercises is to improve the flow of air to the bases of the lungs so that they are well ventilated. This helps to prevent the build-up of fluid or respiratory tract secretions within the lungs and the development of a chest infection. Deep breathing (see Ch. 17) also encourages the coughing reflex, which helps to clear the air passages of sputum and potential pathogens (see Ch. 15). Deep breathing exercises are encouraged in patients/clients who are confined to bed or a chair and in those who can walk only short distances.

Pressure ulcers

This complication of immobility, which is almost always preventable, is discussed in depth in Chapter 25. Nursing intervention is key to the prevention of pressure ulcers.

Constipation

Constipation can be prevented by anticipating the dietary and fluid needs of immobile patients/clients and providing an appropriate intake. Peristalsis (the contraction of smooth muscle that moves contents along the digestive tract) is reduced when mobility is limited, predisposing to constipation. The diet should be high in fibre to stimulate peristalsis. In adults, 1.5–2 litres of fluid are required daily to maintain hydration and achieving this can be a nursing challenge (see Ch. 19). Prevention and management of constipation is discussed in Chapter 21.

Maintaining well-being

Limited mobility will often restrict the social interaction that patients/clients are used to and it is necessary to find out the type of activity that will help to pass the time to prevent boredom and isolation and to maintain social interaction. In children this will include therapeutic play, which is essential to achieving developmental milestones when long-term treatment or intervention is necessary. People of all ages may enjoy watching TV, reading and solving crosswords or jigsaw puzzles.

People adapt to restricted mobility in different ways and patients/clients should be assessed for changes in their usual:

- Emotional reactions to situations
- Behaviour
- Sleep patterns (see Ch. 10).

Coping mechanisms (see Ch. 11) adapt according to circumstances and changes in these and the features above may indicate difficulty in adjusting to a new situation. People should be encouraged to express their experience of limited mobility and interventions can be provided to minimize its impact. Answering the call bell promptly provides social interaction and will reduce feelings of isolation.

Bedmaking

Wrinkled sheets can cause pressure damage (see Ch. 25). As patients/clients confined to bed move around, the sheets tend to become wrinkled. Children tend to wriggle around a lot and therefore their sheets need to be checked at regular intervals to ensure they are dry, flat and wrinkle free. After eating, sheets should be discreetly checked in people of all ages to ensure they are free from crumbs. Bottom sheets should be changed daily, but this may be more difficult in the home environment than in hospitals with laundry facilities. A district nurse or orthopaedic liaison nurse can advise about community laundry facilities. The principles used for making beds, cots and incubators are shown in Box 18.19.

Regaining mobility

A person's independence should always be maximized and therefore nursing care aims to enable people to return to their full capacity as soon as possible. For some people, however, this may be less mobility and independence than they previously enjoyed. For others, chronic conditions such as low back pain may result in ongoing mobility problems. The principles of rehabilitation are explained in Chapter 11. The MDT brings together professions with different skills to help people regain mobility and independence following illness or injury. This section outlines the roles of the different professions that work together to promote mobility, health and well-being.

Physiotherapy

Physiotherapists are the key healthcare professionals involved in assessing which aids should be used to improve mobility and which exercises patients/clients should be practising. Many people attend physiotherapy departments (either as in- or outpatients) where a greater range of equipment is available to facilitate active exercising. This may include hydrotherapy (Box 18.20). Much of the equipment within a hospital physiotherapy department is not available in the community although the physiotherapist may recommend going to a local gym that offers suitable activities.

Physiotherapists are also involved in teaching people with mobility problems or a history of falls how to prevent them in future (see Ch. 13) and how to get themselves up from the floor if they do fall (see p. 523).

Following a stroke, patients are often taught to carry out passive exercises (see p. 525) themselves on their affected limb, e.g. a hand and arm, using their unaffected hand. This helps them to regain their awareness of their affected side, which is often lost as a result of the stroke. Enabling patients to carry out passive exercises means that when they are not working directly with the physiotherapist they can continue to exercise the affected

NURSING SKILLS Box 18.19

Bedmaking, cots and incubator care

- Beds, cots and incubators are always washed and cleaned between use to reduce the spread of infection (see Ch. 15).
- Most clinical areas have height-adjustable beds, cots and incubators and it is important that the mechanisms are used to ensure that staff maintain a good, upright posture while working around the area.
- Brakes, wheels, height-adjusting mechanisms, profiling mechanisms, hydraulics, batteries and hand controls are checked to ensure they are working properly.
- Any faults are reported immediately to prevent accidents (see Ch. 13).
- Before making beds and cots, they are raised to between upper thigh and waist level.
- Preferably, two nurses should make beds with the smaller of the two dictating the height of the bed. All equipment required is brought to the bed area on a trolley, or placed on the extension rail at the bottom of the bed. A linen skip and bag for soiled linen should also be brought to the bedside if the sheets are to be changed. The bed and surrounding area should be cleaned if it is being prepared for a new patient.
- Sheets are unfolded on the surface of the mattress and placed in position before moving to the head end of the bed to fold and secure the corners. Sheets should be free of wrinkles to reduce the potential for skin damage over pressure areas (see Ch. 25).
- It is important to avoid twisting the spine. This is minimized by nurses moving their feet in the direction of intended movement so that their weight is evenly distributed between the soles of their feet while they move from one end of the bed to the other. Nurses should be appropriately close to the end of the bed they are working at without being in a top-heavy position.
- When making cots nurses often work on their own and it is important not to overstretch the spine by stretching across the mattress to fit sheets. Walking round to the cot to make up the opposite side minimizes this risk.
- When making incubators it is often difficult to get all-round access, therefore it is important not to hold one posture too long. Frequent changes of posture allow the upper limb muscles to recover.

HEALTH PROMOTION Box 18.20

Hydrotherapy

Hydrotherapy is the use of water to promote health and wellbeing (Hall et al 1996, Foley et al 2003). The water can be iced, cold, tepid, hot or steam and can also be used as compresses, inhalations or baths. Hydrotherapy has been used since the days of the ancient Greek philosopher Hippocrates who promoted the health benefits of taking a bath.

Cold-based hydrotherapies such as ice packs and cold compresses decrease normal activity, constricting blood vessels and numbing nerve sensation, whereas heat has the opposite effect. Sometimes, treatment involves both cold and heat being applied alternately to a painful area to rapidly promote local circulation.

Exercising painful muscles in a warm hydrotherapy pool is beneficial because water overcomes the effects of gravity, making it easier to move. People do not have to be able to swim to take hydrotherapy. Movements are carried out gently and slowly. The acts of getting into the water and floating, moving the arms or walking through the water help to increase the range of movements and build up muscle strength. A complication of hydrotherapy may be the desire to work too hard! Being in a warm, pain-free environment can lull people into a false sense of security and they may move themselves into a range of movement with which their fascia and muscles are not familiar, causing discomfort. Frequent, short sessions are better than occasional longer sessions.

People with arthritis and chronic back pain benefit from hydrotherapy. Hydrotherapy can also have a calming effect and it is often used for people with learning disabilities and associated dyspraxia.

Student activities

Find out about:

- Hydrotherapy facilities available for patients/clients in your placement.
- Activities for particular groups of people at your local swimming pool.

limb. This also helps to promote independence and gives people a feeling of involvement in their recovery. Passive exercising improves the blood supply to the affected area, helping to keep the muscle tissue and fascia supple. The repeated movements also provide feedback to the nervous system, thereby improving neuromuscular well-being.

Hot wax can be used for exercising the hands, e.g. to increase movement in rheumatoid arthritis. The heat from the wax helps to relieve pain, and as the wax cools and hardens it provides resistance for the muscles, making them work harder to achieve the same movements of extension and flexion. The hands can also be exercised using soft squeezy objects or a bowl of sand.

Occupational therapy

The OT is a healthcare professional who provides activities and exercises to encourage movement and increase independence. OTs help people to regain independence with activities of living such as personal hygiene and dressing as well as carrying out activities in the home, e.g. making tea, washing up and cooking. OTs also provide advice about communication systems that enable people who are at risk of falls to raise the alarm if they fall at home.

Home assessment

Physiotherapists and OTs often carry out home assessment visits together. Patients are taken home and are observed moving and carrying out normal daily activities in their familiar environment. The OT and/or physiotherapist may recommend home modifications including handrails, raised toilet seats, over-bed tables, trolleys on wheels and other gadgets that enable people to continue to live at home safely and independently.

Summary

- Understanding how the musculoskeletal system develops and its involvement in movement and posture underpins the nursing care of people with mobility problems.
- Many conditions can affect the development and maintenance of an upright posture and normal gait.
- People should be encouraged to move themselves whenever possible.
- It is essential to be familiar with the principles of safe EHM before being involved in moving either inanimate loads or people.
- Handling and moving equipment such as hoists, wheelchairs and walking aids should be used appropriately in promoting independence for clients with mobility problems.
- Exercise has many benefits and should be encouraged throughout the lifespan to optimize health.
- Immobility has many associated hazards that can often be prevented by providing appropriate nursing interventions.
- Active and passive exercises should be used to maintain and improve neuromuscular well-being and to promote mobility.
- Nursing care needs to be individualized to enable a person to regain independence in mobility and other aspects of their lives.
- Falls account for a large proportion of mobility problems in the over 65s.
- Each member of the MDT brings a different area of expertise to promoting independence with immobile patients/clients.

Self test

1. State the four areas of the Manual Handling Operations Regulations 1992 (HSE 1998) risk assessment for EHM.
2. Differentiate between active and passive exercises.
3. Outline the role of the MDT in promoting mobility.
4. State the principles of first aid for a person sustaining a fracture.

Key words and phrases for literature searching

Ageing/aging
Cast/Plaster of Paris
Fractures
Immobility
Orthopaedics
Osteoporosis
Traction

Useful websites

Age Concern	www.ageconcernscotland.org.uk Available July 2006
Cross-training	www.physsportsmed.com/issues/1996/09_96/cross.htm Available July 2006
Disabled Living Foundation	www.dlf.org.uk Available July 2006
National Osteoporosis Society	www.nos.org.uk Available July 2006
Royal Society for the Prevention of Accidents (RoSPA)	www.rospa.org.uk Available July 2006
Working-Well	www.working-well.org Available July 2006

References

Alexander MD, Goldberg A 2005 Gait disorders: search for multiple causes. Cleveland Clinical Journal of Medicine 72(7):586–599

Bertolazzi M, Saia B 1999 Risk during manual movement of loads. Giornale Italiano di Medicina del Lavoro ed Ergonomia 21(2): 130–133. Online: www.ncbi.nlm.nih.gov/entrez/query.fcgi?cmd=Retrieve&db=PubMed&list_uids=10771728&dopt=Citation Available July 2006

Brooker C, Nicol M 2003 Nursing adults: the practice of caring. Mosby, Edinburgh

Crozier L, Cozens S 1997 The neuromuscular approach to efficient handling and moving. In: Lloyd P, Fletcher B, Holmes D et al (eds) The guide to the handling of patients. 4th edn. National Back Pain Association/Royal College of Nursing, Middlesex, Chapter 6

Cryer C, Patel S 2001 Falls, fragility and fractures. The Alliance for Better Bone Health, London

Drake RL, Vogt W, Mitchell AWM 2005 Gray's anatomy for medical students. Churchill Livingstone, Edinburgh

Foley A, Halbert J, Hewitt T et al 2003 Does hydrotherapy improve strength and physical function in patients with osteoarthritis? A randomized controlled trial comparing a gym based and hydrotherapy based strengthening programme. Annals of the Rheumatic Diseases 6:1162–1167

Greig J, Rhind J 2002 Riddles's anatomy and physiology. Churchill Livingstone, Edinburgh

Hall J, Skevington SM, Maddison PJ et al 1996 A randomised and controlled trial of hydrotherapy in rheumatoid arthritis. Arthritis Care Research 9(3):206–215

Holmes D 1997 How to move people in bed. In: Lloyd P, Fletcher B, Holmes D et al (eds) The guide to the handling of patients. 4th edn. National Back Pain Association/Royal College of Nursing, Middlesex, Chapter 14

HSE 1998 Manual Handling Operations Regulations 1992: guidance on regulations. HSE, Norwich

Jootun D, MacInnes A 2005 Examining how well students use correct handling procedures. Nursing Times 101(4):38–40

Peattie PI, Walker S 1996 Understanding nursing care, 4th edn. Churchill Livingstone, Edinburgh

Scottish Building Standards Agency 2004 Online: www.sbsa.gov.uk/sbsa_intro.htm Available July 2006

Smith J (ed) 2005 The guide to the handling of people. 5th edn. BackCare, Teddington

Stamford B 1996 Cross-training: giving yourself a whole-body workout. The Physician and Sportsmedicine 24(9):103–104. Online: www.physsportsmed.com/issues/1996/09_96/cross.htm Available July 2006

Tarling C 1997 Sitting and standing. In: Lloyd P, Fletcher B, Holmes D et al (eds) The guide to the handling of patients. 4th edn. National Back Pain Association/Royal College of Nursing, Middlesex, Chapter 14

Thomas S 2005 Sitting to standing. In: Smith J (ed) The guide to the handling of people. 5th edn. BackCare, Teddington

Trew M, Everett T (eds) 2005 Human movement: an introductory text. 5th edn. Churchill Livingstone, Edinburgh

Waugh A, Grant A 2006 Ross and Wilson anatomy and physiology in health and illness. 10th edn. Churchill Livingstone, Edinburgh

Wong DL, Hockenberry-Eaton M, Wilson D et al 2001 Wong's essentials of pediatric nursing. 6th edn. Mosby, St Louis

Further reading

Carr A 2004 Orthopaedics in primary care. Butterworth-Heinemann, London

Crawford Adams J, Hamblen DL 2001 Outline of orthopaedics. 13th edn. Churchill Livingstone, Edinburgh

Dandy DJ, Edwards DJ 2003 Essential orthopaedics and trauma. 4th edn. Churchill Livingstone, Edinburgh

Kneale J, Davis P 2004 Orthopaedic nursing. 2nd edn. Churchill Livingstone, Edinburgh

Petty NJ 2004 Neuromusculoskeletal treatment and management: a guide for therapists. Churchill Livingstone, Edinburgh

19 Promoting hydration and nutrition

Chris Brooker

Glossary terms

Colloid solution

Crystalloid solution

Dehydration

Dysphagia

Electrolyte

Enteral

Hypodermoclysis

Malnutrition

Nausea

Nutrition

Oedema

Parenteral

Learning outcomes

This chapter will help you:

- Apply a basic knowledge of body fluids, electrolytes, fluid compartments and acid–base balance to inform nursing practice
- Outline the *Essence of Care* (NHS Modernisation Agency 2003) best practice benchmarks concerned with eating and drinking
- Describe the assessment of hydration
- Explain the nursing interventions by which fluid balance can be restored and maintained
- Describe the nursing interventions used in caring for a person with fluid and electrolyte imbalance
- Outline the role of the gastrointestinal (GI) tract in the ingestion, digestion and absorption of nutrients
- Describe the nutrients and the principles of a healthy diet
- Describe the nurse's role in assessment of nutritional status
- Explain the ways in which nutrition can be provided
- Describe the nursing interventions used to provide optimum nutrition in people of all ages
- Outline the role of the multidisciplinary team in the promotion of hydration and nutrition.

Introduction

Ensuring that clients and patients have sufficient fluids and nutrition that meets their needs is a basic, but vital role of the nurse. Healthy body function, recovery from illness and eventually life itself depend on being able to access fluids and nutrients. Nurses not only help people to eat and drink during illness but they also have an important role in educating people about eating and drinking for optimum health. Although families, health care assistants (HCAs) and students undertake considerable 'hands on' care, the registered nurse (RN) remains accountable for all nursing interventions (see Ch. 7). The nurse works within a multidisciplinary team (MDT) that includes, amongst others, dietitians, specialist nutrition and intravenous therapy nurses and catering staff, to promote hydration and nutrition.

Inadequate or inappropriate fluid and nutrient intake impedes recovery from illness and surgery, lengthens hospital stay and can lead to complications that include delayed wound healing, pressure ulcers, weight loss, low mood, infection, dehydration and poor oral hygiene.

The importance of providing oral nutrition is emphasized by it forming one of the original *Essence of Care* best practice statements (DH 2001).

Education about and help to eat a healthy balanced diet is imperative given the high prevalence of overweight and obese children and adults in the UK. The House of Commons Select Committee (2004) report that two-thirds of the population in England is overweight or obese.

This chapter is in two parts: maintaining fluid, electrolyte and acid–base balance, and nutrition. However, it is important to understand that all of these are closely linked and that none can ensure well-being without the others.

Skilled promotion of hydration and nutrition is an important nursing role that really can 'make a difference' to the well-being of people in their care.

Maintaining fluid, electrolyte and acid–base balance

This part of the chapter outlines the maintenance of fluid, electrolyte and acid–base balance, some common disorders and investigations. Nursing interventions such as assessment of hydration, helping with drinking and the principles of intravenous infusions are covered in some depth.

The amount of water and electrolytes, e.g. sodium, potassium, in the body compartments and acid–base balance are controlled by interdependent mechanisms that keep levels fairly constant within narrow limits. Normal body function depends on homeostasis, i.e. maintaining water, electrolyte levels and acid–base balance in the internal environment within the normal range. Therefore, dynamic homeostatic mechanisms are required to respond to continually changing conditions within the body.

Body fluids and fluid compartments

The amount of water as a percentage of body weight decreases with age (Fig. 19.1). For example, a newborn baby has around 75% water whereas an average adult male has around 60% and an older adult between 45 and 50%. The amount of body fat and gender also influence water content. Fat (adipose tissue) contains less water than muscle tissue. Body water is lower in older adults because muscle tissue is replaced by fat; people with obesity and women, who generally have more fat than men, also have less body water.

Body water is distributed between two fluid compartments:

- Extracellular fluid (ECF), which comprises the fluid between the cells, also known as interstitial or tissue fluid, plasma (i.e. the fluid part of blood), lymph
- Intracellular fluid (ICF) is present within all body cells.

In adults, the split is approximately two-thirds ICF to one-third ECF (Fig. 19.2). The distribution of fluid in infants and children less than 2 years of age is characterized by more body water in the ECF. The fluid distribution and the increased rate at which ECF is exchanged means that there is very little fluid reserve, hence there is an increased risk of dehydration if an infant or small child loses fluid (Huband & Trigg 2000).

The body surface area also differs in children and infants who have proportionally greater surface areas than adults. Therefore they lose more water through the skin, which has important implications for fluid balance and intravenous (i.v.) fluid therapy (see p. 545). The immature kidneys of infants and small children cannot excrete or conserve the electrolyte sodium, or produce concentrated or dilute urine (Wong et al 1999). In addition, they have a higher metabolic rate that produces more waste products for excretion in the urine. Conditions that increase metabolic rate also increase heat production and hence the amount of water loss through the skin (Wong et al 1999).

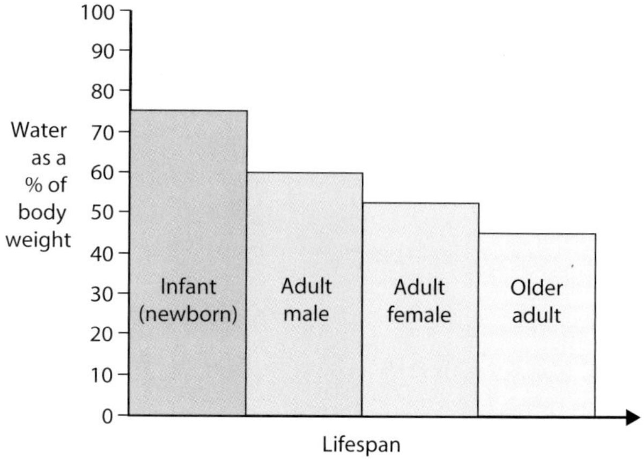

Fig. 19.1 Water as a percentage of body weight (reproduced with permission from Brooker 1998)

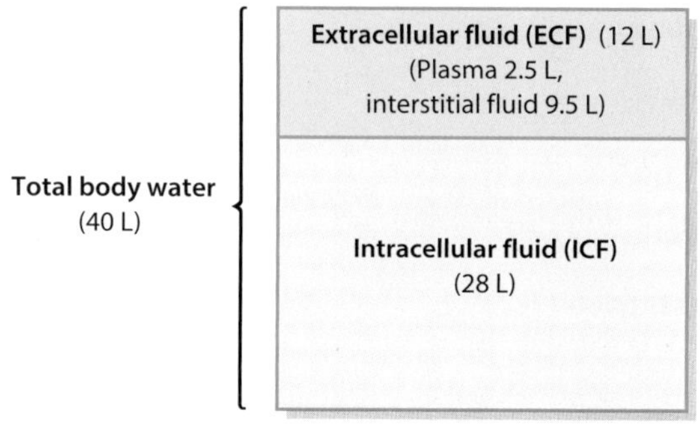

Fig. 19.2 Distribution of body water in a 70 kg adult male (reproduced with permission from Brooker & Nicol 2003)

Electrolytes

Electrolytes are substances such as sodium chloride (described in chemical notation as NaCl), which, when dissolved in water, dissociate into electrically charged particles called ions that conduct electricity. Some ions have a positive charge, e.g. sodium (Na^+), and others are negatively charged, e.g. chloride (Cl^-). In body fluids the main electrolytes are sodium, potassium, calcium and magnesium with a positive charge, and bicarbonate, chloride and phosphate that are negatively charged. The ECF and ICF have different electrolyte compositions; sodium is mainly in the ECF whereas most potassium is in the ICF. Table 19.1 shows the normal range for serum electrolyte levels in adults.

Electrolytes in body fluids and are necessary for:

- Maintaining osmotic pressure, e.g. sodium
- Transmission of nerve impulses and muscle contraction, e.g. sodium, potassium, calcium

Table 19.1 Serum electrolytes – normal reference values (adults)

Electrolyte (chemical notation)	Reference range (serum)
Sodium (Na^+)	135–143 mmol/L
Potassium (K^+)	3.6–5.0 mmol/L
Calcium (Ca^{2+})	2.1–2.6 mmol
Magnesium (Mg^{2+})	0.75–1.0 mmol/L
Chloride (Cl^-)	97–106 mmol/L
Phosphate (PO_4^{2-})	0.8–1.4 mmol/L
Bicarbonate (HCO_3^-)	22–28 mmol/L

Note that the amount of urea (waste product of protein metabolism, normal range 2.5–6.4 mmol/L) is usually measured along with serum electrolytes.

Note that normal ranges may vary slightly on a local basis.

- Blood coagulation, strong healthy bones and teeth, e.g. calcium
- Release of neurotransmitters, e.g. calcium
- Enzyme function, e.g. magnesium
- Acid–base balance, pH homeostasis, e.g. bicarbonate.

Movement of water and electrolytes

Water and electrolytes and other substances continually move between the ECF and ICF in order to:

- Maintain homeostasis of the internal environment
- Allow oxygen (O_2), nutrients and other metabolic substances to enter cells
- Allow waste products to leave cells for excretion by the lungs (see Ch. 17) and kidneys (see Ch. 20).

This movement occurs through a number of processes, including osmosis, diffusion, filtration and active transport.

Osmosis

Osmosis is the movement of water through a semi-permeable membrane. Pores in the membrane allow the movement of water molecules in either direction. Water moves when there is a difference in its concentration on either side of the membrane. The direction of movement is from high water to low water concentration. This means that water will move from a weak solution to a stronger, more concentrated solution until equilibrium is reached, i.e. the water concentrations are the same on either side of the membrane. Osmosis occurs when equilibrium cannot be achieved by the movement of electrolytes or sugars (solutes) across the semi-permeable membrane.

The force required to oppose the movement of water by osmosis is known as the osmotic pressure; this increases with the concentration difference on either side of the membrane. The concentration of particles that contribute to the osmotic pressure in a litre of fluid is termed the osmolality of a solution. The movement of water stops when the opposing pressures (i.e. concentrations) on either side of the membrane are the same. The solutions are then described as being isotonic. In the body, an isotonic solution has the same osmolality as plasma. A solution with a higher osmolality than plasma is described as hypertonic; one with a lower osmolality to plasma is hypotonic. Osmosis is vital in maintaining the correct water distribution within the fluid compartments.

Diffusion

Diffusion involves the movement of gases and solutes from an area of high concentration to an area of lower concentration, i.e. down a concentration gradient. In the body, diffusion down a concentration gradient takes place within cells or body fluids and also across semi-permeable membranes. The latter allow small particles to pass through but hold back larger particles, e.g. proteins.

Diffusion is described as passive because it does not use chemical energy (adenosine triphosphate [ATP]). The end result of diffusion is equal concentrations on both sides of the membrane, i.e. equilibrium. Diffusion is important for the movement of O_2, carbon dioxide (CO_2), electrolytes, nutrients, hormones and waste products such as urea.

Filtration

The passive process of filtration provides another means by which the fluid compartments and the concentration of substances within body fluids are maintained; again there is a gradient difference either side of the membrane, but this time it is pressure rather than concentration. The pressure that forces water and small molecules through membrane pores is known as the hydrostatic (fluid) pressure. Filtration is important in the formation of tissue fluid and urine (see Ch. 20).

Active transport

Active transport is a process requiring chemical energy (ATP) to move substances:

- Against a concentration gradient
- Where no concentration gradient exists
- That are unable to diffuse through membranes.

Substances transported in this way include nutrients and electrolytes, e.g. the sodium–potassium exchange pump in cell membranes where sodium ions (mainly in the ECF) are pumped out of the cell and potassium ions (mainly in the ICF) are pumped into the cell against their concentration gradients.

Acid–base balance

The pH (hydrogen ion concentration or the acidity) of blood and other body fluids must remain within a narrow range for normal cell function. For example, the normal range for the pH of ECF is 7.35–7.45. Small deviations outside this range are associated with serious physiological disruption because pH is a logarithmic scale and a change of 1 represents a 10-fold change in hydrogen ion concentration.

Acids are ingested on a daily basis and metabolic processes continuously produce acidic substances including CO_2 (which, when dissolved, increases the acidity of a solution), lactic acid and ketoacids. Various

Box 19.1 Disorders of acid–base balance

The acid–base disorders alkalosis and acidosis can have either a respiratory or a metabolic cause. Seriously ill patients may develop a mixed disorder.

Alkalosis

- Respiratory alkalosis is due to overbreathing (hyperventilation) that results in a net loss of CO_2. Hyperventilation can be a feature of panic attacks
- Metabolic alkalosis is caused by excessive loss of acids from the GI tract, e.g. vomiting of gastric (stomach) acid, or by excessive ingestion of alkaline indigestion medicines.

Acidosis

- Respiratory acidosis is due to inadequate breathing (hypoventilation) and the build-up of CO_2
- Metabolic acidosis is caused by a failure to excrete H^+ in kidney failure, the production of excess acids or the loss of alkali, e.g. diarrhoea.

[For further information, see Waugh (2003)]

interdependent homeostatic mechanisms function to maintain acid–base balance. These are:

- Chemical buffers (substances that limit pH change) that act immediately to counteract changes in pH (for more information, see Waugh & Grant (2006) in Further reading)
- Excretion of CO_2 by the lungs (respiratory regulation through rate and depth of breathing operates within minutes)
- The kidneys, which provide long-term regulation by excreting hydrogen ions (H^+) and by conserving or excreting bicarbonate ions (HCO_3^-) in processes occurring over many hours.

If these homeostatic mechanisms fail, acid–base balance is disrupted. When the pH of arterial blood rises above 7.45, i.e. becomes more alkaline, this is known as alkalaemia. The process leading to low levels of acid (excess of alkali) is termed alkalosis. When the pH of arterial blood falls below 7.35 this is known as acidaemia. *Note* – the blood is still alkaline but the pH is closer to the acid range. The process that results in the excess acid is termed acidosis.

Homeostatic mechanisms attempt to restore normal blood pH by either excreting more or less CO_2 from the lungs or by changing the amount of H^+ or HCO_3^- excreted in the urine. Acid–base imbalances, which are often associated with fluid or electrolyte imbalances (see p. 535), can be life threatening. Disorders of acid–base balance are outlined in Box 19.1.

Normal fluid and electrolyte balance

The kidneys regulate fluid and electrolyte balance in response to hormone secretion (see below). Healthy people take in most fluid by drinking but there is water in food, e.g. soup, fruit and ice cream, and chemical processes in the body also produce water (metabolic water). Electrolytes are obtained from food and fluids, e.g. sodium from the salt added to processed foods. Fluids and electrolytes are excreted from the body in urine, faeces, sweat, through insensible perspiration and during respiration. Table 19.2 shows average volumes for adults.

Table 19.2 Average water balance over 24 hours in adults

Input (mL)	Output (mL)
Drinks 1700	Urine 1500
Fluid obtained from food 1000	Faeces 100
Metabolic water 300	During respiration 500
	Skin (insensible loss and sweat) 900 in health
Total 3000	Total 3000

REFLECTIVE PRACTICE Box 19.2

Responding to thirst

Think about people you have met during placements.

Student activities

- Identify people who had potential or actual problems in responding to thirst. You might have a list that includes some obvious examples such as small children or a person with poor mobility living at home; however, other examples might be someone with dementia who spends the day wandering in the care home, or a person with severe mental distress (see below).
- Consider whether or not the people you identified received an adequate fluid intake (see Tables 19.2, 19.3, p. 541).
- Think about nursing measures that you have seen used in practice to improve fluid intake (see p. 542).

Factors that regulate normal fluid and electrolyte balance

Hormones such as aldosterone and antidiuretic hormone (ADH) are essential in maintaining fluid and electrolyte homeostasis by their actions on the kidneys (see Ch. 20). Also very important in the regulation of fluid balance is the sensation of thirst. If fluid is lost or intake is inadequate a person feels thirsty and usually remedies the situation by having a drink. However, certain groups of people are unable to respond to thirst: babies, small children, people with mobility problems, unconscious patients, people with a severe learning disability or dementia and older adults (who may not experience thirst) are all at risk of fluid depletion (Box 19.2).

Common disorders of fluid and electrolyte balance

Disorders of fluid and electrolyte balance can cause serious and sometimes life-threatening effects.

Box 19.3 **Common disorders of fluid balance**

Isotonic imbalances

- *Fluid volume deficit* occurs when both water and electrolytes are lost. It can arise through vomiting, diarrhoea, sweating, drainage from the GI tract and the use of diuretic drugs (drugs that increase urine production). Fluid may also move into the 'third space' where it is lost from the ECF but remains in the body, e.g. the abdominal cavity. Note that fluid volume deficit is not dehydration, which correctly describes an osmolar disorder (see below).
- *Fluid volume excess* occurs when there is an increase in both water and electrolytes (usually sodium ions with associated water retention) in the ECF. Fluid moves into the interstitial spaces causing generalized tissue water logging (oedema) (see below) or pulmonary oedema where fluid enters the alveoli of the lungs (see Ch. 17). This can occur when i.v. fluids containing sodium are overinfused and in people with heart failure and liver disease. The mechanisms that give rise to oedema are:
  - decreased plasma proteins leading to a reduction in plasma osmotic pressure which is needed to 'pull' interstitial fluid back into the venous side of the capillary network. This can be a feature of some kidney diseases and occurs when dietary protein is deficient (see p. 554)
  - increased venous hydrostatic pressure caused by venous congestion, e.g. with chronic heart failure, which prevents interstitial fluid returning to the circulation at the venous side of the capillary network
  - 'leaky' capillaries that allow protein to leak out into the interstitial spaces, e.g. as part of the inflammatory process. This increases osmotic pressure in the tissues and because less fluid returns to the bloodstream it collects in the interstitial spaces as oedema
  - impaired lymphatic drainage – some interstitial fluid normally returns to the circulation through the lymphatic system. Obstruction to lymphatic drainage, e.g. from cancer affecting the lymph nodes, means that the excess fluid remains in the interstitial spaces.

Osmolar imbalances

- *Hyperosmolar imbalance (dehydration or water depletion)* occurs when water intake is inadequate or excess fluid is lost from the body. Without a proportional loss of electrolytes it is accompanied by a disturbance in electrolyte balance, especially sodium levels which rise. Loss of water from the extracellular compartment increases the osmolality of the ECF, which becomes hypertonic and fluid moves out of the cells in order to restore the osmotic equilibrium of the ICF and ECF. The overall result is cellular dehydration, which seriously disrupts cell function.
- *Hypo-osmolar imbalance (fluid excess or 'water intoxication')* occurs when ECF water increases without an increase in electrolytes. This can be caused by excessive water intake such as occurs in some severe mental health problems or from inappropriate secretion of ADH. This time the ECF is diluted, its osmolality decreases and, because it is hypotonic compared with the ICF, the movement of fluid is into the cells adversely affecting their function.

Common disorders of fluid balance

Disorders of fluid balance can be divided into two main types:

- *Isotonic imbalances* involving a proportional increase or decrease of both water and electrolytes and hence the osmolality of the ECF may be unchanged
- *Osmolar imbalances* where water only is increased or decreased without a proportional change in electrolyte concentration (mainly sodium) and hence the osmolality of ECF is affected.

An outline of fluid balance disorders is provided in Box 19.3.

Electrolyte imbalances

Disorders of electrolyte balance involve either increases or decreases outside the normal range. Many factors can affect electrolyte levels (Box 19.4).

Frequently more that one electrolyte is affected and is accompanied by a fluid imbalance; sometimes there

CRITICAL THINKING Box 19.4

Factors that can affect electrolyte levels

The next time you are helping to care for a person who has had their electrolytes measured, ask if you can look at the results from the laboratory.

Student activities

- Find out why the investigation was carried out.
- Compare the results with the normal range (see Table 19.1).
- If the results are very different, think about why this has occurred, e.g. has the person been vomiting or have their kidneys stopped functioning (see Box 19.5; see also Ch. 20).
- Discuss your provisional ideas with your mentor.

Box 19.5 **Common causes of abnormal blood electrolyte levels**

Hypernatraemia
Increased blood sodium concentration, caused by excessive loss of water without electrolytes owing to polyuria (increased urinary volume), high salt intake, excessive sweating or inadequate water intake.

Hyponatraemia
Decreased blood sodium concentration, caused by vomiting, diarrhoea, sweating and burns; diuretics, heart failure, kidney disease and diabetes mellitus, or a failure to excrete water or excess intake.

Hyperkalaemia
Increased blood potassium concentration, caused by reduced urine output, e.g. in kidney failure, or excessive prescribed potassium supplements.

Hypokalaemia
Decreased blood potassium concentration, caused by excessive urine output, misuse of laxatives, diarrhoea and vomiting over a prolonged period, starvation.

is also loss of acid–base balance. Box 19.5 outlines some important electrolyte imbalances.

Factors that can lead to fluid and/or electrolyte imbalance

Many physical, psychological and social factors can lead to imbalances in body fluids and electrolytes. The nurse must be able to identify and minimize the impact of factors that increase the risk of people developing problems. These factors include those that prevent a person responding to thirst (see p. 534) as well as the following.

Age
People at the extremes of age are at increased risk of fluid and electrolyte imbalance. In infants and small children this is because of the distribution of fluid in the ECF and ICF, their immature kidneys, greater body surface area and higher metabolic rate (see p. 532). In older adults the risk of imbalances is increased by the reduced percentage of body water, declining kidney function and inability to access fluids or respond to thirst (see p. 534).

Fasting
People who are having investigations or procedures that require a general anaesthetic can develop fluid depletion if they are fasted for unnecessarily lengthy periods (see Ch. 24).

During the religious festival of Ramadan all healthy Muslims over the age of 12 years are required to fast between dawn and sunset (Box 19.6).

REFLECTIVE PRACTICE Box 19.6

Fasting during Ramadan

Although a person who is ill is not required to fast, many devout Muslims want to fast for all or at least part of Ramadan. This observance of faith may be particularly important for the person who is terminally ill or has a life-threatening condition (see Ch. 12).

Muslims who are unwell need special arrangements if they decide to fast during Ramadan. It is important that fluids and a meal are provided before dawn and soon after sunset. The person will also need water and a bowl so that they can rinse their mouth before prayers.

Student activities
- Find out the extent to which the staff on your placement are aware of the needs of people fasting during Ramadan.
- Find out what arrangements are in place for providing meals and/or fluids outside normal meal times in your placement.
- Think about whether the needs of people fasting for religious reasons are fully met and discuss this with your mentor.

Fluid and electrolyte loss
Vomiting and diarrhoea and excessive sweating, such as during heavy work or exercise, lead to problems with fluid and electrolyte balance. In addition, hot weather leads to an increased fluid requirement, especially for those exercising strenuously.

Alcohol and caffeine drinks
Alcohol, tea, coffee, cocoa and 'cola' drinks increase urinary output (diuresis) and cause fluid depletion.

High level of dependency
People with some physical disabilities and/or a severe learning disability may be completely dependent on others for their fluid intake, as they are unable to ask for a drink or make themselves a drink. Some people such as those with cerebral palsy also have problems with chewing, swallowing (see below), muscle tone and posture and the reflexes that protect the airway.

Mental health problems
People experiencing severe mental distress may be unable to maintain an adequate fluid intake because their mood is so profoundly depressed, or they may be experiencing serious manifestations, such as hallucinations, which pervade all aspects of life to the exclusion of self-maintenance activities. Drugs used for some forms of mental distress can lead to fluid and electrolyte imbalances, e.g. lithium carbonate.

People with dementia or confusion may not remember to drink during the day or will have forgotten how to prepare drinks. Lack of fluid worsens confusion and a vicious circle of increasingly severe fluid depletion and worsening confusion ensues.

Immobility and lack of manual dexterity
Older people and those with conditions such as severe arthritis, or following a stroke, may be unable to prepare

Box 19.7 **Routes for the administration of fluid**

Enteral fluids
People who are unable drink sufficient fluids or have swallowing problems, but who have a functioning GI tract, can have their fluid needs met by the enteral route. This may be through a:

- nasogastric tube – passed though the nose and oesophagus into the stomach
- nasoenteric tube – passed into the small intestine via the nose and oesophagus
- gastrostomy tube – inserted through the abdominal wall into the stomach.

The enteral route is usually used to provide both nutrients and fluids and is discussed on page 562.

Subcutaneous fluids
Fluid infused subcutaneously (see p. 543) is known as hypodermoclysis and is increasingly used to provide treatment for mild to moderate dehydration.

Rectal fluids
Fluid infused into the rectum for absorption is known as proctoclysis. The fluid, e.g. tap water or normal saline (sodium chloride 0.9%), is infused and slowly absorbed into the circulation. Proctoclysis is a safe, effective and low cost technique for maintaining hydration in terminally ill patients (Bruera et al 1998).

Intravenous fluids
Sterile intravenous fluids (see p. 545) are infused into a vein to maintain fluid, electrolyte and acid–base balance or to correct imbalances, administer drugs and provide nutrients (see also 'Parenteral nutrition', p. 565).

Intraosseous fluids
The intraosseous route involves the introduction of fluids into the marrow (medullary) cavity of a long bone, e.g. the tibia. It is used for children in some emergency situations (for more information, see Trigg and Mohammed (2006) in Further reading).

drinks safely or to carry them from the kitchen. Dealing with hot drinks can be hazardous, particularly when people find it difficult to hold a cup or mug due severe shaking or deformity of the hands.

Swallowing problems (dysphagia)

Swallowing problems are very common after a stroke and the risk of choking or inhalation of fluids or food into the respiratory tract is present. It is essential that oral fluid and food be withheld until a speech and language therapist (SLT) or specially trained nurse carries out a full assessment. The stages of swallowing are outlined on page 550 and more details about swallowing assessment can be found in Further reading (e.g. Brooker & Nicol 2003).

Fear of incontinence

People may restrict their fluids in an effort to prevent nocturia (passing urine at night) or incontinence (see Ch. 20). Those who limit fluids before bedtime should be encouraged to compensate by increasing intake at other times of the day (Morrison 2000).

Drugs

Drugs – including diuretics, e.g. furosemide (frusemide) – can lead to fluid depletion and loss of electrolytes, especially potassium.

Breathlessness (dyspnoea)

Breathlessness can lead to fluid depletion because insensible water loss increases during mouth breathing. The administration of oxygen without humidification also worsens oral drying. A person with severe breathlessness will have little energy for drinking and will be unable to access fluids.

Serious organ disorders

Heart, liver and kidney failure all lead to severe fluid and electrolyte retention, e.g. sodium and potassium. It may be necessary to restrict the intake of fluids (p. 543) and foods containing particular electrolytes such as sodium (see p. 556).

Lack of access to clean water

Many people in developing countries and those affected by natural disasters or wars do not have clean water piped to individual homes. Often, people spend many hours a day collecting water, or have no alternative to drinking from dirty sources such as rivers contaminated by untreated sewage.

Nursing interventions that aim to help people obtain sufficient fluids are discussed below (pp. 540–543).

Nursing interventions: promoting and maintaining hydration

Although the *Essence of Care* best practice statement 'Patients receive the care and assistance they require with eating and drinking' (NHS Modernisation Agency 2003, p. 1) appears to state the obvious, this does not always happen. This part of the chapter covers the nursing assessment and some investigations used to evaluate fluid and electrolyte status. It also describes how nurses can help people to drink sufficient fluids. Other interventions covered include caring for people with fluid imbalances and those with nausea and vomiting.

Most people maintain hydration and fluid balance with oral fluids. This is the preferred route as it maintains normality, is non-invasive and has fewer complications. Where this is not possible, e.g. due to severe vomiting, unconsciousness or swallowing problems, other ways of

Box 19.8 Common investigations used to assess fluid and electrolyte status

Blood tests

- Measurement of urea and electrolytes in serum (see Table 19.1).
- Serum albumin (normal range 36–47 g/L)
- Packed cell volume (PCV) or haematocrit measures the percentage of red blood cells and from this the amount of fluid in the blood. In fluid loss the PCV may be raised and in fluid gain it can be decreased.

Urine tests

- Routine urinalysis (see Ch. 20)
- Measurement of urine osmolality (normal range 300–1200 mOsml/L)
- 24-hour urine collection for electrolyte estimation.

providing fluid are needed. Box 19.7 outlines other routes and some are discussed more fully below (pp. 543–549).

Assessing hydration

The nursing assessment of hydration is a vital component of holistic assessment, which includes careful observation. It is important to consider all aspects of the person's life such as their normal fluid and food intake and the type of drinks they normally prefer. The nurse needs to be aware of physical, social or psychological factors that may disrupt fluid and electrolyte balance to identify those people who are at risk of potential or actual problems. The nurse documents the findings from this assessment in the nursing records and ensures that any abnormal findings are reported immediately to the RN. Box 19.8 outlines some investigations used to assess hydration.

Skin

Normally when skin is pinched and released it returns at once to its normal position, as the elastic tissue recoils. This feature is termed turgor. People who have a fluid volume deficit may have reduced skin turgor and the pinched up portion remains raised for longer. Skin turgor is not always reliable in the assessment of older people who have less elastic tissue or in people who have recently lost weight. The skin may appear dry.

The presence of oedema (see p. 535) can indicate fluid volume excess with accumulation of fluid in the interstitial spaces. Generalized oedema affects dependent parts of the body, the feet and ankles when standing or sitting and the sacral area in people confined to bed. On waking, some people may have puffiness around the eyes (periorbital oedema) because they have been lying flat. When oedematous tissue is compressed with a finger and stays indented, this is termed 'pitting oedema'.

Fontanelles

Assessment of the anterior fontanelle (often called the 'soft spot' by parents) in the skull is a guide to hydration status in babies. The fontanelles are membranous spaces present between the skull bones in newborn babies. The diamond-shaped anterior fontanelle is located between the frontal and two parietal bones and closes up during the second year of life. A triangular posterior fontanelle is situated at the junction of the occipital and two parietal bones. This closes within weeks of birth.

The anterior fontanelle can be observed and gently felt with the flat part of a finger. In healthy, well-hydrated babies the fontanelle is level with the skull bones. A sunken fontanelle can indicate fluid volume deficit while a bulging fontanelle may suggest fluid volume excess, or it can be due to increased pressure inside the skull (raised intracranial pressure).

Weight

Accurate daily weight (see Ch. 14) can give a good indication of the amount of fluid lost or gained, especially oedema.

Sunken eyes

Sunken eyes can indicate a moderate to severe fluid volume deficit. It occurs because interstitial fluid is lost from the periorbital tissue.

Mouth

The condition of the oral mucosa, which is usually pink and moist, is a good indicator of hydration status (see Ch. 16). Fluid depletion leads to a dry mouth, coated tongue and viscous (thick) saliva. Thirst is an important regulator of fluid balance (see p. 534) and people with fluid depletion will usually say that they are thirsty. It is important to remember that a dry mouth may have other causes, e.g. oxygen therapy, mouth breathing and some drugs.

Behaviour

People's behaviour can give valuable clues about hydration. Lethargy, anxiety or confusion may occur in fluid depletion and acid–base imbalance. Babies and small children may exhibit irritability. Some babies are quiet and show little interest in their surroundings or a favourite toy or game.

Bowel function (see Ch. 21)

Constipation can be caused by fluid volume deficit or dehydration. Severe fluid, electrolyte and acid–base imbalance can result from severe or prolonged diarrhoea.

Urine output and specific gravity (see Ch. 20)

The volume and colour of urine are important indicators of hydration. Small volumes (oliguria) and dark concentrated urine with a high specific gravity (SG >1.030) are features of fluid volume deficit. Infants and toddlers have fewer wet nappies than normal. Concentrated urine may have a stronger odour than usual. Further discussion about fluid balance charts is provided below.

Blood pressure

A fall in blood pressure (BP) accompanies fluid volume deficit. In severe situations the person will have a low BP (hypotension) while lying down. However, in milder cases the fluid volume deficit may only be apparent

NURSING SKILLS — Box 19.9

Maintaining fluid balance charts

Placing a sign above the bed or on the door ensures that the patient, the family, nurses, HCAs and housekeepers are aware that the person is having fluid intake and output measured and recorded.

- All oral intake, including milk on cereals, soup and ice cream in some circumstances
- Nasogastric, gastrostomy, intravenous, subcutaneous and rectal intake are recorded on the intake side of the chart (see Fig. 19.3)
- Fluid output from urine (sometimes measured hourly in seriously ill people), vomit, aspirate from a nasogastric tube, diarrhoea, fluid from a stoma, e.g. ileostomy, ileal conduit (see Chs 20, 21), or wound drain are all recorded on the output side of the chart (see Fig. 19.3). The 'Other' column is used to record output other than urine or vomit and the nature of the fluid should be specified. In order to be accurate it is necessary, in some situations, to weigh articles such as nappies, incontinence pads and wound dressings. The difference between dry and wet weight in grams approximately corresponds to millilitres of urine or drainage
- All measurements of intake and output are charted immediately. This ensures that charts are accurate and up-to-date
- Inappropriate or imprecise terms such as 'up to toilet' should not be used. In a small study of fluid charts, Reid et al (2004) found that inappropriate comments were common
- Many people who are independent in oral fluid intake and elimination take responsibility for noting what they have drunk and measuring their urine. Disposable jugs for measuring urine are placed in the lavatory/sluice
- The nurse monitors all fluid charts at regular intervals, the frequency depending on the person's condition.

Note: Nurses should know the volumes of jugs and drinking vessels such as cups, glasses, mugs, juice cartons and drink cans used in the ward or nursing home (see Fig. 19.4). Patient-friendly charts showing volumes should be provided to encourage people to record their own intake accurately (Reid et al 2004).

because of a marked decrease in BP upon standing up from the sitting position (postural hypotension). An increasing BP may be a feature of fluid overload such as during i.v. fluid therapy (see p. 549).

Pulse

An increase in pulse rate (tachycardia) occurs in fluid volume deficit because there is less fluid in the vascular system (hypovolaemia). Fluid volume excess normally also causes an increase in pulse rate (Carroll 2000).

Respiration

The respiratory rate, effort and depth can change in response to fluid, electrolyte and acid–base imbalance. For example, a person with fluid volume excess can develop pulmonary oedema (see p. 535 and Ch. 19), which causes difficulty in breathing (dyspnoea) and a cough with frothy sputum.

Skin temperature

Cool extremities may indicate a decrease in intravascular volume but there are also many other factors that influence skin temperature (see Ch. 14).

Central venous pressure

Central venous pressure (CVP) estimates the pressure of blood in the right atrium of the heart. CVP is used in seriously ill patients to assess hydration status and inform fluid replacement therapy. It is always interpreted in conjunction with other observations such as pulse, BP, respiration and urine output (for more information, see Further reading, e.g. Metheny 1996).

Fluid balance charts

Fluid balance charts are also known as fluid intake and output charts, or sometimes just fluid charts. They are used to record all fluid intakes and outputs over a 24-hour period (Box 19.9). Normally the amounts for intake and output are totalled daily and the fluid balance calculated at the same time each day, often at midnight, or at 06.00 or 08.00 hours. A positive balance exists where the intake exceeds output. This situation occurs when fluid intake is increased to rectify fluid volume deficit and dehydration (see p. 535), whereas a negative balance exists when output exceeds intake. This occurs, for example, when treatment with diuretics is used to rectify fluid volume excess. A record is also kept of the daily fluid balance over several days so that trends can be assessed.

Oral fluids

The average healthy adult needs a fluid intake of 1.5–2.0 L per day. Most of this fluid should be water, as caffeine-containing drinks such as tea, coffee and colas cause diuresis. There are, however, many situations when more than this is needed such as when a person has a urinary catheter in situ (see Ch. 20), strenuous exercise, sweating and diarrhoea and vomiting.

Older people may need a higher intake because their kidneys become less efficient in the production of concentrated urine. In addition, as mentioned earlier, older people may be less sensitive to and/or responsive to the sensation of thirst. Fluid intake may need to increase further when body temperature is raised and in hot weather to prevent dehydration.

The daily fluid requirements for children are determined by weight. Infants have a greater fluid requirement per kg of body weight than do older children (Table 19.3). Infants and small children have very little fluid reserve and are at increased risk of fluid and electrolyte depletion (see p. 532). For example, infants and children with diarrhoea lose water and the electrolytes sodium and potassium (Box 19.10).

Helping people to drink

Whether a person receives adequate oral fluid or not can depend on simple interventions, advice and encouragement provided by nurses and other members of the MDT. For example, just having a glass of water within reach at all times will influence fluid intake.

Success in achieving the goals set for fluid intake depends on providing individualized care that meets the person's needs. For most people, independence in fluid intake is the norm and nurses must be tactful and sensitive to the feelings of people who need help with drinking. When helping people to drink the nurse should consider points that include the following:

- *Safety in the home, other community settings and in hospital*: This must be assessed. The occupational therapist (OT) can assess the person in their own home to ascertain their ability to safely heat water and prepare hot drinks. Safety and independence can be enhanced by the provision of aids that include tippers for kettles and teapots for pouring, or a small volume kettle that is easier to lift (see Fig. 19.5). The physiotherapist will be involved where people have mobility and balance problems.
- *Swallowing ability*: The SLT or specially trained nurse undertakes swallowing assessment if there

Fluid balance chart

Hospital/Ward: Date:

Hospital number:
Surname:
Forenames:
Date of birth:
Sex:

Fluid intake				Fluid output				
Time (hrs)	Oral	IV	Other (specify route)	Urine	Vomit	Other (specify)		
01.00								
02.00								
03.00								
04.00								
05.00								
06.00								
07.00								
08.00								
09.00								
10.00								
11.00								
12.00								
13.00								
14.00								
15.00								
16.00								
17.00								
18.00								
19.00								
20.00								
21.00								
22.00								
23.00								
24.00								
TOTAL								

Fig. 19.3 A fluid balance chart (reproduced with permission from Nicol et al 2000)

is any doubt about the safety of giving oral fluids (see p. 537).

- *Assessment of the mouth and teeth* (see Ch. 16): A sore mouth, e.g. caused by mouth ulcers, can prevent a person from drinking. Make sure that dentures are clean and in place before offerings drinks.
- *Position*: Where possible the person should sit upright, as this makes swallowing easier.
- *Preferences*: Ask the person about their favourite drinks and the usual timing of these as preferred fluids are usually more acceptable. Always ascertain whether the person takes sugar or milk in their tea or coffee and never put sugar in drinks without asking. Infants and small children should always be offered sugar-free drinks. However, if sugary drinks are consumed children should be helped or encouraged to clean their teeth afterwards (see Ch. 16).
- *Temperature*: Ensure that drinks are served at the correct temperature – that hot drinks are hot and cold drinks are cold. At home, providing hot drinks in a vacuum flask will keep them hot for several hours. This is especially useful if the person has mobility problems and family or carers visit during the day. Adding ice or cooling drinks in the refrigerator increases palatability for some people.
- *Variety*: Tap water can be monotonous; offer variety with carbonated water or water flavoured with fruit juices. People with electrolyte imbalances may need to avoid some fluids, e.g. yeast extract drinks such as Marmite containing high levels of sodium, or a person who needs potassium may be encouraged to drink fruit juices; instant coffee also has high levels of potassium but contains caffeine.
- *Changing water jugs*: This should be done every few hours, as water is not very palatable at room temperature. Try to keep water jugs away from radiators and out of direct sunlight. When jugs are

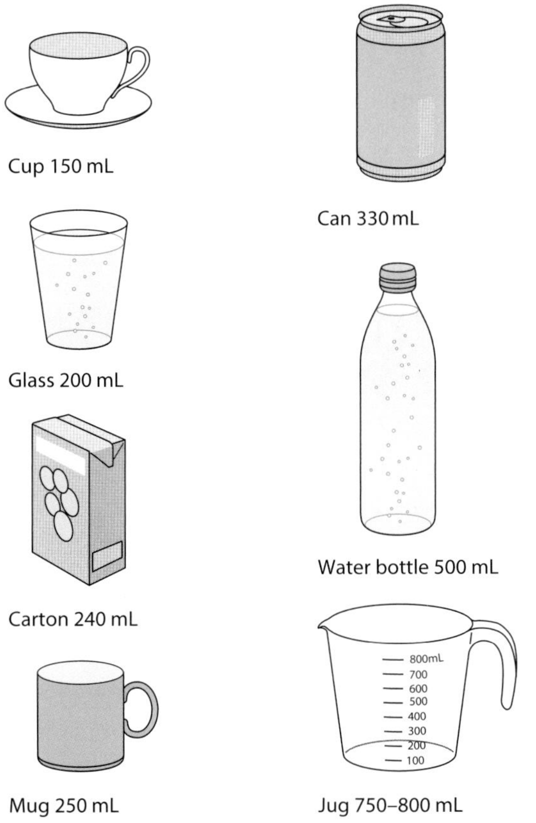

Note - always check the labels and the volume of drinking vessels, as volumes vary

Fig. 19.4 Typical volume of a cup, glass, juice carton, mug, drinks can, water bottle and jug

CRITICAL THINKING Box 19.10

Oral rehydration salts

3-year-old Wayne has had four loose stools in the last 24 hours and he is 'off his food'. When his mother telephoned the local surgery the practice nurse told her that the diarrhoea is likely to stop within 24 hours and gave her advice that included giving Wayne oral rehydration salts (ORS) such as Dioralyte®.

Student activities

- Find out the composition of ORS sold by UK pharmacies.
- Why is glucose or another carbohydrate added to ORS?
- How should Wayne's mother reconstitute the ORS?
- What volume and how frequently should it be given to Wayne?
- How should reconstituted ORS solution be stored?
- What other advice do you think the practice nurse gave Wayne's mother about fluid intake and diet?

[Resources: British National Formulary (BNF) – www.bnf.org.uk; NHS Direct Online/Self Help Guide/Diarrhoea in babies and children – www.nhsdirect.nhs.uk/selfhelp/symptoms/babydiarrhoea/start.asp Available July 2006]

Table 19.3 Daily fluid requirements for children (developed from Wong et al 1999)

Body weight (kg)	Fluid requirement per kg	Worked example
1–10	100 mL/kg	An infant weighing 3.5 kg needs 100 × 3.5 = 350 mL of fluid per day
11–20	1000 mL plus 50 mL/kg for each kg >10 kg	A child of 2½ years weighing 13.5 kg needs 1000 + (50 × 3.5) = 1175 mL of fluid per day
>20	1500 mL plus 20 mL/kg for each kg >20 kg	A child of 10 years weighing 32 kg needs 1500 + (20 × 12) = 1740 mL of fluid per day A teenager weighing 60 kg needs 1500 + (20 × 40) = 2300 mL of fluid per day

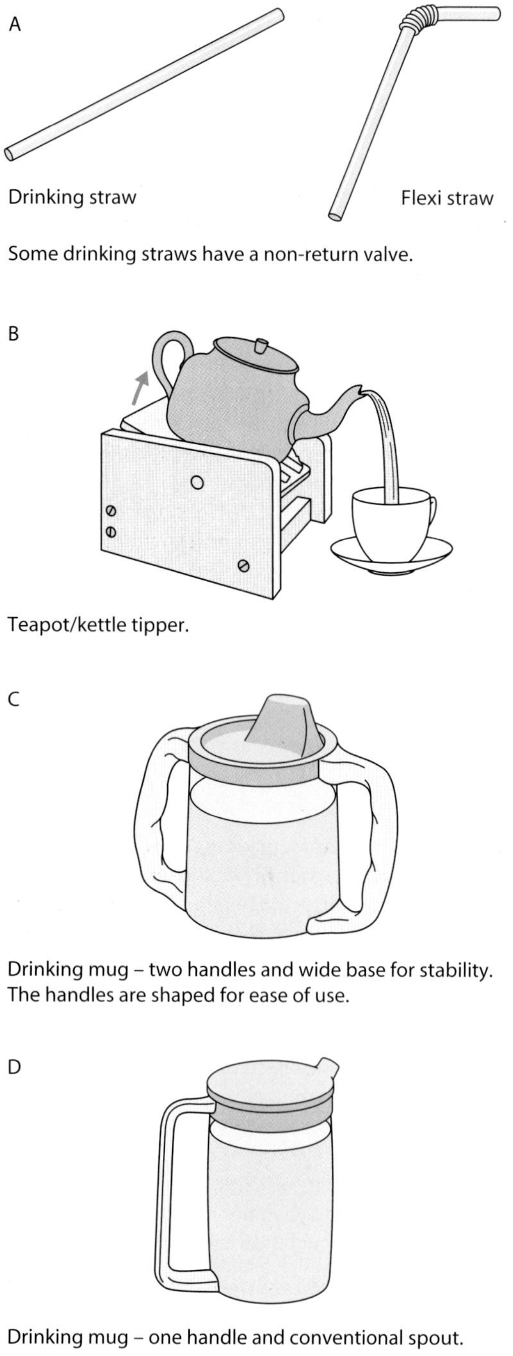

A
Drinking straw
Flexi straw
Some drinking straws have a non-return valve.
B
Teapot/kettle tipper.
C
Drinking mug – two handles and wide base for stability. The handles are shaped for ease of use.
D
Drinking mug – one handle and conventional spout.

Fig. 19.5 Aids to independence in drinking: **A.** Drinking straws. **B.** Teapot/kettle tipper (reproduced with permission from Roper et al 1995). **C.** Drinking mug – two handles. **D.** Drinking mug – one handle

changed, always check that the fluid consumed has been recorded on the fluid chart.

- *Accessibility*: Fluids must be within reach.
- *Providing encouragement and reminders to drink*: This can increase people's fluid intake (Box 19.11).
- *Providing acceptable volumes*: It is often easier for people to have several small drinks from their favourite glass or china cup (Fig. 19.6). Standard vessels full of fluid put off many people.

HEALTH PROMOTION Box 19.11

Encouraging people to obtain sufficient oral fluids

The nurse sets a goal for the daily intake and, together with the patient/client, parent or carer, plans the timing of drinks to achieve this. People need to know how many cups or glasses will provide the daily volume needed, as trying to visualize a specific volume, e.g. 1.5 L, can be difficult (see Fig. 19.6). Encouragement can be as simple as saying, 'Is it time for another drink?' or pouring and offering a drink. Planning an activity that involves a child can encourage them to drink. For example, adding stickers to a card for each drink or by colouring in a chart with the required number of cups or glasses.

Student activities

- Identify a group of patients/clients, e.g. adults with a learning disability, children in a reception class at school (see Table 19.3), people with dementia living in a nursing home, and devise a plan that ensures that they obtain sufficient oral fluids.
- Discuss the plan with your mentor.

[Further reading: Haines L, Rogers J, Dobson P (2000) A study of drinking facilities in schools. Nursing Times 96(40): NTplus Continence 2–4]

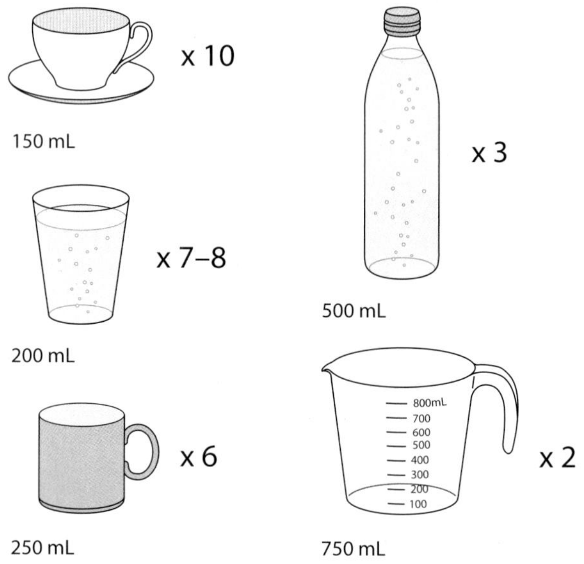

Note – always check the volume of drinking vessels/jugs, as these may vary

Fig. 19.6 How much is 1.5 L?

- *Drinking aids*: These are sometimes needed (see Fig. 19.5) and include:
  - drinking straws (straight, flexible and those with a non-return valve)

- drinking mugs with large handles and wide bases
- mugs that can be used while lying down
- feeding bottle with teat if a small child still has water from a feeding bottle. Although a child usually uses a cup, during illness they may want to use a bottle again.

- *Providing physical help* if needed and ensuring that the appropriate aids are available and sitting level with the patient/client when assisting.
- *Involving specialist nurses*, e.g. nutrition specialists, stroke specialists when appropriate.

Fluid restriction

Sometimes fluid intake is restricted, e.g. in kidney failure. The person needs to know the exact volume prescribed and the reason for the restriction. The points above about helping a person to drink, including timing and spacing of drinks, small vessels, favourite drinks, are especially important in this situation.

A person having restricted fluids is likely to have a dry mouth and complain of being thirsty. The nurse can minimize discomfort by offering crushed ice or an ice cube to suck to moisten their mouth while still adhering to the restriction.

Caring for the person with fluid imbalance

Fluid depletion

A person with fluid volume deficit or dehydration requires specific nursing care. For instance, the skin will be dry and loss of skin turgor (see p. 538) increases the risk of pressure ulcers. Lethargy, which can accompany fluid depletion, can reduce mobility and so increase the risk of skin breakdown. The risk should be assessed using a validated rating scale and appropriate preventive measures put in place (see Ch. 25). Because oral condition is often affected and the mouth is dry, mouth care (see Ch. 16) and mouthwashes are needed until hydration improves. Fluid depletion predisposes to constipation and, when possible, oral fluids, a fibre-rich diet and physical activity are the preferred interventions (see Ch. 21). Lack of fluid can lead to confusion and nurses must be alert to the risks associated with increasing confusion and disorientation, e.g. falls.

Oedema

Oedematous, swollen tissue is easily damaged and this increases the risk of infection and pressure ulcers (see Chs 15, 25). It is important that the risk is minimized by ensuring that neither nurses' nor clients' fingernails, rings or watches damage the skin. People should avoid scratching affected areas. After washing, swollen tissue should be gently patted dry rather than rubbed. People with ankle and leg oedema are advised to elevate the affected part in order to encourage drainage of the excess fluid. Box 19.12 outlines advice for people with long-term ankle oedema.

HEALTH PROMOTION Box 19.12

Helping people with swollen ankles

Nursing advice

- Move about or exercise the ankles and feet when possible because this uses the skeletal muscle 'pump' in the calves to increase return of blood to the heart
- Avoid standing still; always move the feet and contract the calf muscles when this is required
- Putting the feet up when sitting helps drainage of excess fluid
- Use support stockings to promote venous return
- Avoid socks, stockings, trousers with elasticated bottoms and anything else with tight bands that will impair venous return below the constriction
- Wear flat, well-fitting shoes rather than sandals with straps, as excess fluid will collect around the straps.

Student activity

Identify any people in your placement who have ankle oedema and find out what of the above they know about.

[Based on Waugh (2003)]

Caring for the person who is vomiting

Prolonged or excessive vomiting can be distressing and may lead to disruption to fluid, electrolyte and acid–base balance (see p. 535). Prior to vomiting the person often experiences nausea (feeling sick); there may be pallor, sweating and excess watery saliva. The causes of vomiting include:

- GI tract distension or irritants, e.g. bacterial toxins and excess alcohol consumption
- Motion sickness
- Pain (see Ch. 23)
- Drugs, e.g. chemotherapy
- Unpleasant sights or odours
- Fear
- Anxiety.

The care needed by a person who is vomiting is outlined in Box 19.13.

Subcutaneous fluids (hypodermoclysis)

Subcutaneous infusion of fluids is increasingly used for fluid replacement and the maintenance of hydration in older adults and in palliative care (Mansfield et al 1998, Donnelly 1999). It is used to:

- Maintain hydration when people have an inadequate oral intake
- Rehydrate people with mild, short-term fluid deficits who are able to take some oral fluids. Arinzon et al (2004) report that oral intake improved following subcutaneous rehydration.

Suitable infusion sites include the thighs, abdomen, and areas over the scapula and the chest wall. The site

NURSING SKILLS Box 19.13

Nausea and vomiting

Nursing interventions include

- Taking measures to ensure privacy, e.g. drawing screens, shutting cubicle doors
- Providing a vomit bowl and tissues or paper towels. At home an old washing-up bowl can be used to protect bedding, especially with small children
- Providing physical comfort and maintaining dignity by holding the vomit bowl or wiping the person's mouth
- Encouraging the person to sit upright and breathe deeply. People who are lying down or have altered consciousness should be placed in the lateral position to protect their airway (see Fig. 16.17C) and suction equipment should be available close to the patient
- Removing dentures and placing them in a labelled denture container
- Postoperatively, people should be encouraged to support abdominal wounds with their hands to reduce tension on the wound (see Ch. 24)
- Providing a clean vomit bowl before removing the used one
- Assisting with cleaning teeth and/or providing mouthwashes
- Providing a bowl for a hands and face wash, particularly if the person has been sweating
- Changing soiled clothing and bedding as necessary
- Removing the covered vomit bowl to the sluice. Vomit is measured and charted on the fluid balance chart. The vomit is observed for colour, odour, undigested food and presence of blood (haematemesis). The type of vomiting, e.g. projectile, accompanied by nausea, related to drugs or food intake or pain, is reported and documented.

In addition, nurses should ensure that an appropriate antiemetic (drugs that stop vomiting), e.g. metoclopramide, is administered as prescribed. Antiemetics should always be given in anticipation of expected vomiting such as with some anticancer drugs.

Note: Nurses should always wear gloves and a plastic apron if time allows. Vomit is acidic and can damage ('burn') the skin. Damage can occur, if for instance, a baby or unconscious person's face is resting on vomit-stained bedding. Babies who regurgitate may have vomit in the neck creases and nurses must ensure that the skin is washed and gently patted dry.

is only chosen after discussion with the patient and consideration of comfort, ease of access, mobility and skin condition.

Fluid replacement using hypodermoclysis at home or in long-term care establishments can avoid the need to admit frail older people to acute hospitals for rehydration with intravenous fluids (Worobec & Brown 1997, Dasgupta et al 2000).

The infusion is given via a butterfly cannula, inserted by a RN into the subcutaneous tissues (Fig. 19.7). The cannula is secured by covering the area with a transparent occlusive dressing for easy observation. The site is changed according to local policy usually every 24 hours or following infusion of 2L of fluid. Intravenous administration ('giving') sets are used and a RN checks the infusion fluid, e.g. sodium chloride 0.9% or glucose 5%, before commencing a new bag.

The infusion rate depends on individual needs but the recommended maximum is 2L in 24 hours or 125mL/hour into a single site. The prescribed flow rate of subcutaneous fluids can be controlled by using a volumetric infusion pump or regulated by gravity and the roller clamp on the tubing of the administration set.

Fluid overload is unusual but local side-effects include swelling, discomfort or inflammation. The nurse should inspect the infusion site for these, as it might be necessary to change the site.

The advantages of subcutaneous infusion include:

- Suitability for use in most settings, including people's homes

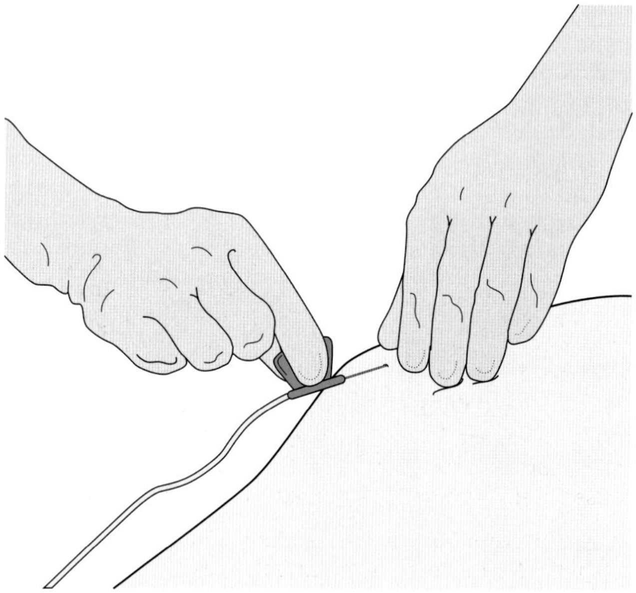

Fig. 19.7 Inserting a butterfly cannula for subcutaneous infusion (reproduced with permission from Nicol et al 2004)

- Convenience, as infusion can be fitted round people's routines, e.g. overnight without disruption to daytime activity
- Cost effectiveness, because nurses, family or the patient themselves can set up and manage the subcutaneous infusion.

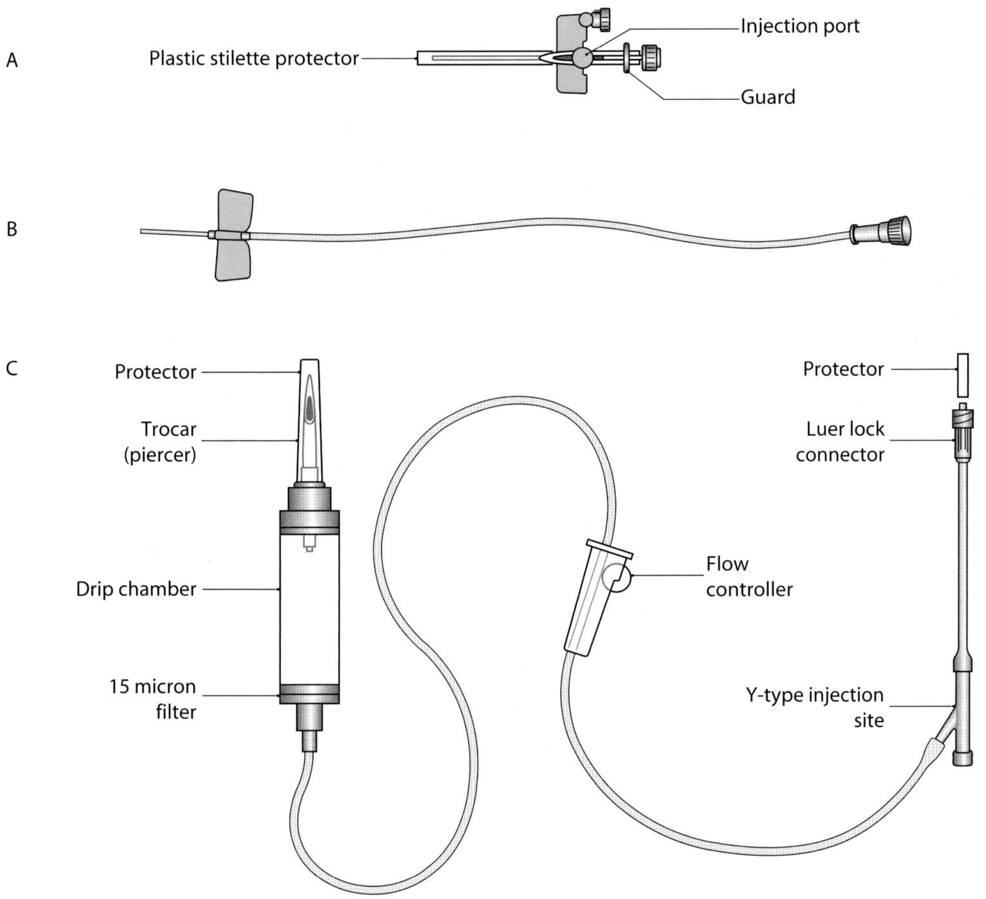

Fig. 19.8 Intravenous cannulae and parts of an administration set: **A.** Cannula used when i.v. drugs are administered with the infusion or post-infusion. **B.** A 'butterfly' cannula used for hypodermoclysis or for short-term i.v. infusion. **C.** Standard administration set for intravenous infusion (reproduced with permission from Jamieson et al 2002)

Intravenous fluids

Intravenous (i.v.) infusion of sterile fluid into the circulation is very common in hospitals and is increasingly used in the community. Most nurses will, at some time, care for patients having i.v. fluids (often referred to as a 'drip'). The principles of i.v. fluid therapy and some of the nursing interventions are outlined in this section. Detailed information about the care of i.v. infusions, including those aspects that only a RN may undertake, is provided in Further reading (Jamieson et al 2002, Dougherty & Lister 2004, Nicol et al 2004).

Intravenous fluid therapy is used when the oral or enteral routes are inappropriate, e.g. following major surgery, serious burns, severe vomiting. Blood transfusion is discussed in Chapter 17. Intravenous fluids are used to:

- Maintain fluid, electrolyte and acid–base balance
- Replace fluids and correct imbalances
- Administer drugs, e.g. pain relief, antibiotics, anticancer drugs
- Provide parenteral nutrition (p. 565).

Most i.v. fluid therapy is short term and can be infused into a peripheral vein in the dorsum (back) of the hand or the forearm, or a scalp vein in infants. Peripheral veins are not suitable for long-term therapy because inflammation can block the vein (see Box 19.16, p. 549). For long-term therapy and when irritant or hypertonic solutions are used, fluid is infused into the superior vena cava (a large central vein) where blood flow is sufficient to dilute the fluid and prevent damage to the vein (see 'Parenteral nutrition', p. 565).

Equipment

Bags or bottles of intravenous fluid are administered through sterile, single-use items of equipment, namely an administration ('giving') set attached to a cannula inserted into the vein. Figure 19.8 illustrates two commonly used cannulae and the parts of a standard administration set.

The type of administration set used depends on the fluid being infused and the safety needs of certain groups. A standard administration set (Fig. 19.9A) is generally used for clear fluids. Blood and blood products are always administered through a set with an integral filter above the drip chamber (Fig. 19.9B; see also Ch. 17). An administration set with a burette (Fig. 19.9C) can be used when drugs or small volumes of fluid are infused. A burette set must always be used with infants, children and others at risk of fluid overload, e.g. frail older people, to prevent accidental infusion of excess fluid (see p. 549). Volumetric infusion pumps (see p. 549) or syringe drivers (Ch. 23) are frequently used and always when precise accuracy is required.

Crystalloids and colloids

Fluids for i.v. infusion are divided into crystalloids and colloids. A crystalloid is a clear solution that moves

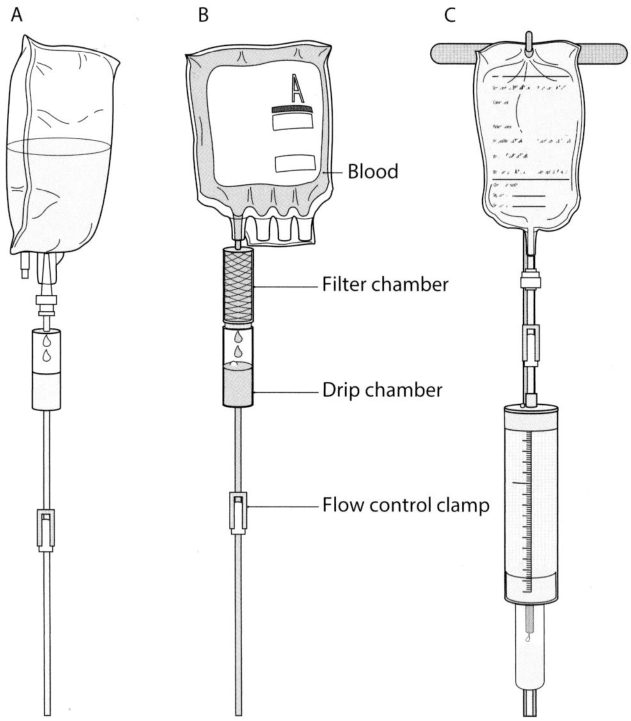

Fig. 19.9 Types of intravenous administration set: **A.** Standard administration set. **B.** Blood administration set. **C.** Burette (paediatric set) (reproduced with permission from Nicol et al 2004)

between the bloodstream and the tissue fluid. They are used intravenously to maintain hydration and electrolyte balance and many are supplied with potassium chloride (KCl) added. Examples of crystalloid solutions include:

- Sodium chloride 0.9% (normal saline)
- Glucose 5%
- Sodium chloride 0.18% and glucose 4%.

Colloid solutions contain particles (solutes) that stay in the blood because they are too large to pass through capillary membranes and are used to increase blood volume. Examples include:

- Synthetic solutions containing gelatin, e.g. Gelofusine®, or starch, e.g. Hepsan®
- Human albumin solution
- Blood and blood products (see Ch. 17).

Principles of care for infusions

The overriding principle is to ensure the safety and comfort of the person having i.v fluids.

The non-dominant arm should be used to site the i.v. infusion whenever possible, thus maximizing independence and minimizing inconvenience. The person may be more comfortable if a pillow with a waterproof cover is used to support the arm or a lightly bandaged single-use splint is applied. The arm may also need to be immobilized with a single-use splint and bandage, according to local policy, if there is a risk of the cannula becoming dislodged such as with small children or adults who are restless or confused.

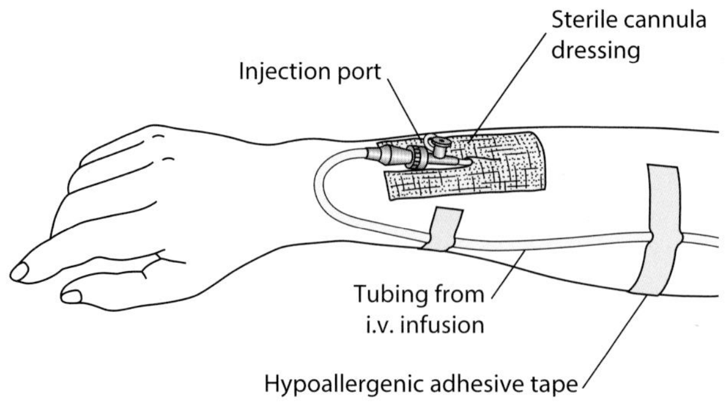

Fig. 19.10 Cannula dressing and securing the tubing (reproduced with permission from Jamieson et al 2002)

It is also important to note that Muslims use the left hand for personal cleansing and the right hand for feeding. This has important implications for the siting of i.v. infusions and the wishes of the patient must be taken into account.

Once the i.v. cannula has been sited, it is secured in place with a sterile cannula dressing (Fig. 19.10). The fluid container is connected to an appropriate administration set and fluid is 'run through' to expel air from the tube before connection to the cannula. The tubing is anchored to the arm (see Fig. 19.10). The date of cannula insertion and type of administration set is recorded in the nursing notes. The cannula is usually changed every 72 hours and even in 24 hours if the cannula has been sited in an emergency as there is some doubt about asepsis during insertion (RCN 2003). This may vary according to local policy.

An i.v. infusion is an invasive procedure so aseptic technique and standard precautions must be in place to prevent the entry of contaminants such as microorganisms, and to protect the staff from potentially infected body fluids (see Ch. 15). The closed system only protects if it is kept closed and when it is necessary to open the system, e.g. to change the fluid bag, it is vital that the nurse adheres to the precautions outlined above. Figure 19.11 illustrates the potential routes for contamination.

Intravenous fluid bags are changed using aseptic technique every 24 hours. Usually administration sets are changed every 72 hours for peripheral i.v. fluids and this is recorded in the nursing notes. The cannula site is inspected regularly for signs of inflammation such as redness, swelling and pain that may indicate the development of phlebitis (inflammation of a vein), infection or other complications (see Box 19.16, p. 549). The dressing around the cannula is changed aseptically if it has become loose, wet or bloodstained. If the dressing is in place, dry and clean, it is usually left undisturbed until the cannula is re-sited or removed (readers should check local policies).

All fluids for i.v. infusion are prescribed and a RN must check that the correct fluid is administered to the correct person. Some areas require that two nurses (one registered) check i.v. fluids. The outer wrapping is removed from the bag and it and the fluid are checked for:

- Expiry date
- Damage or leakage

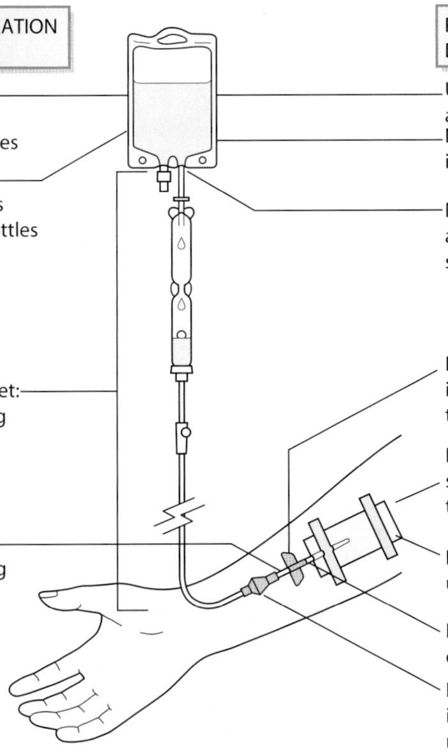

POTENTIAL CONTAMINATION BEFORE USE
Faulty infusion fluid:
• beyond expiry date
• presence of precipitates
Faulty container:
• presence of punctures in bags or cracks in bottles
Faulty administration set:
• puncture in packaging
Faulty cannula:
• puncture in packaging
POTENTIAL CONTAMINATION DURING USE
Using contaminated additives
Not maintaining asepsis when inserting additives
Not maintaining asepsis when attaching the administration set to the container
Not maintaining asepsis when inserting and manipulating the cannula
Inadequately cleansing the skin prior to insertion of the cannula
Leaving soiled dressings unchanged
Not maintaining the integrity of the connections
Not maintaining asepsis when introducing drugs via the rubber bung or 3-way tap

Fig. 19.11 Potential routes for contamination during intravenous infusion (reproduced with permission from Jamieson et al 2002)

NURSING SKILLS Box 19.14

Infusion bag change

Maintaining safety is paramount when undertaking a bag change. The key principles are as follows:

- Changing the infusion bag means that the closed system is breached, thereby increasing the risk of infection
- Thorough handwashing beforehand
- The bag is changed before the fluid level falls below the spike of the administration bag; this prevents air bubbles forming in the tubing leading to the cannula
- The new bag of fluid must be in date and in good condition (see above)
- The fluid type and the person's identity must be checked by a RN.

The bag change is explained and a visual check of the cannula site made, observing for the presence of complications (see Box 19.16).

- Stop the infusion by closing the roller clamp on the administration set
- Take the empty bag from the i.v. stand and remove the administration set from the bag, taking care to avoid contamination of the spike
- Take the protective plastic from the inlet port of the new bag of fluid and insert the spike of the administration set. This is twisted until completely inserted (Fig. 19.12)
- Hang the new bag on the i.v. fluid stand and regulate the roller clamp to administer the prescribed flow rate (see Box 19.15)
- Check the flow rate at least hourly by using a watch with a second hand, if regulated by gravity and the roller clamp (Fig. 19.13)
- Check that the patient has no discomfort at the cannula site and observe for signs of overinfusion causing fluid overload, i.e. rising pulse, BP and respiratory rate (see Box 19.16)
- The used infusion bag and packaging are disposed of safely in the clinical waste
- Wash hands before completing the documentation and the fluid balance chart
- The RN will record and report any problems.

[Based on Nicol et al (2004)]

- Discoloration of the fluid
- Clarity
- Absence of particles.

The type and volume of fluid, e.g. 500 mL of sodium chloride 0.9%, is checked against the prescription sheet and the person's identity band is checked. When a bag of i.v. fluid is commenced the details including the batch number are recorded in the nursing records. In addition, i.v. fluid volumes are recorded on the fluid intake and output chart. The principles of changing infusion bags are outlined in Box 19.14.

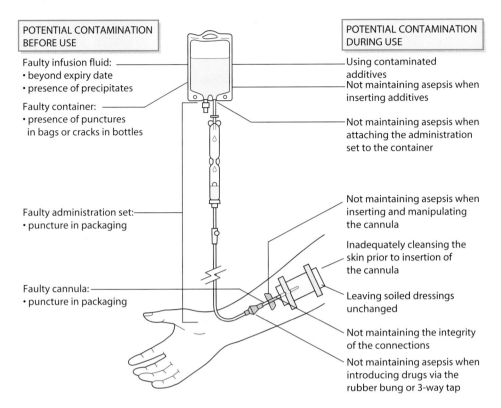

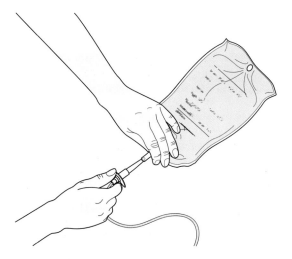

Fig. 19.12 Changing the infusion bag – inserting the administration set spike into a new bag (reproduced with permission from Nicol et al 2004)

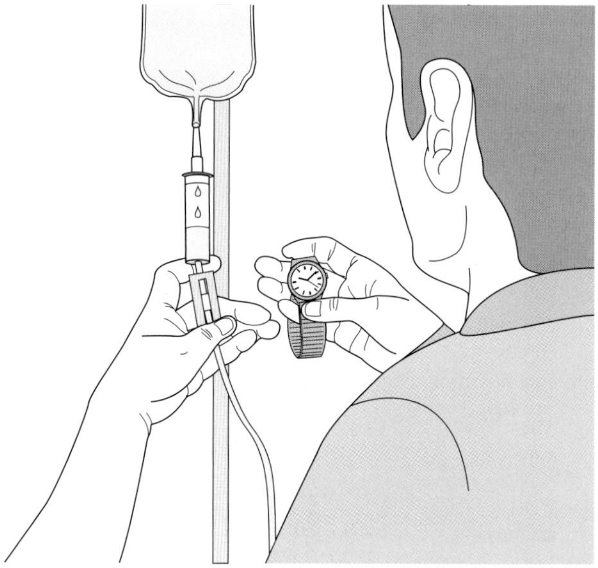

Fig. 19.13 Setting the infusion flow rate (reproduced with permission from Nicol et al 2004)

CRITICAL THINKING Box 19.15

Calculating i.v. flow rates

Infusion flow rates are calculated in one of two ways: drops per minute or millilitres per hour.

Drops per minute

This calculation is used for infusions regulated by gravity and roller clamp on the administration set and for regulatory devices that use drops per minute. In gravity/roller clamp regulation it is vital that the flow rate remains constant. Each type of administration set (see Fig. 19.9) has a specific 'drop factor' (drops per mL):

- Standard administration set = 20 drops/mL for crystalloids
- Standard administration set = 15 drops/mL for colloids
- Blood administration set = 15 drops/mL
- Burette (paediatric set) = 60 drops/mL.

The calculation is:

$$\text{Flow rate (drops per minute)} = \frac{\text{volume of fluid (mL)} \times \text{drop factor (number of drops/mL)}}{\text{time (min)}}$$

Worked example

Tom has been prescribed 1000 mL of sodium chloride 0.9% in 8 hours. A standard administration set will be used.

$$\frac{1000 \times 20}{480} = \frac{20\,000}{480} = 41.6 \text{ drops per minute (rounded up to 42)}$$

Millilitres per hour

Millilitres per hour are used when the i.v. flow rate is to be regulated by a volumetric infusion pump or syringe driver.

The calculation is:

$$\text{Flow rate (mL/hr)} = \frac{\text{volume of fluid (mL)}}{\text{time (hr)}}$$

Worked example

Jyoti has been prescribed 500 mL of glucose 5% in 6 hours via a volumetric infusion pump.

$$\text{Flow rate} = \frac{500}{6} = 83.3 \text{ mL (rounded down to 83)}$$

Student activities

- The next time you are helping to care for a person who is having i.v. fluids, ask if you can be involved in the calculation and regulation of flow rates. Try to do this for flow rates being regulated by both a gravity/roller clamp and an infusion pump.
- Ask your mentor to explain and demonstrate how an infusion pump is set up.

[Resources: Gatford JD, Phillips N 2006 Nursing calculations, 7th edn. Churchill Livingstone, Edinburgh; MacQueen S 2005 The special needs of children receiving intravenous therapy. Nursing Times 101(8):59–64]

Flow rate calculation and regulation

Nurses are responsible for calculating and regulating the flow rate of i.v. fluids. The flow rate can be regulated by gravity and the roller clamp on the administration set tubing, or by an infusion pump.

The flow rate is checked at least hourly. Factors that may reduce the flow rate or stop it completely include:

- Kinking of the administration set tubing
- The fluid container being too low; this is overcome by raising the container

Box 19.16 Complications associated with i.v. therapy

Local complications

- Phlebitis, which is inflammation of the lining of the vein, e.g. chemical irritation from drugs inserted. When inflammation is associated with clot formation it is known as thrombophlebitis
- Infection due to contamination at several sites (see Fig. 19.11). Infection and phlebitis both cause redness, swelling and pain
- Infiltration occurring when fluid infuses into the tissues ('tissuing') instead of the vein. There is swelling around the cannula site, which may be painful. Sometimes, but not always, the infusion stops
- Extravasation is infiltration that causes local tissue damage, including necrosis (death of tissue), which occurs when irritant substances leak out of the vein, e.g. some anticancer drugs.

Systemic complications

- Circulatory overload occurs when fluid, especially sodium chloride 0.9%, is infused too rapidly. The increase in blood volume can lead to heart failure and acute pulmonary oedema (see p. 535 and Ch. 1). The patient's BP, pulse and respiratory rate increase. They have difficulty in breathing and have a cough with frothy sputum. The risk is reduced by regular checks on flow rate as overinfusion often happens when arm position affects the flow rate and through the use of infusion pumps (see above).
- Fluid volume deficit due to inadequate fluid prescription or excessively slow infusion rate
- Septicaemia (multiplication of living bacteria in the bloodstream) due to spread from a local infection at the cannula site
- Rare but life-threatening events that include an air embolism when an air bubble enters the vein and reaches the heart or a pulmonary embolism (a blood clot, known as an 'embolus', travels through the heart to block a pulmonary artery).

[Further information can be found in Further reading, e.g. Dougherty & Lister (2004)]

- The position of the cannula in the vein; this can often be overcome by gently changing the position of the hand or forearm.

Intravenous infusion pumps are increasingly used to regulate the flow rate. They should be used:

- For accuracy when i.v. drugs or small volumes of fluid are prescribed
- When a risk of rapid overinfusion exists or people are at risk of fluid overload, e.g. infants, children, older people and those with heart failure.

Most models have audible alarms that alert the nurse to situations that include 'infusion complete', 'air in line' and when flow is obstructed. It is imperative that alarms are never turned off. RNs are responsible for using pumps safely in accordance with the manufacturer's instructions. RNs receive training for each type of pump used in their area and are competent in their use. Nurses who are unsure about a particular pump must seek help and advice from a more experienced colleague. Student nurses may only deal with pumps when directly supervised by a RN.

Box 19.15 outlines the formulae used to calculate flow rates in drops per minute and millilitres per hour.

Complications of i.v. therapy

Complications associated with an i.v. infusion may be local or systemic and range from minor to serious and life threatening. Box 19.16 provides an overview of common complications; complications specific to blood transfusion are discussed in Chapter 17.

Nutrition

This part of the chapter explores health-promoting activities and nursing interventions such as feeding that help people to obtain the correct nutrients in sufficient quantities to meet individual needs. The importance and scope of these are illustrated in the best practice benchmarks in the *Essence of Care* (NHS Modernisation Agency 2003) (see Box 19.17). In addition, an understanding of digestion and absorption of nutrients, the principles of nutrition and healthy eating throughout the lifespan are important in ensuring that nurses can meet the nutritional needs of people in their care.

The gastrointestinal tract

An overview of structure and function is provided here and readers should consult their own anatomy and physiology book for more detail. In addition, Chapter 16 discusses the structures of the mouth and Chapter 21 the large intestine and defecation.

The general structure of the GI tract comprises four layers:

- Inner lining of mucosa
- Submucosal layer
- Involuntary (smooth) muscle layer
- Outer serous covering or adventitia.

The basic, four-layer structure is modified at various points according to the function of that part. For example, the presence of villi (microscopic projections) in the

REFLECTIVE PRACTICE Box 19.17

Using benchmarks of best practice

Student activities

- During your next placement consider the following benchmark statements in relation to what you observe at mealtimes.
- Discuss your observations with your mentor.

***Benchmarks of Best Practice – Food and Nutrition* (NHS Modernisation Agency 2003, pp. 1–2)**

- Nutritional screening progresses to further assessment for all patients identified as 'at risk'
- Plans of care based on ongoing nutritional assessments are devised, implemented and evaluated
- The environment is conducive to enabling individual patients to eat
- Patients receive the care and assistance they require with eating and drinking
- Patients and/or carers, whatever their communication needs, have sufficient information to enable them to obtain their food
- Food that is provided by the service meets the needs of individual patients
- Patients have set meal times, are offered a replacement meal if a meal is missed and can access snacks at any time
- Food is presented to patients in a way that takes into account what appeals to them as individuals
- The amount of food patients actually eat is monitored, recorded and leads to action when [there is] cause for concern
- All opportunities are used to encourage patients to eat to promote their own health.

mucosa of the small intestine increases the surface area available for the absorption of nutrients.

Parts of the gastrointestinal tract

The GI tract is essentially a long tube that starts at the mouth and ends at the anus (Fig. 19.14). The individual parts are:

- Mouth (see Ch. 16)
- Pharynx
- Oesophagus
- Stomach
- Small intestine (duodenum, jejunum and ileum)
- Large intestine (see Ch. 21)
- Rectum and anal canal (see Ch. 21).

Mouth

The mouth (oral cavity) and accessory structures (teeth, tongue, salivary glands that secrete saliva) are concerned with the ingestion, chewing (mastication), some chemical digestion of food and the first stage of swallowing. Taste sensation is discussed on page 552.

Pharynx

The three-part pharynx (nasopharynx, oropharynx and laryngopharynx) is a cone-shaped, muscular cavity situated behind the nose and mouth. However, only two parts (oropharynx and laryngopharynx) are common routes for food, fluid and air and there are mechanisms that normally keep food or fluids out of the larynx during swallowing. Swallowing involves three stages:

- *Oral stage*: Food is mixed with saliva, chewed and formed into a bolus by the tongue.
- *Pharyngeal stage*: Commences when the bolus enters the posterior pharynx and is enclosed by the muscular walls. At this point swallowing ceases to be under voluntary control. Involuntary control occurs as receptors in the pharynx stimulate the swallowing centre in the brain, which in turn initiates the swallowing reflex. The pharyngeal muscles contract and the food bolus is moved into the oesophagus. During the involuntary phase the bolus should only go in one direction because all other routes are blocked: the soft palate blocks the nasopharynx, the larynx rises and the epiglottis covers the trachea, respiration stops and the mouth is closed. Should these mechanisms fail, the cough reflex functions in a conscious person, clearing the airways if food does enter.
- *Oesophageal stage*: The bolus is moved downwards towards the stomach by waves of smooth muscle contraction and relaxation known as peristalsis.

Oesophagus

The muscular oesophagus is a tube that has no role in digestion or absorption. The oesophagus runs from the laryngopharynx through the thoracic cavity and diaphragm to the stomach. Food and fluid enter the stomach through the gastro-oesophageal (cardiac) sphincter or valve. This is a physiological sphincter where oesophageal muscle contraction keeps the oesophagus closed until swallowing occurs.

Stomach

The stomach is roughly J-shaped and, in adults, can comfortably hold 1.5 L of food and fluids. The mucosa is arranged in folds, or rugae, which greatly increase the surface area for secretion and allow for considerable distension following a meal. However, in infants and children stomach capacity is much smaller. For example, a newborn baby has a capacity of 15–30 mL, which has implications for volumes of feed and frequency of feeding. In addition, the gastro-oesophageal sphincter is underdeveloped, predisposing to regurgitation.

The stomach churns and mixes food with gastric juices to form the semi-fluid chyme. There is some digestion and limited absorption in the stomach (see Table 19.4). Chyme leaves the stomach through the pyloric sphincter, ensuring the coordinated release of gastric contents into the small intestine.

Small intestine

The small intestine has three parts: duodenum, jejunum and ileum. The duodenum is continuous with the stomach

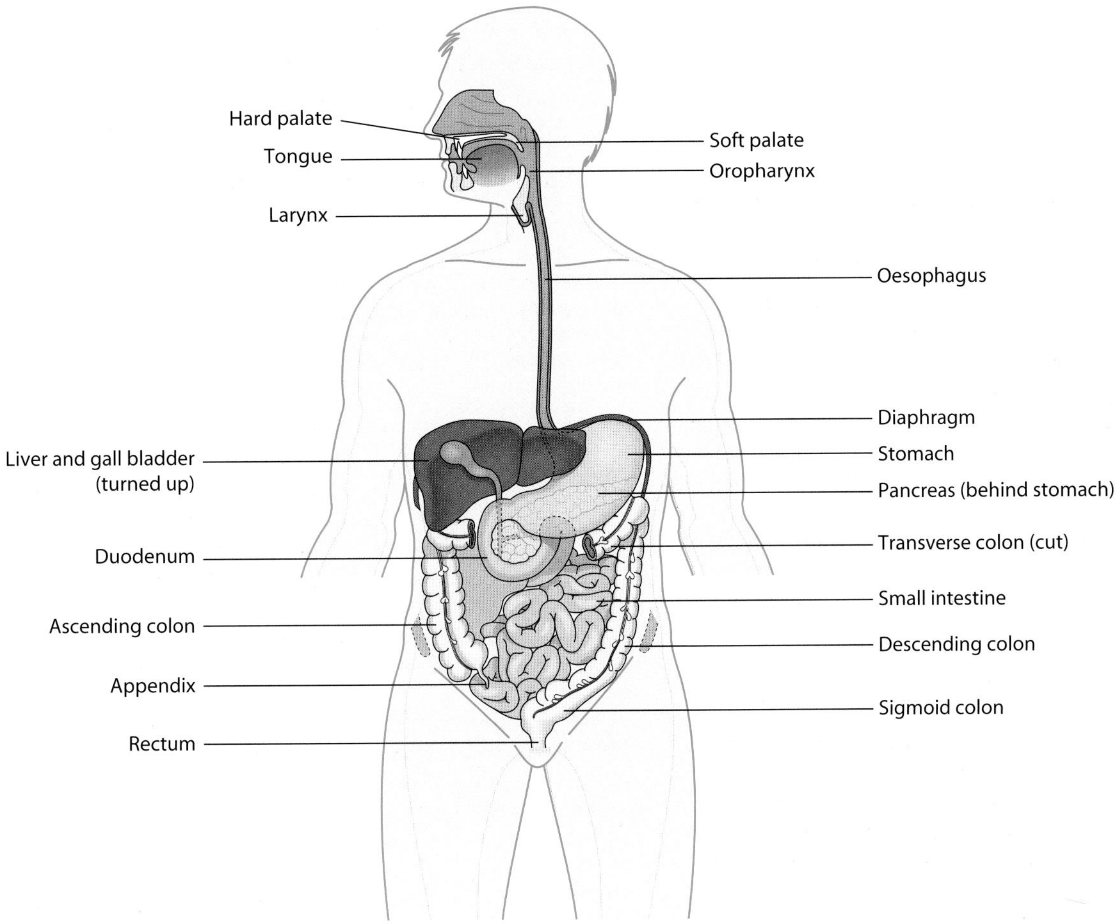

Fig. 19.14 The gastrointestinal tract and some accessory organs (reproduced with permission from Waugh & Grant 2006)

and the ileum leads into the ileocaecal valve where the large intestine starts. Secretions from the pancreas and bile from the gallbladder both enter into the duodenum. Chemical digestion is completed in the small intestine by enzymes from the pancreas and those secreted in the intestinal juice, and nutrients are absorbed (see Table 19.4).

Overview – functions of the gastrointestinal tract

The GI tract, plus the secretions from various accessory organs – three pairs of salivary glands, the liver, gallbladder and bile ducts and the pancreas (see Fig. 19.14) – are concerned with five main activities:

- Ingestion of food
- Movement of food and waste products through the tract by muscular movements called peristalsis
- Digestion of food by mechanical means such as chewing and chemically through the action of enzymes and other chemicals secreted by glands and accessory organs. The chemicals break down the nutrients (protein, carbohydrate and fat) present in food
- Absorption of the end products of digestion, minerals, vitamins and water, mainly through the walls of the small intestine into the blood or lymph vessels
- Elimination of faeces (see Ch. 21).

Table 19.4 provides a summary of the sites of nutrient digestion and absorption.

Smell and taste

The senses of smell and taste are intricately linked and both are important for appetite and nutritional intake. Being able to smell and taste food:

- Increases appetite and enjoyment of food
- Increases the variety of foods eaten and helps to ensure a balanced intake of nutrients
- Stimulates digestive secretions
- Affords some protection against eating food that is 'rotten'. In addition, reflex gagging or vomiting can occur if foul-tasting food is eaten.

Anatomy and physiology of smell

The sense of smell, or olfaction, is provided by specialized nerve endings (chemoreceptors) in the roof of the nasal cavity (Fig. 19.15A). These nerve endings are sensitive to thousands of different chemical odours. Nerve

Table 19.4 Summary showing the sites of digestion and absorption of nutrients

	Mouth	Stomach	Small intestine: Digestion	Small intestine: Absorption	Large intestine
Carbohydrate	*Salivary amylase*: cooked starches to disaccharides	*Acid* denatures and stops action of salivary amylase	*Pancreatic amylase*: cooked and uncooked starches to disaccharides *Sucrase*, *Maltase*, *Lactase* (in enterocytes): disaccharides to monosaccharides (mainly glucose)	Into blood capillaries of villi	–
Proteins	–	*Acid*: pepsinogen to pepsin *Pepsin*: proteins to polypeptides	*Enterokinase* (in intestinal mucosa): chymotrypsinogen and trypsinogen (from pancreas) to chymotrypsin and trypsin *Chymotrypsin and trypsin*: polypeptides to di- and tripeptides *Peptidases* (in enterocytes): di- and tripeptides to amino acids	Into blood capillaries of villi	–
Fats	–	–	*Bile* (from liver): bile salts emulsify fats *Pancreatic lipase:* fats to fatty acids and glycerol *Lipases* (in enterocytes): fats to fatty acids and glycerol	Into the lacteals of the villi	–
Water	–	Small amount absorbed here	–	Most absorbed here	Remainder absorbed here
Vitamins	–	Intrinsic factor secreted for vitamin B_{12} absorption	–	Water-soluble vitamins absorbed into capillaries; fat-soluble ones into lacteals of villi	Bacteria synthesize vitamin K in colon; absorbed here

Reproduced with permission from Waugh and Grant (2006).

fibres transmit impulses to the temporal lobes of the brain for recognition and interpretation.

Anatomy and physiology of taste

The sense of taste, or gustation, is provided by taste buds, which contain sensory receptors (chemoreceptors) (Fig. 19.15B). Most taste buds are located on the tongue and a few on the soft palate and the back of the throat. Chemicals dissolved in saliva activate the chemoreceptors in the taste buds, generating nerve impulses that are transmitted to an area in the parietal lobes of the brain where taste perception occurs.

Four basic taste sensations have been described: salt, sweet, bitter and sour. This is probably too simplistic, as individual perception of taste varies widely.

Alterations to smell and taste

Abnormalities of smell include a reduction in the sense of smell (hyposmia) and complete loss of smell (anosmia). Problems can be temporary, such as with a common cold, or may be permanent, e.g. after head injury (see Box 19.18).

Taste, and hence appetite, can be impaired if a cold affects the olfactory receptors in the nose. Alterations in taste can also occur if the mouth is dry, e.g. fluid deficits (p. 535), and when oral hygiene and/or dental health is poor (see Ch. 16).

The senses of taste and smell change with normal ageing; there is gradual loss of taste and olfactory receptors, which accounts for the diminished sense of taste and smell in older people. Older people may complain

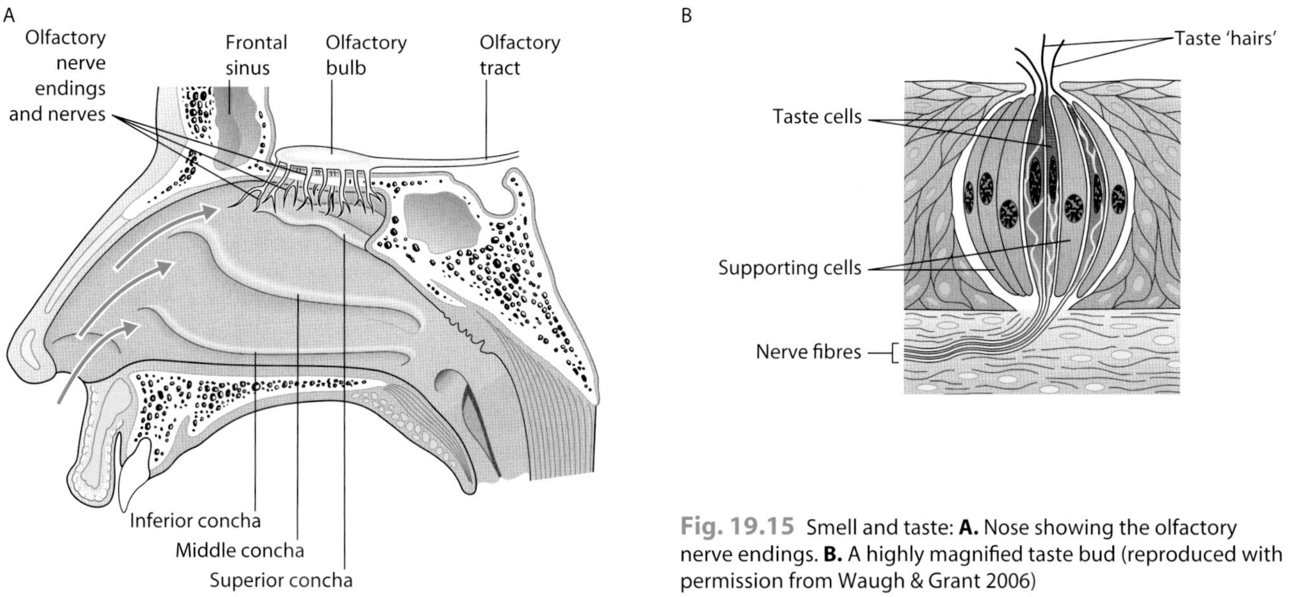

Fig. 19.15 Smell and taste: **A.** Nose showing the olfactory nerve endings. **B.** A highly magnified taste bud (reproduced with permission from Waugh & Grant 2006)

REFLECTIVE PRACTICE Box 19.18

Smell and appetite

Think about situations when your appetite was affected by smell, e.g. a favourite meal being cooked.

Student activities

- Identify situations in placements where an odour or problem with the sense of smell affected people's appetites.
- Think about ways of minimizing the impact of unpleasant odours that may occur in placements affecting people's appetites.

Box 19.19 **Disturbances in smell and taste**

- Some people who have epilepsy experience an aura when they perceive a strange smell or taste immediately before a seizure
- Taste may change in some people with cancers
- Hallucinations (false perceptions) may affect any sense including smell (olfactory) or taste (gustatory), e.g. a person may smell burning or taste 'poison' in their food
- Drugs that may affect taste include lithium, ACE inhibitors such as captopril and the antibiotic metronidazole
- Anticancer drugs can also alter smell.

that 'modern food' has no taste and this can contribute to a reduction in appetite. Nurses can suggest stronger flavours and aromas, seasoning and different textures that may improve the taste of meals.

Disturbances in smell or taste can occur as part of a disease or as a side-effect of some drugs (see Box 19.19).

Nutritional and upper gastrointestinal tract disorders

Some common nutritional disorders, upper GI tract disorders and other conditions that impact on nutrition are outlined in Table 19.5. Related associations and groups also provide useful information (Boxes 19.20, 19.21) and some websites are included at the end of this chapter.

Principles of nutrition and the healthy diet

A healthy diet comprises the correct nutrients in appropriate amounts. This varies during the lifespan and during injury and ill health. For instance, a healthy diet for a toddler differs from that needed by an older adult or someone with diabetes.

Nutrients provide energy for body functions such as muscle contraction, for growth, tissue repair and replacement, and for health maintenance. The nutrients can be divided into:

- The energy-yielding *macronutrients* needed in relatively large quantities – carbohydrates, fat and proteins
- The *micronutrients* needed in relatively small amounts – minerals (including trace elements) and vitamins (water-soluble and fat-soluble)

Many individual foods contain several nutrients, e.g. potato provides carbohydrate, protein, minerals and vitamins and also indigestible fibre.

As water is vital in the ingestion, digestion, absorption and use of nutrients, an adequate fluid intake is also needed (see p. 534 [adults] and p. 541 [children]). In addition, a healthy diet should also contain fibre or non-starch polysaccharide (NSP) (see below).

The energy value of food is measured in the SI unit kilojoules (kJ) but in food labelling the kilocalorie (kcal)

Table 19.5 Common nutritional disorders and other conditions affecting nutrition.

Obesity (see Box 19.20)	Obesity is very common in developed countries and two-thirds of the population in England is overweight or obese (House of Commons Select Committee 2004) Obesity is a major public health problem and can lead to type 2 diabetes, hypertension (increasing the risk of heart attack or stroke), joint problems, psychosocial problems It is a feature of Prader–Willi syndrome, a chromosome disorder characterized by overeating (hyperphagia)
Eating disorders (see Box 19.21)	A range of conditions in which a person's eating behaviour and nutrient intake is inappropriate for their needs: • *Anorexia nervosa* characterized by distorted body image and a deliberate restriction of food intake resulting in severe weight loss, malnutrition, endocrine disorders and electrolyte disturbances (see p. 535) • *Bulimia nervosa* where weight is controlled by periods of restricted eating, vomiting, purging and binge eating. Weight usually remains stable and within normal range • *Binge eating* characterized by periods of binge eating but without periods of food restriction or purging which result in the development of obesity
Nutritional deficiencies	Deficiencies may involve a single nutrient such as poor iron intake leading to anaemia or protein–energy malnutrition (PEM) in which the person has a diet deficient in protein and energy
Failure to thrive	An infant or child fails to develop and grow at the expected rate It may result from a disorder such as cystic fibrosis or have causes that include poor feeding, maternal deprivation or psychosocial problems.
Food intolerance	An abnormal reaction, e.g. colic, diarrhoea, to a food that is not immunological in origin Examples include lactose (milk sugar) intolerance caused by a deficiency in the enzyme lactase
Food allergy	An abnormal immunological response to food, e.g. peanuts, which can be severe and life threatening Signs and symptoms include swelling of the mouth and throat, breathing difficulties, skin rashes and GI tract upsets
Malabsorption	Defective absorption of nutrients from the GI tract caused by diseases of, or surgery to, the small intestine, or lack of digestive enzymes or bile salts There is failure to thrive in children and in adults there is weight loss and fatty stools (steatorrhoea)
Diabetes mellitus (see also Chs 16, 25)	Diabetes mellitus is characterized by hyperglycaemia (elevated blood glucose) and can be due to an absolute or relative deficiency of insulin or a decreased sensitivity to insulin There are two main types: type 1 usually affects people under 40 years of age and is always managed with insulin injections and diet; type 2 (see Obesity above) mainly affects people over 40 years of age and may be managed by diet, oral hypoglycaemic drugs or insulin, or a combination of these
Mouth problems	These include: • congenital abnormalities, e.g. cleft lip and cleft palate • gum hyperplasia (overgrowth), a side-effect of the drug phenytoin used to control epilepsy • abnormal eruption of teeth • infections, e.g. candidiasis (thrush) • mucositis caused by cancer treatment (see also p. 559)
Diaphragmatic hernia (hiatus hernia)	Protrusion of part of the stomach through the diaphragm into the chest May be asymptomatic or cause reflux of stomach contents and oesophagitis (inflammation of the oesophagus) It may be congenital or acquired
Gastro-oesophageal reflux disease (GORD)	An incompetent/malfunctioning gastro-oesophageal sphincter allows the stomach contents to enter the oesophagus on inspiration, resulting in vomiting, oesophagitis, scarring, stricture (narrowing) and possibly aspiration pneumonia GORD can occur with enteral feeding (see p. 564)
Peptic ulceration	A non-malignant ulcer in those parts of the GI tract exposed to gastric juice; usually the duodenum or stomach
Cancer	Cancer can affect the mouth, oesophagus and stomach It rarely occurs in the small intestine (see Ch. 21 for cancer affecting the lower GI tract)

content is often shown too. *Note*: 4.186 kJ (4.2 approx) = 1 kcal or calorie.

The amount of energy needed varies greatly between people and depends on:

- Gender – adult men need approximately 170 kJ (40 kcal) per square metre of body surface area every hour, i.e. 170 kJ/m^2/hour, whereas women need 155 kJ (37 kcal).
- Age
- Size
- Physical activity
- Health status, e.g. major surgery or serious injury increases energy requirements.

Although alcohol is not a nutrient its consumption can substantially increase the total energy intake, as 1 g of alcohol yields 29 kJ (7 kcal). Excessive alcohol intake causes health problems that include:

- Obesity
- Liver damage

Box 19.20

WHO definition of overweight and obesity according to body mass index (BMI)

- Overweight BMI >25
- Pre-obese BMI 25–29.9
- Obese Class 1 BMI 30–34.9
- Obese Class 2 BMI 35–39.9
- Obese Class 3 BMI >40.

Note: BMI is discussed more fully in Box 19.27.

[From WHO (1998)]

CRITICAL THINKING — Box 19.21

Eating disorders

A friend asks you about eating disorders. She wants to know some basic facts and where to get information and help.

Student activities

- Read the information on the BBC website and prepare a summary for your friend.
- Access the Eating Disorders Association website and find out what help is available in your area.

[Resources: BBC Eating disorders – www.bbc.co.uk/health/mental_health/disorders_eating.shtml; Eating Disorders Association – www.edauk.com; NICE 2004 Core interventions in the treatment and management of anorexia nervosa, bulimia nervosa and related eating disorders – www.nice.org.uk Both available July 2006]

HEALTH PROMOTION — Box 19.22

Alcohol 'safe limits'

Men can have up to 3–4 units of alcohol/day and women can have up to 2–3 units/day, without significant risk to health (Food Standards Agency 2005).

Student activities

Access the Food Standards Agency (FSA) website:

- What is the advice about spreading alcohol intake throughout the week?
- Find out how many units of alcohol there are in a glass of wine and in 'alcopops'.
- What health benefits may be associated with having 1–2 units of alcohol/day?
- What advice about reducing alcohol intake is suggested by the FSA?
- Why should women who are trying to conceive or who are pregnant or breastfeeding limit their alcohol intake?

[Resource: Food Standards Agency – www.eatwell.gov.uk/healthydiet/nutritionessentials/drinks/alcohol Available July 2006]

- Hypertension (high blood pressure)
- Damage to other organs such as the heart and brain.

An outline of recommended 'safe limits' for drinking alcohol is provided in Box 19.22.

An outline of the main nutrients and their functions in the body and food sources are provided below but readers should consult Further reading suggestions (e.g. DH 1991) for details of dietary reference values across the lifespan.

Macronutrients

Carbohydrates

Carbohydrates may be sugars – monosaccharides (glucose, fructose and galactose), disaccharides (maltose, lactose and sucrose) or polysaccharides such as starch or glycogen. During digestion available carbohydrates are mainly broken down into glucose, which is used in the body as the major energy source. Each gram of carbohydrate yields 16 kJ (3.75 kcal). Some is used immediately, some stored as glycogen in the liver and skeletal muscles, but any excess is converted to fat.

Carbohydrates are obtained from sugar, pulses, yam, potato and other vegetables, fruit, cereals such as wheat, rice and maize, plus products made from flour, e.g. bread, pasta and chapattis.

NSP is the indigestible plant material, e.g. cellulose and other polysaccharides, that ensures steady absorption of glucose from the intestine, gives a feeling of fullness, adds bulk to the faeces and decreases the time waste remains in the large intestine (see Ch. 21). Good sources of NSP include wholegrain cereals, pulses, vegetables and fruit. An average intake of 18 g/day is suggested for adults. Children should have proportionally lower NSP intakes, and children under 2 years of age should not have NSP-containing foods at the expense of energy-rich foods that are needed for normal growth (DH 1991).

Fats

Fats are formed from glycerol and fatty acids. Fatty acids are classified as saturated, monounsaturated or polyunsaturated according to their chemical structure. Fats are emulsified by bile salts in the small intestine and broken down by fat-digesting enzymes into glycerol and fatty acids. The fatty acids are used as a stored energy source, to form lipid (fat-like) substances such as prostaglandins and phospholipids, and as a source of the fat-soluble vitamins A, D and E and cholesterol. When 1 g of fat is oxidized, it yields 37 kJ (9 kcal). This is twice as much energy as that produced by the same weight of protein or carbohydrate and although this makes it valuable when energy requirements are high, excessive intake in sedentary people leads to obesity. Children under 2 years of age should be given full-fat dairy products.

Fat is obtained from full-fat dairy products, margarine, ghee, cooking oils, fried foods, cakes, biscuits, crisps, pastry, chocolate, meat, oily fish, nuts, pulses and seeds.

Proteins

Like carbohydrates and fats, proteins contain not only carbon, hydrogen and oxygen, but also nitrogen and sometimes sulphur and phosphorus. They are broken down during digestion to provide the amino acids required by the body for protein synthesis, tissue growth and repair and, under certain conditions, for energy (1 g of protein yields 17 kJ or 4 kcal).

Table 19.6 Minerals and dietary sources

Mineral	Dietary sources
Calcium	Hard water, milk and milk products, sardines, bread, soya beans, lentils, sesame seeds
Iodine	Seafood, milk, dairy products, eggs, meat, iodized salt
Iron	Offal, red meat, egg yolk, cereal products, pulses, vegetables, cocoa, dried fruit, potatoes
Magnesium	Nuts, seeds, cereals, cereal products, potatoes, green vegetables
Phosphorus (phosphates)	Many animal and vegetable proteins
Potassium	Vegetables, potatoes, fruit juices, bananas, dried fruit, instant coffee granules, Marmite, meat, fish
Sodium	Common salt, cereal products, meat products, vegetables, cheese, sauces, pickles, snack foods, prepared meals
Zinc	Meat and meat products, milk, eggs, cereals, bread, pulses, nuts

Table 19.7 Vitamins and sources

Vitamins	Sources
Fat-soluble	
Vitamin A	Liver, kidney, oily fish, egg yolk, full fat dairy produce Green, yellow, orange and red fruit and vegetables, e.g. broccoli, carrots, apricots, sweet potatoes, tomatoes
Vitamin D	Oily fish, egg yolk, butter, fortified margarine Action of sunlight on the skin
Vitamin E	Widespread. Best sources are nuts, seeds, vegetable oil, egg yolk and some cereals
Vitamin K	Many vegetables and cereals Also synthesized by intestinal bacteria *Note*: Requires bile in the intestine for absorption
Water-soluble	
Vitamin B_1 – Thiamin	Milk, liver, eggs, pork, fortified breakfast cereals, vegetables, fruit, wholegrain cereals
Vitamin B_2 – Riboflavin	Milk, milk products, offal, fortified breakfast cereals Destroyed by sunlight
Vitamin B_3 – Niacin	Meat, fish, pulses, wholegrains, fortified breakfast cereals Can be synthesized from an amino acid in the body
Vitamin B_5 – Pantothenic acid	Liver, eggs, cereals, yeast, vegetables
Vitamin B_6 – Pyridoxine	Meat, fish, whole cereals, eggs, some vegetables
Biotin (B group)	Widely distributed in many foods, e.g. offal, egg yolk, legumes Can be synthesized by intestinal bacteria
Vitamin B_{12} – Cobalamins	Animal products, meat, eggs, fish, dairy products, yeast extract, fortified breakfast cereals Strict vegetarians and vegans may require dietary supplements *Note*: Requires intrinsic factor secreted by the stomach for absorption
Folates/folic acid (B group)	Green vegetables, fortified breakfast cereals, yeast extract, liver, oranges Supplement recommended prior to conception and during first 3 months of pregnancy to reduce the incidence of spina bifida
Vitamin C – Ascorbic acid	Citrus fruits, blackcurrants; green leafy vegetables; potatoes; strawberries; tomatoes Content decreases with storage Destroyed by cooking in the presence of air and by cutting and grating raw food

The reference nutrient intake for protein in adults is between 45 and 55.5g/day depending upon gender and age (DH 1991). However, this increases during growth, pregnancy, lactation and illness.

Protein may be obtained from both animal and vegetable sources, e.g. meat, milk, cheese, fish, eggs, nuts, pulses, tofu and cereals. It is, however, vital that vegetarians and vegans obtain a balanced intake, as some cereals are deficient in the amino acid lysine and some pulses are deficient in methionine.

Micronutrients

The micronutrients are the minerals (including trace elements) and vitamins required by the body in relatively small amounts. They are necessary for many vital body functions, e.g. iron for haemoglobin synthesis, vitamin K for blood clotting. An outline of minerals is provided in Table 19.6 and vitamins in Table 19.7. Readers should consult their own anatomy and physiology book for details of mineral and vitamin functions.

HEALTH PROMOTION Box 19.23

Healthy packed lunches

The House of Commons Select Committee (2004) report that, in England, 25% of children are overweight and 6% are obese. The promotion of healthy eating in schools, together with other measures, is important in reducing the number of children who are overweight or obese.

Student activities

- Plan 5 days of packed lunches for children aged 9–12 years that provide a balanced intake.
- What other measures in schools can help to promote healthy eating and prevent obesity?

[Resource: www.food.gov.uk/news/newsarchive/2004/sep/lunchbox2 Available July 2006]

Recommendations for a healthy balanced diet

A healthy, balanced diet is one that provides all the nutrients outlined above in the correct proportions (Box 19.23). Eating a variety of different foods is likely to provide a balanced diet. It is convenient to classify foods of similar composition and nutrient content into five food groups:

- Fats, oils and sugars including confectionery – use sparingly
- Proteins – meat, fish, eggs and vegetarian alternatives (serving = 1 egg; 80 g lean meat)
- Milk and dairy products (serving = 50 g hard cheese; 250 mL milk)
- Fruit and vegetables (serving = medium apple; 125 mL orange juice; 1 tablespoon of raisins; 3 heaped tablespoons of peas)
- Starchy foods – cereals, bread and potatoes (serving = 1 slice of bread; 30 g cereal).

The list above starts with foods that should be eaten in small amounts or, in the case of confectionery, only very occasionally and ends with the starchy foods which should provide around a third of the daily energy requirement. Figure 19.16 illustrates the five groups and a balanced diet for most adults.

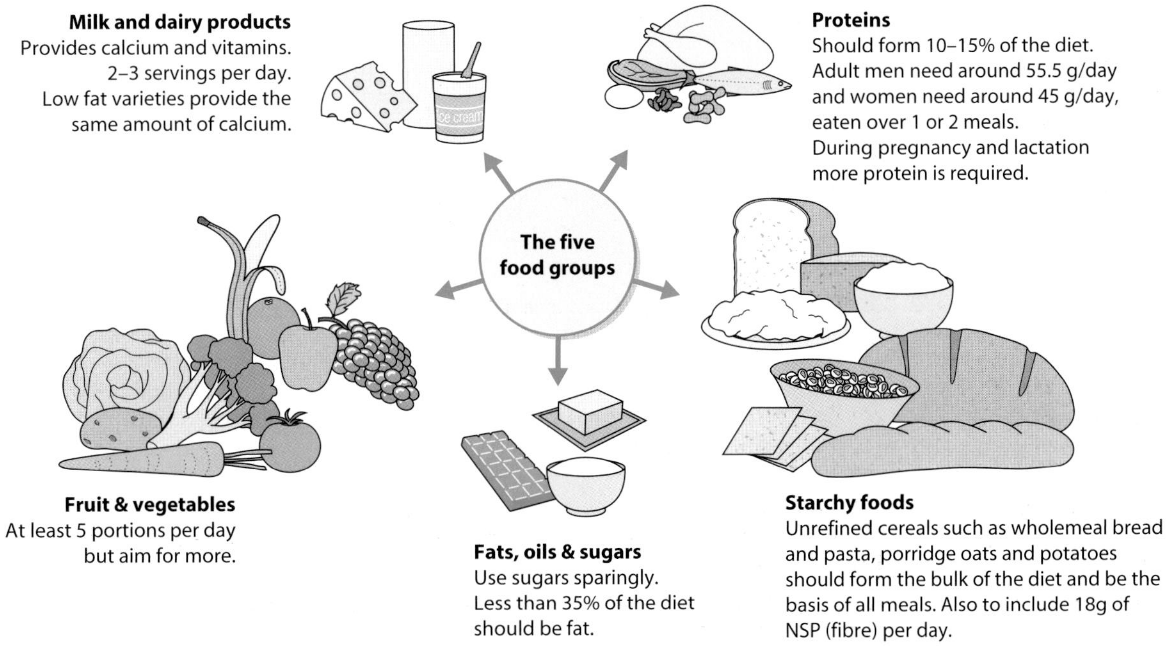

Milk and dairy products
Provides calcium and vitamins.
2–3 servings per day.
Low fat varieties provide the same amount of calcium.
Proteins
Should form 10–15% of the diet.
Adult men need around 55.5 g/day and women need around 45 g/day, eaten over 1 or 2 meals.
During pregnancy and lactation more protein is required.
The five food groups
Fruit & vegetables
At least 5 portions per day but aim for more.
Fats, oils & sugars
Use sugars sparingly.
Less than 35% of the diet should be fat.
Starchy foods
Unrefined cereals such as wholemeal bread and pasta, porridge oats and potatoes should form the bulk of the diet and be the basis of all meals. Also to include 18g of NSP (fibre) per day.

Fig. 19.16 Food groups and proportions in a balanced diet for most adults

HEALTH PROMOTION Box 19.24

Infant feeding

You have been asked to assist with a parent education session about infant feeding with your mentor.

Student activities

- Make a list of important areas to include about breast and bottle-feeding.
- Think about ways in which the information could be presented.

[Resources: Food Standards Agency – www.eatwell.gov.uk/agesandstages/baby; NHS Direct – www.nhsdirect.nhs.uk/en.aspx?ArticleID=63; DH Breastfeeding leaflet 2004 – www.dh.gov.uk/assetRoot/04/13/54/12/04135412.pdf; DH Bottle feeding leaflet 2005 – www.dh.gov.uk/assetRoot/04/12/36/20/04123620.pdf All available July 2006]

The Food Standards Agency (2005) recommends that most adults should:

- Increase intake of vegetables and fruit
- Increase intake of starchy foods such as rice, bread, pasta (wholegrain varieties) and potatoes
- Decrease the amount of salt, fat and sugar in their diet
- Eat some protein-rich foods such as meat, fish, eggs and pulses.

Infant feeding

Breast milk is the perfect food for healthy babies. It contains all the essential nutrients in proportions that meet growth and development needs of babies during the first 6 months. Moreover, breast milk contains maternal antibodies and these help to protect babies while their own immune systems develop. In addition, there are advantages to the mother that include special contact with her baby and ready availability of feeds.

Richardson and Fairbank (2000, p. 42) state 'increasing the initiation of breastfeeding represents an important public health challenge' and that breastfeeding rates in the UK remain low with between 40 and 60% of mothers starting (Box 19.24). Mothers in disadvantaged groups, e.g. teenagers, have the lowest rates.

The milk produced during the first three days after birth is known as colostrum. It contains antibodies and because it is less rich than mature breast milk it meets the needs of newborn babies. Mature breast milk is usually produced by the fourth day.

Artificial bottle-feeding with infant formula milks may be used by choice or where a contraindication exists; for example, a baby who needs special milk or a mother who is severely undernourished. Bottle-feeding has several disadvantages that include increased episodes of diarrhoea and the potential for over- or underfeeding. Maintaining high standards when cleaning and sterilizing bottles and other equipment, and preparing and storing feeds is vital (see Box 19.24).

Weaning is the gradual introduction of solid food to the milk-only diet of babies. Weaning should start when the baby is 6 months old. Breast or formula feeding is continued during weaning. First weaning foods are:

- Puréed fruits and vegetables with no added salt or sugar, e.g. banana, apple, yam, carrot and potato
- Non-wheat gluten-free cereals, e.g. maize, rice and sago, mixed with breast or formula milk.

During the next 6 months the variety, frequency and amount of solid food is increased so that by the age of 1 year the baby is having three family meals a day and around 600 mL of milk. Babies under 12 months of age must not be given cow's, sheep's or goat's milk because it:

- Contains too much protein and salt
- Is not easily digested
- Does not contain sufficient iron and other nutrients.

Factors that affect food intake and appetite

Several physical, psychological, cultural and social factors can affect food intake. The nurse must be able to identify the factors that increase the risk of people developing nutritional problems such as malnutrition caused by inadequate food intake (see p. 554). Many of these factors are outlined below and some are explored further in the section about helping people to eat. These include:

- Limited access to food shops – without a car it is difficult to visit out-of-town supermarkets and take advantage of the large range of foods, special offers and bulk buying
- Cooking facilities may be inadequate, e.g. bed and breakfast accommodation
- Lack of knowledge about what constitutes a balanced diet, menu planning, food shopping and meal preparation and cooking (Box 19.25)
- Poverty reduces the opportunity to eat a balanced diet, as people on a limited income may chose cheaper food that is often high in fat that satisfies hunger in preference to fruit and vegetables
- The environment is important in ensuring adequate food intake. Indeed one of the *Essence of Care* benchmark statements is 'The environment is conducive to enabling the individual patients to eat' (NHS Modernisation Agency 2003; see Box 19.17). For instance, in hospital there should be a dining area, adapted utensils and the ward should be quiet during mealtimes; inappropriate activities, e.g. ward rounds, treatments, should be stopped
- Preferences – if people are offered food that they dislike it is unlikely that their intake will be adequate
- People with specific religious or cultural food needs will not eat properly unless they are confident that the food offered has been prepared in accordance with their faith and that the ingredients are acceptable. For example, Hindus neither eat beef nor other food that has been in contact with beef during cooking or serving, and many vegetarians will refuse foods containing gelatin (Box 19.26).
- Mental health problems, e.g. depression, eating disorders (see p. 554) and dementia, can affect

HEALTH PROMOTION — Box 19.25

Understanding healthy eating

Think about a group of clients you have met while on placement. You might choose:

- Adults with a learning disability in supported living within the community
- Young people leaving the care of the local authority to live independently
- Families with children living in bed and breakfast accommodation
- Homeless people using night shelters.

Student activities

- How would you help your clients to understand what a healthy diet comprises?
- What activities, such as menu planning, shopping and meal preparation, are needed to achieve a balanced intake?

[Resources: Food Standards Agency – www.eatwell.gov.uk/healthydiet/nutritionessentials Available July 2006; Goodman L, Keeton E 2005 Choice in the diet of people with learning difficulties. Nursing Times 101(14):28–29; Grassick S 2001 Nutrition and learning disabilities. Nursing Times 97(32): NTplus Nutrition 48, 50; Kinder H 2004 Implementing nutrition guidelines that will benefit homeless people. Nursing Times 100(24):32–34]

CRITICAL THINKING — Box 19.26

Meeting religious and cultural dietary needs

Vijay Lal Sharma has told the staff in the care home that he does not eat beef. On Sunday the residents are served roast beef for lunch and the care assistant is surprised when Vijay declines to eat the alternative first course provided for him. He explains that he is worried that his meal may have been in contact with the beef in the kitchen or during serving.

Student activities

- When people first come to your placement, what questions are they asked regarding their dietary needs?
- Find out what facilities exist in your placement for preparing meals that are acceptable to people such as Vijay who have special dietary needs.
- Look at the menus for a week – is there always a strict vegetarian choice?

Note: Animal products such as gelatin can be present in foods, e.g. desserts, which might be assumed to meet the needs of vegetarians.

appetite, intake or the motivation to prepare and eat food
- Physical problems with chewing such as a sore mouth, ill-fitting dentures or problems with swallowing (see p. 537)
- Conditions affecting nutrition (see Table 19.5), including nausea and vomiting
- Changes in the senses of taste and smell (see p. 552)
- Immobility, lack of manual dexterity and level of dependency that lead to difficulties with shopping, preparing and cooking food, sitting up to eat, cutting up food and feeding
- Altered consciousness prevents eating.

Malnutrition in vulnerable people

It is a shocking fact that vulnerable people can become malnourished while in hospital and in community settings, including those living at home, but many authors confirm this to be so (Edington et al 1996, McCormack 1997, Corish & Kennedy 2000, Holmes 2003). People whose diets are deficient in protein and energy and/or have increased nutritional needs, e.g. following major surgery, are at risk of protein–energy malnutrition (PEM). It is vital that those at risk of malnutrition are identified on admission and this is discussed below.

Independence in eating

For most children, achieving independence in feeding starts around 9–10 months when they handle food to explore textures and put food in their mouths. During the next 12 months or so children learn to hold a spoon and use it to transfer food into their mouth. Early attempts at feeding are often accompanied by frustration and considerable mess, as food is dropped. It is important to encourage self-feeding while laying the foundation for good habits such as washing the baby's hands prior to eating.

Some people cannot achieve full independence in feeding, e.g. people with dementia or a severe learning and/or physical disability. Nurses must look for ways of maintaining their dignity by ensuring that they have as much independence as is possible. This might be achieved by providing 'finger food', e.g. sandwiches or pieces of fruit or raw vegetable, which the person can hold without requiring cutlery or manual dexterity. This maintains the dignity and independence of these people. The skills required to feed people are discussed on page 560.

Nursing interventions – maintaining nutritional status

Nursing interventions are often vital in helping people maintain or improve their nutritional status. This section explains nursing interventions including:

- Nutritional screening and assessment
- Helping people to eat and feeding
- Nutritional support such as sip feeding and enteral feeding.

In addition, some common investigations used to diagnose upper GI tract disorders that can affect nutrition are outlined.

Nutritional screening and assessment

The assessment of nutritional status requires a holistic approach that embraces physical, social, emotional,

Box 19.27 Body mass index

Body mass index (BMI) is a measurement calculated using body weight and height. It is used to ascertain whether an adult is within a healthy weight range for their height.

BMI is weight (in kg) divided by the height squared (m^2):

$$BMI = \frac{Weight\ (kg)}{Height\ (m^2)}$$

Worked example

Jane weighs 53 kg and is 1.57 m tall:

$$\frac{53}{1.57 \times 1.57} = \frac{53}{2.46} \qquad BMI = 21.5$$

- Normal range is BMI between 18.5 and 24.9
- Underweight is BMI <18.5 (WHO 1998).

Note: BMI <20 is significant in the MUST screening tool (BMI for overweight and obesity is shown in Box 19.20).

Note:
- Sometimes it is not possible to measure a person's height and in these cases other measurements can be used to estimate height, e.g. forearm (ulna) length (BAPEN 2003)
- In situations where neither height nor weight is known, the BMI can be estimated from MUAC, e.g. if the MUAC <23.5 cm the BMI is likely to be <20 (BAPEN 2003).

Box 19.28 Common investigations for upper GI tract disorders

The following investigations may be used to diagnose or evaluate treatment for upper GI tract disorders:

- Blood tests – full blood count, iron and folic acid levels
- X-rays – plain abdominal and chest X-ray, barium meal (swallow) and follow-through
- Endoscopy – pharyngoscopy, oesophagoscopy, gastroscopy, duodenoscopy
- Scans – ultrasound scan (USS), computed tomography (CT), magnetic resonance imaging (MRI)
- Urea breath test for the diagnosis of *Helicobacter pylori* (a bacterium linked with peptic ulceration)
- Gastric acid studies
- Faecal occult blood (see Ch. 21).

A simple explanation of some of these investigations accessed on the BBC website (BBC 2005) will help you provide patient information; more detailed nursing explanation can be found in McGrath (2003). The information about tests needs to take account of the person's ability to understand and retain facts, e.g. modification may be required for a child or a person with a learning disability or dementia.

spiritual and psychological aspects. The *Essence of Care* document states that 'nutritional trigger assessment should always be undertaken at initial contact and the need for reassessment of patients should be continuously considered' (NHS Modernisation Agency 2003, p. 2).

It is essential that people be screened on admission to identify those with existing malnutrition and those at risk of malnutrition (see below). People with a high risk must be referred to a dietitian or specially trained RN for a wide-ranging nutritional assessment. A nutritional assessment includes:

- Anthropometric measurements, e.g. weight, height, skinfold thickness, mid-upper arm circumference (MUAC)
- Use of nutritional screening audit tools (see below)
- Biochemical indicators, e.g. serum albumin.

Nutritional screening audit tool

The Malnutrition Universal Screening Tool (MUST) (BAPEN 2003) is one such screening tool. MUST uses a five-step approach for adults in all settings:

1. Calculation of BMI (Box 19.27).
2. Ascertain the percentage of unplanned weight loss.
3. Estimate the effects of acute illness.
4. Add up the scores for steps 1–2–3 for malnutrition risk score.
5. Implementation of management guidelines and/or local policies to plan care for those at nutritional risk such as frequency of screening or referral.

Stratton et al (2004) suggested a high prevalence of malnutrition in hospital inpatients and outpatients (19–60% using MUST) and agreement beyond chance between MUST and most other tools studied. MUST was quick and easy to use in these patient groups.

Nutritional screening and assessment in children is more specialized and readers are directed to Further reading (Khair & Morton 2000).

Common investigations

There are also many investigations used to identify GI tract disorders affecting nutrition (Box 19.28).

Helping people to eat

Helping people to eat enough to meet their needs may involve the patient/client and their family and appropriate members of the MDT, including dietitians, specialist nurses, doctors, OTs, SLTs, physiotherapists, ward hostesses, porters and laboratory staff.

Making appropriate healthy choices

Nurses should assist people who need help to choose from a menu. Some people may be unable to read or understand the menus. Moreover, a person with a learning disability or dementia may not remember what they had ordered when the meal is served and will need reminders.

Others may need explanations about the most suitable items if they have cultural or religious needs or are prescribed special diets, e.g. reducing or diabetic diets.

Environment and mealtimes

The nurse needs to ensure that the environment is conducive to eating. Basic activities that encourage eating include:

- Encouraging people to eat in a separate dining area away from the bed area
- Encouraging people at home to use mealtimes to socialize by inviting friends to share a meal or attending a day centre
- Ensuring that breastfeeding mothers have support and facilities for washing and privacy as appropriate
- Ensuring that equipment such as bedpans, commodes and vomit bowels are removed
- Ensuring that the ward dining area is quiet and treatments or visitors do not disrupt mealtimes
- Helping people to wash their hands beforehand
- Providing facilities for clients to rinse their mouth or clean dentures if necessary
- Helping people to sit up, ensuring that bed tables are at the correct height and the food is within easy reach. People who are unable to sit up to eat need individual solutions to allow them to eat
- Providing the most appropriate crockery and cutlery such as non-slip mats for plates or plate guards and large handle cutlery for people who only have the use of one arm. The OT can providing appropriate utensils (Fig. 19.17)
- Ensuring that food is served at the correct temperature
- Ensuring that the plate of food looks attractive, for instance by placing food carefully and wiping gravy stains from the edge
- Helping people with poor sight by describing the contents of the plate. Using a clock face, e.g. the meat is at 6 o'clock, can be useful
- Providing help and encouragement, when required, during mealtimes
- Making sure that meals are available if a person misses a mealtime.

Food fortification

This involves measures that modify the nutrient quality of the diet and may be advised for people who have small appetites and find it difficult to consume large volumes of food at a single meal. Fortification can be useful in the care of older people. Measures for people who are malnourished or those at risk of malnutrition may include:

- Having more frequent but smaller meals
- Using full-fat dairy products

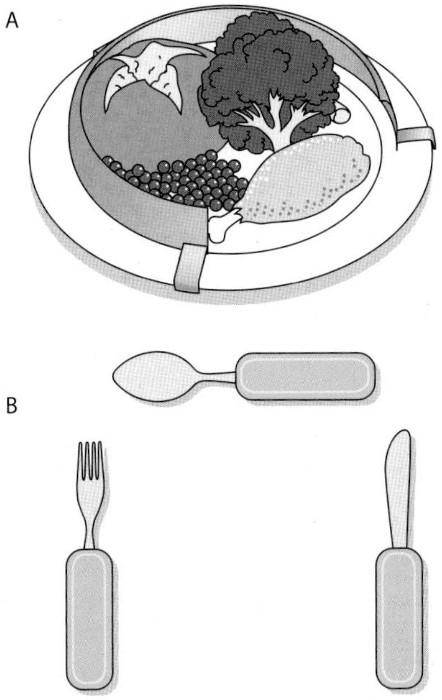

Fig. 19.17 Adaptations for eating: **A.** Plate guard. **B.** Cutlery with large handles

- Using milk powder to fortify full-fat milk, drinks, cereals and puddings
- Fortifying soup by adding milk, milk powder, cream or cheese
- Increasing energy by adding sugar, jam or dried fruit to cereals, porridge and desserts such as rice pudding
- Increasing the number of high-energy protein snacks between meals, e.g. cheese/biscuits, peanut butter.

Feeding

Nurses should only feed older children or adults when all other options have been tried and proved ineffective. Sometimes it is enough to spend time with people at mealtimes to encourage and motivate them to feed themselves, thereby maintaining their independence and dignity.

Independence can be increased for people who are unable to use cutlery or have dementia by providing 'finger foods' (see p. 559). However, there are people who need to be fed and although feeding people is a basic nursing skill it requires time and competence to do well (see Box 19.29). The RN monitors the amounts eaten and, using a nutritional screening audit tool (see p. 560), decides whether nutritional requirements can be maintained by oral feeding alone or whether nutritional support is required (see p. 562).

Clients requiring special diets

Some people are prescribed a special diet as part of managing particular conditions such as reducing, or they may have chosen a particular diet for religious or cultural reasons (see Box 19.30).

People may also require nutritional supplements at particular times during the lifespan or because of lifestyle choices. These include:

- Vitamin D for people who are not exposed to sunlight, e.g. cultures where the entire body is

NURSING SKILLS Box 19.29

Feeding dependent people

Ensure that you have sufficient time to feed the person and that this time is protected.

- Ask the person if they need to go to the lavatory or use a commode
- Prepare the immediate environment and prepare and position the person (see p. 561)
- Offer handwashing facilities and also wash your own hands
- Protect the client's clothing with a napkin, cloth or paper towel. Plastic or towelling bibs compromise people's dignity and should not be used
- Ensure the food is what the person likes and that, where possible, they have chosen it from the menu themselves
- Ensure that food is at the correct temperature and consistency, e.g. puréed for people with dysphagia after a stroke. If it is necessary to purée the meal, each component should be served in separate bowls (Kinloch 2004)
- Only have one course on the tray at a time – people can feel overwhelmed by the sight of several plates of food. Reducing portion sizes or using smaller plates can be less off-putting for those with small appetites
- If the person's mouth is dry, offer sips of water prior to feeding
- Choose appropriate cutlery and try to use the correct utensil for the food. Using a spoon for the entire meal is not conducive to maintaining dignity
- Remember cultural/religious needs, e.g. Muslims use the right hand for eating and to pass anything in the left hand could cause offence
- Sit in a way, e.g. at 90º to and level with the person, that facilitates two-way communication and the provision of appropriate physical assistance
- In situations where communication is difficult, set up a system whereby people can give you information such as 'ready for more'
- Always describe the food prior to feeding for those who cannot see well
- Never use pepper and salt or sauces without first asking the person, and checking any special dietary requirements, such as restricted salt
- Feed small amounts and allow time for chewing and swallowing; offer drinks as appropriate
- Do not hurry the person but do not offer food that has become cold
- Inform the RN about the amount of food and fluid taken and record it in the nursing notes and appropriate charts.

Note: When feeding children the nurse may need to involve play as an activity or therapy, and remember that older children might like to listen to music or watch television.

CRITICAL THINKING Box 19.30

Special diets

Reduced phenylalanine	Low-fibre (low residue)
Gluten-free	Low sodium
Diabetic	Vegan
Reducing	Vegetarian
High-protein	Kosher food
Low-protein	Halal food
High-fibre	

Student activities

- Choose two to three special diets from the list above that you have seen during placements and find out why they were used and what they involved.
- How do you think having a special diet affects people's lifestyles, e.g. a child who has a special diet going to a birthday party?

[For more information, see Further reading, e.g. Barker (2002)]

always covered, older people who are housebound or residents in nursing homes

- Folic acid before conception and during the first 3 months of pregnancy to reduce the incidence of spina bifida
- Iron may be needed during pregnancy or by women who have excessive menstrual loss
- Vegans and some vegetarians need vitamin B_{12}.

Nutritional support

Nutritional support is required to prevent or rectify malnutrition when people cannot eat enough food or absorb or utilize enough nutrients to meet their needs. Box 19.31 outlines different types of nutritional support. However, it is important to maintain normal diet and eating activity as much as possible. The type of nutritional support used depends on:

- Whether the GI tract is functioning
- The underlying reason for malnutrition
- Other factors, e.g. altered consciousness.

The provision of optimal nutritional support requires collaboration between the members of the MDT, especially the specialist nutrition nurse (Box 19.32).

Enteral feeding

It is usual to use a nasogastric (NG) tube for short-term feeding. For long-term feeding a percutaneous endoscopic gastrostomy (PEG) tube is inserted through the abdominal wall into the stomach and held in place by a balloon or flange. PEG tubes are frequently used for

Box 19.31 Types of nutritional support

Texture modification
People who find chewing and/or swallowing difficult may benefit from food that is mashed, liquidized or puréed (see Box 19.29). Thickening fluids may also be helpful. These changes are initiated in collaboration with the SLT and only after a full swallowing assessment (see p. 537).

Sip feeding
This is the provision of nutritious drinks at regular intervals, in place of food, or to supplement the diet in order to meet nutritional needs. Nutritionally complete feeds are produced commercially, e.g. Ensure®, Fortisip®, and may have extra minerals and vitamins. Many proprietary feeds are specially prepared for specific conditions such as kidney failure. When using proprietary feeds it is vital to follow the manufacturer's guidelines for storage and to check the expiry date.

Enteral feeding
This involves the use of a tube to feed people who have some GI tract function, but are unable to swallow or take in sufficient nutrition by the oral route. A nutritionally complete liquid feed is used to meet nutritional requirements (see below).

Parenteral feeding
Parental feeding (outside the GI tract) involves the infusion of sterile nutrient solutions, which require no digestion, directly into the circulatory system (see p. 565).

REFLECTIVE PRACTICE Box 19.32

Role of the specialist nutrition nurse

Think about a person you met on placement who was having nutritional support.

Student activities

- Was a specialist nutrition nurse involved in their care?
- If they were involved, what type of things did they do?
- Arrange to meet the specialist nurse in your area to learn about their role.

home enteral tube feeding (HETF) (Box 19.33). PEG feeding is used in situations that include:

- Dysphagia, e.g. severe learning disability or following a stroke
- Palliative care
- Unconsciousness (see Ch. 16)
- Children with chronic conditions, e.g. cystic fibrosis, cerebral palsy.

Other feeding routes include nasoduodenal or naso-jejunal tubes passed into the small intestine through the

EVIDENCE-BASED PRACTICE Box 19.33

Problems encountered with home enteral tube feeding

Evans et al (2004) identified a number of problems, associated with HETF, experienced by families in the month after their child was discharged from hospital.

Student activities

- Read the abstract or the full article (see Ch. 5 for critical appraisal skills).
- What problems did the authors identify?
- Discuss the article with your mentor and find out what procedures and support are put in place in your area before children are discharged on HETF. The specialist nutrition nurse will be a good source of information.

[Resource: Evans S, Macdonald A, Holden C 2004 Home enteral feeding audit. Journal of Human Nutrition and Diet 17(6):537–542]

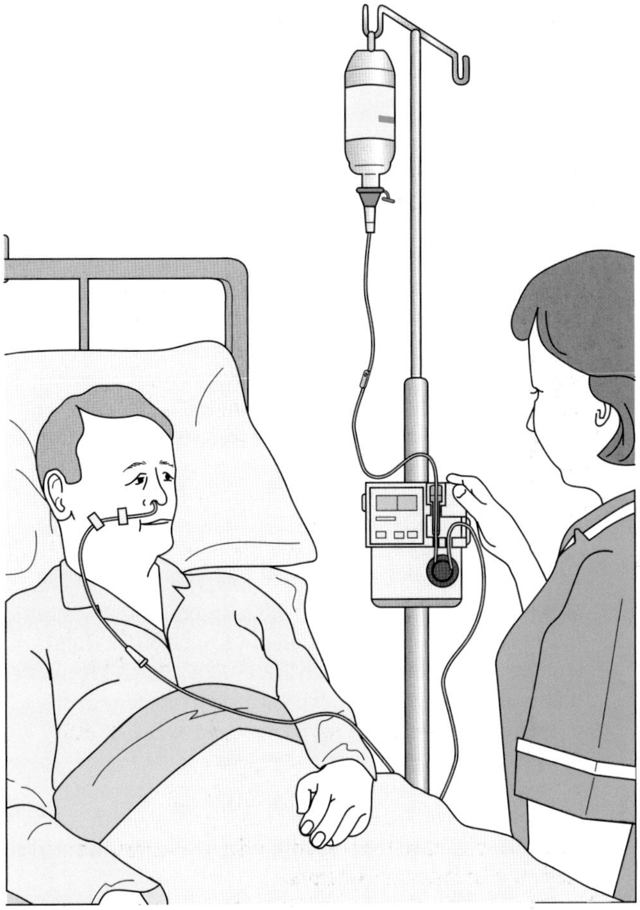

Fig. 19.18 Nasogastric feeding via a pump (reproduced with permission from Nicol et al 2004)

nose, oesophagus and stomach or jejunostomy tubes (inserted into the jejunum through the abdominal wall).

Small-bore NG feeding tubes should be used in preference to wider-bore NG tubes. People find small-bore tubes more comfortable and easier to tolerate. Wider-bore NG tubes are used to empty the stomach, e.g. after gastric surgery or when the bowel is obstructed. The skills needed to insert both types of NG tube are covered in the Further reading suggestions (Burnham 2000, Jamieson et al 2002, Nicol et al 2004).

Enteral feeding in infants and small children is complex and readers are directed to Further reading. In addition, prolonged lack of oral feeding can lead to developmental delay, e.g. problems learning appropriate social behaviour at mealtimes (Huband & Trigg 2000).

Enteral feeding must employ clean procedures to avoid bacterial contamination of the feed and/or administration systems, which can lead to diarrhoea. Nurses must ensure that manufacturers' guidelines are followed in respect of storage, the temperature for administration and the expiry date.

Enteral feeds can be given by bolus, or intermittently or continuously via an administration set with a drip chamber using gravity and a roller clamp, or controlled by a pump (Fig. 19.18).

Bolus feeding

Bolus feeds are given by syringe through a feeding tube at spaced intervals during the day. Although a reliable method, it has disadvantages that include discomfort caused by the volumes needed at each feed to fulfil nutritional needs (200–400 mL in adults). Moreover, large volumes take longer to be absorbed and increase the possibility of high residual volumes being present in the stomach when the next feed is due, which can lead to nausea and vomiting.

Intermittent or continuous gravity feeding

Gravity feeding is delivered by an intermittent or continuous drip method. Very careful monitoring is needed to ensure that the person receives the prescribed amount of feed and that rapid delivery of a large volume does not occur. This can cause gastric distension, which could predispose to gastro-oesophageal reflux disease (GORD) and aspiration of stomach contents into the respiratory tract.

Continuous pump-controlled feeding

Continuous pump-controlled feeding with a 4-hour rest period during the night is the preferred method as it is associated with fewer complications that include

NURSING SKILLS Box 19.34

Nasogastric feeding (adult)

- Explain the procedure and obtain consent
- Wash hands, put on a plastic apron
- Check the person's identity
- Check the nose and face for signs of pressure or soreness
- Check for signs of tube displacement
- Check the feeding tube position according to local protocols before every feed. This should involve aspirating a small volume of gastric contents and checking the pH using a reliable pH testing strip (0–6 with half point graduations) (National Patient Safety Agency [NPSA] 2005). The sample of aspirate should not be obtained within an hour of medication or feeding as this can produce inaccurate results. Some anti-ulcer drugs and previous gastric surgery can also affect results. A 10 mL syringe is used to aspirate a small-bore NG tube whereas a 50 mL catheter-tip syringe is used to aspirate a wide-bore nasogastric (NG) tube (Ryle's type). Avoid creating excess suction when aspirating the tube, otherwise the gastric mucosa could be damaged. A pH of 5.5 or below indicates that the tube is in the stomach (NPSA 2005). When a fine-bore tube is first passed an X-ray is used to confirm the correct position before the guide wire is removed
- Prepare the prescribed feed and enteral administration set according to the manufacturer's guidelines. If a separate container is being used, pour the feed into the bag or reservoir and attach the administration set. Sometimes sterile water is given using this method
- Run the feed through the tubing in order to expel the air and then clamp the tubing using the roller clamp
- Connect the administration set to the NG tube securely
- Commence the feed. In gravity delivery adjust the roller clamp to deliver the prescribed flow rate. If a pump is to be used, insert the administration set according to the manufacturer's instructions and open the roller clamp (Fig. 19.18). The pump is switched on and set at the prescribed rate
- Make the person comfortable and attend to their hygiene needs, e.g. mouth and nostril care
- Observe for signs of GORD, nausea or dyspnoea and diarrhoea
- On completion of the feed, flush the NG tube with 20–30 mL of sterile water to clear feed from the tube
- Record volume of feed given on the fluid chart and document in the nursing records
- The administration set must be changed every 24 hours to minimize the risk of bacterial contamination and growth. Label the new administration set with the date and time and record this in the nursing records
- When a second container of feed is due to start, ensure that the first does not empty completely, allowing air to enter the administration set. Should this occur it would be necessary to disconnect the administration set and run the new feed through as described above.

[Adapted from Nicol et al (2004)]
[Resource: National Patient Safety Agency 2005 Patient safety alert. Reducing the harm caused by misplaced nasogastric feeding tubes. Online: www.npsa.nhs.uk Available July 2006]

diarrhoea and GORD, with the risk of aspiration of stomach contents into the respiratory tract (Martyn 2003).

Nasogastric feeding is outlined in Box 19.34. Caring for the gastrostomy site and PEG tube feeding is outlined in Box 19.35.

Parenteral nutrition

Parenteral feeding into a vein should only be used when enteral feeding is unsuitable, e.g. when the GI tract is non-functional or cannot fully meet nutritional needs. It may be supplemental to oral/enteral feeding, or total (TPN). TPN is also known as i.v. alimentation or hyperalimentation. Sterile nutrient solutions are delivered via a volumetric pump into a central vein; however, a peripheral vein may be used short term, i.e. up to 1 month, for both supplementary parenteral nutrition and TPN. A large central vein is used when hypertonic solutions, e.g. glucose 10–50%, are infused to avoid damaging peripheral veins (see p. 549). Parenteral nutrition is used for people of all ages and enables children with a variety of congenital and acquired conditions to survive. TPN is used in situations that include:

- Conditions causing severe impairment of GI tract function, e.g. major resection of small intestine, severe inflammatory bowel disease, children with short bowel syndrome (SBS)
- People with cancer treated by drugs and radiotherapy
- When metabolic requirements are increased during illness, e.g. severe burns.

Parenteral nutrition requires collaboration between the patient/parents or carer and members of the MDT, in particular the specialist nutrition nurse, specialist i.v. therapy nurse, dietitian, pharmacist, doctor and laboratory staff. It is a complex procedure and readers are directed to Further reading (Hamilton 1999, Trigg & Mohammed 2006, Jamieson et al 2002, Nicol et al 2004).

NURSING SKILLS Box 19.35

Caring for the gastrostomy site and PEG feeding

Caring for the gastrostomy site

- After insertion of a PEG tube the site is treated as a wound (see Chs 15, 25). Local policies vary, but most recommend cleaning with sterile sodium chloride 0.9%, spraying with an iodine-based powder spray and covering the site with a sterile self-adhesive dressing
- Dressings are usually changed twice weekly; however, if the site is discharging it is redressed daily. Once the site has healed, there is no need for a dressing
- Temperature and pulse rate should be monitored for 1 week after tube insertion to detect infection (see Ch. 14)
- The site around the tube is observed daily for signs of inflammation, e.g. redness and swelling, excoriation (soreness), leakage of gastric contents or excessive movement of the tube
- Once the site is healed it is important that the skin disc/guard surrounding the tube (see Fig. 19.19) is lifted daily and slid round the tube so that the area can be washed with warm soapy water, rinsed and then dried thoroughly. The tube should then be rotated to prevent necrosis caused by pressure from the retention balloon in the stomach. The skin disc/guard is then replaced
- People are able to bathe or shower providing the gastrostomy tube is closed. The site is dried thoroughly afterwards.

Note: There are several types of gastrostomy tube, two of which are illustrated in Figure 19.19.

Principles of giving a PEG feed

Many general aspects of care are the same as those needed when giving a nasogastric feed (see Box 19.34).

- Intermittent feeds can be given when others are having a meal in order to create as 'normal' a situation as possible. However, continuous feeding has been shown to reduce the incidence of diarrhoea (Howell 2002)
- It is advisable for the person to be sitting up (unless the feed is given very slowly) to prevent GORD
- Remove the cap from the feed container and, maintaining asepsis (see Box 19.4, p. 547), open the administration set, attach it to the feed container according to the manufacturer's instructions, and close the roller clamp
- Hang the feed container on the infusion stand
- Run the feed through the tubing to expel the air
- Flush the PEG tube according to local policy
- Insert the tubing into the pump, take the plastic cap from the distal end of the tubing and attach it to the PEG tube
- Check that no feed is leaking at the connection of the PEG tube and that the feed is running
- Check at regular intervals that the feed is running as prescribed
- Observe for nausea, vomiting, discomfort or diarrhoea
- When the feed is complete the administration set is disconnected and the PEG tube flushed with sterile water according to local policy
- Document details of the feed in the nursing records and record volume of feed given on the fluid chart
- The administration set must be changed every 24 hours to minimize the risk of bacterial contamination and growth. Label the new administration set with the date and time and record this in the nursing records.

Note: When flushing the PEG tube, care should be taken when attaching the syringe to avoid damaging the connection. A 20 mL (or larger) syringe should be used to flush the tube, as the pressure exerted by smaller syringes is too great. When a PEG tube is not being used for feeding for a period of time, it should be flushed twice a day, to keep it patent (open).

[Adapted from Nicol et al (2004)]

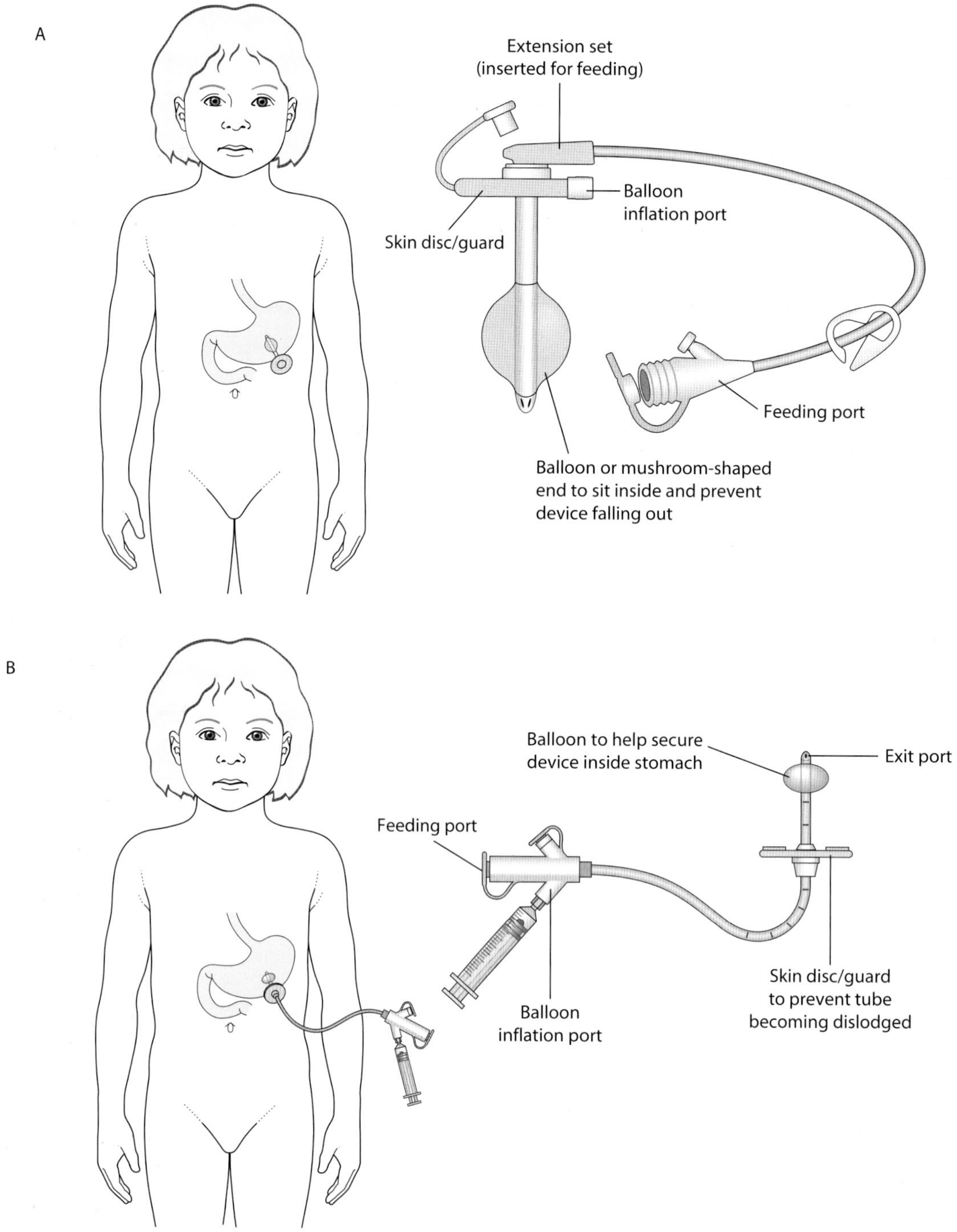

Fig. 19.19 Types of gastrostomy tube: **A.** Skin level 'button' or 'key' device. **B.** Percutaneous endoscopic tube (adapted with permission from Huband & Trigg 2000)

Summary

- Nursing interventions are important in promoting hydration and nutrition.
- *Essence of Care* (NHS Modernisation Agency 2003) best practice benchmarks concerned with eating and drinking are used to underpin nursing practices.
- Nurses have important roles in preventing fluid and electrolyte imbalance and malnutrition, especially in assessment of fluid and nutritional status.
- Nursing interventions for people with problems associated with drinking and eating range from simple nursing interventions to more complex skills.
- The partnership between the person/parents/carers and the MDT is important.
- The importance of promoting hydration and nutrition cannot be overstated; the nurse's role is central in ensuring that people in their care receive sufficient fluids and nutrients.

Self test

1. Why are infants and small children at increased risk of dehydration?
2. What changes occur in the skin of a person with fluid volume deficit? How does observation of the fontanelle help in assessment of fluid status in babies?
3. Stefan is having i.v. fluids and has been prescribed 500 mL glucose 5% in 4 hours. A standard administration set will be used.
   a. Calculate the flow rate in drops per minute
   b. Now do the calculation for mL per hour as if a volumetric pump is in use.
4. Name the energy-yielding macronutrients.
5. What are the recommendations for a healthy diet for most adults?
6. If Frank weighs 56 kg and is 1.75 m tall, what is his BMI? Is Frank underweight, normal or overweight?
7. Outline the principles of feeding a person.

Key words and phrases for literature searching

Dehydration	i.v. therapy
Electrolytes	Malnutrition
Enteral feeding	Nutrition
Fluid balance	Nutritional assessment/support
Hydration	Parenteral feeding/nutrition

Useful websites

BBC	www.bbc.co.uk/health/healthy_living/nutrition Available July 2006
British Association for Parenteral and Enteral Nutrition	www.bapen.org.uk Available July 2006
Food Standards Agency (FSA)	www.food.gov.uk; www.eatwell.gov.uk Available July 2006
Health Education Board for Scotland (HEBS) – *produces many healthy eating leaflets*	www.hebs.scot.nhs.uk/topics/diet/index.htm Available July 2006
La Leche League – *provides support, information and education for breastfeeding mothers*	www.lalecheleague.org Available July 2006
National Obesity Forum	www.nationalobesityforum.org.uk Available July 2006
NHS Quality Improvement Scotland (NHSQIS)	www.nhshealthquality.org Available July 2006
National Institute for Health and Clinical Excellence – *produces guidance*	www.nice.org.uk Available July 2006
Scottish Intercollegiate Guidelines Network (SIGN)	www.sign.ac.uk/guidelines/published/index.html Available July 2006

References

Arinzon Z, Feldman J, Fidelman Z et al 2004 Hypodermoclysis (subcutaneous infusion): effective mode of treatment of dehydration in long-term care patients. Archives of Gerontology and Geriatrics 38(2):167–173

BAPEN 2003 Malnutrition Advisory Group. The malnutrition universal screening tool (MUST). Online: www.bapen.org.uk Available July 2006

BBC 2005 Talking to your doctor – medical tests. Online: www.bbc.co.uk/health/talking/tests Available July 2006

Brooker C 1998 Human structure and function, 2nd edn. Mosby, London

Brooker C, Nicol M (eds) 2003 Nursing adults. The practice of caring. Mosby, Edinburgh

Bruera E, Pruvost M, Schoeller T et al 1998 Proctoclysis for hydration in terminally ill cancer patients. Journal of Pain and Symptom Management 15(4):216–219

Carroll H 2000 Fluid and electrolytes. In: Sheppard M, Wright M (eds) Principles and practice of high dependency nursing. Baillière Tindall, Edinburgh

Corish CA, Kennedy NP 2000 Protein-energy undernutrition in hospital in-patients. British Journal of Nutrition 83(6):575–591

Dasgupta M, Binns MA, Rochon PA 2000 Subcutaneous fluid infusion in a long-term setting. Journal of the American Geriatric Society 48(7):795–799

Department of Health 1991 Dietary reference values for food energy and nutrients for the United Kingdom. HMSO, London

Department of Health 2001 Essence of care. DH, London

Donnelly M 1999 The benefits of hypodermoclysis. Nursing Standard 13(52):44–45

Edington J, Kon P, Martyn C 1996 Prevalence of malnutrition in patients in general practice. Clinical Nutrition 15:60–63

Food Standards Agency 2005 Online: www.eatwell.gov.uk/healthydiet Available July 2006

Holmes S 2003 Undernutrition in hospital patients. Nursing Standard 17(19):45–52

House of Commons Select Committee 2004 Obesity: third report of session 2003–2004; Vol. I. Online: www.phel.gov.uk/search/advanced/fullpolicydetails.asp?recordid=169 Available July 2006

Howell M 2002 Do nurses know enough about percutaneous endoscopic gastrostomy? Nursing Times 98(17):40–42

Huband S, Trigg E (eds) 2000 Practices in children's nursing. Churchill Livingstone, Edinburgh

Jamieson EM, McCall JM, Whyte LA 2002 Clinical nursing practice. 4th edn. Churchill Livingstone, Edinburgh

Kinloch L 2004 Improving the quality and appeal of pureed meals for patients. Nursing Times 100(43):38–42

Mansfield S, Monaghan H, Hall J 1998 Subcutaneous fluid administration and site maintenance. Nursing Standard 13(12):56, 59–62

Martyn K 2003 Nutrition. In: Brooker C, Nicol M (eds) Nursing adults. The practice of caring. Mosby, Edinburgh

McCormack P 1997 Undernutrition in the elderly population living at home in the community: a review of the literature. Journal of Advanced Nursing 26(5):856–863

McGrath A 2003 Nursing patients with gastrointestinal disorders. In: Brooker C, Nicol M (eds) Nursing adults. The practice of caring. Mosby, Edinburgh

Morrison C 2000 Helping patients to maintain a healthy fluid balance. Nursing Times 96(31): NTplus Continence 3–4

NHS Modernisation Agency 2003 Essence of care: patient-focused benchmarks for clinical governance. Online: www.modern.nhs.uk/home/key/docs/Essence%20of%20Care.pdf Available July 2006

Nicol M, Bavin C, Bedford-Turner S et al 2000 Essential nursing skills. Mosby, Edinburgh

Nicol M, Bavin C, Bedford-Turner S et al 2004 Essential nursing skills, 2nd edn. Mosby, Edinburgh

Reid J, Robb E, Stone D et al 2004 Improving the monitoring and assessme nt of fluid balance. Nursing Times 100(20):36–39

Richardson R, Fairbank L 2000 Encouraging mothers to start breast-feeding. Nursing Times 96(34):42–43

Roper N, Logan WW, Tierney AJ 1985 The elements of nursing, 2nd edn. Churchill Livingstone, Edinburgh

Royal College of Nursing 2003 IV therapy forum: standards for infusion therapy. RCN, London

Stratton RJ, Hackston A, Longmore D et al 2004 Malnutrition in hospital outpatients and inpatients: prevalence, concurrent validity and ease of use of the 'malnutrition universal screening tool' ('MUST') for adults. British Journal of Nutrition 92(5):799–808

Trigg E, Mohammed TA 2006 Practices in children's nursing. Guidelines for hospital and community, 2nd edn. Churchill Livingstone, Edinburgh

Waugh A 2003 Problems associated with fluid, electrolyte and acid–base balance. In: Brooker C, Nicol M (eds) Nursing adults. The practice of caring. Mosby, Edinburgh

Waugh A, Grant A 2006 Ross and Wilson anatomy and physiology in health and illness. 10th edn. Churchill Livingstone, Edinburgh

Wong D, Hockenberry-Eaton M, Wilkelstein M et al (eds) 1999 Whaley and Wong's nursing care of infants and children. 6th edn. Mosby, St Louis

World Health Organization 1998 Obesity: preventing and managing the global epidemic. WHO, Geneva

Worobec G and Brown MK 1997 Hypodermoclysis therapy in a chronic care hospital setting. Journal of Gerontological Nursing 23(6):23–28

Further reading

Barker HM 2002 Nutrition/dietetics for healthcare. 10th edn. Churchill Livingstone, Edinburgh

Brooker C, Nicol M (eds) 2003 Nursing adults. The practice of caring. Mosby, Edinburgh

Burnham P 2000 A guide to nasogastric tube insertion. Nursing Times 96(8): NTplus Nutrition 6–7

Department of Health 1991 Dietary reference values for food energy and nutrients for the United Kingdom. HMSO, London

Dougherty L, Lister S 2004 The Royal Marsden Hospital manual of clinical nursing procedures. 6th edn. Blackwell Publishing, Oxford

Hamilton H (ed) 1999 Total parenteral nutrition. A practical guide for nurses. Churchill Livingstone, Edinburgh

Jamieson EM, McCall JM, Whyte LA 2002 Clinical nursing practices. 4th edn. Churchill Livingstone, Edinburgh

Khair J, Morton L 2000 Nutritional assessment and screening in children. Nursing Times 96(49): NTplus Nutrition 2–4

Metheny NM (ed) 1996 Fluids and electrolyte balance. 3rd edn. Lippincott: Philadelphia

National Institute for Health and Clinical Excellence (NICE) 2006 Nutritional support in adults. Clinical guidance 32. Online: www.nice.org.uk/pdf/word/CG032NICEGuidelines.doc Available July 2006

NHS Quality Improvement Scotland (NHSQIS) 2002 Best Practice Statement: Nutrition for physically frail older people. Online: www.nhshealthquality.org/nhsqis/files/BPSNutrition_frail_elderlyMay02.pdf Available July 2006

Nicol M, Bavin C, Bedford-Turner S et al 2004 Essential nursing skills. 2nd edn. Mosby, Edinburgh

Scottish Intercollegiate Guidelines Network (SIGN) Guideline 69: Management of obesity in children and young people. Online: www.sign.ac.uk/guidelines/fulltext/69/index.html Available July 2006

Trigg E, Mohammed TA 2006 Practices in children's nursing. Guidelines for hospital and community, 2nd edition. Churchill Livingstone, Edinburgh

Waugh A, Grant A 2006 Ross and Wilson anatomy and physiology in health and illness. 10th edn. Churchill Livingstone, Edinburgh

20 Elimination – urine

Martin Steggall

Glossary terms

Anuria
Bacteriuria
Catheterization
Dysuria
Frequency
Haematuria
Incontinence
Nocturia
Oliguria
Polyuria
Proteinuria
Pyuria
Retention

Learning outcomes

This chapter will help you:

- Outline the anatomy and physiology of the urinary system and normal micturition
- Understand the common problems with micturition across the lifespan
- Outline the rationale for assessment of urine and micturition
- Describe the composition and characteristics of urine
- Outline the nursing interventions associated with micturition including cultural aspects
- Describe the measures taken to promote continence
- Define the different types of incontinence and the potential management of each
- Outline the care needed for a person who has an indwelling urinary catheter.

Introduction

Continence and bladder (and bowel) care form one of the eight original *Essence of Care* best practice statements from the Department of Health (DH) (2001). The *Essence of Care* benchmarks arose from the commitment in *Making a Difference* (DH 1999), which is the national nursing, midwifery and health visiting strategy.

The *Essence of Care* aims to improve quality in care and has therefore been designed to share good practice amongst health trusts, identifying best practice and remedying poor practice, effectively improving the quality of care that people receive.

Central to this theme, or any that aims to improve care, is a sound understanding of the issues, in this instance related to continence and incontinence. Even though some nurses may not do 'hands-on' care they must understand the processes involved because they are accountable for delegated care (see Chs 6, 7). It is essential therefore to have a thorough grounding in the anatomy and physiology of the urinary system.

Two of the most commonly seen problems associated with urinary elimination are urinary tract infections and loss of continence. The importance of promoting continence cannot be overstated. The report *Making a Difference* (DH 1999) finds that although continence is considered one of the fundamental aspects of care, the provision of that care is below acceptable standards.

The urinary system is an integral component of homeostatic balance, ensuring that there is excretion of unwanted waste products, water balance and assisting with the control of blood pressure, to name a few examples. An understanding of the normal physiology of the urinary system will enable the nurse to care for the patient by anticipating potential problems and understanding the rationale for managing actual problems.

Elimination of urine crosses several traditional specialty boundaries, i.e. renal, urology, continence and gynaecology nursing, although an understanding of how this system works is essential for all nurses, whether children's nurses, mental health or learning disabilities nurses, so that safe and appropriate nursing care can be offered.

The short answer and multiple choice questions have been designed to test your knowledge, and a Further reading section provided for those wishing to gain a greater insight into these common problems.

Overview – anatomy and physiology of the urinary system

The urinary system comprises the kidneys (2), ureters (2), bladder and urethra (Fig. 20.1). Readers should consult their own anatomy and physiology books for further details.

The kidneys

The kidneys are paired organs that lie against the back (dorsal) body wall behind the parietal peritoneum (retroperitoneal) in the superior lumbar region, i.e. they are either side of the spinal column at about the level of the lower ribs, but lying towards the back. When a kidney is cut longitudinally three distinct areas can be seen with the naked eye (Fig. 20.2):

- An outer fibrous capsule
- A cortex
- A medulla, comprising the tissue of the renal pyramids.

The kidneys are key organs with the functions that include:

- Production of urine by filtration of the blood contents, reabsorption of substances that are useful to the body and secretion of waste products
- Control and maintenance of fluid balance (see Ch. 19)
- Maintenance of acid–base balance (see Ch. 19)
- Control and maintenance of electrolyte balance (see Ch. 19)
- Renin production – an enzyme involved with the control of blood pressure
- Erythropoietin production – a hormone that stimulates red blood cell production.

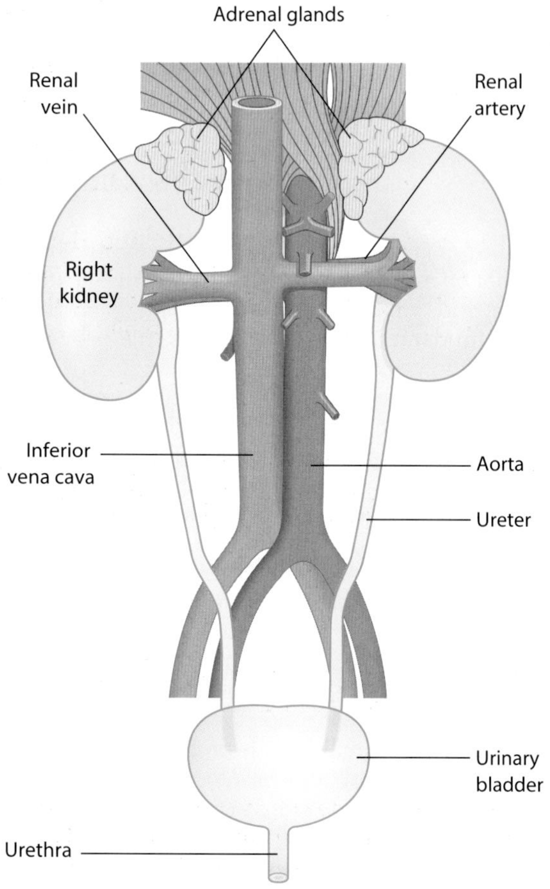

Fig. 20.1 Urinary tract (reproduced with permission from Brooker & Nicol 2003)

In adults, the kidneys receive approximately 625 mL of blood per minute from branches of the renal artery. A high volume of blood supply to the kidneys is required to maintain glomerular filtration rates (GFR) (see below) and to supply oxygen to active cells.

Nephron

Each kidney is composed of approximately one million microscopic, functional units, the nephrons, and a system of collecting ducts that carry urine through the renal pyramids into the calyces and renal pelvis and hence to the ureter.

A nephron has a glomerulus (a knot of arterial capillaries) and a renal tubule that consists of a glomerular (Bowman's) capsule enclosing the glomerulus, a proximal convoluted tubule (PCT), loop of Henle, distal convoluted tubule (DCT) and the accompanying blood vessels (Fig. 20.3).

Blood enters the glomerulus from the afferent arteriole, but this is dependent on blood pressure. Small holes (fenestrations) in the lining of the capillary allow small particles such as glucose to pass through into the renal tubule. However, larger molecules such as proteins cannot normally pass through the glomerular filtration barrier.

Blood leaves the glomerulus in the efferent arteriole, which forms a second capillary network around the renal tubule, the peritubular capillaries and more specialized capillaries called the vasa recta (see Fig. 20.3). The peritubular capillaries form larger and larger veins that carry blood to the renal vein.

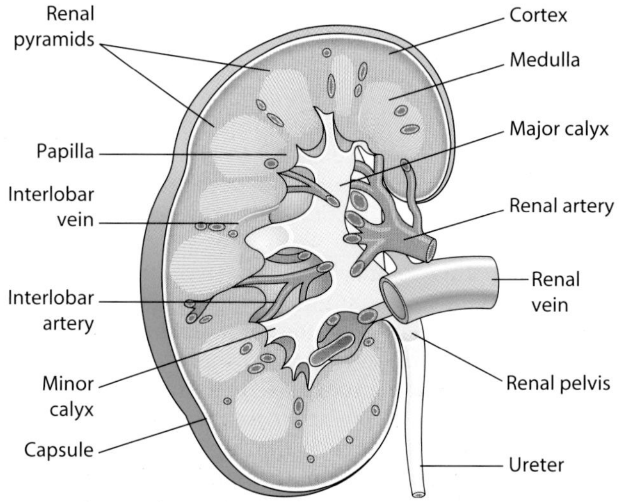

Fig. 20.2 Longitudinal section through a kidney (reproduced with permission from Brooker & Nicol 2003)

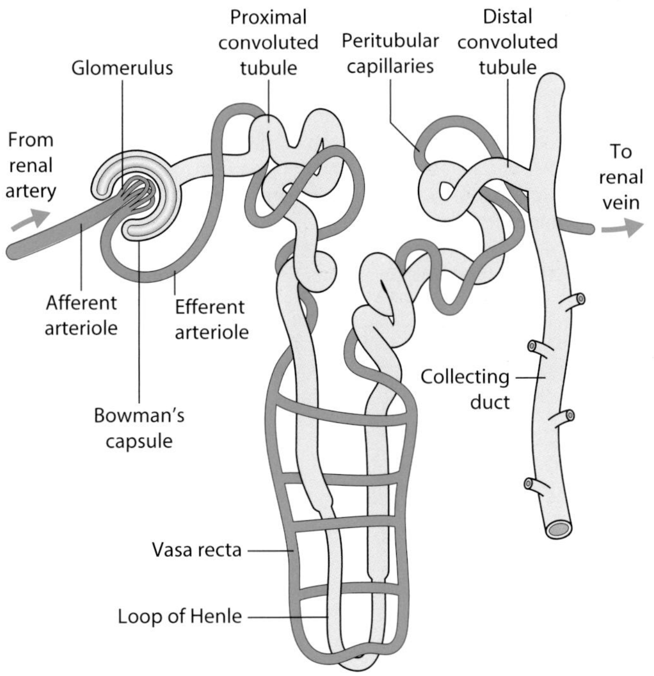

Fig. 20.3 A nephron and blood vessels (simplified)

The filtration membrane allows large quantities of fluid and small molecules such as sodium and glucose to leave the blood and enter the tubule. At this stage the fluid is called filtrate; it will become urine as it passes down the tubule. Substances needed by the body such as glucose are reabsorbed in the PCT and returned to the blood.

Control of blood flow into the glomerulus

The GFR is the volume of plasma filtered through the glomerulus in 1 minute; the adult GFR is about 120 mL/min. Although GFR changes with age, all age groups need to maintain GFR to excrete waste products and balance the amount of water in the body (Box 20.1).

GFR can be controlled to ensure that a constant supply of blood is received at the correct pressure, ensuring that urine is constantly produced. This control is achieved by changing the diameter of the renal arteries and afferent and efferent arterioles by various processes that include:

- The renin–angiotensin–aldosterone mechanism/system. Angiotensin II is an extremely strong vasoconstrictor, i.e. it narrows the diameter of an artery, which results in the pressure inside the artery increasing. The renin–angiotensin–aldosterone system increases blood pressure and therefore GFR through the action of aldosterone, a hormone which allows the kidney to conserve sodium. If sodium is conserved, water will always follow it, so the blood volume increases and therefore the blood pressure.
- Chemicals, e.g. prostaglandins and nitric oxide, which all dilate or widen the diameter of the arterioles, are termed vasodilators.

> **Box 20.1 Glomerular filtration rate at the extremes of the lifespan**
>
> Newborn babies have a low GFR and are therefore vulnerable to fluid overload. Children reach adult GFRs between the first and second years of life. Older people usually have a decreased GFR, and also total body water, and are therefore at increased risk of having adverse drug reactions if a drug, e.g. the heart drug digoxin, accumulates in the body because it is not excreted quickly enough (see Ch. 19).

The amount of urine output is therefore a guide for whether the kidneys are receiving blood at the correct volume and pressure. The minimum urine output, i.e. the smallest volume that will allow the body to excrete waste products, is 0.5 mL/kg/h in both children and adults, although there are exceptions to this rule.

Control of blood volume

The amount of fluid in the body is carefully controlled by many organ systems (see Ch. 19). Several substances help to balance the volume of fluid in the body, particularly antidiuretic hormone (ADH).

ADH, or vasopressin, is released from the brain (stored in the posterior pituitary gland) when blood fluid volumes fall, e.g. as may occur from blood loss. ADH increases the permeability of the renal tubule, increasing water reabsorption. When plasma ADH levels are low, a large volume of urine is excreted (diuresis), and the urine is dilute. When plasma levels are high, a small volume of urine is excreted (antidiuresis), and the urine is concentrated.

Alcohol inhibits the release of ADH and therefore should be avoided when dehydrated (see Ch. 19). Caffeine also acts as a diuretic, i.e. making people pass urine more frequently, by increasing the GFR and inhibiting sodium reabsorption.

Urine production in the nephron

There are three processes involved in the production of urine: filtration (see above), reabsorption and secretion. Table 20.1 (p. 572) outlines the specific functions of each segment of the nephron.

Lower urinary tract

The lower urinary tract comprises two ureters, the urinary bladder and urethra (see Fig. 20.1).

Ureters

The ureters are hollow tubes that convey urine from the renal pelvis to the bladder. They are approximately 30 cm in length and implant into the posterior bladder at the ureteric orifices. Urine moves down the ureters by peristalsis, rhythmic contraction of the smooth muscle layer in the wall of the ureters.

Table 20.1 Summary of the functions of the nephron and collecting ducts

Part of nephron	Processes
Proximal convoluted tubule (PCT)	This is the site of most *reabsorption* – most of the fluid or filtrate that enters the PCT is reabsorbed (approximately 80% of the filtered load) Some water, electrolytes, bicarbonate, glucose, etc. are essential to the body and are reabsorbed and returned to the circulation; the waste products (e.g. urea and creatinine) entering the filtrate are not reabsorbed because they need to be eliminated from the body By the time the filtrate reaches the end of the PCT it has been reduced to 20% of the volume that was filtered. It contains water, electrolytes, urea and other substances that are no longer required by the body
Loop of Henle	Water can leave the descending limb of the loop of Henle via osmosis but sodium is trapped In the ascending limb of the loop of Henle water is now trapped, but sodium can be reabsorbed The loop of Henle can selectively reabsorb water and sodium so that water balance is maintained
Distal convoluted tubule (DCT)	Renin, aldosterone and ADH all act at the DCT (see p. 571) Sodium and chloride can be reabsorbed here There is also reabsorption and/or *secretion* of potassium and hydrogen into the filtrate Secretion is important in acid–base balance Water is only reabsorbed in the presence of ADH
Collecting ducts	It is only in exceptional circumstances that water and electrolytes can be reabsorbed In the absence of ADH, dilute urine enters the collecting tubules When ADH is secreted, the collecting duct becomes more permeable to water and water is removed and the urine becomes more concentrated The fluid that enters the calyces (see Fig. 20.2, p. 570) is urine, which then drains into the renal pelvis and the ureters

Bladder

The bladder is a temporary reservoir for urine. It is a muscular sac lined with transitional epithelial cells (urothelium). When the bladder is empty the lining is arranged in folds called rugae. These folds disappear when urine fills the bladder. The smooth muscle layer is called the detrusor and is an exceptionally strong muscle that contracts to empty the bladder. The three openings in the bladder wall – two ureteric orifices and the urethra – form a triangle called the trigone. The organs associated with the bladder in women and men are illustrated in Figure 20.4.

The bladder is able to distend but when the adult bladder contains around 300–400 mL of urine the urge to pass urine occurs. The volume is much less in children and depends on the child's age, but the bladder wall becomes stretched when approximately 50–200 mL of urine is in the bladder (Kozier et al 2000), although this will be dependent on the infant's feeding regimen, with urine volumes increasing as the child's urinary system matures.

The main defences against infection in the urinary system are the flow of urine, the acidity of urine and, in males, the length of the urethra. Urine is normally acidic (see p. 578) which inhibits bacterial growth.

Urethra

The urethra carries urine from the bladder to the outside. In males, the urethra is around 20–25 cm in length, has several curves and passes through the prostate gland. In addition to carrying urine the male urethra also carries semen. The female urethra is approximately 5–10 cm in length, is straight and not involved in reproduction.

The urethra passes through the muscular pelvic floor where internal and external urethral sphincters are located. The external sphincter is under voluntary control or, more accurately, the external control develops during childhood. Normally the sphincters keep the urethra closed so that urine does not leak from the bladder.

Urinary elimination

Micturition, voiding and urination all refer to the process of passing urine. It is an extremely complex process that involves nerve impulses, coordinated muscle contraction and relaxation of the internal and external urethral sphincters. This process develops over the first few years of life, which explains why babies are not continent. The nerve supply from the bladder to the spinal cord is incomplete until the age of around 2 years when the toddler gradually learns that the sensation in the bladder means that they need to pass urine.

When the infant's bladder fills with urine the bladder wall is stretched and nerve impulses pass to the spinal cord. This initiates a spinal reflex that causes detrusor muscle contraction, internal sphincter relaxation and the baby voids urine (Fig. 20.5A, p. 574).

When development is complete and continence is achieved, the urethral sphincters and the bladder are controlled by a more complex nervous system (Fig. 20.5B, p. 574). As before, the bladder fills with urine and the

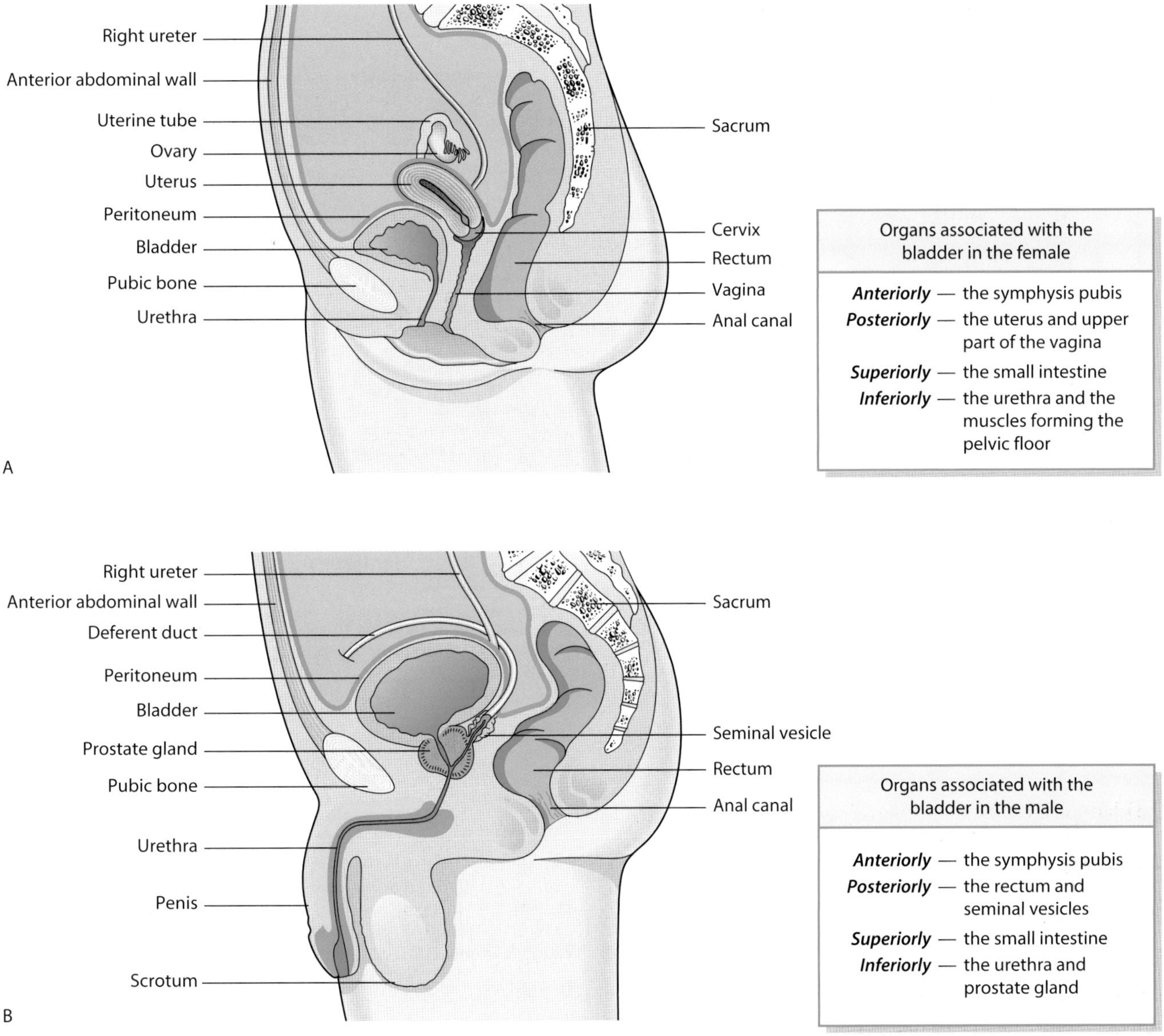

Fig. 20.4 Organs associated with the bladder: A. The female. B. The male (reproduced with permission from Waugh & Grant 2001)

bladder walls are stretched, resulting in a nerve impulse being sent to the spinal cord. Now, however, the nerve impulse is directed upwards to the cerebral cortex of the brain, where the impulse is interpreted as the desire to pass urine. This usually results in a behavioural response, i.e. going into the lavatory or asking the nurse for a bedpan. Conscious inhibition of reflex bladder contraction and sphincter relaxation is possible for a short time when it is not convenient to pass urine such as driving on a motorway until the service station is reached.

The cerebral cortex sends another nerve impulse to the spinal cord, and then on to the bladder and internal urethral sphincter. As the detrusor muscle contracts there is reflex relaxation of the internal sphincter and voluntary relaxation of the external sphincter, allowing urine to pass through the urethra. Once the bladder is empty the nerve impulses stop, the detrusor muscle stops contracting and the sphincters close.

Micturition can be aided by increasing pelvic pressure through contracting the abdominal muscles and lowering the diaphragm (Valsalva manoeuvre).

Factors affecting micturition

There are multiple factors affecting micturition (Box 20.2, p. 574).

Micturition is usually under a degree of conscious control. Usually an adult or older child passes urine alone, at a time determined by them and in surroundings that are usually comfortable and known to them. Hospitalization therefore can be a contributory factor affecting micturition. People can become disorientated or positioned too

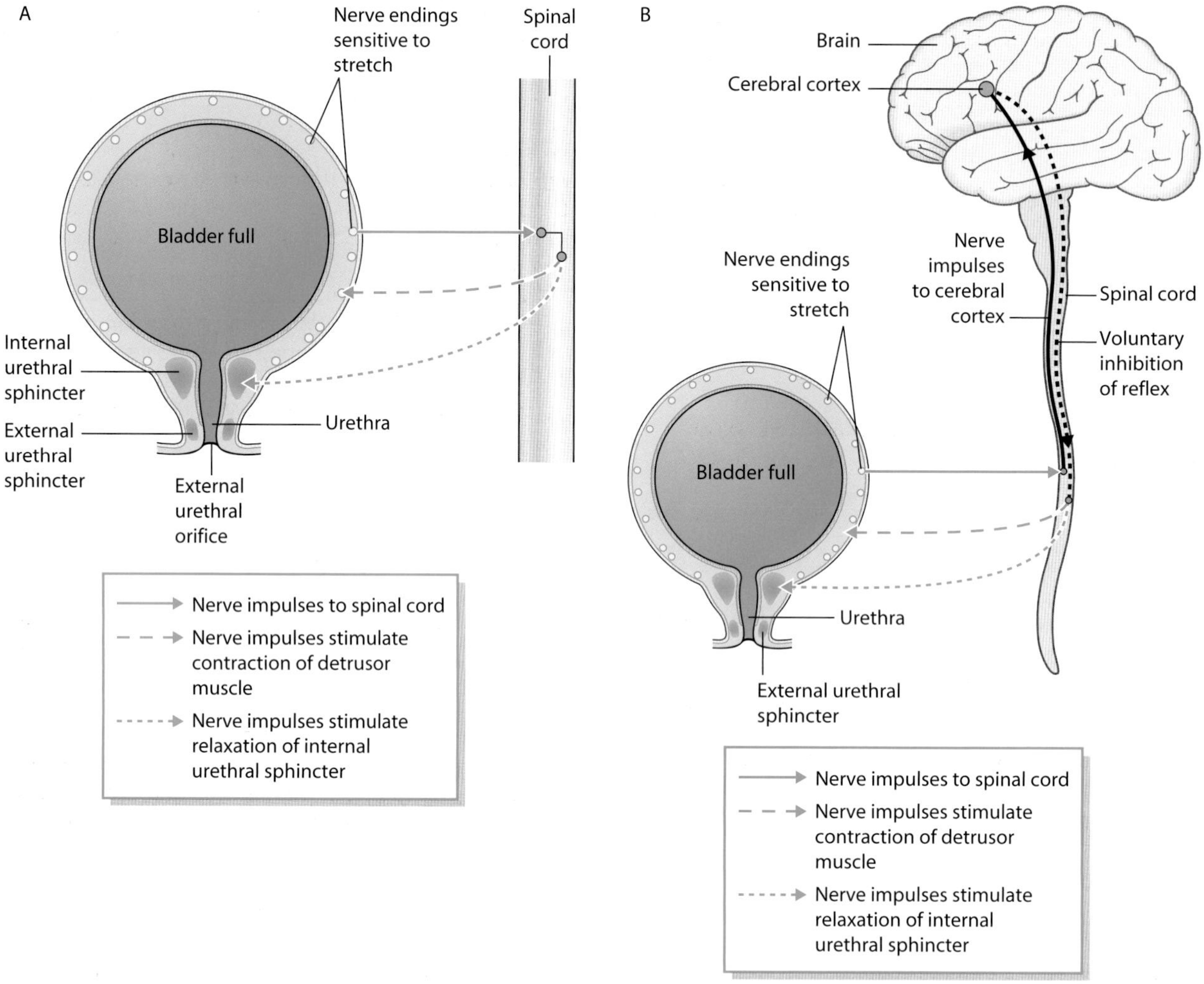

Fig. 20.5 Control of micturition: A. Simple reflex control when conscious effort cannot override the spinal reflex. B. Control of micturition when conscious override is possible (reproduced with permission from Waugh & Grant 2001)

Box 20.2 Factors affecting micturition

- Developmental stage (see Ch. 8)
- Lack of privacy
- Anxiety (see Ch. 11)
- Lack of suitable facilities
- Weather
- Mobility (see Ch. 18)
- Constipation (see Ch. 21)
- Medication (see pp. 583, 584, Ch. 22)
- Fluid intake (see Ch. 19)
- Disease or injury, e.g. cystitis (bladder infection), kidney failure, diabetes mellitus, stroke, spinal injury.

far from the lavatory, which can cause loss of continence. Furthermore, a person's normal urinary habits can be altered by anxiety, following surgery or illness, through constipation or dehydration, and these factors should be considered when caring for people irrespective of age.

Obesity is associated with some types of incontinence (see p. 586) in women but not in men.

Many drugs can also affect the person's ability to urinate normally, from diuretics (e.g. furosemide) which increase urinary volume and frequency, to analgesics that can cause confusion and disorientation. Caffeine, found in tea, coffee and cola-type drinks, as well as performance-enhancing drinks, can have an excitatory effect on the bladder muscle, causing urgency and frequency, as well as being a diuretic. Alcohol acts as a diuretic by affecting ADH release, irrespective of overall hydration. Box 20.3 provides an opportunity to consider how micturition may be affected.

Common urinary disorders

Urinary tract infection (UTI) and loss of continence (incontinence) are very common. These and other conditions that affect the normal urinary elimination are outlined in Table 20.2. Further detail about UTIs is provided in Box 20.4 (p. 576). More information is provided in Cotton et al (2003) and Fanning (2003). Some patient groups also provide useful information and some of their websites are included at the end of this chapter.

Assessment and observation of urine and urinary elimination

Before taking a urine sample, it is essential to ask the person about any problems with micturition and urinary symptoms. Box 20.5 (p. 576) provides an overview of problems with micturition and some urinary symptoms. The key features are the type of symptoms, duration of the problem, what makes it better or worse, and any other circumstances that could exacerbate the problem, e.g. the lavatory is upstairs so the person cannot get to it quickly enough due to arthritis. Bowel habit is also important to assess, since constipation can cause pressure on the urethra/bladder, thereby resulting in urinary symptoms (see Ch. 21).

As well as the focused assessment, the nurse should note how mobile and dextrous the person is. Part of the assessment is gaining a picture of the person and their abilities; this will help guide nursing management and what continence products/support they will need.

REFLECTIVE PRACTICE Box 20.3

Changes to micturition

Think about a situation in which your own micturition was affected, such as being anxious about a new placement, or having a full bladder and being unable to find a public lavatory, or perhaps you needed to pass urine where another person could hear or see you.

Student activities

- Think about how you felt and provide the possible reasons for this.
- Now consider an occasion when a client's or patient's normal pattern of micturition was affected by one of the factors in Box 20.2.
- Reflect on the nursing interventions used to minimize the disruption.

Measuring urine output and observing voiding patterns

This can involve the use of a fluid balance chart, weighing nappies, weighing patients daily and completing frequency–volume charts. In addition, assessment of the skin and mucous membranes and blood pressure monitoring will also enable assessment of hydration (see Chs 17, 19).

Fluid balance chart (see Ch. 19)

Urinary output must be recorded on a 24-hour input and output chart if there are concerns about the elimination of urine or renal function. The minimum amount of urine

Table 20.2 Common urinary disorders

Disorder	Description
Benign prostatic enlargement (BPE)	An enlarged prostate gland caused by increased cell size or growth of new cells occurring mainly in older men Leads to urinary problems such as poor stream, dribbling, frequency and retention (see p. 576)
Cancer – kidney, bladder, prostate	Cancer may affect the kidney, ureter, bladder and prostate gland A cancer affecting the kidney, known as a nephroblastoma (Wilms' tumour), is common during childhood Bladder cancer can cause painless haematuria (blood in the urine) Cancer of the prostate gland is a common male cancer, which can cause symptoms similar to those of BPE
Diabetic nephropathy (kidney disease)	Progressive kidney disease associated with diabetes Caused by damage to the renal blood vessels, loss of glomeruli and renal failure
Glomerulonephritis	Inflammation of the glomerulus (of the nephron), of which there are many different types
Incontinence of urine	An inability to control the voiding of urine The main types are outlined on page 586
Reflux nephropathy (chronic pyelonephritis)	Kidney damage caused by the backflow of infected urine from the bladder up the ureters (vesicoureteric reflux – VUR) (see Box 20.4, p. 576)
Renal (kidney) failure	Renal failure can be acute or chronic: • *Acute renal failure* (ARF) occurs when previously healthy kidneys suddenly fail because of reduced blood supply, e.g. severe haemorrhage; it is potentially reversible • *Chronic renal failure* (CRF) occurs when irreversible and progressive damage, such as from diabetic nephropathy, leads to end stage renal disease (ESRD)
Renal stones (calculi)	Stones can form in the kidney They may move down the ureters to cause intense pain (renal colic), obstruct the flow of urine from the kidney, predispose to infection and may cause renal damage
Urinary tract infection (UTI)	Infection affecting the urinary tract is common across the lifespan (see Box 20.4, p. 576)

Box 20.4 Urinary tract infection

UTIs are more common in females than in males, except in infants under 1 year due to periurethral colonization, breastfeeding or an immature immune system (Dairiki Shortliffe 2002). The site of the infection determines the term used to describe the infection:

- Acute pyelonephritis is an infection in the kidney
- Cystitis is an infection in the bladder.

Urinary tract infections are caused by bacterial invasion, e.g. *Escherichia coli*. Normally the urine does not contain bacteria; the presence of bacteria in the urine is termed bacteriuria. Bacteriuria can be symptomatic, e.g. painful voiding or dysuria, or asymptomatic. Pyuria is the presence of white blood cells (WBCs) in the urine, indicating inflammation of the bladder lining. Bacteriuria without pyuria suggests bacterial colonization, not infection (see Ch. 15).

In children, UTIs tend to be classified into initial infections and recurrent infections. Sometimes the cause of infection can be linked to a congenital abnormality that results in vesicoureteric reflux (VUR) or backflow of urine from the bladder into the ureters or kidney. It is essential to identify the presence of UTI in children so it can be investigated and the cause treated to prevent renal damage in later life. UTI in young children can be particularly difficult to diagnose because of several non-specific signs such as poor feeding, fever, vomiting or failure to thrive, as well as the development of language and children's concepts of health and ill health. This may also be the case in some people with a learning disability.

UTIs in older people are common. The symptoms can range from asymptomatic bacteriuria to life-threatening sepsis. The majority of older people with bacteriuria remain asymptomatic, although symptoms such as lethargy, confusion, anorexia and incontinence may be caused by bacteriuria.

needed to excrete waste from the body was discussed on page 571, i.e. 0.5 mL/kg/h in both children and adults.

Therefore, an infant weighing 5 kg must produce 2.5 mL/h (60 mL in 24 hours) whereas an adult weighing 55 kg must produce 27.5 mL/h (660 mL in 24 hours). Obviously these are minimum amounts and people produce much larger volumes of urine under everyday conditions, approximately 1 mL/kg/h but up to 2 mL/kg/h (Box 20.6). The volume of urine produced depends on many factors that include fluid intake, fluid loss and renal function, but a healthy adult should aim to pass more than 1000 mL daily, with an 'ideal' urinary volume of 2000 mL. This ensures that the kidney and lower urinary tract are 'flushed' regularly, thus reducing the risk of UTI.

Box 20.5 Problems with micturition and urinary symptoms

- *Dribbling*: Occurs with bladder outflow obstruction such as benign prostatic enlargement (BPE) or damage to the pelvic floor (more common in women who have had children)
- *Dysuria*: Pain on passing urine. Often a feature of UTI
- *Enuresis*: Incontinence of urine (see p. 585)
- *Frequency*: The need to pass urine more often than is usual or acceptable for the person. Usually small amounts of urine are passed. Often associated with UTI but can be due to anxiety, bladder outflow obstruction or bladder irritability caused by infection or injury
- *Hesitancy*: A delay in starting to pass urine. Could be a result of bladder outflow obstruction, hypersensitivity or instability
- *Incomplete emptying*: Indicates a failure of the bladder to empty completely; results in acute urinary retention
- *Poor urinary flow*: May be due to bladder outflow obstruction
- *Retention*: Inability to pass urine due to obstruction or bladder failure such as BPE
- *Strangury*: Frequent painful desire to void small amounts of urine, due to muscle spasm associated with irritation or inflammation such as UTI
- *Urgency*: Strong desire to pass urine, which, if not acted upon immediately, may lead to urge incontinence. Associated with detrusor instability or UTI.

CRITICAL THINKING Box 20.6

Variations in urinary volume

Measure your own urine output for 24 hours and calculate how much this is in terms of mL/kg/h.

Student activities

- How close were you to the approximate 1 mL/kg/h?
- Think about the factors that might have influenced the volume on that particular day.
- When you are next helping to care for a person who is having their fluid intake and output measured, calculate how much urine they are producing per kg per hour. Try to do this for a child and an adult.
- Discuss the findings and factors affecting them with your mentor.

Weighing nappies

Accurate measurement of urine volume in babies and young children is more difficult but can be achieved by weighing wet nappies. The known dry weight of the nappy is subtracted from the weight of the nappy after the baby or child has passed urine. The difference in weight in grams approximately corresponds to millilitres of urine voided.

Frequency–volume charts
Frequency–volume charts can be completed by the person or carer at home and brought to the clinic to be assessed. They are particularly helpful in gaining an insight into voiding patterns. The volume of fluid taken in, the urine output, and occasions when the person had an episode of incontinence should all be recorded. Although frequency–volume charts are widely advocated for assessing urinary incontinence (see p. 585), they can focus the person's attention on their urinary symptoms, leading to inaccuracies and additional distress. To minimize this, the charts should be completed for at least 5 days, and when the person is seen again, time should be taken to discuss how they feel about their condition.

Observation of urine and urinalysis

Observation of urine and routine urinalysis by the nurse are both important in the routine screening for abnormalities and possible disease. Any abnormal findings should prompt further urinary analysis by the laboratory, e.g. by sending a midstream specimen of urine (MSU) (see p. 581).

Urine normally contains:

- Water (96%)
- Electrolytes (2%)
- Waste (2%) – urea, creatinine, uric acid, drugs and food residues and small amounts of urobilinogen (note that both a reduction in or excessive amounts of urobilinogen are abnormal).

The urine used for routine testing (urinalysis) should be a fresh 'midstream' sample. This can pose problems for many people who are unable to stop and start their urine and 'catch' the middle part of the flow. People can be assisted in catching the stream by use of a clean funnel. A 'clean catch' sample may the best alternative in babies, small children, some adults with dementia and some people with learning disabilities. Urine samples should not be the first void of the day unless the urine is being tested for renal tuberculosis (TB). Before performing the urinalysis the nurse should always observe the sample for colour, clarity and odour (Table 20.3, pp. 578–579) as these physical characteristics can give valuable clues about potential abnormalities.

Urinalysis using a reagent test strip is a quick and simple test for assessment of renal function, hydration and nutritional state (Fig. 20.6, p. 579). Urine reagent sticks usually test for the following:

- Specific gravity (SG)
- pH
- Protein
- Blood
- Glucose
- Ketones
- Urobilinogen
- Bilirubin.

Some reagent sticks also include a test for nitrites and leucocytes (white blood cells), the presence of which might indicate bacteriuria and UTI, respectively. Since the kidneys excrete waste, the presence of substances not normally excreted, e.g. protein, glucose, can help with diagnosis of renal disease, diabetes mellitus, infection, etc. (see Table 20.3, pp . 578–579).

This test is relatively simple and accurate to use, although nurses should be familiar with the manufacturer's recommendations for use (Box 20.7, p. 580). Care should be exercised to avoid contaminating samples, e.g. from menstrual blood that could give rise to inaccurate results.

Collection of urine samples for the laboratory

When a urine sample is required, the person or parents/carers of children should be advised why that sample is necessary, e.g. to confirm an infection etc. The accuracy of any test and subsequent diagnosis of urinary tract abnormality can be influenced by many factors, e.g. the amount of bacterial contamination when the urine is collected (see Ch. 15).

The options for urine collection from babies and young children are outlined in Box 20.8 (p. 580). In adults, most samples are voided midstream urine (MSU) (Box 20.9, p. 581) or a catheter specimen of urine (CSU) (see Box 20.28, p. 594). In order to identify infection, urine is sent to the laboratory for microscopy, culture and sensitivity (MC&S). The scientist will confirm the presence of microorganisms on microscopy, these will be grown on an appropriate culture medium and sensitivity tests will determine the most effective antibiotic to treat the infection. Urine may also be collected for cytology, looking for abnormal cells, such as cancer cells from the urinary system, that are passed in the urine. Urine samples, often collected over 24 hours, may be analysed for electrolyte levels, protein and various hormones and other chemicals (Box 20.10).

Voided urine specimens are the most acceptable and simplest form of collection for people. A midstream sample is used because it does not contain any debris that may be in the urethra, thus preventing a false result. It is essential for the external urethral meatus to be cleaned before collection of the sample. This helps to reduce the amount of contaminants in the sample.

Common urinary investigations

There are many different investigations used to identify disorders affecting the urinary tract and elimination (Box 20.11, p. 582).

Nursing interventions – micturition

Assisting people with urinary elimination starts with ensuring that adequate hydration has been provided (see Ch. 19). For many people their fluid requirements are

Table 20.3 Normal characteristics of urine and the significance of abnormalities*

Physical and chemical characteristics	Normal findings – observation and urinalysis	Possible significance of abnormal findings
Colour	Pale straw colour to deep amber depending on the concentration	Dark urine may indicate dehydration Blood in the urine (haematuria) can be bright red or can give the urine a smoky appearance Bilirubin turns the urine a brown/green colour or the urine may even be frothy Certain foods or drugs may also influence colour: eating red beet (beetroot) can produce 'pinkish' urine; the drug rifampicin can cause orange/red urine
Clarity (need urine in a clear container)	Usually clear with possible turbidity caused by mucus	Cloudiness or debris can indicate the presence of pus, protein or white cells and would need further investigation
Odour	Freshly voided urine may have a slight aromatic odour but does not usually smell, whereas stale urine can smell of ammonia	A 'fishy' smell would indicate an infection and a 'pear-drop' smell indicates ketones in the urine Certain foods such as asparagus produce a characteristic odour
Specific gravity (SG) – the density of a substance as compared with an equal quantity of distilled water, the latter being represented by 1.000	It is impossible to urinate pure water because the urinary system is 'designed' to remove waste products from the body The normal SG range of urine is 1.001–1.035, depending on the solids contained in the urine, i.e. a high SG indicates a high level of solids Small children tend to have a relatively fixed SG of 1.008 because their renal system is relatively immature and the kidneys are unable to concentrated urine (Kozier et al 2000)	A high SG is found if the urine is concentrated; this may indicate that the person is dehydrated (see Ch. 19) High levels of glucose or other abnormal substances can also result in a high SG Conversely, dilute urine will have a low SG, which occurs normally when the fluid intake is increased, but can occur during a stage of renal failure When assessing SG, the ambient or environmental temperature should be considered; individuals can very quickly become dehydrated in hot conditions
pH	The pH of urine is normally acidic, but within the pH range of 5–8 urine is considered normal Urinary pH is influenced by dietary intake – high meat intake produces acid urine whereas a vegetarian diet produces alkaline urine	Very acidic urine may suggest urinary stone formation, whereas alkaline urine suggests an infection with certain types of bacteria such as *Proteus mirabilis*
Protein	Negative	Normally protein (albumin) molecules are too large to pass through the glomerular filtration barrier, therefore the presence of protein in the urine is abnormal and is called *proteinuria* or *albuminuria* It can indicate glomerular/renal damage, although a urinary tract infection can cause proteinuria Transient proteinuria can occur in children during febrile illnesses or exercise, and would not normally require further investigation, although persistent proteinuria would necessitate a 24-hour urine collection (see p. 581)
Blood	Negative	Blood in the urine (haematuria) is abnormal Haematuria usually indicates problems somewhere in the urinary tract, e.g. cancers, renal damage, stones, or it can be due to causes outside the urinary tract, e.g. as a side-effect of anticoagulant drugs or a blood clotting problem Haematuria can be 'frank', i.e. the urine clearly contains blood, smoky or microscopic It is important to eliminate the possibility that haematuria is due to contamination with menstrual blood In young baby boys, haematuria may be due to crystals forming in the urethra. The haematuria should only be

(Continued)

Table 20.3 (*Continued*)

Physical and chemical characteristics	Normal findings – observation and urinalysis	Possible significance of abnormal findings
		slight and resolve within the first few weeks. Any concerns should be referred to the appropriate health professional
Glucose	Negative	Glucose is not normally present in the urine because in health it is reabsorbed in the nephron (see p. 572) Glucose in the urine is termed *glycosuria* Glycosuria can indicate diabetes mellitus but also can occur during pregnancy, in physiological stress and in people taking corticosteroids Glycosuria can be accompanied by a high urine output, because the glucose molecules draw water with it, resulting in high volume urine output and subsequent dehydration
Ketones	Negative	The presence of ketones in the urine is called *ketonuria* Ketones are acidic chemicals that are formed during the abnormal breakdown of fat in certain situations that include prolonged vomiting, fasting, starvation and poorly controlled diabetes mellitus
Urobilinogen	Small amounts of urobilinogen are normally found in the urine	Elevated levels may indicate liver damage or abnormal breakdown of red blood cells (haemolysis) Urine that contains high levels turns dark when left to stand A reduction or absence occurs in biliary obstruction, i.e. when bile does not reach the intestine
Bilirubin	Negative	The presence of bilirubin can indicate liver disease or biliary obstruction
White blood cells	None	The presence of white cells is associated with UTI, but may indicate more severe renal problems
Nitrites	Negative	A positive test for nitrite is associated with bacteriuria (see p. 576)

Note: All abnormal findings must be reported.

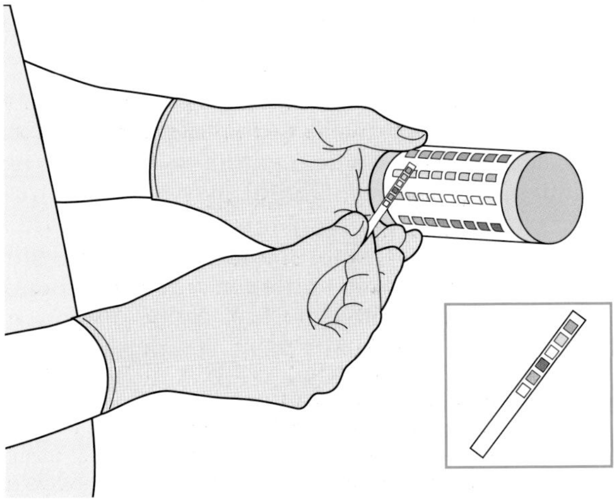

Fig. 20.6 Urine testing (reproduced with permission from Nicol et al 2004)

higher when hospitalized than at home, e.g. people may be sweating, vomiting, have diarrhoea, blood loss, etc., all of which lead to fluid loss from the body.

People may also be weakened by their condition or treatment and may well require assistance in meeting their elimination needs. Many people will feel more comfortable using the lavatory on the ward rather than a urinal, commode or bedpan, and should be escorted or assisted to the lavatory by the nursing staff, to assess their mobility and maintain safety (see Chs 13, 18). For those unable to use the lavatory, a urinal, bedpan, potty or commode will need to be provided. This should be provided quickly and efficiently to limit any embarrassment that the person may have. The nurse should ensure privacy and maintain the person's dignity at all times. The nurse must consider cultural needs, e.g. Hindus and Muslims require that nurses of the same sex meet their intimate care needs (see Ch. 16).

NURSING SKILLS Box 20.7

Testing urine

Equipment

- Lavatory, urinal or bedpan
- Urine in a clean disposable container or a wet nappy
- Reagent test sticks in original container
- Watch with a second hand.

Preparation

Explain what you are going to do and seek verbal consent; maintain respect and dignity at all times. The nurse washes and dries hands and puts on non-sterile gloves, plus plastic apron if assisting the person to collect the sample (see below).

Procedure

- Check the expiry date on the container of reagent strips and make sure that the container has not been left open (to prevent contamination)
- Dip the reagent strip into the urine, so that all the reagents are covered with urine. Remove the test strip from the urine. Remove excess urine by tapping the stick against the inside of the urine container
- Check the time on your watch as accurate timing is imperative
- Wait for the recommended time before reading the test strip against the reference guide on the outside of the container. Remember the results
- Put the used stick in the clinical waste and dispose of the urine safely in the sluice or lavatory
- Discard the disposable container as per local policy
- Remove gloves and wash hands (see Ch. 15)
- Record the results on the nursing observation chart and in the nursing notes. This is an important part of the process of urinalysis because it forms an integral component of holistic care. If any abnormalities are detected, refer to the registered nurse for advice. The registered nurse will discuss the result with the person as appropriate.

Note: Some hospital units or GP centres have automatic urine testing machines. It is essential to gain training in how to use these machines to ensure that accurate results are obtained.

[Further reading: Cook R 1996 Urinalysis: ensuring accurate urine testing. Nursing Standard 10(46):49–54]

Box 20.8 **Collecting urine samples from babies and young children**

Urinary specimens are the main method used to diagnose UTI, but it is particularly difficult to obtain an uncontaminated sample from children, and the reliability of the test is related to the quality of the urine sample collected. The four ways in which to obtain a urine sample in children are:

- A 'bagged' sample obtained by attaching the correct size plastic bag to the perineum
- A 'clean catch'
- A midstream void
- Suprapubic bladder aspiration.

The plastic bag specimen is least favoured because of the high degree of contamination of the sample from the perineum and rectum. For non-emergency urinary specimens the baby or child can be sat over a sterile receptacle and the urine collected and tested. This is referred to as a 'clean catch'. The midstream urine sample is the most reliable but not always possible in young children. Girls must be encouraged to part the labia and in older boys the foreskin should be retracted to prevent contamination.

Suprapubic bladder aspiration is only performed when the sample is needed urgently in children less than 2 years of age. It is an advanced role undertaken by specially trained nurses who have demonstrated competence in this technique.

[Further reading: Huband S, Trigg E 2000 Practices in children's nursing. Churchill Livingstone, Edinburgh, pp. 263–264, 307–308]

Use of urinal, bedpan and commode

Passing urine is usually a private experience and therefore asking people to pass urine in an outpatient department or ward can put them under considerable pressure, especially when they have a longstanding continence problem. The person should be assured that there would be a bedpan/urinal/commode or a lavatory available for them, that they will not be interrupted, and that the nurse will assist them as much as they want, provided that their safety can be maintained.

If the person is unable to walk to or be taken to the lavatory, a commode/bedpan (see Ch. 21) or urinal will be required. Respect and dignity need to be maintained by ensuring the curtains are completely closed round the bed space and the person allowed time to pass urine without interruption. It is also important to ensure that other members of staff and visitors are aware that the person requires privacy.

For males, using a urinal is relatively simple, provided they are able to sit up. Some men find it difficult to pass urine unless they are standing. It may be necessary to help the person position the penis and hold the urinal. Once completed, the urinal should be covered with a paper towel and removed. The person should then be provided with handwashing facilities. Some cultures, e.g. Muslims, wash their genitalia using running water after passing urine or faeces. A jug of water for washing is provided if the person is confined to bed.

The use of a slipper bedpan (Fig. 20.8, p. 583) for women is easier and more comfortable to use, since it can be inserted from the side. If the woman is immobile, assistance with mobilizing will require additional staff and handling aids (see Chs 13, 18).

NURSING SKILLS — Box 20.9

Collecting a midstream specimen of urine

Equipment

- Lavatory, urinal or bedpan
- Sterile specimen pot
- Soap and water
- Paper towels
- Gauze swabs.

Preparation

Explain what you are going to do and seek verbal consent; maintain respect and dignity at all times. The nurse washes and dries hands and puts on non-sterile gloves, plus plastic apron if assisting the person to collect the sample.

Procedure

- The person should clean around the external urethral opening with the warm soapy water. In older boys and adult males, the foreskin (if present) should be retracted, and the glans cleaned with the swab, using each swab once only. In females, the swabs should also be used singly, and the perineal area should be cleaned from front to back (see Ch. 16)
- The person should start to pass urine, directing the middle part of the stream into the sterile pot
- After the sample has been obtained, the person should be offered handwashing facilities
- The specimen should be labelled with the person's details, put into the plastic specimen bag along with the laboratory request form and placed in the specimen fridge ready for transporting to the laboratory (Fig. 20.7, p. 582). If a red-topped specimen bottle is used the specimen can be stored at room temperature until it is taken to the laboratory.
- Finally, the date, time and type of sample taken should be documented in the nursing notes.

NURSING SKILLS — Box 20.10

24-hour urine collection

Equipment

- Lavatory, urinal or bedpan
- Correct container(s) supplied by the laboratory
- Jug and/or funnel
- A sign for the bed or door that alerts staff that all urine is being collected, with start and finish times.

Preparation

- Explain the collection to the person – most people or their carers will take responsibility for managing the 24-hour collection at home. In hospital an ambulant person will often do the collection
- The container is labelled with the person's details before the collection is started
- Ensure that all staff know that the collection is about to start and when it will finish
- Attach sign to the bed or door.

Procedure

- 24-hour collections normally start after the first void of the day and continue for the next 24 hours. It is important that the finish time is planned to coincide with a time when the laboratory is open
- The use of a jug and/or funnel may be needed to transfer urine each time it is passed into the container, which is kept in the sluice. It is important that the person and staff know that if fluid intake and output are being monitored then all urine is measured and recorded before being added to the container
- When the person does the collection the nurse needs to make sure that the person has fully understood and that all urine is collected during the 24 hours
- The person should be encouraged to empty their bladder just prior to the finish time to ensure that the sample represents the whole 24 hours
- If the nurse is collecting the urine, non-sterile gloves and plastic apron are worn
- On completion, the container and the request form are taken to the laboratory
- The date, time and type of sample taken should be documented in the nursing notes
- Staff are informed when the collection is complete and the sign removed.

Tissues/lavatory roll is provided but should not be placed in the bedpan if the person's fluid intake and output is being recorded because this will give an inaccurate result. Used tissue should be placed in a separate receptacle (disposable or a specific bowl that can be sterilized before use); the used tissue is disposed of by flushing it down the sluice. The use of an incontinence pad will catch any urine that accidentally spills from the bedpan, but should on no account be left under the person once they have been assisted off the bedpan because 'inco' pads can contribute to the development of pressure ulcers (see Ch. 25) and are uncomfortable to sit on.

Again, the person should be allowed privacy and time to pass urine. The person is provided with handwashing facilities and the necessary assistance to clean and dry the perianal area to remove urine, which can contribute to the development of pressure ulcers (see Ch. 25).

If the person is able to use a commode, this can often assist with passing urine. For most people, voiding when lying flat is extremely difficult (Box 20.13, p. 583). Using the commode can help the person by returning a degree of 'normality' to passing urine. Before giving the commode to the person, it must be thoroughly cleaned with soap and warm water and carefully dried (see Ch. 15). Attention should be paid to safety, ensuring the bed space is free from obstruction. The wheel brakes on the commode should be in working order and applied to maintain the person's safety. Lavatory tissue must be provided in a separate receptacle for the person to use. In all instances the nurse call bell must be left within easy reach of the

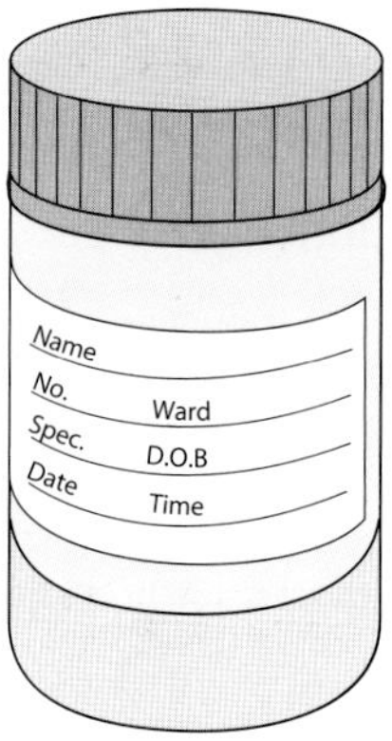

DO NOT WRITE IN THIS SPACE

Dr/Mr	Hospital	Last name	Mr/Mrs/Miss
Specimen		First name	
		Address	
Date		Unit no.	Date of birth
		Patient's label to be attached here and not on copy	
Clinical diagnosis			

Sensitivity to	1	2	3	Sensitivity to	1	2	3
Penicillin				Metronidazole			
Flucloxacilin				Chloramphenicol			
Erythromycin				Gentamicin			
Tetracycline				Aziocillin			
Cefalexin				Cefolaxime			
Ampicillin							
Augmentin							
Nitrofurantoin							

Lab. No.	Date received		Bacteriology

Fig. 20.7 Urine specimen and request form (reproduced with permission from Nicol et al 2004)

person. If a fluid balance chart is being kept, do not assess the volume of urine at the bedside, but make a note of the volume in the sluice room before discarding. The nurse must dispose of gloves and wash their hands before recording the voided volume on the person's chart.

Readers are directed to Nicol et al (2004) for comprehensive information about helping people who require bedpans, urinals or commodes for urinary elimination.

Promoting continence

Incontinence is not uncommon, particularly in women. Although the actual number of women with incontinence is unknown, approximately 6 million women in the UK are estimated to be affected annually by some form of incontinence (The Continence Foundation 2004). It is often preventable, and can be improved in many cases. However, maintaining continence is always the preferred option and nursing care should be individualized to meet the person's needs, in accordance with the *Essence of Care* benchmarking statements (DH 2001). Loss of continence affects all age groups and includes school-aged children, new 'mums', postmenopausal women, older men with prostate problems, etc.

Box 20.11 Common urinary investigations

The following investigations may be used to diagnose or evaluate treatment for disorders of the urinary tract and elimination:

- *Urine tests*: Urinalysis, midstream urine for MC&S, cytology, 24-hour collection for protein, electrolytes, hormones and other chemicals
- *Blood tests*: Full blood count, urea and electrolytes (U&Es), creatinine, prostate specific antigen (PSA)
- *Endoscopy*: Flexible cystoscopy
- *Ultrasound*: Urinary tract (kidneys, ureters and bladder [KUB]), renal ultrasound, post-void residual volume
- *Biopsy*: Renal, bladder (during cystoscopy)
- *X-rays*: Intravenous urogram (IVU), cystogram (or cystourethrogram), angiography
- *Computed tomography* (CT scan)
- *Magnetic resonance imaging* (MRI)
- *Urodynamic tests*: Cystometry, uroflowmetry to evaluate voiding pattern
- *Pad testing* to assess whether urine is voided or assess leaking.

The simple explanation of some these investigations as provided on the BBC website (BBC 2004) will help you provide patient information (Box 20.12); more detailed nursing explanation can be found in Further reading, Cotton et al (2003), Fanning (2003) and Wells (2003).

CRITICAL THINKING Box 20.12

Intravenous urogram

Brian is 22 years old and has a mild learning disability. He lives at home with his parents and his younger sister. Brian has had several UTIs and is to have an intravenous urogram (IVU) in order to identify any abnormalities of his urinary tract.

Student activities

- Find out about what happens before, during and after an IVU.
- Identify the key information needed by Brian so that he is well prepared psychologically and physically for the IVU.
- Consider how to provide Brian with information that meets his needs.
- Find out if there is a learning disabilities liaison nurse in your area.

When assessing the person using a model of nursing, elimination must be included. As discussed above, there are many factors that can affect micturition, but nurses themselves cause some of these. People should feel confident that their request for a commode, urinal or bedpan will be promptly met, or that assistance in

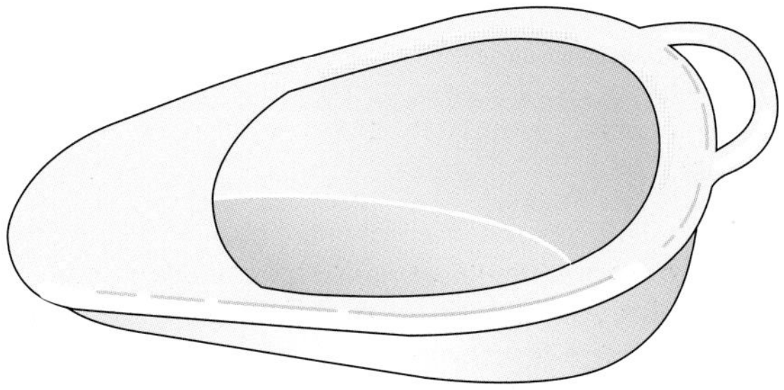

Fig. 20.8 Slipper bedpan (reproduced with permission from Nicol et al 2004)

REFLECTIVE PRACTICE Box 20.13

Position for passing urine

Think about a person you have helped to care for who had difficulty passing urine because of their position or lack of mobility.

Student activities

- What made the position difficult?
- What measures were taken to minimize the problem?

getting to the lavatory will be swiftly provided so that their anxiety about hospitalization is not worsened.

Consideration should also be given to the proximity of the lavatory to the person's bed space, i.e. a person who has difficulty in mobilizing should not be situated at the end of a ward. Accessibility of the lavatory is also important at home. A commode may be used at home if the person is unable to climb stairs to the lavatory. Adaptations to the lavatory, such as a raised seat and handrails, can increase independence and help to maintain continence (see Fig. 21.5).

Making appropriate choices or small changes to clothing can help people to remain continent. For example, a woman with poor manual dexterity may be unable to remove trousers, tights and pants in time but a wrap-around skirt allows her to use the lavatory (Fig. 20.9). The use of Velcro fastenings instead of buttons and zips can also be helpful.

Furthermore, the nurse should consider the effects of medication on elimination. Many drugs can affect the ability to urinate normally, from diuretics ('water tablets') that increase urinary volume and frequency, to analgesics and sedatives that can cause confusion and disorientation (Box 20.14).

Box 20.15 (p. 584) outlines some factors that affect the person's ability to maintain continence. Many of these factors can cause urinary incontinence (involuntary loss of urine).

Normal voiding habits

Essentially there is no 'normal' pattern of voiding; however, there are clearly abnormal patterns. Between the ages of 18 months and 3 years, children become aware

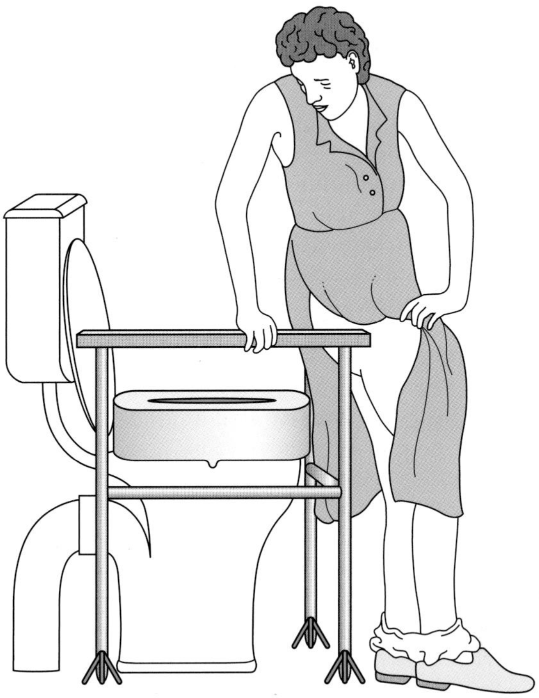

Fig. 20.9 Adaptation of clothing (adapted with permission from Jamieson et al 2002)

REFLECTIVE PRACTICE Box 20.14

Diuretics – maintaining continence

Arrange to talk to a person who takes a loop diuretic such as furosemide (these affect processes in the loop of Henle). This might be a client, friend or relative.

Student activities

- Ask if the person has made any changes to lifestyle or routine since taking a loop diuretic, i.e. a change that helps to maintain continence.
- Think about your own routines. How would they be affected by passing more urine more often? For example, you might think about needing to know the location of all the lavatories in a new placement or regularly having to leave a lecture to pass urine.

of the sensations to pass urine as their nervous system develops (see below). It would still be within the range of 'normal' for children to wet the bed until the age of 5 years. Daytime wetting decreases as the child ages and the majority of children over 5 should be continent during the daytime. Only 1% of girls and 0.8% of boys wet during the day (Cook 1999).

As the child ages, voiding volumes increase, estimated to be:

$$\text{age in years} \times 30 + 30 = \text{volume in mL}$$

until they reach the adult range of around 400 mL every 4–6 hours or so (Cook 1999). The normal voided volume for babies is approximately 60 mL per day, increasing to 500 mL in the first year, and rising steadily to the adult

Box 20.15 Factors affecting ability to maintain continence

- Caffeine in tea, coffee and 'cola' drinks has an excitatory effect on the bladder muscle, causing urgency and frequency, as well as being a diuretic
- Alcohol has sedative and diuretic properties
- Medication side-effects, e.g. diuretics, antipsychotics, anticholinergics, analgesics, sedatives, can affect continence by causing retention of urine, or changes in behaviours that can affect continence. Diuretics – particularly loop diuretics, e.g. furosemide – can cause frequency or urgency, or worsen incontinence
- Older people often take many prescribed medicines (polypharmacy) including diuretics that increase urine volume and therefore can affect continence
- Obesity is associated with stress and urge incontinence (see p. 586)
- Constipation, faecal impaction
- Lack of mobility
- Lack of accessible facilities, e.g. lavatory upstairs
- Inability to remove/undo clothing
- Cognitive impairment such as dementia
- Pregnancy and childbirth (mainly stress incontinence) that may be caused by a hormone imbalance, but usually resolves postnatally (Getliffe & Dolman 2003)
- After the menopause due to oestrogen deficiency causing loss of collagen, and to previous damage to the pelvic floor
- Neurological conditions, e.g. strokes, multiple sclerosis, Parkinson's disease, spinal cord damage, affect the central inhibition of micturition (see pp. 572–574)
- Diabetes causing autonomic nerve damage
- Urinary tract problems – UTI, prostate enlargement, bladder stones, bladder cancer.

NURSING SKILLS Box 20.16

Potty training

- Make sure the potty is in a prominent position so the child notices it and gets to know what it is for
- Try to potty train at the same time every day. If, for example, the child is soiled immediately after mealtimes, start potty training immediately after the meal and suggest they try the potty. If they do not, postpone potty training for a few weeks
- If they void in the potty, praise them (verbally – not by using sweets)
- Eventually the child will ask for the potty. Consider having at least two potties (one downstairs and one upstairs) to help avoid accidents
- Try to instil a toileting regimen, e.g. after meals. This will help in establishing a set routine and overcome problems in encouraging the child to use the potty when they are busy playing
- Finally, encourage the child to wash their hands after each use of the potty.

norm of approximately 1500 mL every 24 hours (Kozier et al 2000).

The main feature, however, is that the amount voided is dependent on the amount of fluid consumed and whether the kidneys are functioning properly. People with voiding problems often reduce their fluid intake, which almost universally worsens the situation by increasing the risk of UTI and reducing the benefits of flushing the urinary system.

Achieving urinary continence during childhood

Continence is achieved by socialization of the child and maturation of the nervous system (which usually occurs between the age of 2 and 3 years) (Rogers 2002).

For a child to develop continence, they must:

- Be aware that they are wetting
- Be getting a sensation to void
- Understand that they must tell someone when they want the potty or to go to the lavatory (this can be quite difficult if the child is enjoying playing or is 'busy' with activities)
- Be able to release the urine when they are using the lavatory (Cook 1999).

Introducing the child to the potty at a time when a routine is often already established, e.g. before a bath at bedtime, can facilitate this learning. The child is encouraged to sit on the potty. It can be helpful to bring a book to read with the child, so that their concentration can be maintained. Once the child has passed urine (or faeces) it is essential to reward them in the form of praise. This helps the child to understand what the potty is for, and that passing urine/faeces in the potty is 'good'. The 'right' time to start potty training depends on each child, but once the child notices that they are wet or soiled is an indication of maturity and therefore a good time to start. Children can control their bowels before their bladders. It may take a long time, many months, before the child notices the desire to void, but a toileting routine will help in establishing some patterns that will promote continence (Box 20.16).

Boys need to learn to stand to pass urine, that it is acceptable to pass urine in front of other males, but not females, and that the whole process is usually conducted behind closed doors. This will take some time; the essential element is not to make this too stressful or put too much pressure on the child since they will not cope with the extra demand. In addition, both boys and girls need to be able to undo buttons or zips, pull down pants or tights, wipe themselves afterwards and flush the lavatory (Rogers 2002).

CRITICAL THINKING Box 20.17

Spina bifida

Spina bifida is a neural tube defect (NTD). During the first few weeks of the pregnancy, folic acid helps to 'build' the vertebrae of the developing fetus. Women who have diets low in folic acid, or whose partners may have spina bifida, need additional folic acid to prevent this condition. The child can be born with a hole or opening in their back, with exposure of the spinal cord where the spinal vertebrae have failed to close.

The defect is surgically closed, but it is only after closure, and as the child develops, that the extent of damage to the spinal cord is noted. Since the nerves that control the bladder (and bowel) connect with the spinal cord, there can be persistent incontinence.

Student activities

- Find out the current advice about folic acid supplements for women planning to become pregnant.
- How long during their pregnancy should women take extra folic acid?

[Resources: Association for Spina Bifida and Hydrocephalus – www.asbah.org Available July 2006]

'Accidents' should be anticipated until the age of 5 years or so. These include episodes when the child is too engrossed in playing, for example, to pay attention to the signals from the bladder, or not sure where the lavatory is located, introduction of a new baby or just starting school.

Enuresis is leakage of urine occurring on regular basis (at least once per week). It is important to check physical causes, such as proximity to a lavatory, as well as physical disabilities that may interfere with manual dexterity or movement.

Nocturnal enuresis is the passing of urine involuntarily at nighttime. Again, for a diagnosis, the child will be older than 5 years and not have any congenital abnormality that may affect the nervous or urinary system, e.g. spina bifida (Box 20.17).

Enuresis is often subdivided into types, which include diurnal enuresis, true or 'giggle' incontinence and functional incontinence (Box 20.18).

Box 20.18 **Enuresis**

The aetiology of enuresis is complex, but includes genetics, bladder structure and function, congenital abnormalities (e.g. spina bifida), UTI and sleep patterns (Lukeman 2003). There is also thought to be a behavioural/emotional component to enuresis. Separation from the family or tension in the family, such as a new sibling, may provoke or maintain enuresis; furthermore, poor self-esteem in the child will exacerbate bedwetting.

Types

- Diurnal enuresis, or day and night wetting, can be caused by lack of attention to the sensation to void
- Nocturnal enuresis is nighttime bedwetting. In some children there is delay in learning to control emptying of the bladder and this may be associated with unusually deep sleep. The problem may be 'primary' or 'persistent' and refers to a scenario when a child has never been dry (Lukeman 2003)
- 'Giggle' incontinence is uncommon, but characterized by complete bladder emptying when the child laughs or giggles, and this can persist into adulthood. There is usually normal function of the bladder and sphincters
- Functional incontinence results from a problem with the urinary sphincter or bladder (or both).

Management

The management of enuresis is aimed at keeping the child dry throughout the day and night, and is often achieved through change in behaviours (Box 20.19, p. 586).

Devices can be used that sense when urine has leaked which then sound an alarm that wakes the child. On waking, the urinary sphincters tend to close, which allows the child to empty their bladder in the lavatory or potty. It can take time for the child to get used to these devices (Cook 1999).

Nurses should support parents or carers by providing information about treatment and support groups (see 'Useful websites', p. 597).

Pelvic floor awareness and exercise

Pelvic floor exercises or Kegel exercises are designed to 'retrain' the pelvic floor muscles after injury/childbirth (Dorey 2003) or after trauma to the bladder after prostate surgery. They are useful in men and women with bladder/continence problems. The exercises involve contracting the pelvic floor to strengthen it, therefore strengthening the muscles that surround the internal and external urinary sphincters (Box 20.20, p. 586).

Use of frequency–volume charts

Frequency–volume charts can assist in the promotion of continence (see p. 577). The chart can be used to prompt the person to attempt to void every couple of hours to prevent 'accidents', then gradually increase the time between voids. This timing would need to be titrated to the fluid input; a high fluid input will result in increased urine output if renal function is normal, so more voids would be required.

Types of urinary incontinence

The major types of incontinence with causes are outlined in Table 20.4 (p. 586) (see also Box 20.18).

Common findings of the effects of incontinence can include isolation and feelings of loneliness, threatening self-image and disrupting usual activities of living.

HEALTH PROMOTION Box 20.19

Behavioural programme for enuresis

As with any behavioural programme, it is essential to establish a baseline from which to compare change. A chart could be used to record episodes of bedwetting and rewards given for goals achieved, e.g. using a potty, or keeping dry overnight.

The child is taught how to sit on the lavatory, with feet flat on the floor to promote a relaxed position that limits abdominal straining. This allows the detrusor muscle to work properly. The child should be encouraged to pass their urine in one go, not to stop and start the flow. Occasionally the child cannot completely empty their bladder. They should be encouraged to pass urine, then wait for a few minutes, and then try again. Fluids are encouraged because reducing fluid intake can lead to infections and dehydration.

Finally it is essential to reward the child, e.g. by making a chart and affixing self-adhesive stars to it, to show how the child is progressing. In addition, positive rewarding, such as simple praise, can also help the child.

[Further reading: Rogers J 2002 Managing daytime and nighttime enuresis. Nursing Standard 16(32):45–52]

HEALTH PROMOTION Box 20.20

Pelvic floor awareness and exercises

The individual should imagine that they are trying to stop passing flatus. They squeeze and lift the muscles around the rectum, holding this contraction for as long as possible (up to 10 seconds). The contraction is then released, and then repeated as often as possible.

This should not be tried when micturating because the detrusor will merely strengthen to overcome the resistance, which will make the incontinence worse.

Pelvic floor exercises require training and therefore referral for specialist advice from the continence nurse specialist. As it can be particularly difficult to exercise the 'correct' muscle group, individuals may need an invasive investigation to assess the strength of the muscles. For men, this will involve the continence nurse specialist inserting a finger into the rectum and assessing muscle tone. For women, there may be assessment of the rectal and/or vaginal muscles.

[Further reading: Getliffe K, Dolman M 2003 Promoting continence: a clinical research resource. Baillière Tindall, Edinburgh]

Table 20.4 Types and causes of incontinence

Type of incontinence	Causes
Enuresis	See Box 20.18 (p. 585)
Stress incontinence – leaking when coughing, laughing, sneezing or during physical activity (increases intra-abdominal pressure)	More common in women and is often associated with damage to the pelvic floor following childbirth Symptoms of stress incontinence worsen with age and are aggravated by obesity Stress incontinence rarely occurs in men, but may occur following prostate surgery
Urge incontinence (overactive bladder/ detrusor instability) – rushing to the lavatory, frequency, leaking urine	More common in women, again in part caused by anatomical changes related to childbirth, but also because of the shorter urethra and weaker pelvic floor, compared to men Neurological conditions Commonest type of incontinence in older people
Voiding difficulties (inefficiency) – incomplete bladder emptying, hesitancy	Commonly occurs in neurological conditions such as stroke, multiple sclerosis, etc. Occurs in women with a prolapse and men with prostatic enlargement
Overflow incontinence – involuntary leak of urine from an overdistended bladder	Occurs in both men and women (less common) Causes include obstruction of the urethra or bladder outlet, e.g. BPE Can occur in women with pelvic prolapse or as a complication of surgery to correct the prolapse Can be caused by underactive detrusor muscle that is associated with conditions such as multiple sclerosis and strokes or as a side-effect of some medicines
Reflex incontinence – incontinence without warning	Can be caused by urethral strictures (narrowing) or an enlarged prostate
Functional incontinence – as an impairment of physical or mental ability	Causes include spina bifida, muscular dystrophy, etc.
Mixed with both urge and stress	Common in postmenopausal women

However, for some, accessing healthcare can be problematic, especially if English is not their first language. Wilkinson (2001) contends that culture, religion and ethnicity can all impact on delivery and access to healthcare for certain groups, recommending a higher profile of continence services, particularly in areas where there is a high immigrant population who may not know how to access healthcare.

Management of urinary incontinence

The aim of management is to promote continence, ideally without surgical means. Simple interventions include the following:

- The first therapy in assisting an individual in becoming continent is to adopt a behavioural programme. Behavioural changes start with the reduction of dietary irritants, e.g. caffeine drinks, and an increase in water intake, i.e. up to 1500 mL per day. People should be encouraged to build up the volume input over time (i.e. weeks), but must drink enough to avoid urine concentration that may predispose to UTI. Additional strategies include drinking less fluid before retiring to bed.
- Pelvic floor exercises (see pp. 585, 586).
- Keeping a voiding diary or charting fluid input/output may help in reminding people to void, thereby achieving regular bladder emptying, resulting in fewer episodes of incontinence.
- Passing urine just before retiring to bed.

Information about other treatment options such as bladder retraining, biofeedback, electrical stimulation, medication, e.g. trospium chloride, solifenacin succinate, duloxetine, etc. and surgery can be found in Further reading suggestions (e.g. Fillingham & Douglas 2004).

Continence nurse specialist

The management of urinary incontinence requires a multidisciplinary approach to care, i.e. specialist continence nurse, doctor (hospital doctor or GP), physiotherapist and pharmacist. An accurate diagnosis of the type of incontinence is essential. A registered practitioner should prescribe pharmacologic management options and a multidisciplinary plan devised for each person.

The specialist nurse will coordinate and manage these approaches, forming longstanding links with the person (Boxes 20.21 and 20.22, p. 588).

REFLECTIVE PRACTICE Box 20.21

Specialist continence services

Think about a person you have met on placement who was unable to achieve continence.

Student activities

- Did the specialist nurse see them?
- If yes, what interventions did the specialist nurse suggest?
- Find out what specialist continence services are available in your area (community and hospital).

[Resources: Shields N, Thomas C, Benson K, Major K, Tree J 1998 Development of a community nurse-led continence service. British Journal of Nursing 7(14):824–826, 828–830; Scottish Intercollegiate Guidelines Network (SIGN) Management of urinary incontinence in primary care (Guideline 79, Dec 2004). Online: www.sign.ac.uk/guidelines/published/index.html Available July 2006]

Continence aids (devices)

When the person, despite every effort, cannot achieve continence, the use of appropriate pads and other devices may be indicated. Devices can either be to contain the urine, e.g. with a pad that absorbs the urine, or devices that carry the urine away from the body, e.g. urinary sheaths (Conveen®) or a pubic pressure urinal, catheters (see pp. 588–592), urological stomas (see p. 596) or implantation of artificial sphincters (Sanders 2002).

Pads

Protective pads to keep clothing or bed linen dry decrease the person's embarrassment, the risk of pressure ulcers (see Ch. 25) and the amount of laundry needed. It is important to select the most suitable pad for the person. A woman who only has stress incontinence when she exercises can often manage with a slim pad worn inside her normal underwear, whereas a person who is incontinent of all urine may need to wear a body pad (similar in shape to a nappy) that will absorb more urine (Fig. 20.10, p. 588).

If pads are worn, particular attention should be paid to skin care. It is better to protect the skin rather than treat sore or damaged skin (Sanders 2002); this is particularly problematic in children. The perianal region is the site most commonly affected, along with the thighs and legs. To limit damage to the skin, personal hygiene should be considered a priority and advice sought from the tissue viability nurse specialist (see Chs 16, 25).

Urinary sheath

A urinary sheath (also called external catheter or condom catheter) is a sleeve of latex or silicone that fits over the penis and is attached to a night drainage or, preferably, a leg drainage bag to aid mobility. They can remain on the penis for between 24 and 48 hours and are used to promote continence where the use of pads is unwanted.

The urinary sheath is similar to a condom except that there is a short tube on the tip that allows urine to escape (Fig. 20.11, p. 588). Like most devices, urinary sheaths come in varying sizes (based on the diameter of the flaccid penis) and it is essential that the correct size be used to allow some natural movement in the penis, but not too loose that the sheath becomes detached or leaks urine (Box 20.23, p. 589). Most manufacturers of sheaths provide a 'size' guide to assist in correct selection of the sheath. There are various types of sheath available: self-adhesive or ones where there is a separate adhesive, some come with an applicator, whereas others depend on correct positioning manually, but they do not suit all men. Commonly reported problems include leakage, detachment or sore skin, due to the adhesive damaging the skin on the shaft of the penis, or constant irritation of the skin due to prolonged contact with urine (Sander 1999).

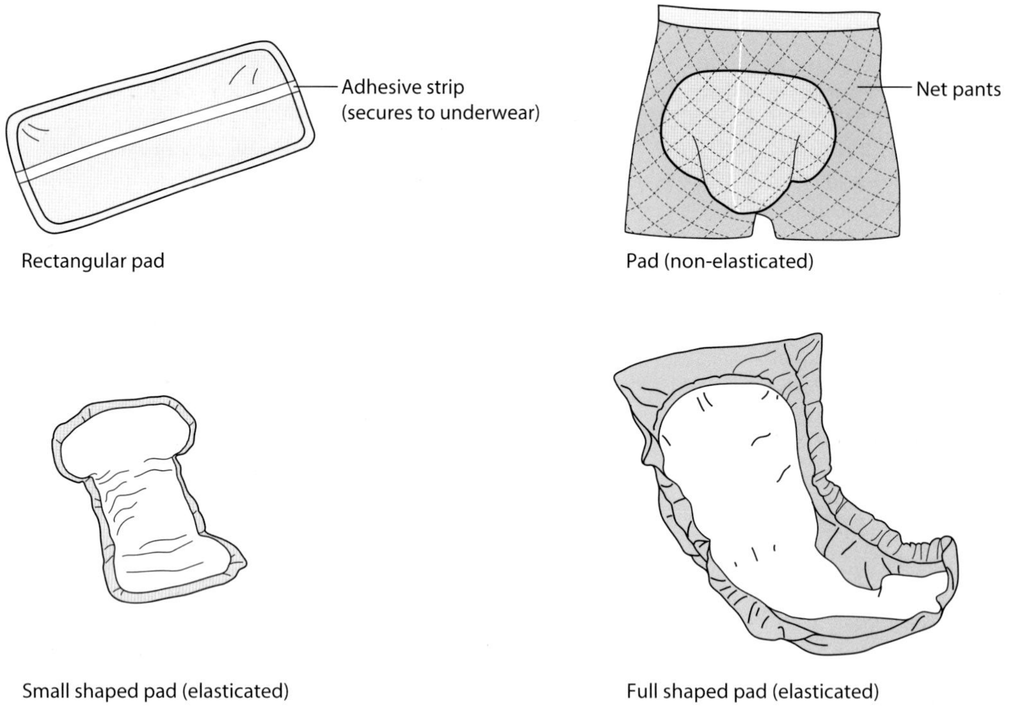

Fig. 20.10 Disposable pads

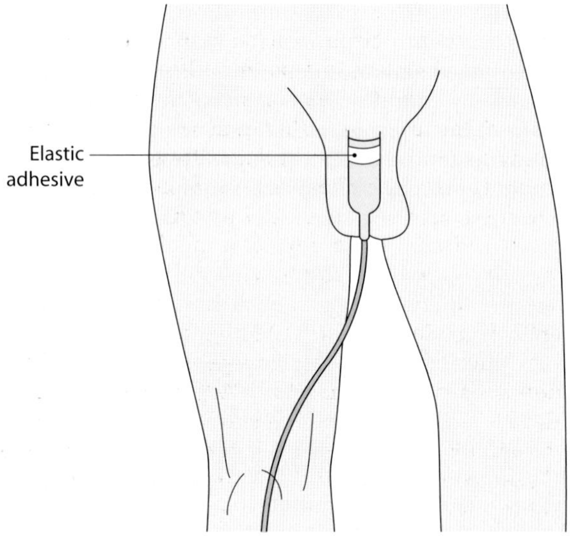

Fig. 20.11 Urinary sheath (reproduced with permission from Nicol et al 2004)

> **CRITICAL THINKING** Box 20.22
>
> **Mrs Begum**
>
> Mrs Begum is a 65-year-old Muslim woman who has had five children. She attends the outpatient clinic and gives a history of incontinence when she coughs or sneezes and when she holds on to her urine for too long. This has been getting worse for several years, and she admits to staying at home rather than risk incontinence. She is extremely embarrassed. Her relationship with her husband has also deteriorated.
>
> **Student activities**
>
> - What type of incontinence do you think Mrs Begum has?
> - What practical interventions might be helpful for Mrs Begum?
> - What are the likely tests and investigations that she may need to undergo?
> - What other issues may there be for Mrs Begum? Consider the modesty issues/need for interpreter/female staff/special hygiene requirement? She will need to pray five times a day and may choose to fast during Ramadan (see Ch. 19). Will this affect her ability to try behavioural changes?
> - Which members of the multidisciplinary team will support her?

Care of people with a urinary catheter

Catheterization is common and all nurses will care for a person who has a catheter. Therefore this section will deal, in some depth, with the care involved. There are many reasons why a person would require catheterization, but the most common are:

- Relieve retention of urine
- Determine residual volume of urine
- Accurate measurement of urine output in critically ill people
- Bypass obstruction
- Introduce drugs, e.g. cytotoxic drugs
- Enable bladder function tests to be performed, e.g. urodynamics

NURSING SKILLS Box 20.23

Application of a urinary sheath

Equipment
- Penile sheath with adhesive
- Measuring disc
- Catheter bag (night drainage or a leg bag)
- Warm water, soap, disposable cloth and towel.

Preparation

Explain what you are going to do and seek verbal consent; maintain respect and dignity at all times. The nurse washes and dries hands, then puts on non-sterile gloves and plastic apron.

All equipment should be taken to the bedside. Curtains must be drawn to maintain dignity. Assist the man into a sitting position.

Procedure
- The penis (including the glans penis) must be socially clean before the sheath is applied. Avoid using creams, sprays or powder on the penis since this may affect adhesion of the device. The man should retract his foreskin and wash the glans penis, then, moving from the end of the penis to his body, clean the shaft of the penis. The foreskin should be returned to its normal position after washing. If he is unable to meet his own penile hygiene needs, the nurse will need to assist. Pubic hair needs to be away from the site of attachment and may need to be trimmed so that the hair does not interfere with the adhesive
- Using the size guide provided, assess the diameter of the penis. This will ensure that the correct size of sheath is used. The correct size is important to avoid problems with leaking and skin irritation
- To apply the sheath, hold the penis and roll the sheath down the shaft of the penis. Some sheaths come with applicators which should be used
- At the base of the penis, the sheath should be secured. This depends on the type of sheath. If it is a self-adhesive type, make sure that you secure the device to the base of the penis. If it is a 'two-piece' type, apply the adhesive approximately 1–2 cm from the base of the penis, making sure that the adhesive is not too tight, then roll the sheath onto the adhesive
- The sheath should be attached to a leg bag during the day (to promote mobility) and a night drainage bag overnight, making sure that the tube does not become twisted
- Once the sheath is attached, make sure that the man is comfortable and that his dignity is maintained by replacing loose clothing or bedding
- Dispose of any clinical material in the clinical waste bins, remove gloves and wash and dry your hands, then document your actions in the nursing notes
- A care plan should be prepared to ensure that signs of infection, irritation, pain, discomfort or failure of the device are noted immediately. The sheath should be checked twice a day, but must be removed after 24–48 hours.

Box 20.24 **Intermittent self-catheterization**

The person or their carer passes a catheter into the bladder to drain residual urine, preventing damage to the bladder by overstretching (distension), reducing infection and minimizing incontinence (Barton 2000). ISC can be used for people with, for example, multiple sclerosis, spina bifida or spinal injury.

ISC can enhance independence, since there are no obvious signs of a urinary catheter and the person can 'control' when they void (of great benefit to children and adults who wish to remain active), but the major advantage of ISC from a clinical perspective is that the incidence of UTI is reduced compared to indwelling urethral catheters. Additional benefits of ISC (for adults) include maintenance of sexual activity (Naish 2003).

The frequency of ISC is dependent on the person's needs, although it is important that the amount of urine drained from the bladder does not exceed 400–500 mL because this can cause nerve damage from overstretching (Barton 2000).

- Allow irrigation of the bladder
- Management of incontinence as a last resort.

The introduction of infection (see p. 576), thereby causing harm to the person, is a potentially serious problem that can occur whenever a person is catheterized. For these reasons, catheterization should never be undertaken without consideration of the potential risks and alternatives to catheterization. The most common cause of hospital-acquired infections in the urinary tract is urethral instrumentation and catheterization. The incidence of UTIs in people with indwelling catheters is directly related to the duration of catheterization (Sedor & Mulholland 1999), with an average daily rate of infection of 4% for men and 10% for women; the calculated chance of remaining free of infection is only 50% (Schaeffer 2002). Hospital-acquired UTI leads to prolonged hospital stay and increased treatment costs. Once the catheter is in the bladder, the person should be encouraged to drink as much as they can, if possible more than 2 L per day. This will help to 'flush' the urinary tract and limit the chances of UTI.

Catheters are hollow tubes that are usually inserted through the urethra into the urinary bladder, and are normally used to let urine drain from the bladder as part of medical treatment or instilling fluids (Pomfret 1996).

Occasionally a catheter will be inserted suprapubically through an artificial tract in the abdomen, above the pubic bone, into the top of the bladder. For some people, particularly those with an enlarged prostate gland or urethral stricture (narrowing), suprapubic catheterization may be the preferred option for draining urine from the bladder. The insertion of a suprapubic catheter tends to be completed by medical staff, although some senior nurses have been trained in this procedure.

Clean intermittent self-catheterization (ISC) is another method of draining urine from the bladder (Box 20.24).

NURSING SKILLS Box 20.25

Female catheterization

Equipment

- Catheterization pack
- Sterile local anaesthetic (6 mL)
- 1 pair of sterile gloves, 1 pair of non-sterile gloves
- Sachet of sodium chloride 0.9% (normal saline) for cleansing
- A good light source
- A clinical waste bag
- A sterile 10 mL syringe and 10 mL sterile water for injection
- Two catheters (in case one becomes contaminated) of the correct size and for the correct duration of use
- Catheter bag and catheter bag stand
- Absorbent sheet
- Plastic apron.

Preparation

Explain what you are going to do and seek verbal consent; maintain respect and dignity at all times. Ask the woman to wash and dry genitalia, assist as necessary. The nurse washes and dries hands.

Procedure

- Assist the woman into a recumbent (lying down on her back) position
- Place the absorbent sheet underneath the woman's buttocks. This will help to protect the bedding and therefore avoid unnecessary moving of the woman
- Wash hands and, using aseptic technique (see Ch. 15), open the sterile catheterization pack, remove the sterile drape and put the normal saline in the sterile pot inside the pack
- Cover the woman with the sterile drape that is found in the catheterization pack
- Put on non-sterile gloves and apron. The woman should bend her knees and open (abduct) her hips to allow thorough cleaning of the vulval area with normal saline. The vulva should be cleaned from the labia minora then the vestibule (and wiped from front to back). Dispose of gauze swabs used to clean the vulva into the contaminated waste bag
- Apply the local anaesthetic to the urethra and wait 3–5 minutes, allowing the anaesthetic time to work
- Remove non-sterile gloves, wash hands or use alcohol hand-rub
- Open all sterile equipment onto sterile field. Draw up the 10 mL of water into the syringe. Open the sterile catheter bag. Remove the catheter from the outer packet. Note that catheters come with two covers; the outer cover should be discarded. Put on sterile gloves (see Ch. 15)
- Open the catheter along the perforations, making sure that you do not touch the catheter itself. Using your non-dominant hand, part the labia minora using a piece of sterile gauze or your gloved fingers (Fig. 20.12)
- Insert the tip of the catheter into the urethral opening. Gently continue to insert the catheter into the urethra. This is a difficult skill and will need practice. Do not touch the catheter, but as the catheter goes into the urethra, remove the outer sterile covering of the catheter (see Fig. 20.12)
- The catheter should be inserted to the fullest extent, i.e. the 'y' junction. Urine should flow from the catheter. This can be collected in the kidney tray that is in the catheterization pack
- Once the catheter is fully in, inflate the balloon using the sterile syringe and inflation port (Fig. 20.13)
- Once inflated, gently pull the catheter back until resistance is felt. This confirms that that catheter is in the correct place
- Attach the catheter bag to the catheter, then to the catheter stand
- Clear away all equipment and make sure that the woman is comfortable
- Consider obtaining a urine sample from the collection port
- Record the insertion date, size of the catheter and balloon volume, reason for catheterization and amount of anaesthetic used in the medical and nursing notes. Make sure that the catheter does not remain in the bladder for longer than the recommended time.

[Resource: British Association of Urological Nurses – www.baun.co.uk Available July 2006]

In general, catheterization is an aseptic technique (see Ch. 15) although ISC may be a clean procedure. Catheterization of females is a basic nursing skill. Before nurses can perform female catheterization they must have training and supervised practice and be assessed as competent. Once assessed as competent, then female catheterization can be performed as a student nurse (Box 20.25). Male urethral catheterization is a skill that requires further training after registration. This is due to the potential harm, i.e. damage to the urethra or prostate gland, that can occur when catheterizing a male.

Types of catheter

Selection of the catheter needs to be based on the indications for catheterization and the length of time it will be in situ – this will determine whether an intermittent, short- or long-term self-retaining catheter will be used. Self-retaining Foley catheters have a balloon at the end of the catheter that is inflated after it has been inserted (Fig. 20.14). The balloon stops the catheter from falling out.

The types of catheter and their uses are:

- *Intermittent*: Balloon-less, very small and used for insertion of drugs or to release urine stored in the bladder
- *Short-term self-retaining*: Typically used in hospital for assessment of postoperative urine output
- *Long-term self-retaining*: Used for people who need to have a catheter in situ for more than 2 weeks.

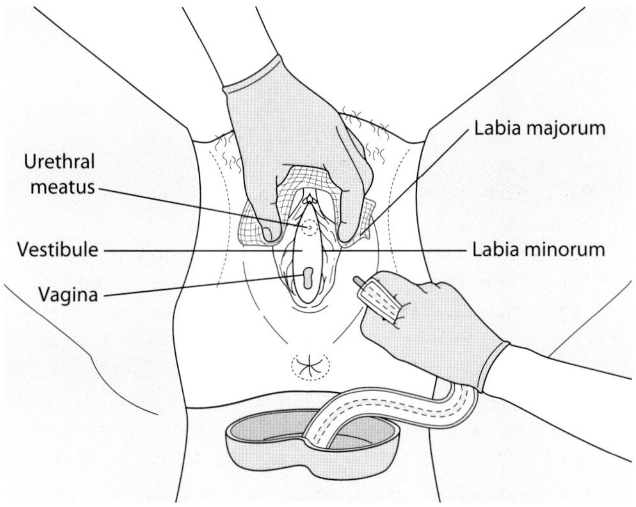

Fig. 20.12 Female catheterization (reproduced with permission from Nicol et al 2004)

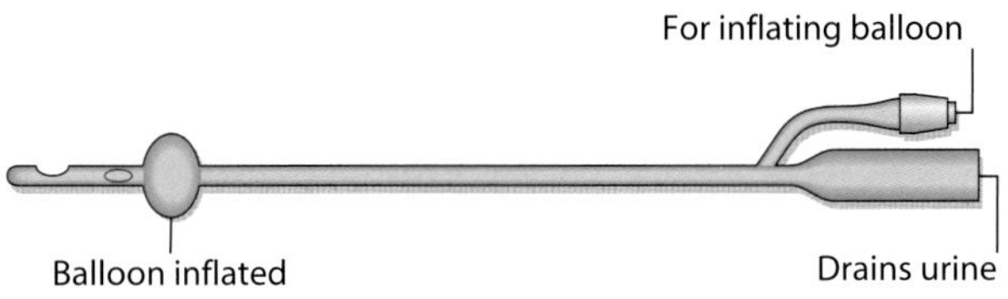

Fig. 20.14 Self-retaining catheter (double-lumen Foley)

Box 20.26 Catheter length

- Female: 23–26 cm
- Standard, more commonly known as male length: 40–44 cm.

[From Robinson (2001)]

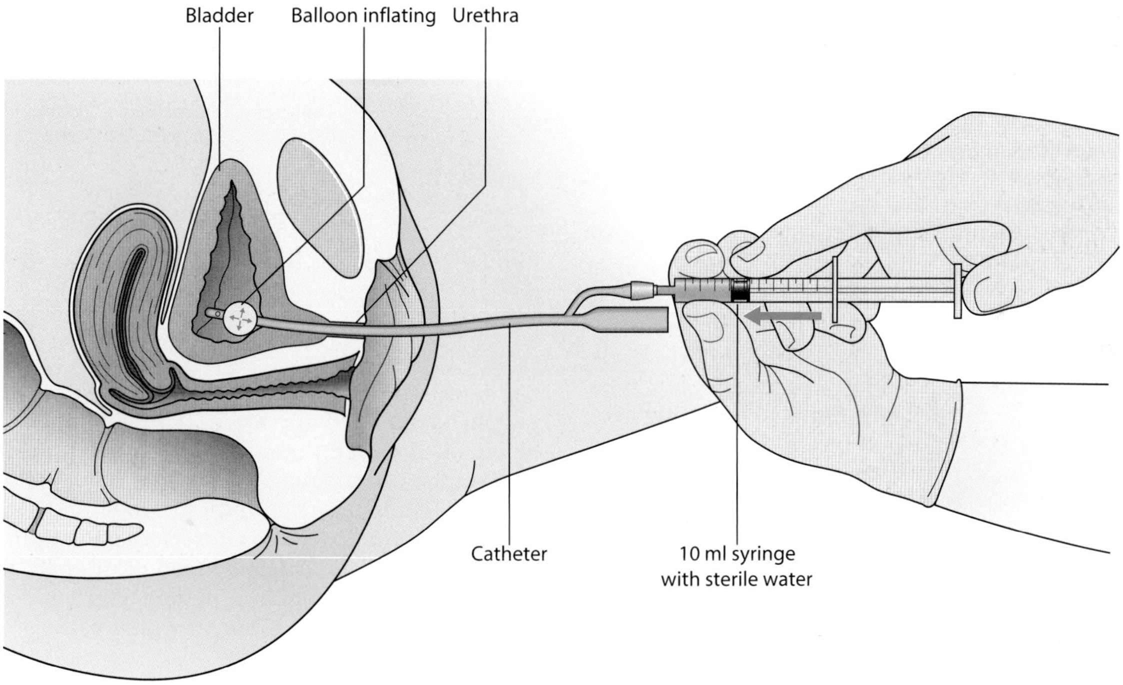

Fig. 20.13 Inflating the catheter balloon

Catheter length

Catheters come in different lengths for men and women (Box 20.26). The 'male' length catheter is almost twice as long as the 'female' length catheter. No attempt should be made to insert a female length catheter into a male.

Catheter materials

The length of time that a catheter can remain in situ is dependent on the material that it is made from (Table 20.5, p. 592).

The 'short-term' catheters easily become encrusted or coated with the debris from the urine in the bladder. Longer-term catheters, e.g. the silicone- or hydrogel-coated catheters, tend to encrust at much slower rates than short-term catheters, and are therefore used in people who need a catheter in situ for more than 2 weeks.

Catheter lumen size

Each type of catheter is produced in different sizes. The size of the internal diameter is measured in Charrière scale (Ch) or French Gauge (FG). One Ch or FG equals 0.3 mm, so a 12Ch catheter is approximately 4 mm in diameter. The important point here is that the larger the Ch/FG size, the more the urethra will be dilated or stretched when a catheter is in situ.

Table 20.5 Types of catheter

Length of use	Catheter material
Short term (0–14 days)	Polyvinyl chloride (PVC) Latex – check for allergies (both person and staff)
Short term (0–4 weeks)	Polytetrafluoroethylene (PTFE)-coated latex
Long term (0–12 weeks)	Silicone-coated latex Hydrogel-coated latex 100% silicone

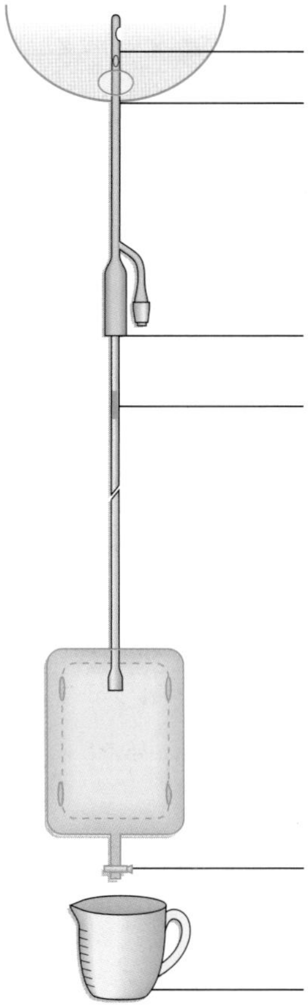

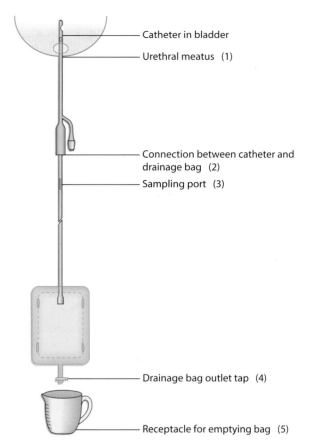

Fig. 20.15 Closed drainage system showing potential entry points (1–5) for pathogenic microorganisms

The 'golden rule' for catheterization is always to select the smallest size catheter to do the job. Examples include:

- For retention of urine, a catheter between Ch/FG 10–12 is used for women, and 12–14 for men
- If haematuria is evident, a large bore catheter or an irrigation catheter will be required, at a size of Ch/FG 18–30
- For infants and children, a size Ch/FG 6–8 would normally be used, but again depends on the reason for catheterization and the age and size of the child.

Balloon size

A self-retaining catheter will come with instructions of how much to inflate the balloon once it is in situ. It is normally inflated with 10 mL of sterile water, but there is a chance that, over time, some of this fluid will leech out. The importance of filling the balloon with the correct volume is that the drainage ports in the catheter should be level; underfilling of the balloon results in a leaning over of the catheter tip, preventing drainage.

Overfilling the balloon can worsen detrusor instability or cause urine to bypass. In addition, the added volume will put pressure onto the bladder neck that can result in necrosis of the bladder neck and incontinence.

Drainage systems

The selection of a closed drainage system should be on an individual basis, but the main consideration should be whether the person is mobile or not. Leg bags are available in 350, 500 and 700 mL sizes. Women usually wear the leg bags on their thigh and men usually wear their leg bags around their calf region. The bags are secured with Velcro tapes or leg straps. Irrespective of leg bag size or location used, it is important to make sure the tubing does not become kinked, because this will prevent drainage. Dragging on the catheter, which can cause injury to the urethra and external urethral opening, must be avoided by securing the bag.

If a person is mobile they should not be encumbered by carrying a catheter bag round with them. This limits their ability to mobilize safely because they are carrying the catheter bag (see Chs 13, 18). A leg bag *must* be used. This allows the person to have both hands free to assist them with mobility. It also confers dignity since a leg bag is relatively discrete. Immobile or non-ambulatory people would normally use a 2 L 'night-bag', which must be attached directly to a catheter stand to prevent dragging on the urethra and cross-infection from the floor.

All catheter drainage bags are a 'closed system' and should be carefully looked after in order to minimize infection. Each time the bag is opened or drained, the potential for infection increases. Figure 20.15 illustrates the points in the 'closed system' at which pathogenic microorganisms can gain entry.

If the person is using a 2 L drainage bag at night, they could use a 500 mL drainage bag during the day. The 2 L night bag is capped using a sterile spigot (bung) and not allowed to touch the floor as this is a potential source of infection. At all times the urine bag should be kept below the level of the bladder to prevent urine from tracking back into the bladder and causing infection. Although the catheter bags have one-way filters to prevent backflow of urine, they should be changed weekly (Drug Tariff 2003) to prevent harbouring bacteria that could cause UTI. The simplest way to ensure that this is completed is to put the date that the bag was opened on the drainage bag and record the date in the nursing notes; alternatively, the date that the bag needs to be changed can be recorded on the bag itself. Essentially, the most important aspect is that the bag is changed once per week if the individual is in hospital.

NURSING SKILLS Box 20.27

Emptying the catheter bag

Equipment

- Disposable measuring jug or a sterile jug that is used *only* once
- Cover or paper towel
- Alcohol swab.

Preparation

Explain what you are going to do and seek verbal consent; maintain respect and dignity at all times. The nurse washes and dries hands, then puts on non-sterile gloves and plastic apron.

Procedure

All equipment should be taken to the bedside. If the drainage bag is a 2 L bag, then it should already be attached to a catheter bag stand. The bag will not need to be removed.

- Hold the bag over the disposable jug, making sure the drainage port does not touch the jug. Open the drainage port and allow the urine to flow into the jug. Do not let the jug become more than three-quarters full to minimize the risk of spillage (Fig. 20.16)
- When the urine bag is empty, wipe the drainage port with the alcohol swab to stop urine from dropping onto the floor
- Reposition the catheter bag, making sure that the catheter tube has not become kinked or tangled
- The jug should then be covered and taken to the sluice. The amount of urine should be measured then disposed of in the sluice. According to local policy the disposable jug is discarded and a non-disposable jug is resterilized by the sterile supplies department
- Gloves and aprons are removed and the hands thoroughly cleaned and dried before attending to the next person
- Fluid balance charts are completed as necessary.

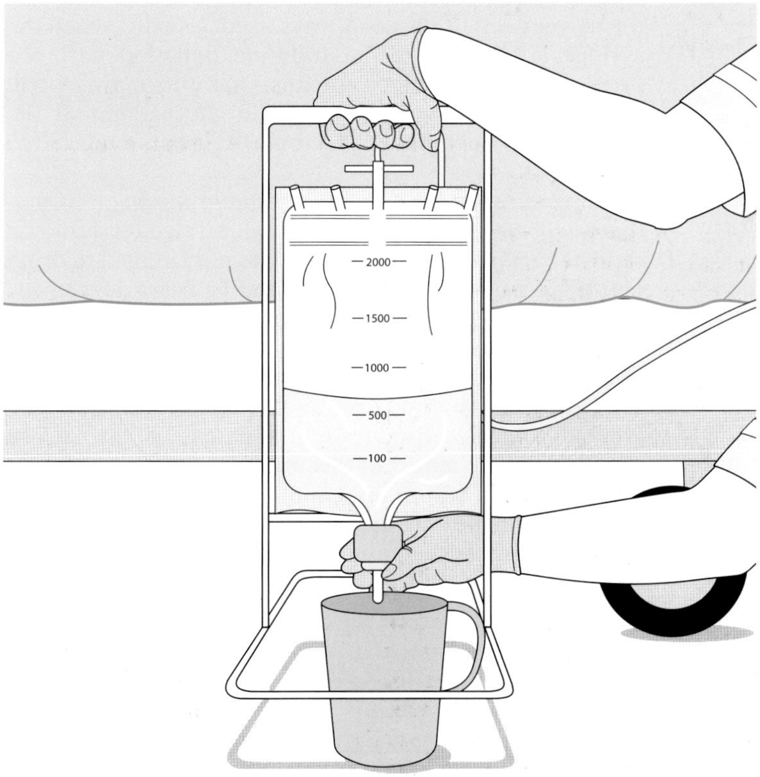

Fig. 20.16 Emptying the catheter bag (reproduced with permission from Nicol et al 2004)

As emptying the drainage bag breaches the 'closed' system and increases the infection risk, it must be done carefully (Box 20.27).

Collecting a catheter specimen of urine

A catheter specimen of urine (CSU) for bacteriological investigation is obtained from the sampling port on the drainage tubing using a sterile syringe (Box 20.28, p. 594).

Catheter hygiene

Urinary tract infection is almost inevitable with a catheter in situ (Penfold 1999). This is because the normal protective measures, e.g. closed urethra, are bypassed. To limit the chance of infection, twice daily catheter care should be completed, e.g. during personal hygiene in the morning and before going to bed. The person who is able

NURSING SKILLS Box 20.28

Collecting a catheter specimen of urine

Equipment
- 10 mL sterile syringe
- Sterile specimen container with screw-top lid
- Alcohol swab.

Preparation
Explain what you are going to do and seek verbal consent; maintain respect and dignity at all times. The nurse washes and dries hands, then puts on non-sterile gloves and plastic apron.

Procedure
- Draw the curtains round the bed space to maintain the person's privacy
- Expose the section of the catheter bag tubing with the sampling port. Swab the port with the alcohol swab and wait 30 seconds for the alcohol to dry. If there is no urine in the tubing, the catheter bag tube can be clamped to allow collection of urine
- Insert the syringe into the port; if a needle is used, make sure it does not perforate the catheter tubing. Withdraw approximately 10 mL of urine from the catheter tubing. Remove the syringe. Unscrew the sterile specimen container and transfer the contents of the syringe into the container slowly to prevent spillage. Screw the top back onto the container, and then write the person's details on the container. Replace bedding before opening the curtains
- Take the specimen to the sluice; remove gloves and wash hands before putting the sample into a plastic specimen bag. The specimen should be placed in the specimen fridge, along with the laboratory request form ready for transport to the laboratory as soon as possible. If a red-topped specimen bottle is used the specimen can be stored at room temperature until it is taken to the laboratory
- Finally, the date, time and type of sample taken should be documented in the nursing notes.

to use their hands and see the catheter can be taught to carry out their own catheter care.

Warm soapy water should be used to clean around the catheter where it enters the urethra. In uncircumcised males, this also involves retracting the foreskin, cleaning the glans penis and replacing the foreskin. This should be completed at least twice per day, thus preventing encrustation around the urethral meatus and removing a potential source of infection. If the person wants a bath it is important to ensure that all wounds have completely healed so that infection is not introduced or spread. In someone with a long-term catheter who wants a bath, the catheter must be disconnected from the catheter bag and a spigot used to prevent water from entering the catheter, or urine exiting the catheter when the person is in the bath. After the bath, the catheter spigot can be removed and the catheter bag reattached. It is important to ensure that the catheter bag does not touch the floor while the person is having their bath as this would allow bacteria to enter the bag and become a potential cause of infection.

The principles of care of a person with a catheter in situ are summarized in Box 20.29.

Removal of a self-retaining catheter

A registered nurse or doctor will decide on the removal of a self-retaining catheter. They will also decide if a catheter specimen of urine is required. If a specimen is required, collect a CSU before removing the catheter. The technique for removal is clean rather than aseptic but sterile syringes must be used. As with all procedures, the nurse must wash their hands and prepare their equipment before attempting the procedure.

All catheters should have the balloon deflated before removing the catheter, using a sterile 10 mL syringe for short-term self-retaining catheters or three sterile 10 mL syringes for long-term self-retaining catheters. It is essential to check the medical/nursing notes to see how much water was used to inflate the balloon. Although the catheter itself indicates how much water should be inserted, the correct amount is not always used. Usually, when the syringe is attached to the inflation/deflation port, the pressure in the balloon means that the syringe will automatically fill with the fluid in the balloon. If the balloon does not deflate then report this to the registered nurse.

Depending on how long the catheter has been in situ, there will be a period of time before bladder function returns to normal. People should be encouraged to drink plenty (2–3 L) of fluid per day and to use a measuring jug to check how much urine has been voided at each attempt. Although the amount of urine voided varies according to age, adults should not be discharged home until they are voiding a minimum of 150 mL. The catheter can cause localized trauma or damage to the urethra and bladder. The effect of this trauma can be haematuria, but this should be minimal and resolve after a few days. People should be encouraged to seek advice from a nurse or doctor if they have any deterioration in their urinary function or if haematuria persists for more than a couple of days.

Sexual activity and urethral catheterization

There is no reason why people should abstain from sexual activity if they have a catheter in situ. The key point is that sexual activity does not have to end if one partner has been catheterized. As people will not be sure how to broach this issue with the nurses caring for them, the registered nurse should adopt a proactive approach. A simple statement such as, 'Some people feel their sex lives change once they are catheterized, but this does not need to be the case. If you would like to discuss this, let me know and I can go through the options with you', can help in broaching the subject, although any discussion should be with your mentor initially (Box 20.30).

Box 20.29 **Care of a person with a catheter in situ**

Problem

A catheter is in situ for . . . . reason.

Goal

To reduce the risk of infection, blockage (i.e. urine not flowing, low abdominal pain, spraying of urine from the urethra), trauma and discomfort.

Nursing actions

- Record urine output and perform dipstick urinalysis a minimum of once per week. Ensure that urine output is greater than 0.5 mL/kg/h. If there are any positive indicators on urinalysis, such as blood, protein, leucocytes, nitrites, etc., a catheter specimen of urine should be sent for MC&S if it is a short-term catheter. If long-term, refer to the district nurse/GP
- Encourage fluid intake of between 2 and 3 L per day. If oral fluids cannot be taken, or are taken in insufficient quantity, consider other routes (see Ch. 19)
- Check temperature, pulse, BP and respiratory rate as condition dictates (for those in hospital)
- Observe for signs of infection, i.e. pyrexia, but also sepsis, i.e. hypotension, increase in pulse and respiratory rates, and pyrexia. Smelly, cloudy or bloody urine will indicate an infection. Advice should be sought from the senior nurse/doctor immediately
- Catheter care must be performed twice a day with warm soapy water
- Encourage the use of leg bags during the day to promote mobility
- Only empty the catheter bag when three-quarters full, unless the person is having a shower/bath
- Keep the urine drainage bag below the level of the bladder. Use a stand to ensure that the drainage tap does not touch the floor
- Encourage a high fibre diet to minimize constipation; administer prescribed aperients where necessary. Impacted faeces can block the outflow of urine, causing urinary retention
- Perform bladder washouts if the catheter is bypassing (Nicol et al 2004). The catheter may need to be changed
- If the person is going home with a catheter in situ, ensure that the catheter is a long-term catheter and provide a district nurse referral after assessing the person's/carer's ability to self-care. Educate the person about the importance of handwashing before and after catheter care or emptying or changing the bag
- Arrangements for emergency changes of the catheter should be prearranged via the district nursing team/GP, or the local policy may be to refer directly to the local Emergency Department
- With regards to sexual activity, drainage bags should be capped off. Men can use a condom to secure the catheter along the underside of the penis. Women can tape the catheter to the abdomen (see Box 20.30).

[Further reading: Atkinson K 1997 Incorporating sexual health into catheter care. Professional Nurse 13(3):146–148; Getliffe K 1995 Care of urinary catheters. Nursing Standard 11(11):47–50; Penfold P 1999 UTI in patients with urethral catheters. British Journal of Nursing 8(6):362–374]

REFLECTIVE PRACTICE Box 20.30

Discussing sexuality

Discussing sexuality with people can be anxiety provoking for nurses – but consider their journey. For example, they might be anxious about loss of continence, undergoing invasive tests and then being 'saddled' with a urethral catheter. This is likely to have profound effects on their relationship with their partner.

Student activities

- Is discussing the issue of sexuality really so difficult?
- Why do nurses feel anxious about talking to people about sexuality?
- Talk to your mentor about who you could ask for advice about broaching this subject, e.g. specialist nurses in erectile dysfunction, continence specialist nurses.

[Resource: Milligan F 1999 Male sexuality and urethral catheterisation: a review of the literature. Nursing Standard 13(38):43–47]

Table 20.6 Complications of catheterization

Complication	Cause	Solution
Infection	Incorrect insertion, size, poor technique	Only undertake catheterization when assessed as competent Use strict aseptic technique Observe the urine for signs of infection Change the catheter in accordance with manufacturer's instructions Change the catheter bag weekly, or more frequently if the person's condition dictates
Pain	Detrusor spasm due to irritation; irritation to urethra/external meatus	Ensure the correct size catheter is used – large catheters will cause more pain Make sure the catheter has not been in too long Provide analgesia as prescribed and note efficacy Medication to reduce detrusor spasm, e.g. oxybutynin Local anaesthetic gel may be applied on the glans or external urethral meatus to reduce irritation
Blockage	Debris, e.g. blood clots, bladder tissue; catheter tubing may be kinked or the catheter bag blocked	Ensure that the catheter or drainage tube is not twisted or caught up with any equipment Make sure the catheter has not been in too long Observe the urine for blood or debris The catheter may need to be 'flushed' or a bladder washout performed If these measures fail, the catheter will need to be changed
Bypassing	Detrusor instability	Make sure the catheter has not been in too long If possible, put in a smaller size catheter Detrusor muscle relaxants, e.g. oxybutynin
Urethral strictures	Damage to the urethra	Medical management or either surgery or dilatation of the urethra, followed by a period of intermittent self-catheterization to keep the urethra open
Trauma to urethra	Can occur when the catheter and catheter bag are not secured properly Causes tension on the catheter by weight of urine in the bag, resulting in damage to the bladder, urethra and external urethral meatus	Ensure that the catheter is correctly secured to either a catheter bag stand or the person's leg
Encrustation	Leaving the catheter in the urinary bladder for longer than the manufacturer's instructions	Change catheter as per manufacturer's instructions; see also Table 20.5

Complications of catheterization

The complications of catheterization are outlined in Table 20.6.

Urinary stomas

Urinary stomas are openings in the skin that drain urine from the urinary system. Some people may have had their bladders removed (cystectomy) or find that the bladder muscle does not work, resulting in potential harm to the kidneys. For these people the urine needs to be diverted, or a passageway (conduit) formed, to help drain the urine from the urinary system. The main reasons for urinary diversion include cancers in the urinary system, congenital abnormalities, e.g. spina bifida, and complete bladder failure.

There are many different ways in which urine can be diverted from the bladder; collectively they are called urostomies (see Further reading, e.g. Fillingham & Douglas 2004).

Summary

- This chapter covers basic but essential aspects of nursing interventions in relation to promoting continence and urinary elimination.
- The *Essence of Care* (NHS Modernisation Agency 2003) best practice benchmarks concerned with continence and urinary elimination is included and used to underpin the nursing practices that you will see during placements.
- The nurse's role in preventing incontinence is discussed, especially the assessment of urinary function across the lifespan, and the subsequent effects that incontinence can cause.
- Nursing interventions for people with problems associated with incontinence have been considered. The emphasis has been on simple nursing interventions such as ensuring that people can access the lavatory easily, but more complex interventions have been outlined.
- The partnership between the person/parents/carers and the MDT is stressed.
- The importance of promoting continence cannot be overstated; the nurse's role is central in ensuring that people in their care receive sufficient assistance in maintaining continence/promoting continence. UTIs are common and are encountered in all areas of practice.

Self test

1. List the three renal processes involved in urine production.
2. What are the physical and chemical characteristics of normal urine?
3. What factors affect micturition?
4. How are urine samples collected from infants?
5. What measures can you adopt to improve continence in adults?
6. How would you advise parents to potty train their child?
7. List three types of incontinence.
8. What is the normal catheter size (length and diameter) for women?
9. How can nurses reduce trauma caused by a catheter?

Key words and phrases for literature searching

Catheters
Continence
Elimination
Urinary
Urinary tract infection

Useful websites

Association for Continence Advice	www.aca.uk.com Available July 2006
British Association of Urological Nurses	www.baun.co.uk Available July 2006
Continence worldwide – *website of the Continence Promotion Committee of the International Continence Society*	www.continenceworldwide.com Available July 2006
Assist UK	www.assist_uk.org Available July 2006
Enuresis Resource Information Centre (ERIC)	www.eric.org.uk Available July 2006
Ileostomy and Internal Pouch Support Group	www.the-ia.org.uk Available July 2006
Incontact – *provides support and information for people with bladder and bowel problems*	www.incontact.org Available July 2006
Royal Association for Disability and Rehabilitation (RADAR)	www.radar.org.uk Available July 2006
The Continence Foundation	www.continence-foundation.org.uk Available July 2006

References

Barton R 2000 Intermittent self-catheterisation. Nursing Standard 15(9):47–52

BBC 2004 Talking to your doctor – medical tests. Online: www.bbc.co.uk/health/talking Available July 2006

Brooker C, Nicol M (eds) 2003 Nursing adults. The practice of caring. Mosby, Edinburgh

Cook E 1999 Assessing continence needs in children. Nursing Standard 13(38):48–52

Dairiki Shortliffe LM 2002 Urinary tract infections in infants and children. In: Walsh PC, Retik AB, Vaughan ED, Wein AJ (eds) Campbell's urology. 8th edn. Saunders, Philadelphia, Ch. 54

Department of Health 1999 Making a difference – strengthening the nursing, midwifery and health visiting contribution to health and health care. DH, London

Department of Health 2001 Essence of care – patient focused benchmarking for health care practitioners. DH, London

Dorey G 2003 Pelvic floor muscle exercises for men. Nursing Times 99(19):46–48

Drug Tariff 2003 Part 1xb. Department of Health, National Assembly for Wales. TSO, London. In Association for Continence Advice: Notes on good practice

Getliffe K, Dolman M (eds) 2003 Incontinence in perspective. In: Promoting continence: a clinical research resource. Bailliére Tindall, Edinburgh, Ch. 1

Jamieson EM, McCall JM, Whyte LA 2002 Clinical nursing practice. 4th edn. Churchill Livingstone, Edinburgh

Kozier B, Erb G, Berman AJ, Burke K (eds) 2000 Urinary elimination. In: Fundamentals of nursing: concepts, process and practice. Prentice Hall Health, Upper Saddle River, NJ, Ch. 46

Lukeman D 2003 Mainly children: childhood enuresis and encopresis. In: Getliffe K, Dolman M (eds) Promoting continence: a clinical research resource. Baillière Tindall, Edinburgh, Ch. 5

Naish W 2003 Intermittent self-catheterisation for managing urinary problems. Professional Nurse 18(10):7–9

NHS Modernisation Agency 2003 Essence of care guidance – patient-focused benchmarks for clinical governance. Online: www.dh.gov.uk/PublicationsAndStatistics Available September 2006

Nicol M, Bavin C, Bedford-Turner S, Cronin P, Rawlings-Anderson K 2004 Essential nursing skills. 2nd edn. Mosby, Edinburgh

Penfold P 1999 UTI in patients with urethral catheters. British Journal of Nursing 8(6):362–374

Pomfret IJ 1996 Catheters: design, selection and management. British Journal of Nursing 5(4):245–251

Robinson J 2001 Urethral catheter selection. Nursing Standard 15(25):39–42

Rogers J. 2002 Managing daytime and nighttime enuresis. Nursing Standard 16(32):45–52

Sander R 1999 Promoting urinary continence in residential care. Nursing Standard 14(13–15):49–53

Sanders C 2002 Choosing continence products for children. Nursing Standard 16(32):39–43

Schaeffer AJ 2002 Infections of the urinary tract. In: Walsh PC, Retik AB, Vaughan ED, Wein AJ (eds) Campbell's urology. 8th edn. Saunders, Philadelphia, Ch. 14

Sedor J, Mulholland SG 1999 Hospital-acquired urinary tract infections associated with the indwelling catheter. Urology Clinics of North America 26:821–828

The Continence Foundation 2004 Online: www.continence-foundation.org.uk Available September 2006

Waugh A, Grant A 2001 Ross and Wilson anatomy and physiology. 9th edn. Churchill Livingstone, Edinburgh

Wilkinson K 2001 Pakistani women's perceptions and experiences of incontinence. Nursing Standard 16(5):33–39

Further reading

Cotton J, Jones M, Steggall M 2003 Nursing patients with sexual health and reproductive problems. In: Brooker C, Nicol M (eds) Nursing adults. The practice of caring. Mosby, Edinburgh, Ch. 25

Department of Health 2000 Good practice in continence services. DH, London

Edwards S 2001 Regulation of water, sodium and potassium: implications for practice. Nursing Standard 15(22):36–42

Fanning H 2003 Nursing patients with urinary disorders. In: Brooker C, Nicol M (eds) Nursing adults. The practice of caring. Mosby, Edinburgh, Ch. 24

Fillingham S, Douglas J 2004 Urological nursing. 3rd edn. Baillière Tindall, Edinburgh

Getliffe K, Dolman M (eds) 2003 Promoting continence: a clinical research resource. Bailliére Tindall, Edinburgh

McMahon-Parkes K 1998 Management of supra-pubic catheters. Nursing Times 94(25):49–51

Nicol M, Bavin C, Bedford-Turner S, Cronin P, Rawlings-Anderson K 2004 Essential nursing skills. 2nd edn. Mosby, Edinburgh

Rigby D 2001 Integrated continence services. Nursing Standard 16(8):46–52

Sanders C 2002 Choosing continence products for children. Nursing Standard 16(32):39–43

SIGN 2006 SIGN 88 Management of suspected bacterial urinary tract infection in adults. Quick reference guide. Online: www.sign.ac.uk/pdf/qrg88.pdf Available September 2006

Wells M 2003 Maintaining continence. In: Brooker C, Nicol M (eds) Nursing adults. The practice of caring. Mosby, Edinburgh

21

Elimination – faeces

Susan Walker

Glossary terms

Constipation

Diarrhoea

Encopresis

Enema

Faecal incontinence

Flatus

Laxative

Melaena

Stool

Stoma

Suppository

Learning outcomes

This chapter will help you:

- Understand the structure and function of the large intestine, rectum and the anal canal
- Describe normal defecation in the child and the adult
- Outline factors which affect bowel habit
- Demonstrate an awareness of holistic assessment and history taking
- Outline the *Essence of Care* (NHS Modernisation Agency 2003) best practice benchmarks concerned with bowel care
- Describe nursing interventions that maintain or restore normal defecation
- Outline some common conditions affecting the large intestine, rectum and the anal canal
- Outline some common diagnostic procedures
- Develop an understanding of the assessment and nursing management of constipation, diarrhoea and faecal incontinence.

Introduction

The elimination of faeces (defecation), which requires proper functioning of the gastrointestinal (GI) tract, is vital in the maintenance of homeostasis. When defecation is disrupted it can adversely affect the person's quality of life and ultimately their health. Unfortunately, many people still choose to ignore symptoms that may be indicative of disease because they are too embarrassed to discuss their bowel habit or fear the prospect of undergoing physical examination.

Meeting patients' bowel needs was included in the original *Essence of Care* document in 2001, which detailed patient-focused benchmarks to assist health professionals in raising standards for basic but essential aspects of care. Bowel care is part of the *Benchmark for Continence and Bladder and Bowel Care* (NHS Modernisation Agency 2003). This chapter contributes to the attainment of those standards for patients/clients who require assistance with bowel care and defecation.

The chapter covers basic anatomy and physiology of normal defecation and the factors that affect it. The nursing interventions needed to assist patients with defecation, including relevant health promotion, are discussed in detail. The importance of a holistic approach to care is illustrated in the section dealing with patients/clients who experience a range of problems with defecation. The nurse's knowledge and skill is fundamental in the assessment of bowel habit and the delivery of holistic care based on best evidence.

The nurse must work in partnership with the patient/client/parents and other health and social care professionals in the multidisciplinary team (MDT) to achieve independence of faecal elimination for the patient/client wherever possible, and to promote personal dignity when assistance is required.

An overview of defecation

This section covers the anatomy and physiology of the large intestine and defecation and the factors that affect it. In addition, holistic assessment of faecal elimination is explored and an outline of common conditions and investigations is provided.

One of the characteristics of a simple cell is that of excretion of waste products. An inability to excrete waste

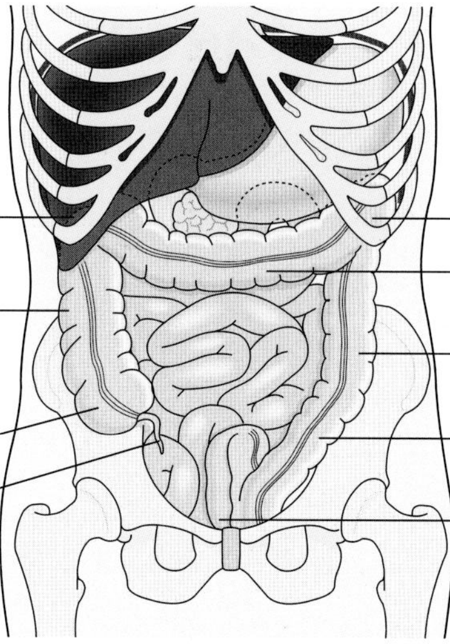

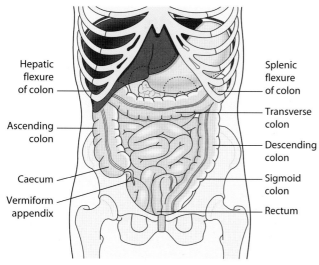

Fig. 21.1 Parts of the large intestine and their positions (reproduced with permission from Waugh & Grant 2001)

leads to a loss of homeostasis and disruption of cellular function. In the body, the large intestine (bowel) plays the major role in the elimination of solid waste (faeces). The elimination of faeces is known as defecation.

The gastrointestinal (GI) tract is a coiled muscular tube. It includes the:

- Mouth
- Pharynx
- Oesophagus
- Stomach
- Small intestine (duodenum, jejunum and ileum)
- Large intestine (colon, rectum and anal canal) (Fig. 21.1).

(For further detail, see Chs 16, 19 and your anatomy and physiology book.)

Large intestine, rectum and anal canal

Much of the absorption of nutrients from the diet takes place within the small intestine (see Ch. 19). The remaining waste material then passes into the large intestine where it gradually solidifies as water is reabsorbed into the bloodstream through the bowel mucosa. The resultant material, faeces, is normally a semi-solid brown mass. Despite absorption of water, 60–70% of the weight of faeces is water. Among other constituents (see Table 21.1, p. 605), faeces contains undigested fibre residues and mucus which help lubricate the faeces or stool, aiding defecation.

Structure

Four layers of tissue form the walls of the large intestine:

- Adventitia – serous outer layer
- Muscle layer – longitudinal and circular muscle fibres concerned with moving intestinal contents by peristalsis (rhythmic wave-like contraction and dilatation)
- Submucosal layer
- Mucosal lining.

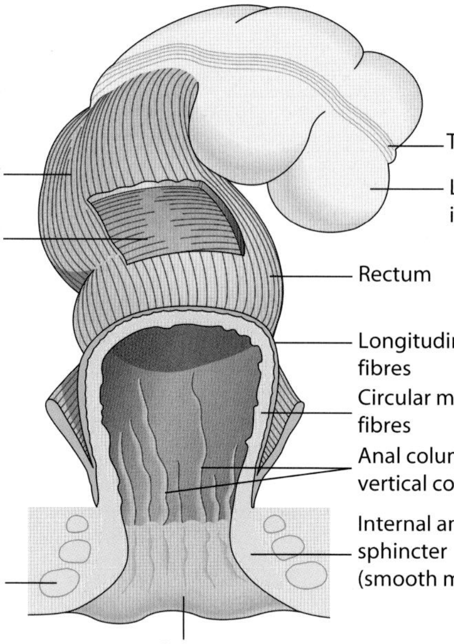

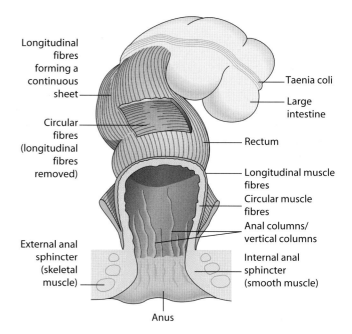

Fig. 21.2 Rectum and anus (adapted with permission from Waugh & Grant 2001)

There are several modifications to the muscle layer. Two folds of the circular muscle layer form the ileocaecal valve, which controls the passage of material from the ileum to the caecum (first part of the large intestine). The circular muscle layer also forms the anal sphincters: the internal (involuntary, smooth muscle) and the external (voluntary, skeletal muscle). The longitudinal muscle layer in the colon consists of three bands called taeniae coli (Fig. 21.2). As the bands are shorter than the colon they produce a puckered or sacculated appearance. The sacculations are known as haustrations. The rectum and anal canal are completely surrounded by longitudinal muscle fibres, so there are no haustrations.

The submucosal layer contains lymphoid tissue that provides some defence from invading microbes. The mucosal lining of the colon and upper part of the rectum has a large number of mucus-secreting cells.

The mucosa in the upper part of the anal canal is arranged in vertical folds, known as the anal or vertical columns (see Fig. 21.2). Each column contains a terminal branch of the superior rectal vein and artery. The anus is lined with stratified squamous epithelium, which is continuous with the rectal mucosa above and merges with the perianal skin outside the external sphincter.

The large intestine is about 1.5 metres in length. It comprises the caecum, colon (ascending, transverse, descending and sigmoid), rectum and anal canal (see Fig. 21.1).

The caecum is the dilated first part of the large intestine. It has a worm-like appendix – the vermiform appendix – that extends from it. The appendix has a blind end and contains lymphoid tissue. Just above the lower end of the caecum there is a T-junction where the ileocaecal valve opens into it.

The colon is divided into the ascending, transverse, and descending colon in relation to its anatomical position (see Fig. 21.1). The ascending colon runs from the caecum, up the right side of the abdominal cavity. When it reaches just below the liver, it makes a 90° turn to form the hepatic (right colic) flexure. It then becomes the transverse colon where it crosses the body below the stomach until it reaches the spleen. It turns again at the splenic (left colic) flexure and becomes the descending colon as it passes down the left side of the abdominal cavity, moving towards the midline. As the descending colon enters the pelvis it becomes the sigmoid colon and then the rectum. The rectum is a slightly dilated section of colon, about 3 cm in length in infants, growing to 13 cm in adults, terminating at the anal canal.

The anal canal leads from the rectum to the exterior. It has two muscular sphincters, one internal, one external, which are involved in the process of defecation (see Fig. 21.2 and below).

Functions

Functions of the large intestine, rectum and anal canal include:

- Microbial activity
- Absorption
- Mass movement of faeces.

The waste material that reaches the large intestine normally remains there for approximately 12–24 hours prior to expulsion from the body as faeces. There is some digestion of the waste products by the bacteria that colonize the large intestine, but no further food breakdown occurs. The bacteria include *Escherichia coli*, *Enterobacter aerogenes*, *Streptococcus faecalis* and *Clostridium perfringens*. Many colonic bacteria have the capability to become pathogens should they be transferred to another part of the body (see Ch. 15). The bacteria metabolize remaining carbohydrates and amino acids, releasing gases, e.g. hydrogen, which contribute to faecal odour. Normally the build-up of gas is expelled from the anus as flatus. People vary but some foods such as onions tend to produce excessive flatus. Flatus has an offensive odour due to bacterial decomposition of food residues in the colon. In Western society the passing of flatus is considered as a natural bodily function, but offensive and unacceptable in public.

There is some microbial vitamin production, mostly vitamins K and B group. Absorption in the large intestine is mostly of these vitamins, some electrolytes and water.

The remaining faecal mass is propelled towards the rectum by mass movements, long, slow and powerful contractile waves that move over large areas of the colon three or four times daily. These movements usually occur during or just after eating, indicating that it is the presence of food in the stomach and small intestine that activates the gastrocolic and duodenocolic reflexes. This may then lead to defecation.

Normal process of defecation

Involuntary, reflex or automatic defecation occurs in infancy because the infant has not yet developed voluntary control of their external anal sphincter. It is usual in the second or third year of life for the child to develop the ability to override the defecation reflex (Box 21.1).

Box 21.1 Developing control of defecation in healthy children

In order to control defecation a child needs to:

- Have control over the anal sphincter
- Recognize the sensation to defecate and associate this with feeling clean, dry and comfortable
- Have the motor skills needed for sitting on a 'potty' or lavatory
- Have the ability to convey the need to defecate so the child can be provided with a potty or taken to the lavatory. The lavatory then becomes recognized and associated with defecation
- Associate the positive feedback of parents/carers with the activity of successful defecation.

  This is assessed by an ability to convey the need to defecate, recognize an appropriate place, maintain a position for successful defecation and associate this with a positive response from grown-ups and the comfortable feeling of being clean and dry.

The rectum is normally empty, and the defecation reflex is initiated when faeces moves into it, causing stretching of the rectal walls. The defecation reflex is mediated through the spinal cord and causes the walls of the sigmoid colon and the rectum to contract and the anal sphincter to relax, allowing faeces to pass into the anal canal. These contractions bring with them a feeling of fullness.

Once control has been achieved it is usually possible to delay the opening of the external anal sphincter (controlled through the pudendal nerve). Defecation is aided by voluntary contraction of the diaphragm and abdominal muscles to increase intra-abdominal pressure and force faeces down. This is achieved by the Valsalva manoeuvre – a forced expiration against a closed glottis (opening between the vocal cords). If defecation is delayed, the feeling of fullness will diminish as the rectal walls relax, until the next defecation reflex is initiated.

Reflex defecation may occur after a stroke, with sacral spinal cord damage or damage to the pudendal nerve.

Factors affecting defecation

Many psychological, social, cultural and physical factors can affect defecation and bowel habit; some of these are discussed below and others are outlined in Box 21.2 (p. 602).

Despite the fact that faecal elimination is a normal bodily function, it carries a great taboo (Small 1999). In Western society this can be related to sociocultural factors, where both the anal region and the process of elimination are 'private'.

Infants have no control over their bowel and defecation occurs involuntarily. Milk-fed infants normally have yellowish, malodorous faeces. Infants have small stomachs, reduced enzyme secretion and material moves rapidly through the GI tract, which means that four to six soiled nappies in 24 hours is not uncommon. Faecal

Box 21.2 Factors that affect defecation and bowel habit

Physical factors

- Age – particularly at the extremes of age (see p. 603)
- Ignoring the urge to defecate – leads to constipation (alteration in normal bowel movements, resulting in the less frequent and uncomfortable passage of hard stools)
- Reduced physical activity/immobility – leading to constipation
- Mobility – lack of mobility can prevent the person accessing the lavatory
- Diet/type, amount of food, eating habits – lack of fibre causes constipation; some foods in excess, e.g. fruit, lead to diarrhoea (a loose watery stool that occurs frequently)
- Fluid intake – dehydration (see Ch. 19) causes constipation
- Hormones – constipation can occur during pregnancy.

Emotional/psychological factors

- Anxiety and stress – causes diarrhoea
- Low mood, depression and dementia – leading to constipation
- Life events such as bereavement or new sibling, etc. can affect bowel habit.

Facilities and environment

- Poor facilities (cold, dirty, dark, too far away)
- Lack of privacy
- Admission to hospital and use of a bedpan/commode.

All the above can cause people to ignore the urge to defecate, leading to constipation.

Bowel conditions (see Table 21.2, p. 606)
Congenital and acquired bowel conditions both affect defecation, e.g. gastroenteritis; inflammatory bowel disease (IBD) causes diarrhoea; intestinal obstruction and diverticular disease cause constipation; colorectal cancer causes a change in bowel habit (alternating diarrhoea/constipation) and painful anorectal conditions, e.g. haemorrhoids, cause people to 'put off' defecation.

Neurological conditions
Many neurological conditions can affect the bowel or sphincter control, e.g. multiple sclerosis, paraplegia or stroke. Multiple sclerosis and paraplegia can cause constipation.

Systemic conditions

- Underactive thyroid gland – constipation
- Overactive thyroid gland – diarrhoea
- Electrolyte imbalance (see Ch. 19) – e.g. low potassium level in the blood (hypokalaemia) causes constipation
- Food sensitivities and intolerance cause diarrhoea
- Infection causes diarrhoea.

Medication (Box 21.3)

- Opioids, e.g. morphine, codeine (see Ch. 23) – constipation
- Antibiotics – diarrhoea
- Laxatives (drugs that stimulate or increase evacuation of faeces from the bowel) – cause diarrhoea, especially if misused such as in eating disorders, or paradoxically constipation when overused
- Diuretics (see Ch. 20) can lead to excess fluid and potassium loss and cause constipation
- Antidepressants, e.g. amitriptyline, can cause constipation; fluoxetine can cause change in bowel habit
- Iron – causes altered bowel habit (constipation or diarrhoea)
- Antimuscarinics (anticholinergics), e.g. oxybutynin, causes constipation.

REFLECTIVE PRACTICE Box 21.3

Medication and bowel habit

Think about common medications used for the patient/client group in your placement.

Student activities

- Find out if any of the common medications used were likely to cause constipation or diarrhoea.
- Are patients/clients routinely informed of this side-effect?

[Resource: *British National Formulary* – www.bnf.org.uk Available July 2006]

soiling, if left in contact with the skin for a prolonged time, will lead to discomfort, distress and soreness.

The infant is dependent upon parents/carers to attend to their elimination needs until they have reached the stage of psychosocial and motor development that allows them to gain control over defecation. Parents/carers will wash the infant, change nappies and bedding in order to promote comfort. But those around the infant often show distaste when the odour of a full nappy is recognized. Potty training normally commences when the child is between 18 months and 2 years of age. However, for some children who have a motor or learning disability this may not be possible (Box 21.4).

Potty training is seen as a normal stage of development and parents will often produce a potty for the child to use in communal areas of the home (see also Ch. 20), sometimes encouraging the child to 'perform' in front of visitors and grandparents, and positively praising the successful result when the potty is used. Parents/carers often take great pride in their child's successful potty training. As soon as potty training is achieved the child will progress to the lavatory and suddenly asking to use a potty or removing underwear in front of others results in a reprimand for the child, as this behaviour

REFLECTIVE PRACTICE Box 21.4

Children with a learning disability – development in relation to defecation

Think about how this aspect of development in children with a learning disability may be different from that in other children.

Student activity

- Find out what services are available in your area to support parents/carers of children with learning disabilities with this aspect of motor and psychosocial development.

REFLECTIVE PRACTICE Box 21.5

Assessing bowel habit

How would you feel if you were asked how often you have your bowels open, and details about colour and consistency?

Student activities

- What questions are asked about bowel habit in your placement?
- Discuss with your mentor how you can ensure that intimate questions are asked with sensitivity.

is now unacceptable. Elimination has become a private function, and this part of the body is no longer revealed to others. Behaviours learned as a child will continue to influence attitudes and behaviours related to defecation throughout life.

During childhood, experiences associated with defecation can influence a child's toilet habits. For example, a child may refuse to use a school lavatory, or they develop a fear of a dark lavatory, which may lead to regression (return to behaviour associated with an earlier stage of development), resulting in soiling underclothes with urine and faeces as an alternative to visiting the lavatory. Constipation (see pp. 610–613) can develop if a child does not respond to the urge to defecate during school hours, retaining faeces within the bowel until they can go to their own lavatory. In a young child, control over the bladder and bowel may be lost if the child is engrossed in a game, greatly exited or experiences great fear.

During adolescence the large intestine grows rapidly to reach adult size. The lifestyle choices adopted during childhood and adolescence will influence health as an adult. For example, habits acquired during adolescence such as poor diet and inactivity can persist into adulthood, despite these being factors that a person has choice and control over in adult life.

Age changes can affect defecation. A reduction in muscle strength and mobility can make older people become susceptible to problems associated with elimination, e.g. constipation. In addition, the external sphincter may weaken or people can have reduced sensation, which may give rise to faecal soiling, e.g. when passing flatus. Older people are also more likely to take medications that affect bowel habit, e.g. non-steroidal anti-inflammatory drugs (NSAIDs) can cause diarrhoea, which may result in loss of continence.

There is also a greater risk of developing bowel (colorectal) cancer in those over 50 years of age (see p. 607). An older person is often reluctant to seek help, due to embarrassment, concern over possible cancer diagnosis, and may associate faecal incontinence with child-like behaviour and dependence (van Dongen 2001).

Holistic assessment of faecal elimination

Many patients are embarrassed to discuss their elimination difficulties and the assessment interview requires privacy and a sensitive and skilled approach (Box 21.5). It is important to use age-appropriate language; for example, a child or indeed an adult with learning disabilities may have special names for faeces (e.g. 'number 2' or 'poo') and the nurse should always ask the parents/carers for this information.

Assessing normal bowel habit – patterns of defecation and characteristics of faeces

Normal bowel habit varies from person to person and changes during the lifespan. However, in a study of adults admitted to hospital, the usual bowel habit prior to admission was five to seven stools weekly (Wright 1974).

The assessment of stool type can be enhanced by the use of a pictorial assessment tool such as the Bristol Stool Form Scale (Fig. 21.3A, p. 604) or the Children's Bristol Stool Form Scale, which uses child-friendly language to describe stool type (Fig. 21.3B, p. 604). In addition, the nurse should measure fluid stools and record the volume lost on the fluid intake and output chart (see Ch. 19). Table 21.1 (p. 605) outlines the normal characteristics of faeces and defecation and some abnormalities.

Nursing history

When assessing and taking a history of a person's bowel habit the nurse must ask about normal bowel habit and any changes that have occurred. It is important to note when any changes first occurred and for how long they have been present, as unexplained changes may indicate diseases such as cancer. The nursing history typically includes information about the following:

- Usual bowel habit: how often, time of day, relation to mealtimes/hot drinks
- Does the person feel that their bowel habit is normal?
- Measures taken to promote defecation such as trying at the same time, after breakfast/hot drink, eating specific foods (e.g. dried apricots), avoiding foods that affect bowel habit, laxatives (see pp. 611–612)
- Does the person always respond to the urge for defecation
- The normal/usual stool colour, shape and consistency

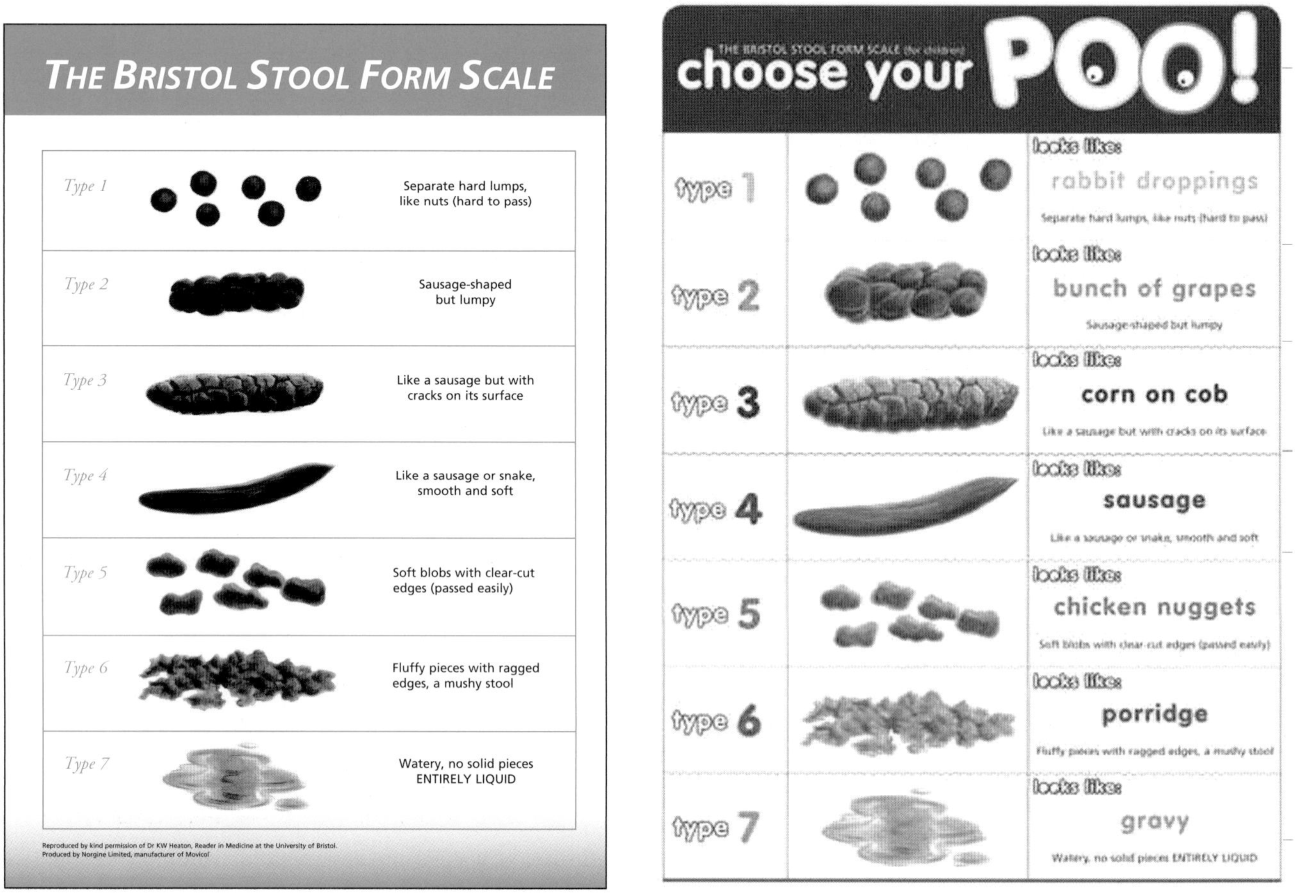

Fig. 21.3 **A.** Bristol Stool Form Scale (reproduced by kind permission of Dr KW Heaton, Reader in Medicine at the University of Bristol. ©2000 Norgine Ltd). **B.** Children's Bristol Stool Form Scale (Concept by Professor DCA Candy and Emma Davey, based on the Bristol Stool Form Scale by Dr KW Heaton, Reader in Medicine at the University of Bristol. ©2005 Norgine Ltd) For further copies of the Bristol Stool Form Scales please freephone Norgine on 0800 269865 or email mss@norgine.com

- Usual fluid intake, types of food and preferences, amount of fibre, meal frequency and when main meal taken (see Ch. 19)
- How emotions affect defecation, e.g. anxiety about using a public lavatory
- Oral health, own teeth; if dentures are used are they well fitting? (see Ch. 16)
- Usual level of mobility, manual dexterity and exercise pattern
- Whether they use the lavatory, commode, bedpan or potty
- Is the person's lavatory modified, e.g. handrails or raised seat?
- Is the person independent for bowel care or do they need help?
- History of faecal soiling/incontinence
- Usual medication (over-the-counter and prescribed) and use of illegal drugs
- History of conditions, e.g. irritable bowel syndrome, spinal injury, or surgery that might affect defecation
- The presence of a stoma that discharges faeces and, if so, the frequency and nature of discharge. Is the person self-caring?
- Changes in behaviour, e.g. a child who develops faecal incontinence after the birth of a sibling
- Increasing confusion or aggression in an older adult with dementia
- Change of environment such as moving into a care home
- Changes to routine or elimination habits
- Change in the mode of eliminating, e.g. frequency, pain, straining, increased flatus, etc.
- Changes to colour, consistency, shape or amount of faeces
- Have dietary habits altered? If so, how?
- Recent changes in health status.

A holistic assessment will also ascertain how culture, beliefs and religious practices influence defecation (see p. 609). Acknowledging this individuality will ensure that the person's needs are met.

Table 21.1 Characteristics of faeces and defecation

Characteristic	Normal	Abnormal
Frequency	Infants vary: breast milk 4–6 times/day or less; formula milk 1–3 times/day Adults: daily to 2/3 times/week	More than 6 times/day or less than once every 1–2 days More than 3 times/day or less than once a week
Consistency (see Fig. 21.3)	Soft, formed	A range between the two extremes of: • Separate hard lumps in constipation • Completely liquid in diarrhoea
Amount	Adults: depends on fibre intake, e.g. stool weight 39–223 g with refined/processed diet and 71–488 g with vegetarian mixed diet (Burkitt et al 1972)	Reduced volume with frequent stools
Colour	Infant: yellow Adult: brown	Clay/putty colour – absence of bile Green – gastroenteritis Red – eating beetroot Blood: • Bright red if lower GI bleeding • Melaena – characteristic offensive odour, black and tarry if bleeding from higher up GI tract Black/grey with oral iron Pale if contains undigested fat
Shape	Resembles rectal diameter	Narrow 'ribbon stools' such as with increased peristalsis
Odour	Characteristic – depends on diet	Offensive if pus or blood is present
Constituents	Water Epithelial cells from the intestine Mucus Microorganisms Undigested fibre (non-starch polysaccharide [NSP]) Electrolytes Fat Stercobilin – pigment that colours faeces Various chemicals	Less water in constipation More water in diarrhoea Excess mucus and pus with inflammatory bowel disease Blood – see above Foreign bodies Parasites, e.g. threadworms (see Box 21.6), tapeworm segments
Flatus	Depends on diet, e.g. increases after beans, onions, etc.	May be reduced if the bowel is obstructed
Pain/discomfort on defecation (dyschezia)	Normally no pain or straining	Abdominal pain relieved by defecation Pain in the rectum (proctalgia) and anus during defecation Straining with constipation

HEALTH PROMOTION Box 21.6

Threadworms

You have been asked by your mentor to help prepare an information sheet about threadworms (*Enterobius vermicularis*).

Student activity
Access the website below and prepare a summary of the main points concerning threadworm infestation in children and preventing reinfestation.

[Resource: Prodigy Guidance – www.prodigy.nhs.uk/guidance.asp?gt=Threadworm Available July 2006]

Some people will resist the urge to defecate if this means using a lavatory other than their own and individual bowel assessment must incorporate any psychological and environmental factors affecting bowel habit.

It can be helpful for patients/parents to keep a diary of bowel actions to establish a pattern; this is particularly helpful when bowel-training programmes are in progress. Nurses should record bowel actions in the nursing notes and on the appropriate charts, e.g. a stool record chart (Fig. 21.4, p. 606) and episodes of diarrhoea are measured and recorded on the fluid intake and output chart.

Common conditions affecting the bowel

Before considering individualized nursing care, nurses need some knowledge of conditions that can affect bowel habit. Some congenital and acquired conditions are outlined in Table 21.2. Readers requiring more information should consult the Further reading suggestions (e.g. McGrath 2003).

Common investigations

There are many different investigations used to identify disorders affecting the large bowel and elimination of faeces (Box 21.8, p. 607; see also Ch. 19).

Name: Hospital number:				Department/ward:			Consultant:	
Date	Time	Amount	Colour	Consistency (Bristol Scale 1–7)	Blood	Mucus	Comments, e.g. pain, flatus, straining, etc	Nurse's signature

Fig. 21.4 Stool record chart

Table 21.2 Common bowel conditions

Condition	Description
Appendicitis	Inflammation of the appendix
Irritable bowel syndrome (IBS)	A common condition of bowel dysfunction for which no organic cause can be found There is pain and passage of mucus rectally, with alternating diarrhoea and constipation
Inflammatory bowel disease (IBD): Crohn's disease and ulcerative colitis	Depending on the type and severity there is pain, diarrhoea, blood and mucus passed rectally, malabsorption, anaemia, weight loss and fever Complications include bowel obstruction and perforation, toxic dilatation, fluid and electrolyte disturbances (see Ch. 19) and colorectal cancer
Diverticular disease	The presence of sacs (diverticula) in the wall of the colon Increases with age May be asymptomatic, may bleed, or become inflamed to cause diverticulitis, or perforate
Cancer of the colon or rectum (colorectal)	A common cancer in the UK (see Box 21.7)
Rectal prolapse	The rectum is displaced downward and the mucosa may be visible outside the anus Associated with chronic constipation and straining to defecate
Haemorrhoids (piles)	Varicosities in the rectum/anus; may be internal or external Caused by increased venous pressure and may occur with chronic constipation and straining There may be itching, burning, pain and bleeding during defecation
Anal fissure	Break in the skin or anal mucosa, associated with constipation Causes pain/bleeding when passing faeces
Imperforate anus	Congenital anomaly where an infant does not have a patent anal opening or the anus does not communicate with the bowel above Corrected surgically
Hirschsprung's disease	Congenital megacolon Defective nerve supply to the terminal colon leads to defective peristalsis, build-up of faeces, massive dilatation and bowel obstruction

HEALTH PROMOTION Box 21.7

Colorectal cancer – early detection

Over 34 500 people per year in the UK are diagnosed with colorectal cancer (Cancer Research UK 2005). It is essential to seek professional advice early if any of the following occur:

- A change in bowel habit, constipation and/or diarrhoea that lasts
- Blood and mucus passed with faeces
- Feeling of incomplete emptying after defecation
- Pain in the rectum or abdomen
- Weight loss
- Signs/symptoms of anaemia such as tiredness.

A screening programme for colorectal cancer, using faecal occult blood (FOB) samples, is being introduced in England. All people aged 60–69 years will be included by 2009 and will be screened every 2 years. People aged 70 years or over can request screening.

[Reference: Cancer Research UK 2005 – www.cancerresearchuk.org Available July 2006]

Box 21.8 **Common investigations**

The following investigations may be used to diagnose or evaluate treatment for large bowel disorders:

- Blood tests – full blood count, urea and electrolytes
- X-rays – plain abdominal X-ray, barium enema
- Digital rectal examination
- Endoscopy including biopsy and treatments – rigid or flexible sigmoidoscopy (screening test), colonoscopy
- Ultrasound scan (USS), computed tomography (CT), magnetic resonance imaging (MRI)
- Stool/faecal samples – for microscopy, culture and sensitivity for infection, faecal occult blood (FOB) (screening – see Box 21.7), fat content (3–5 day sample) and parasites
- Adhesive tape slides for threadworms.

A simple explanation of some of these investigations accessed on the BBC or the National Institutes of Health websites will help you provide patient information (see Box 21.9).

[Resources: BBC Talking to your doctor: medical tests – www.bbc.co.uk/health/talking/tests; National Institutes of Health – http://digestive.niddk.nih.gov/ddiseases/a-z.asp
Both available July 2006]

CRITICAL THINKING Box 21.9

Mary – preparation for colonoscopy

Mary noticed blood on the tissue after defecation and eventually plucked up courage to see her GP who referred Mary to the hospital for a colonoscopy.

Student activities

- Find out what happens during a colonoscopy.
- Obtain a copy of the local patient information sheet about bowel preparation prior to colonoscopy, other bowel investigations and surgery.
- Identify the information needed by Mary so that she is physically and mentally well prepared for her investigation.

[Resource: Bulmer F 2000 Bowel preparation for rectal and colonic investigation. Nursing Standard 14(20):32–35]

Nursing interventions to promote defecation

This part of the chapter considers how nurses can assist people by promoting normal defecation (Box 21.10, p. 608), providing a suitable environment and facilities, preventing or dealing effectively with alterations such as constipation or diarrhoea and ensuring that privacy and dignity are maintained.

Alterations in defecation can include changes in frequency or consistency, loss of continence and the care needed following the formation of a stoma. Many alterations can be anticipated by the nurse and either prevented or at least minimized, such as being aware that people who have to use a bedpan or commode (see pp. 609–610) are more likely to become constipated (Box 21.12, p. 608).

Many patients will require assistance in meeting their faecal elimination needs and nurses must give full explanations and obtain consent prior to interventions. If possible, most people will want to use the lavatory. For those unable to use the lavatory, a bedpan, potty or commode will need to be provided promptly and efficiently to limit worries about 'accidents' and any embarrassment that the person may have. For example, where there is embarrassment about malodorous stools, the nurse can provide an air freshener to keep in the locker, which can be discretely sprayed following the use of the bedpan/commode or carried to the lavatory in a dressing gown pocket. However, the nurse must first check that the patient and those close by have no breathing difficulties or allergies.

Environment and facilities for faecal elimination

The importance of a suitable environment for bowel care is illustrated by it being a benchmark of best practice in

Box 21.10 Promoting normal defecation

- Assessment of bowel habit and reassessment as required (see pp. 603–605)
- Encouraging regular habits, e.g. responding to the urge to defecate (see Box 21.11)
- Promoting exercise and mobility (see Ch. 18); involve the MDT
- Encouraging a balanced, high-fibre diet (see Ch. 19)
- Maintaining or increasing fluid intake (see Ch. 19)
- Reviewing medication that may affect defecation (see Chs 12, 22, 23)
- Relieving pain associated with defecation (see Ch. 23)
- Minimizing patient embarrassment through interpersonal skills (see Ch. 9)
- Providing suitable facilities for defecation
- Meeting privacy and dignity needs
- Being aware that the nurse's attitudes (comments or facial expressions when dealing with faeces) can affect a patient's bowel habit
- Meeting cultural or religious needs
- Anticipating and, where possible, preventing problems such as constipation
- Maintaining faecal continence
- Ensuring that nursing interventions are evidence-based (see Ch. 5)
- Contributing to a multiprofessional approach to patient management.

HEALTH PROMOTION Box 21.11

Promoting good habits in children

Children should be encouraged to use the lavatory prior to leaving home for school. They should be encouraged to use the school lavatory during play and lunch times but to always respond to the urge to defecate by asking to be excused if it occurs during class time. However, some children may be reluctant to defecate in the school lavatory.

Student activities

- Make a list of factors that might make a child reluctant to use the school lavatory.
- Select one of the factors and think about how the problem might be solved.

the *Essence of Care Guidance*: *Benchmark for Continence and Bladder and Bowel Care* (NHS Modernisation Agency 2003) (Box 21.13).

Patients/clients must be informed about where the lavatory facilities are located. The nurse should always show them and assess whether they need help to access the lavatory. In addition, the patient is told how to call for help: verbally or by the use of the call system.

EVIDENCE-BASED PRACTICE Box 21.12

Bedpans, commodes and constipation

A study by Wright (1974) confirmed that use of a bedpan or commode increased the incidence of constipation in patients admitted to hospital. Wright found that 44% of people who used a bedpan or commode developed constipation whereas only 26% of patients able to use the lavatory became constipated.

Student activities

- Access Wright's study and consider other findings regarding constipation.
- Consider how these might be used in practice to prevent constipation associated with immobility.

REFLECTIVE PRACTICE Box 21.13

Benchmarks of best practice in bowel care

'All bladder and bowel care is given in an environment conducive to the patient's individual needs' (NHS Modernisation Agency 2003, p. 3).

Student activities

- Think about an experience from a recent placement or when you were a patient and compare the care given against the benchmark above.
- Discuss with your mentor how this aspect of bowel care could be improved.

It is vital that the environment for elimination is suitable for the purpose. This requires a lavatory area to be clean, warm, dry, comfortable and private, with appropriate handwashing facilities to reduce the risk of infection (see Ch. 15). Comfortable, effective lavatory tissue must be available and, for some people, running water to wash the perianal area. The provision of adequate ventilation and/or air fresheners can reduce potential embarrassment regarding odour.

The normal position for defecation is sitting or squatting, leaning slightly forward to increase the intra-abdominal pressure with the Valsalva manoeuvre (see p. 601). The height of a standard lavatory will need to be adapted for a child in order to aid hip flexion, normally by using a footstool. A higher lavatory seat may be better for people with reduced mobility as rising from a low lavatory will be difficult; again a footstool may be needed to aid correct positioning for defecation. The provision of a higher seat and handrails can maintain independence for many people (Fig. 21.5).

Space may be an issue for a person with a disability who requires assistance to transfer to and from the lavatory. Handles fixed to the lavatory wall are a cheap and effective means of assisting with transfer. The availability

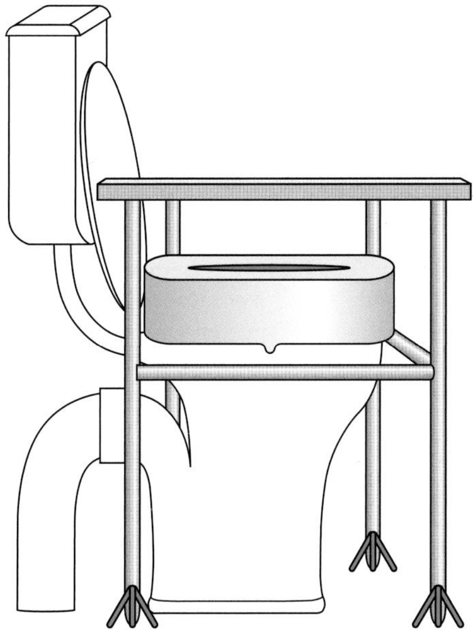

Fig. 21.5 Use of raised seat and hand rails to promote independence (reproduced with permission from Jamieson et al 2002)

of disabled lavatories is now a legal requirement in all buildings to which the public have access.

A change in environment, e.g. change in diet, being away from home, can compromise bowel habit, particularly if accompanied by a change in the person's level of dependence. Becoming reliant on another to assist in meeting elimination needs is an area of great concern for people, and this can be directly associated with the facilities provided.

Some people will need assistance to use the lavatory (Box 21.14) or help with clothing. People may be unable to remove clothing before using the lavatory due to lack of mobility or dexterity, or lack of understanding. Various adaptations to clothing may need to be considered by the nurse in order to maintain the person's independence and dignity (Box 21.15).

The nurse must consider cultural needs. Many people, e.g. Sikhs, Hindus and Muslims, require that nurses of the same sex meet their intimate hygiene needs (see Ch. 16). Personal hygiene is very important and washing with water after using the lavatory is normal practice for many groups. In Islam a cleansing ritual is performed before prayers and this becomes void after urination, defecation, passing flatus or vomiting and needs to be repeated (Akhtar 2002). Muslims also prefer to wash their genitalia and perianal area with running water after using the lavatory. Offering a jug of water following elimination will meet this need. The left hand is used for personal cleansing.

Bedpans and commodes

Some patients will need to use a bedpan or commode (Fig. 21.6, p. 610). Most people will find this embarrassing and nurses must be aware of these worries and take all necessary steps to maintain the person's privacy and dignity and provide culturally sensitive care.

NURSING SKILLS Box 21.14

Taking a patient to the lavatory

- Respond immediately to the patient's request
- Put on plastic apron and non-sterile gloves if help is needed with personal hygiene
- Ascertain whether a stool specimen is required (see p. 617)
- Assist the patient from the bed or chair as required (see Ch. 18)
- Ensure patient is wearing slippers and dressing gown to promote a safe environment and promote dignity
- Collect any personal items such as toiletries, sanitary towels, fresh underwear
- Guide to the lavatory cubicle or take in a wheelchair
- Offer assistance with clothing if required
- Remain in the immediate vicinity if the patient requests/requires and maintain privacy
- Once the patient has defecated, offer assistance with personal hygiene, ensuring perianal area is clean and dry, and help with clothing. Consider cultural preferences for running water for hygiene purposes. When assisting females with personal hygiene, wipe from front to back to avoid bacterial contamination of the urethra (see Chs 16, 20)
- Offer handwashing facilities to the patient
- Remove gloves if you have assisted with personal hygiene and wash your hands
- Escort back to bed/chair, make sure that the patient is comfortable and has everything they need, e.g. call bell, drink, within reach
- Document bowel movement in patient records.

REFLECTIVE PRACTICE Box 21.15

Adaptation to clothing

Think about a person who had difficulty removing clothing in order to use the lavatory. They may have had a learning disability or dementia, or had poor dexterity following a stroke, etc.

Student activities

- What particular difficulties did they experience?
- Find out about adaptations that might have helped.

[Resources: Disabled Living Foundation – www.dlf.org.uk Available July 2006]

Using a bedpan may lead to worries over spillage in the bed or the escape of offensive sounds or smells in the ward. Bedpans are difficult to balance on, and getting a patient on a bedpan requires the nurse to complete an appropriate risk assessment for moving and handling (see Chs 13, 18), ensuring that neither patient nor nurse safety is compromised. Box 21.16 (p. 610) outlines how the nurse can provide a bedpan or commode safely while maintaining privacy and dignity.

A

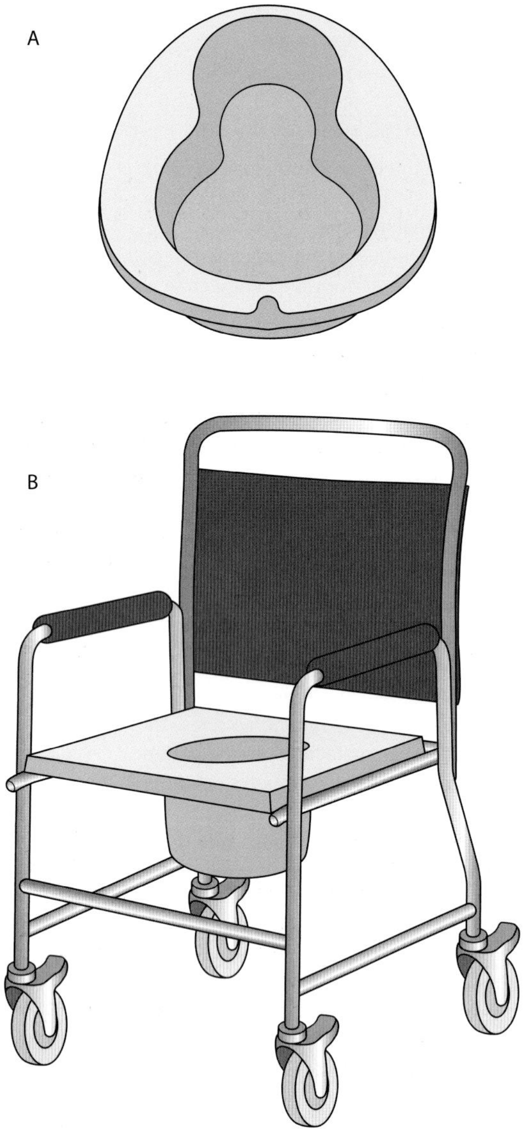

B

Fig. 21.6 **A.** Bedpan. **B.** Commode

A commode can be used for patients with more mobility. It has the advantage of providing a more normal position for defecation and can be used in the lavatory for greater privacy. The commode can be used beside the bed, if privacy and dignity can be ensured (see Box 21.16). Alternatively, the patient may be transferred from the bed to a wheelchair, taken to the lavatory and there transferred to the commode, which may then be moved over the lavatory. Again a risk assessment is undertaken and safe moving and handling procedures adhered to (see Chs 13, 18). The commode should never be used for transport between the bed and lavatory due to the risk of cross-infection.

Constipation

Constipation can be difficult to define. There is no accepted definition for constipation as it depends on individual interpretation (Winney 1998). For example,

NURSING SKILLS Box 21.16

Providing a bedpan or commode

- Respond immediately to request
- Put on plastic apron and non-sterile gloves (Ch. 15)
- Collect either the clean bedpan and a bedpan cover, or the commode from the sluice. The commode is first checked to ensure that the brakes are in working order and the commode seat, handles and foot rests are clean
- Take the bedpan or commode to the bedside; if using the commode, position and apply the brakes
- Draw curtains around the bed to promote privacy and dignity
- Ensure wipes and tissues are readily available
- Assist the patient onto the bedpan, if possible well supported in an upright position. Offer assistance if needed to remove/move clothing. Placing a disposable incontinence sheet under the bedpan will aid personal cleansing following defecation.

  If a commode is used, ensure that slippers are worn by the patient to prevent slipping. Assist the patient from the bed to the commode, offering assistance to remove/move clothing. Once the patient is safely seated on the commode cover their knees with a blanket to promote dignity and keep them warm
- Once the patient is safely seated on the bedpan or commode ensure support with balance is offered as required
- Instruct the patient not to remove themselves from the bedpan unaided as this may lead to injury or spillage of contents, or not to attempt to transfer themselves from commode to bed unaided
- Stay with the patient if they wish or require constant supervision, or ensure that the patient can reach the call bell to indicate when defecation is completed
- Remove the commode or bedpan and ensure that the protective sheet is in place
- Offer assistance with personal cleansing as required and remove the incontinence sheet from beneath the patient. When assisting females, wipe from front to back to avoid bacterial contamination of the urethra (see Chs 16, 20)
- Remove the commode or covered bedpan with protective sheet to the sluice
- Observe the colour, amount and consistency of the stool passed (see p. 605)
- Take any required samples before disposing of the stool (see p. 617)
- Wash/sterilize/dispose of the bedpan, or clean the commode according to local policy (see Ch. 15)
- Remove and dispose of apron and gloves and wash hands (see Ch. 15)
- Return to the patient to offer handwashing equipment: wet and dry wipes, or a bowl, jug of water and hand towels (see Ch. 15). Respect cultural preferences
- Ensure that the patient is comfortable and has everything they need, e.g. call bell, drink, within reach
- Make sure the immediate environment is tidy, use air-freshener as necessary and open the curtains
- Document bowel action in patient records and report any abnormalities.

some people may pass stools more frequently than others. Normal bowel movement can occur anything from three times a day to twice a week (Crouch 2003). A useful definition may be 'an alteration in normal bowel movements, resulting in the less frequent and uncomfortable passage of hard stools'.

For the most part, constipation is a temporary condition and not life threatening. People often treat it with over-the-counter laxatives without any advice from a healthcare professional. This, however, can lead to recurrence of the condition and a key part in the management of constipation is education for prevention (see Box 21.10, p. 608). When there is no underlying medical cause for recurrent episodes of constipation, the term chronic idiopathic constipation is used. Many people do seek medical advice, with constipation accounting for approximately three million general practitioner (GP) consultations each year in the UK, with an estimated 10% of the population taking laxatives regularly (Moayyeddi 1998).

Constipation may be secondary to systemic or bowel disease and a thorough assessment on presentation is undertaken to ensure that underlying disease is detected.

Box 21.17 The effects of constipation

- Abdominal colic
- Flatulence
- Bloating
- Lethargy and feeling generally unwell
- Irritability and fretfulness in children, e.g. no interest in play
- Excessive straining during defecation
- Headache
- Nausea
- Halitosis ('bad breath')
- Faecal impaction with overflow diarrhoea (spurious). This may be mistakenly diagnosed as diarrhoea. If antidiarrhoeal drugs are prescribed, this will exacerbate the constipation
- An abdominal mass
- Increased confusion in people with dementia
- Changes in behaviour and distress in people with a learning disability
- Sudden or worsening urinary incontinence due to hard faeces pressing on the bladder or urethra.

Contributing factors and causes of constipation

The dry, hard stools of constipation occur when the colon absorbs too much water. This happens when the muscular contractions of the colon are sluggish, causing the stool to move too slowly through the colon. Lack of fibre in the diet reduces bulk, slowing down motility. Most people will experience an episode of constipation at some time or another such as following childbirth or surgery.

Constipation affects all age groups but it is the very young and older adults who are affected most. People worry more about their bowels as they age, but ageing does not in itself slow down stool movement in the colon (Norton 1996). This is usually due to other factors such as lack of exercise and a reduction in the consumption of fruit, vegetables and bread, increasing the risk of constipation. Fibre intake is positively associated with increased frequency of bowel movement and faecal mass (Bennett & Cerda 1996). The prevalence of constipation may be increasing as modern food processing methods have produced a refined fibre-free diet (Taylor 1997). Other risk factors contributing to the development of constipation may be reduced fluid intake. Older people may drink less in an attempt to control urinary incontinence (see Ch. 20), particularly if mobility is poor and assistance with reaching the lavatory is required.

Box 21.2 (p. 602) outlines the many factors that affect defecation and bowel habit, including those that cause constipation. However, nurses should always be aware of situations when constipation is likely to occur and anticipate the need for interventions, e.g. laxatives when opioid drugs are used for pain relief (see Ch. 23).

Effects of constipation

The effects of constipation are outlined in Box 21.17.

Assessment of constipation

A thorough and complete assessment and history are essential to determine the normal bowel habit for the person (see pp. 603–605) and to identify contributing factors or causes for the condition (see Box 21.2, p. 602). Constipation can be a chronic problem for many individuals.

Self-assessment of bowel habit is also helpful and the person or parent can be taught the use of the Bristol Stool Form Scale (see Fig. 21.3, p. 604). The person may be asked to log their dietary and fluid intake and keep a record of daily exercise.

A doctor or a registered nurse who is appropriately trained and competent will perform a physical examination. This will include:

- Abdominal palpation, which may reveal the presence of a faecal mass
- Digital rectal examination involving the insertion of a lubricated gloved finger into the rectum. It can be performed to assess tone of the anal sphincter and rectal contents. Normally the rectum is empty but can often contain hard stools in constipation. Explicit consent must be obtained from the patient/parent, and documented in nursing and medical records.

Management of constipation

Most people who experience constipation will not require extensive investigation and can be successfully treated with lifestyle changes that include increasing fluid intake, exercise and fibre content of the diet (Box 21.18, p. 612).

In the short term, laxatives may be prescribed to relieve constipation. They are only used if the person is constipated and the cause is not an undiagnosed condition such as intestinal obstruction. Laxatives (or aperients) are drugs that cause the bowel to empty in a variety of ways. There are four basic types, plus bowel cleansing solutions (Table 21.3):

- Bulking agents
- Faecal softeners
- Stimulants
- Osmotic.

Laxatives can be administered orally, rectally as suppositories or as an enema for severe constipation. Many patients will be able to self-administer enemas or suppositories and parents/carers can also be shown how to administer them to children and others. However, it does require a degree of mobility and manual dexterity. People who self-administer should be directed to the manufacturer's instructions and advised to contact their practice nurse or general practitioner if problems arise.

Bowel cleansing solutions are used to empty the lower bowel before investigations that include colonoscopy and barium enema X-ray (see Boxes 21.8 and 21.9, p. 607) and before surgery. Laxatives are also prescribed to prevent constipation, e.g. when people are receiving morphine or other opioid drugs to relieve pain.

Readers requiring more information about a specific laxative are directed to the *British National Formulary* (www.bnf.org.uk).

HEALTH PROMOTION Box 21.18

Increasing fibre intake

Increasing fibre intake is necessary to prevent constipation and is also part of any care plan for the management of constipation. Fibre contributes to the formation of a bulkier stool, as it is not digested. The bulkier stool stimulates the colon to produce a strong peristaltic movement leading to the need to defecate (Crouch 2003).

The following foods contain high levels of fibre (see Ch. 19):

- Wholegrain cereals and bread
- Fruit
- Vegetables
- Pulses and beans.

Enemas

An enema is the introduction of fluid into the rectum or lower bowel for the purpose of producing a bowel movement or instilling medication. The drugs administered rectally include corticosteroids used in inflammatory bowel disease, etc. (see Ch. 22).

The are two types of enema available for the management of constipation: evacuant and retention.

- *Evacuant*, e.g. phosphate enemas supplied in single-dose packs with a standard or long rectal tube, or sodium citrate micro enema (Fig. 21.7). These are used to evacuate the rectum and lower colon of flatus and faecal matter. The enema solution is retained for a short time only (always follow the manufacturer's recommendations and local policy) and is then expelled from the bowel along with faeces and flatus

Table 21.3 Laxatives – oral and rectal

Type	Examples and routes	Action/comments
Bulking agents	Bran, ispaghula and methylcellulose (also a faecal softener) – oral	Increase fibre in the stool, thereby increasing the water absorption by the stool Produces softer, bulkier stool, which stimulates peristalsis and is easier to pass *Note*: Sufficient oral fluids are required to prevent intestinal obstruction
Faecal softeners	Arachis oil retention enema *Note*: Rectal Arachis oil is obtained from peanut/groundnut oil and must never be administered to a person with peanut allergy	Softens the stool and also lubricates the hard stool, making it easier to pass
Stimulants	Senna – oral Bisacodyl – oral and rectal (suppositories) Docusate sodium (also a softener) – oral and rectal (micro-enema) Dantron – oral Glycerol suppositories (rectal) Sodium picosulfate – oral	Stimulate the nerves in the colon and increase intestinal motility
Osmotic laxatives	Lactulose – oral Phosphate and sodium citrate enemas, e.g. Fleet® Ready-to-use Enema, Micralax® Micro enema® – rectal Macrogols, e.g. Idrolax®, Movicol®, Movicol® Paediatric Plain – oral	Act by drawing water into the colon or retaining water in the colon by osmosis, thus distending the colon and stimulating peristalsis
Bowel cleansing solutions	Various preparations, e.g. Fleet Phospho-soda®, Picolax®	Used before examination, barium enema or bowel

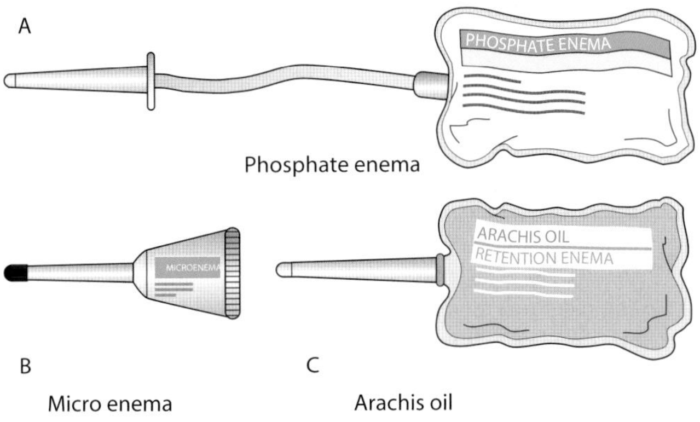

Fig. 21.7 Types of enema (reproduced with permission from Nicol et al 2004).

- *Retention*, e.g. single-dose arachis oil enema (see Fig. 21.7). Retention enemas are usually retained in the bowel for a longer period of time than an evacuant enema in order to soften and lubricate impacted faeces, making it easier to pass.

Before administering an enema it is necessary to obtain informed patient/parent consent.

In order to give informed consent the patient must understand what an enema involves. A clear explanation is required so that the patient understands what is required of them, i.e. retention of the enema solution. The patient must understand the benefits and risks of the intervention in relation to symptom relief, and that this will be short term. The nurse should also consider who is best to administer the enema. For example, a nurse of the same gender as the patient may minimize embarrassment and should be offered whenever possible.

There are contraindications to giving an enema. These include:

- Intestinal obstruction
- Paralytic ileus – lack of peristalsis, common after surgery when the bowel has been handled
- Where there is risk of circulatory overload (see Ch. 19)
- Following certain types of gastrointestinal or gynaecological surgery unless written medical consent is given
- Inflammatory bowel disease (IBD).

The enema must be prescribed by an appropriately qualified practitioner and local policy followed regarding checks on medication and patient identity for the administration of medicines (see Ch. 22). Box 21.19 (p. 614) outlines how the nurse can administer an enema safely and effectively while maintaining privacy and dignity.

Suppositories

Rectal suppositories, like enemas, are used to evacuate the lower bowel. They are also used to administer medications, e.g. bronchodilators, antibiotics and analgesics (see Chs 22, 23). More commonly they are used to relieve constipation. Lubricant suppositories such as glycerol can be purchased without prescription (see Table 21.3).

The procedure for administering suppositories is similar to that for an enema in respect of physical and psychological preparation (Box 21.20, p. 615). If administering a medicated suppository, the patient should be encouraged to first empty their bowel, as this enables better retention of the suppository while the drug is released and absorption is more effective if the rectum is clear of faeces.

There are contraindications to giving suppositories. These include:

- Intestinal obstruction
- Paralytic ileus
- Following certain types of gynaecological or gastrointestinal surgery unless written medical consent is given.

Manual faecal evacuation

For patients who suffer chronic constipation a manual faecal evacuation may be required. Manual faecal evacuation must only be undertaken by a registered practitioner who is trained and competent in the procedure. Prior to this procedure, the patient's pulse rate is recorded, noting rhythm, regularity and strength as well as rate (see Chs 14, 17). This will serve as a baseline, as it is important to respond to changes in the patient's condition during this procedure, as manual evacuation can cause vagal stimulation and slow the heart rate. The presence of a second person allows for constant monitoring during the procedure, and provides reassurance for the patient. Privacy and dignity for the patient must be maintained at all times.

Diarrhoea

Diarrhoea is defined as an abnormal faecal discharge, usually characterized by the frequency at which it occurs and its watery appearance (King 2002), i.e. a loose watery stool that occurs more frequently than normal. Diarrhoea occurs in many gastrointestinal disturbances and may be acute or chronic. Loose stools indicate that the bowel mucosa is irritated and is not absorbing enough water from the stool. There can be rapid transit of material through the bowel.

Contributing factors and causes of diarrhoea

Chronic diarrhoea may be associated with underlying pathology such as IBD (see Table 21.2, p. 606) or malabsorption due to lactose intolerance. The causes of acute diarrhoea include:

- Side-effects of treatment (e.g. radiotherapy), medication (e.g. antibiotics) or enteral feeding via a nasogastric tube (see Ch. 19)
- Infections, e.g. bacterial or viral gastroenteritis, which are a common cause of diarrhoea in babies and small children (see Ch. 15)
- The use of broad-spectrum antibiotics which can predispose to superinfection with the bacterium *Clostridium difficile*; this leads to pseudomembranous colitis and is responsible for outbreaks of diarrhoea in many clinical areas and care settings

NURSING SKILLS Box 21.19

Enema administration – adults

Equipment

- Incontinence pads to protect bed/trolley
- Disposable gloves and apron
- Disposable wipes and tissues
- Prescribed enema/prescription chart
- Jug of water at required temperature, bath thermometer
- Lubricating gel
- Commode or bedpan and tissue, or access to a lavatory.

Preparation

- Explain the procedure to ensure informed consent
- Check that patient does not have a peanut/groundnut allergy before giving an arachis oil enema
- Ensure privacy by using a treatment room or pull curtains around the bed. Ask other staff to avoid interruptions
- Warm the enema in a jug of warm water until the required temperature is reached. Follow the manufacturer's recommendations for single, pre-prepared products. Mallet and Doherty (2000) recommend that the enema be warmed to body temperature, or just above. Oil retention enemas are warmed to 37.8°C
- Assist the patient into the left lateral position, with knees flexed (Fig. 21.8). This allows the nozzle or tubing of the enema to follow the natural anatomy of the colon and gravity will also help flow and/or retention of any solution used (Mallet & Doherty 2000)
- Place an incontinence pad/sheets under the patient's hips and buttocks to protect the bedding and relieve potential distress if fluid is expelled from the anus
- Cover the lower body with a blanket to maintain dignity
- Put on a protective apron, wash hands and put on non-sterile gloves (see Ch. 15).

Procedure

- Lubricate the enema nozzle to minimize anal/rectal trauma
- Separate the patient's buttocks and observe for soreness or other abnormalities
- Introduce the nozzle into the anal canal, which is approximately 3.8 cm in length in adults, and then advance to approximately 10 cm to ensure the tip reaches the rectum. This is normally the full length of the nozzle for pre-prepared enemas
- To administer an evacuant enema, roll the packaging slowly from bottom to top to prevent backflow of the solution into the packet
- Remove the nozzle slowly while still keeping the bag rolled, and encourage the patient to hold onto the solution for as long as possible; however, the effect can be rapid and the patient should not be left without easy access to a nurse call bell
- A retention enema should also be introduced slowly. Again the patient is encouraged to hold onto the solution for as long as prescribed. If possible, this may be aided by raising the foot of the bed against gravity
- Wipe the patient's perianal/perineal area and leave them clean and dry. Cover the patient
- Ensure access to a nurse call bell, a bedpan, a commode or lavatory. When called, give any assistance required (see Box 21.16, p. 610)
- Take the commode or covered bedpan with protective sheet to the sluice
- Observe the colour, amount and consistency of the stool passed (see p. 605)
- Collect faecal specimen if required (see Box 21.22, p. 617)
- Wash/sterilize/dispose of the bedpan, or clean the commode according to local policy (see Ch. 15)
- Remove and dispose of apron and gloves and wash hands (see Ch. 15)
- Return to the patient to offer facilities for personal hygiene and handwashing: wet and dry wipes, or a bowl, jug of water and hand towels (see Ch. 15). Respect cultural preferences
- Ensure that the patient is comfortable and has everything they need, e.g. call bell, drink, within reach
- Make sure the immediate environment is tidy, use air-freshener as necessary and open the curtains
- Document the type of enema given, the resultant bowel action and any specimens collected in patient records and report any abnormalities
- Continue to monitor bowel function, along with reassessment and evaluation of the patient's presenting symptoms.

- Food intolerance or allergic reaction
- Stress and anxiety
- Change in diet or excesses, e.g. alcohol or fatty food.

Box 21.2 (p. 602) outlines other factors that cause diarrhoea. Nurses should always be aware of situations when diarrhoea may occur and anticipate the need for interventions that include ensuring the person's bed/room is close to the lavatory.

Effects of diarrhoea

The effects of diarrhoea are outlined in Box 21.21 (p. 616).

Assessment of diarrhoea

A thorough and complete assessment and history are essential to determine the normal bowel habit for the person (see pp. 603–605) and to identify any contributing factors or causes for the diarrhoea (see Box 21.2, p. 602).

Episodes of diarrhoea are recorded on a stool chart (see Fig. 21.4, p. 606). Frequent, loose watery stools should be measured and recorded on the fluid intake/output chart in order to assess fluid loss. Self-assessment of bowel habit using, for example, the Bristol Stool Form Scale (see Fig. 21.3, p. 604) can be helpful. The person may also be asked to record their dietary intake.

NURSING SKILLS — Box 21.20

Administration of suppositories

Equipment
- Incontinence pads to protect bed/trolley
- Disposable gloves and apron
- Disposable wipes and tissues
- Prescribed suppositories/prescription chart
- Lubricating gel
- Commode or bedpan and lavatory tissue, or easy access to a lavatory.

Preparation
- Explain the procedure to ensure informed consent
- Ensure privacy by using a treatment room or pull curtains around the bed. Ask other staff to avoid interruptions
- Assist the patient into the left lateral position, with knees flexed (see Fig. 21.8)
- Place an incontinence pad/sheets under the patient's hips and buttocks to protect the bedding and relieve potential distress if fluid is expelled from the anus
- Cover the lower body with a blanket to maintain dignity
- Put on a protective apron, wash hands and put on non-sterile gloves (see Ch. 15).

Procedure
- Lubricate the blunt end of the suppository to reduce anal trauma on insertion
- Separate the patient's buttocks and insert the suppository blunt-end first (Fig. 21.9, p. 616), using your index finger to advance the suppository. Repeat for a second suppository. *Note*: Inserting suppositories blunt-end foremost aids retention (Abd-el-Maeboud et al 1991).
- Wipe the patient's perianal/perineal area and leave them clean and dry. Cover the patient
- Ask the patient to retain the suppositories for as long as possible, up to 20 minutes, for suppositories to melt and soften the stool, making it easier to pass
- Ensure access to a nurse call bell, a bedpan, a commode or lavatory. Give assistance as required (see Box 21.16, p. 610)
- Remove commode or covered bedpan with protective sheet to the sluice
- Observe the colour, amount and consistency of the stool passed (see p. 605)
- Collect faecal specimen if required (see Box 21.22, p. 617)
- Wash/sterilize/dispose of the bedpan, or clean the commode according to local policy (see Ch. 15)
- Remove and dispose of apron and gloves and wash hands (see Ch. 15)
- Return to the patient to offer facilities for personal hygiene and handwashing: wet and dry wipes, or a bowl, jug of water and hand towels (see Ch. 15). Respect cultural preferences
- Ensure that the patient is comfortable and has everything they need, e.g. call bell, drink, within reach
- Make sure the immediate environment is tidy, use air-freshener as necessary and open the curtains
- Document the type of suppositories given, the resultant bowel action and any specimens obtained in patient records and report any abnormalities
- Continue to monitor bowel function, along with reassessment and evaluation of the patient's presenting symptoms

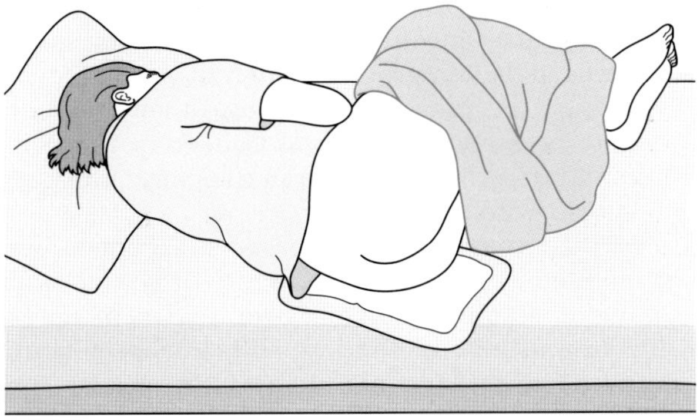

Fig. 21.8 Left lateral position for administration of enemas and suppositories

A specimen of faeces may be collected for microbiological examination (Box 21.22, p. 617).

Management of diarrhoea

Management depends on whether the diarrhoea is acute or chronic. It is important to prevent dehydration and adults and children are advised to take frequent sips of water. Oral dehydration salts can be purchased over-the-counter following advice from the pharmacist (see Ch. 19).

The advice about eating has changed and both adults and children are encouraged to eat high carbohydrate foods, e.g. rice, pasta, etc. if they feel well enough (NHS Direct 2005). Where people do not feel like eating they should continue to drink and try to eat when they feel able.

Babies with diarrhoea should be fed as normal if they will breastfeed or take formula milk. The formula feed should be made up at the usual strength. If oral rehydration preparations are used, breast or formula milk should continue to be offered between oral rehydration fluids (*British National Formulary* 2005).

Adults may use antidiarrhoeal drugs, e.g. loperamide. However, anyone with a high temperature, or blood or mucus in their stool, should first seek medical advice. Parents and carers should not give over-the-counter antidiarrhoeal drugs to children. If symptoms persist, or signs of dehydration are present, medical advice must be sought.

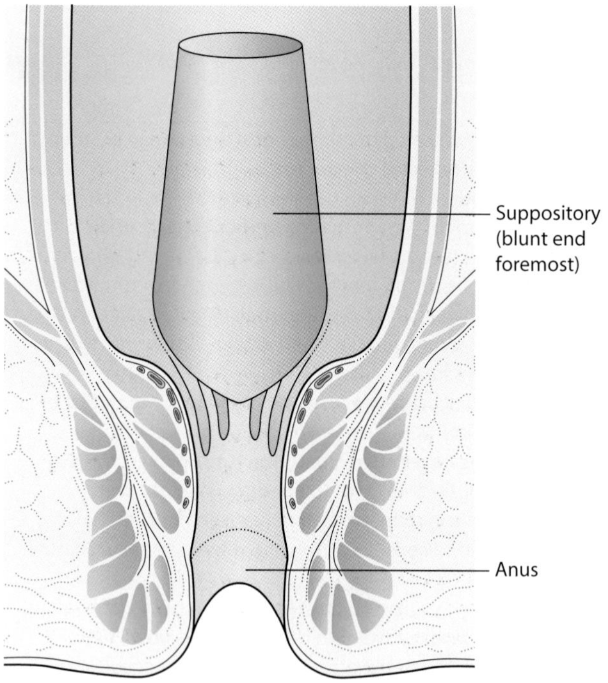

Fig. 21.9 Position of suppository – blunt-end foremost

Box 21.21 **Effects of diarrhoea**

- Watery stools without solid matter
- Increased frequency, more than five times in a 24-hour period
- Loss of fluid and electrolytes – potentially life threatening, e.g. in babies, children and frail older people (see Ch. 19)
- Loss of nutrients in watery stools
- Perianal soreness
- Flatulence
- Abdominal pains and cramps
- Nausea and vomiting, e.g. with infective diarrhoea
- Poor appetite
- Increased body temperature if infective
- Headache
- Foul-smelling stools
- Embarrassment
- Urgency, need to get to a lavatory quickly
- Loss of continence in previously continent children and adults
- Faecal soiling.

Note: It is vital to exclude faecal impaction with faecal leakage (spurious diarrhoea) (see p. 611).

Other nursing interventions for a person with diarrhoea include the following:

- Ensure that the person is located close to the lavatory, has an en-suite side ward or a bedpan/commode readily available
- Provide adequate ventilation and/or air fresheners to minimize embarrassment
- Provide soft tissue or wet wipes
- Provide assistance with perianal hygiene and change pads or napkins promptly to prevent skin damage
- Observe for soreness, excoriation, nappy rash and apply barrier cream as appropriate
- Provide clean clothes and bed linen
- Observe for signs of fluid depletion (see Ch. 19)
- Ensure adequate fluid replacement (see p. 615 and Ch. 19)
- Implement infection control measure such as handwashing and seek advice from Infection Control Nurses (see Ch. 15)
- Collect a faecal sample for microbiological examination (see Box 21.22)
- Provide appropriate dietary and food hygiene advice (Box 21.23)

Faecal incontinence

There is a lack of consensus about a definition for faecal incontinence, but it can be described as the inappropriate or involuntary passage of faeces (Royal College of Physicians 1995). The defining characteristics for faecal incontinence include:

- Faecal soiling
- Involuntary passage of faeces (in a socially inappropriate place)
- Lack of awareness of the urge to defecate, or muddling the sense with that of passing flatus.

Faecal incontinence is a taboo subject with a high degree of social stigma; it is often associated with regression and lack of control. Faecal incontinence tends to be underreported because people find it repugnant and are often reluctant to seek help. The reluctance to report faecal incontinence means that prevalence is underestimated. Faecal incontinence is more common in older people and affects more women than men. Studies have reported the prevalence amongst those aged over 65 years to be higher. The Royal College of Physicians (1995) found that 15% of people in the community aged over 65 years were affected.

Faecal incontinence in children is referred to as encopresis, defined as repeated involuntary or voluntary faecal soiling of clothing by a child over 4 years of age (see p. 619). Around 1.5% of children still lack bowel control by their 7th birthday (Royal College of Physicians 1995).

Continence services are available, and need to be accessible for all and this is made clear in the benchmark of best practice: 'Patients have direct access to professionals who can meet their continence needs and their services are actively promoted' (NHS Modernisation Agency 2003). There is a need for an integrated continence service that spans both primary and secondary care settings, focusing on healthy living and ensuring specialist continence advice for maintaining both faecal and urinary continence and care if continence is lost (Box 21.24). The philosophy underpinning such services is that promoting continence will reduce the incidence of incontinence.

NURSING SKILLS Box 21.22

Collection of stool/faecal sample

The patient or parent/carer often collects the sample at home and should follow the instructions provided with the sample container. Stool samples are also collected for faecal occult blood testing and for the presence of parasites.

Equipment

- Disposable gloves and apron
- Bedpan or commode
- Sterile stool sample container (with integral spatula) and specimen bag
- Request form for microbiology.

Preparation

- Explain the procedure to the patient to ensure informed consent
- Collect the specimen container, request form and transport bag
- Put on plastic apron and non-sterile gloves (see Ch. 15)
- Ensure privacy. Where possible the person should go to the lavatory to produce a sample; where this is not possible the person is offered a bedpan or the commode
- Ensure that a nurse call bell is available and assist as required
- Place a clinically clean bedpan beneath the lavatory seat
- Ideally the person should void urine separately, but if this is not possible lavatory tissue in the bedpan will absorb most of the urine
- The bedpan/commode is removed to the sluice and the stool examined for colour and consistency, and evidence of parasites (see p. 605)
- Open the faecal sample container and use the integral spatula (fixed in the lid) to collect a small amount of faeces from the bedpan and place the faeces and spatula in the container. Make sure that the sample container lid is securely closed
- Dispose of the remaining excreta in line with local policy
- Wash/sterilize/dispose of the bedpan, or clean the commode according to local policy (see Ch. 15)
- Assist with hygiene needs if required
- Remove gloves and apron and wash hands
- Label the specimen container with the correct patient information and enclose in a specimen bag with the completed request form
- Arrange for transfer to the laboratory
- Document the observation made of the faecal matter on the stool chart
- Record date and time the specimen was collected in patient records.

HEALTH PROMOTION Box 21.23

Preventing traveller's diarrhoea

Traveller's diarrhoea is usually caused by viruses and as such does not respond to antibiotics. The source is often the water supply in areas where sanitation and general hygiene are poor.

Advice to travellers about preventing diarrhoea includes:

- Using bottled water (sealed bottles) for drinking and teeth cleaning
- Avoiding ice cubes in cold drinks
- Avoiding salads and uncooked foods
- Washing hands after using the lavatory and before eating
- Obtaining necessary vaccinations before travelling
- Carrying a supply of antidiarrhoeal drugs and oral rehydration salts.

REFLECTIVE PRACTICE Box 21.24

Continence services

Think about a patient/client or a relative who had faecal incontinence.

Student activities

- Did this person have support from the continence service?
- Is there an integrated continence service in your area?
- Is a specialist continence nurse available?

Contributing factors and causes of faecal incontinence

The causes of faecal incontinence include:

- Constipation – among the commonest causes of faecal incontinence in older people
- Diarrhoea such as IBD
- Pelvic floor problems, including loss of sensation, weak muscles or rectal prolapse in older people. May be caused by damage during childbirth many decades earlier
- Loss of sensation in the anal area caused by damage to nerves controlling sphincter/rectum, e.g. long-term straining to defecate, stroke, spina bifida and conditions such as multiple sclerosis, which damage the nerves
- Sphincter abnormalities or damage, e.g. after haemorrhoid surgery, or reduced rectal capacity caused by chronic inflammation, surgery, etc.

Factors that contribute to faecal incontinence include dementia, lack of facilities or poor access, immobility and poor manual dexterity.

Box 21.2 (p. 602) outlines factors that affect bowel habit, many of which can lead to loss of continence, e.g. faecal impaction with overflow (spurious) diarrhoea. Nurses should always be aware of situations when continence may be lost and anticipate the need for interventions that include the use of laxatives to minimize constipation when patients are prescribed opioids.

Effects of faecal incontinence

The effects of faecal incontinence are outlined in Box 21.25.

Access to a lavatory or other facility is a major concern for all patients who experience urgency to defecate. This is a common problem for people with IBD who also have bowel actions that are explosive, noisy and malodorous (Box 21.26).

Assessment of faecal incontinence

A full patient history and physical assessment are essential to determine the normal bowel habit for the person (see pp. 603–605), and to identify any contributing factors or causes for faecal incontinence (see Box 21.2, p. 602). Physical factors such as mobility and manual dexterity and access to appropriate facilities for defecation must form part of any assessment, along with assessment of factors such as cognition and motivation.

Episodes of incontinence can be recorded on a stool chart (see Fig. 21.4, p. 606) and self-assessment of bowel habit using, for example, the Bristol Stool Form Scale (see Fig. 21.3, p. 604) can be helpful. The person, parent or carer may also be asked to record food and fluid intake and regular exercise pattern.

Box 21.25 Effects of faecal incontinence

- Embarrassment caused by odour and noisy/explosive defecation
- Low self-esteem
- Urgency to defecate
- Perianal soreness
- Risk of pressure ulcer development (see Ch. 25)
- Behaviours to keep problem hidden, e.g. hiding soiled underwear
- Financial – clothing/pads/laundry
- Social – isolation and loneliness, need for proximity to lavatory.

REFLECTIVE PRACTICE Box 21.26

Urgency and defecation

23-year-old Rosa has IBD and needs to plan any journeys very carefully because if she is unable to respond at once to the urge to defecate she will soil her underwear. She needs to know the location of every public lavatory and always has clean underwear, a bag for soiled pants and wet wipes in her bag.

Student activities

- Consider the psychological and social impact of the potential for faecal incontinence on this young woman's life.
- How would you feel about the possibility of being 'caught short' in a public place?

Managing faecal incontinence

The management of faecal incontinence will depend upon the cause. It is often secondary to constipation and may be resolved through the following:

- Treatment of constipation with laxatives, including rectal preparations to empty the bowel (see p. 612)
- Increases in fibre and fluid intake
- Planned regular meal times
- Increased exercise to stimulate gastrointestinal motility
- Immediate response to the urge to defecate when normal sensation and sphincter muscle function is present.

A toileting programme that closely follows the person's previous normal bowel habit, such as sitting on the lavatory after breakfast, can be very helpful. For patients requiring assistance to the lavatory, an immediate response from the nurse to the patient's request is essential before the gastrocolic reflex subsides.

The specialist continence nurse/adviser can provide information and education about prevention of faecal incontinence and measures to regain continence (see Further reading, e.g. Wells 2003).

When patients have impairment of both sensation and sphincter control, as in conditions such as multiple sclerosis, the bowel is usually emptied by routine administration of enemas or suppositories (see pp. 214, 215). The National Institute for Health and Clinical Excellence provide guidance for the management of bowel problems for people with chronic conditions which recommend that the patient be assessed and considered for the routine use of enemas or suppositories (NICE 2003).

Antidiarrhoeal drugs such as loperamide may be used to produce a more formed stool if the faecal incontinence is due to a very liquid stool.

More advanced methods such as biofeedback may be used by specialist nurses and physiotherapists to retrain the anal sphincter muscles that control release of bowel movement. Other methods for managing faecal incontinence may be more radical and involve surgery; these interventions will be specific to the cause, i.e. rectal prolapse.

Continence may not be achievable and nurses will need to plan care that minimizes the effects while continuing to promote continence. The care will include:

- Advice regarding suitable underwear, e.g. for use with small pads
- Providing appropriate pads
- Protection for bedding/chairs
- Skin care, cleanliness and use of barrier cream
- Checking for skin damage (see Ch. 25)
- Education about safe disposal of pads, etc.

- Ensuring that patients are aware of entitlement to state benefits such as attendance allowance
- Providing contact details of support groups (see 'Useful websites', p. 625)
- Maintaining dignity and privacy.

Encopresis

There is sometimes confusion caused in diagnosis of encopresis and faecal soiling with other childhood problems. For example, fear associated with using the lavatory may lead to a child soiling their clothes. Children who are isolated and lonely may smear faeces; however, this is different from encopresis, as they have control of their bowel and their behaviour is a symptom of an emotional disorder (Heins & Ritchie 1985).

In most cases of encopresis, prolonged constipation and faecal impaction is the most likely cause. Stretch receptors in the rectum are continually stimulated because the rectum is full of faeces and this leads to the prohibition of signals and loss of the normal response of muscle contraction. It can take 2–6 months for an overstretched rectum to return to normal functioning (Heins & Ritchie 1985).

For a school-age child, social acceptance is important; a feeling of belonging and inclusion among peers will aid development of self-esteem and confidence (Gross 2001). A child with encopresis is likely to experience difficulties (Box 21.27). The child may be unable to wash/change in privacy after faecal soiling and this may lead to 'being smelly' and a focus of fun for other children. The child may avoid activities such as games where there is a need to undress in public. Opportunities to go on school trips and sleepovers may be rejected to avoid embarrassing situations. The response from parents/carers is important, as family support is vital; reprisal and rejection from constant criticism and telling off will only lead to further isolation and lowering of self-esteem (Gross 2001).

The MDT will usually be involved in planning strategies and supporting the child and family in resolving the problem. The composition of the team will depend on the cause of the child's encopresis. They may include the specialist continence nurse, GP, psychologist, school nurse, community nurse and dietitian.

Strategies used to resolve encopresis will include dealing with constipation and education (see pp. 611–612) about diet and exercise to avoid recurrence once the current episode has been relieved.

The bowel has to regain the ability to respond to stretch receptor signals, and also to contract and relax to expel faeces from the bowel. Recording the times that faecal soiling occurs will give some indication of when the child should be encouraged to visit the lavatory. Visiting the lavatory each morning will reduce the amount of faeces left in the bowel and hence the risk of soiling later in the day. A breakfast comprising a high-fibre cereal such as porridge will help but a laxative may be necessary.

Choosing high-fibre options such as fruit and vegetables from school dinner menus or healthy sandwiches made with granary bread with salad and a fruit snack, plus sufficient water for the day, is essential. Again, visiting the lavatory after meals (usually 20 minutes) when the bowel muscles begin to respond to the feeling of fullness is important. Informing teachers of the need to access lavatory facilities, even though this may disrupt lessons, is important, as is access to somewhere private to change for physical education lessons.

REFLECTIVE PRACTICE Box 21.27

Encopresis – the emotional and social effects

Sam is 8 years old and attends primary school. Over the last few months Sam has developed faecal soiling.

Student activities

- Consider some of the emotional and social difficulties Sam may experience.
- Discuss with your mentor how these difficulties may affect Sam's relationships with his classmates and his ability to fully engage in school and social activities.

Caring for a person with a stoma

A stoma is an artificial opening of an internal organ, such as the bowel discharging faeces onto the surface of the body (Fig. 21.10). An outline of stoma care is provided here but more information is available in the Further reading suggestions (e.g. Bruce & Finlay 1997).

Types of stomas include:

- Colostomy – the colon opens onto the abdominal wall
- Ileostomy – the ileum opens onto the abdominal wall
- Urostomy – a stoma that drains urine (see Ch. 20).

Approximately 80000–100000 people in the UK have a stoma. Colostomy patients form the largest proportion of patients requiring a stoma (Black 2000).

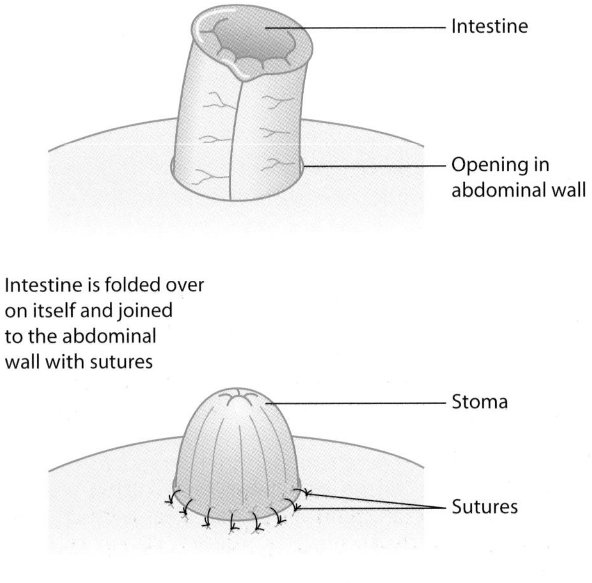

Fig. 21.10 Stoma formation

A colostomy may be performed as a temporary measure to divert faeces away from a healing anastomosis (join) or diseased area, allowing bowel continuity to be restored at a later date. When this is not possible the colostomy will be permanent.

The anatomical position of the stoma will determine the consistency of faecal output. An ascending colostomy will produce soft/liquid stool, while transverse and descending colostomies produce an increasingly formed stool because a greater length of colon is available to absorb water from the faeces. Some patients may require an ileostomy, in which the end of the ileum or a loop of the ileum is brought out to the surface of the abdominal wall. The stool from an ileostomy will be a liquid/soft stool.

Stoma formation may be undertaken for a variety of conditions. These include:

- Colorectal cancer
- Trauma
- Bowel ischaemia (poor blood supply)
- Congenital bowel malformations; stoma surgery is usually carried out within hours of birth
- Hirschsprung's disease
- Diverticular disease
- Inflammatory bowel disease
- Faecal incontinence
- Bowel obstruction
- Intestinal inflammation following radiation.

Specific preoperative care for patients having a stoma

Preparation for stoma formation will depend on the reason for surgery, and whether it is planned or undertaken as an emergency. Readers are directed to Chapter 24 for details of general preoperative care.

Physical and psychological preparation should include:

- A full explanation of all aspects of the surgery, the immediate aftercare, e.g. intravenous fluids, nasogastric tube for aspiration, drains, etc., and gradual reintroduction of oral fluids and diet
- Details about the stoma such as that, in some types, the patient will still have some mucus discharge rectally despite faeces being discharged through the stoma
- Administration of prophylactic antibiotics to minimize the risk of infection
- The opportunity for the patient and family members to talk about issues of altered body image, relationships and activities such as sport and work. The factors that affect the patient's ability to adapt to an alteration in body image are the disease process, diagnosis, treatment and the professional care received within the primary and secondary health care setting (Black 2000). Adaptation to changes in body image is often associated with the grieving process and recovery time is individual, eventually each person reaching an acceptance of what is gone and adapting to life with its absence (see Ch. 12).
- Dietary modification – normal diet up to 24 hours before surgery then clear fluids only. A bowel cleansing solution such as Picolax® may also be administered to clear solid material from the bowel. These measures help to ensure a clear bowel, which will aid visibility for the surgeon and reduce the risk of infection
- Input from the specialist stoma care nurse to provide information, education and support to the patient, family and the nursing team (Boxes 21.28, 21.29). The stoma nurse will provide diagrams and photographs of what a stoma looks like, and information including written or audio/video material about managing the stoma. It can be helpful for patients to have the opportunity to meet and talk with a person who has a stoma. Knowledge of the type of stoma and the expected output will influence the appliance

Box 21.28 **Role of the specialist stoma care nurse**

The stoma care nurse is part of the MDT involved in supporting adults, children and families in their preparation and adaptation to life with a stoma. They work in acute hospitals and the community.

The role involves the following:

- Education and support for the person and their family
- Counselling regarding lifestyle adaptations, relationships, body image and expressing sexuality
- Acting as patient advocate when necessary
- Education of other healthcare professionals
- Updating knowledge of developments and evidence to support best practice
- Participation in clinical audit and research.

Manufacturers of stoma care products often employ stoma care advisers (not to be confused with specialist stoma care nurses) to support patients and professionals but also to promote particular products.

CRITICAL THINKING Box 21.29

Mary – information needs before stoma formation

Mary has been diagnosed with colorectal cancer. The position and extent of Mary's cancer means that the colon cannot be joined together (an anastomosis) and a permanent colostomy is necessary.

Student activities

- What aspects of the planned surgery are likely to cause Mary most anxiety?
- Access some information about stoma formation for cancer from a support group (see 'Useful websites', p. 625)
- Find out if there is a specialist stoma care nurse working in your locality.

(pouch/bag) chosen. The presence of allergies also needs to be considered, as most stoma appliances have a flange that adheres directly to the skin

- The position of the stoma should be carefully planned with the involvement of the patient/carer, the surgeon and the stoma nurse to ensure optimum self-care in daily living activities. For example, will the patient be able to see and reach the stoma for pouch emptying? Knowledge of any difficulties with manual dexterity or disability will also influence the choice of appliance.

Specific postoperative care for a patient having a stoma

Postoperative care following stoma formation is also influenced by the reason for surgery, and whether it was planned or undertaken as an emergency. Readers are directed to Chapter 24 for details of general postoperative care.

Specific postoperative care should include:

- Ensuring that intravenous fluids (see Ch. 19) are maintained until oral fluids and diet can be reintroduced. Following bowel surgery peristalsis is reduced (paralytic ileus) due to the handling during surgery and the anaesthetic. Peristalsis normally starts to return after 48 hours and small amounts of oral fluid are introduced, increasing in amount if tolerated, and progressing to a light diet, usually within 5 days if the stoma begins to function. The amount of observed flatus and audible bowel sounds give an indication that the stoma is starting to work
- Ensuring that the nasogastric tube is draining or gastric contents are aspirated by syringe at regular intervals to reduce the risk of nausea and vomiting until peristalsis returns
- Administration of prophylactic antibiotics
- Early postoperative observation of the stoma to include colour, length, location, size, etc. Colour is very important; normally the stoma is red and moist and signs of a poor blood supply such as a dark red or dusky appearance must be reported at once and recorded in the nursing notes. Failure to deal with this can lead to bowel necrosis.

Appliances and skin care

It is usually 48 hours postoperatively that the drainable appliance put on in theatre is changed for the first time (Black 2000). It is usual practice to use a clear plastic pouch when in hospital as this allows the nurses to observe the stoma and any output directly. Patients are initially very distressed by the odour produced when the pouch is emptied or changed, and should be reassured that this will decrease as diet is reintroduced (Black 2000). Pouches that are opaque and have flatus filters and contain charcoal to reduce odour can be introduced later should they be required (see p. 622).

Appliances may be either one- or two-piece, with a flange, sealed or drainable (Fig. 21.11). A two-piece appliance allows the flange to remain in contact with the skin and the pouch can be removed and changed without

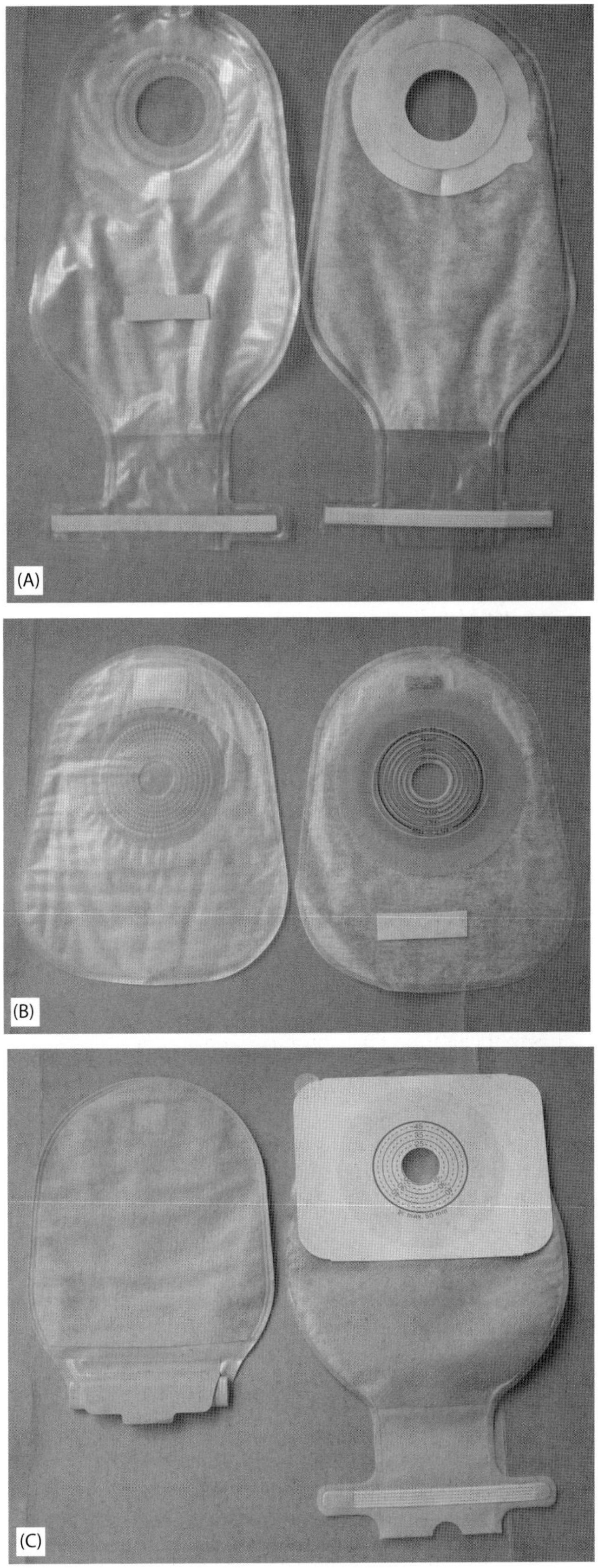

Fig. 21.11 Selection of stoma pouches/bags – front and back views: **A.** Drainable pouch/bag. **B.** Sealed pouch/bag. **C.** Opaque pouch/bag (drainable).

disturbing the flange. The flange is usually changed every 2–3 days; however, it may be left for longer when skin is sore to avoid further irritation (manufacturer's guidelines must always be followed). Sealed pouches are often used with a colostomy, and although the contents can be flushed down the lavatory, the bags must be placed in a plastic disposal bag and disposed of with normal household waste.

Patients with an ileostomy generally use a drainable pouch. Patients are encouraged to protect the skin around the stoma with a barrier cream.

Skin must be kept in optimum condition to tolerate the stoma appliance. Karaya, a natural absorbent rubber, revolutionized stoma care in the 1950s. However, some patients developed allergies and difficulties with adherence (Black 2000). It is still used by some patients who have had a stoma for many years.

In 1972 Stomahesive® was introduced. It is a flat wafer that is resistant to temperature, perspiration and the gastrointestinal fluids which come into direct contact with it. Stomahesive can be tolerated by inflamed and weepy skin and can be left in place for up to 15 days without requiring change.

When appliances are changed the skin should be cleansed and dried. Protective wafers should be used to fix appliances to the skin. If skin is prone to inflammation the longer the wafer can remain in situ the better, meaning a two-piece appliance would be worn.

The therapeutic relationship between the patient and the healthcare team is important in assisting the patient in accepting the stoma. By seeing the nurses at ease when providing early stoma care, patients/parents and carers are more likely to accept the changes to their physical appearance. Box 21.30 outlines the procedure for changing a stoma pouch.

Continuing stoma care – advice and support for patients

Various designs and colours of pouches are available, including some designed specifically for children. Pouches and appliances are designed to lie flat, be odour-free, rustle-free and to be unnoticeable under clothing. Some pouches

NURSING SKILLS Box 21.30

Changing a stoma pouch

A planned teaching programme ensures that the patient does not feel rushed and has the opportunity to develop confidence and dexterity with the procedure. Initially, pouch changes are managed by the bedside but the aim is for the patient to change the appliance in the bathroom. This will increase confidence for coping at home. In the case of a child, the parents/carers will be taught to care for the stoma until the child is able to self-care.

Equipment

- Bowl of warm water
- Gauze wipes
- Barrier cream
- Clean stoma appliance – one- or two-piece
- Stoma template/measurement tool (Fig. 21.12)
- Scissors and a pen if a new flange for a two-piece appliance is required or to customize a one-piece appliance to the patient's stoma
- Clinical waste disposal bag
- Protective sheet
- Disposable gloves and apron
- Disposable jug for the used appliance or the faecal drainage from a drainable bag. If supporting a patient/client in the bathroom the contents of a drainable bag may be emptied directly into the lavatory.

Preparation

- Prepare the patient for the procedure, remembering that many patients will be anxious and distressed about seeing the stoma
- Explain the procedure to the patient to ensure informed consent
- Wash and dry hands and put on protective gloves and apron
- Ensure privacy
- Protect the bedding
- Empty contents from a drainable appliance bag
- Gently remove the used pouch from top to bottom. Support the surrounding skin to avoid pulling and patient discomfort
- Use the soft gauze to wash the skin around the stoma and dry thoroughly. Dispose of used wipes in the clinical waste bag
- Observe skin condition for redness or excoriation
- If necessary, measure the stoma by placing the curved edges of the measurement tool around the stoma until an exact measurement is achieved. This provides a template for cutting the flange in the new appliance to the correct size, ensuring a good fit to prevent excoriation of the surrounding skin by contact with faecal material
- When applying the new flange, ensure the lower edge fits with the bottom of the stoma, folding the top half over the stoma and pressing firmly to the skin. Attach the new pouch, remembering to apply clip if appropriate (Fig. 21.13)
- Remove equipment to the sluice. Measure the faecal material if fluid output is being recorded. The used pouch or disposable jug should be emptied into the sluice or lavatory. The pouch and disposable jug are disposed of in the clinical waste
- Remove protective gloves and apron and wash hands (see Ch. 15)
- Return to the patient to offer handwashing facilities if the patient assisted with the pouch change. Respect cultural preferences
- Ensure that the patient is comfortable and has everything they need, e.g. call bell, drink, within reach
- Make sure the immediate environment is tidy, use air-freshener as necessary and open the curtains
- Document the procedure in the nursing notes, including the appearance of the stoma, skin condition and the faecal matter produced. Record output as appropriate.

have an inner lining that can be flushed with the contents down the lavatory, and soft cloth covers are available for some pouches. Appliances can be left in place or removed during bathing/showering. Once the patient has found a suitable appliance, the stoma care nurse will advise them about obtaining supplies after discharge.

Prior to discharge all stoma patients should be given contact numbers/email address for the stoma care nurse. When patients are discharged from hospital they are supplied with sufficient appliances for at least the first week with extra to cover any public holidays. The district nurse or GP will provide prescriptions for appliances. Continuation of supplies may be direct from the manufacturer or from the local pharmacy.

Following discharge, the GP, district nurse and the stoma care nurse who works between the hospital and community assist the patient/parent to prevent or overcome any problems that arise. Other members of the MDT such as the dietitian may also provide specialist advice. In the case of children the specialist community public health nurse (health visitor) and school nurses will also be involved in their ongoing care.

Clothing which has some stretch and give provides most comfort by avoiding the restrictions of waistbands and belts.

Most patients will quickly discover any food or drink that upsets the function of their stoma, e.g. changes in stool consistency, odour, blockage or excess flatus. However, they should be given advice regarding eating a balanced diet (see Ch. 19) and informed about food and drink that are known to cause problems. For example, beer and onions can cause flatus, and eggs and onions are associated with odour. Many patients find that a bulkier stool is more manageable and will want to increase their intake of fibre with, for example, bananas, boiled rice, pasta, etc.

Support groups are very useful sources of information and support (see 'Useful websites', p. 625). These groups provide information about travelling and holidays, special appliances for sports and swimming for adults and children, etc. Patients whose stomas function at regular times can use a special cap while swimming instead of a pouch.

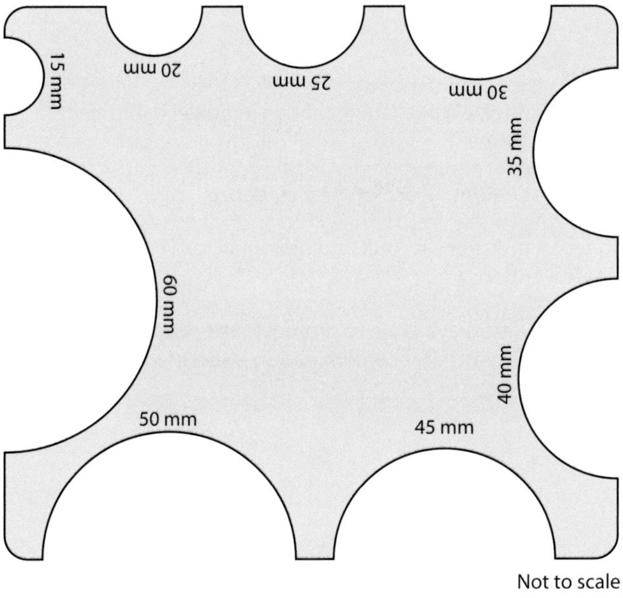

Fig. 21.12 Stoma measurement tool

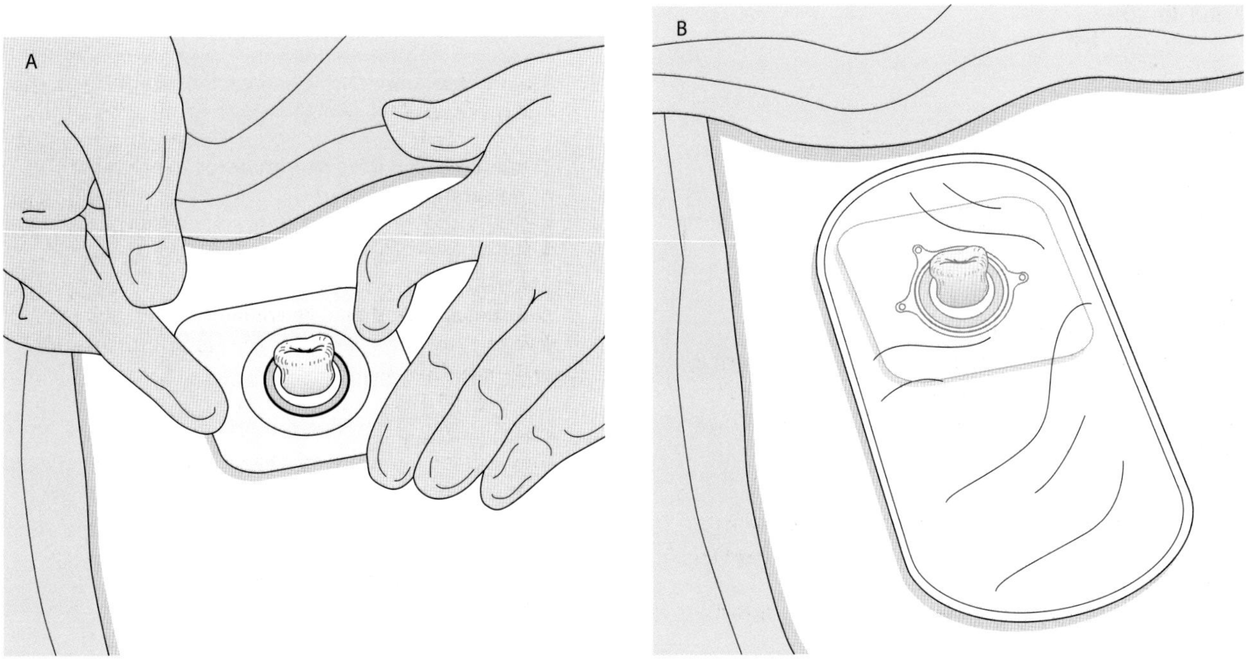

Fig. 21.13 Changing a stoma pouch/bag: **A.** Fitting the flange. **B.** Stoma pouch/bag in place (reproduced with permission from Nicol et al 2004)

Summary

- Defecation is a normal bodily function, yet it carries great taboo.
- The inability to defecate normally can impact on the person's physical, psychological, social, spiritual and emotional well-being.
- Symptoms of disease are often ignored due to the embarrassment and fear of cancer and physical examination.
- Holistic assessment is necessary to ensure that health professionals work together in partnership with patients, setting achievable and attainable goals as part of the nursing process, in any care setting. Thorough bowel assessment will enable care to be planned and implemented that takes into account individual lifestyle, culture, beliefs and behaviours.
- Education about reporting changes in bowel habit is an essential part of the nurse's role.
- Bowel care is far from basic; it requires a skilled and knowledgeable practitioner.
- Bowel care should be viewed as essential care. For those individuals who recognize a persistent change in bowel habit, and actively seek help and advice, much can be done to resolve distressing symptoms.
- The nurse requires knowledge of common bowel conditions and their management, based on best evidence.
- Skill is required in eliciting information, as many patients will be inhibited in this process. Tact and diplomacy are essential, as is the need to provide privacy and promote dignity during any nursing interventions.
- Equity in access to services ensures individuals receive the best advice and support available to promote independence in faecal elimination wherever possible, and to promote personal dignity when assistance with faecal elimination is required.

Self test

1. How much water makes up the weight of faeces?
   a. 10–20%
   b. 30–40%
   c. 40–50%
   d. 60–70%
2. At what age is it most appropriate to commence potty/lavatory training for a child?
   a. 3–6 months
   b. 12–18 months
   c. 18–24 months
   d. 36–48 months
3. List three drugs that can alter bowel habit.
4. During assessment, which characteristics of faeces should the nurse note?
5. What position is used to administer an enema or suppositories and why?
6. List four causes of faecal incontinence.

Key words and phrases for literature searching

Bowel care
Constipation
Diarrhoea
Faecal incontinence
Stoma care

Useful websites

BBC	www.bbc.co.uk/health Available July 2006
Ileostomy and Internal Pouch Support Group	www.the-ia.org.uk Available July 2006
National Advisory Service for Parents of Children with a Stoma (NASPCS)	www.patient.co.uk/showdoc/267391771 Available July 2006
National Association for Colitis and Crohn's disease	www.nacc.org.uk Available July 2006
National Digestive Diseases Information Clearing House	http://digestive.niddk.nih.gov Available July 2006
National Institute for Health and Clinical Excellence	www.nice.org.uk Available July 2006
Prodigy – *practical support for clinical governance*	www.prodigy.nhs.uk Available July 2006
The Continence Foundation	www.continence-foundation.org.uk Available July 2006

References

Abd-el-Maeboud KH, el-Naggar T, el-Hawi EM et al 1991 Rectal suppositories: commonsense mode of insertion. Lancet 338(8770):798–800

Akhtar SG 2002 Nursing with dignity – Islam. Nursing Times 98(16):40

Bennett WG, Cerda JJ 1996 Dietary fibre: fact and fiction. Digestive Disorders 14:43–58

Black P 2000 Continuing professional development. Stoma care. Nursing Standard 14(41):47–53

British National Formulary 2005 Online: www.bnf.org.uk Available July 2006

Burkitt D, Walker A, Painter N 1972 Effect of dietary fibre on stool and transit time and its role in the causation of disease. Lancet 2(7792):1408–1412

Crouch D 2003 Easing the pain of constipation. Nursing Times 99(11):23–25

Gross RD 2001 Psychology: the science of mind and behaviour. 4th edn. Hodder and Stoughton, London

Heins T, Ritchie K 1985 Beating sneaky poo. ACT Health Authority, Canberra Publishing and Printing Co. (available from NASPCS, see Useful websites)

Jamieson E, McCall J, Whyte L 2002 Clinical nursing practice. 4th edn. Churchill Livingstone, Edinburgh

King D 2002 Determining the cause of diarrhoea. Nursing Times 98(23):47–48

Mallet J, Doherty L (eds) 2000 The Royal Marsden Hospital manual of clinical nursing procedures. 5th edn. Blackwell Science, London

Moayyeddi P 1998 The patient with constipation. Nursing Update 24 June:1302–1306

National Institute for Clinical Excellence 2003 Multiple sclerosis: management of multiple sclerosis in primary and secondary care. Clinical Guideline No 8. NICE, London

NHS Direct 2005 Health Encyclopaedia. Online: www.nhsdirect.nhs.uk/en.aspx?ArticleID=131 Available July 2006

NHS Modernisation Agency 2003 Essence of care guidance – patient-focused benchmarks for clinical governance. Online: www.modern.nhs.uk/home/key/docs/Essence%20of%20Care.pdf Available July 2006

Nicol M, Bavin C, Bedford-Turner S, Cronin P, Rawlings-Anderson K 2004 Essential nursing skills. 2nd edn. Mosby, Edinburgh

Norton C 1996 The causes and nursing management of constipation. British Journal of Nursing 5(20):1252–1258

Royal College of Physicians 1995 Incontinence: causes, management and provision of services. Journal of the Royal College of Physicians London 29(4):272–274

Small A 1999 Are you sitting comfortably? Nursing Times 95(1):24–25

Taylor C 1997 Constipation and diarrhoea. In: Bruce L, Finley TMD (eds) Nursing in gastroenterology. Churchill Livingstone, Edinburgh

van Dongen E 2001 It isn't something to yodel about, but it exists! Faeces, nurses, social relations and status within a mental hospital. Aging and Mental Health 5(3):205–215

Waugh A, Grant A (eds) 2001 Ross and Wilson anatomy and physiology. 9th edn. Churchill Livingstone, Edinburgh

Winney J 1998 Constipation. Elderly Care 10(4):26–31

Wright L 1974 Bowel function in hospital patients. Royal College of Nursing Research Project Series 1, number 4. RCN, London

Further reading

Bruce L, Finlay T (eds) 1997 Nursing in gastroenterology. Churchill Livingstone, Edinburgh

Colley W 1999 Practical procedures for nurses. Constipation – 1: Causes and assessment. Nursing Times 95(20) Supplement 27.1

Colley W 1999 Practical procedures for nurses. Constipation – 2: Treatment. Nursing Times 95(21) Supplement 27.2

Jooton D 2002 Nursing with dignity – Hinduism. Nursing Times 98(15):38.

Kaur Gill B 2002 Nursing with dignity – Sikhism. Nursing Times 98(14):39–41

McGrath A 2003 Nursing patients with gastrointestinal disorders. In: Brooker C, Nicol M (eds) Nursing adults. The practice of caring. Mosby, Edinburgh

Wells M 2003 Maintaining continence. In: Brooker C, Nicol M (eds) Nursing adults. The practice of caring. Mosby, Edinburgh

22 Promoting the safe administration of medicines

Christine Burton and Jayne Donaldson

Glossary

Adverse drug reaction

Compliance

Concordance

Pharmacology

Polypharmacy

Learning outcomes

This chapter will help you:

- Outline the legal and professional principles governing the use of medicines
- Explain how medicines must be stored, ordered and prescribed in hospital and community settings
- Outline common groups of drugs and their actions
- Explain the nurse's role in the safe administration of prescribed drugs
- Describe the nursing skills used to administer drugs by commonly used routes
- Discuss the nurse's role in promoting concordance/compliance
- Describe factors that contribute to drug errors and how such incidents are handled.

Introduction

Safe administration of medicines is of paramount importance to ensure patient/client safety. The legislation and professional guidance (Nursing and Midwifery Council [NMC] 2004a, 2004b) that should enable this are explored at the beginning of this chapter. The requirements for safe storage, ordering and prescribing of medicines in hospital and community settings are then reviewed.

In order to understand how drugs act, some pharmacological principles are explained and their implications for nursing practice are illustrated. Commonly used groups of drugs and their effects are listed. Adverse drug reactions, or side effects, and the safeguards that apply to newly marketed medicines are considered. Medications that come in several forms and are administered by a variety of routes are described later in this chapter.

This chapter discusses the essential checks that must be carried out before administering medicines and how to obtain valid consent. An overview of calculating drug doses is provided. The nursing skills needed to administer medication by several common routes are explained in detail using an evidence-based approach. Towards the end of the chapter polypharmacy and the nurse's role in maximizing concordance and compliance are explored. This is important in maintaining patient/client safety and maximizing effective use of NHS financial resources. Finally, drug errors, the factors that may predispose to these incidents and how they are dealt with are considered.

Legislation concerning medicines

All medicines are potentially harmful and nurses must be fully aware of the importance of safe storage, ordering and prescribing of drugs, which are explained later in this section. The manufacture, safe storage, prescription and sales of medicines within the UK are subject to Acts of Parliament and guiding regulations with which every nurse should be familiar:

- The Medicines Act 1968
- The Misuse of Drugs Act 1971
- The Misuse of Drugs Regulations 1985.

Additional legislation governs prescribing by appropriately qualified registered nurses. Nurses also need to be familiar with the professional guidance from the NMC.

The Medicines Act 1968

This act protects manufacturers, prescribers and recipients of medicines. It controls licensing, manufacturing and distribution of medicines, the registration of retail pharmacists, and identifies three classes of medicinal products:

- Prescription only medicines (PoMs) – potent medicines that can be sold or supplied on prescription only, e.g. antibiotics

- Pharmacy only medicines (P) – may only be sold only under the supervision of a pharmacist, e.g. antihistamines
- General sales list medicines (GSL) – can be sold in any retail outlet, e.g. supermarkets. Examples include aspirin and paracetamol.

The Act stipulated that only doctors, dentists and veterinary surgeons could prescribe medicines; however, later legislation has since extended prescribing to appropriately qualified registered nurses (RNs) (see below) and other healthcare professionals such as some pharmacists. The Act outlines:

- How drugs should be labelled
- The types of container to be used to contain drugs between the factory and the patient/client
- Controls that govern the writing of prescriptions (see Box 22.3, p. 631).

Many medicinal products not governed by legislation are widely available, e.g. homeopathic and herbal preparations. In addition, GSL medicines – often referred to as 'over-the-counter drugs', such as aspirin and medicines for indigestion – are widely believed to be safe. However, they can have serious side effects and may interact with each other and with prescribed medicines. Additionally, the use of alcohol and recreational drugs can have harmful effects and they too can interact with prescribed medication.

The Misuse of Drugs Act 1971

This Act identified controlled drugs that are likely to cause dependence and other harmful effects if misused. It aims to prevent the misuse of these drugs and protects public safety by controlling their importation, exportation, supply and possession. Controlled drugs are widely known as CDs and were previously known as 'dangerous drugs of addiction'. The Act classifies CDs according to the harm they may cause if misused.

- *Class A* (most harm) includes cocaine, diamorphine (heroin), methadone, morphine, ecstasy and lysergide (LSD) and also injectable forms of Class B drugs
- *Class B* (intermediate) includes oral amfetamines, barbiturates and codeine
- *Class C* (least harm) includes cannabis, most benzodiazepines, androgenic and anabolic steroids, and growth hormone.

The Misuse of Drugs Regulations 1985

This divides controlled drugs into five schedules, which have specific requirements regarding their supply, possession, prescribing and record keeping. There is a legal requirement to keep a controlled drug register for drugs in Schedule 2, which includes the most addictive drugs used in practice such as morphine and pethidine. Further information can be found in the *British National Formulary* (BNF; see Useful websites, p. 651). Storage, ordering, prescribing and administration of CDs are described later.

Nurse prescribing

The Medicinal Products: Prescription by Nurses Act 1992 and The Health and Social Care Act 2001 contain the primary legislation that allows nurse prescribing and its subsequent extension to 'non-medical prescribing'. Increasingly, RNs who have undertaken further specific training are prescribing many drugs in a range of settings.

Professional advice that affects nurses

In relation to the administration and prescribing of medicines, nurses are not only constrained by the legislation above but also by *Guidelines for the Administration of Medicines* (NMC 2004a). These outline nurses' professional accountability (see Ch. 7) in relation to knowledge of drugs and their actions, and the safe administration of medicines. Nurses must also be familiar with the *Code of Professional Conduct: Standards for Conduct, Performance and Ethics* (NMC 2004b) and *Guidelines for Records and Record Keeping* (NMC 2005).

The NMC (2004a) recommend that only RNs, midwives and specialist community public health nurses should be involved in the administration of medicines. Practitioners must always be aware of local policy as it may vary regarding the number of practitioners involved. For example, in some placements the second checker will also require to be a registered practitioner whereas in others this may be a student nurse.

The *Standards of Proficiency for Pre-registration Nursing Education* (NMC 2004c) state that student nurses must be able to demonstrate competence in essential skills including administration of medicines. Student nurses undertaking administration of medicines must do so only under the direct supervision of a RN. The RN must countersign the signature of a student who administers any prescription (NMC 2004a).

Storage of medicines

In clinical settings all drugs, not just CDs and including GSL medicines, are 'controlled' by the legislation outlined above. Storage depends on the type of drug and the setting involved.

Storage of non-controlled medicines in hospitals and nursing homes

The Duthie report (Department of Health [DH] 1988) set out precautions concerning the storage of medicines in hospitals to safeguard staff and patients/clients. The nurse in charge of a clinical area is responsible for the safe storage of all medicines (Box 22.1). Safe storage requires that:

1. Medicines are always stored in:
   - A locked cupboard
   - A locked medicine trolley (Fig. 22.1A)
   - A locked section of the patient's/client's bedside locker (Fig. 22.1B), or
   - A locked refrigerator that is only used for drugs

2. Some medicines are stored at room temperature (between 15 and 25°C), others require to be kept in a cool dark cupboard and some are stored in a refrigerator (between 1 and 4°C), e.g. vaccines and reconstituted antibiotics

REFLECTIVE PRACTICE Box 22.1

Storage of medicinal products

Medicinal products are stored in different parts of placements and under different conditions.

Student activities

1. In your placement, identify at least one medicine that is stored:
   - At room temperature
   - In the drugs refrigerator.
2. Find out where the following are stored:
   - Disinfectants
   - Urine testing materials
   - Creams and ointments
   - i.v. fluids.

3. Disinfectants/antiseptics such as chlorhexidine, intravenous (i.v.) fluids such as 0.9% sodium chloride, clinical reagents such as urine testing materials and topical substances, including creams and ointments, should be stored in locked cupboards and separately from other medicines
4. Medicines should always be kept in their original packaging, e.g. blister packaging is designed to reduce decomposition of the drugs by moisture.

Storage of controlled drugs in hospitals and nursing homes

Because of their potential to cause harm if misused, there are specific legal requirements concerning the ordering, storage and dispensing of controlled drugs. Controlled drugs are the responsibility of the charge nurse. They are kept locked in an inner cupboard within a cupboard (Fig. 22.2). The keys for both cupboards are held in the sole custody of the charge nurse or a designated RN or other healthcare professional. The contents of the cupboard and the controlled drug register are checked regularly according to local policy. This may be at each change of shift, daily or weekly. The controlled drug register is kept as an accurate record of the contents of the controlled drugs cupboard. Once completed, the registers are kept in the clinical area for 2 years.

Storage of medicines in the home

The strict regulations used in hospitals cannot be maintained in people's homes. A family member may collect any medicine if the person for whom the drug is

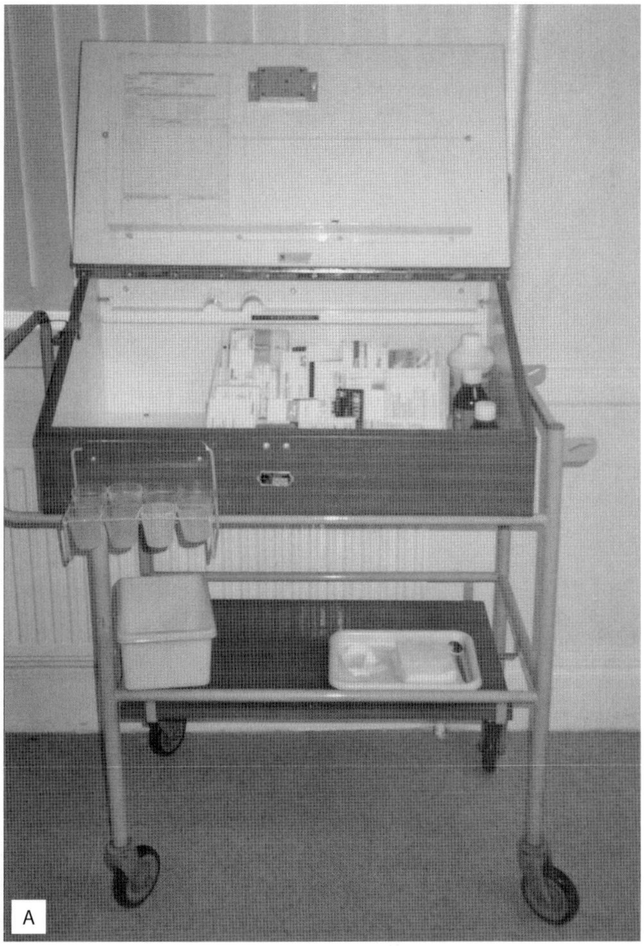

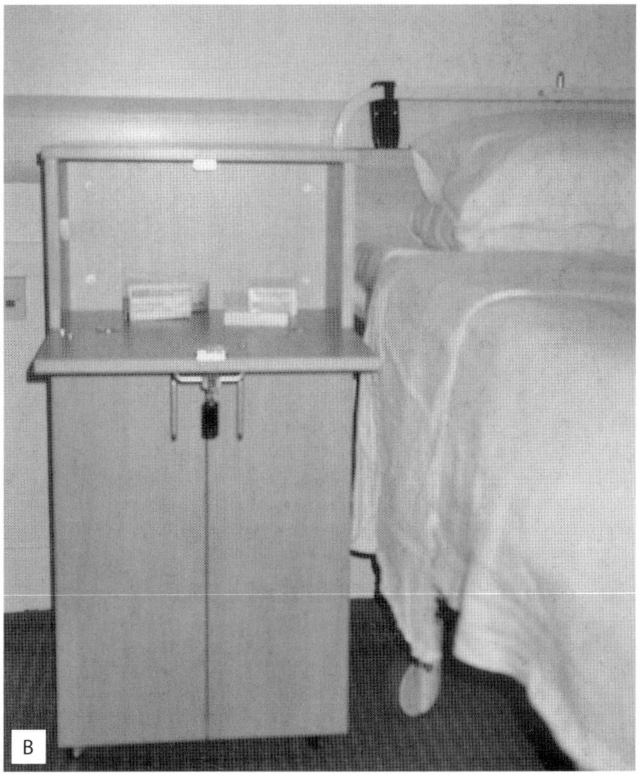

Fig. 22.1 Storage of medicines: **A.** Medicine trolley. **B.** Locked section of bedside locker

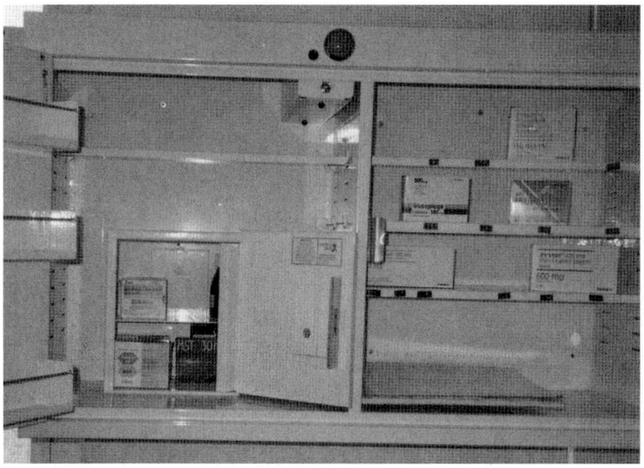

Fig. 22.2 Drug cupboard with an inner controlled drugs cupboard

prescribed is unable to do so. In general, patients/clients should be advised to:

- Check the manufacturer's instructions concerning storage
- Keep medicines that require refrigeration away from raw food
- Keep medicines out of reach of children.

Controlled drugs are dispensed from the pharmacy in the normal way. However, the pharmacist keeps a register of controlled drugs ordered, the amount delivered to the pharmacy and the volume or amount dispensed.

Ordering drugs in hospitals

This depends on the type of drug to be ordered.

Controlled drugs

In hospitals, qualified practitioners order controlled drugs in a specific way (Box 22.2).

Non-controlled drugs

In hospitals, this is usually the responsibility of the RN and/or pharmacist. Upon receipt, the order sheet is checked by a RN to ensure that the correct medicines have been supplied.

Principles of prescribing

It is essential to ensure that the prescription meets the principles laid down in the *Guidelines for the Administration of Medicines* (NMC 2004a). In order to safeguard both the public and practitioners, specific guidelines govern the prescribing of medicines (Box 22.3). Drugs may be prescribed:

- Regularly, i.e. for administration at particular times each day
- 'As required', e.g. painkillers, when the dose interval, maximum number of daily doses and reason for administration must be included
- Once only, e.g. for preoperative medication.

Box 22.2 **Ordering controlled drugs**

- A specific controlled drug order book with carbonized order sheets is used
- Qualified practitioners sign the controlled drugs ordering book using a separate page for each drug.
- This is sent to pharmacy in the normal way unless it is non-stock or needed urgently, in which case a member of staff may take the controlled drug order book to the pharmacy
- A pharmacist dispenses controlled drugs
- The signature of the member of staff responsible for their safe delivery to the ward/department is required before leaving the pharmacy
- They are transported to the ward/department in a sealed package
- Controlled drugs are accepted on the ward/department by an RN and the package is checked to ensure that it is still intact
- Two RNs or one RN and the pharmacist check the drug packaging
- The drug is checked against the order form
- The total number of tablets, ampoules of the drug or volume of liquid is checked and added to the stock in the controlled drug register.

If the prescription does not meet the required standards for safe practice, the nurse should contact the prescriber to amend their prescription before proceeding further. An example of a prescription sheet is provided in Figure 22.3.

Introduction to pharmacology

Pharmacology is the science of chemical substances, e.g. drugs, medications and other substances such as herbal and homeopathic preparations (see Ch. 10) that interact with the body. These interactions are divided into:

- *Pharmacodynamics*, which considers the effect of drugs on the body or 'what the drug does to the body'
- *Pharmacokinetics*, which explains how the body affects a drug with time, i.e. 'what the body does to the drug'.

This section provides an overview of important processes; further information can be found in pharmacology textbooks (e.g. Downie et al 2003, Greenstein 2004).

Pharmacodynamics

Receptors on cell membranes often act as recognition sites for substances produced by the body to regulate or mediate specific functions. Substances that act on cell membrane receptors include hormones and neurotransmitters – chemicals that transmit nerve impulses across the tiny gaps (synapses) between nerve cells. Many

Box 22.3 **Good practice in relation to prescriptions**

Prescriptions must:

- Wherever possible, be based on the patient's/client's informed consent and awareness of the purpose of the treatment
- Be clearly written, typed or computer generated and indelible, and for controlled drugs be handwritten in ink although controlled drugs prescriptions may now also be computer generated and signed in ink
- Clearly identify the patient using their full name
- Record the weight of the patient/client on the prescription sheet where the dose is related to weight
- Clearly specify the substance to be administered using its generic name (see p. 634) together with the strength, dosage, timing, frequency, start and finish dates, and route for administration
- Be signed and dated by the prescriber
- Not be for a substance to which the patient/client is known to be allergic
- Avoid decimal points as far as possible to prevent errors
- Use only acceptable abbreviations. Internationally recognized abbreviations can be found in the BNF and some are listed below.

(Adapted from NMC 2004a)

The practitioner administering the medicine should be aware that:

- Telephone instruction to administer previously unprescribed medication is not acceptable (DH 1988)
- Administration by the patient and/or carer must only be performed if the individual is competent (see Ch. 6).

Specific to hospital

- Each medication is individually signed
- In hospital, several controlled drug prescriptions may be prescribed on the same chart
- Two nurses, one of whom must be qualified, must administer controlled drugs (although local policies may differ).

Specific to community

- Two drugs can be prescribed on each prescription
- Prescriptions for each controlled drug must be handwritten in full using ink or computer generated and signed in ink
- Controlled drugs may be administered by a carer or taken by patients themselves
- Where controlled drugs are administered via a medical device a RN or medical practitioner should set up and administer the preparation.

Accepted abbreviations for drug routes

- i.m. – intramuscular
- INHAL – inhalation
- i.v. – intravenous
- p.r. – per rectum
- p.v. – per vaginam
- s.c. – subcutaneous
- s.l. – sublingual
- TOP – topical

Notes: depending on local policy, abbreviations may also be written in upper case letters without punctuation, e.g. i.m., i.v., p.r., etc.

Units

SI units are normally used in prescriptions avoiding the use of decimal points:

- *Mass*: 1 kilogram (kg) = 1000 grams; 1 gram (g) = 1000 milligrams; 1 milligram (mg) = 1000 micrograms*
- *Volume*: 1 litre (L) = 1000 millilitres; 1 millilitre (mL) = 1000 microlitres*.

International units (IU) are used for some preparations, e.g. heparin, insulin (see Table 22.1).

* This must not be abbreviated.

drugs produce their effects because they are structurally similar to the naturally occurring substances that act on receptors (Fig. 22.4A). Drugs that act on receptor sites in a similar way to natural body substances are known as agonists, whereas those that prevent (block) their normal action are known as antagonists. Therefore, by attaching to specific receptor sites on target cells, some drugs act by stimulating or blocking the storage, manufacture or release of naturally produced substances.

However, not all drugs act on receptor sites, e.g. antacids reduce indigestion by neutralizing gastric acid. Many other drugs act by inhibiting the actions of enzymes (Fig. 22.4B), e.g. non-steroidal anti-inflammatory drugs (NSAIDs), or by blocking ion channels in cell membranes (Fig. 22.4C), e.g. local anaesthetics.

Pharmacokinetics

Important processes influence plasma levels of a drug within the body, in particular absorption, distribution, metabolism and excretion (Fig. 22.5). Knowledge of pharmacokinetic principles is useful when considering factors that determine how much of a drug is needed to maintain appropriate (therapeutic) blood levels.

Absorption

The oral route is most commonly used for administration of drugs (see p. 639). In order to exert its action at the desired site, the drug must be absorbed from the digestive tract into the blood, which then travels through the liver before entering the systemic circulation (see 'First

PRESCRIPTION AND ADMINISTRATION RECORD
Standard Chart

Hospital/Ward: 17	**Consultant:** DR BROWN	**Name of Patient:** DAVID BURTON
Weight: 72Kg	**Height:**	**Patient Number:** 01234567
If re-written, date:		**D.O.B.** 13/12/45
DISCHARGE PRESCRIPTION		
Date completed:-	**Completed by:-**	(Attach printed label here)

A. **ONCE ONLY**

Date	Time	Medicine (Approved Name)	Dose	Route	Prescriber - Sign + Print	Time Given	Given By
13/03/07	11:10	PETHIDINE	50mg	I.M	RaReid R.A.REID	11:20	CB

B. **REGULAR THERAPY**

PRESCRIPTION		Patient's Own Medicine	Date → / Time ↓	06/03	07/03	08/03	09/03	10/03	11/03	12/03	13/03	14/03
Medicine (Approved Name) DIGOXIN		For use	6									
Dose 125 MICROGRAMS	Route ORAL		(8)	HB	CB	HB	HB	HR	CB	HR	HB	CB
		Quantity	12									
Notes	Start Date 06/03/07	Date	14									
			18									
Prescriber - sign + print RaReid R.A.REID		Pharmacy SK	22									
Medicine (Approved Name) FUROSEMIDE		For use	6									
Dose 40mg	Route ORAL		(8)	HB	CB	HB	HB	HR	CB	HC	HB	CB
		Quantity	12									
Notes	Start Date 06/03/07	Date	14									
			18									
Prescriber - sign + print RaReid R.A.REID		Pharmacy SK	22									

C. **AS REQUIRED THERAPY**

PRESCRIPTION		Patient's Own Medicine				
Medicine (Approved Name) SALBUTAMOL		For use	Date	07/03	11/03	14/03
			Time	08:05	18:35	21:10
Dose 2 PUFFS	Route INHAL	Quantity	Dose	2 puffs	2 puffs	2 puffs
			Initials	CB	CB	CB
Notes For breathlessness MAX - 4 x dose/per day	Start Date 07/03/07	Date	Date			
			Time			
Prescriber - sign + print RaReid R.A.REID		Pharmacy SK	Dose			
			Initials			

Fig. 22.3 Prescription chart (reproduced with permission from NHS Lothian 2005)

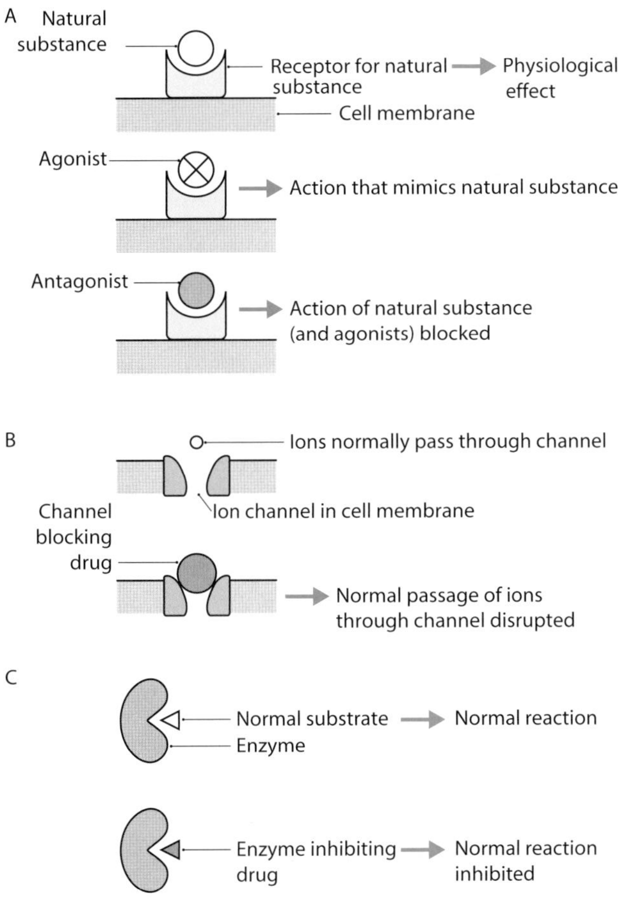

Fig. 22.4 Sites of drug action: **A.** Receptors. **B.** Ion channels. **C.** Enzymes (adapted with permission from Rang et al 2003)

pass metabolism', below). The rate of absorption can be affected by several factors including the presence or absence of food in the stomach. It is recommended that some drugs are taken half an hour before meals, e.g. some antibiotics are absorbed more effectively from an empty stomach.

First pass metabolism

Drugs taken orally are usually absorbed in the small intestine and then transported to the liver via the hepatic portal vein before reaching the systemic circulation. Many drugs are broken down, or metabolized, as they pass through the liver and when this is extensive only a small amount enters the systemic circulation and even less reaches the site of action. This effect is called first pass metabolism.

Glyceryl trinitrate, which is given to provide very rapid relief from cardiac pain in angina, is almost completely broken down in the liver. It is administered sublingually (placed under the tongue) or as a spray to the oral mucosa. The oral mucosa has an extensive blood supply that facilitates rapid absorption and therefore the action of glyceryl trinitrate is also very rapid. The blood from the oral mucosa does not travel through the liver before entering the systemic circulation and therefore first pass metabolism is avoided.

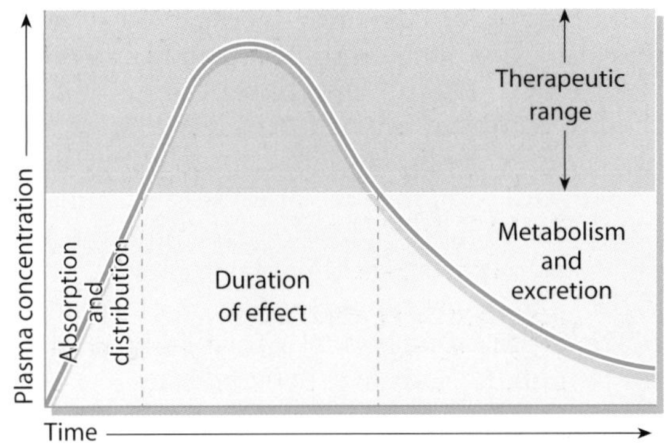

Fig. 22.5 Effects of absorption, distribution, metabolism and excretion on the plasma concentrations of an administered drug (reproduced with permission from Downie et al 2003)

Other drugs are given by injection or as transdermal patches (see p. 647) to avoid first pass metabolism. In people suffering from liver disorders, first pass metabolism is reduced, and therefore drug doses must be reduced to take this into account.

Distribution

After entering the bloodstream, the drug is transported throughout the body. In the capillaries drugs diffuse out of the bloodstream to reach their site(s) of action. Movement from the bloodstream into the tissues may be influenced by several factors such as the extent of plasma binding (see below), the quality and quantity of plasma proteins and blood flow. Where there is good systemic blood flow, drugs are transported more rapidly into the tissues. In some cardiac conditions, where the cardiac output is reduced (see Ch. 17), drug distribution will also be reduced. Many drugs cross the placenta, causing abnormal fetal development, and must therefore be avoided during pregnancy.

Plasma binding

Many drugs bind to plasma proteins in the blood. Some of the drug is bound and the remainder is unbound; however, only the unbound form is active. People who have a liver disorder or malnutrition have fewer plasma proteins available for binding and therefore more of the drug remains unbound and is available to act. In such situations, the dosage must be reduced to avoid excessive plasma levels, e.g. warfarin (see Table 22.1), which may cause severe bleeding.

Metabolism

Metabolism includes processes that often involve specific enzymes which may break down the drug, combine it with another chemical (conjugation) or increase its solubility in water. In these states drugs are usually more active and can be easily eliminated by the kidneys. Some drugs are already water soluble and so do not require to be metabolized. Most drugs are metabolized in the liver.

Half-life

This is also referred to as $T_{1/2}$ and is the time taken for the concentration of a drug in the bloodstream to fall by half of its original value. The half-life determines the length of time a drug is available within the body and the intensity of its action. The plasma concentration of a drug at one half-life is 50%, at two half-lives it is 25%, etc. By five half-lives most of the drug will have been eliminated from the body regardless of the dose or route of administration. The half-life is therefore used to determine the number of daily doses required for drug plasma levels to remain within the therapeutic range (see Fig. 22.5). It can also be useful when estimating how long it will take for a drug to be cleared from the body, e.g. in overdosage.

Excretion

The kidneys excrete most drugs from the body. The more water soluble the substance, the more easily it is excreted by the kidneys. People with kidney failure or impaired renal function may suffer toxic effects as elimination of drugs is reduced. Digoxin is a commonly used cardiac drug that can be toxic in older adults because kidney function is often reduced in this age group. The kidneys can reabsorb those drugs that are lipid soluble, making them available within the body for longer. Some drugs are excreted by the lungs or from the digestive tract.

Therapeutic range

To achieve optimal concentrations at the target tissue the correct dose must be given. If this is too low drug action will be ineffective; if too much is administered it may produce side effects that might be toxic. The therapeutic range refers to the plasma levels of a drug that must be maintained so that it can exert its optimal response without producing side effects (Fig. 22.6). Some drugs have a narrow therapeutic range while for others this is wider. Nurses need to recognize the implications of this in relation to drug administration, i.e. if drugs are omitted or given at times other than those prescribed, plasma drug levels will not be maintained in the therapeutic range.

Measurement of plasma drug levels is carried out when drugs with a narrow therapeutic range are used, e.g. gentamicin (an antibiotic) causes irreversible kidney damage and hearing impairment when therapeutic levels are exceeded. Children, until their liver and kidneys are fully mature, older adults whose kidney and liver function may be declining and people with a liver or kidney disorder are at greatest risk of drug toxicity.

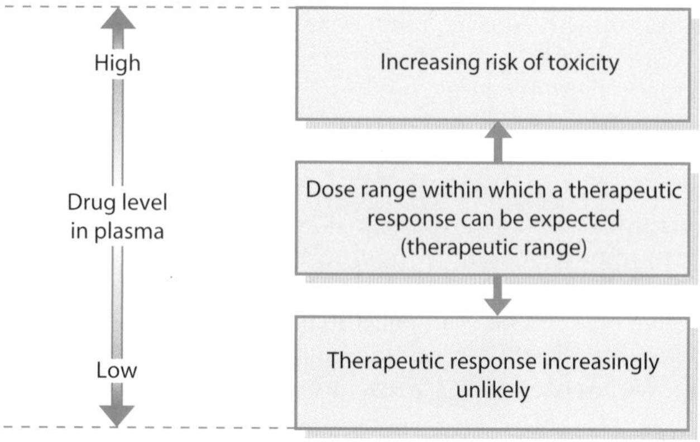

Fig. 22.6 Therapeutic range (reproduced with permission from Hopkins & Kelly 1999)

Adverse drug reactions

All medicines have the potential to cause harm including over-the-counter medication. Interactions increase with the number of drugs used, including homeopathic and herbal preparations, recreational drugs and alcohol. It is important, therefore, that nurses know about and recognize potential adverse effects of drugs they administer. Adverse drug reactions (ADRs) include any unwanted effects of drugs, which range from minor side effects to those that are harmful, serious and sometimes fatal. They can be classified into five groups, of which the two outlined below are the most common (DH 2001).

Type A

These are predictable, dose dependent and can be anticipated. They are related to the physiological effects of the drug, e.g. constipation that occurs in people receiving morphine.

Type B

These types are bizarre or idiosyncratic, unexpected and rare reactions, which are not dose related. However, they are generally severe, causing serious and sometimes fatal consequences such as severe allergic responses. Genetic, host and environmental factors are thought to contribute to their occurrence.

Surveillance for ADRs

Potential new drugs must undergo approved and staged clinical trials that report to the Committee on Safety of Medicines to ensure that they are as safe as possible before being granted a product licence. Once marketed, they become more widely available and the Committee on Safety of Medicines keeps them under surveillance so that the occurrence and incidence of ADRs can be monitored. Drugs under surveillance have the symbol ▼ in their BNF listing (see Useful websites, p. 651).

Healthcare practitioners, including nurses, and patients/relatives should report all adverse or unexpected reactions, however minor. Yellow cards, which can be found in the BNF, and online reporting are used to report ADRs so that they can be systematically evaluated and a drug withdrawn if there are safety concerns.

Naming of drugs and common groups

Drugs that have similar functions are classified into groups and there is more than one name for each drug. Some names reflect drug actions more clearly than others.

Naming of drugs

The recommended International Non-proprietary Name (rINN) of a drug is also referred to as the generic, non-proprietary or British Approved Name (BAN). This name may start with a lower case letter, e.g. 'p' in paracetamol.

The manufacturer gives the trade or proprietary name to a particular preparation. This is recognized by the symbol ® denoting its registered trademark, which follows its name on the packaging. Proprietary names start with a capital letter, e.g. 'P' in Panadol®, which is a trade name for paracetamol. The manufacturer who has registered a drug has exclusive rights to market it for up to 10 years, during which time they can recover the development costs. Different drug companies often manufacture similar or identical generic preparations and may give them similar names.

To avoid errors, and because manufacturers price drugs differently, the Department of Health (1999) recommended that drugs be prescribed by their generic name (e.g. paracetamol) and that trade names (e.g. Panadol®) should only be specified if a particular manufacturer's drug has different effects. Lists of drugs can be found in the BNF.

Common groups of drugs and their actions

Common drug groups are listed in Table 22.1 together with their effects and examples. Nurses must understand how commonly used drugs in their practice area act and be familiar with their side effects and contraindications in order to maintain patient/client safety (Box 22.4). This information can be found in the BNF/Children's BNF.

Table 22.1 Common drug groups and their actions

Group	Effect	Common examples (generic names)
Analgesics:	Reduce or prevent pain	
Opioids		Morphine
Non-opioids		Aspirin, paracetamol
(see also NSAIDs and Ch. 23)		
Antacids	Counteract gastric acidity in indigestion	Aluminium hydroxide, magnesium trisilicate
Antibiotics (antibacterials)	Kill bacteria (bactericidal) or arrest their growth (bacteriostatic)	Ampicillin, erythromycin, gentamicin
Anticoagulants	Prevent and/or break down blood clots in the circulation	Warfarin (oral), heparin (parenteral)
Anticonvulsants (antiepileptic)	Control and prevent seizures	Phenytoin, sodium valproate
Antidepressants:	Improve low mood	
Monoamine oxidase inhibitors (MAOIs)		Phenelzine
Selective serotonin reuptake inhibitors (SSRIs)		Fluoxetine
Tricyclic antidepressants		Amitriptyline
Antidiarrhoeals	Reduce intestinal motility	Codeine phosphate, loperamide
Antiemetics	Alleviate nausea and/or vomiting	Metoclopramide, cyclizine
Antifungals	Combat fungal infection	Nystatin, fluconazole
Antihistamines	Treat and prevent allergic reactions	Chlorphenamine (chlorpheniramine)
Antihypertensives	Several groups that act in different ways to reduce high blood pressure, e.g.:	
	Beta-blockers	Atenolol, propranolol
	Angiotensin-converting enzyme (ACE) inhibitors	Captopril, enalapril
Antipsychotics (neuroleptics):	Alleviate symptoms of psychotic illness	
Typical		Haloperidol
Atypical		Clozapine
Antipyretics	Lower raised body temperature	Aspirin
Anxiolytics	Alleviate anxiety and related symptoms	Diazepam
Aperients, laxatives	Promote emptying/evacuation of the bowel	Lactulose, bisacodyl
Bronchodilators	Relax bronchial smooth muscle, thus increasing air entry to lungs	Salbutamol
Diuretics	Groups of drugs that increase production of urine	Bendroflumethiazide, furosemide (frusemide)

(Continued)

Table 22.1 (*Continued*)

Group	Effect	Common examples (generic names)
Hypoglycaemic agents (antidiabetic):	Lower raised blood glucose levels in diabetes mellitus	
Oral		Metformin, glipizide
Parenteral, usually given by subcutaneous injection (see p. 642)		Insulin – short-, intermediate- and long-acting preparations
Hypnotics	Promote sleep	Zopiclone
Non-steroidal anti-inflammatory drugs (NSAIDs)	Reduce inflammation (see Ch. 23)	Ibuprofen, aspirin
Thrombolytics ('clot busting' drugs)	Disintegrate blood clots in, e.g., myocardial infarction, deep vein thrombosis (DVT), pulmonary embolism	Streptokinase, alteplase

CRITICAL THINKING Box 22.4

Drug groups, their actions and routes of administration

Under the supervision of your mentor, you are to be involved in drug administration. In order to do this safely, preparation is required.

Student activities

1. Within your placement:
   - Identify commonly used drugs and the groups to which they belong (see Table 22.1).
   - For these drugs, consider their intended effects and relate them to the patient's/client's clinical condition.
   - Find out about the side effects of each drug.
2. There are many different routes used to administer medicines. Find out:
   - What routes are used.
   - If there is more than one route that could be used for administering any of the drugs identified above.

Medicinal preparations and routes of administration

Medicines are manufactured in different forms for administration by particular routes. The different forms and their characteristics are summarized in Table 22.2. The prescribed route is determined by which will provide the optimal effect and minimize side effects, and the preparations available.

Routes of administration can be divided into two categories: systemic and local (Table 22.3). Following systemic administration, the drug circulates throughout the whole body. Use of local routes, e.g. inhalation or per vagina, involves giving lower doses directly to the site of action. As a result, the amount of the drug elsewhere in the body is relatively low and side effects are less likely. The term 'parenteral' includes all routes of administration except the oral route.

Oral medication

Once swallowed, drugs are usually absorbed from the small intestine. Oral preparations include tablets, capsules and liquids (see Table 22.2). Some tablets are manufactured to exert their effect over long periods and are described as 'slow release' (SR) or 'extended release' (XR). Other tablets are covered in an enteric coating (e/c). For example, NSAIDs are potential gastric irritants and are enteric coated so that they travel through the stomach unchanged before entering the small intestine where they are absorbed, thus avoiding gastric irritation. People should therefore swallow these tablets whole and not crush or chew them, so that the enteric coating and/or extended release action is maintained. Crushing tablets increases the risk of adverse drug reactions and toxicity (Miller & Miller 2000). Bending (2001) cautions that when controlled release tablets are crushed the whole dose may be released within 5–15 minutes instead of over the 24-hour period intended. Manufacturers' instructions warn against the crushing of tablets or opening of capsules as this is outwith the marketing licence (Wright 2003). When available, it is safer to use liquid preparations when swallowing tablets is difficult or impossible.

Sublingual and buccal routes

Some preparations put into the mouth are not intended for swallowing, including those for sublingual and buccal administration which avoids first pass metabolism, e.g. glyceryl trinitrate (see p. 633). Prochlorperazine (an antiemetic) can be administered via the buccal route. The tablet is placed between the upper lip and the gum to avoid swallowing the drug when nausea or vomiting is present.

Table 22.2 Drug preparations for administration by specific routes

Type	Characteristics
Oral preparations	
Tablets	Powdered substances compressed or moulded into solid forms Many are covered or sugar-coated to assist swallowing or to prevent them dissolving in the stomach, which may result in release or disintegration of the drug causing gastric irritation Some tablets should be swallowed when fully dissolved in water and are labelled: soluble, dispersible or effervescent
Capsules	Medication contained within a soluble shell, usually made of gelatin to aid swallowing and which carries the drug to the small intestine where it is absorbed
Lozenges	A solid form intended for sucking until fully dissolved; absorption is through the oral mucosa
Solutions	Medication is dissolved in a solvent, usually water
Suspensions	Contain solid particles that are dispersed in a liquid, not necessarily water
Syrup	A thick concentrated solution of medication that may include sugar (see Box 22.6) and flavouring
Emulsion	Minute globules of one liquid dispersed through another liquid
Preparations administered by other routes	
Pessaries	Moulded or compressed form of medication inserted into the vagina
Suppositories	Medicated solid bodies inserted into the rectum
Enemas	Medicated suspensions, oils or foam solutions administered into the rectum
Nebulized solutions	Minute liquid particles inhaled into the lungs as a vapour using a nebulizer (see Ch. 17)
Dry powder inhaler	A solid that is converted to minute particles, which are inhaled
Metered dose inhaler	A pressurized device that delivers a preset dose of tiny medicated particles into the lungs

Table 22.3 Common routes of drug administration

Route	Systemic/local	Site of administration
Oral	Systemic	Taken by mouth and swallowed, or given via a nasogastric tube (see Ch. 19)
Sublingual/buccal	Systemic	Sprayed into the mouth or allowed to dissolve under the tongue or in the cheek
Topical	Can be local and/or systemic	Applied onto the skin, e.g. ointments, creams (local, p. 647), transdermal patches (systemic, p. 647) or mucous membranes, e.g. eyes (local, p. 642), ears (local, p. 643), vagina (usually local, p. 644), rectum (may be either local or systemic, p. 644)
Inhalation	Local	Inhaled into the lungs, e.g. metered-dose inhalers (with or without a spacer device), nebulizers, steam inhalations
Injections:	Systemic	
Intradermal		Into the skin
Subcutaneous (s.c.)		Into the subcutaneous tissue under the skin (see Fig. 22.9A)
Intramuscular (i.m.)		Into a skeletal muscle (see Fig. 22.9B)
Intravenous (i.v.)		Into a vein by a trained registered practitioner
Intraosseous		Into a bone by a trained registered practitioner
Intrathecal		Into the subarachnoid space (within the meninges) via a lumbar puncture by a trained registered practitioner

Parenteral medication

Parenteral medication includes those given by any route other than the alimentary tract. This includes preparations that are:

- Given by injection (see p. 640)
- Inserted into body orifices, e.g. pessaries and suppositories (see p. 644)
- Instilled, e.g. into the eye, nose or ear (see pp. 642–643)
- Inhaled through the mouth (see Ch. 17) or nasal passages, e.g. bronchodilators or nasal decongestants.

Administering prescribed medication

Nurses should exercise professional judgement when administering medicines (NMC 2004a) and bear in mind

CRITICAL THINKING Box 22.5

Drug administration policies and obtaining consent

Drug administration policies may very between care settings.

Student activities

1. Within your placement, locate and read the local drug administration policy and identify:
   - Who must be involved in administration of controlled drugs.
   - Who must be involved in administration of non-controlled drugs.
2. Bana is a client with a moderate learning disability who attends a day centre 3 days a week. She receives regular medication to prevent seizures.
   - Think about how you would explain a change in the dose of Bana's medication to her.
   - Discuss with your mentor the ways in which you could gain valid consent from Bana before administering her medication.

that they are accountable when carrying out medical instructions (NMC 2004b; see also Ch. 7). Medicines must always be administered in accordance with legislation (see p. 627) and local policies. It is every nurse's duty to be familiar with these policies and student nurses should refer to these in each new placement (NMC 2004a, 2005). The importance of gaining consent and situations in which covert administration may be appropriate are considered below; calculation of drug doses is explained. The later parts of this section explain how nurses administer drugs by a number of routes.

Consent

It is important that healthcare professionals are aware of the individual's right to refuse treatment, including medication, and must always respect their decisions (NMC 2004b). Adults must always be presumed to have the mental capacity (see Ch. 6) to consent to, or refuse, treatment, including taking medication, and no medication should be given without their agreement.

However, there are many situations when people may not be capable of providing valid consent. People with mental health problems, including dementia, or a learning disability may lack the capacity to make the decision whether or not to take medication (Box 22.5). When patients/clients are incapable of providing consent, or their wishes are contrary to their best interests (see Ch. 6), a registered practitioner should consult relevant people such as the family, carers or members of the multidisciplinary team (MDT). Assessment of capacity is primarily a matter for the treating clinicians but nurses as members of the MDT should be involved in such discussions.

For people detained under mental health legislation the principles of consent still apply to medications prescribed for other conditions. In other words, only medicines prescribed for mental health problems can be administered without the client's consent.

The Children Act 1989 ensures that children's wishes and feelings are taken into account, that they should always be consulted (subject to age and understanding) and kept informed about what is planned (see Ch. 6). The age of consent to medical treatment varies across the UK:

> If the child is under the age of 16 in England and Wales, 12 in Scotland and 17 in Northern Ireland, you must be aware of legislation and local protocols relating to consent.
>
> NMC 2004b (Clause 3.9, p. 7)

Covert administration of medicines

The United Kingdom Central Council (2001) states that the practice of covert, or 'hidden', administration of medicines may be only carried out in some specific instances. This should only be necessary or appropriate in the case of individuals who actively refuse medication and who are judged not to have the capacity to understand the consequences of their refusal. Treloar et al (2001) state that, in these cases, there is a duty to care and practitioners should be protected by transparent procedures which are framed in local policy. The following principles must always apply:

- The best interests of the individual is considered at all times
- The medication must be considered essential
- The decision to administer in this way is not considered as routine
- Consensus agreement has been reached after full discussion between staff and relatives
- The method of administration has been discussed and agreed with the pharmacist
- The decision, action and names of all involved in administering/agreeing to the procedure involved is accurately documented
- Regular attempts are made to encourage the individual to take medicines as prescribed
- There are written local policies in place.

Calculation of drug doses

The units used for drug doses and accepted abbreviations are shown in Box 22.3. Most drugs are manufactured in a form that enables straightforward administration, and some are found in a variety of strengths. This helps to ensure that the prescribed dose can be provided accurately and easily calculated.

Accurate calculation of drug doses requires practice. Student nurses must always have their drug calculations checked by a RN.

Tablets and capsules

In order to calculate the number of tablets or capsules required, the nurse needs to know the dose prescribed and the strength of tablets/capsules available.

The following formula is then used:

$$\frac{\text{dose prescribed}}{\text{dose available}} = \text{number of tablets or capsules to be given}$$

For example: An adult is prescribed 1 g of paracetamol, for which 500 mg tablets are available.

Using the above formula:

$$\frac{1000\text{ mg (or 1 g)}}{500\text{ mg}} = 2\text{ tablets.}$$

If the calculation reveals that a tablet requires to be halved, a scored tablet is halved using a tablet splitter. Only scored tablets must be split to provide the correct dose and prevent potentially serious consequences. If the tablet cannot be halved, the medication should be withheld and advice should be sought from the prescriber and/or pharmacist.

Liquid preparations

In the case of liquid preparations the nurse needs to know the prescribed dose and the amount or weight of drug in a given amount of solution.

The following formula is used:

$$\frac{\text{dose prescribed} \times \text{volume available}}{\text{dose available}} = \text{volume to be given (mL)}$$

For example: An adult is prescribed 500 mg of penicillin. The stock is syrup containing 125 mg/5 mL.

Using the above formula:

$$\frac{500\text{ mg} \times 5}{125\text{ mg}} = 20\text{ mL of syrup to be given}$$

Calculations based on body weight or surface area

These are used for some drugs in adults (e.g. chemotherapy treatment for cancer) and also in children.

Body weight

Body weight is often used for calculating doses for children and also for older adults. The following formula is used:

$$\frac{\text{Weight (kg)} \times \text{dosage per day}}{\text{Number of doses per day}} = \text{mg per dose}$$

For example: A child weighing 16 kg is prescribed intravenous erythromycin for a severe infection. The dosage is 50 mg/kg/day in four doses.

Using the above formula:

$$\frac{16\text{ kg} \times 50\text{ mg/kg/day}}{4\text{ doses/day}} = 200\text{ mg/dose}$$

In other words, a 200 mg injection would be administered every 6 hours.

Surface area

Doses are calculated according to body surface area, which is estimated in square metres (m^2) using a nomogram (a graph that determines surface area from measurements of height and weight). This may be used for chemotherapy (drug treatment for cancers) in people of all ages. Drug doses are calculated using the following formula:

$$\text{surface area} \times \text{prescribed dosage} = \text{dose required}$$

For example: A child is prescribed cytarabine. The recommended dosage is 120 mg/m^2 and their surface area is 0.5 m^2.

Using the above formula:

$$0.5\text{ m}^2 \times 120\text{ mg/m}^2 = 60\text{ mg}$$

(For more examples of drug calculations, see Gatford & Phillips 2002.)

Preparation for the administration of medications

Nurses must be familiar with both the procedure and the drugs(s) to be given in order to answer any questions the patient/client may ask about their medication and to administer it safely. It is important to explain to the patient/client how the drug works and how it is to be administered. Explanation may be either verbal, using language appropriate to the individual, and/or in writing, and must include the reason why the drug has been prescribed. Before receiving a new medicine, people may feel anxious about its administration and/or their reaction to it.

It is essential to ensure that any allergies are written in the medical/nursing notes and on the prescription sheet to ensure that people are not given drugs to which they are allergic.

There are several additional and specific precautions that must be adhered to when prescribing and administering drugs to children and also points of good practice (see Box 22.6).

Checks are carried out to ensure that the correct patient/client is given the right medication (correct dose via the right route and the correct preparation) at the right time and that the correct documentation is accurately completed afterwards. It is essential to adopt a systematic approach to ensure that medicines are administered safely (Box 22.7).

Administration of oral medications

When possible the patient/client is assisted to sit upright as this makes swallowing easier. The person should be offered a glass of water, which moistens the mouth, prevents tablets or capsules sticking to the oral or oesophageal mucosa and aids their transport to the stomach. Principles for administering oral preparations are shown in Box 22.8. Some medications should be given at specific times. For example, nystatin pastilles given to treat an oral fungal infection should be taken after food as the drug would be removed by food and drink. Nurses administering medicines should be aware of specific instructions.

Box 22.6 Administering medicines to children

Specific precautions for children

- In both hospital and community settings medications must always be kept out of reach of children
- Most paediatric drug dosages, which includes children under 50 kg or before puberty, are prescribed according to age, body weight, body surface area or a combination of these parameters
- Student nurses must always have their calculations checked by a RN
- When calculating any dose for children, a RN must also have their calculations checked by another RN as accurate doses are very important since even small discrepancies can be dangerous and overdosage fatal.

Points of good practice

- As children may experience difficulty in swallowing solid medications, transdermal patches (see p. 647) or liquid forms may be prescribed
- Some liquid preparations contain sugar to make them more palatable. Where a liquid preparation is required over a long period, a sugar-free version should be prescribed to reduce the incidence of dental caries. This is also important in children with diabetes
- If the dose is less than 1 mL, oral syringes should be used. This avoids the possibility of the preparation being injected and allows accurate dose measurement
- Medications should not be diluted in bottle feeds or other liquids as the drug may interact with milk or other liquid and the dose cannot be guaranteed if the drink is not completely finished
- Injections should be avoided whenever possible. Guidance on injection techniques in children can be found in the *Position Statement on Injection Technique* (Royal College of Paediatrics and Child Health 2002; see also p. 642).

NURSING SKILLS Box 22.7

Principles of drug administration

- If administering medicines to a group of patients/clients the medicine round should begin with the first individual and move on to the next in order
- Accurate identification of the person to whom the medicine is to be administered is paramount. Local policy regarding identification of patients/clients, especially for children, older adults, people with mental health problems or a learning disability and those who are unconscious, must be followed
- The prescription chart (see Fig. 22.3) is checked carefully and if there are any doubts about its accuracy, the procedure must be stopped and clarification sought
- The medication is checked against the written prescription and the expiry date checked to ensure it is in date
- The recording section of the prescription chart is checked to ensure that the medication has not already been administered
- The medicine is selected and carefully checked against the prescription
- This procedure is repeated for all medicines to be administered together. Care must be taken to ensure that medications given together are compatible, i.e. they will not interact with one another, using the BNF if necessary.
- Immediately after administration, the recording section on the prescription chart is initialled.

NURSING SKILLS Box 22.8

Administration of oral preparations

- Medication is dispensed directly from its original packaging without touching it (Fig. 22.7)
- All tablets and capsules are dispensed into medicine containers
- Liquid medication is dispensed into separate containers
- Medicine containers are placed on a tray and taken to the patient/client
- The person's identity is confirmed according to local policy and they are consulted as to how they wish to take their medication: some people prefer to swallow tablets or capsules from the container, some like to lift them out of the container and others prefer the tablets placed into their hand to swallow either all together or one by one. If a person is unable to manipulate the medications then they are delivered into their mouth using a spoon to avoid cross-infection
- Immediately after administration, each medicine is signed as given on the recording sheet.

Injections

Injections are considered the appropriate route of administration when:

- Fast onset of action is required
- Fasting is required
- Digestive enzymes would inactivate the drug, e.g. insulin
- Long-term release of the drug is necessary, e.g. depot injections (see 'Z track technique', p. 642 and Fig. 22.12).

Injections can be given via the intradermal, subcutaneous, intramuscular, intravenous, intraosseous and intrathecal routes (see Table 22.3). Student nurses are normally only involved in administering injections by the subcutaneous and intramuscular routes.

Preparing and giving injections

Preparation of injections is carried out in accordance with local policies and the *Good Practice Statement* (Clinical Resource and Audit Group 2002). Box 22.9 outlines the steps in preparing or 'drawing up' injections. This section also considers intramuscular (i.m.) and subcutaneous (s.c.) injections, and the sites used. As i.m. injections are given into muscles and s.c. injections into the more superficial subcutaneous tissue, the depth of these injections is different.

Skin cleansing prior to injections

There is some controversy about the need to cleanse the skin prior to injections. The skin should be cleansed using an alcohol wipe only if local policy recommends this. Some local policies state that if the patient is physically clean, and the nurse has good hand hygiene and uses a non-touch technique during the procedure (see Ch. 15), skin cleansing with an alcohol-impregnated wipe is not required. If used, the skin should be cleansed for 30 seconds and then allowed to dry for another 30 seconds in order that adequate skin disinfection is achieved (Workman 1999).

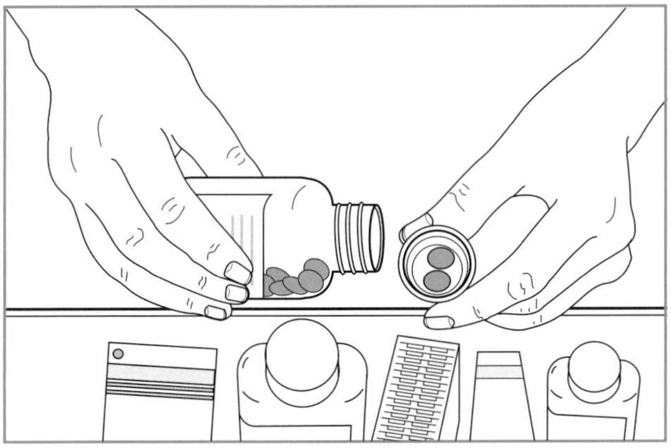

Fig. 22.7 Non-touch technique for dispensing oral medication (reproduced with permission from Nicol et al 2004)

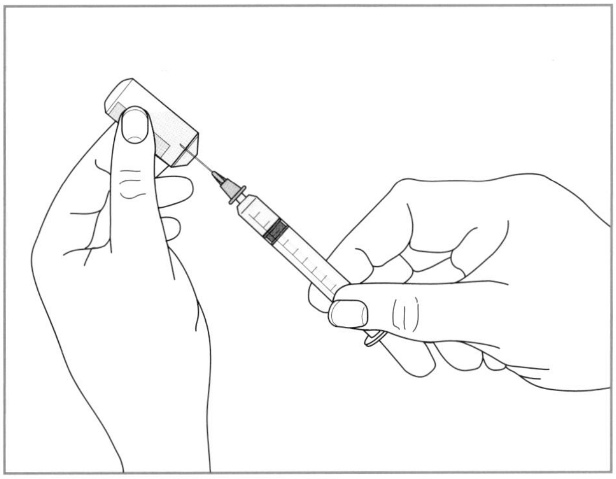

Fig. 22.8 Drawing up an injection (reproduced with permission from Nicol et al 2004)

NURSING SKILLS Box 22.9

Drawing up injections

- Collect the equipment required, i.e. a suitable tray to hold the materials, an appropriately sized syringe, two appropriately sized needles, an alcohol-impregnated wipe and the ampoules(s) containing the correct medication
- Clean the surface where preparation will take place according to local policy
- The hands are thoroughly washed and dried, and gloves worn as per local policy (see Ch. 15)
- The prescription is checked
- The integrity of the needle and syringe packaging and their expiry dates are checked
- Peel apart the packaging as directed by the manufacturer to expose the plunger end of the syringe
- Lift the syringe out by the barrel taking care to ensure that the nozzle does not become contaminated
- Peel apart the packaging to expose the hub of the needle
- Assemble the needle and syringe, and place in the tray
- Open the ampoule according to the manufacturer's instructions
- If an ampoule with a rubber or plastic top is used then the top is cleansed with the alcohol-impregnated wipe for 30 seconds and allowed to air dry for 30 seconds
- The needle sheath is removed and carefully inserted into the ampoule at a 45° angle. The prescribed dose is carefully withdrawn using a non-touch technique (Fig. 22.8). Care must be taken to ensure that the needle does not hit the bottom of the ampoule as this would blunt the tip
- Gently tap the syringe barrel to encourage any air bubbles to rise towards the air space
- Push the barrel slowly upwards, expelling any air from the syringe; this is complete when droplets of liquid are seen at the top of the needle. The syringe is now primed ready for use
- At this point the unsheathed needle is discarded and a second needle used to reduce the risk of needlestick injuries (National Institute for Health and Clinical Excellence [NICE] 2003, NHS Education for Scotland [NES] 2004) (see local policy).
- The tray containing the drawn-up injection and empty ampoule, and the prescription chart are taken to the patient/client.

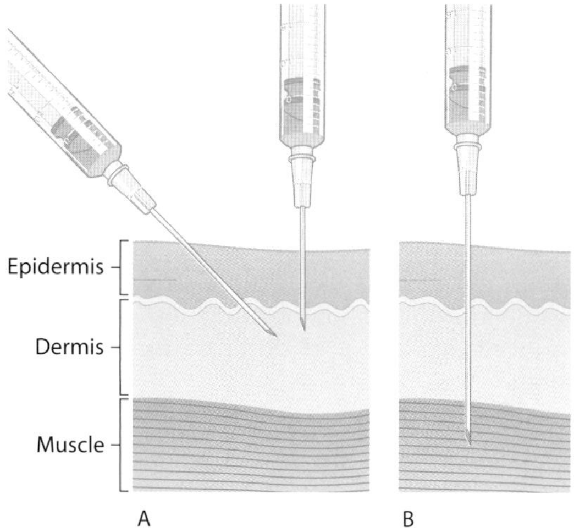

Fig. 22.9 Skin layers and needle insertion for injections: **A.** Subcutaneous. **B.** Intramuscular (reproduced with permission from Downie et al 2003)

The intramuscular route

Intramuscular injections are delivered into the muscles below the skin. Figure 22.9B shows the needle angle used to access the muscle layer. There are several sites that can be used for i.m. injections. The person's general health and age are considered before deciding upon the most appropriate site. Older and emaciated people are likely to have less muscle than those who are young and active. The proposed site should be inspected for signs of swelling, inflammation, infection and skin lesions; affected areas should be avoided.

Deltoid muscle

The deltoid muscle is commonly used for vaccinations and for older children (Royal College of Paediatrics and Child Health 2002) (Fig. 22.10C).

Dorsogluteal site

The dorsogluteal site, also known as 'the upper outer quadrant' of the buttock, uses the gluteus maximus muscle (Fig. 22.10A). Studies have shown that there is relatively slow uptake of medication from this site (Rodger & King 2000). This is due to the large amount of adipose tissue located there, even in mildly obese patients, and means that the medication often ends up in the adipose tissue rather than the muscle (Workman 1999, Greenway & Hainsworth 2004). The nurse must therefore choose an appropriate length of needle depending on the size of the adult. There is also a risk of damaging the sciatic nerve if the site is not carefully located.

The Royal College of Paediatrics and Child Health (2002) do not advocate this site for children, except when a large volume of fluid is to be injected.

Ventrogluteal site

The ventrogluteal site accesses the gluteus medius muscle (Fig. 22.10D). Following an extensive literature review, Beyea and Nicoll (1995) promote the use of this site as it avoids potential sciatic nerve damage and the adipose tissue in the area is of relatively consistent thickness, thus ensuring the medication is administered into the muscle tissue (Greenway 2004). Workman (1999) suggests that a standard 21G (green) needle could be used in most adults of any size due to the consistent thickness of adipose tissue over this site.

Vastus lateralis muscle

This muscle is on the outer aspect of the thigh (Fig. 22.10B) and can be used for children, including infants (Royal College of Paediatrics and Child Health 2002). However Beyea and Nicoll (1996) suggest that, after 7 months of age, the ventrogluteal site should be the site of choice.

Rectus femoris

The rectus femoris is the anterior quadriceps muscle of the thigh. This is rarely used in adults, but can be easily accessed for self-administration or for infants (Workman 1999).

Administering intramuscular injections

The principles of administering i.m. injections are shown in Box 22.10.

The Z-track technique, formerly used exclusively for medications that stain the skin, is now widely recommended for all i.m. injections, as it is believed to reduce pain and leakage of medicine from the injection site. This technique involves gently pulling the skin and subcutaneous tissue so that it is no longer directly over the underlying muscle before carrying out the injection (Fig. 22.12) (Workman 1999). This is widely used for depot injections, commonly given to people with mental health problems.

Subcutaneous injections

These are given into the subcutaneous fat or connective tissue that lies between the muscles and the skin (see Fig. 22.9A). A short fine needle is used, e.g. 25G orange (Workman 1999). This route is suitable for drugs such as insulin that require slow and steady release. If a needle longer than 9 mm (25G orange) is used, an angle of 45° is recommended. When a shorter needle is required, e.g. for the administration of insulin, an angle of 90° is recommended (Workman 1999).

Some s.c. injections are pre-filled with the drug (such as heparin, given to prevent deep venous thrombosis), which means that there is no need to draw up the injection and therefore reduces the risk of needlestick injury. When using a shorter needle, it is not necessary to aspirate before injecting (Peragallo-Dittko 1997).

Figure 22.13 shows the sites that can be used for s.c. injections. People who require frequent s.c. injections, e.g. those with diabetes, should rotate injection sites and avoid using alcohol-impregnated wipes, which harden the skin. The principles of giving s.c. injections are shown in Box 22.11.

Administration of medication into the eye

People who regularly receive eye drops or ointment may prefer to have the medication instilled either while lying

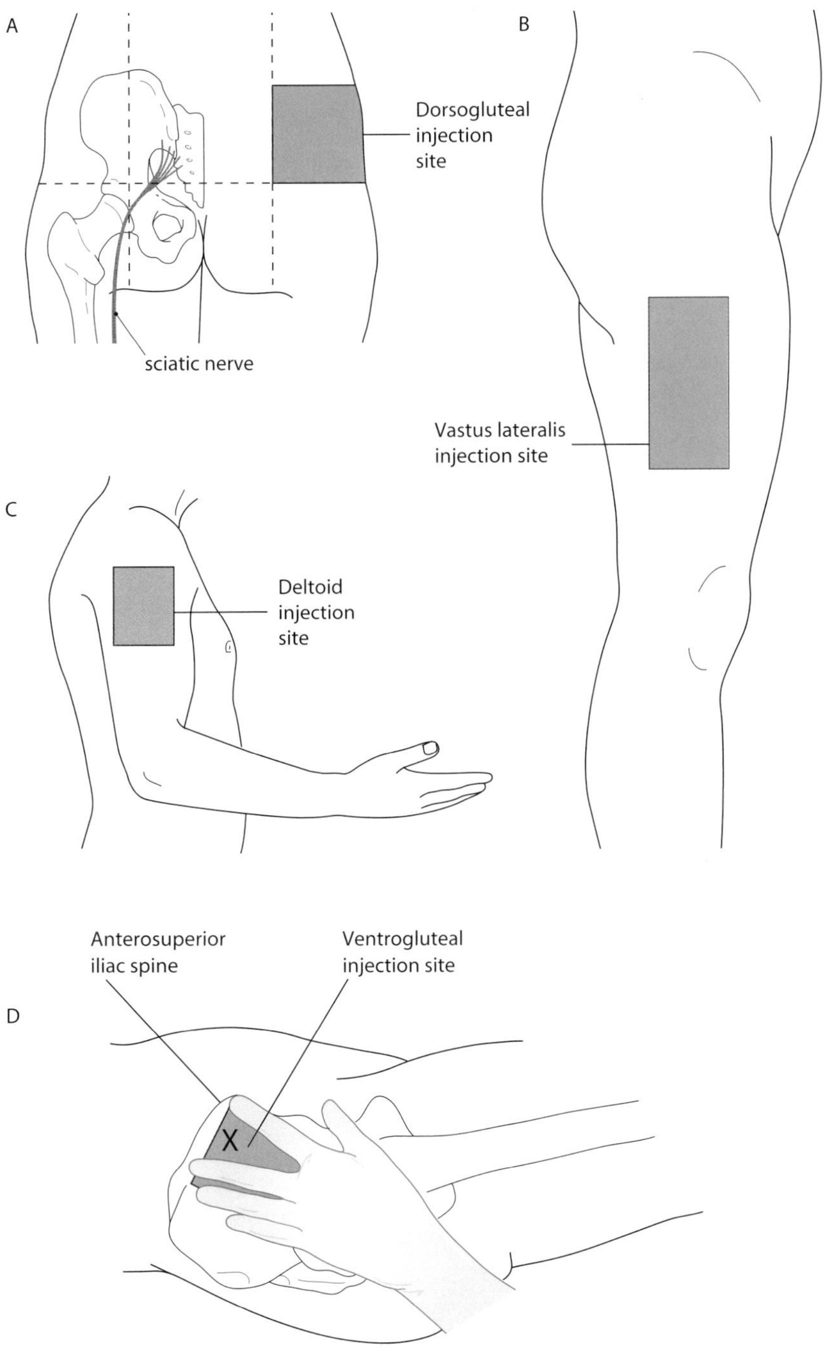

Fig. 22.10 Intramuscular injection sites (A, B, C reproduced with permission of Nicol et al 2004; D reproduced with permission from Wong et al 2001)

down or sitting upright and their wishes should be taken into account. This may be for an eye condition (e.g. glaucoma), after eye surgery or in preparation for examination of the eye. Postoperatively it may be essential that the patient is lying down while eye drops are instilled. The patient/client is prepared to receive medication following the principles outlined on page 639. Box 22.12 lists the principles of administering eye medication.

Administration of medicines into the ear

The patient is prepared to receive medication following the principles outlined on page 639. Ear drops may be instilled (Box 22.13, p. 646) to soften earwax prior to irrigation or syringing, or to relieve inflammatory or infective conditions of the outer ear.

Administration of medication into the nose

The patient is prepared to receive medication following the principles outlined on page 639. Box 22.14 lists the principles of administering nose drops.

NURSING SKILLS — Box 22.10

Administration of intramuscular injections

Principles

- The technique is explained to the person and their agreement is sought
- Handwashing is carried out according to local policy (see Ch. 15) and gloves worn
- The injection is drawn up as outlined in Box 22.9
- Privacy is ensured and the injection site exposed
- The skin is cleaned according to local policy
- The normal needle size for adults is 21G (green) (Nicol et al 2004). Local policy may recommend the use of smaller needles (23G blue) in, for example, very thin individuals or children
- The skin is stretched or pulled apart (Fig. 22.11) using the non-dominant hand. Alternatively, the Z-track technique (Fig. 22.12) should be used
- The syringe barrel is held like a dart or pencil in the dominant hand
- The patient/client is informed and the needle inserted swiftly and firmly into the skin at an angle of 90° (see Fig. 22.11). The plunger is inserted until about only 1 cm of the needle is showing (Nicol et al 2004)
- The plunger is withdrawn slightly to check that the needle is not in a blood vessel. Nicol et al (2004) recommend that if blood is present at this stage, the needle should be withdrawn, the needle and syringe discarded and the injection drawn up again using fresh equipment
- The plunger is then firmly and steadily depressed until all the fluid has been expelled
- The syringe is quickly removed and the alcohol-impregnated wipe held firmly over the puncture site until any bleeding stops
- The syringe and unsheathed needle are disposed of immediately into the designated sharps bin (NICE 2003, NES 2004)
- The remaining equipment is discarded
- Handwashing is carried out according to local policy
- The recording sheet is signed.

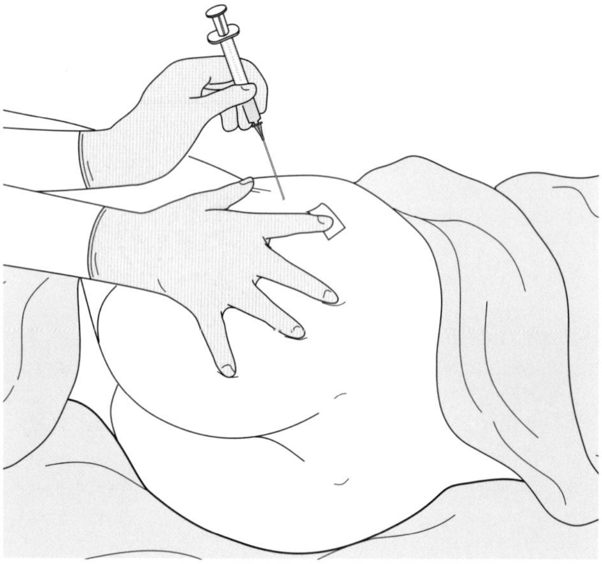

Fig. 22.11 Intramuscular injection technique (reproduced with permission from Nicol et al 2004)

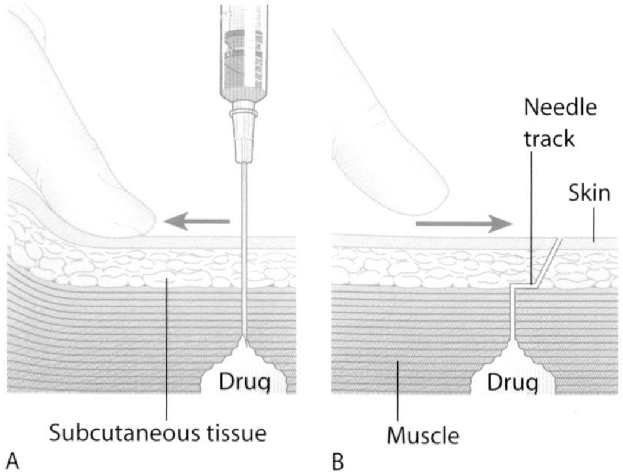

Fig. 22.12 Administering a Z-track injection (reproduced with permission from Downie et al 2003)

Rectal administration

This route is selected when:

- A person is unable to swallow oral preparations or during nausea and/or vomiting
- Medication may cause irritation of the upper gastrointestinal tract
- Drug delivery is required near to a diseased site, e.g. corticosteroids for inflammatory bowel disease
- Evacuation of the rectum is required i.e. a laxative effect.

Medication can be inserted into the rectum as suppositories and enemas (see Ch. 21). When this route is used for therapeutic drug administration (rather than for evacuation of the rectum), it must be explained that the medication should be retained, as many people associate suppositories and enemas with evacuation of the bowel. Ready access to lavatory facilities is necessary following administration of evacuant medication.

Administration of pessaries

The patient should be prepared to receive medication following the principles outlined on page 639. Box 22.15 (p. 647) provides the principles of administering a pessary into the vagina. Nurses must remember that most women find insertion of anything into the vagina very

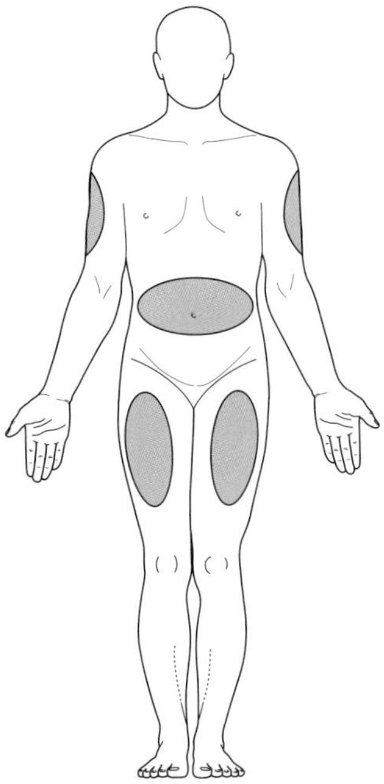

Fig. 22.13 Sites for subcutaneous injection (reproduced with permission from Nicol et al 2004)

NURSING SKILLS Box 22.11

Administering subcutaneous injections

Principles

- The technique is explained to the person and their agreement is sought
- Privacy is ensured by, for example, closing the cubicle door or pulling the screens
- Handwashing is carried out according to local policy (see Ch. 15) and gloves worn
- The injection is drawn up as outlined in Box 22.9
- Select a suitable site
- Skin cleansing is not usually required if the skin is clean
- The site is exposed and the skin fold pinched
- The drug is injected using the desired angle (see Fig. 22.9). For a 90° angle, the syringe is held in a 'pencil' grip and the needle is stabbed through the skin. For a 45° angle, the syringe is cradled across all four fingers, steadied with the thumb and, with the needle bevel uppermost, is pushed gently through the skin
- The syringe and unsheathed needle are disposed of immediately into the designated sharps bin (NICE 2003, NES 2004)
- The remaining equipment is discarded
- Handwashing is carried out according to local policy
- The recording sheet is signed.

NURSING SKILLS Box 22.12

Instillation of eye medication

Principles

- The technique is explained to the person who is advised that some eye medications cause discomfort when instilled
- Privacy is ensured by, for example, closing the cubicle door or pulling the screens
- Handwashing is carried out according to local policy (see Ch. 15)
- Medication is stored according to the manufacturer's instructions (usually refrigerated)
- If both eyes require medication, two containers are labelled (left and right), i.e. medication from one container is administered to the left eye and the other container used for the right eye to prevent cross-infection
- Remove the cap from the medication container
- Using the index finger of the non-dominant hand, gently pull down the lower eyelid while holding a tissue under the eye (Nicol et al 2004)
- The medicine container should be held in the dominant hand between the thumb and forefinger, about 2–3 cm from the eye and the person asked to look straight ahead.

For eye drops

- The container is gently squeezed and one drop inserted into the eye (Fig. 22.14A)
- The individual is asked to blink
- Further drops are instilled as prescribed.

For eye ointment

- The tube is squeezed gently until approximately 1–2 cm of ointment is expelled
- The 'ribbon' of ointment is placed inside the lower eyelid (Fig. 22.14B) from the inner to the outer canthus
- There should be no contact between the nozzle of the tube and any part of the eye.

Afterwards, in either case

- The person should close their eye gently for a few seconds to allow the drops to disperse or the ointment to dissolve
- Excess medication is wiped away with a clean tissue
- The cap is replaced
- Where more than one drug is prescribed, instillation of another drug should not be undertaken until 2 or 3 minutes have elapsed, ensuring that different preparations are compatible for administration at the same time (see BNF)
- Blurring of vision may occur following instillation and people are advised to wait until their vision returns to normal before moving about, to prevent falls or accidents
- Handwashing is carried out according to local policy (see Ch. 15).

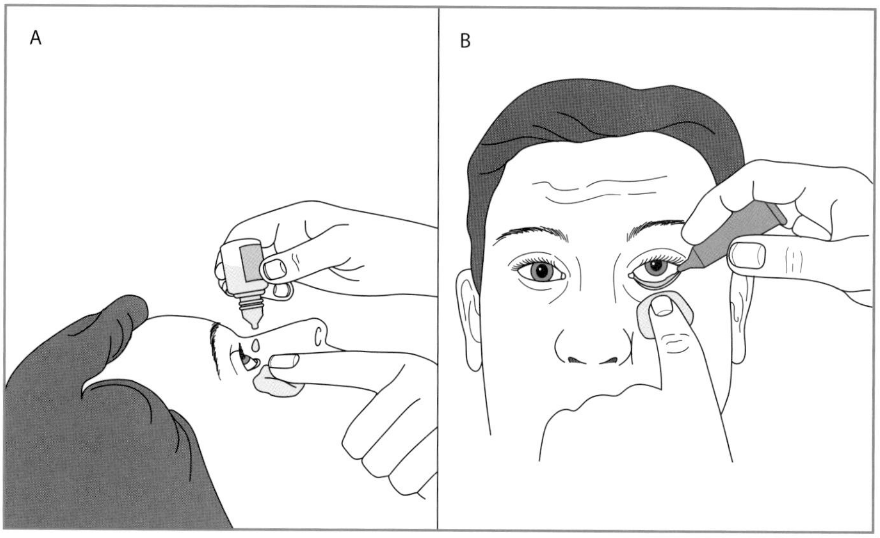

Fig. 22.14 Administration of eye medication: **A**. Drops. **B**. Ointment (reproduced with permission from Nicol et al 2004)

NURSING SKILLS Box 22.13

Instillation of medication into the ear

Principles

- The technique is explained to the person and their agreement is sought
- Handwashing is carried out according to local policy (see Ch. 15)
- The container is opened and the correct ear selected
- The person is asked to put their head down to the opposite shoulder and the projecting part of the external ear (the pinna) is pulled upward and back for an adult and down and back for a child
- Care should be taken to prevent contamination by ensuring that neither the nozzle of the container nor the dropper makes contact with the skin
- The container or dropper is gently squeezed, allowing the correct number of drops to be instilled into the ear
- The pinna is released and the container lid replaced
- The person should remain in this position for 1–2 minutes until the drug has travelled down the external auditory canal to the eardrum (Nicol et al 2004)
- When the individual resumes an upright position, any excess visible fluid is wiped away with a clean tissue
- If the prescription is to be delivered into both ears, 5–10 minutes should elapse between instillations. Two containers are labelled, one for each ear, so that medication from one container is administered into the left ear and from the other into the right ear, to prevent cross-infection.

NURSING SKILLS Box 22.14

Instillation of nasal drops

Principles

- The technique is explained to the person and their agreement is sought
- Handwashing is carried out according to local policy (see Ch. 15)
- Instillation may be performed with the person either lying down or sitting in a chair with their neck hyperextended, i.e. as far back the neck will allow
- With the cap of the container removed, the drops are administered into the nostril(s). A dropper is usually supplied with nose drops to ensure that the correct number of drops can be delivered in a controlled manner
- Care should be taken to ensure that the dropper does not make contact with the skin and become contaminated
- The person should be encouraged to remain in the same position for 1–2 minutes after insertion of the medication (Nicol et al 2004)
- Excess medication visible when the person sits upright again is wiped away with a clean tissue
- Handwashing is carried out according to local policy (see Ch. 15)
- The individual is advised not to blow their nose for approximately 20 minutes after instillation of medication into the nose (Nicol et al 2004).

embarrassing and when possible the patient/client should be encouraged to do this themselves. Nystatin pessaries may be prescribed for vaginal thrush (*Candida albicans*).

Inhaled medication

Medications can be introduced directly into the airways for local action (e.g. bronchodilators to relieve bronchospasm, corticosteroids to reduce inflammation) in respiratory conditions such as asthma and chronic bronchitis. Action via this route is fast and high concentrations can be delivered. There are various types of inhaler devices and their use is explained in Chapter 17. These include:

- Metered dose inhalers
- Dry powder inhalers
- Nebulizers.

NURSING SKILLS Box 22.15

Administration of pessaries

Principles

- The technique is explained and the woman's agreement is sought
- Handwashing is carried out according to local policy (see Ch. 15)
- Protective clothing, i.e. gloves and an apron, is worn
- The patient may require assistance to lie on her back, with her knees up and her legs apart
- Medication is inserted using an applicator that may be either preloaded or loaded following the manufacturer's instructions
- The applicator is introduced along the posterior wall of the vagina in an upward and backward direction and fully inserted (Fig. 22.15)
- The pessary is then ejected from the applicator
- The individual is given wipes to clean and dry the vulval area
- Sanitary protection should be worn afterwards, e.g. a panty liner or pad, as staining of underwear and bedding can occur after the pessary has melted
- Vaginal preparations are best administered at bedtime, when the person will be recumbent for several hours, thus allowing maximum absorption of the medication
- Handwashing is carried out according to local policy (see Ch. 15).

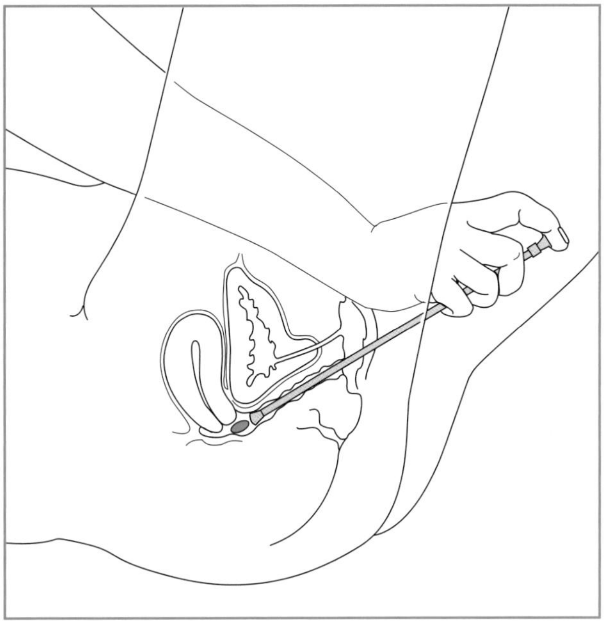

Fig. 22.15 Insertion of a vaginal pessary (reproduced with permission from Nicol et al 2004)

Administration of topical medication

The patient should be prepared to receive medication following the principles outlined on page 639. Box 22.16 provides the principles involved in administering topical creams, ointments or lotions that are usually prescribed for skin conditions.

NURSING SKILLS Box 22.16

Administration of creams, ointments and lotions

Principles

- The technique is explained to the person and their agreement is sought
- Handwashing is carried out according to local policy (see Ch. 15)
- An apron and gloves (to prevent absorption through the skin) are worn
- Creams, ointments or lotions are applied to clean, dry skin using sterile, strand-free gauze (Nicol et al 2004)
- Handwashing is carried out according to local policy
- The skin and/or any lesions are assessed and changes documented in the nursing notes.

Transdermal patches

Transdermal patches are used to deliver medication such as hormones, opioids and nicotine replacement therapy (Fig. 22.16). In these situations topical application is used to provide systemic effects, usually for a prolonged period. The old patch is removed, the skin cleaned and a new patch is applied, usually to a different area. The skin is observed for redness, soreness and other signs of a reaction to either the drug or the adhesive. Patches are placed on non-hairy areas according to the prescription and the manufacturer's instructions.

Post-drug administration measures

After administration of any medication, the nurse must always ensure that:

- The patient/client is comfortable
- Any equipment is removed and disposed of appropriately
- Administration has been recorded in line with professional and legal requirements (NMC 2004a, 2004b) and local policy.

The nurse must ensure that the patient/client knows:

- Why the medication has been given
- When the medicine should take effect, e.g. around 20 minutes for i.m. injections
- Any potential side effects and to report these if they occur.

The RN must check that:

- The prescription chart has been signed/initialled according to local policy if the medicine has been

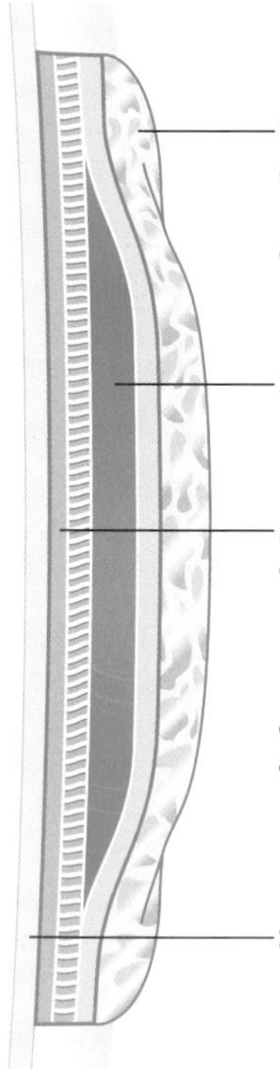

Fig. 22.16 Transdermal patch (adapted with permission from Downie et al 2003)

administered. If medication has not been administered, the reason for this must be documented
- The controlled drugs register has been completed, where appropriate, in accordance with local policy
- Medicines administered by student nurses have been countersigned
- Any adverse drug reactions are reported to the prescriber and/or charge nurse.

It should be noted that if the patient has been unable to swallow medicines, this should be reported immediately to the pharmacist and prescriber. A suitable alternative may be prescribed and dispensed.

Concordance, compliance and polypharmacy

The success of any medication regimen is most likely when it is completed according to the prescription. In this section, compliance, concordance and polypharmacy are considered.

Compliance

In order that medication can achieve its intended benefit it is important that people complete the prescribed course or continue to take it when a chronic condition is present. Compliance refers to the extent to which people follow health advice or other prescribed regimens, including drug treatment. It may be assumed that most people comply with prescribed drug treatment; however, this is often not the case and there are many reasons for this, including polypharmacy (see below) and difficulty in:

- Understanding why the medication is necessary
- Understanding what benefits the medication may have
- Remembering advice given to them
- Accepting disruption to their lifestyle
- Accepting that they have a condition that requires treatment.

There may be complex emotional, motivational or physical reasons (such as difficulty in swallowing) why a person does not or cannot take their medication as prescribed. People may have religious or cultural beliefs about taking drugs or a specific treatment; for example, vegetarians and people who do not eat beef (e.g. Hindus) may refuse to take gelatin capsules. Some patients/clients have difficulty in remembering when to take the medicine or if they have taken it. Sensory and/or motor difficulties can make opening the packaging difficult or impossible. Others may stop taking their medication when their symptoms are alleviated or if side effects (actual or perceived) occur. Downie et al (2003) highlight that there is usually more than one reason behind non-compliance.

Bending (2002) found that approximately 50% of older people do not take their medication as directed. This not only incurs wastage in relation to the drugs and their costs to the NHS but also results in incomplete or inappropriate treatment.

Concordance

Because the term compliance is considered to suggest a degree of compulsion, it is beginning to be replaced by the term concordance, especially in mental health nursing. Concordance involves a partnership approach to treatment such as medicine taking where an agreement between the patient/client and the healthcare professional is negotiated in relation to the use of prescribed medication (DH 2001). This is a person-centred approach where an individual's beliefs and wishes concerning their decision about medicine taking are paramount.

Polypharmacy

The Department of Health (2001) define polypharmacy as being prescribed four or more drugs. This is associated with more adverse drug reactions, predisposes to readmission of older adults following discharge from hospital and increases non-compliance. The Department of Health (2001) reviewed medicine-related aspects in the care of older adults and highlighted that medicine use increases with age:

- 80% people over the age of 75 took at least one prescribed drug
- 36% took more than four medications.

Bending (2002) highlighted that up to 17% of all hospital admissions relate to ADRs, which illustrates the immensity of this problem.

People may forget to mention any over-the-counter medicines that they take regularly, assuming that they

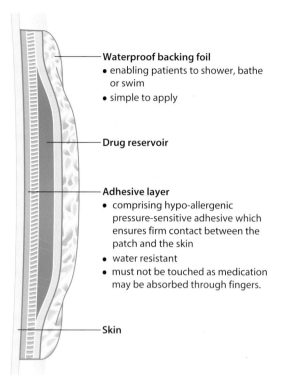

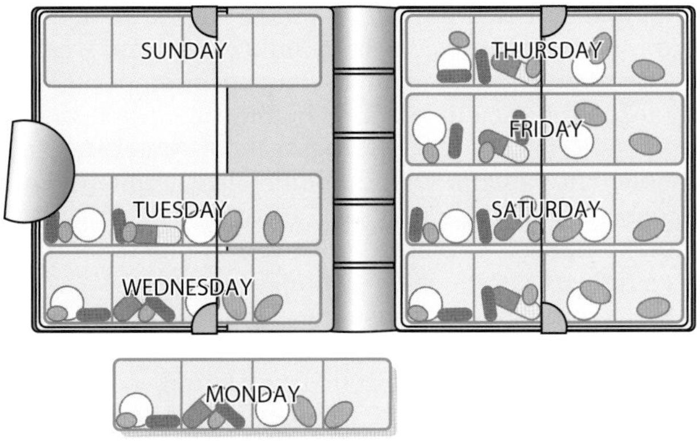

Fig. 22.17 Dosette box

are not 'real' medications, and the nurse should therefore ask patients/clients about these products as their use is widespread.

Nurses should be aware that both under- and over-medication can arise from personal beliefs, forgetfulness, impatience, improvement in a person's condition, lack of knowledge and/or misunderstanding about the drugs and that these should be considered when assessing compliance and monitoring response to treatment.

Improving compliance and concordance

Many people will require considerable support if compliance and concordance are to be achieved. Nurses must take the individual's physical and psychological state into account when explaining, demonstrating and teaching people about medication. Relatives and carers may also become involved in education about drug treatment in, for example, children and people with a learning disability. Individuals who lack manual dexterity, e.g. due to arthritis, may require medications to be organized in a Dosette box or supplied in easy-to-open containers. For people with visual impairment large-print labels help with compliance. In Scotland, written instruction leaflets must be supplied with all medicines (Scottish Executive Health Department 2002). Overcoming the factors that may predispose to poor compliance/concordance forms the basis of enabling people to follow their drug treatment.

Dosette boxes

These contain sections for each day of the week, which are further divided to correspond with the times of day when the patient/client takes their medication, e.g. 8 am, 12 midday, 6 pm, 10 pm. Each daily column has a sliding lid that can be opened to expose only the drugs to be taken at a particular time (Fig. 22.17). Individuals, carers, pharmacists or other healthcare professionals can fill these boxes with the appropriate prescribed medications. There may, however, be a loss of efficacy if tablets are removed from blister packs and put into these boxes.

Self-medication

Deeks and Byatt (2000) reported that compliance may improve if patients/clients are encouraged to self-medicate. Self-medication has long been performed in the individual's own home and now, increasingly, patients administer their own drugs in hospital. Since the introduction of lockable medicine cabinets (see Fig. 22.1B, p. 629) at each hospital bedside, self-administration has been discussed widely (Scottish Executive Health Department 2002). However, successful self-administration and ultimately compliance relies not only on nurses providing adequate education and support but also patient cooperation (Nicol et al 2004).

HEALTH PROMOTION Box 22.17

Medication in older adults

Mary is 79 years old and was admitted to hospital in a confused state. Investigations revealed she had a chest infection. She takes regular medication for high blood pressure and arthritis and has been prescribed antibiotics for her chest infection.

Student activities

Looking at the factors that may influence a person's concordance/compliance with their drug regimen, think about those that may apply to Mary:

1. Identify the nursing interventions that will help maximize compliance and concordance after Mary is discharged.
2. Find out from the pharmacist what aids to compliance are available in your placement.
3. Speak to some patients/clients in your placement and find out:
   - How much they know about drugs they take regularly.
   - The likely extent to which they comply with prescribed treatment.
   - What medications they often buy for themselves in a shop or pharmacy.

Patient-centred drug administration

Many patients/clients successfully adhere to complex medication regimens at home, but in the past people almost universally gave up control of this aspect of their care when admitted to hospital. Today many clinical areas have introduced an individual-centred drug administration system where all a person's drugs are stored locked in their bedside locker. These include their own drugs brought in on admission and/or new ones prescribed following admission.

In many clinical areas the nurse caring for a patient/client will administer their own drugs from the bedside locker according to the prescription sheet. This is a step towards complete individual-centred medicine administration where the patient/client administers their own medication from their bedside locker. One of the reasons behind this government-backed system is an effort to reduce the cost of medicines in both primary and secondary healthcare settings. Additionally, this system provides opportunities for patient education about drug treatment and assessment of people's understanding and likely compliance after discharge.

Drug errors

Much has been done to make drug administration safe and yet errors do still sometimes occur. The extent of drug errors has been the subject of much attention from the government, hospital management, pharmacists and healthcare professionals, all of whom consider the safe administration of medicines to be an essential nursing skill.

Following studies into how errors occur, changes to drug administration policies have been made in an effort to make this as safe as possible. Student nurses are taught how to administer drugs safely in university, then supervised carrying this out in practice and later assessed as competent before gaining registration. Thereafter nurses are expected to continually update their knowledge of the drugs they administer. In spite of this, errors sometimes still occur and the consequences for a patient/client can be fatal. The consequences for nurses can result in disciplinary action, an investigation of professional misconduct, criminal charges or a civil case for negligence (see Ch. 6). Most importantly, however, being involved in drug errors significantly reduces their confidence as practitioners.

Minimizing drug errors

There are many models aimed at minimizing the occurrence of drug errors. Smetzer (2001) suggested a 10-step model to safeguard the recipient, the nurse (administrator), the pharmacist (dispenser) and the doctor (prescriber). She maintains that all involved should know:

- The patient/client
- The drugs
- How to communicate clearly (see Ch. 9)
- Drug names that look and/or sound alike.

The storage and distribution of drugs should be restricted and standardized, and any drug delivery systems should be assessed for safety and be user friendly. The care environment should be conducive to safe working practices that include nurses having appropriate education and sufficient practice before being assessed as competent to administer drugs safely. Smetzer (2001) advises that patients/clients should also be involved and become part of the safety net. In order to reduce drug errors, emphasis is placed on drug administration processes rather than the practitioners involved.

Many authors have considered factors that predispose to drug errors. These include omission of the drug, administration of an unauthorized drug, wrong dose given, wrong delivery route used, wrongly completed prescription forms (see Box 22.3), wrong time of administration, wrong preparation given and incorrect administration technique. Contributing factors identified in nurses and nursing practices that have been implicated in drug errors include:

- Poor mathematical skills
- Lack of knowledge of medications
- Tiredness caused by, e.g. long shifts and shift patterns
- High workload
- Interruptions during drug administration.

Dealing with drug errors

When a drug error occurs it must be reported immediately. An incident form is completed and an investigation is undertaken (see Chs 6, 13). The NMC (2004a) recommend that this is undertaken by a multidisciplinary critical incident panel and staff should feel that they will be supported throughout the investigation. Information about reporting and developing a 'no blame' culture can be found on the National Patient Safety website (see p. 651).

Summary

- Nursing practice is underpinned by legislation that governs the safe storage, ordering and prescribing of medicines.
- Pharmacodynamic principles are used to explain 'what drugs do to the body'.
- Pharmacokinetic principles help to explain 'what the body does to drugs'.
- Nurses must be familiar with actions and side effects of drugs commonly used in each placement.
- Safe administration of medicines requires a methodical approach that follows local policies.
- Nurses need to be familiar with a range of routes used for drug administration.

- Patient/client education about prescribed drug is important.
- Polypharmacy is the prescribing of more than four drugs and is associated with poorer concordance and compliance.
- Awareness of predisposing factors may reduce drug errors.
- Drug errors should be approached using a 'no blame' culture.

Self test

1. A patient is prescribed 50 mg of clozapine. The tablets available are 25 mg. Calculate the number of tablets required.

2. A patient is prescribed 125 micrograms of digoxin. The stock on hand is 0.25 mg. Calculate the number of tablets required. *Tip*: Look carefully at both weights.

3. A patient is prescribed 500 mg of erythromycin. The department stock is 250 mg/5 mL. Calculate the volume of mixture required.

4. A child is prescribed flucloxacillin. The dosage is 50 mg/kg/day, four doses daily. If the child weighs 36 kg, calculate the size of a single dose.

5. a. A child is prescribed vincristine. The recommended dosage is 1.5 mg/m^2. The child's surface area is 0.6 m^2. Calculate the dose required.
   b. The stock available is 1 mg/mL. Now calculate the volume required.

6. Identify whether each statement is TRUE or FALSE:
   a. A student nurse's signature must always be countersigned by a RN.
   b. The ventrogluteal site can be used for i.m. injections.
   c. A prescription-only medicine can only be supplied when it is prescribed.
   d. Nurses are not responsible for the administration of medicines.
   e. Medicines can sometimes be stored in an unlocked area within hospital areas.

7. Identify whether the following statements refer to subcutaneous or intramuscular injections:
   a. The normal size of needle used for adults is a 21G (green).
   b. The Z-track technique may be used.
   c. The skin fold is pinched prior to needle insertion.

8. If cleaning the skin prior to an injection is advocated by the local policy, for how long should the skin be cleansed?

Key words and phrases for literature searching

Compliance
Concordance
Drug administration
Drug calculations
Injections
Medicines
Parenteral
Prescribing
Self-medication

Useful websites

British National Formulary	www.bnf.org.uk/bnf Available July 2006
British National Formulary for Children	http://bnfc.org/bnfc Available July 2006
Medicines and Healthcare Products Regulatory Agency	www.mhra.gov.uk/home/idcplg?IdcService=SS_GET_PAGE&nodeId=5 Available July 2006
National Patient Safety Agency	www.npsa.nhs.uk Available July 2006

References

Bending A 2001 Hiding medicines. Primary Health Care 11(8):24–25

Bending A 2002 Just how do you make sure the medicine goes down? Nursing in Practice March:426–428

Beyea S, Nicoll L 1995 Administration of medications via the intramuscular route: an integrative review of the literature and research-based protocol for the procedure. Applied Nursing Research 8(1):23–33

Beyea S, Nicoll L 1996 Administering IM injections the right way. American Journal of Nursing 96(1):34–37

Clinical Resource and Audit Group 2002 Good practice statement for the preparation of injections in near-patient areas, including clinical and home environments. Online: www.show.scot.nhs.uk/crag/publications/inpa.pdf Available July 2006

Deeks PA, Byatt K 2000 Are patients who self-administer their medicines in hospital more satisfied with their care? Journal of Advanced Nursing 13(2):395–400

Department of Health 1988 Guidelines for the safe and secure handling of medicines (The Duthie Report). HMSO, London

Department of Health 1999 Review of prescribing: supply and administration of medicines. TSO, London

Department of Health 2001 Medicines and older people: implementing medicine-related aspects of the National Service Framework. TSO, London

Downie G, Mackenzie J, Williams A 2003 Pharmacology and medicines management for nurses. 3rd edn. Churchill Livingstone, Edinburgh

Gatford JD, Phillips N 2002 Nursing calculations. 6th edn. Churchill Livingstone, Edinburgh

Greenstein B (ed) 2004 Trounce's clinical pharmacology for nurses. 17th edn. Churchill Livingstone, Edinburgh

Greenway K 2004 Using the ventrogluteal site for intramuscular injection. Nursing Standard 18(25):39–42

Greenway K, Hainsworth T 2004 Is it right to be injecting the dorsogluteal site? NT practical procedures. Nursing Times 100(47):16

Hopkins SJ, Kelly JC 1999 Drugs and pharmacology for nurses. 13th edn. Churchill Livingstone, Edinburgh

Miller D, Miller H 2000 To crush or not to crush. Nursing 30(2):51, 52

National Institute for Health and Clinical Excellence 2003 Infection control: prevention of healthcare-associated infections in primary and community care. Online: www.nice.org.uk/pdf/Infection_control_fullguideline.pdf Available July 2006

NHS Education for Scotland 2004 Healthcare associated infection. Online: www.space4.me.uk/hai/index.html Available July 2006

Nicol M, Bavin C, Bedford-Turner S et al 2004 Essential nursing skills. 2nd edn. Mosby, Edinburgh

Nursing and Midwifery Council 2004a Guidelines for the administration of medicines. Online: www.nmc-uk.org/aFrameDisplay.aspx?DocumentID=610 Available July 2006

Nursing and Midwifery Council 2004b Code of professional conduct: standards for conduct, performance and ethics. Online: www.nmc-uk.org/aFrameDisplay.aspx?DocumentID=201 Available July 2006

Nursing and Midwifery Council 2004c Standards of proficiency for pre-registration nursing education. Online: www.nmc-uk.org/aFrameDisplay.aspx?DocumentID=328 Available July 2006

Nursing and Midwifery Council 2005 Guidelines for records and record keeping. Online: www.nmc-uk.org/aFrameDisplay.aspx?DocumentID=609 Available July 2006

Peragallo-Dittko V 1997 Re-thinking subcutaneous injection technique. American Journal of Nursing 97(5):71–72

Rang HP, Dale MM, Ritter J, Moore P 2003 Pharmacology. 5th edn. Churchill Livingstone, Edinburgh

Rodger MA, King L 2000 Drawing up and administering intramuscular injections: a review of the literature. Journal of Advanced Nursing 31(3):574–582

Royal College of Paediatrics and Child Health 2002 Position statement on injection technique. Online: www.rcpch.ac.uk Available July 2006

Scottish Executive Health Department 2002 The right medicine: a strategy for pharmaceutical care in Scotland. TSO, Edinburgh

Smetzer J 2001 Take 10 giant steps to medication safety. Nursing 31(11):49–53

Treloar A, Beats B, Philpot M 2001 Concealing medication in patients' food. Lancet 357(9249):62–64

United Kingdom Central Council for Nursing, Midwifery and Health Visiting 2001 UKCC position statement on the covert administration of medicines – disguising medicine in food and drink. Online: www.nmc-uk.org/aFrameDisplay.aspx?DocumentID=623 Available July 2006

Wong DL, Hockenberry-Eaton M 2001 Wong's essentials of pediatric nursing. 6th edn. Mosby, St Louis

Workman B 1999 Safe injection technique. Nursing Standard 13(39):47–53

Wright D J 2003 Altering medication forms: what you should know. Nursing and Residential Care 5(8):372–375

Further reading

Chernecky CC et al 2002 Drug calculations and drug administration. Saunders, Philadelphia

Dougherty L, Lister S (eds) 2004 Drug administration: general principles. The Royal Marsden Hospital Manual of Clinical Nursing Procedures. 6th edn. Blackwell, Oxford, pp. 184–227

Dunning G 2005 The choice, application and review of topical treatments for skin conditions. Nursing Times 101(4):55–56

Gabriel J, Dailly S, Keyley J 2004 Needlestick and sharps injuries: avoiding the risk in clinical practice. Professional Nurse 20(1):25–26

Hopkins SJ, Kelly JC 1999 Drugs and pharmacology for nurses. 13th edn. Churchill Livingstone, Edinburgh

Nicoll LH, Hesby A 2002 Intramuscular injection: an integrative research review and guideline for evidence-based practice. Applied Nursing Research 15(3):149–162

Pickering K 2003 Nutrition: the administration of drugs via enteral feeding tubes. Nursing Times 99(46):46–47, 49

Small SP 2004 Preventing sciatic nerve injury from intramuscular injections: literature review. Journal of Advanced Nursing 47(3):287–296

Trim J 2004 Clinical skills: a practical guide to working out drug calculations. British Journal of Nursing 13(10):602–606

23

Pain management – minimizing the pain experience

Carol Chamley and Gay James

Glossary terms

Acute pain

Adjuvants

Analgesics

Chronic pain

Gate control theory

Neuropathic pain

Nociceptive pain

Pain modulation

Pain threshold

Pain tolerance

Learning outcomes

This chapter will help you:

- Explain the biopsychosocial effects of pain on people throughout the lifespan
- Outline different types of pain
- Explore the subjective and individual impact of pain on people
- Discuss how the gate control theory of pain influences nursing management of pain
- Demonstrate an awareness of holistic pain assessment
- Describe the principles of pharmacological management of pain
- Outline non-pharmacological approaches to pain management.

Introduction

Pain is a common experience throughout life and often it was seen as a burden to be endured because little treatment was available. It may be argued that people start life with acute pain following birth, though this may only recently have been acknowledged. As people age, degenerative disorders of the musculoskeletal system often lead them to accept pain as a natural consequence of the ageing process. This acceptance can limit quality of life, an important issue in the ageing population. Over the past 50 years advances in pain management have been possible due to an improved understanding of the multidimensional nature of pain and subsequent advances in treatments available.

Pain is recognized as a useful indicator of tissue damage and, from childhood, pain 'hurt' is associated with injury. The pain experience is not just a sensory signal; pain triggers complex physiological, emotional and social responses. These are influenced by many factors that include pain type, age, past experiences, emotional state, environment, culture and cognitive appraisal.

Although pain is often a useful warning of tissue injury that allows people to respond to external harm or internal changes, it may also cause physiological stress and emotional distress, which can harm the individual if unrelieved. Indeed some diseases, e.g. cancer, are not associated with pain as a presenting feature though it is commonly associated and feared in advanced disease. Even trauma may not initially be associated with pain at the time of injury; often a sports injury is not recognized until the game is over unless it is serious.

Poor pain management can lead to physical and emotional problems; postoperatively it is linked to complications and delayed recovery. In children, pain may lead to regression; a poor experience can have serious implications for future contact with healthcare personnel and settings in adult life.

Nurses are frequently key workers in the management of pain. Pain recognition and prioritization are important aspects of patient care. Pain is a common experience across all care settings, both hospital and community based. An elementary understanding of pain and its management is relevant to foundation studies and central to all branches of nursing.

The nature of pain

This part of the chapter outlines the different types of pain, gate control theory, pain physiology and psychological and cultural aspects of pain.

Pain is a subjective, complex and multidimensional experience that has physical, psychosocial, emotional and spiritual elements. Due to its complexity, a simple

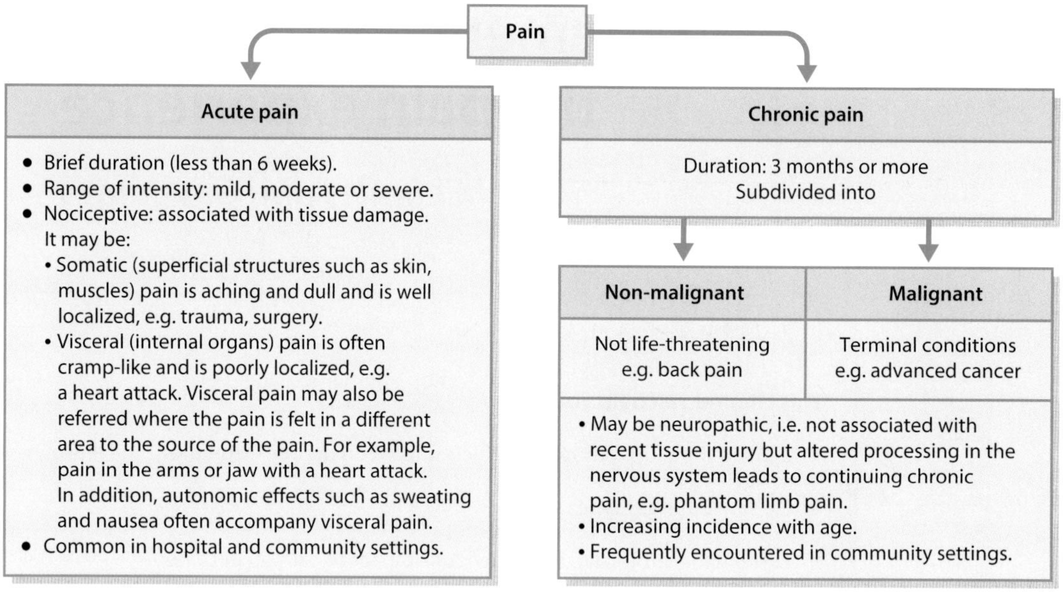

Fig. 23.1 Types of pain

agreed definition for pain is elusive. The International Association for the Study of Pain (IASP) (Merskey & Bogduk 1994) defines pain as 'an unpleasant sensory and emotional experience associated with actual or potential tissue damage, or described in terms of such damage'. In 1968, McCaffery proposed a simple statement which is widely accepted in nursing as it emphasizes the individual nature of pain and the patient is clearly identified as the key person in pain assessment – 'Pain is: whatever the experiencing person says it is, existing whenever he says it does' (McCaffery & Pasero 1999).

Types and characteristics of pain

Clear distinctions between types may not be possible (McCaffery & Pasero 1999). However, general categories can help to identify suitable evidence on which to base care. One of the broadest categories is acute or chronic, which classifies pain according to a timescale (Fig. 23.1). This chapter will concentrate on acute and chronic pain; however, pain can be categorized in other ways that include:

- Cause related to pathology
- Nociceptive or neuropathic
- Clinical specialty/client group.

In order to provide appropriate care, nurses need to appreciate the type of pain experienced as this influences assessment and suitability of pharmacological and non-pharmacological interventions.

Acute pain (Fig. 23.1)

Acute pain is usually of brief duration (less than 6 weeks) and is commonly nociceptive, associated with tissue injury such as surgery, which subsides as healing takes place (Box 23.1). Acute pain is very common; it can range in intensity from transitory pain felt after a minor bump or a mild headache to severe pain associated with trauma or disease, e.g. fractures or heart attack. Mild acute pain may be managed successfully with patient/parent-initiated interventions at home. However, the pain may also indicate problems and motivate the person to seek medical advice.

> **REFLECTIVE PRACTICE** Box 23.1
>
> **Acute pain**
>
> Think about a recent minor injury you had, such as a cut or a bruise.
>
> **Student activities**
>
> - Consider the intensity of pain you experienced at the time of injury.
> - How long was it before the pain subsided to soreness or an ache?
> - How long did it take for the pain to cease?

Acute nociceptive pain may be referred; this is when pain arises in internal organs (viscera) but is experienced some distance from the source of the pain. For example, a heart attack frequently causes pain down the arms (usually the left) and up the neck and jaw, despite there being no tissue injury in those areas. Sensory impulses from the left arm and heart enter the spinal cord at the same level. Normally, few sensory impulses are processed from the heart so when more impulses are received for processing, this results in perception of pain arising from the arm. Another example of referred pain is the initial pain of acute appendicitis, which is felt around the umbilicus, despite the appendix being sited in the right lower part of the abdomen (Fig. 23.2).

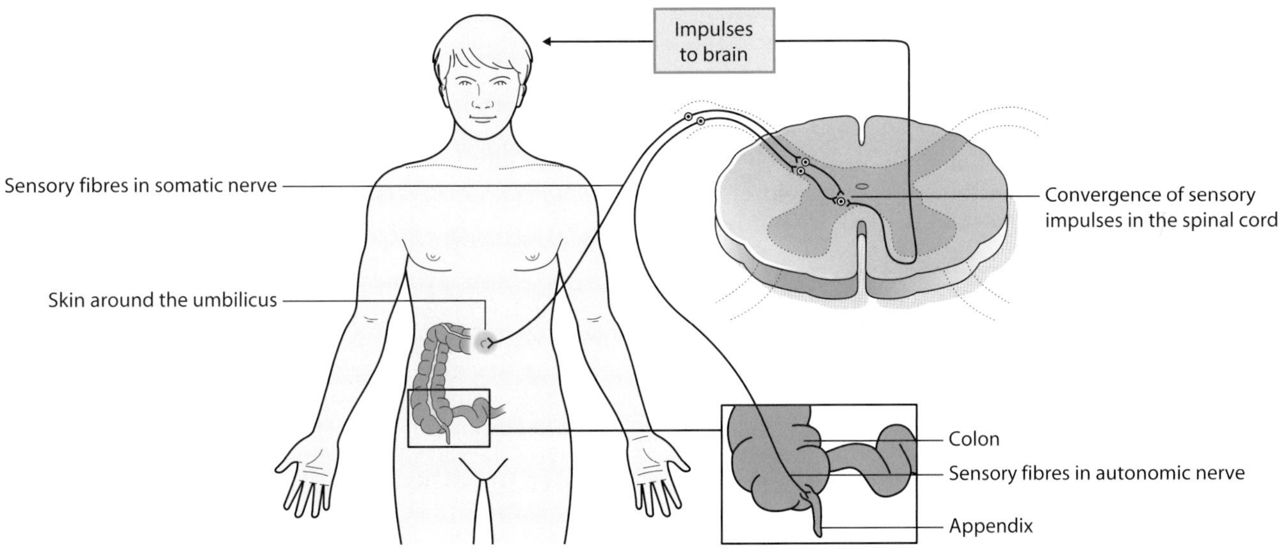

Fig. 23.2 Referred pain – acute appendicitis (adapted with permission from Rutishauser 1994)

Chronic pain (Fig. 23.1)

When pain does not resolve and becomes chronic (usually lasting longer than 3 months) the effect on a person's quality of life can lead to depression and social isolation. In a child this may seriously influence their education and their future potential as adults. In adults it can cause relationship problems, isolation and financial difficulties and it may be a cause of mental health problems including suicidal ideation. Chronic pain is further subdivided into non-malignant and malignant (life-threatening) pain.

Chronic non-malignant pain

Chronic non-malignant pain is not life threatening and may be due to continuing tissue injury, e.g. rheumatoid arthritis, where the degeneration may continue for the rest of a person's life. The two most common reasons for this type of pain were identified as back pain in all age groups and arthritis, which increased proportionally with age (Elliot et al 1999). This research estimates that 46.5% of the general population suffers chronic pain, though for many this was mild pain (Elliot et al 1999). This has implications for support required by this group in the community. However, when back pain first occurs it could be considered as acute, its failure to subside can then lead it to become chronic. Effective management of acute back pain may reduce the risk of people developing chronic back pain. Horn and Munafo (1997) discuss pain dimensions and propose that acute and chronic pain may be usefully regarded as at the ends of a spectrum, rather than fundamentally separate conditions.

Chronic non-malignant pain can involve alterations in pain processing by the nervous system, which results in pain memories. This is known as neuropathic pain, e.g. phantom limb pain where pain is perceived as coming from the amputated part, or the nerve pain (neuralgia) after shingles (Box 23.2). Neuropathic pain may exist without any identifiable tissue damage.

> Box 23.2 **Neuropathic pain after shingles**
>
> The acute pain of shingles (herpes zoster) can also lead to chronic pain known as postherpetic neuralgia if the pain is not well managed. The chronic continuing pain becomes typical of neuralgia with:
>
> - Abnormal skin sensitivity in the area (allodynia)
> - Continuous burning or aching pain with additional shooting pain (McCaffery & Pasero 1999, p. 562).
>
> This can have serious effects on quality of life, affecting sleep, normal mobility and social interaction, particularly a concern in older people. The aggressive management of the acute pain with appropriate drugs reduces the risk of postherpetic neuralgia developing.

It is suggested that the initial tissue or nerve damage can lead to persistent changes in the central nervous system (CNS). It is then argued that failure to effectively manage acute pain can lead to an increased sensitivity known as 'wind-up' in the CNS, which can be responsible for chronic pain (Carr & Mann 2000). Evidence supports this in the example of phantom limb pain, where the incidence is greater in patients who had pain prior to amputation, and incidence of neuropathic pain that has been reduced with the use of effective preoperative pain management (McCaffery & Pasero 1999).

Neuropathic pain is difficult to treat and can be particularly baffling for patients and carers as it does not follow the more familiar acute pain pattern and may continue for many years. In the past the person was often referred to mental health professionals, particularly if an organic cause (tissue injury) could not be identified.

It is now recognized that all pain involves psychological and physiological factors, and that the role of psychological factors increases when the condition is long lasting (Sarafino 2002).

All pain experiences may be modified by psychological factors so treatment and management should incorporate this knowledge for both acute and chronic pain. Chronic pain can impact on the following:

- The person's behaviour causing disability
- Their psychological state causing emotional distress
- Social interaction (loss of confidence).

This can be destructive to normal quality of life for the individual and their carers, and management should focus on all these areas to provide holistic care. For these people, pain management often involves more specialized pharmacological approaches. Many people with chronic pain are in the community and may require support from the primary care team (see Ch. 3) with referral to specialist multidisciplinary teams (MDT) (see p. 668) to achieve the best in pain management.

Chronic malignant pain

Chronic malignant pain is associated with terminal conditions, often linked to cancer, where the progression and spread of the disease lead to pain. However, pain is rarely a presenting symptom of cancer. Initially the 'cancer journey' involves acute pain (nociceptive) associated with diagnostic procedures and treatments, e.g. surgery. If the cancer spreads, pain can then become chronic and more complex, involving nociceptive, neuropathic and psychological components that require regular review and adjustment of treatment to meet the person's needs (see Ch. 12). This is recognized as 'total pain' and requires skills across the MDT (Paz & Seymour 2004). The patient with cancer pain can also suffer acute pain episodes, e.g. pain following a pathological fracture.

Gate control theory

In 1965, Melzack and Wall devised the gate control theory which proposed that the pain sensation is modulated (processed) in the spinal cord by a gate-like mechanism. The gate theory proposed that active processing of nerve impulses occurs in the spinal cord where the pain sensation first enters the CNS. The proposed 'gates' are thought to be in a region of the spinal cord known as the dorsal horn. The gate is opened or closed depending on the combination of sensory ascending impulses from the periphery or descending impulses from the brain. Pain will only be appreciated if the gate is open. This recognized the psychological influences on pain such as anxiety and proved a sound theory on which to explain clinical observations of pain perception. The theory is proving to be robust and has been refined by further research. The subsequent discovery of endogenous opioids, e.g. endorphins, in the 1970s enabled the actual mechanism of modulation to be understood in more detail. The gate control theory is acknowledged as providing a good theoretical basis for understanding pain perception in individuals as it recognizes factors that open or close the gate and guides approaches taken to managing pain (Fig. 23.3).

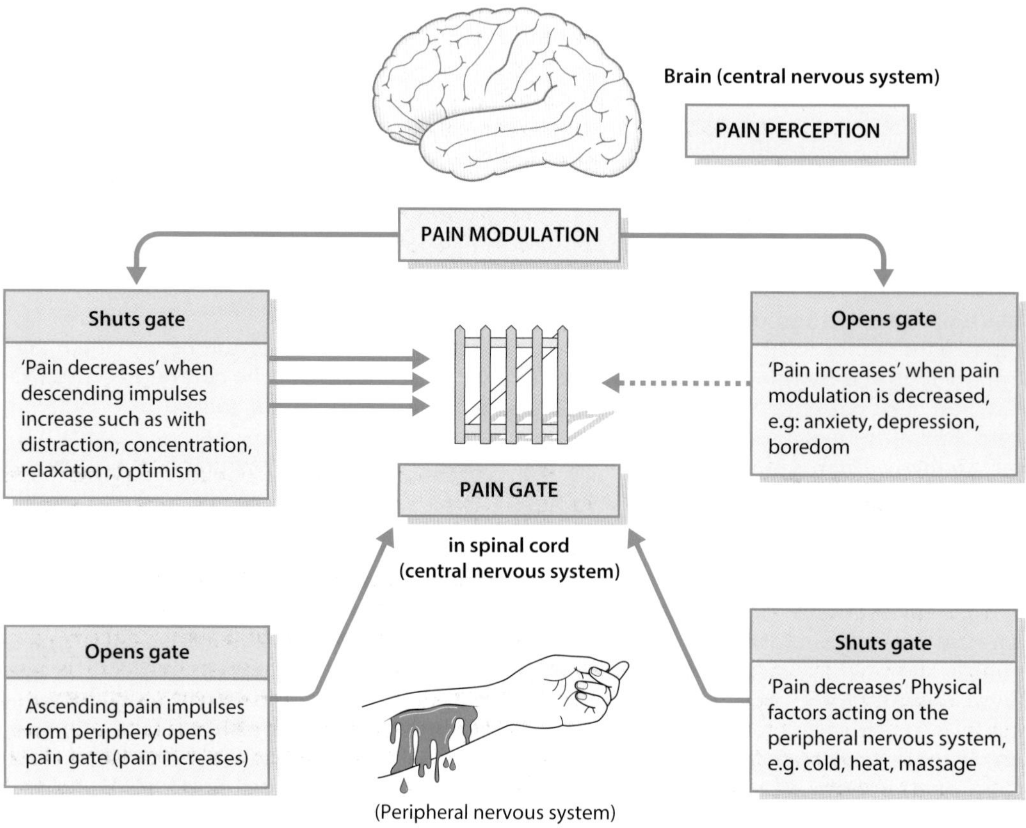
Brain (central nervous system)
PAIN PERCEPTION
PAIN MODULATION
Shuts gate
'Pain decreases' when descending impulses increase such as with distraction, concentration, relaxation, optimism
Opens gate
'Pain increases' when pain modulation is decreased, e.g: anxiety, depression, boredom
PAIN GATE
in spinal cord (central nervous system)
Opens gate
Ascending pain impulses from periphery opens pain gate (pain increases)
Shuts gate
'Pain decreases' Physical factors acting on the peripheral nervous system, e.g. cold, heat, massage
(Peripheral nervous system)

Fig. 23.3
Gate control theory

Conditions	Conditions which may open the gate *'Make the pain worse'*	Conditions which may close the gate *'Make the pain better'*
Physical	Extent of injury Inappropriate activity levels Fatigue	Medication Heat, cold, massage, transcutaneous electrical nerve stimulation (TENS) Exercise including sexual intercourse
Emotional	Anxiety Depression	Positive emotions (happiness or optimism) Relaxation, rest
Mental	Boredom Focusing on pain	Intense concentration Distraction

Table 23.1 Factors known to influence the 'pain gate' (summarized from Sarafino 2002, p. 347)

The theory recognizes the multidimensional nature of pain and explains the many aspects of pain that are known to influence pain perception and can be used in pain management. As psychological (emotional) and cognitive (evaluative) aspects appear to influence the opening and closing of the 'pain gate', it encourages nurses to take a holistic approach to pain management, which acknowledges these components. This supports the unique nature of a person's pain experience; even when pain physiology appears to be closely matched, the emotional state and cognitive appraisal (past experience and meaning) of the experience can result in different pain perception by individuals. Table 23.1 summarizes the factors known to influence the 'pain gate'. Some examples of the influences on a person's perception of pain are provided in Box 23.3 and the effects of chronic pain in Box 23.4.

Physiology of pain

The experience of pain results from integrated processes involving chemicals, sensory receptors, nerve fibres, spinal cord with the 'pain gates' and various areas in the brain. Knowledge of pain physiology enables the nurse to understand how pain can be relieved and how analgesics (drugs that relieve pain) act. Acute (nociceptive) pain is described as involving four processes:

- Transduction
- Transmission
- Modulation
- Perception

The four processes are outlined and shown diagrammatically in Figure 23.4 (p. 658).

Transduction

Injury causes the release of inflammatory chemicals such as prostaglandins and 5-hydroxytryptamine (5-HT) that form an 'algesic soup' (meaning pain causing). These chemicals stimulate nociceptors (receptors that respond to stimuli that are harmful and cause pain) on sensory nerves, which transmit impulses from somatic areas (skin, joints, bone) and the viscera (internal organs). Prostaglandins are among the key chemicals released by damaged tissues. Drugs collectively known as non-steroidal

REFLECTIVE PRACTICE Box 23.3

Influences on pain perception

Pain is influenced by a number of factors such as knowing the cause or not. Read the statements below and then carry out the activities.

- Pain of known cause such as a migraine compared with sudden chest pain
- Pain after planned, curative surgery compared with pain following emergency surgery or trauma
- Child in pain following a tumble during a football game compared with a scald from boiling water
- Mild toothache that appears to increase when trying to sleep compared with it appearing to diminish when watching an exciting film.

Student activities

- How might knowing the cause of pain influence perception?
- Think about how reasons for surgery can influence pain perception.
- How can these events be explained by the gate control theory of pain?

REFLECTIVE PRACTICE Box 23.4

Chronic pain – biopsychosocial perspective

Think about a patient, client or someone you know who has chronic pain, e.g. back pain.

Student activities

- How do you think the person might feel about having no identifiable reason for the pain?
- Consider how emotions may affect the 'pain gate' for this type of pain.
- How much empathy and support do you think the person received from health professionals and family?
- What impact would chronic pain have on normal activities of daily living?

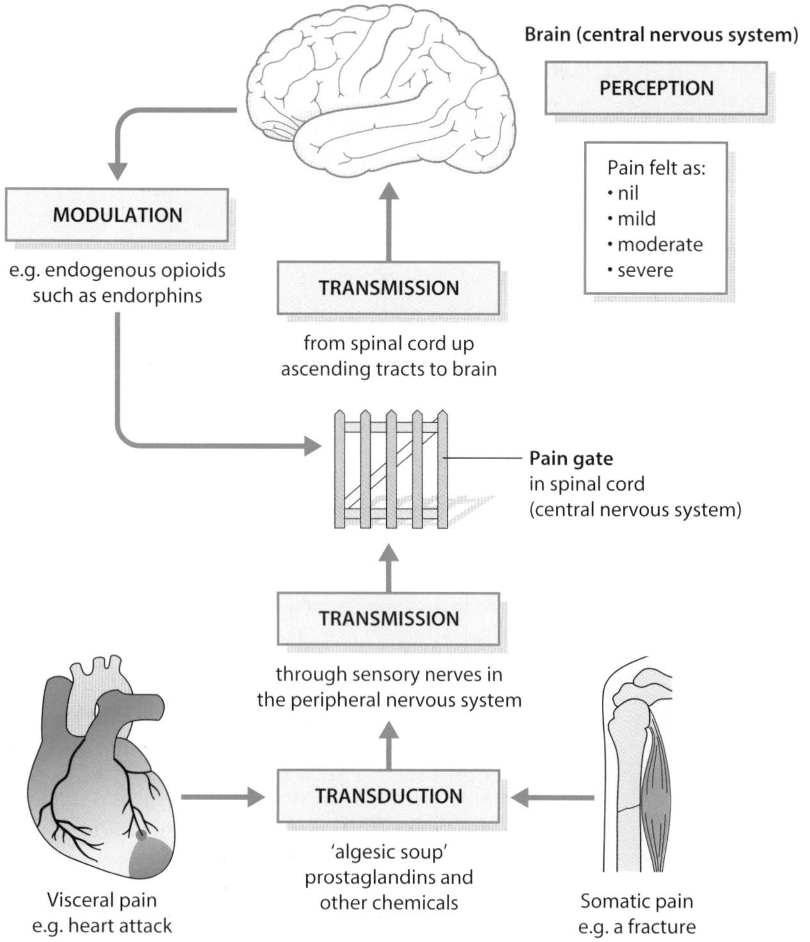

Fig. 23.4 Pain physiology

anti-inflammatory drugs (NSAIDs) relieve pain by inhibiting prostaglandin production.

Transmission

Transmission is the spread of pain impulses through sensory nerves of various types in the peripheral nervous system (PNS) to the spinal cord and up the ascending tracts to the brain. Some pain nerve fibres are classified as fast fibres and others as slow fibres. Fast fibres, found in skin and mucous membranes, transmit pain that is sharp and well defined, whereas slow fibres conduct impulses more slowly and pain appears to grow in intensity. It is described as dull, diffuse and aching, and continues after the event, such as the pain felt after removing a foot from a bath that is too hot.

The nerve impulses are processed in the 'pain gates' in the spinal cord. Other fast fibres that transmit touch or pressure impulses from receptors in the periphery and descending impulses from the brain both influence the 'pain gate', which may remain open to transmit pain or close and prevent pain transmission. If the dominant sensation is from touch receptors that release inhibitory chemicals, the 'pain gate' may close. This is the basis for the use of local pressure, massage and other non-pharmacological coping strategies used by patients to help shut the 'pain gate' (see pp. 673–677).

Many of the pharmacological treatments for pain act by interfering with the transmission of pain impulses along the pathway between the tissue injury and the cortex of the brain, e.g. local anaesthetic drugs administered as topical cream or gel.

Modulation

Modulation describes the inhibition of pain impulses by neural and chemical influences on the 'pain gate'. Nerves that descend from the brain stem to the spinal cord close the gate by releasing endogenous opioids, e.g. endorphins (Box 23.5). This is why nociceptive pain is responsive to opioids such as morphine. Endogenous opioid modulation may also explain the variation in pain perception seen in clinical practice. Some individuals have more effective modulation than others (McCaffery & Pasero 1999). In experimental studies, the *placebo effect* is identified where subjects show an analgesic response to a masked inert drug (e.g. sugar pill versus analgesic). Some subjects respond, whereas others are non-responders. Placebo responders represent a group with a highly developed endogenous opioid system.

Other modulating substances identified are the neurotransmitters 5-HT and noradrenaline (norepinephrine). Drugs such as amitriptyline can be used as adjuvants to assist the action of other analgesics for neuropathic

Box 23.5 **Endogenous opioids**

- From animal studies it appears that the endogenous opioid system develops after birth and declines with age. This could have implications for human subjects, particularly babies and older people
- Individual variations in pain tolerance and opioid analgesia response may indicate differences in endogenous opioid activity
- Opioids are released in response to extended physical exertion, e.g. 'runners high'
- Acupuncture appears to stimulate the endogenous opioid system (see Ch. 10)
- Major trauma is accompanied by release of endogenous opioids, which may explain the initial absence of pain in some people at the time of trauma
- Endorphin levels are lower in some people with chronic pain. This may explain why their pain worsens and why they are highly sensitive to acute pain.

pain by preventing the reuptake of released 5-HT and noradrenaline (norepinephrine).

Modulation is triggered from higher brain centres and allows the psychological influences on pain perception to be explained. For example, negative or positive past experiences – anxiety, fear and depression, or relaxation and optimism – all influence pain modulation, either opening or closing the 'pain gate'. Modulation may also be influenced by genetic factors, age and pain type, which could influence the endogenous opioid mechanisms.

Perception

There is no central pain centre within the brain but opioid-binding sites have been found in several areas in the brain, indicating that they are involved in pain perception. Pain perception is a complex process involving the sensory impulses relayed from the 'pain gates' and activation of pain responses via the limbic ('primitive' area of the brain that influences feelings and emotions) and autonomic nervous system (ANS) to develop a pain experience that includes emotional and subjective sensory components. Immediate responses associated with acute pain and activation of the sympathetic nervous system include heightened awareness and anxiety. Longer-term responses to chronic pain involve behavioural adaptations, and psychological and social changes.

Psychological factors influence pain perception; for example, emotional distress, anxiety and helplessness are recognized as increasing the pain experience and are of significance in clinical practice. Sarafino (2002) notes the importance of psychological, social and behavioural factors that become more dominant in chronic pain. Cognitive behavioural therapy (Morley et al 1999) may be used in chronic pain to change people's thoughts and behaviour and to enhance coping skills, so improving quality of life.

Individual pain responses are influenced by appraisal and past experiences. Responses are also modified by culture and social conditions and children learn during their upbringing about acceptable pain behaviour for their social group. McCaffery and Pasero (1999) note that some societies value a stoic response to pain, probably closely aligned with valuing high pain tolerance (see p. 660). This can lead to judgemental, negative attitudes to less stoic histrionic expression of pain. This is why the patient's direct communication of their pain experience must be encouraged, as it is the most valid assessment. Individual differences lead to great variations in the pain experienced and in how it is expressed by similar pain-provoking stimuli. An individual's pain cannot be predicted with accuracy.

Physiological and behavioural responses to acute pain

It is important for nurses to understand common physiological and behavioural responses to acute pain. This is important as part of pain assessment (see pp. 661–667), particularly so in patients or clients unable to describe their pain, e.g. babies, people with dementia or people with learning disabilities and associated communication problems. The responses may be:

- Physiological, e.g. sweating, increased heart rate, respiratory rate and blood pressure
- Behavioural, e.g. anxious, poor concentration (focused on the pain), grimaces/frowns, moans/cries/screams, reports pain if able, rubs or holds painful part, may thrash about or keep very still, may be withdrawn (see also Box 23.11, p. 663). Note that in a person with learning disability it can lead to changes in behaviour which staff may attribute to the person rather than the pain.

Pain threshold and pain tolerance

Pain threshold, or pain perception, is described as the lowest intensity at which a stimulus is experienced as pain. This relates to the point at which the painful stimulus is first felt and the amount of pain that subsequently ensues. The pain perception threshold is relatively constant and not, as is commonly thought, something that varies widely between individuals and cultures (Davies & Taylor 2003).

Pain tolerance relates to intensity or duration of pain and the maximum amount of pain that an individual is willing, or capable, of enduring. Pain tolerance may vary between and within individuals at different times, and may be influenced by emotional and cultural factors (see p. 660); pain tolerance is often referred to as being high or low (Box 23.6, p. 660). Thus an individual with high pain tolerance can withstand intense or protracted pain over an extended period before requiring pain relief. Conversely, the opposite is likely to be true for those individuals with low pain tolerance. There is little evidence to suggest that children have different pain tolerance from adults

REFLECTIVE PRACTICE Box 23.6

Pain tolerance

Think about a client or patient who experiences chronic pain.

Student activities

- Is their pain tolerance always the same?
- Do they need the same amount of medication each day?
- If there are differences, consider what factors might be affecting their tolerance.

although there may be a link between the age of the child and their pain threshold.

Pain psychology – personal and sociocultural influences

The pain experience is the end result of a number of dynamic interrelated factors. Recent thinking has moved away from the notion of personality and overt pain behaviours to focus interest on the mental processes, e.g. comprehension and memory, that mediate pain behaviours. It is now recognized that children can and do remember their pain experiences and learn from modifying their responses to future episodes, e.g. injections or visits to the dentist. There has been a view that neonates were unable to remember pain; however, there is now increasing evidence to support the fact that infants do remember pain (Carter 1994). Furthermore, the interrelationship between pain, fear and anxiety has been extensively investigated over time and evidence suggests that anxiety and fear undoubtedly magnify pain perceptions, particularly in children. Recent studies have included other variables including memory, locus of control, self-efficacy, coping mechanisms/styles and depression (Box 23.7).

The influence of culture on the perception of pain has been extensively documented. There is evidence to support the fact that pain and culture are closely linked, especially when responses and behaviours are closely aligned to culturally specific traditions, rules and rites of passage associated with a particular culture. For example, in Africa the men of the Kikuya or Masai tribes are expected to respond to pain with dignity and composure, whereas it is acceptable for the women to wail and cry. There is some evidence to suggest that the further that an individual is away from the original immigrant population, the less culturally specific the behaviours become. Therefore, a pain response may be modified or diluted according to the multicultural society in which the person lives. Zborowski (1952) reported differences in pain responses between 'old' Americans and more recent Jewish or Italian immigrants: the 'old' Americans were unemotional and generally optimistic, whereas newer immigrants were frank in their pain expression and sought more sympathy.

Studies related to children, culture and pain found similar features to those found in adults. However, nurses view the child and family as part of a sociocultural group

EVIDENCE-BASED PRACTICE Box 23.7

Depression and chronic pain

Depression associated with chronic pain has been the subject of much research over the years. Lin et al (2003) report that treating depression in older people with arthritis can reduce their pain and improve functional status and quality of life.

Student activities

- Access the study by Lin et al (2003).
- Discuss their findings with your mentor and consider how they could be used to improve the management of chronic pain in your area.

[Reference: Lin EHB, Katon W, Von Korff M et al 2003 Effect of improving depression care on pain and functional outcomes among older adults with arthritis. JAMA 290(18):2428–2429]

REFLECTIVE PRACTICE Box 23.8

Values, beliefs and attitudes towards pain

Think about your own values, beliefs and attitudes towards pain and the episodes that formed these. For example, can you remember people saying 'rub it better' when you fell over as a child?

Student activity

Consider how your feelings about pain might influence your response to a patient or client who reports having unbearable pain.

and a multicultural approach to pain management is crucial to manage the child's pain experience effectively. Of equal importance are the implications of culture and ethnicity for nurses who will all have their own values, attitudes, beliefs and explanatory models of health and illness (see Ch. 1) (Box 23.8).

Myths, misconceptions and facts about pain

The complexity of pain makes it difficult to define, describe, explain and measure, thus increasing the likelihood that pain is underdetermined and undertreated. However, there is a school of thought which proposes that complete relief from pain is not achievable or necessarily desirable, especially after minor injury or surgery where low intensity pain limits overexertion. Moreover, pain is a valuable diagnostic tool and can be a learning mechanism. However, pain that is severe and prolonged, or which limits activity and movement, can be detrimental to recovery and general well-being (Box 23.9).

Moreover, enduring myths, misconceptions relating to false judgements, mistaken beliefs or misunderstandings surrounding pain all reflect prejudice, outmoded beliefs and lack of knowledge and understanding. Collectively

Box 23.9 **Detrimental effects of pain**

Respiratory effects (see Ch. 17)

- Reduced lung capacity and ineffective coughing, leading to retention of secretions and chest infections
- Reduced oxygen to the tissues and respiratory failure.

Cardiovascular effects (see Ch. 17)

- Rapid heart rate and high blood pressure may reduce the blood supply (ischaemia) to the heart muscle, leading to a heart attack, particularly in susceptible patients.

Gastrointestinal effects

- Decreased bowel motility leading to constipation, nausea and vomiting and prolonged need for intravenous fluids (see Chs 19, 21)
- Nausea caused by inappropriate analgesia may lead to dehydration and poor dietary intake.

Nervous system and hormones

- Increased secretion of catecholamines such as adrenaline (epinephrine) and stress hormones, e.g. corticosteroids, which in turn increase metabolism and oxygen consumption and promote sodium and water retention (see Chs 17, 19). These changes are not caused exclusively by pain, but unrelieved pain may increase the extent of the changes

Poor/reduced mobility (see Ch. 18)

- Deep vein thrombosis (see Chs 18, 24)
- Reduced musculoskeletal function (see Ch. 18), e.g. joint stiffness
- Pressure ulcers (see Ch. 25).

Psychological effects (see Ch. 11)

- Fear and anxiety
- Helplessness
- Depression
- Fatigue.

Social effects

- Isolation and withdrawal from family/friends
- Inability to function within the family unit or maintain normal roles within society.

[Based on Davies & Taylor (2003)]

these present healthcare professionals with enormous challenges to manage pain effectively, as knowledge and beliefs relating to pain and its subsequent management are the foundations upon which healthcare professionals make judgements and decisions.

A number of myths and misconceptions flourish, despite these having been disproved by sound evidence. In particular, two such myths that continue to perpetuate the undertreatment of pain relate to fears about respiratory depression and addiction from the use of strong opioid analgesics, e.g. morphine. Box 23.10 (p. 662) outlines some pain myths and facts.

In order to dispel myths and misconceptions, nurses need to attain and maintain up-to-date evidence-based knowledge about pain and practical experience of relating this knowledge to preventing and managing pain. According to Davies and Taylor (2003), nurses require knowledge about:

- Causes of pain and major influences on pain perception
- Effects of unalleviated pain
- Pain assessment across the lifespan
- Pharmacological interventions according to individual needs
- Potential complications of pain-relieving interventions
- Appropriate non-pharmacological interventions.

Pain assessment

There are several good reasons why objective and systematic assessment of pain is necessary. Article 3 of the Human Rights Act (1998) states that 'no one shall be subjected to torture or to inhuman or degrading treatment or punishment'. This part of the chapter provides an outline of how pain is assessed.

McCaffery and Pasero (1999) summarize the essential message about pain assessment as:

- Ask the patient about their pain
- Accept and respect what they have to say
- Intervene to relieve their pain
- Ask them again about their pain.

Pain assessment is cyclical, involving assessment, intervention and reassessment.

Pain assessment therefore sets the tone for the therapeutic relationship formed with the patient/client/family in the assessment and treatment process, and underpins the respect and concern of the healthcare team. Furthermore, assessment is the foundation for therapeutic pain management. In acute pain the objective of assessment might be to evaluate the need for and effectiveness of medication, whereas in chronic pain the focus is on how the pain affects the person's ability to function normally. One of the purposes of assessment is to facilitate objective clinical decision-making in pain management.

Pain is not a unitary phenomenon; it is multidimensional and a holistic assessment needs to address all aspects of the pain experience, the critical components of which are:

- *Physiological*: Primarily concerned with the aetiology (cause) of pain
- *Sensory*: How the pain feels to the person and its characteristics, e.g. location, intensity and quality
- *Affective*: How the pain makes the individual feel and is related to mood and their well-being

Box 23.10 Pain myths – fact or fiction

Myths (false)

- *Pain is the earliest symptom of cancer*. Not true – except in cancers involving nerve tissue or bone. Pain is usually a late symptom of advanced cancer
- *Older adults may believe that chronic pain is inevitable during ageing, that nothing can be done, and it is a sign of serious illness or impending death*. Not true – but this myth is firmly embedded in sociocultural beliefs and poses significant barriers to pain relief for older people
- *Infants cannot feel pain*. Not true – complete development of nerves is not required for pain perception, and neonates exhibit both behavioural and physiological responses to pain
- *Infants and children experience less pain than adults*. Not true – younger children may perceive a greater intensity of pain than older children and adults
- *Infants', children's and adults' behaviour accurately reflects their pain*. Not true – children and adults who are sleeping, or who are active, playing, reading, etc., may still be experiencing pain but coping with it
- *Psychological dependence and respiratory depression are common side-effects of opioid analgesics*. Not true – these are uncommon but fear of them by nurses and patients can hamper effective pain management.

Facts (true)

- *Adults and children with severe motor problems or a learning disability are particularly prone to pain, e.g. earache, muscle spasm, and may be unable to articulate their pain clearly*. True
- *Protective pain is that which alerts the body to potential danger*. True – protective pain is usually accompanied by reflex withdrawal of the part of the body in contact with the noxious stimulus, and may be accompanied by a cry, grimace, shout or tears
- *Treatment for depression improves pain in older people*. True – treating depression in older people helps them cope with the pain associated with chronic illnesses and improves quality of life.
- *Complementary and alternative therapies have an important role in pain management*. True – various techniques can be used by patients/clients as coping strategies for managing pain (see pp. 673–677, Ch. 10).

- *Cognitive*: The manner in which the pain affects the person's thought processes. Also embraces the individual's values, beliefs and coping strategies related to the pain experience and how they perceive themselves as individuals
- *Behavioural*: How the pain experience affects the person's behaviour. Certain behaviours may be adopted in order to reduce pain and may also relate to elements of physical activity, medication and treatments. Behaviours may also be adopted because the person does not understand the pain or indeed cannot communicate to others that they are in pain
- *Sociocultural*: Relates to age/gender, transcultural issues, folk law, spiritual and other factors relating to the individual's pain experience.

Holistic pain assessment

Determining the level of pain that an individual may experience is one of the most challenging yet common tasks that nurses undertake. However, it is important to distinguish between pain measurement and holistic pain assessment. Pain measurement measures pain on a scale relating to the intensity of pain without considering any of the other components of pain. In contrast, pain assessment is a broader notion that requires different knowledge and skills including pain measurement.

When assessing pain, nurses should be measuring not only the severity of the pain but also what the experience means to that person. However, it is notable that there is a difference between pain measurement and assessment, and when these definitions are applied to human suffering it requires the nurse to evaluate the whole experience and what it means to the person. Melzack and Katz (1994) proposed that the main aims of pain assessment are to:

- Determine the intensity, quality and duration
- Aid diagnosis
- Determine the most appropriate therapy
- Evaluate the relative effectiveness of different therapies
- Monitor standards of clinical practice.

The assessment of pain is important because it provides the person with the opportunity to verbalize their pain (if able), takes account of the personal pain experience (Davies & Taylor 2003) and engages the person and/or their family with healthcare systems.

The 'gold standard' is always to ask the person about their pain experience. Assessment will be influenced by the person's ability to respond and the type of pain will also influence assessment priorities, e.g. priorities will be different in the following situations:

- Acute pain after a heart attack
- Chronic back pain
- Pain in a person with cancer.

Communication skills are essential for effective pain assessment; the person needs to be encouraged to report their pain (see Ch. 9). If the person's condition allows, use open questions that allow them to elaborate upon their pain episode. For example:

- How would you describe your pain or discomfort? (see 'Pain language')
- When did you first feel the pain?
- Is there anything that makes the pain worse or better?
- How does the pain affect your daily activities?

The potential barriers and differences in pain expression, e.g. due to culture, age, personality, gender and cognitive ability, need to be acknowledged by the nurse. However, for some people verbal communication may be difficult, absent or not yet developed. Furthermore, cultural and language difficulties may hamper the assessment process.

Behavioural responses to pain

Behavioural responses to pain are important in the assessment of all patients/clients but can be especially relevant when people are unable to verbalize their pain. Although there are only limited pain assessment tools available for vulnerable groups, it is important to understand that people with special needs experience pain the same as everyone else. It is vital that nurses recognize that they may be unable to verbalize their pain or explain it clearly. Vulnerable people include the following:

- People whose thinking processes are impaired, e.g. confusion
- People with dementia
- People experiencing mental distress
- People with severe physical and/or learning disability
- People who have suffered a stroke or brain damage
- Unconscious patients
- Neonates, infants and children (especially pre-verbal)
- Older people
- People with language and speech problems.

Certain behaviours are useful for identifying patients/clients who may be experiencing pain (Box 23.11; see also p. 659). In situations where verbal communication is limited or impossible, observations of behaviour alone can be used.

In addition to the limited availability of assessment tools for vulnerable groups, there may also be a culture where lack of assessment hampers effective evaluation of pain management. Furthermore, pain assessment can fail if there is poor communication between the nurse and the patient/client or family.

Pain language

There are many words used to describe the pain experience (Box 23.12). Many patients/clients and children develop their own pain language and behaviours that communicate pain. Instead of the word pain, depending upon the age and stage of development, children may use words such as 'baddie', 'nasty' or 'hurt' (Carter 1994). Descriptions of pain expressions may have little or no meaning outside the family and reinforce the need for partnerships and child and family-centred care in pain management with infants and children and others with communication difficulties. Therefore, identifying pain language in children and adults, including those with a learning disability or older people, is important for the delivery of high quality care and also informs the assessment process.

CRITICAL THINKING Box 23.11

Behaviours that may indicate pain

Abusive	Disjointed
Aggressive	Moaning
Agitated	Mute
Attention seeking	Picking at clothes/bedding
Babbling	Refusing food
Being quiet	Rocking
Calling out	Rubbing/holding the site of the pain
Cries easily	Uncooperative
Difficulty breathing	Withdrawn

Student activities

- Consider the list above and think about patients/clients who have displayed any of these behaviours.
- Is observation of behaviour part of pain assessment in your placement?
- Is the family asked about how the person usually expresses that they have pain?

Box 23.12 **Words used to describe pain**

Aching	Penetrating
Boring	Piercing
Burning/hot	Pounding
Bursting	Pressing
Colicky	Punishing
Cramping/crampy	Scalding
Cruel	Sharp
Cutting	Shooting
Discomfort	Smarting
Dragging	Sore
Dull	Spasms
Exhausting/tiring	Stabbing
Exploding	Tearing
Gnawing	Tender
Gripping	Throbbing
Heavy	Tingling
Hurting	Twinge

Assessing children's pain

Until recently, pain in children was not recognized or prioritized, resulting in poor pain management (Twycross et al 1998). Infants and children have the right to careful consideration as they may experience pain differently from adults. The child's experience of pain is often separate from their experience of their illness or disease. As with adults, children have different experiences and reactions to pain from the same stimulus, and the relationship between the pain stimulus and the response is neither direct nor simple.

An understanding of how children develop their understanding of health and illness will enhance the quality of care offered to each child (see Chs 1, 8). Evidence suggests that most health professionals do not approach children according to their developmental level but rather address all children according to Piaget's (1924) concrete operational stage of development (see Ch. 8). Therefore, knowledge about how a child's understanding of illness develops will mean that age-specific explanations can be given to the child, thus reducing the anxiety and distress that children suffer during hospitalization (Twycross et al 1998). A child's developmental stage affects their perception and ability to adequately report or express the pain they are feeling.

Children have the right to feel secure and to be nursed in an atmosphere where compassion, trust and caring are at the centre of all decisions. These principles must underpin the child's pain assessment and management, with the child central to all considerations and decisions.

The QUESTT model (Baker & Wong 1987) encompasses many important features of assessment and involves:

- **Q**uestioning the child (where appropriate)
- **U**sing pain rating scales (see pp. 664–666)
- **E**valuating behaviour and physiological changes
- **S**ecuring parental involvement
- **T**aking the cause of pain into account
- **T**aking action and evaluating the results.

This model provides a comprehensive overview of the child's pain and informs the treatment and therapeutic management.

Pain history

Establishing a pain history is important as it will not only identify previous pain experiences, but may also offer insights into how the person's knowledge and perception have influenced and shaped coping strategies, and how this may influence the current situation. This is particularly important for vulnerable groups, e.g. older or confused clients. Children can be better prepared for painful procedures by comparing the previous experience with the new experience and often children develop strategies that compare one situation with another. Furthermore, pain behaviours may be an integral part of the pain history and behavioural cues may be important pain indicators. Being sensitive to pain indicators may mean that practitioners can intervene at an early stage before pain is fully established. It is also useful to establish if there are separate behaviours relating to sudden acute pain compared to chronic pain. Again this is important in patient/client populations where there may be difficulties in articulating pain.

Pain diaries

These are useful tools for the assessment of chronic pain and a means of reflecting upon the many components of pain, e.g. physical, emotional, social. They can also include numerical ratings and descriptions of pain (see Box 23.12, p. 663).

Pain maps

The patient, if able, is asked to identify, mark or sketch areas on a body outline or 'body map' that reflects the area(s) of pain (see p. 667). Pain maps are used increasingly as part of the assessment process, especially for patients with complex chronic pain. Pain maps can empower the patient during the assessment process; they can be used across the lifespan and are important tools for informing decisions about pain management and providing a basis for evaluating the effectiveness of treatment.

Pain assessment tools

A pain assessment tool must be reliable and valid. The term reliability relates to the issues of consistency, stability and the repeatability of measurements made by different nurses; validity refers to the appropriateness, applicability and the representativeness of measurements made as true findings of an individual's pain at any given time. There are different types of pain assessment tools that can be classified as follows:

- Self-report scales – what people say
- Observation techniques – what people do
- Physiological measurements such as heart rate.

There are wide variations in the levels of sophistication of these tools and also between approaches to pain assessment. Pain assessment tool selection must be based on the patient's age and ability, a child's developmental stage, patient preferences, amount of time available to teach the patient about the scale and the knowledge of the nurse (Box 23.13).

Self-report scales

Self-report assessment scales include visual analogue scales (VAS), verbal numerical rating scales and categorical verbal rating scales but can also include pain interviews or questionnaires that incorporate variables such as coping skills (Fig. 23.5). Self-report scales can be modified; for example, the pain 'thermometer' scale or by using a child's own words on the scale, e.g. 'worst hurt' (Box 23.14, p. 666). They can also be used with pain maps or pain diaries.

Visual analogue scale

The visual analogue scale (VAS) is usually a 10cm horizontal line with indicators of severity such as 'no pain' at one end to 'worst pain possible' at the other end (Fig. 23.5A). Patients mark the position on the scale that best reflects their current pain. This is also a useful tool for children, but the child needs the ability to translate their experience into an analogue format and to be able to understand proportions (from 9 or 10 years).

Verbal numerical rating scales

Verbal numerical rating scales are based upon the VAS but use a scale where 0 is 'no pain' and 10 is 'worst possible pain' (Fig. 23.5B). These usually provide a more reliable means of measuring pain and can be used with descriptions as well as numbers.

EVIDENCE-BASED PRACTICE Box 23.13

Choosing the most appropriate pain assessment tool

Studies have identified that patient preference is important with practical acceptability of tools.

- Visual impairment in older people may limit practicality for self-report scales. The presentation of tools is recommended in bold Arial font on buff-coloured paper to accommodate visual difficulties (Herr & Mobily 1993)
- The pain 'thermometer' – a 0–10/100 scale represented as a picture of a thermometer – has been well received by older people (Benesh et al 1997)
- Within pain assessment the nurse should evaluate patient fears and concerns regarding analgesics since this may be an important issue in successful pain management. Fear of analgesic drugs and their side-effects or acceptance of pain as inevitable can be barriers to effective pain management
- Self-expression may be limited, thus requiring the nurse to use alternative aspects such as behavioural indicators. Observing the facial expressions and vocalizations of people with advanced dementia is seen as an accurate means for assessing the presence of pain, but not its intensity (Manfredi et al 2003).

Student activity

Access one of the articles and discuss with your mentor how the findings could be used effectively with your patient/client group.

[References: Benesh L, Szigrti E, Ferraro R, Naismith Gullicks J 1997 Tools for assessing chronic pain in rural elderly women. Home Healthcare Nurse 15(3):207–211; Herr K, Mobily P 1993 Comparison of selected pain assessment tools for use with the elderly. Applied Nursing Research 6(1):39–46; Manfredi P, Breuer B, Meier D, Libow L 2003 Pain assessment in elderly patients with severe dementia. Journal of Pain and Symptom Management 25:48–52]

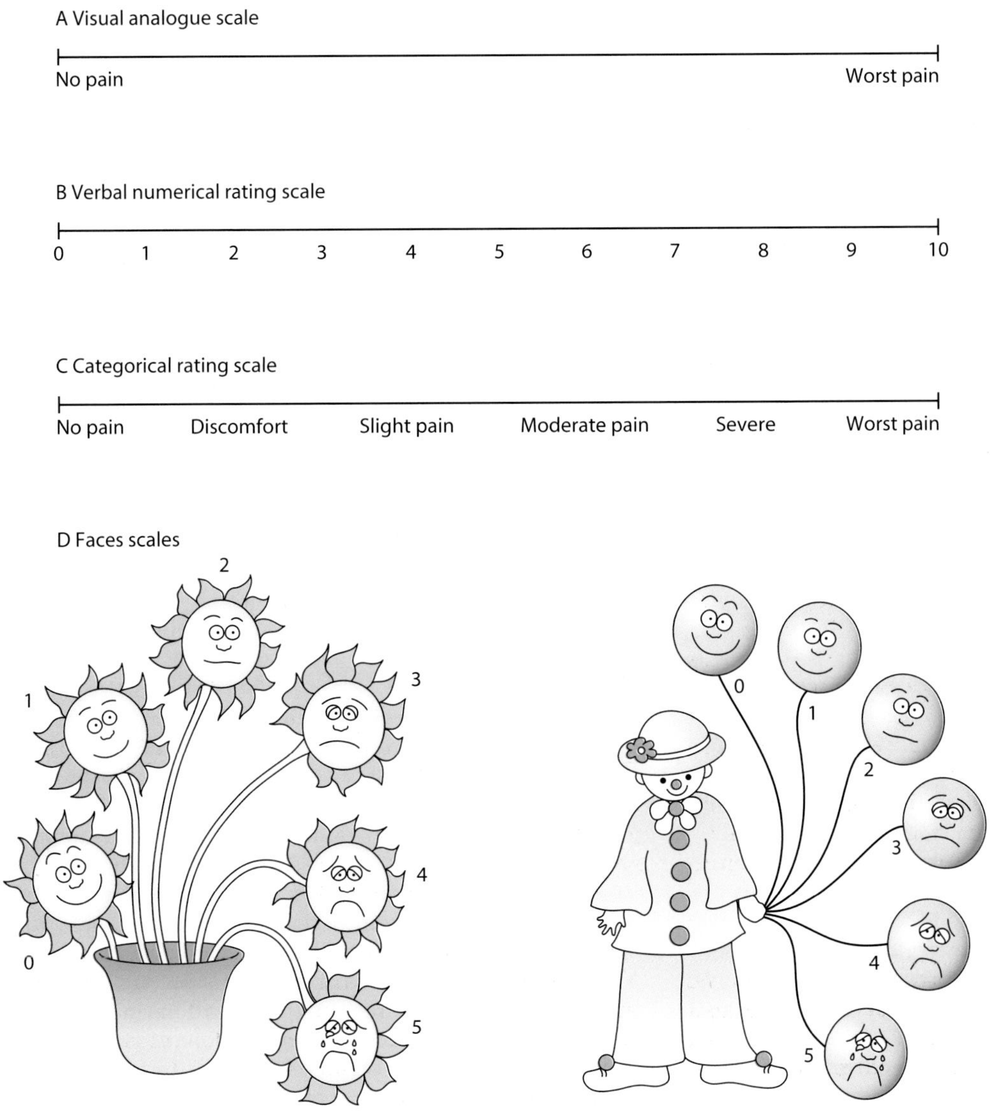

Fig. 23.5 Self-report pain scales: **A.** Visual analogue scale. **B.** Verbal numerical rating scale. **C.** Categorical rating scale. **D.** Faces scales

REFLECTIVE PRACTICE Box 23.14

Using self-report scales

Think about a placement where self-report scales are in use.

Student activities

- Were the scales in use suitable for all patients/clients?
- Were existing scales modified to increase their suitability?
- Discuss with your mentor how sociocultural factors may influence a person's use of self-report scales.

CRITICAL THINKING Box 23.15

Physiological measurements and changes

Marie has just fallen and broken her arm. She does not speak English and is unable to tell you about her pain.

Student activities

- What changes in Marie's blood pressure, pulse rate and respiratory rate may indicate that she has pain? (see p. 659).
- How might Marie's pain be observed from non-verbal expressions of pain?

Categorical rating scale

One of the most commonly used tools in the postoperative period, it offers the patient a series of terms that best describes their pain (Fig. 23.5C). It has been found to be simple and effective to use in clinical practice and can be incorporated into an observation chart. Pain on movement rather than at rest is an important area to assess. Pain intensity at rest is not a reliable indicator of effective pain management, especially postoperative pain.

Self-report scales for children

Self-report scales for children include:

- 'Faces' scale (from 3 years) – series of faces depicting a smile through neutral to total misery (Fig. 23.5D)
- Pain thermometer
- Colour scale (4–10 years) – used in conjunction with a body map it provides information about pain intensity and location. It has a series of colours from which the child chooses the colour that best represents their pain to create a 'key'. Once the key has been created the child is encouraged to colour in the outline of where it hurts
- Poker chip (4–8 years) – the child rates their pain in a concrete manner using the chips that are described as 'pieces of hurt'.

For a comprehensive account of pain assessment tools for infants, children and adolescents, see Further reading (e.g. Hockenberry et al 2002).

Observation techniques

This involves recording variables that may include:

- Sleep patterns
- Periods of rest
- Pain behaviours
- Verbal and motor responses.

Observational tools used for adult pain assessment and measurement show potential when trained observers are used and there are clearly defined terms and boundaries. A number of observational tools have been developed to assess the pain of children aged 0–5 years, who are unable or less able to use self-report scales. Observation may also be useful in cases where self-report tools may be unreliable or unsuitable, as with people with a learning disability and those with communication or language difficulties.

Physiological measurements

The quest for objectivity in pain assessment has led some researchers to measure functions such as increased heart rate, feeling faint, etc. or disease activity as equivalents for the experience of pain (Box 23.15).

Physiological measurements such as respiratory rate, blood pressure, heart rate and oxygen saturation (see Ch. 17) have their limitations. However, they are used for neonatal pain assessment because there are few other comprehensive neonatal assessment tools available.

Multimethod approaches to pain assessment

These approaches give richer information regarding the pain experience of the patient/client and often pain assessment tools combine quantitative and qualitative elements (see Ch. 5). One such tool is the Pain Anxiety Symptoms Scale (PASS) which incorporates three modes: cognitive, overt behaviour and physiological, including reports of changes, e.g. sweating, feeling faint and dizzy, etc. Various multimethod approaches exist for assessing pain in children and young people (see Further reading), e.g. the Pain Assessment Tool for Children (PATCh) which includes:

- Faces
- Body maps
- VAS
- Descriptive words
- Behaviour.

Assessment for different types of pain

The choice of assessment method must be appropriate for the person and the pain type. In acute pain a self-report scale such as the categorical rating scale, which concentrates on pain intensity alone, is often sufficient for evaluation of interventions, especially if there is a single pain location.

However, with chronic pain a body map is frequently required to improve multidisciplinary recognition and communication of pain location and pattern. For patients with cancer-related pain, a body map is essential because as the cancer advances several pain locations may develop (see Ch. 12). The different pains locations require regular reassessment as the disease progresses. In addition, the impact of the pain on mood and behaviour are important

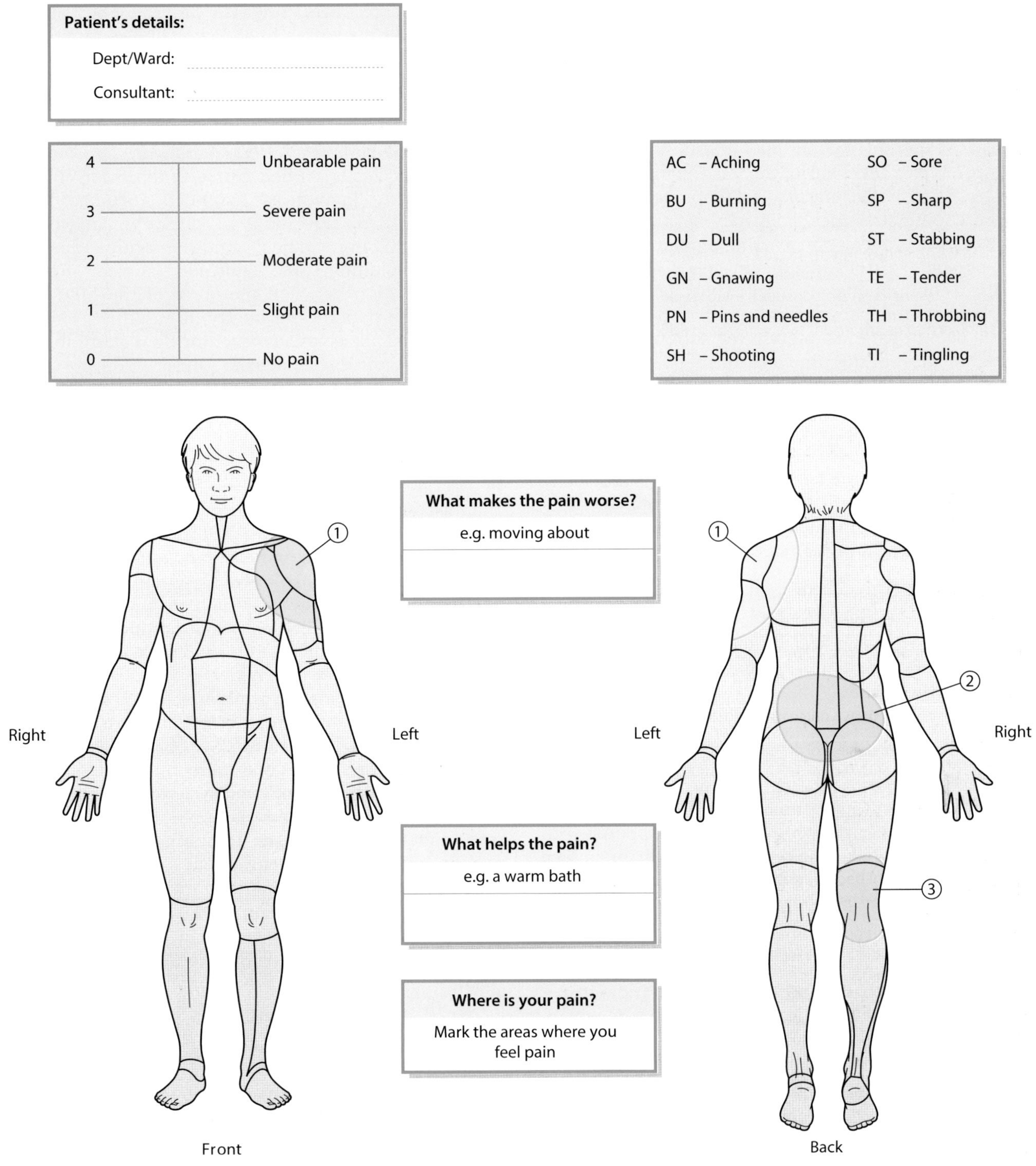
Patient's details:
Dept/Ward:
Consultant:
4 Unbearable pain
3 Severe pain
2 Moderate pain
1 Slight pain
0 No pain
AC – Aching
BU – Burning
DU – Dull
GN – Gnawing
PN – Pins and needles
SH – Shooting
SO – Sore
SP – Sharp
ST – Stabbing
TE – Tender
TH – Throbbing
TI – Tingling
What makes the pain worse?
e.g. moving about
What helps the pain?
e.g. a warm bath
Where is your pain?
Mark the areas where you feel pain
Right
Left
Left
Right
1
1
2
3
Front
Back

Fig. 23.6 Pain assessment tool (reproduced with permission from Brooker & Nicol 2003)

considerations. These will be missed if a simple self-report scale is used.

Questions that explore quality of sleep and the impact of pain on mobility and social interaction are valuable. Patients are asked about what makes the pain better or worse, thus helping to identify characteristics that may be of value in evaluating treatment options and coping skills that people may have developed. The quality and character of pain may guide pharmacological management, e.g. a pain described as 'shooting' may be neuropathic such as after shingles (see p. 655). Pain clinics and specialist nurse practitioners use detailed tools and may ask people to complete pain diaries in order to evaluate the pain experience comprehensively.

Figure 23.6 illustrates an example of a more comprehensive assessment tool that combines a body map, self-report scale and description of the type of pain with factors that increase or decrease pain.

Pain management

This part of the chapter outlines holistic pain management, principles of pharmacological pain relief and a variety of non-pharmacological approaches used to enhance coping strategies. Pain may be a primary reason for care or it may be an existing problem not related to the person's current healthcare needs. Bruster et al (1994), in a comprehensive survey of hospital experiences in England, found pain management to be an area of concern: 61% of patients interviewed suffered pain, 33% had it all or most of the time and for many the pain was severe or moderate.

Effective pain management is complex and requires a holistic approach, starting with a thorough assessment (see pp. 661–667). The type of pain and the person's response are important factors to consider when planning strategies for pain management. Pain management usually involves a combination of pharmacological and non-pharmacological measures.

Mild acute pain following minor injury may be easy to resolve with simple painkillers, measures such as an ice pack and sympathetic listening and support from the nurse. Many hospitals now have acute pain teams to support pain management following surgery and act as a resource to clinical staff.

However, for chronic pain a multidisciplinary approach is most effective and that management takes place in hospital and in the community. The MDT may involve pain specialist consultants, pain nurse specialists (Box 23.16), physiotherapists, occupational therapists, clinical psychologists and pharmacists. Support for patients with chronic pain depends on the cause of the pain, but advice and help are available from palliative care specialists (see Ch. 12) and specialist pain clinics.

Pharmacological management

Depending on the pain type, patient's age and setting, there are a range of pharmacological approaches available including the use of analgesics (widely described as painkillers). The nurse has a key role in teaching patients and family about the safe management of drugs including analgesics (Box 23.17; see also Ch. 22). The variability in individual responses to analgesics gives nurses a key responsibility in monitoring effects and side-effects in order to achieve successful pain management.

Increasingly, registered nurses (RNs) who have completed additional training are able to prescribe analgesics from the *Nurse Prescribers' Formulary for Community Practitioners* and 'qualified Nurse Independent Prescribers (formerly known as Extended Formulary Nurse Prescribers) are now able to prescribe any licensed medicine for any medical condition within their competence, including some Controlled Drugs' (DH 2006). Communication between members of the MDT, which includes the patient and family, is essential. The nurse may need to act as an advocate for the patient to ensure adjustment of the analgesic prescription to achieve acceptable pain management.

Age and analgesic drugs

The patient's age is an important consideration when analgesics are chosen: the drug type, dose required and the most suitable administration route. Infants, children, adults and older people have different body compositions (see Ch. 19) and the metabolism and elimination of drugs are affected by the stage of development.

The amount of water as a percentage of body weight decreases during the lifespan. For example, a neonate has around 75% water whereas an adult male has around 60% and an older adult between 45 and 50%.

Infants and children metabolize and eliminate drugs differently from adults and this must be considered in the dose calculations. For example, neonates and premature infants are particularly vulnerable to the harmful effects of drugs because liver enzyme systems and kidney function are immature and plasma protein concentrations are low. In children, weight, height and age are important in calculating drug doses (see Ch. 22).

REFLECTIVE PRACTICE — Box 23.16

Role of the pain nurse specialist

Think about a person you met on placement who had pain.

Student activities

- Was a pain specialist nurse involved in their care?
- If they were involved, what type of things did they do?
- Arrange to meet the specialist nurse in your area to learn about their role.

HEALTH PROMOTION — Box 23.17

Aspirin and Reye's syndrome

A friend asks you why he should not give aspirin to his 8-year-old son. He has heard someone talking about a serious side-effect and is confused about which over-the-counter painkillers are safe for children. He wants to know some basic facts and where to get information.

Student activities

- Access the *British National Formulary* online (www.bnf.org.uk) *BNF for Children* and find some basic facts about aspirin and Reye's syndrome.
- What is the advice about when young people can take aspirin?
- Find out where your friend can get information about painkillers for children.

[Resource: http://www.mhra.gov.uk/home/idcplg?IdcService=SS_GET_PAGE&nodeId=132 Available July 2006]

There are also important considerations for the older person as reduced metabolism and excretion of drugs can result in accumulated effect and reduced doses may be required. In addition, polypharmacy causes concern with drug interactions. Poor pain management can significantly reduce quality of life, particularly in chronic pain. Effective pain management is essential in maintaining optimum independence and mobility in older people. This is a particular concern for older people with dementia who are more likely to suffer chronic pain but be unable to express their pain.

Drugs used in pain management

These can be divided into three groups: non-opioids, opioids and adjuvants (Table 23.2).

Nurses need to develop an adequate knowledge of analgesic action and potential side-effects (Box 23.18). Unfortunately there are no perfect analgesics; all drugs that relieve pain also have side-effects. These range from mild light-headedness to more troublesome problems that occur with opioids that include constipation, nausea and sedation, up to life-threatening respiratory depression, or NSAID-induced gastric ulceration or kidney failure. The nurse is responsible not only for the evaluation of pain reduction but also the occurrence of side-effects.

Mild sedation can be a useful side-effect in the management of acute pain, e.g. following major trauma, surgery or heart attack, as it will reduce anxiety and distress. However, for chronic pain management, independence with minimum disruption to daily living is important; frequent administration is therefore undesirable and side-effect management is essential, e.g. minimal sedation.

With opioid analgesics such as morphine, the higher the dose, the greater the risk of side-effects. The dose is therefore increased in graduated amounts known as titration, which allows optimum pain relief without adverse side-effects (Fig. 23.7, p. 670). However, knowledge of likely side-effects allows pre-emptive action to be taken, e.g. ensuring that laxatives are always prescribed for patients who are having regular long-term codeine or morphine.

When an adjuvant drug, e.g. amitriptyline, is prescribed it may take days or weeks before there is a therapeutic effect. This must be explained, as patients will be disappointed if they were expecting a prompt response and may discontinue the therapy. Starting adjuvants at a low dose and gradually increasing the dose helps to reduce side-effects and improves patient tolerance.

Routes of administration

The routes used for the administration of analgesic drugs include:

- Oral (p.o.) – either swallowed or mucosal absorption (e.g. sublingually dissolved under the tongue or spray, or absorbed through the buccal mucosa)
- Intranasal sprays
- Topical/transdermal as creams, gels or patches
- Rectal
- Subcutaneous (s.c.)
- Intramuscular (i.m.)
- Intravenous (i.v.)

CRITICAL THINKING Box 23.18

Side-effects of analgesic drugs

Select two or three examples from each group in Table 23.2 (non-opioids, opioids and adjuvants).

Student activities

- Access the *British National Formulary* (www.bnf.org.uk) and make some notes about the side-effects of the drugs chosen.
- Add to your notes as other analgesic drugs are encountered in placements.

Table 23.2 Drug groups used in pain management

Drug group	Examples	Details
Non-opioid	Aspirin, paracetamol, NSAIDs, e.g. ibuprofen, diclofenac, and local anaesthetics, e.g. lidocaine	Non-opioids work in a variety of ways, e.g. NSAIDs inhibit the production of 'algesic' chemicals such as prostaglandins that stimulate the pain-sensitive nociceptors which mediate the inflammatory response
Opioid	Buprenorphine, codeine, dihydrocodeine, diamorphine, fentanyl, methadone, morphine, pethidine, tramadol	Opioids are a group of naturally occurring (extracted from opium poppies) and synthetic analgesics They act on opioid receptors in the central nervous system and block pain transmission by mimicking the effects of naturally occurring endorphins at the receptors, thus making pain feel less They range in strength and efficacy from the weak opioid codeine to morphine
Adjuvant	These include: • Anticonvulsants, e.g. carbamazepine • Antidepressants, e.g. amitriptyline • Antispasmodics, e.g. hyoscine butylbromide • Capsaicin (derived from chillies) • Corticosteroids, e.g. dexamethasone	Adjuvants act to enhance the action of analgesics, e.g. amitriptyline enhances pain modulation and is useful for neuropathic pain

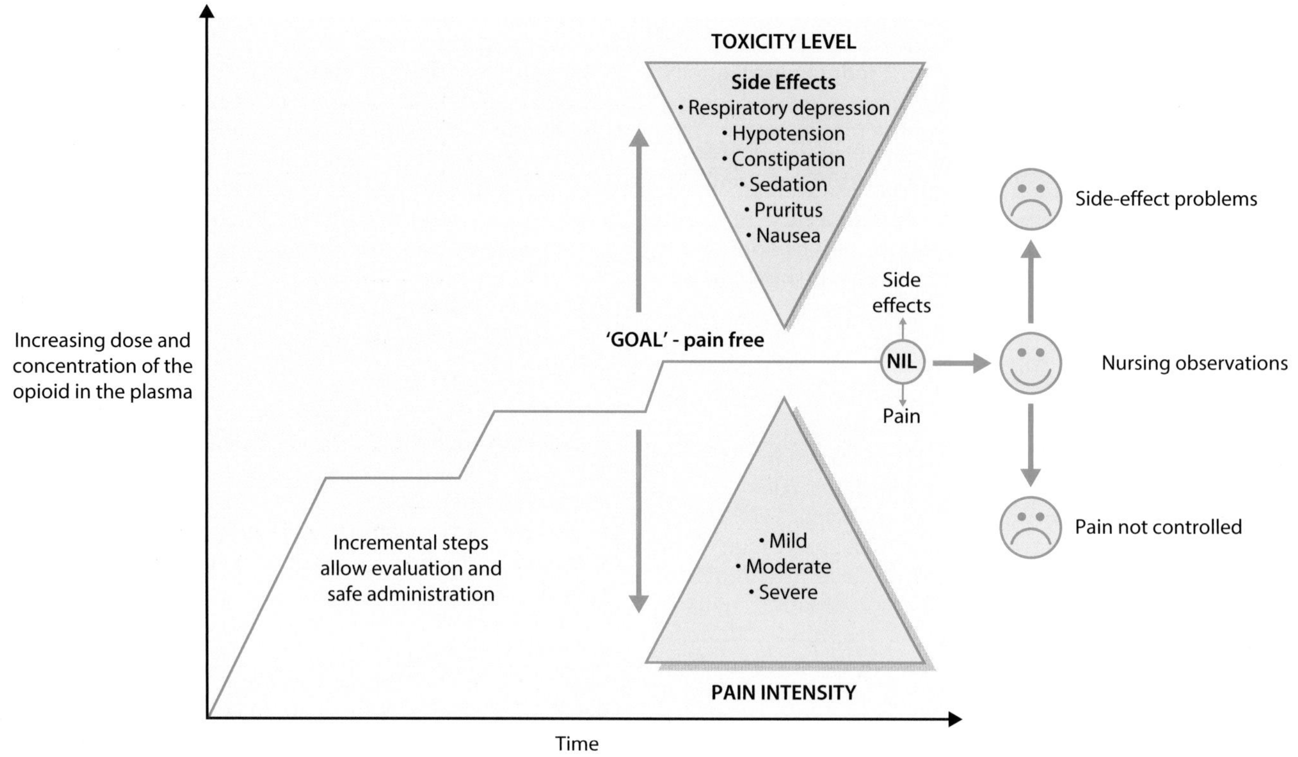

Fig. 23.7 Titration of opioids

- Inhalation
- Epidural
- Nerve blocks using local anaesthetics such as bupivacaine
- Intraspinal drug delivery via an intraspinal catheter and a pump.

Nurses need to know about different routes of administration and should be familiar with relative advantages and disadvantages of each route (Ch. 22). Analgesic administration may be low technology, e.g. independent self-administration of oral drugs at home where the nurse's role is educational, or – in contrast – invasive, high technology approaches where drugs are introduced into the epidural space outside the dura mater (the outer meningeal layer covering the spinal cord; Fig. 23.8), used in clinical areas to manage severe pain with additional staff training and support from pain teams. In general, the analgesic approach should be appropriate for the pain type and intensity, and should suit the person concerned.

An important consideration is the flexibility and availability provided by different routes of administration. In acute severe pain the route needs to be fast acting and the dose easily adjustable to allow optimum effect without development of adverse side-effects. The most widely available routes for adults are i.m. and s.c. opioid administration; the effectiveness of these routes has been greatly improved by the use of algorithms by RNs to provide greater flexibility to meet individual patients needs. Readers requiring more information about the use of algorithms for postoperative pain relief are directed to Davies and Taylor (2003).

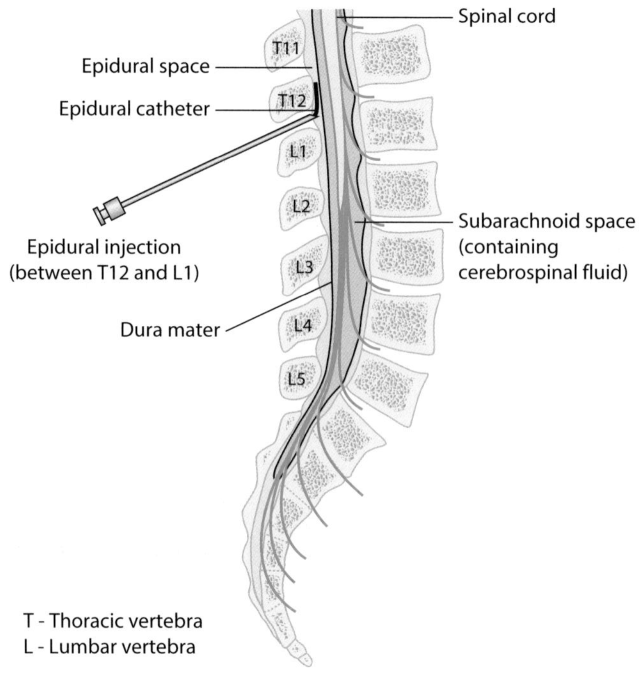

Fig. 23.8 Epidural analgesia

Opioids may be required for chronic severe pain, e.g. modified release morphine given twice daily or transdermal fentanyl (patch). Transdermal fentanyl takes 12 hours to reach therapeutic levels but lasts 3 days, thereby

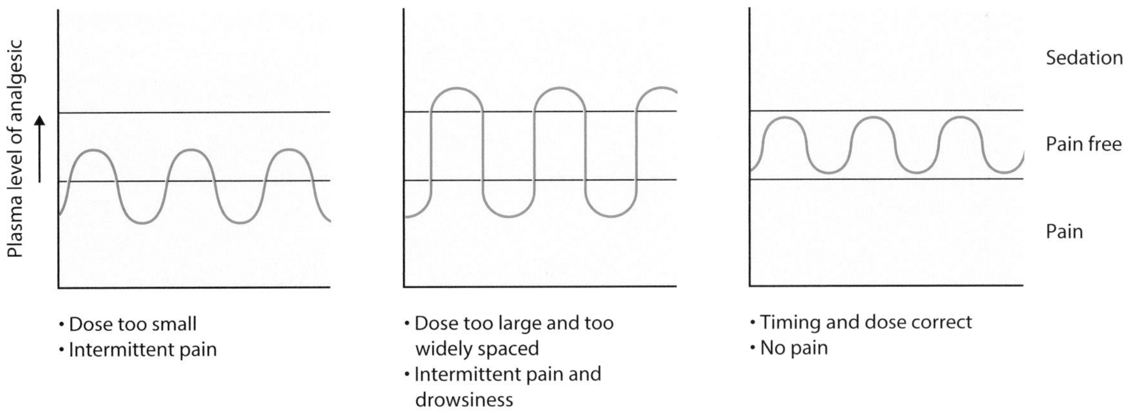

Fig. 23.9 Adjusting the dose to keep the patient pain-free (reproduced with permission from Greenstein & Gould 2004)

avoiding the inconvenience of frequent administration and allowing the patient to get on with their life.

The most common routes of administration (p.o., i.m., i.v.) rely upon sufficient quantity of the drug reaching the circulation to achieve therapeutic effect. An injection is not necessarily more powerful than an oral drug, a common misconception; the analgesic should be matched to pain intensity and a suitable route chosen. The i.v. route allows for rapid therapeutic effect to be achieved within 5 minutes, which makes patient-controlled i.v. administration a fast and flexible method of managing acute pain. Intramuscular and s.c. routes have a delayed onset as the drug has to be absorbed from the muscle or fat before it can reach the circulation.

The oral route can be as fast as i.m. if the drug is designed for rapid absorption. Avoidance of painful injection is essential in children and often desirable in adults because treating pain with injections can lead to reluctance to report pain. It is important to note that oral morphine is subject to first pass effect/metabolism in the liver (see Ch. 22), thus explaining why the oral route requires a dose higher than that given by i.v. or i.m. injection. This has important safety issues for the nurse (see www.bnf.org.uk).

Patient-controlled analgesia

Patient-controlled analgesia (PCA) usually means i.v. administration but also includes inhaled nitrous oxide and oxygen (Entonox®), and s.c. or epidural administration (Ch. 24). Specialized equipment is needed for safe administration of analgesics by these routes and PCA requires patient education and reassurance. Children can safely self-administer inhalation, i.v. or s.c. PCA.

Because PCA administration relies on the fact that a sedated patient will not be able to administer more analgesia, so therefore cannot overdose; carers and staff must understand they should not administer for the patient.

Regular assessment and management of nausea, a common side-effect of opioids, is important. This is particularly so with i.v. PCA, as the patient is unlikely to use it effectively if they feel sick every time they press the button. It is important that there is regular assessment of postoperative nausea and vomiting (see Ch. 24).

Readers requiring more information about PCA are directed to Davies and Taylor (2003) and Greenstein and Gould (2004).

Administration of analgesic drugs

Analgesics with a fast onset and short duration of action need to be administered frequently to maintain therapeutic effect and prevent pain, e.g. oral morphine liquid 4-hourly. This is why the 'as required' (p.r.n.) approach to pain management, which relies on patients reporting pain, is criticized; the intermittent administration results in regular pain with periods of relief. Good pain management requires regular administration of a suitable analgesic to avoid pain (Fig. 23.9). Regular administration 'by the clock', or techniques which allow the patient to administer as soon as pain is present, e.g. by using i.v. PCA, have greatly improved pain management. Many patients manage pain at home following early discharge or day case surgery. Advice is required about taking painkillers regularly to avoid pain at first and how to step down the 'analgesic ladder' (see below) to milder analgesics as the pain subsides. Advice regarding avoidance of constipation (see Ch. 21) should also be included if opioids are prescribed.

Analgesic potency

Pain management is achieved by administration of the most suitable analgesic drug combination. The pain type (acute or chronic) and intensity (mild, moderate or severe), the patient's age and individual sensitivities are all important considerations. A useful tool when considering the choice of analgesic is the 'analgesic ladder' (World Health Organization [WHO] 2005), which groups drugs into categories that match analgesic potency with pain intensity (Fig. 23.10, p. 672; see also Ch. 12):

- *Mild pain*: Drugs at the bottom of the analgesic ladder are useful for mild pain; these include the non-opioids, e.g. paracetamol and adjuvants
- *Moderate pain*: Step 1 drugs are administered at the correct dose and interval; if pain is not controlled, then a drug from the Step 2 is considered, e.g. co-codamol (paracetamol + the weak opioid codeine)

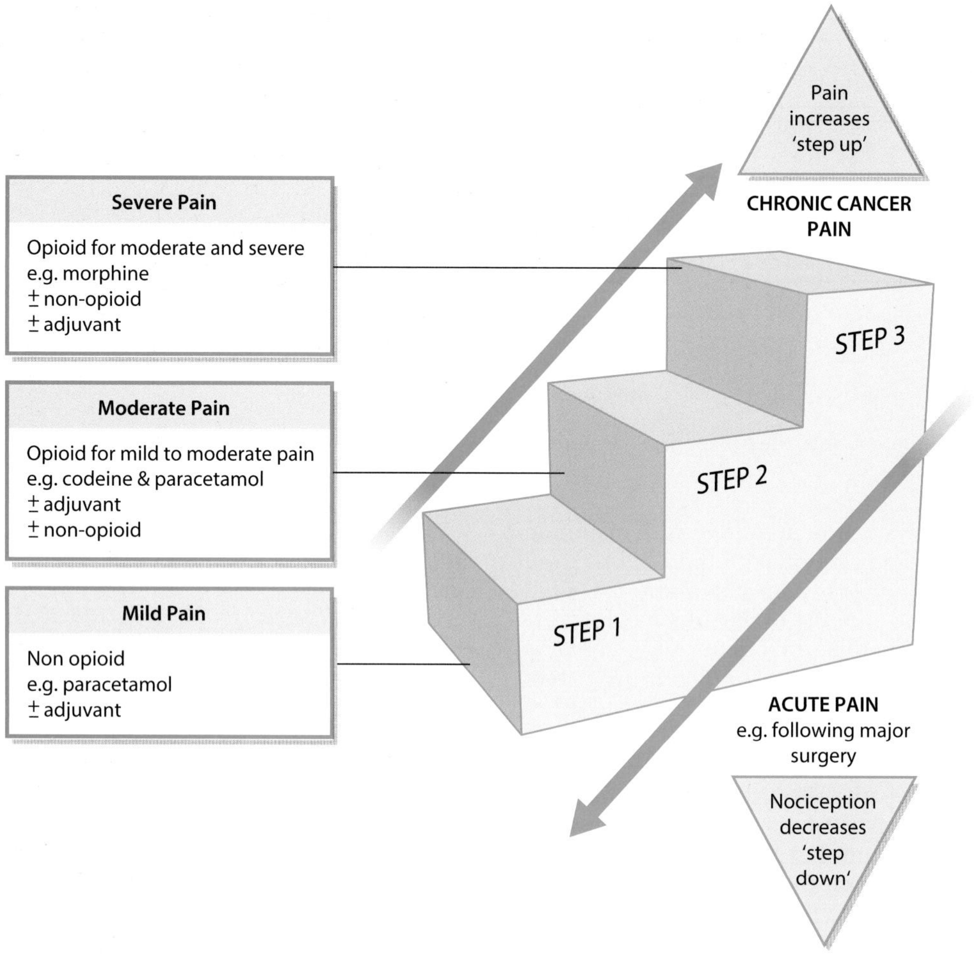

Fig. 23.10 Analgesic ladder (based on WHO 2005)

- *Severe pain*: When pain is not relieved by Step 2 drugs, then a strong opioid, e.g. morphine, is recommended in combination with non-opioid and adjuvant drugs.

This ladder was first proposed for use by the World Health Organization in the management of cancer pain in the 1980s; however, it is also useful to consider when matching analgesic prescription to pain intensity for other pain types. It can be used to guide analgesic prescribing in any patient setting, e.g. community, Emergency Department and hospital. Postoperative pain relief often starts at the top of the ladder and steps down as pain subsides. In contrast, for chronic malignant cancer pain the analgesia will be adjusted as pain intensity increases with advancing disease; for many patients this approach has been successful in achieving good pain control (see Ch. 12).

Box 23.19 outlines a study by Moore et al (2003) that compared analgesic effectiveness in acute pain.

A combination of analgesic drugs, known as the balanced or multimodal approach, may be required for effective pain management. This can enhance pain management because less opioid is required (opioid sparing) when given in combination with other drugs and thus reduces side-effects (Broadbent 2000). Examples include

EVIDENCE-BASED PRACTICE Box 23.19

Analgesic effectiveness

Moore et al (2003) compared the effects of various analgesics used in acute pain management. Their findings include:

- The most effective drugs for acute pain are NSAIDs
- The mild opioid codeine did not evaluate well when used alone; however, in combination with paracetamol it was much more effective
- Paracetamol evaluated well in the study, which is important as patients and parents often perceive this as a weak drug for use with mild pain only.

Student activities

- Consider the finding regarding the effectiveness of paracetamol.
- Discuss with your mentor how this finding could be used to achieve more effective pain management in your placement.

[From Moore et al (2003)]

oral co-codamol (paracetamol and codeine) and epidural administration of an opioid with local anaesthetic. In combination, the drugs target different areas involved in pain physiology (see pp. 657–659), which appears to improve the analgesic effect.

Pre-emptive and procedural pain management

The principle of providing analgesia before tissue injury to minimize pain is generally accepted as good practice. Some patients require repeat procedures and previous poor pain management can make patients fearful and reluctant to participate again. This is a particularly important issue for children and leads to further distress. Furthermore, poorly managed procedural pain is thought to contribute to physiological changes, which in some patients have been linked to chronic pain development (Carr & Mann 2000). Certain procedures in clinical practice, e.g. taking blood samples, cannulation, painful dressings and postoperative physiotherapy, are recognized as causing pain, and planning care to minimize this is essential. Both pharmacological treatment and psychological support are required. The management of procedural or transitory pain can be achieved by a variety of techniques:

1. Blocking pain transmission with local anaesthetics:
   - Topical application of creams containing a eutectic mixture of local anaesthetics (EMLA), e.g. lidocaine with prilocaine prior to venepuncture, etc. (Box 23.20)
   - Instillation of lidocaine gel into the urethra prior to catheterization (see Ch. 20)
   - Subcutaneous infiltration of lidocaine prior to wound suturing in the Emergency Department.
2. Nitrous oxide 50% + oxygen 50% (Entonox®) inhalation by self-administration, e.g. during a painful dressing. Note that it is widely used during labour.
3. Administration of a short-acting strong opioid, which allows for rapid recovery.

Drug tolerance and dependence

The use of analgesics is influenced by drug tolerance, dependence and addiction. A common misperception that opioid analgesics lead to addiction has a negative influence on pain management. Several authors (Carr & Mann 2000, Mann 2003) identify that nurses and patients have exaggerated fears about addiction risk with opioids. This affects drug prescribing by medical staff, pain reporting by patients and drug administration by nurses leading to unrelieved pain.

- Physiological tolerance occurs when a patient becomes used to a drug and may require larger doses for the same effect. Tolerance to some side-effects of opioids is a useful adaptation. Initially, central side-effects such as sedation and nausea and vomiting occur, but tolerance to these side-effects develops with time. Unfortunately, tolerance to peripheral side-effects, e.g. constipation, does not occur and so must be prevented.
- Physical dependence is described as an adaptive state (Mann 2003). Physical disturbance with 'withdrawal symptoms' occurs in a physically dependent person if opioids are suddenly stopped (Carr & Mann 2000); opioids are therefore gradually reduced.
- Addiction is a disorder of psychological dependence and craving when the person is not using the drug for analgesia. The risk of addiction with the use of opioids for pain relief is below 1% (Carr & Mann 2000). Acute pain has minimal risk. Evidence from the management of chronic malignant pain shows that people can maintain normal activities without demonstrating features of addiction. Increasingly, opioids are being used for severe chronic non-malignant pain. The Pain Society (2003) has published recommendations about the appropriate use of opioids for this group of people (see Further reading).

The management of pain in people who misuse drugs often requires support from the acute pain team, as drug tolerance means that larger doses will be needed. The route of administration also requires careful consideration: regular i.m. administration, for example, would not be desirable, as it encourages dependence on an invasive approach (Box 23.21, p. 674).

CRITICAL THINKING Box 23.20

Topical local anaesthesia before cannulation

Sophie, who is 19 years old and has a learning disability, needs to have an i.v. cannula sited for drug administration.

Student activities

- Find out how local anaesthetic cream is used to reduce pain before cannulation.
- Discuss with your mentor the factors that must be considered before deciding that local anaesthetic cream should be offered to Sophie.
- Think about the need to provide appropriate information and support for Sophie and her family.

Non-pharmacological methods of pain control

Over recent years non-pharmacological methods of pain control such as massage and the use of essential oils have become more widely accepted within conventional healthcare systems, although many still lack robust evidence of efficacy. Information giving is pivotal in pain control, as fear of pain increases pain perception (see pp. 659, 675). An outline of some methods is provided here but readers are directed to Further reading (e.g. Rankin-Box 2001).

It is vital that nurses understand the importance of simple (but by no means trivial) comfort measures that can be initiated as part of pain management, e.g. a carefully placed pillow (Box 23.22, p. 674).

Pain type, severity and the patient's age are important factors to consider when planning the use of non-pharmacological approaches to pain management. It is

CRITICAL THINKING Box 23.21

Opioid misuse and pain relief

Leo has been admitted for major surgery but providing postoperative pain relief is complicated by his regular misuse of heroin. The acute pain team is able to prescribe an analgesic regimen to relieve his pain. Although the focus of immediate care remains effective postoperative pain management, rehabilitation will hopefully become a goal for the future. Drug rehabilitation requires skilled specialist support.

Student activities

- Discuss the role of the acute pain team in the care of people such as Leo with your mentor.
- Find out what services are available in your area for community-based drug rehabilitation, e.g. Community Alcohol and Drug Service.

REFLECTIVE PRACTICE Box 23.22

Comfort measures

Think about the comfort measures that you use to decrease pain and discomfort. For example, after a busy shift you may rest your aching legs on a chair or in a warm bath, or use a hot water bottle to relieve 'period pain'.

Student activities

- Think about your most recent placement – were there opportunities for you to initiate simple comfort measures for people in pain?
- Discuss with your mentor how you might increase the use of comfort measures in pain management.

Box 23.23

Examples of non-pharmacological methods – psychological and physical (counterirritation)

Psychological methods (central stimulation and enhanced pain modulation of the 'pain gate')

- Relaxation
- Distraction (cognitive strategy)
- Music therapy
- Humour
- Guided imagery
- Cognitive behaviour therapy – hypnosis, biofeedback.

Physical (counterirritation) methods (peripheral stimulation of the 'pain gate')

- Heat and cold
- Chemicals – topical applications that cause skin irritation, e.g. products containing combinations of eucalyptus oil, menthol, methylsalicylate, etc.
- Massage
- Transcutaneous electrical nerve stimulation (TENS)
- Acupuncture.

also important to note that the patient's mental and emotional state are important in pain management and, as these are likely to vary over time, can affect the severity, tolerance and expression of pain.

Non-pharmacological methods can be classified into two groups: physical (counterirritation) and psychological. However, some methods, such as massage, have both physical and psychological benefits. Box 23.23 outlines some physical and psychological methods.

Many non-pharmacological methods are complementary therapies or alternative therapies and more detailed coverage of some of these is provided in Chapter 10 and in Further reading suggestions (e.g. Rankin-Box 2001).

Effective holistic pain management usually requires a combined pharmacological and non-pharmacological approach. In acute severe pain the dominant intervention is usually pharmacological along with explanation, anxiety reduction, emotional support and appropriate touch. Distraction and relaxation require patient participation as well as energy, which may limit their usefulness in severe pain. Relaxation is further limited in acute severe pain as there may be insufficient time to teach relaxation techniques. However, appropriate techniques can be taught in advance, e.g. prior to planned surgery.

Non-pharmacological methods of pain control (e.g. a visit to the hydrotherapy pool), which reduce pain perception by closing the 'pain gate', are probably most effective as coping strategies in chronic non-malignant pain rather than for reducing the intensity of pain (see Fig. 23.3, p. 656 and Table 23.1, p. 657). There are some exceptions to this, such as cold applications, but the most likely outcome of techniques such as relaxation and distraction is that the pain may become more bearable but not necessarily less severe in intensity. Specialized practitioners may be available via the pain specialist services for chronic pain or for cancer patients.

Despite the obvious benefits of pain relief achieved by using non-pharmacological methods, nurses must ensure that they possess the appropriate knowledge and skills to deliver such techniques (NMC 2004; see also Ch. 7). It is also important to note that non-pharmacological methods may be overused in some circumstances and with certain people. For example, clients and patients who are cooperative and adapt to techniques such as distraction may suffer their pain in silence and not be provided with appropriate or adequate analgesia.

Simple comfort measures

These can improve the experience of the person in pain and include:

- Careful positioning and changes in position as required. Analgesia may be needed if the repositioning itself is likely to cause pain
- Ensuring that people have sufficient rest and sleep (see Ch. 10) can enhance coping strategies

EVIDENCE-BASED PRACTICE Box 23.24

Information and pain

Over 30 years ago, Hayward (1975) published the seminal study that considered how the provision of information affects pain.

Hayward's study concluded that information about pain and its duration given preoperatively reduced the need for analgesic drugs after surgery.

Student activities

- Access a copy of Hayward's study and read about other findings.
- Think about other findings from the study that you have seen in practice.

[Reference: Hayward J 1975 Information, a prescription against pain. RCN, London]

- Pillows and footstools for support and a bed cage to keep heavy bedding off the legs
- Warmth with heated pads or warm baths, or cold applications/ice packs. Nurses must follow local safety guidelines when using heat or cold to prevent injury (see Ch. 13)
- Attention to proper bed/cot making is important, e.g. ensuring that bed sheets are not creased (see Ch. 18)
- Providing comfort for infants by swaddling or 'nesting', which means to snuggle, cuddle or cradle the infant.

These measures are also valuable for patient/clients and their carers who can become actively involved, especially in the management of chronic pain.

Information giving

Effective communication (see Ch. 9) and the provision of high quality information are vital components of holistic pain management. Inadequate information leads to the fear of pain, especially when the cause is unknown, or fear of not coping and poor understanding of pain relief methods, which can all worsen pain (Box 23.24). RNs must ensure that patients/clients/parents have sufficient information about pain and pain relief. They should discuss options, give explanations and provide written information about methods of managing pain, all of which can help to minimize anxiety and fear. There are also many self-help books designed to help patients cope with pain.

Relaxation

Relaxation may provide relief from pain and/or reduce anxiety. It may not lessen pain intensity but may decrease the distress associated with the pain. A patient/client cannot usually be relaxed and anxious at the same time. Relaxation aims to decrease skeletal muscle tension, as muscle pain can heighten painful stimuli, and the gate control theory predicts that decreasing muscle tension will reduce pain sensation. Relaxation is an effective coping mechanism for chronic or procedural pain. It can be initiated with music therapy, and relaxation techniques (see Ch. 11) can be taught prior to, and in preparation for, painful procedures. A warm bath can also aid relaxation. For infants, holding them in a well-supported comfortable position and/or rocking them rhythmically can facilitate relaxation.

Snoezelen multisensory room/environments, initially developed for people with a learning disability to create an environment for sensory stimulation, have recently been used to promote rest and relaxation for patients with chronic pain as a way to promote their coping strategies (Schofield 1996).

Hypnosis

Hypnosis is defined as focused attention, an altered state of consciousness or a trance that is followed by a period of relaxation. Hypnosis is one way of achieving relaxation and is useful in relieving the distress caused by pain and improving confidence. It may not take the pain away but reduces or removes pain perception by stimulating the higher centres of the brain so that they inhibit opening of the 'gate'.

Distraction

Distraction is a means of putting the pain at the periphery of awareness (McCaffery 1990) and focusing attention on something other than the pain. The focus of attention is diverted to the 'distracter' rather than the pain. Distracters include:

- Company and conversation, especially when humour and laughter are involved
- Television, video/DVD, radio, personal music players
- Hobbies
- Exercise, activity and sport (also linked to endorphin production)
- Caring for pet animals
- Reading
- Computer games – these are valuable distracters for children, particularly if activity is limited
- Play (see below).

Children in particular tend to be talented at using distracters as a means of pain relief. Additional distracters for children include:

- Having stories read to them
- Music, singing, and tapping to the rhythms of the song
- Talking books, especially via headphones, as active listening is a strong distracter
- Watching a favourite video/DVD or a television programme
- Blowing bubbles
- Visits from role models such as the local football team
- Shouting or yelling.

The distracter can be increased or reduced according to the intensity of the pain (Box 23.25, p. 676).

In children's wards a play specialist may be available to support nurses with 'play as distraction'. This is

CRITICAL THINKING Box 23.25

Distraction in children

The use of play is important to help children bring some familiarity to an unfamiliar situation, such as the experience of illness and pain and the healthcare environment. Therapeutic play is structured by adults and followed through by the child who is given the opportunity to overcome fears and anxieties by bringing unconscious feelings to the surface such as in needle phobia (Trigg & Mohammed 2006).

Student activities

- Read Appendix 1: Play in Trigg & Mohammed (2006)
- Think about how you could use some of their ideas, e.g. puppets, a distraction box, etc. in your practice.

[Reference: Trigg E, Mohammed T 2006 Practices in children's nursing: guidelines for hospital and community, 2nd edn. Churchill Livingstone, Edinburgh]

REFLECTIVE PRACTICE Box 23.26

Therapeutic touch

When you are in pain, what sort of touch, e.g. a light touch on the arm, can help you to cope?

Student activities

- Think about how often you use therapeutic touch with patients or clients.
- During your next placement discuss with your mentor how therapeutic touch can be used to help a person who has mental distress, dementia or a learning disability to manage their pain.

beneficial, as boredom can be a factor that opens the 'pain gate'. Similarly, an activities coordinator working in a care home can arrange outings and social events that act as distracters for residents with pain.

Older people who live alone may find that social isolation is a negative influence on pain perception, as it is likely to open the 'pain gate'. Therefore, encouraging social interaction and hobbies, e.g. lunch clubs, day centres, reading groups, that stimulate and distract may be valuable strategies in pain management

Imagery

Imagery is the use of imagination to modify pain responses and involves using sensory images to modify the pain – for example, that the pain is a balloon and the person is trying to blow the balloon (pain) as far away as possible. In doing so it makes the pain more bearable by providing a focus or substitution and organizes energies that facilitate the healing process. Imagery provides relief through relaxation, distraction and producing an image of the pain. Imagery can also empower patients/clients to take some control over their pain.

Imagery can be used in a guided way with children and is usually described as *guided therapeutic imagery*. The child imagines something about their pain that will help to reduce it, e.g. their pain flowing out of their bodies.

Massage

Massage may modify the pain experience by stimulating the nerve fibres responsible for inhibiting pain perception by closing the gate and potentially stimulating endorphin production. The relief obtained by rubbing an area after a minor knock demonstrates this.

Where possible, the patient/client/parents should be involved in the decision-making process and appropriate permission should be sought. Using massage involves a level of physical contact that is an essential element of the therapy. Massage can provide carers with a useful role and make them feel that they are contributing something positive to the experience, e.g. the carer or relative can massage their loved one's back and shoulders. Older adults especially may be deprived of physical contact and massage can have a dual effect of contact with another human being and lead to relaxation.

Massage provides healing and relaxes tightly contracted muscles that may result from pain-induced stress. Therefore, massage can lead to relaxation and provide renewed energy needed for coping strategies.

Therapeutic touch

Touch is a means of communication (see Ch. 9). It is normally a two-way process involving feelings and sensation, and indicates a caring or loving relationship; on the other hand, touch used therapeutically aims to aid healing.

Therapeutic touch is a non-invasive means by which the nurse can help to manage a person's pain. This is particularly important for certain groups such as children, people with mental distress or those with a learning disability. Some patients in hospital are deprived of therapeutic touch even though they are exposed to high levels of touch, especially in relation to observations and technical procedures (Box 23.26). In fact parents, especially those of children who are severely ill, touch their children more than the nursing staff.

Acupuncture (see Ch. 10)

Acupuncture aims to treat the person and not the disease or the symptoms. Using acupuncture for the treatment of painful conditions is based upon a greater understanding of physiological mechanisms involved in the pain transmission and modulation (Henderson 2002). There is also some evidence to suggest that acupuncture encourages the production of endorphins (see pp. 656, 658, 659).

Transcutaneous electrical nerve stimulation

Transcutaneous electrical nerve stimulation (TENS) is useful in localized pain and is thought to increase endorphin levels and act as a counterirritant. Ideally TENS should be used in combination with other treatments. The non-invasive device delivers controlled low-voltage electricity to the body via electrodes placed on the skin (Fig. 23.11). People using TENS often describe a tingling sensation when the device is active. It is useful for both acute and chronic pain and is used in labour (Box 23.27).

In chronic pain management TENS provides a modality with fewer side-effects than other treatments and is attractive because it is controlled by the patient and does not limit mobility. However, some people may be unable to tolerate the electrodes on their skin.

Aromatherapy (see Ch. 10)

Aromatherapy is a holistic form of healing using essential oils extracted from aromatic plants. The oils can be used in massage, in the bath, through inhalation and compresses. Aromatherapy massage can offer several ways of reducing the experience of pain, e.g. by acting on the 'pain gate' mechanism, positively affecting the cognitive control mechanisms and by the release of endorphins. Aromatherapy is frequently used to reduce stress, promote relaxation, treat symptoms and relieve pain.

Aromatherapy must only be practised by trained practitioners, although once the oils have been made safe into an effective blend patients/clients/parents can use them as prescribed by the therapist. However, nurses must consult local guidelines and polices before using essential oils.

CRITICAL THINKING Box 23.27

Non-pharmacological pain relief during labour

Women may choose to use TENS or other non-pharmacological methods as part of the management of labour pain.

Student activities

- What non-pharmacological methods have you seen used during labour?
- How did these methods affect the woman's pain experience and the experience of her partner/supporter?
- Did women choose to combine the method with drug-based pain relief?

Surgical intervention

Sometimes this is necessary for intractable pain. Surgical interventions include:

- Nerve ablation or destruction – temporary or permanent
- Spinal cord stimulation
- Brain stimulation using s.c. pulse generators.

These interventions are only used when other pain control methods have proved unsuccessful and usually fall within the remit of the specialist pain clinic.

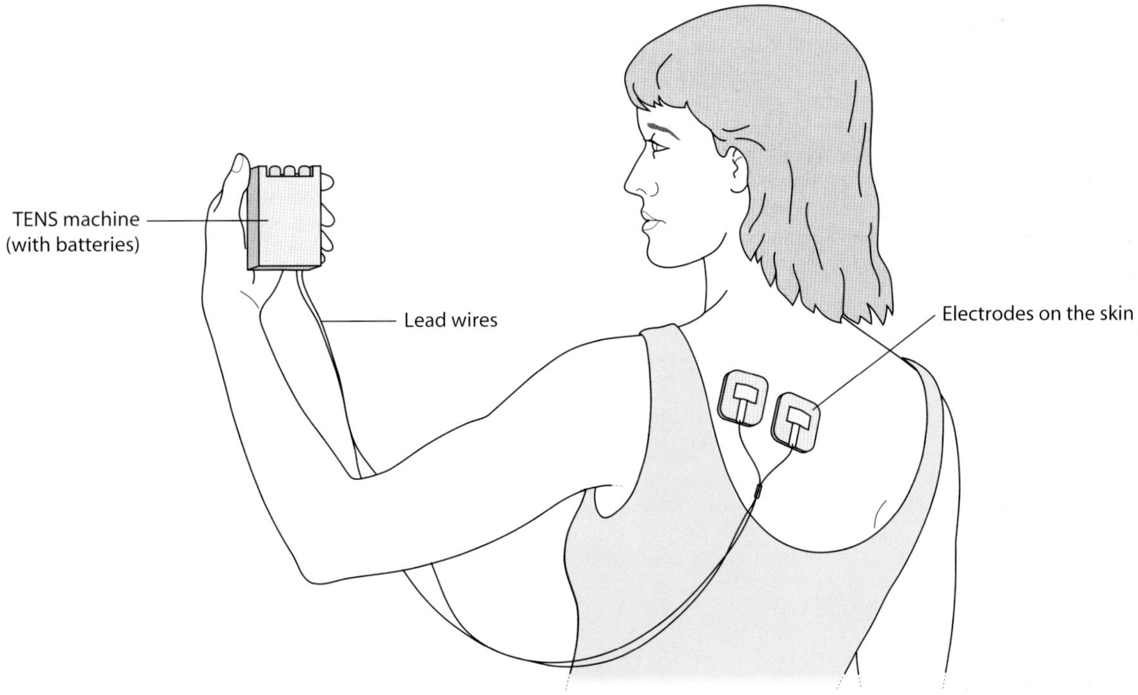

Fig. 23.11 Transcutaneous electrical nerve stimulation

Summary

- Pain is a subjective, complex and multidimensional experience that has physical, psychosocial, emotional, cultural and spiritual elements.
- Accurate pain assessment is essential for effective management and requires good communication skills and an awareness of possible barriers to effective communication.
- Recognition of vulnerable people who cannot express pain easily is vital.
- Assessment tools improve the objectivity of pain assessment; the appropriate choice of tools requires the nurse to have an awareness of suitability for pain type and client group.
- The recognition that pain is multidimensional has encouraged holistic care, which recognizes the importance of pharmacological and non-pharmacological approaches.
- For those people who are suffering from chronic pain, empowerment to encourage independence and coping skills is important.
- Ineffective pain management can seriously hamper rehabilitation following surgery and trauma and may lead to depression and disability if it becomes unrelieved chronic pain.
- Effective pain management is an important quality issue in nursing care across the lifespan and in all branches of nursing.
- Lastly, it is vital to remember that pain is 'whatever the experiencing person says it is, existing whenever he says it does' (McCaffery & Pasero 1999).

Self test

1. Outline the characteristics of acute and chronic pain.
2. What is the gate control theory of pain?
3. Codeine is a weak opioid. True/false?
4. What modifications can be made to self-report pain scales to make them more appropriate for children?
5. Which side-effects do not diminish when morphine is used long term for chronic pain?
6. Regular administration of analgesics is required to prevent pain following surgery or trauma. True/false?
7. Which of the following factors is likely to open the 'pain gate' and increase pain?
   a. Watching a favourite TV programme
   b. Listening to music
   c. Disturbed sleep pattern
   d. Relaxation with guided imagery

Key words and phrases for literature searching

Acute pain
Analgesics
Chronic pain
Neuropathic pain
Nociceptive pain
Pain clinics
Pain relief

Useful websites

Bandolier – *The Oxford Pain Internet Site*	www.jr2.ox.ac.uk/bandolier/booth/painpag/index2.html Available July 2006
British National Formulary	www.bnf.org.uk Available July 2006
Cancerbackup	www.cancerbackup.org.uk Available July 2006
National Institute for Health and Clinical Excellence	www.nice.org.uk Available July 2006
Pain site	www.pain-talk.co.uk Available July 2006
Scottish Intercollegiate Guidelines Network	www.sign.ac.uk Available July 2006
The British Pain Society	www.britishpainsociety.org Available July 2006

References

Baker C, Wong D 1987 QUESTT: a process of pain assessment in children. Orthopaedic Nurse 6(1):9–11

Broadbent C 2000 The pharmacology of acute pain. Nursing Times 96(26):39–41

Brooker C, Nicol M (eds) 2003 Nursing adults. The practice of caring. Mosby, Edinburgh

Bruster S, Jarman B, Bosanquet N et al 1994 National survey of hospital patients. British Medical Journal 309:1542–1549

Carr E, Mann E 2000 Pain: creative approaches to effective management. Macmillan, Basingstoke

Carter B 1994 Child and infant pain. Principles of nursing care and management. Chapman & Hall, London

Davies K, Taylor A 2003 Pain. In: Brooker C, Nicol M (eds) Nursing adults. The practice of caring. Mosby, Edinburgh

Department of Health 2006 Non-Medical Prescribing Programme. Online: www.dh.gov.uk/PolicyandGuidance Available September 2006

Elliot A, Smith B, Penny K et al 1999 The epidemiology of chronic pain in the community. Lancet 354:1248–1252

Greenstein B, Gould D 2004 Trounce's clinical pharmacology for nurses, 17th edn. Churchill Livingstone, Edinburgh

Henderson H 2002 Acupuncture evidence base for its use in low back pain. British Journal of Nursing 11(21):1395–1403

Horn S, Munafo M 1997 Pain theory, research and intervention. Open University Press, Buckingham

Human Rights Act 1998 TSO, London. Online: www.opsi.gov.uk/acts/acts1998/19980042.htm Available July 2006

Mann E 2003 Chronic pain and opioids: dispelling myths and exploring the facts. Professional Nurse 18(7):408–411

McCaffery M 1990 Nursing approaches to nonpharmacological pain control. International Journal of Nursing Studies 27(1):1–5

McCaffery M, Pasero C 1999 Pain clinical manual. 2nd edn. Mosby, St Louis

Melzack R, Katz J 1994 Measurement in persons in pain. In: Wall P, Melzack R (eds) Textbook of pain. 3rd edn. Churchill Livingstone, Edinburgh

Melzack R, Wall P 1965 Pain mechanisms: a new theory. Science 150:971–979

Merskey H, Bogduk N (eds) 1994 Classification of chronic pain: descriptions of chronic pain syndromes and definitions of pain terms. Report by the International Association for the Study of Pain, 2nd edn. IASP Press, Seattle

Moore A, Edwards J, Barden J, McQuay H 2003 League table of analgesia in acute pain. In: Bandoliers little book of pain. Oxford University Press, New York

Morley S, Eccleston C, Williams A 1999 Systematic review and meta-analysis of randomized controlled trials of cognitive behavior therapy and behavior therapy for chronic pain in adults excluding headache. Pain 80:1–13

Nursing and Midwifery Council 2004 The NMC code of professional conduct: standards for conduct, performance and ethics. NMC, London

Paz S, Seymour J 2004 Pain theories, evaluation and management In: Payne S, Seymour J, Ingleton C (eds) Palliative care nursing. Open University Press, New York

Piaget J 1924 Judgement and reasoning in the child. Routledge, London

Rutishauser S 1994 Physiology and anatomy. Churchill Livingstone, Edinburgh

Sarafino E 2002 Health psychology. 4th edn. Wiley, New York

Schofield P 1996 Snoezelen. Its potential for people with chronic pain. Complementary Therapies in Nursing and Midwifery 2(1):9–12

Twycross A, Moriarty A, Betts T 1998 Paediatric pain management a multidisciplinary approach. Radcliffe Medical Press, Oxon

World Health Organization 2005 Pain ladder. Online: www.who.int/cancer/palliative/painladder/en Available July 2006

Zborowski M 1952 Cultural components of pain. Journal of Sociological Issues 8:16–30

Further reading

Adams N, Field L 2001 Pain management: psychological and social aspects of nursing. British Journal of Nursing 10(14):903–911

Bruce A 2001 Pain experienced by older people. Professional Nurse 16(11):1481–1485

Clinical Standards Advisory Group 2000 Services for patients with pain. DH, London

Day R 2002 The management of acute and chronic pain in the community. Professional Nurse 17(6):386–388

Department of Health 2004 National Service Framework for children, young people and maternity services. Online: www.dh.gov.uk/childrensnsf Available July 2006

Field L, Adams N 2001 Pain management 2: use of psychological approaches to pain. British Journal of Nursing 10(15):971–974

Hockenberry MJ, Wilson D, Winkelstein ML, Kline N 2002 Wong's nursing care of infants and children. 7th edn. Mosby, St Louis

Needham J 2004 Issues relating to effective pain management in young people. Professional Nurse 19(7):406–408

NHS Quality Improvement Scotland (NHSQIS) 2004 Best Practice Statement: Postoperative pain management. Online: www.nhshealthquality.org/nhsqis/files/Post_Pain_COMPLETE.pdf Available July 2006

Rankin-Box D (ed) 2001 The nurse's handbook of complementary therapies. 2nd edn. Baillière Tindall, Edinburgh

Royal College of Nursing 1999 The recognition and assessment of acute pain in children: recommendations. RCN, London

Sofaer B 1998 Pain: principles, practice and patients. 3rd edn. Stanley Thornes, Cheltenham

The Pain Society 2003 Provisional recommendations for appropriate use of opioids in patients with chronic non-cancer related pain. The Pain Society, London

24

Caring for the person having surgery

Aurea Amos and Anne Waugh

Glossary terms

Anaesthesia

Biopsy

Elective surgery

Endoscopy

Perioperative care

Postoperative care

Preoperative care

Prophylactic

Prosthesis

Learning outcomes

This chapter will help you:

- Explain the differences between elective and emergency surgery
- Describe preoperative preparation of a patient
- Understand the nursing interventions needed to maintain the safety and dignity of people undergoing surgery
- Explain the principles of postoperative care
- Describe potential postoperative complications and their prevention
- Understand the principles of effective discharge planning.

Introduction

A person who has to undergo a surgical procedure or invasive investigation is likely to experience both psychological and physiological stress (see Ch. 11). Stressors can be reduced by careful planning and considered nursing intervention. Preoperative care is that carried out before an operation and postoperative care begins after surgery. Perioperative care is a nursing speciality that includes the care provided from arrival in the anaesthetic room, during an operation and in the recovery area afterwards, although this term is sometimes extended to include all the care given to a surgical patient during their admission to hospital or a treatment centre (specializing in certain types of surgery such as joint replacement) (see Ch. 3). Examples of invasive procedures, day surgery and inpatient stays are outlined, together with different reasons for and aims of surgery. The importance of the nurse's role in preoperative and postoperative care is explored within this chapter. Maintaining patients' safety and dignity is paramount in surgical nursing. Discharge planning usually begins before admission for surgery and is explained in the final section. Surgical nursing care should be seamless, despite it being carried out in several different settings, and the factors that facilitate this are considered.

Types of surgery

This section considers the different approaches to surgical interventions. There have been great advances in the way people can receive surgical treatment, including:

- Pre-assessment clinics prior to admission for surgery
- Day surgery (also known as ambulatory surgery) – the development of less, and minimally, invasive surgical procedures have reduced patients' stay in hospital from days to a few hours
- Improvements in anaesthesia.

The expected outcome of surgery varies depending on the reason for intervention. This may be:

- A *curative* procedure which involves the removal of diseased or damaged tissues that aims to restore health and may use radical methods, e.g. removal of an inflamed appendix or amputation following a crush injury
- A *conservative* procedure that involves the removal of diseased or damaged tissues using non-radical methods to improve health and preserve function, e.g. debulking/removal of a cancer
- A *palliative* procedure which is undertaken to relieve unpleasant or distressing symptoms when curative

Table 24.1 Terminology used to describe surgical procedures

	Meaning	Example
Prefixes		
Angio~	Of a vessel	Angiography
Chol~	Bile	Cholecystectomy
Cysto~	Of the bladder	Cystectomy
Gastro~	Of the stomach	Gastrostomy
Laparo~	Abdominal	Laparotomy
Suffixes		
~ectomy	Removal of	Appendicectomy
~oscopy	View of	Laparoscopy
~ostomy	Opening of	Ileostomy
~otomy	Incision into	Osteotomy
~plasty	Reconstruction of	Angioplasty
~therm	Heat	Diathermy

or conservative procedures are not possible, e.g. insertion of a hollow tube into the oesophagus to relieve an obstruction caused by a cancer.

There is a wide range of terminology used to describe surgical procedures. By understanding the meaning of some commonly used prefixes and suffixes this becomes logical and much easier to understand (see Table 24.1). It is good practice to look up the meanings of new terms encountered in practice. Surgery and invasive procedures take place in a wide range of specialities (see Table 2.4, p. 61).

Surgical interventions may be classified as:

- *Elective* – this is planned beforehand and includes day surgery. It aims to improve a person's health and/or promote comfort and can be curative, conservative, radical or palliative
- *Emergency* – this is unplanned and necessary for the person's survival and may be curative, conservative, radical or, occasionally, palliative.

Elective surgery

People who undergo elective surgery are usually admitted on the day of surgery having already had pre-assessment and the necessary investigations (see below). Careful preparation ensures patients are in optimal health for their operation. This minimizes cancellation when further investigations are needed or unforeseen problems arise, thereby reducing the likelihood of postoperative complications. The type and extent of surgery, together with the individual's state of health before, during and after surgery, will determine the length of stay in hospital. When day surgery is undertaken the patient goes home again the same day, whereas inpatient surgery usually requires several days in hospital postoperatively. Some patients need a series of surgical interventions, e.g. reconstructive surgery following severe or disfiguring injuries.

Day surgery

Day surgery, which started with children, has increased steadily in the treatment of adults. Many minor surgical procedures, such as cataract extraction, hernia repair, vasectomy or endoscopy, may be carried out as day cases.

Day surgery patients are admitted for elective procedures, invasive investigations, minor operations or endoscopy (Box 24.1) and the majority return home again the same evening. Some day surgery units provide care for up to 23 hours. Many people prefer to have the shortest stay possible in hospital for several reasons, including:

- Dislike of hospitals and sick people
- Less disruption to their personal lives
- Recovery within familiar surroundings.

The Audit Commission (2001) outlined advantages of day surgery for the NHS, which include:

- Economy, in that more inpatient beds are available for patients requiring specialized management
- Fewer postoperative complications due to early mobilization, thus reducing bed occupancy due to complications
- Shorter waiting times
- Reduced stress that can build up during the waiting period.

There are also disadvantages of day surgery. Some procedures are not suitable for day surgery and neither are some patients. For example, some people may not be fit enough, or not fit enough on the day of surgery, due to exacerbation of an underlying medical condition, e.g. hypertension (high blood pressure). Each unit has its own criteria for acceptable travelling distance and availability of medical assistance should complications arise, and therefore people who live far from the unit may not be suitable candidates for day surgery. Some people, who although fit for day surgery, may refuse it for several reasons, including:

- Having to cope with postoperative pain management by themselves
- Fear of possible complications
- Being a burden to their relatives.

On discharge after day surgery, all patients – adults and children – must have a responsible adult to care for them for at least 24 hours afterwards. The patient must also have a suitable home environment within which to recover and no need to use public transport. The need for care by a significant other can cause financial hardship due to loss of earnings or high travel costs.

Emergency surgery

This is sudden and unplanned. Patients may find this very stressful for many reasons, including fear of the unknown, fear of pain or dying, fear of hospitals and fear that far-reaching lifestyle changes may be needed. Bearing this in mind, the nurse must assess not only patients' physiological needs but also their psychological and emotional needs. In this situation social needs are also very important, e.g. children may be waiting at the school gate or older adults or pet animals may depend on the person being at home at certain times. It is very important to

Box 24.1 **Endoscopy and laparoscopy**

Endoscopy

Endoscopy is examination of internal structures using an endoscope. This instrument enables visualization of hollow organs and body cavities including the:

- Upper gastrointestinal tract – oesophagogastroduodenoscopy (OGD), gastroscopy
- Lower gastrointestinal tract – colonoscopy, sigmoidoscopy
- Urinary tract – cystoscopy
- Bronchial tree – bronchoscopy
- Uterus – hysteroscopy
- Joints – arthroscopy.

Endoscopes are usually made from flexible fibreoptic material but are sometimes rigid metal devices. Endoscopy is used for:

- Diagnosis
- Taking tissue samples, known as biopsies, and/or fluid for diagnostic purposes
- Performing interventions such as sealing off bleeding points, e.g. peptic ulcers, removal of polyps from the large intestine, gallstones from the common bile duct or bone pieces from joints
- Photography of findings
- Surgery, e.g. laparoscopic cholecystectomy (removal of the gallbladder, see below).

Endoscopy may cause pain and discomfort and is usually carried out under light sedation or anaesthesia (general or local).

Laparoscopy

The laparoscope is an endoscope used for investigations or 'keyhole' surgery within the peritoneal cavity, e.g. laparoscopic cholecystectomy. Laparoscopic surgery is carried out under general anaesthesia and the immediate postoperative care is the same as that following conventional surgery (see p. 692).

Advantages of laparoscopic surgery

- Small wound sites (around 12 mm)
- Less postoperative pain
- Early mobilization and discharge
- Fewer postoperative complications associated with immobility, e.g. chest infections, deep vein thrombosis (see p. 698).

Disadvantages of laparoscopic surgery

- Costly equipment required
- Training of practitioners is expensive.

establish a trusting nurse/patient relationship quickly. This relationship can be enhanced by the way the nurse informs and involves the patient during admission and preparation for urgent surgery. Effective communication skills (see Ch. 9) are therefore essential.

Preoperative care

The aim of preoperative care is to ensure that each patient receives holistic preparation for a safe and dignified surgical experience. For emergency admissions this is accelerated and takes place very soon after admission; however, the principles are the same. It involves assessment, planning, intervention and evaluation. Preparation usually beginswith referral from the general practitioner (GP) for elective procedures. In the future this will become better organized as patients are able to provisionally pre-book admission dates through their GP.

Investigations

Some investigations are carried out routinely on all patients; others are used to confirm the diagnosis or are specific to the type of intervention being considered. Routine investigations include:

- Blood samples – full blood count, urea and electrolyte levels, liver function tests, coagulation studies, and grouping and cross-matching if a blood transfusion (see Ch. 17) may be required
- Chest X-ray
- Electrocardiogram (ECG)
- Urinalysis.

Depending on the type of surgery, some of the following may also be carried out:

- Respiratory function tests (see Ch. 17)
- Microbiology tests, e.g. sputum, urine to exclude infection
- Other X-rays
- Computed tomography (CT) scan
- Magnetic resonance imaging (MRI) scan
- Ultrasound scanning
- Barium studies
- Angiography.

A simple explanation of some of these investigations that will help you provide patient information can be found on the BBC website (see 'Useful websites', p. 701). More detailed information can be found in Brooker and Nicol (2003).

Pre-assessment clinics

Pre-assessment clinics enable both healthcare staff and patients to plan and prepare for elective interventions involving day surgery or an inpatient stay. This means that on admission for surgery, staff know that the patient has been well prepared and has an understanding of their care before, during and after surgery, and also following discharge. Some rural areas have pre-assessment outreach clinics that reduce time and expense for patients.

Many pre-assessment clinics are nurse led and provide a point of contact should the person/parent/carer require more information or subsequent clarification. Patients of all ages are encouraged, if they wish, to have a friend, partner or carer with them during the consultation. Children should be accompanied by their parent or legal

Box 24.2 Preoperative considerations for children

Paediatric pre-assessment clinics are a time for nurses to gather information about the child and for children and their parents to visit the ward and meet staff. Pre-assessment clinics are usually run as clubs, often on Saturdays, instead of formal clinics. At these clubs parents and children gain insight into the proposed intervention by learning through, for example, play (see Ch. 9) and stories with pictures. Pre-assessment visits also provide the opportunity for nurses to correct any misconceptions and allay potential fears or anxieties. Booklets are sometimes used to reinforce information and children may be sent special letters from a character that has been adopted by a ward.

Action for Sick Children (2006) highlights the value of play in hospital to reduce anxiety about surgery or invasive procedures. This website also provides useful information for parents about what to expect during hospitalization for any reason. Trigg and Mohammed (2006) suggest that clubs include not only the child and their parents but also siblings, thus involving the whole family. Once in hospital, family links can be maintained by visits and use of the telephone, text messaging or the Internet.

guardian during the pre-assessment process. However, there are some circumstances in which this may not be case, e.g. where an older child is deemed mature enough to understand the procedure and its implications and is competent to make their own decisions about their care, for example, a girl of 15 years with sufficient maturity having a termination of pregnancy without her parents' knowledge (see Ch. 6). Pre-assessment clinics for children are described in Box 24.2.

At the pre-assessment clinic patients have the opportunity to:

- Discuss their treatment options
- Identify whether day surgery or inpatient surgery is more appropriate
- Undergo all, or some, of the investigations required on the same day.

Physical health is assessed to ensure the patient will be fit for the proposed intervention. Working together, nurses and patients discuss:

- Available options and what they involve. Nurses can provide information so that the experience is not threatening and anxieties can be worked through in a holistic manner. This is especially important in the case of children and those who lack mental capacity (see Ch. 6). Therapeutic play is central to the planning of children's care
- Lifestyle changes that will improve postoperative recovery, e.g. weight reduction, smoking cessation (see below)
- The surgical experience
- Local fasting policy (see p. 686) so that the patient understands what is required
- The patient's personal and domestic circumstances to ensure their discharge, aftercare and convalescence can be managed appropriately. Those who will be at home after discharge or who have an older partner may need support and assistance. Members of the multidisciplinary team (MDT), e.g. social worker, home help or the community health team, may be included to provide specialist advice and help
- Local policy regarding routine medicines, e.g. a patient may be advised to cease taking warfarin (medication which thins the blood) a few days prior to the invention or surgery.

It is important that everyone, including both children and parents, is provided with information in a way that is understood (see below).

Smoking cessation

Patients who smoke should be advised to give up as smoking is a risk factor for many postoperative complications, e.g. chest infections, deep vein thrombosis (DVT, p. 698), poor wound healing and pressure ulcers (see Ch. 25). Smoking cessation should start at least 2 weeks before surgery; however, this advice can have either a negative or a positive effect as withdrawal of nicotine can increase people's stress levels. Some people find nicotine replacement therapy helpful. Nurses must not be judgemental or critical if a patient cannot heed this advice; however, information about potential postoperative complications related to smoking should always be provided.

Communication

Psychological preparation for investigative procedures or surgery requires effective communication skills that form an essential part of holistic care. This begins at the pre-assessment clinic where patients and their relatives are able to have information clarified and questions answered using language that they understand. On the other hand, poor communication – both verbal and written – can adversely affect the way people respond and may result in abnormal behaviour, people feeling threatened and increased anxiety levels.

The nurse explains to the patient what to expect, both immediately afterwards and during the convalescent period; this can vary considerably depending on the surgery to be performed. The immediate aftercare may involve equipment including intravenous (i.v.) infusions, a wound with skin closures, etc. There may also be exercises to be carried out and dietary or mobility considerations. The steps involved in returning to previous fitness are also discussed in detail. Even when patients appear to be fully informed, they often find the preoperative waiting period stressful. Some surgery may not have a favourable outcome and this may add to people's fears and impair their ability to cope with bad news (see Ch. 9).

Written material can reduce misunderstanding and reinforces verbal and other sources of information from health professionals; CD-ROMs and videos may also be used. This allows people to read or watch when they feel able to concentrate and is a useful reminder of what to expect. For those for whom English is not their first language, material in their own language should be provided whenever possible; sometimes an interpreter may be needed (see Ch. 9).

When faced with an impending operation, some people seek information from other sources including the Internet although there may be difficulty in fully understanding the information found there. Nurses are in an ideal position to help patients work through information from any source and ensure that their understanding is accurate. Information may have been provided, but people's perceptions can be that it is too much, duplicated or not enough. Patients are also at risk of overlooking important information because they are selective in what they read (Otte 1996).

Benefits of providing preoperative information

Lin and Wang (2005) studied the effect of pain information given before abdominal surgery, and concluded that this information-giving could reduce pain intensity experienced in the immediate postoperative period (at 4 and 24 hours). Several authors have noted other postoperative benefits of providing preoperative information, including fewer postoperative complications and reduced patient anxiety (Hayward 1975, Boore 1978, Wilson-Barnett 1979, Bysshe 1988, Devine 1992), as well as improved job satisfaction for nurses who were given the opportunity to meet their patients before the day of surgery (Crawford 1999, Holmes 2005).

REFLECTIVE PRACTICE Box 24.3

Preoperative anxiety

Some patients undergoing surgery report anxiety about having an anaesthetic, the possibility of waking up during the operation and being unable to tell anyone, not recovering from the anaesthetic or that they may behave inappropriately under the anaesthetic. Anxiety may also be increased when the potential prognosis is poor. Patients in unfamiliar surroundings, who have had bad previous experiences or little technical knowledge, may feel powerless.

Franklin (1974) found that anxious patients needed more information about their treatment, progress and surroundings, and also reassurance from the care team. Patients who have communication difficulties may become frustrated or upset when they are not understood (Ashworth 1980).

Student activities

1. What would be your greatest anxiety if you needed to have (or have had) an anaesthetic?
2. Observe your mentor speaking to a patient preoperatively to identify potential sources of anxiety:
   - Think about the communication skills used
   - List the anxieties identified.
3. Identify the communication skills that you might use to reduce feelings of powerlessness.

Common sources of preoperative anxiety

Patients are encouraged to express their fears and concerns using good interpersonal communication skills (see Ch. 9). It is important to recognize that apprehension can build up while waiting for an operation despite effective planning (Box 24.3). Fear of the unknown and loss of independence are common anxieties that can cause a person to develop either introverted or extroverted behaviour. In children, this may manifest itself by a change in behaviour, e.g. withdrawal, regression, overactivity or parent dependence. Reduced contact with family and changes in daily routines can instil a feeling of loss or abandonment, especially in young children and older adults. These feelings can become exaggerated, especially if someone will have few, or no, visitors. The nurse can discuss these potential problems and offer suggestions such as making phone calls to their friends and family from the ward.

Sometimes a recovery room nurse visits patients on the ward preoperatively. These visits facilitate seamless care from the ward to theatre and back again, and help the patient cope with an essentially unpleasant experience (Weins 1998). The nurse can talk to the patient about any fears about the anaesthetic or other issues they would like clarified, e.g. relating to fear of needles or the wearing of dentures and hearing aids until induction of anaesthesia. Patients who need initial postoperative care in a high dependency or intensive care unit may find visiting the area useful but this should not be imposed as it may increase their anxiety (Skacel & McKenna 1990).

Many people prefer to have intimate care carried out by professionals of the same gender. Cultural norms can be a source of anxiety, especially to older women, who may have had little personal contact with men, and those whose religion or culture dictates restriction of physical contact with a male who is not their husband. Nurses need to be sensitive to people's needs and preferences by ensuring they are taken into account whenever possible. For women, a female chaperone is arranged when this is not possible. Similarly, many men prefer not to have intimate care carried out by female staff.

Surgery that changes body appearance will affect people's body image (see Ch. 11), e.g. removal of a breast due to cancer is often a source of great preoperative anxiety. However, to other people the same surgery may bring positive outcomes despite postoperative discomfort, e.g. breast reduction or amputation of a painful gangrenous extremity.

Mitchell (2000) advocates that ideally the amount of information provided for a patient should match their preferred coping strategies (see Ch. 11). Some patients use their spirituality to help them cope. Coping strategies can be observed and discussed at the pre-assessment clinic and also at the time of admission (see Box 24.4). Identifying postoperative coping strategies beforehand may help patients to work through postoperative problems using their own stress-reducing mechanisms, e.g. yoga exercises

REFLECTIVE PRACTICE Box 24.4

Coping mechanisms

As we go through life we are faced with many challenges, pleasant and unpleasant. We generally learn coping mechanisms that help us to deal with challenging situations. However, our usual coping mechanisms are sometimes inadequate in abnormal circumstances (see Chs 9, 11).

Student activities

- Recall the coping mechanisms that you use to reduce your anxiety.
- Think about how you could use some of them to help anxious patients.
- Find out about a support group or network that could help to reduce a patient's preoperative anxiety.

that reduce tension may be used to assist postoperative pain management (see Ch. 23). Other strategies may include arranging a meeting with an ex-patient who has undergone the same type of surgery or a parent may be put in contact with another family that has been in the same situation. This can be of great help, as many people benefit from a personal approach.

Obtaining consent

Prior to any operation or invasive investigation people must sign a consent form for both legal and ethical reasons (see Chs 6, 7). For consent to be valid it is essential that three criteria are satisfied: that it is voluntary, that it is informed and that there is mental capacity to make the decision (see Ch. 6). Rigge (1997) reminds readers that patients have the right to ask the surgeon about their success rates, and the likelihood and nature of potential complications. The patient not only agrees in writing to the proposed invasive investigation or surgery but also to the type of anaesthesia used.

The surgeon undertaking the procedure must mark the site of operation when a limb or paired organ is involved. This is usually performed on the day of, or evening before, the operation to safeguard against later errors regarding the correct surgical site. A waterproof marker pen prevents removal of the marks during bathing or showering. The patient must be in agreement with the correct site.

While discussing impending surgery, if there is any doubt that a particular procedure may not be possible, for example when a more extensive procedure might be required, the patient should also sign for the proposed variation. Nurses must be aware that it is a patient's right to withdraw their consent at any time. If this occurs, the charge nurse must be informed immediately. The Nursing and Midwifery Council (NMC) *Code of Professional Conduct: Standards for Conduct, Performance and Ethics* (2004) points out that nurses must always respect patients' wishes, however frustrating this may be. Consent may also be withheld in relation to an aspect of treatment (Box 24.5).

CRITICAL THINKING Box 24.5

Obtaining consent

Mrs George signs a consent form for a laparoscopic cholecystectomy. During the operation complications arise and a more invasive procedure (laparotomy) is carried out to complete the surgery safely. Mrs George had been well prepared for this eventuality. She had already agreed and signed the consent form indicating that she understood and was prepared to have the more invasive procedure if the need arose.

Student activities (1)

- Negotiate an opportunity to observe a practitioner obtaining consent.
- Ask a patient how effectively the consent interview prepared them for their experience.

Sometimes consent may not be given, e.g. a patient may refuse a blood transfusion due to personal or religious beliefs or the fear of infection from blood-borne viruses.

Student activities (2)

- Find out which group of people may refuse a blood transfusion.
- Why might someone not consent to a blood transfusion?
- Consider how you might support a patient who has refused a blood transfusion.

In an emergency situation, a surgeon might operate on an unconscious patient without formal signed consent. In the absence of this the intervention must be justifiable and carried out on the basis that it is in the patient's best interests.

Preoperative fasting

Usually patients can eat and drink normally until 2–6 hours before surgery unless the surgery involves the gastrointestinal (GI) tract. The Royal College of Nursing (RCN 2005) suggests that:

- Clear fluids (water) can be taken up to 2 hours prior to surgery
- Breast milk can be given up to 4 hours prior to surgery
- Solids, cow's milk, formula milk and milky drinks can be given up to 6 hours prior to surgery.

The reason for fasting is to ensure safety during induction of general anaesthesia by preventing inhalation of acid stomach contents into the lungs when the gag reflex is lost. Some patients, including those who are having day surgery, are admitted having fasted overnight for surgery in the morning although this is significantly longer than the RCN (2005) suggests is necessary.

Fasting (see Box 24.6) is also known as 'nil by mouth'. Before fasting begins the local policy is explained, including the safety reasons outlined above. Water jugs

EVIDENCE-BASED PRACTICE Box 24.6

Preoperative fasting

Hamilton Smith (1972) demonstrated that preoperative fasting time was based on ritual rather than evidenced-based practice. Recent evidence demonstrates that many patients still fast for longer than necessary (O'Callaghan 2002). The reasons for this include ritualistic practice, poor communication between theatre and ward staff and resistance to change.

Prolonged fasting can lead to fluid and electrolyte imbalance (see Ch. 19). Nausea is sometimes reported while fasting and may be due to the stress of being unable to have oral fluids, a dry mouth or the smell of food (Cronin 1996). Dean and Fawcett (2002) suggested that long periods of fasting might be a cause of postoperative nausea and vomiting. The RCN (2005) suggests that patients should normally be allowed clear fluids up to 2 hours preoperatively.

Student activities

Select a small group of postoperative patients or those who have undergone invasive investigations:

- Find out for how long they fasted.
- Find out if they experienced nausea and vomiting.
- If the fasting time is longer than suggested, discuss the possible reasons for this with your mentor.

EVIDENCE-BASED PRACTICE Box 24.7

Preoperative hair removal

AORN (2002) recommend that the site should be inspected for potential problems such as warts, rashes or acne prior to choosing the method of hair removal. Depilatory cream can be used but a small area (test patch) must be tested first to ensure there is no allergy. In areas where the hair is particularly thick, cream may not be effective. Wet shaving with warm soapy water softens the hair, making it easier to remove and reduces microabrasions. Hair can also be removed using clippers with disposable heads, thus reducing the incidence of cross-infection. McIntyre and McCloy (1994) stated that using razors carried a higher risk of infection than depilatory creams or clippers and that hair removal should take place not more than 2–3 hours before surgery to reduce bacterial colonization within microabrasions. In some specialities, e.g. orthopaedics and plastic surgery, preoperative skincare following hair removal is carried out using antiseptic solutions such as chlorhexidine. AORN (2002) stated that topical antiseptics should be chosen carefully to prevent hypersensitivity reactions such as blisters and rashes.

Student activities

- Find out about skin preparation in your placement.
- Discuss the practices with your mentor.

and other fluids are removed from the bedside and, in the case of children, sweets and biscuits should also be removed. A sign is put above the bed or the side room door to remind those fasting and to inform others that someone is 'nil by mouth'. Some patients may require an i.v. infusion during fasting to prevent or correct dehydration (see Ch. 19). Some patients are admitted to hospital so that their fasting regime may be monitored, e.g. people with diabetes.

If someone who is meant to be fasting is found to have taken anything orally, this must be reported promptly to the charge nurse or anaesthetist who will decide whether it is safe for the intervention to go ahead.

Some patients who are having surgery under local anaesthesia, e.g. removal of a toenail, may not need to fast. However, if sedation, e.g. midazolam, is required for a procedure, fasting may be necessary to avoid the risk of aspiration (inhalation of gastric contents into the respiratory tract).

In children and those who have communication problems, the nurse should also discuss effective ways of maintaining fasting with the parent or carer during pre-assessment and reinforce this on admission. Fasting should be implemented without causing undue stress, otherwise it may become an issue.

When a patient is admitted as an emergency, the last time they had food or fluids must be clearly established. In emergency situations a tube may be passed into the patient's stomach to aspirate the contents, thereby reducing the risks from inhalation of gastric contents.

Skin preparation

Preoperative skincare involves cleaning the skin and sometimes removing hair from the surgical site. The aim is to reduce the normal flora but also potentially harmful (pathogenic) microorganisms (see Ch. 15) that may be present on the skin or hair. Practice in these respects varies and the available evidence is largely inconclusive.

If the person is fit, a warm shower is preferable to a bath as running water rinses off loose hair and dead skin cells more readily and showering is also a cultural requirement for many people. Care is taken not to wash off any marks indicating the operation site. The patient is encouraged to wash their hair, as some may be unable to wash their hair for several days postoperatively. People undergoing head and neck or eye (ophthalmic) surgery may be given specific instructions for hair washing.

Hair removal

Nurses must be sensitive to patients' dignity and recognize that body hair contributes to people's body image and cultural identity, and therefore hair removal may be distressing. The reasons for hair removal are explained and patients should be encouraged to do this themselves when possible, although the outcome should be checked prior to the final preparations for surgery (Box 24.7).

Preventing potential postoperative complications

Many postoperative complications can be prevented or minimized by effective preoperative care. This section explains nursing interventions undertaken to achieve this.

Chest infection

This can be both life threatening and debilitating, and people at increased risk include:

- Those who are overweight
- Cigarette smokers
- Patients undergoing thoracic or major abdominal surgery
- Those with chronic respiratory disease, e.g. bronchitis (see Ch. 17)
- Older adults.

At the pre-assessment clinic patients are given information about deep breathing exercises that minimize the risk of chest infection (see Ch. 17). Some people attend physiotherapy classes to learn these exercises and how to support their wounds when they need to cough postoperatively. Others are provided with written instructions to follow at home. People's knowledge is assessed on admission to ensure it is adequate and appropriate.

Deep vein thrombosis

A deep vein thrombosis (DVT) is the formation of a thrombus (clot) in the deep veins of the legs or pelvic veins (see Ch. 17). Pulmonary embolism (blockage of a pulmonary artery by a detached thrombus that has travelled there in the bloodstream) is a potentially fatal consequence of DVT that must be prevented when possible and is the reason for the care described below.

Several aspects of surgical treatment increase the risk of DVT. Immobility is a major risk factor that occurs during invasive procedures and surgery, and also postoperatively to a greater or lesser extent depending on the nature and length of the intervention. The nurse explains the leg exercises that will reduce the incidence of a DVT (see Ch. 18) so that patients can practise them preoperatively and implement them postoperatively to improve and maintain venous return and also to prevent stiffness of the joints. Further measures, e.g. stopping hormone replacement therapy (HRT), prophylactic heparin and anti-embolism stockings (see Box 24.8) may also be implemented to minimize occurrence of a DVT.

NURSING SKILLS Box 24.8

Anti-embolism stockings

- Establish whether knee, thigh or full-length stockings are needed. This depends on local policy, the operation and its aftercare
- Explain why the stockings are worn and for how long
- Using a tape measure, measure the widest circumference of the calf on both legs and the widest circumference of both thighs. (It may also be necessary to measure the patient's leg length if they are very tall or large, as the size may have to be adjusted to ensure the correct fit.)
- Select the correct size of stockings following the manufacturer's instructions
- Apply the stockings, ensuring that the toes are able to move freely and that the rest of the stocking fits the contours of the leg. It is important to ensure that stockings are not rolled over at the top; any excess should be eased back into the stocking to make a perfect fit
- The stockings are carefully removed prior to bathing or showering
- Written instructions about correct application, wearing and washing are provided when they are to be worn after discharge.

Bowel preparation

Bowel preparation prior to surgery aims to prevent:

- Defecation during anaesthesia
- Faecal contamination during surgery, particularly for surgery on the GI tract
- Postoperative stress on the wound
- Postoperative discomfort or constipation due to a full rectum.

Emptying of the bowel can be achieved by administration of oral or rectal laxatives (see Chs 21, 22). For procedures involving the lower GI tract, specific bowel cleansing laxatives, such as sodium picosulfate, may be prescribed, together with prophylactic antibiotic therapy. These patients may undertake some of their bowel preparation in the comfort of their own homes.

Any bowel preparation can cause distress, which can be greatly reduced by effective nursing intervention. Good communication is essential to ensure that the patient receives the correct preparation and understands why it is necessary (Finlay 1996). The patient's ability to reach the lavatory promptly and safely is assessed (other nursing considerations are discussed in Ch. 21). Dehydration can occur during extensive bowel preparation, even when patients have achieved the recommended fluid intake. It is therefore important to be aware that headaches or changes in behaviour, such as loss of concentration, can be signs of dehydration. When extensive bowel preparation is carried out it may be necessary to commence an i.v. infusion to:

- Prevent dehydration
- Restore fluid balance prior to surgery
- Reduce the incidence of postoperative nausea and vomiting (Dean & Fawcett 2002).

Final preoperative care

The nurse must implement local policies to prepare the patient safely for theatre. A checklist of specific measures is often used (Fig. 24.1).

NAME:	Consultant
Date of birth:	
Unit number:	
Weight:	

Please tick	Yes	No	Please tick	Yes	No
Allergies, state:			Case notes including latest laboratory results		
Consent form signed			X-rays		
Identiband on wrist/ankle			Fluid balance chart		
Operation site identified			Medicine records		
Hair removed from operation site			Nursing notes		
Make up/nail varnish removed			Manual handling risk assessment form completed and with records		
Fasted			Antiembolism stockings applied		
Premedication given			Bladder emptied/Catheterized		
EMLA cream applied			Jewellery removed/taped		
Dentures removed			Body piercings and other metal objects removed		
Hearing aid in situ			Modesty pants		
Spectacles with patient			Menstruating Pad/Tampon in situ		
Contact lenses removed			Crowns/loose teeth present, if yes, where?		
Other prosthesis in situ (state):			Pressure ulcer risk assessment score		

Ward Nurse: Printed Name	Signature
Theatre Nurse: Printed Name	Signature

Fig. 24.1 Preoperative checklist

Emptying the bladder

The bladder is emptied before showering so that the perineal area is clean. An empty bladder will prevent urinary incontinence during surgery and damage to the bladder during pelvic surgery. For patients having extensive surgery, pelvic surgery and epidural or spinal anaesthesia, a urinary catheter is passed (usually in theatre) to ensure that the bladder remains empty and that urinary output can be measured accurately postoperatively (see Ch. 20). However, if there is a long delay and/or the patient becomes anxious, they may need to pass urine again before transfer to theatre.

Theatre clothing

After showering or bathing, the patient wears a clean hospital gown. As the skin continuously sheds dead surface cells and commensal bacteria (see Ch. 15), a clean gown ensures that the skin is exposed to the minimum possible number of bacteria after showering. The bed is made using clean sheets for the same reason. Theatre gowns usually open down the back so that they can be easily removed during surgery if necessary. Female patients can wear disposable paper pants or clean cotton knickers for some procedures, depending on local policy. If antiembolism stockings are needed, the correct size should be used (see Box 24.8).

James (1995) advocates that children should be able to choose what to wear, arguing that theatre gowns are not necessary and removal of underwear can be distressing and bewildering.

Removal of cosmetics, jewellery and prostheses

Cosmetics are removed so that skin colour changes, e.g. pallor, can easily be observed. Nail varnish is also removed so that the nail beds can be assessed for early signs of cyanosis (see Ch. 17).

Jewellery, hairclips or ornaments are removed and stored safely according to hospital policy and taking into consideration cultural and religious needs. Plain rings that cannot be removed, or for patients who prefer them not to be removed, are taped securely to the finger using hypoallergenic tape. Removal of metal objects prevents:

- Contact burns from diathermy equipment (electrical equipment used during surgery to minimize bleeding)
- Their loss
- Damage to jewellery
- Damage to the patient if it is caught on a piece of equipment.

Patients may be asked to remove prostheses such as wigs, false eyes or artificial limbs on the ward to prevent their damage or loss. Removing a wig may cause embarrassment and a patient's dignity can be maintained by allowing it to be worn until after they are anaesthetized. If the wig has to be removed, the patient should be offered a paper cap to cover their head. Patients who have long hair should have this tied back on the top of their head so that it does not hinder extension of the neck during induction of anaesthesia.

Contact lenses are removed to prevent corneal abrasions during anaesthesia and are stored safely on the ward. Spectacles may also be removed and stored on the ward although many people are less anxious if any prosthesis can be worn to the anaesthetic room.

Hearing aids are worn to theatre to maintain effective communication and only removed after the patient is anaesthetized, when they are carefully removed, labelled and stored in the recovery room until consciousness is regained.

The presence of loose teeth, caps or bridges is written on the preoperative checklist as these can be damaged or dislodged during intubation or insertion of an airway. Removal of dentures can be a source of embarrassment and dignity should be considered by offering patients the option of keeping them in place until they are anaesthetized (Wood 2002). Dyke (2000) also considers their removal on the ward to be unnecessary as they maintain effective interpersonal communication.

Allergies

Any allergies must be checked with the patient and clearly entered on the preoperative checklist to prevent administration of harmful medication or skin preparations. Common allergies include adhesive tape, antibiotics (especially penicillin), iodine and anaesthetic gases.

Identity bands

These are worn to ensure that patients can always be easily identified, especially when they are unable to communicate effectively, e.g. due to anaesthesia or sedation. Sometimes local policy requires identity bands on both wrists, ensuring that if one is cut off, a patient can still be easily identified. Identity bands must be checked for legibility and accuracy each time a patient is moved between environments and when medication is administered. Patients having upper limb surgery may have identity bands round their ankles.

Premedication

Premedication is rarely used before day surgery. Other patients may be prescribed premedication, usually a light sedative or hypnotic (see Ch. 22), to reduce preoperative anxiety. Sometimes an anticholinergic drug such as hyoscine is given to reduce oral and bronchial secretions and vagal overactivity. Reducing secretions lessens the incidence of their inhalation during induction of anaesthesia when the gag reflex is lost. Premedication is administered approximately 1 hour before transfer to the anaesthetic room. When preoperative prophylactic heparin is prescribed, it is administered at the same time as the premedication.

Patients who have been given sedative drugs must remain in bed afterwards as the effects can make them unstable should they stand up. It is essential to check that the patient has signed their consent form before administering sedation. The call button is placed within easy reach and bedrails may be raised depending on local policy. When bedrails are used, the nurse must explain that this is for safety reasons as use of bedrails for restraint is unethical (see Ch. 7).

Preparation for intravenous cannulation

Preparation for i.v. cannulation is especially important in children and those who have needle phobia. Topical anaesthetic cream such as EMLA (eutectic mixture of local anaesthetic) minimizes pain during i.v. cannulation and takes approximately an hour to act (Fitzsimmons 2001; also see Ch. 23).

Final preoperative checks

The completed preoperative checklist and the patient's documentation, including their current observation charts, are collected together so that they are ready to accompany the patient to theatre. Doctors are responsible for preparation of the medical notes, which must include the signed consent form, relevant blood test results and X-rays. The nurse may also check that these are available on the day of surgery. The nursing records include the completed preoperative nursing checklist, nursing care plan and medicine records. Patients who have an i.v. infusion in progress or specific medication such as insulin may also have other records, e.g. a fluid balance chart.

NURSING SKILLS Box 24.9

Preparation of the bed space

This enables straightforward monitoring of postoperative progress and may involve moving the bed nearer to the nurses' station and assembling equipment, including:

- A sphygmomanometer (automated or manual) to record blood pressure
- A drip stand to suspend bags of i.v. fluids
- An observation chart to record temperature, pulse, respirations, blood pressure and oxygen saturation levels (see Chs 14, 17)
- A fluid balance chart to record fluid inputs and outputs (see Ch. 19)
- A vomit bowl and tissues
- A pulse oximeter to record oxygen saturation, if appropriate (see Ch. 17)
- Checking the oxygen supply and attaching clean tubing and mask (see Ch. 17)
- Checking and preparing suction equipment
- Additional equipment depending on the nature of the surgery.

CRITICAL THINKING Box 24.10

Perioperative care

Student activities

Select a patient who is to undergo surgery and negotiate their permission for the activities below. Ask your mentor if you can follow them from your placement to theatre, recovery and back to the ward.

1. Assist with their preoperative preparation.
2. Accompany the patient to the anaesthetic room and observe:
   - The handover from the ward nurse
   - The patient's reactions to the experience
   - Who is involved in the anaesthetic room.
3. In theatre, observe who does what during the operation.
4. In the recovery room, observe:
   - The nursing care carried out
   - The handover to the ward nurse.
5. Back on the ward, observe the immediate postoperative care.

Consider the extent to which preparation was effective in providing the patient with a realistic expectation of their perioperative experience.

Prior to transfer to the operating theatre the registered nurse and the theatre porter ensure that the correct patient is taken by checking their identity band for the correct:

- Name
- Unit number
- Date of birth.

The bed space is then prepared to receive the patient on their return from surgery (see Box 24.9). Carrying out the activities in Box 24.10 will help you understand a patient's perioperative experience.

Perioperative care

Adults are usually transferred to theatre on their beds or theatre trolleys. In day surgery settings, patients may be able to walk to the operating theatre if they have not been given premedication. Children are usually accompanied to the anaesthetic room by a parent and they may be transferred on child-friendly equipment, e.g. a Thomas the tank engine truck. They often take something personal and comforting with them such as their favourite teddy, doll, toy or comfort blanket. Small children may be carried by a parent or taken on a trolley depending on local policy.

Anaesthetic room

On arrival the receiving nurse checks the name, unit number, date of birth and the proposed surgery with the patient. The preoperative checklist is checked again and countersigned by the receiving nurse to ensure that all the measures required to protect the patient have been carried out. The patient is transferred to the operating table in preparation for the operation and is then ready for their anaesthetic.

Anaesthesia

Anaesthetics block sensation from the operative site so that surgery or investigations are not painful. There are three different types:

- *General anaesthesia*: Several drugs are used to induce unconsciousness, analgesia and muscle relaxation
- *Regional anaesthesia*: Techniques include spinal and epidural anaesthesia (see Ch. 23) where a local anaesthetic agent, e.g. lidocaine, is used to induce loss of sensation from a region of the body
- *Local anaesthesia*: A local anaesthetic agent, e.g. lidocaine, is used to induce loss of sensation from a small area around the site of administration.

Theatre

In theatre all care is provided by experience practitioners. More information about what is involved can be found in Further reading suggestions (e.g. Morris & Ward 2003).

Recovery room

Postoperative care is carried out to ensure safe recovery from the anaesthetic and operation or invasive procedure, and to minimize potential postoperative complications. Parents are encouraged to come to the recovery room to be with their child as they wake up after surgery.

Information about the patient's anaesthetic including all drugs, i.v. fluids and blood given during surgery is given to the recovery room nurse by the anaesthetist. Oxygen is often prescribed at this time. The surgeon explains the details of the operation including the type of skin closures, wound drains used and any specific care required. This information enables the recovery room nurse to plan the immediate postoperative care. The priorities of postoperative recovery (Scottish Intercollegiate Guidelines Network 2004) are to maintain:

- Airway
- Breathing
- Circulation (see Table 24.2 and below).

The patient is orientated and made comfortable in the recovery position (see Fig. 16.17) until they are fully conscious again. Pain is assessed and analgesia given if required. Personal effects such as a hearing aid, wig, false eye or facial prosthesis worn from the ward are returned to maintain dignity.

After a spinal or epidural anaesthetic the patient will have loss of sensation in their lower limbs for several hours. Positioning and support of the legs is important. Blood pressure recordings may also be affected during this period.

Discharge from the recovery room

A scoring system is normally used to assess when patients are fit enough to be transferred safely from the recovery room. Prior to discharge the equipment needed for safe transfer back to the ward is assembled, e.g. a portable oxygen system or drip stand. Extra blankets may be needed to prevent heat loss. The notes are checked and assembled, ensuring prescriptions for oxygen, i.v. fluids and analgesia, if needed, are completed. The ward nurse identifies the correct patient. The recovery room nurse provides a handover to the ward nurse prior to transfer.

Postoperative care

Postoperative care begins in the high dependency setting of the recovery room (see above) and continues through discharge from hospital until convalescence is complete. Its aims are to promote recovery and minimize postoperative complications. The principles and milestones after return to the ward are explored in this section.

Postoperative baseline assessment

On return to the ward a registered nurse completes the initial assessment of the patient's condition, which forms the basis of their postoperative care. This starts with airway, breathing and circulation, and comprises a new set of observations, which include:

- Temperature, pulse, respiratory rate (see Ch. 14)
- Blood pressure (see Ch. 14)
- Oxygen saturation levels (see Ch. 17), skin colour
- Inspection of wound site/dressing and drains (if present) and any signs of leakage on the bed clothing, especially under the patient.

Any abnormal trends or readings are reported to the charge nurse immediately.

Airway

Assessment begins with checking that the airway is clear and that breathing is quiet. The airway is maintained by ensuring that the head is positioned so that air entry into the lungs is not impeded. The position of the head should allow the tongue to drop forward so that secretions can drain or pool in the side of the mouth where they can be removed using suction. Adequate oxygenation is assessed using a pulse oximeter to measure oxygen saturation levels. Patients are not discharged from the recovery room until they can maintain their own airway.

Breathing

Respiratory rate is recorded every 15 minutes initially to ensure that it is stable, regular and within acceptable limits for the particular patient.

Circulation

This is assessed by feeling the skin, which should be warm to touch, and observing the nail beds, which should be pink. Insufficient oxygen in the blood (hypoxaemia) can give the skin a bluish tinge, especially around the lips and nail beds.

Measurement of blood pressure and pulse also indicate whether the circulation is adequate. Changes that suggest development of shock are:

- Hypotension (low blood pressure) due to excess blood loss, e.g. from the wound/drain
- Tachycardia (pulse over 100 bpm in adults)
- Cold clammy skin.

There are different causes of shock but postoperatively the most common is due to hypovolaemia, which occurs when the circulating blood volume is reduced following excessive blood loss. For more detail, see Further reading suggestions (e.g. Adam 2003).

Observations

The intervals between recordings (see above) must be clearly stated on the care plan. Initially these may be every 15 minutes for the first hour then adjusted when they are within an acceptable range for that patient.

Drains should be supported to avoid traction on the tubing and to prevent potential dislodgement or poor drainage. The amount, consistency and type of drainage into the drain, as well as any fresh staining on the theatre dressing, are noted during the initial postoperative assessment so that subsequent loss can be measured. Drains are checked for flow and patency if a vacuum system is used (see Fig. 24.2). If patency is lost, leakage from the wound may increase. The type of drain and volumes draining dictate the frequency of checking.

Urinary catheter drainage tubing should be positioned to allow free drainage, ensuring that the collecting bag does not come in contact with the floor (see Ch. 20). Urinary output may be measured hourly depending on the patient's

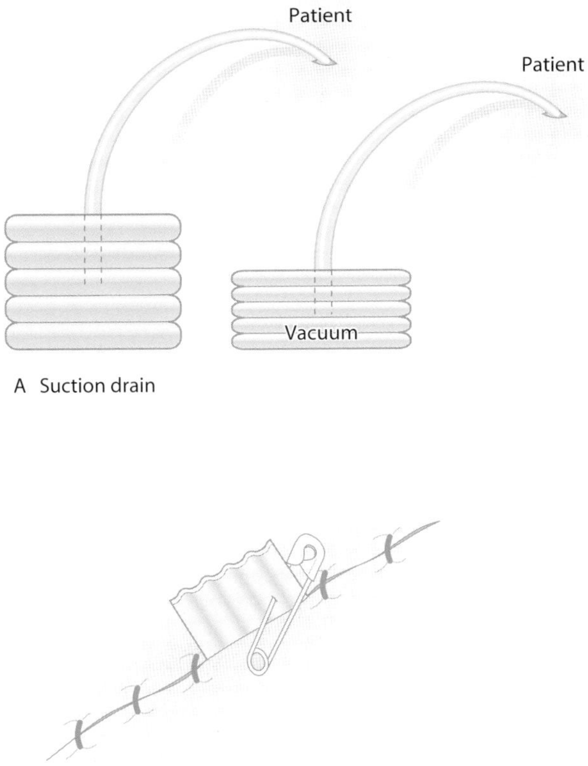

Fig. 24.2 Wound drains (reproduced with permission from Brooker & Nicol 2003)

condition and the type of surgery. All drainage is recorded on the fluid balance chart as per local protocol.

Postoperative care is outlined in Table 24.2, the most important principles of which are explored in more detail below.

Communication

When the patient is safely settled, the nurse reorientates them to the ward and explains that the procedure is complete. The environment may be full of unfamiliar sounds which will have been explained preoperatively but this is often forgotten in the immediate postoperative period and should be included in the reorientation information. For patients who wear hearing aids, it is important to check that they have been reinserted and are working correctly. Hearing is the first of the senses to return after a period of unconsciousness and for this reason staff must avoid discussing patients' conditions near the bedside. At this stage, children often ask for their parents. The sound of the parent's voice gives reassurance and comfort that allows a child to rest and recover.

Maintaining dignity

Patients are vulnerable postoperatively and it is important to maintain their dignity at all times. Replacing a patient's prosthesis aids their dignity and also improves their body image. Dentures are usually returned in the recovery room when the patient regains consciousness. However, if this was not the case, then oral hygiene should be given and their freshly rinsed dentures returned. Xavier (2000) points out that people who have worn dentures for a long time are able to manoeuvre them into the correct place even when they are very drowsy.

Pain management

Chapter 23 addresses this topic in depth and should be consulted for further information about all aspects of pain management. Postoperative pain management begins preoperatively when the available options are discussed with the patient. Postoperatively, the nurse must ensure the patient is comfortable and given adequate pain relief. Effective pain management reduces postoperative anxiety (Hayward 1975) and aids mobility. Patients expect to encounter some pain following a surgical intervention but only to their degree of tolerance. Carr and Thomas (1997) found that although patients expected to have pain following day surgery, some stated this was significantly greater than expected. Furthermore, Coll and Ameen (2006) found that many patients have inadequate pain relief after discharge. Pain is not necessarily wound related and can be due to dehydration, a full bladder or the after-effects of being on the operating table. Pain may adversely affect postoperative recovery and is assessed and documented using a pain assessment chart.

Individual coping mechanisms in relation to pain vary widely. Some people lie as still as possible, hoping that the pain will subside, whereas others become very vocal. Other people cannot verbalize their pain, e.g. young children and those with learning disabilities, and nurses need to be alert to behavioural cues. Drugs used in pain management range from mild analgesics such as ibuprofen for mild pain to opioids, e.g. morphine, for moderate to severe pain. Several routes may also be used, including:

- Oral
- Subcutaneous
- Intravenous, including patient-controlled analgesia (PCA)
- Intramuscular
- Rectal.

PCA devices deliver preset doses of analgesic drugs and allow patients to give themselves analgesia by pressing a button on the handset. Tye and Gell-Walker (2000) suggest that PCA reduces patients' anxiety about experiencing postoperative pain. It can be used by people of all ages provided they have sufficient understanding and the manual dexterity to push the delivery button. Some patients may use non-pharmacological methods of pain relief, such as visual imaging or yoga exercises (see Chs 10, 23), which may reduce the amount of analgesic drugs needed. The activities in Box 24.11 will help you understand postoperative pain management.

By anticipating the need for analgesia and speaking to patients about their pain levels well before increased activity is needed, e.g. chest physiotherapy, bed bathing/

Table 24.2 Care plan: principles of postoperative care (adapted from Peattie & Walker 1995)

Actual/potential problem	Aim	Nursing action	Rationale
		BREATHING	
1. Airway obstruction	To prevent or detect, and report promptly	• Nurse patient in the recovery position until conscious	Maintains airway patency and prevents the tongue occluding it
		• Observe for stridor (Chs 14, 17)	Indicates partial airway obstruction
2. Inadequate breathing	To detect and report promptly	• Observe rate, depth and effort of breathing	Changes may indicate inadequate respiratory function
		• Observe skin for pallor or cyanosis	Indicates hypoxia
3. Potential hypoxia	To maintain normal oxygenation	• Administer oxygen therapy as prescribed (Ch. 17)	Additional oxygen will increase level of oxygen available to tissues, thus preventing hypoxia
4. Development of haemorrhage or hypovolaemic shock	To detect early signs and report promptly	• Record blood pressure, pulse, respiration as instructed	These would be detected by falling blood pressure readings and a rising pulse rate
		• Observe the patient's skin and report pale, cold, clammy skin	Indicates the presence of shock
		• Observe wound site for signs of oozing or leakage	Increasing leakage can indicate haemorrhage. May require the application of pressure dressing or further attention from the surgeon
		• Observe drain(s) for nature and volume of drainage	Increasing drainage can indicate haemorrhage
		COMMUNICATING	
5. Anxiety and fear following surgery	To reassure patient by explaining all procedures at a level of the patient's understanding	• Explain all procedures prior to them being performed using terms the patient understands	Continues philosophy of having a well-informed patient who is more likely to have an uncomplicated and speedy postoperative recovery
		• Repeat explanations as necessary	Disorientation is common in the immediate postoperative period after general anaesthesia
6. Postoperative pain	To control pain by effective use of analgesia	• Give analgesia as prescribed, particularly prior to painful events, e.g. physiotherapy	Patient who is pain free will be able to cooperate with physiotherapy and move more easily in bed. Pain-free patient will also benefit psychologically
		• Monitor effect of analgesia with the aid of a pain chart (Ch. 23)	If analgesia is not controlling pain, the medical staff should be asked to review prescription
		EATING AND DRINKING	
7. Dehydration or fluid overload	To maintain fluid balance	• Maintain accurate record of fluid intakes and outputs	Enables evaluation of fluid balance
		• Monitor rate and flow of intravenous infusion if present	Important to ensure that the correct amount of fluid is administered
		• Monitor intravenous cannula site for signs of infiltration (Ch. 19)	If infiltration occurs, the infusion may be resited
		• Observe for presence of, and report increasing dyspnoea, cyanosis, tachycardia and expectorating frothy sputum (Ch. 17)	These indicate pulmonary oedema which can arise from fluid overload
		• Offer patient sips of water when permitted	Increases oral comfort. When fluids are well tolerated intravenous infusion can be discontinued
8. Postoperative nausea	To minimize or alleviate	• Administer antiemetics as prescribed	Recognize that opioid analgesia and anaesthetic drugs cause nausea
		• Aspirate nasogastric tube if present	Minimizes gastric contents

(Continued)

Table 24.2 *(Continued)*

Actual/potential problem	Aim	Nursing action	Rationale
9. Impaired nutritional status caused by prolonged fasting	To regain nutritional status	• Introduce easily digested diet when fluids are tolerated	Re-establishes oral intake, providing energy and protein required for wound healing
		MAINTAINING BODY TEMPERATURE	
10. Wound or other infection	To prevent infection occurring	• Administer prophylactic antibiotics as prescribed	Reduces the possibility of infection after major surgery
		• Monitor patient's temperature 4 hourly. Note and report pyrexia, confusion and restlessness	These are signs of infection Early identification and reporting allows prompt treatment
		• Observe wound and other susceptible sites for signs of infection; local pain, redness, increased warmth, presence of purulent exudate. Send specimen for culture and sensitivity if infection is suspected	Any infection must be identified and treated promptly
		• When fully conscious and vital signs are stabilized, patient should be assisted into an upright position well supported by pillows	The upright position aids fuller chest expansion and minimizes stasis of secretions which predisposes to chest infection
		• Encourage patient to perform deep breathing hourly as taught preoperatively by physiotherapist	
		• Encourage patient to support abdominal or thoracic wound when coughing	Stress on the wound is painful
		PERSONAL CLEANSING AND DRESSING	
11. Patient unable to maintain his own hygiene in the short term	To maintain a good standard of hygiene	• On return from theatre once vital signs are stable, patient is assisted to wash his face and hands, and helped into own nightclothes	Helps the patient to feel fresher and more comfortable
		• Patient may require a bed bath on the first day. Attention paid to all his hygiene needs	Patient too ill to have shower or immersion bath. Maintains the usual standard of personal hygiene
		• Patient can begin to take a more active part in his personal hygiene as his condition improves	Restores a feeling of being more in control of events, and therefore improves morale
		• As the patient's condition improves, patient can progress to a shower or immersion bath	A shower is preferable as there is less risk of infection through sitting in potentially contaminated water
		MOBILIZING	
12. Patient immobile and prone to complications until he is able to resume full mobility	To prevent the complications of immobility	• Prevent DVT:	
		i. on return from theatre, implement passive leg exercises until the patient is able to exercise his legs independently	Encourages venous return by use of calf muscle pump. Prevents stasis of blood in deep veins and DVT
		ii. Encourage deep breathing	Facilitates the removal of anaesthetic gases from lungs and aids venous return
		iii. Administer heparin if prescribed	Prevents the formation of clots in the blood vessels
		iv. Apply antiembolism stockings if prescribed	Aids venous return from the legs

(Continued)

Table 24.2 (*Continued*)

Actual/potential problem	Aim	Nursing action	Rationale
		v. Observe calves and report swelling, complaints of calf tenderness or pain, redness or increased heat	These are indicative of DVT
		• Prevent the formation of pressure ulcers:	Allows evaluation of nursing action and reassessment and planning as required
		i. perform pressure area care identified by risk assessment score (see Ch. 25)	Prevents formation of pressure ulcers
		ii. use pressure-relieving aids as appropriate	
		• The patient is helped to sit out of bed when his condition permits, and encouraged to mobilize gradually thereafter (Fig. 24.3)	Improves morale and improved expansion of lungs reducing the risk of chest infection. Promotes increased independence
		ELIMINATING	
13. Urinary retention	To prevent or detect	• Monitor and record urine output	To monitor fluid balance
		• Report to medical staff if patient has not passed urine 6–8 hours postoperatively	Patient may be underhydrated or have retention of urine. Recognition of either allows prompt treatment
		• Encourage patient to pass urine regularly	Reduces stasis time in bladder, which predisposes to urinary tract infection

CRITICAL THINKING Box 24.11

Postoperative pain management

Student activities

In your placement:

- Identify analgesic drugs used postoperatively and find out about their side effects.
- Identify the routes used to administer them.
- Identify non-pharmacological methods of postoperative pain relief.
- Speak to a patient about their postoperative pain management.
- Discuss your findings with your mentor.

showering, getting out of bed and mobilizing, nurses can minimize pain experienced during these activities.

Patients should be encouraged to change their position in bed and to carry out their therapeutic exercises, e.g. leg and deep breathing exercises. This helps to reduce general discomfort and enables people to feel more in control of their postoperative recovery. The nurse will help the patient feel safe at all times by leaving the call button within reach and answering it promptly.

Fluid balance

All intakes and outputs are recorded accurately on the fluid balance chart until urine output and oral fluids are re-established. Fluid balance charts are explained fully in Chapter 19 and this section outlines the fluid intakes and outputs recorded postoperatively.

Fluid intake

Re-establishing oral fluids following surgical interventions depends on the type of procedure and local policy. Some day surgery patients or those who have had a spinal or epidural anaesthetic may be able to drink immediately they are fully orientated. Those who have had anaesthetic throat spray administered prior to upper endoscopic investigations or ear, nose and throat procedures must remain 'nil by mouth' until the swallowing reflex returns (usually around 2 hours afterwards). When there has been handling of the intestines, the period of fasting is more prolonged due to paralytic ileus (see p. 699).

The site of an i.v. infusion can reduce mobility and manual dexterity such as cleaning the teeth. Once an adequate oral intake is re-established without complications, the i.v. infusion can be discontinued but a fluid balance chart is still required until the patient can maintain the required fluid intake.

For adults, an i.v. fluid regime over a 24-hour period normally comprises approximately 3 L of fluid consisting of 0.9% saline (normal saline) and 5% dextrose. Smaller volumes are required for children, older adults and those with cardiovascular problems (see Ch. 19). Adequate i.v. fluids ensure an adequate blood supply to the kidneys that maintains renal perfusion and urinary output (see below). This is essential to prevent kidney failure. Intravenous fluids are administered to replace fluid deficits due to:

- Preoperative or postoperative fasting
- Excess loss through a wound or fistula
- Pyrexia (excessively raised temperature) caused by inflammation or sepsis.

Infusion pumps may be used to administer prescribed i.v. fluids but nurses using them must have a working knowledge of their use and the potential complications (see Ch. 19).

Intravenous medications, e.g. antibiotics, are also recorded on the fluid balance chart as they can be a significant part of fluid intake. The fluid balance is reviewed regularly to ensure that the patient is not in negative balance or fluid overloaded (see Ch. 19).

Nausea and vomiting

Nausea and vomiting sometimes occur following an anaesthetic or handling of the viscera during abdominal surgery, and also when people are in pain or anxious about the future (Jolley 2000). Postoperative nausea and vomiting may be due to accumulation of gas within the GI tract or from hiccups due to the irritation of the diaphragm. Fluid loss due to vomiting is measured and recorded on the fluid balance chart. Vomiting can cause depletion of water and electrolytes.

Postoperative nausea and vomiting can be reduced if the patient is administered a prophylactic antiemetic, e.g. domperidone, before or during surgery. However, even if an antiemetic has been given, some patients may still continue to experience nausea for several days postoperatively. They can be reassured that the feeling will subside and there are several nursing interventions that may help:

- Moving the patient into a more upright position, well supported by pillows, to assist drainage and reduce reflux of gastric secretions
- Reviewing analgesic drugs used as opioids, e.g. morphine, stimulate the vomiting centre in the brain
- Providing oral hygiene at least 3–4 hourly or more often if necessary
- Giving ice chips to suck if indicated on the care plan
- Reviewing the nasogastric drainage regime if present (see below and also Box 20.13).

Urine output

Adults, including those who have an indwelling urinary catheter, should pass a minimum of 30 mL of urine per hour. Smaller volumes are normal in children (see Ch. 20). The well-hydrated patient should be able to void urine within 6–8 hours following a general anaesthetic. Inability to void following surgery may be due to:

- The site of operation, especially when within the pelvic region, e.g. hysterectomy
- Spinal or epidural anaesthesia
- Muscle relaxant drugs administered during surgery – these can reduce the ability to void or cause voiding of small, frequent volumes
- Dehydration due to prolonged preoperative fasting, inadequate postoperative fluid intake or excessive loss, e.g. vomiting
- Poor pain control
- Embarrassment, lack of privacy or unusual position required for voiding.

When there is failure to pass urine following surgery or a significant drop in hourly urine output, this is reported to the charge nurse. It is important to note that small volumes may represent overflow due to a full bladder and urinary retention (see Ch. 20) or negative fluid balance (see Ch. 19). If there is difficulty in passing urine and the patient is in pain, analgesia should be administered as this may help them to relax and void. If all these interventions fail, it may become necessary to pass a catheter to drain the bladder. This is retained until hydration is satisfactory and urine volumes are sustained. The closed catheter system must be allowed to drain freely and specific nursing care is required (see Ch. 20). Urine output is recorded on the fluid balance chart.

Nasogastric aspirate

Wide-bore nasogastric tubes are used postoperatively to withdraw (aspirate) gastric secretions that accumulate when paralytic ileus (see p. 699) is present, e.g. following surgery that involves the stomach or the small or large bowel. The frequency of aspiration is dictated by the type of surgery and patient discomfort. This may be continuous using a low-pressure suction unit or intermittent using a suction unit or syringe. The nasogastric tube may be attached to a collecting bag to allow the free passage of gas and drainage of gastric secretions. These may increase with abdominal pressure, e.g. when the patient coughs, breathes deeply or moves around to change position.

The colour and presence of blood of each aspirate is noted and the volume recorded on the fluid balance chart. Sometimes the consistency is also recorded.

The disadvantages of a nasogastric tube include:

- Restriction of the nasal passage reducing air entry
- Patient discomfort and embarrassment due to excess secretions if the tube irritates the mucous membranes lining the nose
- Inability to blow the nose adequately
- Pressure and soreness around the nose or face
- Difficulty coughing.

The nursing care required by a patient with a nasogastric tube is shown in Box 24.12.

Wound drainage

Wound drains (see Fig. 24.2) are used to drain fluid away from surgical sites, especially vascular areas. Fluid may be:

- Sanguineous – heavily bloodstained
- Serosanguineous – blood and serum
- Serous – clear
- Purulent – cloudy.

NURSING SKILLS Box 24.12

Care of a patient with a nasogastric tube

- The nasogastric tube is firmly attached to the patient's nose using hypoallergenic tape to prevent it from sliding in and out of the nasal passage or becoming dislodged
- The tape is checked frequently to ensure that it remains adherent, as the nose can become moist and greasy, allowing the tape and/or the tube to move
- The nose, nostrils and face are checked for signs of pressure or soreness
- The skin around the nose and mouth is kept dry to prevent excoriation and infection
- Oral hygiene and/or mouthwashes keep the oral mucosa moist and prevent infections such as *Candida albicans* (thrush)
- Patients may be offered ice chips to moisten the oral mucosa if appropriate
- The nasogastric tube is aspirated continuously or intermittently as indicated on the care plan
- The colour, consistency and volumes of aspirate are observed and recorded on the fluid balance chart.

A collection of fluid in a confined space causes pain, acts as a potential source of infection and impairs wound healing (see Ch. 25). The function of the drain is explained to the patient preoperatively and also the need to avoid putting traction (pulling) on it, especially when moving around in bed and up walking.

- *Vacuum drains*: These draw fluid out from the drain tip, usually adjacent to the site of the operation, preventing accumulation of fluid and formation of a haematoma (blood clot). The drainage volume is recorded on the fluid balance chart and its characteristics entered in the nursing notes. An accurate record of the drainage will assist the decision about when to remove the drain. Prior to removal, the vacuum is released to prevent tissue damage and minimize patient discomfort. A small sterile dressing is applied over the drain site to absorb residual drainage and protect the area from infection.
- *Gravity drains*: These allow drainage of fluid into a collection bag, e.g. a corrugated drain.

Preventing chest infections

Patients are encouraged to take deep breaths hourly postoperatively and to cough as necessary to aid lung expansion and to expel anaesthetic gases and pooled respiratory tract secretions. Poor lung expansion and pooling of secretions predispose to chest infections. The physiotherapist educates patients preoperatively (see p. 688) about these exercises. Chest physiotherapy and/or early mobilization can help to reduce the incidence of chest infection and the need for antibiotics (see Ch. 17). In order to carry out deep breathing and coughing, the patient should have enough pain relief and support for chest or abdominal wounds. Placing a hand or pillow firmly over the wound can provide support.

Signs of chest infection include:

- A raised temperature that may vary over a 24-hour period
- Increased pulse rate
- Skin that is hot and damp to touch
- A productive cough with expectoration of purulent sputum (see Ch. 17).

A sputum specimen may be required for culture and testing of sensitivity to an appropriate antibiotic (see Ch. 17).

Prevention of deep vein thrombosis

Preoperative preparation helps to reduce the incidence of DVT (see p. 688). Preventative postoperative measures include:

- Administration of prophylactic anticoagulants, e.g. subcutaneous heparin
- Wearing of anti-embolism stockings (see p. 688)
- Maintaining adequate hydration
- Effective pain management to assist mobilization
- Carrying out active or passive leg exercises (see Ch. 18)
- Early mobilization (see Ch. 18).

The incidence of DVT is higher after major surgery of the lower abdomen, pelvis and hip joints than other surgery. Not all patients who undergo surgery need these interventions as early mobilization and day surgery reduce the incidence of DVT.

The presence of pain, swelling or redness in the lower limbs is reported urgently, as these may be early signs of a DVT. It is important, however, to realize that the majority of DVTs cause no local signs and that some arise in the pelvic veins.

Nutrition

Preoperative nutritional assessment is carried out so that nutritional intake can be adjusted to meet each patient's needs. Poor nutrition affects many body processes and has widespread postoperative consequences, including:

- Delayed wound healing and potential infection
- Loss of muscle tone that may adversely affect mobilization
- Skin fragility, slow repair and development of pressure ulcers
- Impaired immune response
- Depression.

Patients who are not undergoing major surgery are usually able to eat normally again within 12 hours. Those who have been fasting for some time may be reluctant to recommence solid food for fear that their preoperative symptoms will return. Patients may need assistance to select a diet that meets their nutritional needs in the postoperative period. Meals and snacks should be served appropriately, taking people's medical and cultural needs into consideration (see Ch. 19).

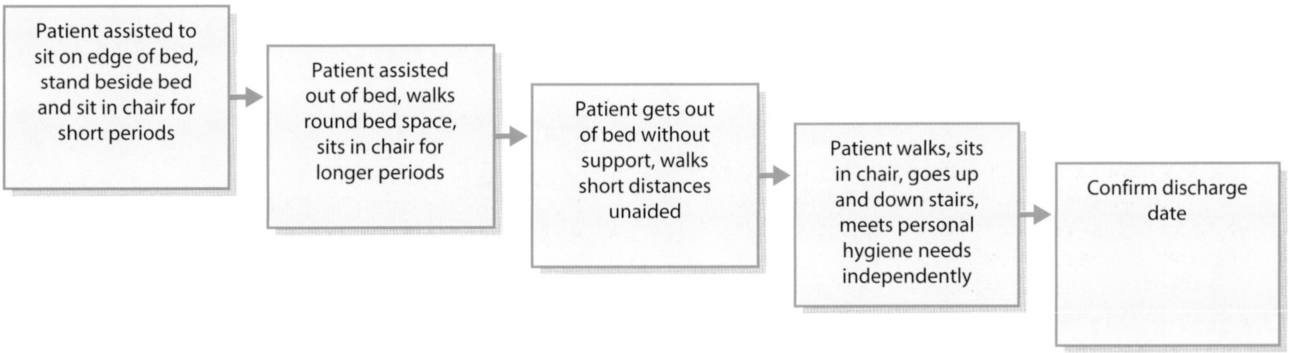

Fig. 24.3 Steps of mobility

Sometimes it will not be possible for patients to eat for several days or even weeks, such as after removal of large parts of the GI tract, and a preoperative referral to the dietitian should be made. Others cannot eat sufficient food to meet their energy requirements and food fortification or nutritional support may be used to prevent malnutrition (see Ch. 19).

Preventing constipation

Patients may not pass faeces or flatus (gas) for several days postoperatively, especially when there is paralytic ileus or following preoperative bowel cleansing. Paralytic ileus occurs after surgery that involves extensive handling of the bowel when peristalsis (the muscular movements that normally move contents along the intestines) is temporarily lost. Flatus is passed when peristalsis returns. Before then many patients experience discomfort caused by trapped wind.

Opioid drugs predispose to firm stools or constipation. Postoperative passing of faeces is recorded in the nursing notes. The faeces may be watery at first and stools may take time to form normally again, even after a normal diet has been re-established. Laxatives (oral or rectal, see Ch. 21) are not normally necessary when patients are well hydrated, eating normally and ambulant again.

Regaining mobility

The type of surgery dictates the level of mobility and the timescale over which this can be achieved. Nurses must be aware of a patient's preoperative mobility when planning their postoperative mobility goals. Patients having day surgery are mobilized soon after the procedure is completed. Those who undergo major surgery without complications can usually walk to the bathroom the day after surgery; however, following some specific types of surgery, e.g. major vascular surgery (femoral popliteal bypass), bed rest for 24–48 hours may be required.

Preoperatively, patients are supplied with information about exercises that they can practise and implement soon after surgery (see p. 688). The nurse should encourage the patient to carry out these exercises to reduce limb stiffness and aid venous return. When patients are unable to exercise by themselves the physiotherapist and nurse perform passive exercises (see Ch. 18).

Postoperative mobility extends from moving around in bed to walking independently and being able to climb stairs. Gradual mobilization (Fig. 24.3) may start with a short walk from the bed to a chair when the patient is able to sit out of bed for short periods. When a patient stands up too quickly, this can cause faintness due to postural hypotension (a rapid drop in blood pressure on standing upright). The patient should be moved slowly from a semi-recumbent position to the edge of the bed before being helped to stand up (see Ch. 18). Moving from the bed to a chair must be assessed and carefully planned, especially when assistance of nurses or a hoist is needed (see Ch. 18). Walking distances and periods spent out of bed are increased gradually as the patient's condition allows until independence is regained. Patients who have had orthopaedic surgery may have specific mobilization programmes. The physiotherapist implements the planned activities with the nurse in a supporting role until the patient is confident and can mobilize safely.

Wound care

On completion of surgery, the incision is usually covered with a light dressing that consists of a thin non-adherent pad with a hypoallergenic adhesive cover if the skin is healthy and intact. The pad absorbs any exudate, which is usually minimal in a surgical wound and may be bloodstained initially. The dressing provides an ideal environment for healing and protects the wound from minor trauma and entry of bacteria (see Ch. 25). The aim of wound care is to promote healing and prevent infection. Healing can be compromised by many factors, including:

- Poor nutritional status
- Impaired local circulation
- Metabolic abnormalities, e.g. diabetes mellitus.

According to local protocol, the theatre dressing should be left in situ for at least 24–72 hours unless there is excessive staining as this has been shown to reduce infection rates following surgical interventions. If the wound is clean and dry after the initial dressing has been removed, the patient can shower and carefully pat the wound area dry with a clean towel to prevent trauma or potential infection.

Surgical wounds normally heal by primary intention because skin closures, e.g. sutures, staples, glue or clips

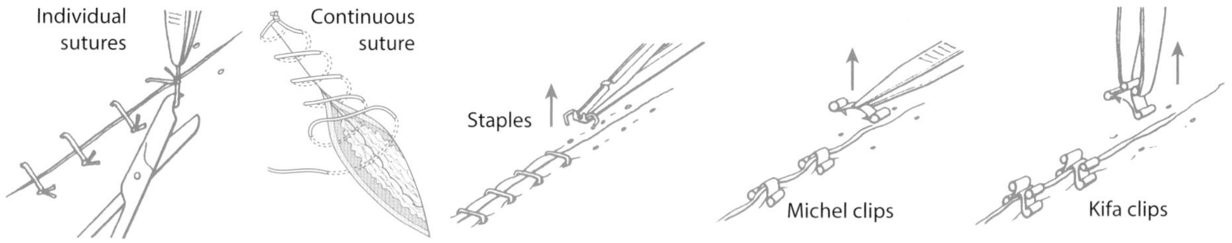

Fig. 24.4 Removal of skin closures

(Fig. 24.4), are used to hold and support the skin edges together as healing takes place. The superficial layers close within 24–72 hours as epithelial cells migrate across the wound and initially the wound may appear inflamed, e.g. red and swollen. Wound healing is discussed in detail in Chapter 25.

Both adults and children may find the removal of skin closures frightening and the procedure is explained to reduce fear and anxiety. Distraction, e.g. talking to the patient while removing skin closures, often greatly reduces anxiety.

Sutures are usually removed after 5–10 days unless they are absorbable whereas staples are normally removed after 2–5 days. More specifically, their removal depends on the reason for surgery, its location and the patient's age and general condition. If a patient is discharged before skin closures are removed, then arrangements must be made for their removal by a community nurse.

Wound complications

- *Wound infection*: Early signs of a wound infection include pyrexia and/or pain in or around the wound. An inflamed area may appear red and swollen, and look quite different from a non-inflamed area. If an infection is superficial, a suture may be removed to allow purulent exudate (pus) to escape. A wound swab or sample of pus is sent to microbiology for microscopy, culture and sensitivity testing (see Ch. 15)
- *Haematoma*: A small collection will gradually resolve spontaneously but larger collections cause pain, discomfort and predispose to infection. They may be evacuated by aspiration using a needle and syringe, or through a small incision
- *Dehiscence*: This is the splitting open of a wound exposing the abdominal contents that occurs only rarely (see Fig. 25.1). The causes include wound infection, poor nutrition, compromised immunity and increased tension on the wound by, for example, abdominal distension or excessive coughing. The warning signs may be serosanguineous (serum and blood) discharge from a previously dry wound and/or the patient saying that they 'felt something go'.

Discharge planning

Discharge planning should begin at the pre-assessment clinic or on admission to hospital in emergency situations. Successful discharge planning provides a seamless transition between day or inpatient care and primary health care. Attending a pre-assessment clinic facilitates planning and enables patients, their families and carers to understand planned interventions, the likely aftercare and its implications. Care required after discharge is planned in partnership with the patient and their family or carers, the primary healthcare team and social services. Many factors must be taken into account, including:

- Transport home
- Ascertaining who is at home and available to help with aftercare
- Removal of skin closures
- Availability of the patient's medicines, including analgesics, and instructions about taking them
- Date and time of follow-up appointment
- Other appointments required, e.g. specialist nurse, physiotherapist
- Specific advice about recovery and likely timescale
- Support groups, counselling services
- Nutritional advice
- Need for aids or prosthesis
- Phone numbers or email addresses for advice after discharge
- Information about when to seek help, e.g. chest pain, feeling hot
- Information booklets to reinforce verbal information
- Community services, e.g. meals on wheels.

Some patients may be too distressed to think about their aftercare due to fear of an adverse postoperative outcome; in such cases the nurse can talk through potential scenarios to provide insight into potential needs.

Following surgery, including day surgery, people need at least a short period of convalescence. Planning an admission date helps patients to organize help at home during their convalescence. People with specific needs may have a home assessment arranged. Occupational therapists (OTs) can assess the patient's home environment and postoperative needs. They can then provide advice and supply aids, e.g. raised toilet seats or walking frames to assist following surgery such as hip replacement.

Other members of the MDT, such as social workers, may also be involved in discharge planning as some patients will be unable to care for themselves independently following surgery and therefore require a package of short- or long-term aftercare. Sometimes a period of rehabilitation (see Ch. 11) or convalescence in a care home is arranged until the patient can safely return home. Delayed discharge planning prolongs hospital admission until suitable arrangements can be completed and inadequate planning not infrequently results in readmission. Hospitals usually have discharge policies working in partnership with other agencies such as primary healthcare and social services to provide a seamless return home from hospital.

Discharge planning is important for all patients, but especially following day surgery and those who require arranged transport home and/or assistance from community services after discharge.

Before discharge surgical patients are given information about mobility, pain and wound management. This should be both verbal and in writing as this gives the patient a point of reference after discharge. Time should be spent discussing lifestyle issues including:

- Driving
- Increasing exercise, including housework
- Resuming sexual relationships
- Returning to work/school.

Having this information before discharge reduces stress and gives patients the opportunity to plan their convalescence and resumption of their normal activities and routines.

Summary

- Pre-assessment clinics facilitate preoperative preparation and enable individual needs to be planned for.
- Preoperative anxiety is alleviated by effective communication and provision of information about the surgical experience.
- The aim of preoperative preparation is to ensure patient safety during the intraoperative and postoperative periods.
- Postoperative care aims to promote recovery and minimize postoperative complications.
- Effective discharge planning should start at the pre-assessment clinic and facilitates a seamless transition from home to hospital and home again.

Self test

1. List three benefits of pre-assessment/assessment clinics.
2. List some common anxieties that people have about general anaesthesia and surgery.
3. Why is it important for patients to remove dentures, nail polish and make-up prior to theatre?
4. What are the priorities of care in the recovery area?
5. What observations are carried out on the ward after major abdominal surgery?
6. Describe the postoperative measures taken to minimize the risk of DVT.
7. What factors are considered in discharge planning?

Key words and phrases for literature searching

Consent
Discharge planning
Patient communication
Perioperative care
Postoperative nausea and vomiting
Surgery
Surgical nursing

Useful websites

Ethnic minority groups	www.minorityhealth.gov.uk Available July 2006
Investigations BBC 2005	www.bbc.co.uk/health/talking/tests Available July 2006
Patient information leaflets	www.patient.co.uk/pils.asp Available July 2006
Surgery	www.yoursurgery.com Available July 2006
Wound care	www.smtl.co.uk Available July 2006

References

Action for Sick Children 2006 What to do when your child goes into hospital. Online: www.actionforsickchildren.org/parentshospital.html Available July 2006

AORN 2002 Recommended principles for skin preparation of patients. AORN Journal 75(1):184–188

Ashworth PM 1980 Care to communicate. RCN, London

Audit Commission 2001 Audit Commission for Local Authorities and the National Health Service in England: A short cut to better services: day surgery in England and Wales. TSO, London

Boore JRP 1978 Prescription for recovery. RCN, London

Brooker C, Nicol M (eds) 2003 Nursing adults. The practice of caring. Mosby, Edinburgh

Bysshe J 1988 The effect of giving information to patients before surgery. Nursing 3(30):36–39

Carr CJ, Thomas VJ 1997 Anticipating and experiencing postoperative pain: the patient's perspective. Journal of Clinical Nursing 6:191–201

Coll A, Ameen J 2006 Profiles of pain after day surgery: patient's experience of three different operation types. Journal of Advanced Nursing 53(2):178–187

Crawford B 1999 Highlighting the role of the perioperative nurse – is preoperative assessment necessary? British Journal of Theatre Nursing 9(7):309–311

Cronin P 1996 How it feels to be nil by mouth. Nursing Times 96(46):44

Dean A, Fawcett T 2002 Nurses' use of evidence in preoperative fasting. Nursing Standard 17(12):33–37

Devine EC 1992 Effects of psychological care for adult surgical patients: a meta-analysis of 191 studies. Patient Education and Counselling 19(2):129–142

Dyke M 2000 Pre-operative communication. In: Hind M, Wicker P (eds) Principles of perioperative practice. Churchill Livingstone, Edinburgh, pp. 66–76

Finlay T 1996 Making sense of bowel preparation. Nursing Times 92(45):38–39

Fitzsimmons R 2001 Intravenous cannulation. Paediatric Nursing 13(3):21–22

Franklin B 1974 Patient anxiety on admission to hospital. RCN, London

Hamilton Smith S 1972 Nil by mouth. RCN, London

Hayward J 1975 Information: a prescription against pain. RCN, London

Holmes J 2005 Preoperative visiting: landmarks of the journey. British Journal of Perioperative Nursing 15(10):434–443

James J 1995 Day care admission. Paediatric Nursing 7(1):25–29

Jamieson EM, McCall JM, Whyte LA (eds) 2002 Clinical nursing practices. Churchill Livingstone, Edinburgh

Jolley BA 2000 Postoperative nausea and vomiting: a survey of nurses' knowledge. Nursing Standard 14(23):32–34

Lin L, Wang R 2005 Abdominal surgery, pain and anxiety: preoperative nursing intervention. Journal of Advanced Nursing 51(3):252–260

McIntyre FJ, McCloy R 1994 Shaving patients before operation: a dangerous myth? Annals of the Royal College of Surgeons of England 76:3–4

Mitchell M 2000 Nursing intervention for preoperative anxiety. Nursing Standard 14(37):40–43

Nursing and Midwifery Council 2004 Code of professional conduct: standards for conduct, performance and ethics. NMC, London

O'Callaghan O 2002 Pre-operative fasting. Nursing Standard 16(36):33–37

Otte DI 1996 Patients' perspective and experiences of day case surgery. Journal of Advanced Nursing 23:1228–1237

Peattie PI, Walker S (eds) 1995 Understanding nursing care, 3rd edn. Churchill Livingstone, Edinburgh

Rigge M 1997 Dr. Who? The Health Service Journal 107(5570):24–26

Royal College of Nursing 2005 Perioperative fasting for adults and children. Online: www.rcn.org.uk/publications/pdf/guidelines/PerioperativeFastingAdultsandChildren-002779.pdf Available July 2006

Scottish Intercollegiate Guidelines Network (SIGN) 2004 Postoperative management in adults. Guideline No. 77. SIGN, Edinburgh

Skacel C, McKenna F 1990 Patients' perception of orientation to the intensive therapy unit pre-operatively. Nursing Monograph 10

Trigg E, Mohammed T 2006 Practices in children's nursing. Guidelines for hospital and community. 2nd edn. Churchill Livingstone, Edinburgh

Tye T, Gell-Walker V 2000 Patient controlled analgesia. Nursing Times 96(25):38–39

Weins A 1998 Preoperative anxiety in women. AORN 68(1):74–88

Wilson-Barnett J 1979 Stress in hospital: patients' psychological reactions to illness and healthcare. Churchill Livingstone, Edinburgh

Wood M 2002 What do patients want to happen to their dentures before surgery? British Journal of Nursing 11(15):1027–1031

Xavier G 2000 The importance of mouth care in preventing infection. Nursing Standard 14(18):47–52

Further reading

Adam S 2003 Shock, systemic inflammatory response and multiorgan dysfunction. In: Brooker C, Nicol M (eds) Nursing adults. The practice of caring. Mosby, Edinburgh, Ch. 9

Greenstein B, Gould D 2004 Trounce's clinical pharmacology for nurses. 17th edn. Churchill Livingstone, Edinburgh

Jamieson EM, McCall JM, Whyte LA (eds) 2002 Clinical nursing practices. 4th edn. Churchill Livingstone, Edinburgh

Morris D, Ward K 2003 Perioperative nursing. In: Brooker C, Nicol M (eds) Nursing adults. The practice of caring. Mosby, Edinburgh

Nicol M, Bavin C, Bedford-Turner S, Cronin P, Rawlings-Anderson K (eds) 2004 Essential nursing skills. 2nd edn. Mosby, Edinburgh

Peattie PI, Walker S 1995 Understanding nursing care. 3rd edn. Churchill Livingstone, Edinburgh

Sheppard M, Wright M (eds) 2006 Principles and practice of high dependency nursing. 2nd edn. Baillière Tindall, Edinburgh

Stott R 2002 Pre-op visiting – revisited (1). British Journal of Theatre Nursing 12(8):306

Wound management

25

Irene Anderson and Jacqui Fletcher

Glossary terms

Acute wound
Chronic wound
Compression therapy
Débridement
Dehiscence
Epithelialization
Exudate
Granulation
Leg ulcer
Necrosis
Pressure ulcer
Primary intention healing
Secondary intention healing
Slough
Tissue viability

Learning outcomes

This chapter will help you:

- Describe the various types of wound
- Describe the stages of wound healing
- Identify local and patient-related factors that delay healing
- Describe wound assessment, cleansing and débridement
- Identify treatment objectives when selecting wound dressings
- List the main dressing categories
- Identify risk factors for pressure ulceration
- Outline the prevention of pressure ulcers
- Describe the assessment and management of pressure ulcers
- Outline how venous leg ulceration occurs and the signs of venous insufficiency
- Outline the assessment and management of venous leg ulcers.

Introduction

Tissue viability encompasses a variety of clinical issues/problems. Although primarily related to the management of wounds, the term also includes preventing tissue damage and care of vulnerable skin. Skin can become damaged for many reasons, including trauma such as cuts, as a result of problems such as incontinence or during surgery, or may arise from an underlying disease, e.g. leg ulceration.

Although many aspects of wound care have been traditionally deemed a nursing role, good tissue viability care depends upon holistic assessment of the patient/client and involvement of the relevant members of the multidisciplinary team (MDT).

In order to care for patients/clients with the potential for or compromised tissue viability, healthcare professionals must understand the normal structure and role of the skin and changes during the lifespan (see Ch. 16). This knowledge assists in determining deviations from the normal processes and helps to inform appropriate care plans and management.

Tissue viability includes the whole spectrum of patient/client care, including all age groups and all branches of nursing. Specific issues and problems may arise in particular areas of nursing, e.g. babies, older people with dementia or people with limited mobility, but a broad understanding of the fundamental principles gives a basis from which any nurse can begin to provide appropriate care.

Types of wound

The many different types of wound are classified in a variety of ways. This may relate to the aetiology (cause), the amount of tissue loss, whether they heal by primary or secondary intention (see p. 705) or the length of time they usually take to heal. There are also many subcategories within the definitions which provide a more accurate description and assessment of the wound.

Table 25.1 Common wound types

Type of wound	Acute or chronic	Primary or secondary healing
Surgical wound	Acute	Primary
Donor sites where skin has been removed for a skin graft	Acute	Secondary
Traumatic wound	Acute	Primary or secondary
Burn	Acute	Secondary
Fungating wound which occurs as cancer infiltrates the skin	Chronic	Secondary
Pressure ulcer (see pp. 714, 716–721)	Chronic	Secondary
Leg ulcer (see pp. 721–725)	Chronic	Secondary
Diabetic foot ulcer	Chronic	Secondary

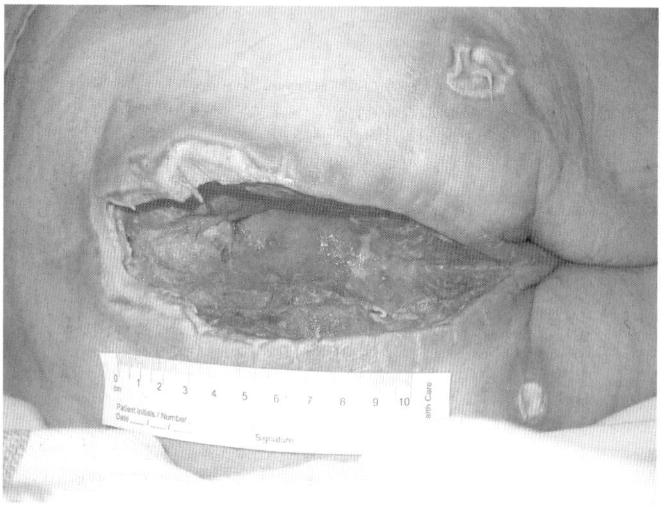

Fig. 25.1 Wound dehiscence

Wound classification and categories

Most commonly wounds are described as being either acute or chronic (Table 25.1). Acute wounds are those where healing is straightforward and follows an orderly sequence, whereas chronic wounds are slow to heal with some delay in the healing process. Chronic wounds – pressure ulcers and venous leg ulcers – are covered later in the chapter (see pp. 714–725). This definition of what is acute or chronic is overly simplified and there are many examples where these definitions are inappropriate. For example, a surgical wound that becomes infected, dehisces (bursts open) and fails to heal for many months does not fit the definition of an acute wound (Fig. 25.1); equally a laceration of the leg in an older woman with underlying venous disease is unlikely to heal in a straightforward way unless the underlying disease is also treated (Box 25.1).

REFLECTIVE PRACTICE Box 25.1

Common wounds

There will be patients/clients with wounds, wherever you practise.

Student activities

- Reflect on the types of wound that you have seen. Which types were common?
- Were the wounds mainly acute or chronic, or specific to a particular patient/client group?

Acute wounds

Acute wounds may be categorized by type and cause of the injury. They include:

- *Incised wound* – caused by cutting with a sharp instrument. Examples include a surgical incision or trauma caused by glass
- A *laceration* is a wound where tissues are torn, usually with a blunt instrument or pressure
- A *contusion* is caused by high-energy impact, usually with a blunt instrument (may also include bullet wounds). Contusions are usually more severe than lacerations; there is tissue layer separation and considerable tissue loss
- An *abrasion* is caused when the skin is forced against a resistant surface in a rubbing/scraping fashion. The resulting wound may resemble a burn (abrasions are sometimes known as friction burns). Most commonly they are superficial and expose the nerve endings so they can be extremely painful. An abrasion is frequently contaminated by particles of the surface against which it was abraded, most commonly gravel/grit but often clothing fabric may be embedded in the wound
- *Shearing wounds* occur when the skin is subjected to a twisting or tearing mechanism, the most severe example being a 'degloving' injury where the skin is peeled back, usually from a hand or foot, exposing the underlying structures
- *Puncture wounds* such as those caused by a bite have a small opening, which penetrates to the underlying tissues, frequently driving microorganisms into the wound
- *Crush injuries* occur when the tissues are trapped between an external surface and the underlying bone. Considerable internal damage may be present without a visible break in the skin.

Burn wounds are classified according to the depth and surface area of the skin affected (see Ch. 13).

Surgical wound categories (see Ch. 24)

The most common acute wounds result from surgical procedures that are frequently an elective (planned) event. Surgical wounds are further subdivided into categories based on the risk of wound infection occurring. Leaper and Harding (1998) describe four risk categories which relate to the reason for surgery and the organs involved, as follows:

- *Clean*: Wounds are non-traumatic, i.e. elective surgery using aseptic technique (see Ch. 15) and without any septic focus or internal organ (viscus) being opened, e.g. a skin graft
- *Clean–contaminated*: Non-traumatic wounds, i.e. elective surgery with only a minor breach in aseptic technique or entry into a viscus without significant spillage, e.g. elective cholecystectomy (removal of gallbladder)
- *Contaminated*: Traumatic wounds from a relatively clean source, or with a major breach in aseptic technique or significant spillage from an open viscus, or when acute non-purulent infection (without pus) is encountered, e.g. surgery for appendicitis
- *Dirty*: Traumatic wounds from a dirty source, or following a delayed treatment, or when acute bacterial contamination or release of pus (dead white cells and bacteria, cell debris and tissue fluid) occurs, e.g. surgery following trauma or where there is passage through the viscera such as following peritonitis (inflammation of the peritoneum).

Wound healing

In order to deliver appropriate care to patients/clients it is vital that nurses understand the processes by which wounds heal. The process involves a sequence of overlapping events or stages. It is important to link the theory to clinical practice so that recognition of the stage of wound healing informs treatment objectives. This is particularly important when documenting assessment findings and clinical decisions. It is logical to understand normal wound healing before considering abnormal and compromised healing.

Some injured tissue heals by regeneration and this can be seen in very superficial wounds affecting only the epidermal layer of the skin because these wounds heal without leaving any visible signs on the skin. Wounds affecting deeper layers of the skin are not able to do this and heal by a process of repair. New connective tissue is formed and healing occurs by fibrosis with scarring.

There are major differences in the healing process within fetal tissue. Wounds heal without scarring during the first 6 months of gestation; thereafter, healing resembles that occurring after birth. Fetal tissue heals by regeneration characterized by little inflammation, fibrosis or scarring.

Wounds can heal by primary or secondary intention. Primary intention healing occurs where there is minimal tissue loss and it is possible to draw the wound edges together with sutures (stitches) or clips. Secondary intention healing occurs where there is tissue loss and it is not possible or desirable to draw the wound edges together. Wounds subject to extensive tissue loss usually heal by a process of granulation (formation of new capillaries and the growth of new healthy moist, red tissue in the wound bed), contraction and epithelialization (epithelial cells move across the wound once it is filled with granulation tissue to resurface the wound).

Stages of wound healing

Wound healing is often described in four stages. These are:

- Vascular response
- Inflammation/inflammatory response
- Proliferation
- Maturation.

The four stages are considered separately but it is important to remember that the stages overlap, and progress and regress according to the circumstances of the patient's environment, lifestyle and underlying conditions (Fig. 25.2, p. 706).

Stage 1 – Vascular response (0–3 days)

Stage 1 involves processes that stop bleeding (haemostasis) and encourage migration of the cells that initiate healing. The blood vessels constrict initially and platelets accumulate at the breach in the vessel and stick together (aggregate), forming a plug to stop the bleeding for a short time. This is followed by blood coagulation whereby coagulation factors cause the formation of a fibrin (insoluble substance formed from the soluble protein fibrinogen) clot. Bleeding ceases as blood cells are trapped in the fibrin mesh to form the clot, which eventually dries to a scab.

Stage 2 – Inflammation/inflammatory response (1–6 days)

Once the clot has formed and bleeding stopped, the blood vessels dilate (vasodilatation). This is caused by the release of histamine by mast cells (a type of white blood cell [WBC]) that migrate to the wound. Gaps open up between the cells in the capillary walls and fluid leaks out into the tissues. The extra fluid and increased blood supply from the dilated capillaries result in redness, heat, swelling and pain, with some loss of function/movement in the area. This response can continue for some days. Therefore it is important that wound assessment (see p. 708) includes wound history, otherwise these signs may lead to an assumption of wound infection.

Vasodilatation and increased blood flow in the area mean that other WBCs (neutrophils and monocytes, which become macrophages) are attracted to the area by protein growth factors, which stimulate specific cell division and proliferation. The WBCs migrate to the site by a process called chemotaxis in order to defend the body against bacteria and remove debris from the wound. The neutrophils and macrophages do this by engulfing bacteria and debris, a process known as phagocytosis.

Other growth factors released by WBCs stimulate fibroblasts (immature cells that form connective tissue) and the growth of new blood vessels (angiogenesis) in the wound. Fibroblasts present in the fibrin clot begin to form collagen, a protein that provides the supportive framework in connective tissue. The wound contains fibrin debris known as slough (soft, creamy yellow tissue comprising cellular debris, which rises to the surface of the wound). Once enzymes in the wound fluid liquefy the slough, granulation tissue is visible in the wound bed. Increased capillary permeability leads to fluid loss, or exudate (fluid containing serum, nutrients such as proteins, proteolytic enzymes and cell debris), from the wound.

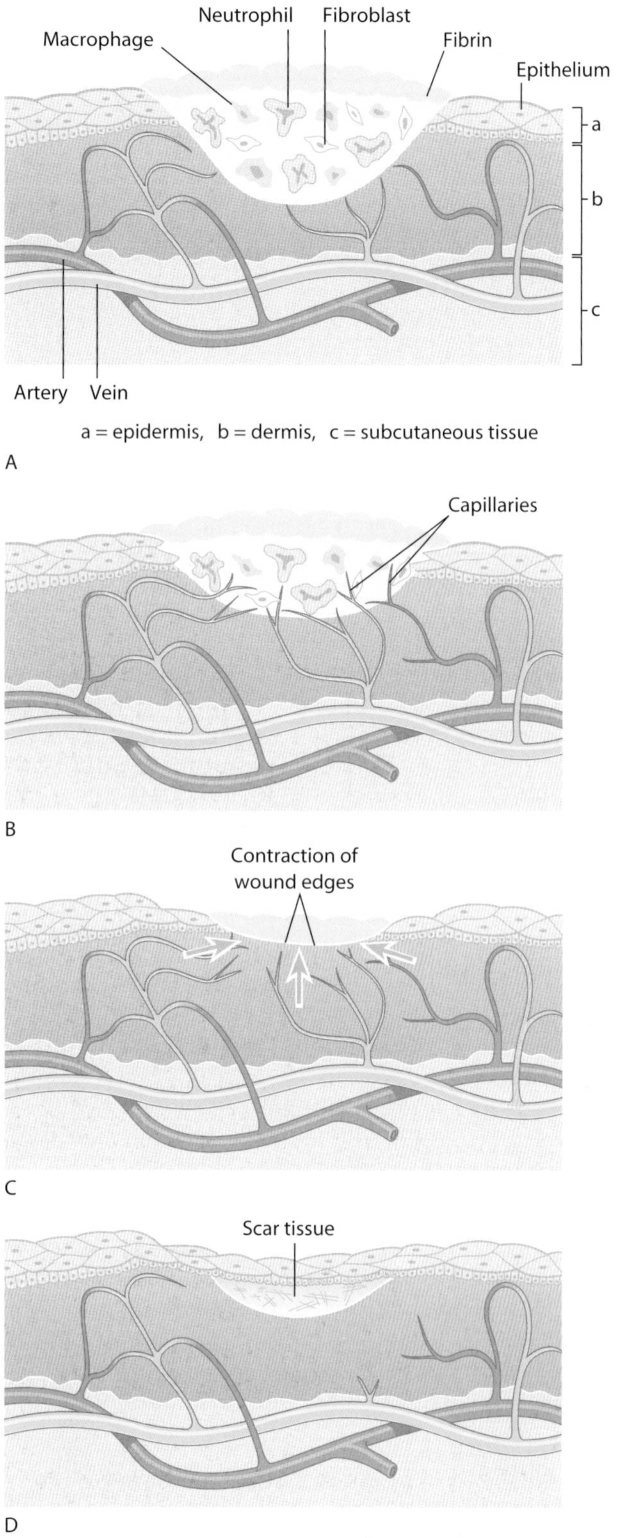

Fig. 25.2 Stages of wound healing: **A.** Inflammatory. **B.** Proliferative. **C.** Maturation. **D.** Mature (early) (reproduced with permission from Brooker & Nicol 2003)

An extracellular matrix (ECM) is formed in the wound, which serves as a platform over and through which cells can move and be supported as they act in the wound. The ECM constantly breaks down and reforms during healing and serves as a scaffold for new blood vessels.

Stage 3 – Proliferation (3–20 days)

Growth factors continue to stimulate fibroblasts and the ECM supports the new tissue. Other growth factors encourage angiogenesis and epithelial cell proliferation and migration. The deficit resulting from tissue loss is filled with new blood vessels and granulation tissue. At the same time, fibroblasts change shape, link with other fibroblasts and form a net-like structure. The changes result in fibres of collagen which give the elasticity needed to retain shape and resist injury. The collagen fibres begin to contract, each cell pulling on others. The wound shrinks in size and now has a covering of new, paler epithelial tissue (epithelialization). The wound is healing by granulation, contraction and epithelialization.

Stage 4 – Maturation (21 days to >1 year)

In normal, healthy people this stage often begins at about 21 days. The wound appears 'healed' because it has a covering of epithelial tissue (new skin). The collagen matures, gains strength and has a more orderly structure, and the new blood vessels mature. Capillary dilatation reduces and the number of fibroblasts decreases. Because healing occurs by repair rather than regeneration, the healed wound leaves the skin looking different. This is scar tissue and, depending on the wound and the individual, takes a variety of forms. Scars are formed from fibrous tissue, which initially appears red and slightly raised, and are itchy. Eventually this will settle to an area commensurate with the original wound dimensions and flattens. Scar tissue takes a long time to mature, possibly up to 2 years, during which tissue is remodelling. Scars have little elasticity and are generally paler than surrounding skin once they have matured.

Factors influencing healing

The prerequisites for normal wound healing include:

- A diet containing sufficient protein, energy, vitamin C, iron, zinc and copper
- An adequate blood supply of oxygen and nutrients, and removal of waste
- The absence of contaminants, e.g. microorganisms, toxins, foreign bodies
- Freedom from wound trauma
- A healthy immune system
- Adequate rest and sleep.

Healing is influenced by a variety of factors and circumstances. Some factors that delay healing are local to the wound, including wound complications, whereas others are systemic or patient-related.

Local wound factors

A variety of local wound factors can impair or delay healing (Box 25.2), as follows:

- Poor surgical technique, e.g. rough handling, can damage tissues and delay healing
- Mechanical disruption caused by:
  - recurring trauma from scratching, deliberate self-harm, falls, inappropriate use of adherent dressings or careless dressing removal, all of which may damage delicate granulation tissue
  - lack of protection during the maturation stage – patients/clients should be informed that the wound continues to heal and new tissue needs protection and should be kept moisturized and supple
- Foreign bodies, e.g. gravel, grit, sutures, etc., may set up a prolonged inflammatory response if not removed from the wound
- Toxic agents, e.g. inappropriate antiseptic use, can damage fragile tissue
- Reduced wound temperature caused by cold cleansing solutions or prolonged wound exposure reduces cellular activity
- Presence of excess slough and necrotic tissue (dead tissue caused by lack of oxygen to the local area) inhibits the cell migration required for healing and increases the risk of infection
- Proteolytic enzymes in exudate from chronic wounds can damage intact skin. Although the presence of exudate is vital for cellular activity, there needs to be management of the fluid if the wound and surrounding skin are not to suffer damage (Fletcher 2002)
- Local hypoxia (lack of oxygen in the tissues) caused by unrelieved pressure or prolonged oedema (abnormal collection of tissue fluid within the tissues) prevents cells from receiving sufficient oxygen for healing and delays granulation
- Dehydration of the wound bed caused by inappropriate dressings or exposure inhibits cellular activity.

Inappropriate wound management, poor assessment and clinical decision-making, and failure to set treatment objectives can all contribute to delayed and impaired wound healing.

> **CRITICAL THINKING** — Box 25.2
>
> ### Amina
>
> 3-year-old Amina has had surgery and her mother asks why she needs a dressing over the wound.
>
> **Student activity**
>
> What reasons do you think the registered nurse will give?

Problems with wound healing may compromise scar formation. The scar, which remains proud of skin level, can be dry, flaky and itchy. In some darker skin types keloid scarring can occur. This is a hard, raised overgrowth of scar outside the proportions of the original wound, which can cause the person considerable emotional and physical problems.

Wound complications

Wound healing is seriously affected by complications that include:

- *Infection*: Bacteria compete with body cells for oxygen and nutrients. The wound is considered infected when increasing bacterial numbers induce a host reaction (normally heat, redness, pain and swelling) (see Ch. 15). Exudate and pain may increase and wound healing slows
- *Haematoma*: Bleeding and the collection of blood within a wound, which has been closed (by primary intention) or covered with a skin graft. This causes tension in the wound, leading to tissue damage and possibly infection
- *Dehiscence*: Partial or total breakdown of the wound. This can be due to increased tension on the wound edges or, more commonly, to infection (see Fig. 25.1, p. 704).

Systemic or patient-related factors

Many patient-related factors have an impact on healing, e.g. age and nutritional status. Patient-related factors that may affect healing should be considered during the holistic assessment (see pp. 708–712). Factors may impact directly on the healing process, e.g. severe malnutrition, or may impact on the planned objectives of care, e.g. for a patient/client with arterial disease it may not be possible to heal the wound and an alternative objective would be determined or the suggested time to healing modified (see pp. 713–714).

Age

The skin of older people often thins and becomes more vulnerable to damage (Norman 2004). When trauma occurs, healing may be delayed because of slower cell turnover, reduced collagen synthesis and age-related poor circulation (Box 25.3).

> **REFLECTIVE PRACTICE** — Box 25.3
>
> ### Wound healing rates
>
> Think about the people with wounds you have met during placements.
>
> **Student activities**
>
> - What differences in healing rate did you observe between people of different ages?
> - Discuss the observations with your mentor and consider other factors that influenced healing in the group you observed.

Nutritional status (see Ch. 19)
Many individual nutrients are vital in wound healing (see p. 706) and a deficiency in any can affect healing. Protein–energy malnutrition (PEM), for example, results in insufficient resource for the increased needs of a healing wound.

Dehydration (see Ch. 19)
Dehydrated cells are not able to function efficiently and cell replication will be impaired. All cells need a moist environment for survival and movement.

Systemic diseases
Many diseases impair or delay wound healing. These include:

- Clotting disorders, e.g. haemophilia, disrupt clotting and delay the arrest of bleeding
- Poor circulation resulting from cardiovascular disease means that the wound area will be poorly perfused with oxygen and have a reduced supply of nutrients (see Ch. 17). Poor venous return results in venous congestion and collection of cellular debris within the wound area. Impaired venous return may also lead to localized oedema and increased exudate
- Poor oxygenation resulting from chronic respiratory diseases, cardiovascular diseases and anaemia (see Ch. 17) impairs collagen synthesis and epithelial growth, and also increases susceptibility to infection
- Cancer and its treatment with chemotherapy, e.g. methotrexate, or radiotherapy reduce the body's ability to heal. Chemotherapy, for example, adversely affects the inflammatory response and impedes cell proliferation. In addition, the reduction in WBCs affects immunity and increases the risk of infection
- Diabetes mellitus is associated with arterial disease, which impairs healing. Diabetes also damages peripheral nerves (neuropathy) and people may be unaware of tissue damage
- Impaired mobility and sensation can impact on wound healing. Reduced mobility, such as after a stroke, leads to reduced circulation and the associated problems.

Medication (see Ch. 22)
Several commonly used drugs have a negative impact on wound healing (Box 25.4). These include:

- Cancer chemotherapy, e.g. vincristine (see above)
- Non-steroidal anti-inflammatory drugs (NSAIDs), e.g. ibuprofen, affect the inflammatory response
- Corticosteroids, e.g. prednisolone, reduce the inflammatory and immune responses; reduced levels of immunity increase the risk of infection
- Anticoagulant drugs, e.g. warfarin, or long-term use of aspirin delay platelet aggregation, vasodilatation and attraction of cells. They affect the inflammatory response and healing is delayed.

Smoking
The adverse effects of smoking tobacco on wound healing include local hypoxia and altered platelet aggregation, which increase the risk of thrombus (clot) formation.

REFLECTIVE PRACTICE Box 25.4

Drugs that affect wound healing

Think about the drugs commonly prescribed in your placement.

Student activities

- Are people asked if they are taking over-the-counter drugs, e.g. aspirin?
- Find out what people are told about the potential effects of their prescribed medication on healing.

Stress
Psychological factors affecting patients/clients also influence wound healing. Stress and anxiety result in the production of glucocorticoid hormones, e.g. cortisol (see Ch. 11). These are anti-inflammatory and may inhibit fibroblasts, collagen synthesis and granulation (Keicolt-Glaser et al 1995). They may also reduce blood supply. Everything possible should be done to relieve stress and anxiety, including ensuring adequate sleep and rest (see Ch. 10).

Wound management

This part of the chapter outlines wound assessment, cleansing, débridement and dressing products.

Good wound management is dependent on a thorough holistic assessment of the patient/client and their wound. This is followed by the setting of appropriate patient/client-centred objectives and the use of evidence-based wound care to encourage healing or, where this is not possible, to manage the symptoms appropriately.

Wound assessment

Assessment of the wound is only one part of holistic assessment and should never be carried out in isolation. A full history is taken to identify any systemic patient-related factors which may influence healing, e.g. malnutrition, and also the causation and time scale of the wound.

Wound assessment is a multifaceted process and, in order to make best use of the information, it should be documented systematically and objectively. A variety of wound assessment charts exist but, whichever chart is selected, it should address all the elements of a holistic assessment outlined below. Reassessments should be carried out at least weekly but may be more frequent depending on the individual wound characteristics (see Ch. 14).

Wound characteristics

When assessing a wound, several characteristics should be considered, including:

- Cause
- Location

> **CRITICAL THINKING** Box 25.5
>
> **Self-harm emergency care**
>
> A friend has told you that her daughter is cutting herself. On occasions the injury has bled for some time but the girl was too frightened to go to the Emergency Department. Your friend asks you what will happen if they seek help.
>
> **Student activity**
>
> - Find out what treatment and help would be offered if your friend persuades her daughter to attend the Emergency Department.
>
> [Resource: National Institute for Clinical Excellence (NICE) 2004 Self harm: short-term treatment and management. Online: www.nice.org.uk/pdf/CG016publicinfoenglish.pdf Available July 2006]

- Condition of the surrounding skin
- Size
- Type of tissue present in the wound
- Exudate – type and amount
- Odour
- Wound pain.

Cause of the wound

The cause may impact on further assessment and care planning. The cause will also help determine the risk of complications. For example, if the knife causing the wound is contaminated with soil, the risk of infection is much higher than if it was a clean knife from a dishwasher. Sometimes the cause is immediately obvious, but in other cases the cause may only be determined by careful and systematic history taking and in some instances sensitive questioning (see Ch. 9).

Particular consideration should be given to patients/clients whose wounds are self-inflicted, as their need for psychological support may be greater than an immediate need for wound care (Box 25.5). Frequently a MDT approach to care is required, with involvement of mental health teams, psychologists and social services. The MDT is also important in managing patients with other types of wound and their individual input should always be considered. Many traumatic wounds require input from both physiotherapists and occupational therapists to maintain function and mobility; equally these team members help to manage chronic wounds such as venous leg ulcers where increased mobility may accelerate healing.

Location

Initially wound location is considered in relation to its proximity to vital structures, as life-saving care takes priority. Location may provide clues to the cause of the wound. Buttock wounds tend to be automatically classified as pressure ulcers but this is often incorrect, as pressure ulcers usually (but not exclusively) occur over bony prominences (see pp. 719–720). Wounds appearing on or between the buttocks are more frequently caused by incontinence (see Chs 20, 21).

The position of the wound may also impact on the dressing choice (see p. 714), e.g. keeping a dressing on the sacrum is notoriously difficult because it is subject to shear and friction forces. Equally if the wound is easily visible, such as on the face or hand, the cosmetic impact of the dressing may be the overriding consideration. When managing wounds over or close to joints, consideration must be given to maintaining mobility and joint function.

Condition of the surrounding skin

The condition of the surrounding skin may indicate the patient's/client's general health or the presence of problems, e.g. eczema. This impacts on dressing choices; for example, if the surrounding skin is very fragile it may not be possible to use adhesive dressings. If there is gross oedema present there may be seepage of fluid onto the skin, which will lead to maceration (damage caused by excess moisture leading to overhydration and increased susceptibility to trauma) if not adequately managed. Fluid is trapped on the skin surface when the dressing used does not manage the exudate adequately or is not changed frequently enough. Maceration also increases the risk of infection.

Size

The size of the wound is accurately measured and recorded in order to evaluate progress. Sometimes wounds appear to get bigger during healing; this may be because the full extent was previously masked by necrotic tissue or thick slough.

Measurement can be undertaken by using a disposable paper ruler to record the length and width. However, as most wounds are irregular in shape this does not record the overall size.

More frequently a tracing is taken of the outline of the wound using a transparent overlay (Box 25.6, p. 710). An overlay may be either a commercial wound tracing sheet (Fig. 25.3) or the clear part of a dressing packet. As the packet contained a sterile dressing the inside should be sterile and therefore safe to put in contact with the wound. This outline may then be traced onto paper and stored in the notes. If commercial tracing sheets are used, the backing film that had contact with the wound is removed and the initial tracing stored in the notes.

A tracing can also be used to record areas of different tissue types, e.g. slough or necrosis (Fig. 25.4, p. 710 and p. 713). The change in percentages of these tissues may indicate wound progress as much as a change in overall size.

If tracing materials are not available, a simple line drawing can be made with measurements marked on, as well as the areas of different tissues. Alternatively, a photographic record of wound size and condition can be obtained. If photography is used, written consent must be obtained from the person (see Chs 6, 7) and this must detail what the photograph may be used for, i.e. for use in the records or used for teaching purposes or for publication, when further written consent will be required by the publisher.

Types of tissue present in wounds

In addition to the size of the wound, it is important to record the type of tissue visible in the wound bed. For example:

- *Necrotic tissue* is black and hard or leathery; however, as it softens, it may become grey or brown

NURSING SKILLS Box 25.6

Measuring wounds

Equipment

- Tracing grid
- Permanent marker pen.

Preparation

Ensure the patient/client understands what is happening and has given consent. If necessary, ensure that appropriate analgesia is administered. Ensure privacy. It may be necessary to clean the wound to remove any surface debris (see p. 713). Mark the grid with head and foot, left and right.

Procedure

- Apply the grid lightly to the surface of the wound
- Ensure the patient is in the same position each time the wound is measured – this should be documented within the care plan
- Trace the outline of the wound, taking care not to apply too much pressure as this may cause pain. Mark on the proportion of different types of tissue present in the wound
- Carefully peel the grid away from the wound
- Remove the backing film that has been in contact with the wound and dispose of in a yellow bag
- Place the tracing safely to one side until the dressing procedure is completed and the patient is comfortable
- Place the dated tracing in the patient's/client's nursing notes and record findings
- Compare the tracing to those done previously, noting any changes in the wound.

- *Slough* is usually soft and stringy and may vary in colour from creamy yellow through brownish grey as the wound progresses. Despite removal of thick slough, a thin layer of creamy-coloured slough remains closely adherent to the wound surface, almost until healing is complete; this is not a cause for concern
- *Granulation tissue* contains many new capillaries and is bright red, moist and uneven in texture. Overgranulation occurs where the granulation tissue becomes overexuberant and grows above the surrounding tissue. This type of tissue is friable and may bleed easily. Unhealthy granulation tissue is a dull, deep red; it may be gelatinous and appear to be less well attached to the wound. Although

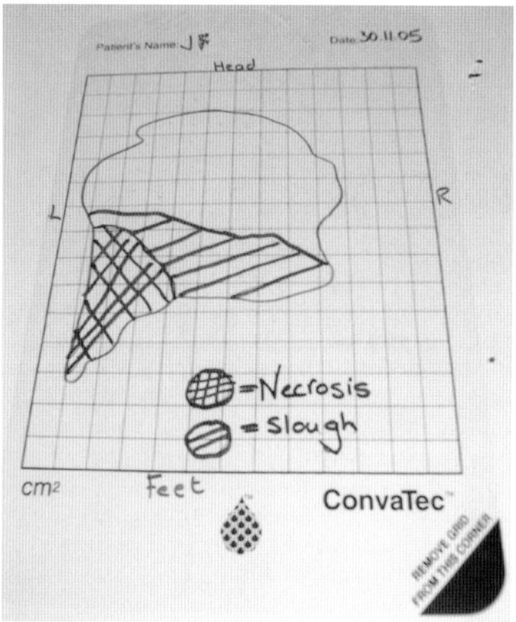

Fig. 25.4 Wound trace of a sacral pressure ulcer showing different types of tissue

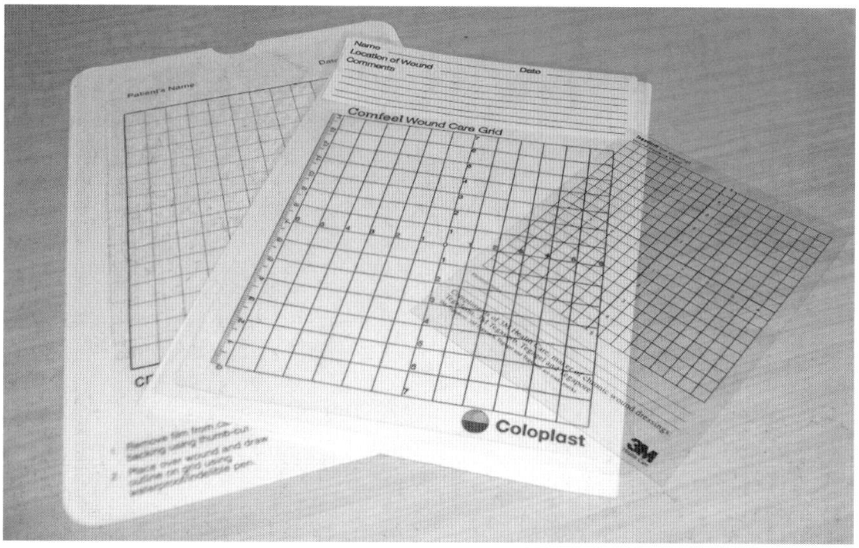

Fig. 25.3 Wound tracing sheet

its presence may indicate infection or poor blood supply, it is generally seen as an indicator of poor wound healing
- *Epithelial tissue* is pale pink or silvery white tissue, which denotes wound resurfacing. It develops from the wound margins and also as islands in partial thickness wounds where remnants of hair follicles and sebaceous glands remain.

Exudate

All wounds produce protein-rich exudate throughout the healing process. Exudate bathes the wound, keeping it moist and supplying the substances needed for healing (see p. 706). In acute wounds, the level of exudate decreases as healing progresses; however, in chronic wounds exudate may persist or increase.

It is important to monitor the quantity of exudate but in practice this is not easy. Most wound assessment charts use subjective assessment of exudate quantity, e.g. low, moderate or high level, or symbols (+, ++, +++). While most experienced nurses would claim to understand the meaning of these descriptions, they are not objective measurements and different nurses may have differing views of what constitutes a particular level. For this reason it is better to use an objective descriptor.

It is not usually possible to record the volume of exudate unless a wound drainage bag or vacuum-assisted closure system is being used (Fig. 25.5). What can be recorded is the frequency with which the dressing becomes saturated and requires changing. For example, if initially the dressing requires changing twice daily and later progresses to once every 2 days, a clear reduction in exudate can be recorded or vice versa. This is dependent upon the same dressing type and size being used for consistency.

When observing for differences in exudate volume it is important to consider what else is happening to the wound. There may be an apparent increase in exudate but this may be due to the presence other fluid, e.g. that produced by some dressings.

The type, colour and consistency of the exudate should also be recorded. Changes in the exudate are often the first signs of changes occurring within the wound. Exudate may be described as:

- *Serous* – clear, straw-coloured fluid
- *Serosanguineous* – usually clear but with streaks of blood. Becomes pink/pale red in colour as the fluids mix. May be observed prior to wound dehiscence
- *Sanguineous* – bloody fluid
- *Seropurulent* – serous fluid and pus
- *Purulent* – thick, pus-filled fluid of varying colour.

The consistency may vary from watery to thick and almost semi-solid.

Odour

Most wounds produce a typical smell, and odour within the wound is not necessarily abnormal. However, changes or increase in odour may suggest the presence of infection or progress within the wound. The odour normally becomes stronger and less pleasant as necrotic tissue is rehydrated and liquefies. Equally, some dressing products produce a typical odour. Assessment of odour is subjective and is often recorded as +, ++ or +++, but again this does not allow for comparison. One way of objectively describing the odour is to record when it is first detectable. For example:

- Very strong – odour obvious on entering the room with dressing intact
- Strong – odour obvious on entering the room when the dressing is leaking or removed
- Moderate – odour obvious within 2 metres with dressing intact
- Minimal – odour obvious within 2 metres when the dressing is leaking or removed

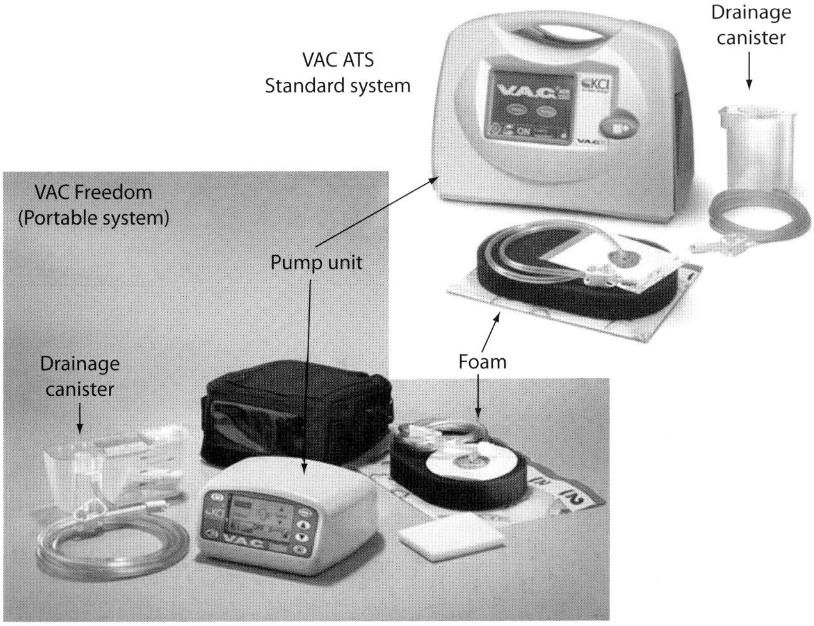

Fig. 25.5 Vacuum-assisted closure system (reproduced with permission from KCI Medical Ltd)

- Scant – odour obvious when standing next to the patient with dressing intact
- None – no odour obvious even when the dressing is removed.

Wound pain

It is only recently that pain has been widely acknowledged as being a problem in all wound types (see Ch. 23). A recent consensus document (World Union of Wound Healing Societies 2004) suggests that nurses:

- Assume that all wounds are painful
- Appreciate that they may become more painful
- Know that the surrounding skin can become sensitive and painful
- Realize that, for some patients, the lightest touch or even moving air over the wound can be intensely painful
- Know when to refer for appropriate specialist advice. The pain team may be helpful.

When assessing wound pain, the type, nature and intensity should be determined. The type of pain relates to what causes the pain: is it constant background pain, related to procedures such as dressing changes, or incident pain related to things such as coughing? This is important, as it influences the type of analgesic required. The patient should be encouraged to describe the nature of the pain; common words include dull or aching (e.g. with venous leg ulcers), burning, itching pain (with skin reactions) or sharp, stabbing pain. Pain should be assessed using an appropriate pain-rating scale (see Ch. 23).

Social factors

Wounds may impact on social aspects of life, and social factors may influence a person's wound and its management. For example, many older adults with leg ulcers become socially isolated, as they stay at home because of pain and embarrassment about the look and/or odour of the ulcer. Other groups have difficulty accessing services for wound care due to social circumstances, e.g. homeless people and people with wounds related to drug misuse where there is considerable stigma associated with the cause.

In children, older adults and other vulnerable groups such as people with a learning disability, the presence of traumatic wounds should alert the nurse to the possibility of non-accidental injury; however, it should be borne in mind that children, for example, frequently injure themselves (see Chs 3, 6).

Most dressing products and care from a tissue viability nurse are increasingly available in both hospital and community settings. However, some products remain non-prescribable in the community.

Environmental factors

The care environment may influence the management and also the risk factors such as infection. In hospital, the patient/client is vulnerable to cross-infection from contact with other patients and exposure to different microorganisms, which are more virulent/pathogenic than typical microorganisms found outside hospital (see Ch. 15). At home, the infection risk differs and there is less risk of cross-infection; however, the home environment is not always ideal. Many people have pet animals and both personal hygiene and general cleanliness vary considerably.

If the person is well and mobile, consideration must be given to where they go and what they do and what impact this will have on their wound. Children need a dressing that will withstand play and school activities. Work environments, e.g. where dressings are likely to become wet or contaminated, are considered in planning wound management. Caring for people with mental health problems presents particular difficulties and many usual nursing interventions cannot be used. For example, it may be judged unsafe to use a compression bandage for a patient with suicidal ideation or if other patients in close proximity are at similar risk.

Organizational factors

Nurses in both community and hospital usually deliver wound care. Care delivery should be at a time that meets the needs of both the patient/client and the need to provide appropriate care. Patients and families should be as fully involved as possible in the care provided. Involvement requires that they receive adequate and appropriate information, at an appropriate level and in a language they understand.

For children and those with ongoing care needs, the family and/or friends are frequently involved in providing wound care; this relies upon the carer being both willing and able to do this. For children, involvement of the family or their own participation in care of the wound can help to reduce pain and relieve anxiety. Family or patient participation in wound care, especially at home, means that the care can be provided at the most appropriate time and is not dependent on a nurse visiting. However, additional support is required to ensure that ongoing wound assessment is maintained and that the family feels fully supported and confident to call for nursing assistance when it is needed.

The need for input from other healthcare workers should be assessed. These include:

- Tissue viability nurse
- Doctor
- Healthcare assistant
- Dietitian
- Physiotherapist
- Occupational therapist
- Podiatrist
- Nurse specialists, e.g. diabetes, infection control, etc.
- Equipment/wound product suppliers
- Patients/clients and their carers, etc.

Input from most of these groups is equally important in caring for patients/clients with any type of wound. Other individuals whose participation may be needed include pharmacists, vascular surgeons and plastic surgeons, as well as domestic staff whose role in maintaining cleanliness is crucial.

Wound cleansing

Cleansing is important to clear loose debris from the wound. Frequently this must be undertaken to facilitate wound assessment, particularly in acute traumatic wounds where the area may be obscured by blood or debris. However, in the absence of debris, it is not always essential to cleanse the wound each time the dressing is changed (Flanagan 1997). Wound healing occurs in a warm, moist environment and cleansing may cool the wound. The surrounding skin should always be cleansed to remove dressing material or exudate which has a detrimental effect on the skin. Wound cleansing is achieved by irrigating the wound with warm fluid, either normal saline or tap water to prevent cooling. Aseptic technique is used when there is an invasive component, such as in theatre, but otherwise a clean technique is used (see Ch. 15).

Many people cleanse their wounds by showering or by irrigating/soaking in warm tap water (Günnewicht & Dunford 2004). Soaking is particularly suitable for leg wounds as the limb can be immersed in a bucket or bowl lined with a new plastic liner for each patient/client to reduce the risk of cross-infection.

Cotton wool/fibrous material must not be used to cleanse wounds as debris can become incorporated into the wound bed, causing inflammation. Slough or necrotic tissue may persist in the wound and this should be removed or débrided (see below). Dead tissue may act as a focus for infection, physically impede wound healing and cause, or increase, odour.

Wound débridement

Débridement is the removal of devitalized (dead) tissue which is adherent to the wound bed or the removal of foreign material from the wound. There are various methods that include:

- Surgical débridement in theatre
- Sharp débridement using scalpel and scissors. This is a highly skilled procedure and must only be undertaken by specially trained healthcare professionals who have been assessed as competent
- Chemical débridement using enzymes, e.g. streptokinase, to remove dead tissue. There may be discomfort and the potential for damaging the surrounding skin (Singhal et al 2001)
- Providing a moist wound environment by using dressings, e.g. hydrocolloids, to enhance natural débridement mechanisms whereby debris is liquefied by enzymes by autolysis. This is slower than sharp or surgical débridement but may be appropriate for some patients/clients
- Larval therapy (maggot therapy) is used for wound débridement. Hydrocolloid is placed around the wound to protect the surrounding skin. Sterile blowfly (*Lucilia sericata*) larvae are put on the wound and covered by a fine nylon net, which is held in place by Sleek® tape. Moist gauze may be placed on top to hydrate the larvae if required. Light padding is applied to absorb the liquefied debris. The maggots are left in place for 48–72 hours and a second application may be required. Larval enzymes break down slough and necrotic material, and the surrounding skin must be protected as the enzymes may irritate intact skin. Larval therapy can be used in the presence of infection but is unsuitable for wounds producing high levels of exudate or where the larvae may be squashed (Thomas et al 1996).

REFLECTIVE PRACTICE Box 25.7

Larval therapy

Patients/clients, carers and nurses often have anxieties about having or using larval therapy.

Student activities

- How would you feel about a suggestion that 'maggots' could be used on your chronic wound?
- Ask the tissue viability nurse about patient preparation for larval therapy and what support is available during the treatment.
- Discuss with your mentor the measures needed to ensure that nurses feel confident in using larval therapy.

Patients/clients require careful preparation for larval therapy. The practitioner must be confident in handling the larvae and be able to reassure and support the patient/client and their carers (Box 25.7).

Wound dressings

Given the huge variety of wound dressings it is important to know how dressings work so that appropriate choices can be made. No single dressing will be appropriate for all wound types so nurses need know the wound circumstances for which each dressing is designed.

Aims of treatment

Following assessment, it is usual to develop a care plan to meet specific wound objectives. While it is tempting to set the overall aim of 'to heal the wound', this is too long term and lacks guidance for immediate wound management. More detailed objectives for specific wounds would typically include:

- For a *dry black necrotic wound* – débridement and rehydration. Dry, devitalized tissue is softened, liquefied and removed
- For a *yellow sloughy wound* – remove slough. Débridement and cleansing as above. If the wound bed is already wet, the treatment objective is to control fluid and encourage autolysis
- For a *red granulating wound* – protect and maintain moisture balance. There should be enough exudate to keep the wound moist and promote cell movement, but not so much that the wound and surrounding skin are damaged by the enzymes or by the constant wetness, and to promote healing
- For a *pink epithelializing wound* – protect and maintain moisture balance.

Additional objectives may be required for the prevention or management of infection. Specific objectives related to the wound aetiology should also be set, e.g. pressure reduction in the management of a pressure ulcer. These objectives must be considered together with other aspects of patient care and may have to be modified to meet more pressing objectives, e.g. increasing mobility.

Choosing an appropriate dressing

Essentially the choice of dressing is determined by assessment findings, the aims of treatment and patient/client preferences. However, three key factors must be considered in dressing selection:

- Amount of exudate
- Condition of the surrounding skin
- Patient/client preference.

An estimation of exudate level (see p. 711) can assist in dressing choice. Selecting a dressing designed for low levels of exudate, e.g. film dressing, may cause maceration and leakage on a wet wound, whereas choosing a dressing designed to cope with high exudate levels may allow drying of a wound with only minimal exudate.

The condition of the surrounding skin helps in determining the dressing type. Adhesive dressings may cause trauma on removal if applied to fragile skin. Where infection or copious exudate necessitates frequent dressing changes, it would be inappropriate to use adhesive dressings as these are designed to remain in place for a few days. The surrounding skin may be macerated or excoriated due to damage from excess fluid and for this reason the selected dressing should be designed to hold exudate within its structure away from the skin. It is important to read the manufacturer's instructions for use, as some dressings are cut to the shape of the wound and some to lie over the wound and surrounding skin.

Patient preference is an important consideration when assessing the patient, the wound and selecting dressings (Box 25.8). Before using any product there must be explanation for, and negotiation with, the patient who is to wear the dressing.

It is vital that the manufacturer's instructions for dressing use are read and understood before the final decision is made to apply any dressing. These instructions state at least:

- The structure of the dressing
- The wound types and circumstances for which it is designed
- The circumstances when it should not be used or when particular caution should be exercised.

If nurses have questions about a dressing they should seek the advice of the tissue viability nurse who may contact the manufacturer directly. Nurses must read professional literature and other sources information in addition to that from manufacturers. It is vital to appraise the clinical use of products and consider carefully the evidence base to support them. Manufacturers provide telephone and email facilities to answer questions.

ETHICAL ISSUES Box 25.8

Ethical and religious considerations

Some dressings may contain human and/or cow or pig tissue. It is important that nurses provide full information about a particular dressing and ensure that patients/clients or carers give informed consent prior to its use.

Student activities

- Read the article by Enoch et al (2005).
- Find out if any dressings used in your placement contain human or animal products.
- What information is given to patient/clients or carers about dressing products?

[Resource: Enoch S, Shaaban H, Dunn KW 2005 Informed consent should be obtained from patients to use products (skin substitutes) and dressing containing biological material. Journal of Medical Ethics 31(1):2–6]

Types of dressing

The main dressing categories and their functions are summarized in Table 25.2. Some are primary (applied directly onto the wound surface), some are secondary (cover a primary dressing) and some can be used as either a primary or a secondary dressing.

In addition, there are ancillary products used in wound management. These include:

- Tubular gauze – fix and retain dressings, particularly in awkward areas or where the skin is unsuitable for adhesive products
- Tape – there are many products available to suit different skin types and circumstances
- Paste bandages – cotton bandages coated with substances such as zinc oxide used to treat skin conditions.

Chronic wounds

Chronic wounds are those where healing is delayed or interrupted for some reason; most have persistent or recurrent inflammation and tend to have high levels of exudate. Most chronic wounds, including pressure ulcers and leg ulcers, will heal by secondary intention. Management of these wounds depends as much on management of the underlying cause as care of localized wound factors.

Pressure ulcers

Pressure ulcers (pressure sores, decubitus ulcers) are an area of localized damage to the skin and underlying tissue caused by pressure, shear or friction, or a combination of these (European Pressure Ulcer Advisory Panel [EPUAP] 1999) (Fig. 25.6, p. 716). They are common and a survey suggests that, on average, 22% of hospitalized patients develop pressure ulcers (EPUAP 2002).

Table 25.2 Dressing types

Dressing	Function	Notes
Gauze type/padding	Secondary dressing Extra absorption Protection	Not for primary dressings May adhere and shed fibres into granulation tissue
Low adherent (film with thin layer of padding)	Primary dressing Protection Absorption	No dressing can be guaranteed non-adherent Secondary dressing required in some cases Generally used in low exudate wounds and/or in the final stages of healing Exudate may become trapped under the dressing and cause skin damage May require frequent dressing changes
Paraffin gauze (gauze mesh coated with white soft paraffin and sometimes other substances, e.g. chlorhexidine)	Primary dressing Protection	Risk of adherence, as the mesh can trap exudate, which dries Granulation tissue may grow into the dressing resulting in wound trauma when removed It needs to be used in multilayers and changed frequently Secondary dressing required
Silicone (thin layers of netting coated with soft silicone gel)	Primary dressing Low adherent Sometimes used for control/management of scarring	Modern materials reduce risk of adherence or the growth of granulation tissue into the dressing May be used on highly exuding wounds with an absorbent secondary dressing
Hydrogel (soft amorphous gel, squeezed from a tube onto the wound bed or available in sheets)	Primary dressing Rehydration Débridement in low exudate wounds Promotion of moisture in dry wounds	Because hydrogels contain water they should not be used when the wound is already wet Protect the surrounding skin if used to liquefy slough Secondary dressing needed to keep gel in place and maintain moisture Sheet hydrogel has a film backing and is useful for minor burns and painful wounds
Film (adhesive polyurethane film)	Primary/secondary dressing Protection Promotion of moisture	Use on wounds with low exudate if surrounding skin is suitable for adhesive dressings May cause maceration if used as a primary dressing on a wet wound If the exudate level increases, a more absorbent dressing must be considered Films are also used as secondary dressings, e.g. over a hydrogel or absorbent pad
Foam (polyurethane foams that absorb exudate but hold fluid away from the skin to minimize maceration)	Primary/secondary dressing Protection Absorption	Available as adhesive and non-adhesive Different shapes are available and some can be cut to shape Use on wounds with low to moderate or high exudate levels depending on the manufacturer Available in different absorbency levels
Hydrocolloid (mixture of components that include cellulose, gelatin and/or pectin combined with adhesives and other materials)	Primary/secondary dressing Protection Débridement Absorption	Use on wounds with low to moderate exudate As they are adhesive, the skin must be suitable for an adhesive dressing They are intended to stay in place for a few days and frequent removal may cause skin redness and discomfort Different shapes are available and the dressings can be cut to shape Thin hydrocolloid dressings are available and can be used for low exudate levels, when the skin is less robust or when greater conformability of the dressing material is required May be used as secondary dressings, especially as an outer waterproof layer

(*Continued*)

Table 25.2 (*Continued*)

Dressing	Function	Notes
Alginate (derived from seaweed; available in flat sheets or ribbons/ropes for use in cavity wounds)	Primary dressing Absorption Débridement in high exudate wounds Control of minor bleeding (some products)	Absorbent material for use on wet wounds Forms a soft gel on contact with exudate Some alginates absorb fluid vertically and do not need to be cut to shape; others use the whole surface area of the dressing (horizontal wicking) and should not cover the surrounding skin Not for low exudate wounds, as adherence may occur Secondary dressing required
Hydrofibre (cellulose spun to produce sheet and ribbon forms)	Primary dressing Absorption Débridement in high exudate wounds	Designed to absorb high levels of exudate; the fibre becomes a gel when wet The fluid is absorbed vertically into the dressing, which helps to prevent maceration of surrounding skin May adhere if used on low exudate wounds Secondary dressing required
Topical antimicrobials (dressings containing silver or iodine)	Infected wounds (with appropriate antibiotic therapy) Wounds at significant risk of infection Wounds that are failing to heal Controlling malodour	Dressing material, e.g. foam, hydrocolloids, etc. containing iodine or silver Careful wound assessment and monitoring is required It is important to follow the manufacturer's instructions for correct use and recommended wear times Secondary dressings required with some products
Deodorizing dressings (dressings containing carbon/charcoal which attracts chemicals causing malodour)	Primary/secondary dressings Control of malodour Protection	Use on malodorous wounds, e.g. those containing dead tissue, fungating or infected wounds
Honey (Manuka) sometimes mixed with waxes/oils (a paste squeezed from a tube or as dressing material coated with honey)	Primary dressings Wet wounds Infected wounds Débridement	Honey (especially Manuka) has antibacterial properties It is important that honey products used are specifically indicated for wound use May require frequent dressing changes in wet wounds to ensure sufficient honey is in contact with the wound Patients may experience pain/discomfort and honey dressings may need to be discontinued
Vacuum-assisted closure (topical negative pressure; see Fig. 25.5, p. 711)		Uniform negative pressure to the wound bed Removes excess fluid and therefore bacteria and substances which may delay healing

Note: Always refer to the manufacturer's application instructions.

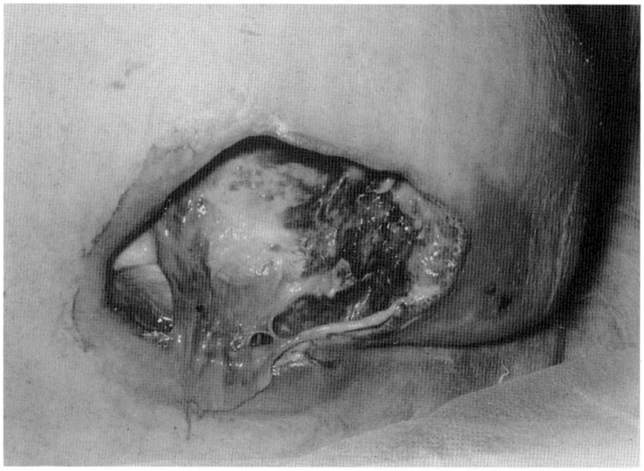

Fig. 25.6 Pressure ulcer (reproduced with permission from Brooker & Nicol 2003)

All grade 2 and above pressure ulcers should be documented as a clinical incident and the circumstances thoroughly investigated (NICE 2005). They occur in all age groups and across all specialities and care settings. They cause patients and carers distress, pain and embarrassment; they increase morbidity and increasingly are recorded as a cause of death. In addition, they are costly, as management requires specialist equipment and dressings. Real costs are difficult to quantify, as costs also arise from the extra time that patients are hospitalized for what is an eminently preventable condition.

Risk factors for pressure ulcers

Several factors increase the risk of pressure ulcer development; these may be extrinsic (external to the patient, related to their environment) and intrinsic (directly about the patient).

Extrinsic factors

The extrinsic risk factors are (Fig. 25.7):

- *Pressure* – the direct application of force to the skin, usually the weight of the patient's body pressing down on a surface such as a bed or chair. The underlying blood vessels are compressed and blood supply to the area is reduced. This results in local tissue damage and, if the pressure is sustained, necrosis occurs
- *Friction* occurs when the skin is moved in a direction opposite to the surface with which it has contact. For example, if the patient/client slides down in bed, their skin drags along the sheet, which can result in removal of the superficial layer of the skin (epidermis)
- *Shear* is an internal force that occurs when the body slides down in bed or a chair. Before friction is overcome and the body moves, the bony skeleton moves inside the skin. Where the underlying blood supply is attached, it becomes stretched and twisted, eventually tearing or cutting off the local blood supply.

The role of moisture is less clear. However, when moisture is trapped against the skin, the skin becomes macerated, thus increasing susceptibility to trauma, e.g. from nurses'/carers' nails, rings, etc., and friction forces.

Intrinsic factors

Intrinsic factors are numerous and individual to the patient:

- Increasing age is associated with changes in skin resilience and thinning, which increases susceptibility to trauma. Similar changes occur with some medications, e.g. long-term corticosteroids
- Concurrent disease that reduces blood flow or tissue oxygenation, e.g. arterial disease, chronic respiratory disease or anaemia
- Reduced mobility, such as after a stroke, or related to hospitalization, e.g. during surgery, or altered conscious, physical disabilities or pain. Immobility may be associated with depression or caused by drugs, particularly night sedation, which reduces spontaneous movements
- Poor nutrition, particularly PEM (see Ch. 19), as nutrients are needed for cell replacement and to fuel activity. Recent weight loss is usually thought to be of greater importance than actual weight (EPUAP 2003)
- Sensory loss impairs the response to pain normally associated with prolonged pressure. Without pain/discomfort the person is unaware of the need to move, thereby increasing their susceptibility to prolonged pressure
- Incontinence is a risk factor, both because of the effect of moisture on the skin and because urine and faeces may damage the skin, thereby reducing resistance to extrinsic factors
- Build/weight for height. Both extremes – being underweight or overweight – increase the risk of pressure ulceration. Underweight individuals have little subcutaneous tissue to buffer the impact of pressure. Overweight individuals, while they have additional padding over which to distribute the pressure, are sustaining much higher levels of pressure because of their additional weight.

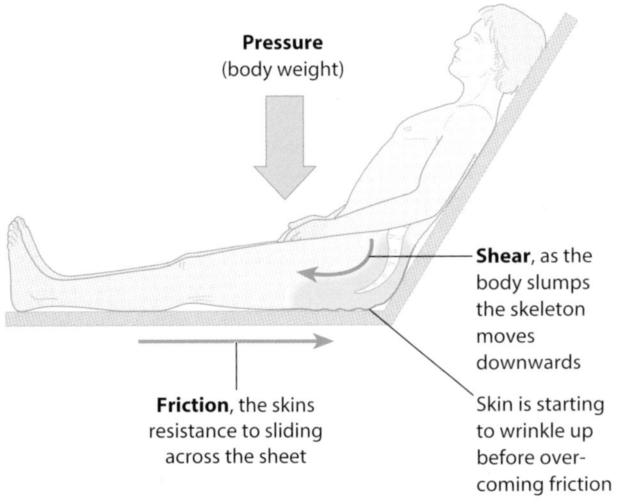

Fig. 25.7 Relationship between pressure, shear and friction (reproduced with permission from Brooker & Nicol 2003)

Pressure ulcer risk assessment tools

In order to identify which patients/clients may be at risk of developing a pressure ulcer, a risk assessment tool is used (Table 25.3, p. 718). Many such tools exist, e.g. Waterlow (see Fig. 14.3, p. 357), Braden, etc.

The tools are based on a list of risk factors, each of which is allocated a numerical score. The numbers are summed to reach a total which defines the patient's level of risk, e.g. low, medium or high. Differences exist between the tools, perhaps the most crucial of which is the way the numbers relate to risk. In the Braden score, the lower the number, the higher the risk; however, in the majority of such tools, the higher the score, the higher the risk of developing a pressure ulcer. Each tool and its risk factors were designed for a particular area of care, e.g. the Walsall tool for use in the community. Therefore the risk factors in each tool vary to take account of the particular issues associated with either a speciality such as intensive care or a particular care setting such as community (Table 25.3).

Although risk assessment tools cannot replace clinical assessment, they do provide a structure for recording the factors which together determine whether the patient/client is 'at risk' or not. Once a level of risk has been identified, appropriate preventative actions are implemented (see pp. 718–719). For example, if sections are scored indicating that the patient has discoloured skin, the care plan should include regular repositioning, skin assessment and skin care. Evaluation of risk should be carried out on a regular basis determined by the patient's overall condition; in acute care this will usually be at least weekly, but may be less frequent in a care home where the resident's condition is stable (Box 25.9, p. 718). Assessment must be carried out if the patient's condition changes (deterioration/improvement) and on transfer to another care setting.

Table 25.3 Risk factors included in different pressure ulcer risk assessment tools

Risk factor	Risk assessment tool						
	Norton (Norton 1989)	Braden (Bergastrom et al 1987)	Waterlow (Waterlow 2005)	Gosnell (Gosnell 1982)	Maelor (Williams & Fonseca 1993)	Walsall (Chaloner & Franks 2000)	Andersen (McClemont et al 1992)
Physical condition	✓				✓	✓	
Mental condition	✓			✓			
Activity	✓	✓		✓	✓		
Mobility	✓	✓	✓	✓	✓	✓	✓
Continence	✓		✓	✓	✓	✓	✓
Nutrition		✓	✓	✓	✓	✓	✓
Build/weight for height			✓				
Skin condition			✓		✓	✓	✓
Age			✓				✓
Sex			✓				
Sensory perception		✓	✓				
Moisture		✓					
Friction and shear		✓					
Conscious level					✓	✓	✓
Tissue malnutrition			✓				
Major surgery			✓				✓
Medication			✓				
Carer involvement						✓	
Dehydrated							✓
Pain					✓	✓	

REFLECTIVE PRACTICE Box 25.9

Evaluating pressure ulcer risk

Which pressure ulcer risk assessment tool is used in your placement?

Student activities

- Is this tool appropriate for the patient/client group?
- Is pressure ulcer risk evaluated for all patients/clients on admission?
- How frequently is the risk re-evaluated?

[Resource: NHS Modernisation Agency 2003 Essence of care: patient-focused benchmarks for clinical governance. Online: www.modern.nhs.uk/home/key/docs/Essence%20of%20Care.pdf Available July 2006]

Pressure ulcer prevention

The prevention of pressure ulceration requires multidisciplinary working. The patient/client should, where necessary, have input from the appropriate health professional. These include:

- Nurses – assessment and evaluation of risk, positioning, holistic care, coordinating the MDT
- Tissue viability nurse – expert advice and education
- Specialist nutrition nurse, dietitian – nutritional needs (see Ch. 19)
- Physiotherapist – improving mobility
- Moving and handling coordinator – expert advice and education about correct techniques (see Ch. 18)
- Occupational therapist – providing aids to independence and increasing mobility
- Specialist continence nurse – expert advice and education (see Chs 20, 21)
- Medical staff, nurse prescribers and pharmacists – review medication.

Repositioning

Where equipment is neither available nor suitable, it is still possible to prevent pressure damage by regular manual repositioning (see Ch. 18). Even when using specialist beds and mattresses, the patient should be regularly repositioned as this serves other functions, e.g. preventing

> **CRITICAL THINKING** Box 25.10
>
> **Preventing pressure ulcers**
>
> Consider the following scenarios:
>
> - Shami has a learning disability and limited mobility. She uses a wheelchair.
> - Mick, who is fully mobile, has dementia. He sits by the TV all day and is reluctant to move around unless reminded.
>
> **Student activity**
>
> Discuss with your mentor which pressure-reduction/relieving strategies would be appropriate for Shami and Mick?

sputum retention (see Ch. 17) and providing the patient with a changing view.

The skin should be examined at regular intervals and at every repositioning for the first signs of pressure damage (see below). Repositioning schedules should be tailored to the individual and should take account of when they may need to be in a particular position, e.g. sitting upright at mealtimes. While traditionally patients are repositioned from side to side and on their back, this increases the risk as they are being placed directly onto bony prominences. A more appropriate way of repositioning is to use the 30° tilt, where the patient's weight is supported on areas of large muscle bulk such as the buttocks. If the patient/client can tolerate the prone position it should be considered, as it gives full pressure relief to the back and increases the number of positions available and therefore the body surface area used to distribute pressure.

Pressure-redistributing equipment

This may include any type of equipment that enables the patient/client to maintain their independence, e.g. specialist seating, electric bed frames, etc., but more commonly includes a wide range of pressure area care mattresses and seating. Pressure-redistributing equipment is available to help reduce susceptibility to pressure ulcers and it is important that an appropriate product is chosen to meet individual patient's needs (Box 25.10). Particular problems may arise when supplying equipment for use at home, especially if the patient sleeps in a double bed with their partner. Very few pieces of equipment are designed for this situation, with most mattresses taking up more than half the bed, leaving the carer with insufficient sleeping space; however, some do exist and must be considered. Equally, there are far fewer products for use with infants and children; most mattresses fit a standard hospital bed.

Equipment must be provided for both bed and chair. Pressure ulcer prevention is required throughout the 24 hours, as when seated there is increased risk of pressure damage as the body weight is supported on a much smaller area.

Skin assessment

Skin assessment is essential in preventing pressure damage. Key areas of the body are at greater risk of developing pressure damage because of an underlying bony prominence (Fig. 25.8, p. 720). These include the:

- Sacrum
- Heels
- Ischial tuberosities (part of pelvis that supports the body when seated)
- Trochanters (at the hip)
- Between the knees
- Elbows
- Head
- Ears.

The most common place for pressure ulcers is the sacrum (approximately 29%), with the heels as the second most common location (EPUAP 2002). There is, however, some variation; for example, in people who sit for long periods the ischial tuberosities are the most at-risk area. At-risk areas are different in babies whose head to bodyweight ratio differs from adults, making the head the most vulnerable area. Where pressure damage occurs over non-bony prominences it is usually caused by equipment, e.g. urinary catheter or oxygen mask/tubing (see Chs 17, 20).

Pressure ulcer grading

While it is estimated that 95% of all pressure ulcers are preventable, some people because of their poor general condition will develop one. Where a patient is admitted with existing pressure damage it is vital that this is clearly and comprehensively documented and, where possible, photographed.

The extent of damage is usually described as the depth of tissue damage using a grading/classification system. Several grading tools exist, the most common of which are the Stirling grading tool (Reid & Morison 1994) and the EPUAP grading tool (EPUAP 1999) (Fig. 25.9, p. 720).

Although the tools may appear straightforward, training is required to ensure reliability between users in describing the extent of damage. This is particularly so with the lesser degrees of damage where differentiating between blanching and non-blanching erythema (redness) may be difficult, and in people with darker skin. Blanching erythema is a patch of redness that resolves once the pressure is removed. Blanching refers to the test used to differentiate between this and persistent redness. Light finger pressure is applied to the reddened area. Where the microcirculation is intact the area blanches (whitens). However, if the microcirculation is damaged, the colour does not change. Non-blanching erythema is a prime warning sign of imminent skin breakdown.

Another difficulty arises when the area is covered with necrotic tissue. It is not possible to see the full extent of damage and so the area is classified as probably EPUAP grade 4. To assist with these difficulties, the EPUAP has recently proposed additional criteria for identifying the grade of damage and also to exclude damage due primarily to moisture (Defloor et al 2005). As the pressure ulcer heals, it is usual practice to refer to its original grade but designated as healing, e.g. healing grade 4.

The grading tools indicate the extent of the damage but provide little information about the appearance of

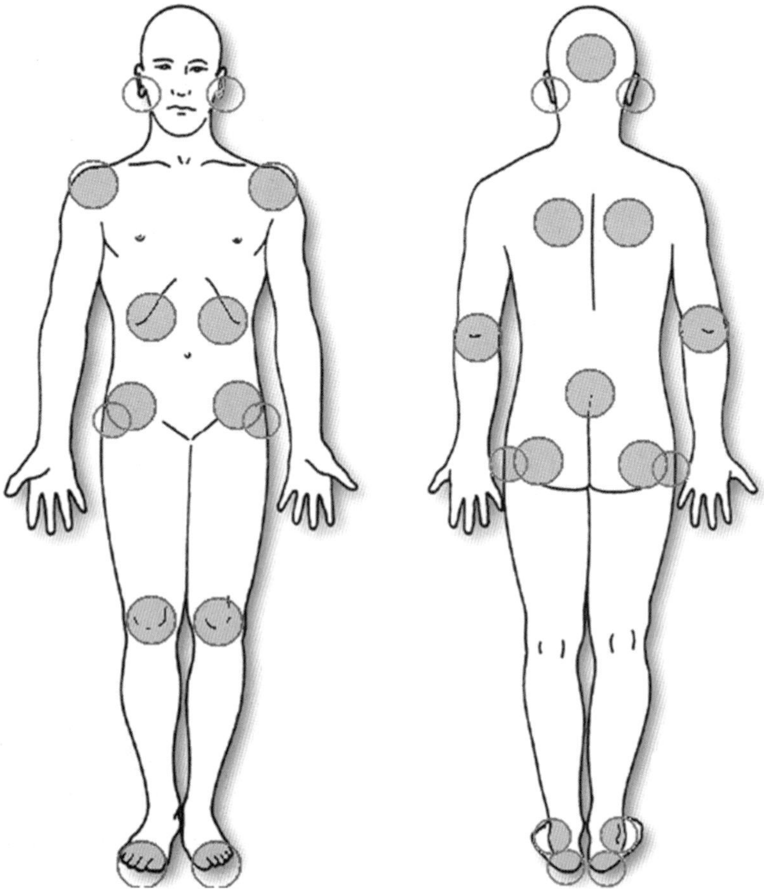

Fig. 25.8 Areas of the body most at risk from pressure damage (reproduced with permission from the European Pressure Ulcer Advisory Panel)

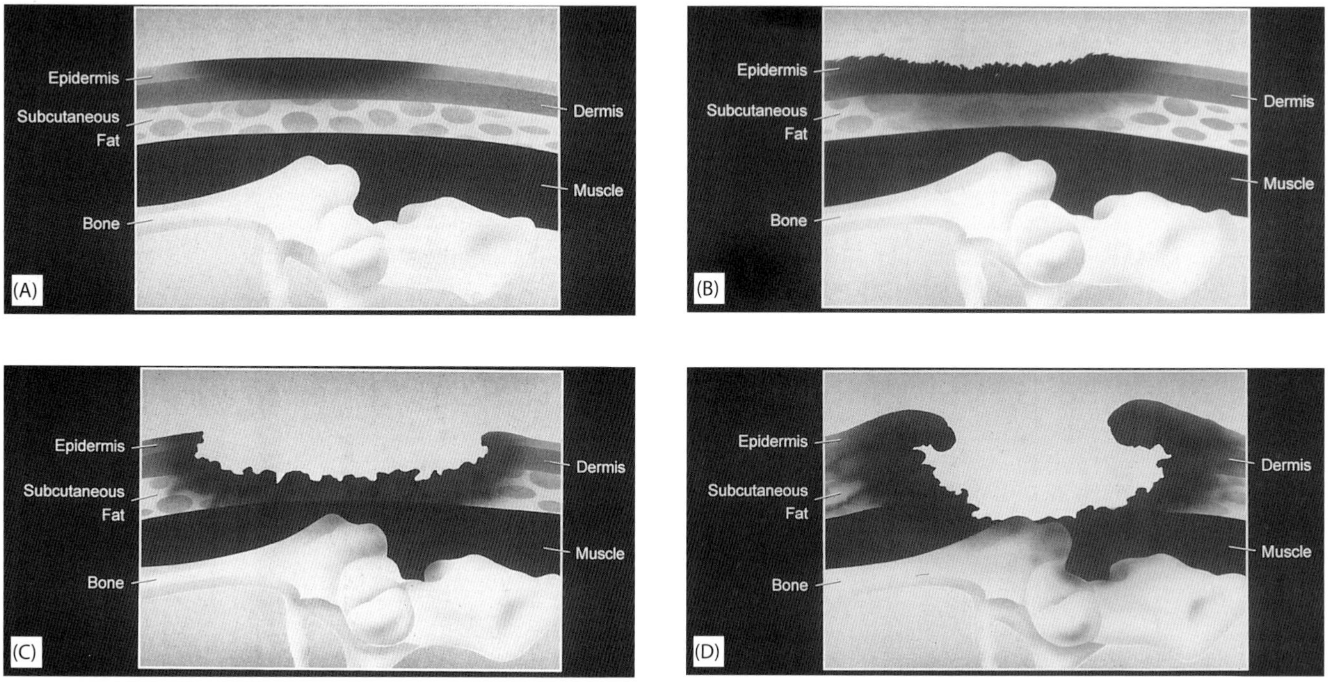

Fig. 25.9 EPUAP four-grade classification tool: **A.** Grade 1: non-blanchable erythema of intact skin. Discoloration of skin, warmth, oedema, induration (hardness) may also be used as indicators, particularly in people with darker skin. **B.** Grade 2: partial-thickness skin loss involving the epidermis or dermis, or both. The ulcer is superficial, which presents as an abrasion or blister. **C.** Grade 3: full-thickness skin loss involving damage to, or necrosis of, subcutaneous tissue that may extend down to, but not through, the underlying fascia. **D.** Grade 4: extensive destruction, tissue necrosis or damage to muscle, bone or supporting structures with or without full-thickness skin loss (reproduced with permission from Huntleigh Healthcare)

the pressure ulcer and therefore cannot be used alone to set care objectives or to describe the wound. A thorough description should be supported by holistic wound assessment including a photograph (see pp. 708–712). Pressure ulcer management follows the wound care guidelines and dressing selection outlined above (see pp. 712–716) but with the additional objective of relieving pressure (Box 25.11).

EVIDENCE-BASED PRACTICE Box 25.11

Management of pressure ulcers

NICE (2003, 2005) has evidence-based guidelines which summarize the evidence supporting assessment and holistic management of pressure ulcers.

General findings and recommendations

1. Patients with grade 1 pressure ulcers are at significant risk of developing more severe ulcers and should receive interventions to prevent deterioration.
2. The most benefit for patients with pressure ulcers is likely to be achieved with a multi-interventional interdisciplinary approach which includes:
   - Local wound management using modern or advanced dressings and other technologies
   - Pressure-relieving support surfaces such as beds, mattresses, overlays or cushions
   - Repositioning the person
   - Treatment of concurrent conditions, which may delay healing.
3. All grade 2 and above pressure ulcers should be documented as a clinical incident and the circumstances thoroughly investigated.

Student activities

- How are pressure ulcers recorded in your placement?
- Does your clinical area have a guideline for pressure-relieving equipment selection?
- Do local guidelines include how to identify grade 1 pressure ulceration?

Leg ulcers

Leg ulcers are a huge economic burden on NHS budgets. It is estimated that 1–2% of the UK population will experience a leg ulcer at some time, with the higher figure more likely in older people. Seventy percent of leg ulcers have a venous aetiology, arterial disease accounts for 8–10%, some have a mixed venous and arterial cause (10–15%) and others are secondary to other diseases (2–5%), (Günnewicht & Dunford 2004). As nurses in the community usually manage venous leg ulcers, the emphasis here is on the principles of managing venous leg ulcers. Readers requiring more information should consult Further reading suggestions (e.g. Morison et al 2006). The management of venous leg ulcers entails increasingly sophisticated care pathways involving the MDT and improved wound care products and bandaging techniques. Importantly, the impact of leg ulceration on quality of life is well recognized.

Causation of venous leg ulceration

It is important to understand how venous leg ulceration occurs in order to carry out assessment and make safe and effective clinical decisions.

Blood returning to the heart in the leg veins is aided by the pressure changes occurring in the abdomen and thorax during respiration ('respiratory pump') and by muscle contraction in the lower limbs ('calf muscle pump'). The legs contain deep (high pressure) veins and superficial (low pressure) veins connected by perforating veins (Fig. 25.10A). Some blood returns to the heart through superficial veins but most drains from the superficial to the deep veins through the perforating veins and on to the heart. The calf and foot 'pumps' squeeze blood along the veins. The lining of the limb veins is modified to form valves which allow flow in one direction only and normally prevent backflow and pooling of blood in the legs.

The valves can be damaged by trauma or surgery, and by deep vein thrombosis (DVT) (see Chs 17, 24). Once the valve is damaged, it malfunctions and backflow occurs (Fig. 25.10B). Backflow between the high and low pressure veins results in increased blood volume in the

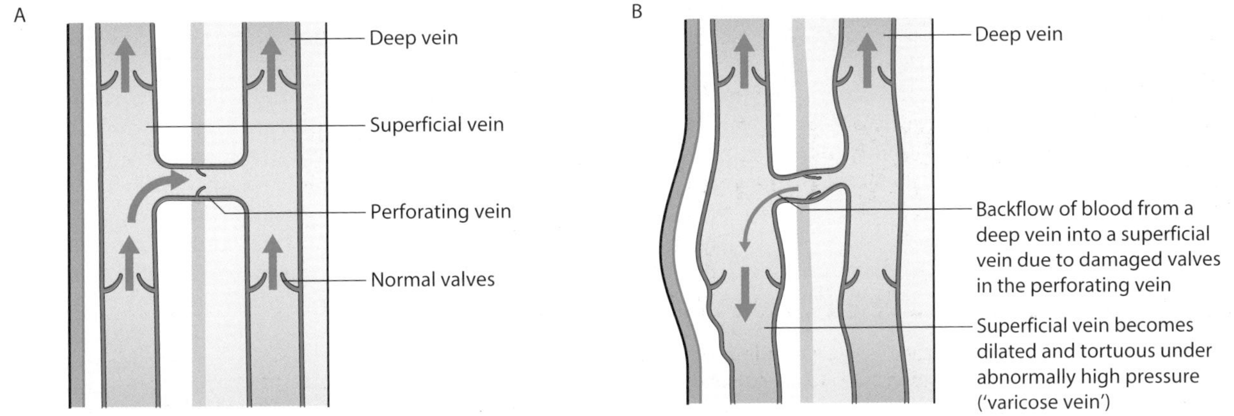

Fig. 25.10 A. Deep, superficial and perforating veins of the leg. **B.** Valve damage and backflow (reproduced with permission from Bale & Jones 1997)

leg and increased pressure in the thin-walled superficial veins; this is called venous hypertension. Further stretching of the vein and valve occurs, and if backflow continues, signs and symptoms of venous insufficiency and ulceration develop.

Characteristics of venous ulceration

The physical characteristics and symptoms of venous ulceration are outlined in Box 25.12; Figure 25.11 shows a 'typical' venous ulcer. However, it is very important to remember that ulcer appearance can vary significantly and it is impossible to determine ulcer aetiology on appearance alone.

Specific assessment

Assessment and documentation are vital in identifying the factors contributing to the ulcer; knowledge of underlying aetiology leads to safer management decisions.

The physical characteristics outlined in Box 25.12 are associated with venous disease and are important to consider during assessment. Their presence indicates risk of ulceration through trauma, however trivial.

The assessment of a person with a leg ulcer must take account of factors influencing healing and general wound assessment, including description, wound measurement and photography, etc. (see pp. 708–712). In addition, specific factors include:

- History of venous or arterial disease
- Existing medical conditions and medication which may influence wound healing
- Family history of venous disease
- History of current ulcer, any previous ulceration and treatment(s)
- Members of the MDT involved in the care of the patient/client and the outcomes of any investigation or intervention
- Lifestyle factors, e.g. mobility, and activities such as standing for long periods or sleeping in a chair. This provides valuable information about action of the calf muscle pump and the likely pattern of oedema
- Nutritional assessment (see Ch. 19)
- Health beliefs – repeated episodes of leg ulceration are often associated with reduced quality of life. Understanding the patient's/client's perception

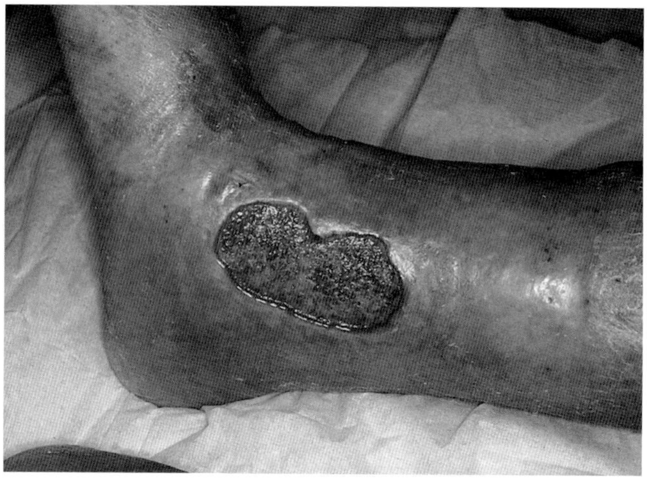

Fig. 25.11 Venous leg ulcer (reproduced with permission from Brooker & Nicol 2003)

Box 25.12 Physical characteristics of venous ulceration

- Usual location – gaiter area of the leg (ankle/lower calf), commonly above the medial malleolus
- Appearance – shallow with ill-defined edges, often quite widespread
- High exudate level
- Aching legs due to oedema
- Oedema – excess fluid in the subcutaneous tissues around the foot and ankle. Caused by increased capillary pressure, stretching and increased permeability of the capillary walls. Elevating the feet higher than the hips reduces oedema because venous pressure reduces and gravity helps blood flow back to the heart
- Ankle flare – increased capillary pressure resulting from venous hypertension means that capillaries are visible through the skin as red, broken vessels (Moffatt & Harper 1997)
- Brown staining of the skin – red blood cells leak from the capillaries and staining results from a pigment (haemosiderin) released when the red cells disintegrate
- Varicose veins occur when the valves fail. There is backflow of blood from the deep veins and high-pressure blood enters the superficial veins, which are stretched and damaged. The vein becomes dilated and tortuous and is visible through the skin. The 'varicose' vein can be felt (palpated) and will often be tender or painful to touch, particularly after standing for a while
- Local skin changes:
  - dry, flaky skin due to reduced cell turnover and lack of natural 'moisturization' as congestion reduces the nutrients reaching the cells
  - hypersensitivity and inflammation caused by exudate
  - itching caused by dryness and inflammation; scratching can then lead to breaks in the skin and increased risk of infection
  - skin hardening (lipodermatosclerosis) – the skin loses elasticity, taking on a hard 'woody' appearance and feel. It also leaves tissue very vulnerable to trauma (Morison et al 1999).

of their ulcer is vital for partnership working. Involvement of the patient/client as a partner in care (concordance) is much more likely where there are agreed goals and treatment strategies (Edwards 2003).

Once comprehensive knowledge is available, decisions can be made about further investigations that may be required. These include:

- Urinalysis to exclude undiagnosed diabetes and protein loss in the urine, etc.
- Blood tests – full blood count (FBC) used to detect anaemia or infection; a raised erythrocyte sedimentation rate (ESR) may indicate inflammation or infection and blood glucose testing will confirm diabetes
- Skin tests for hypersensitivity or allergy.

A vascular assessment using Doppler ultrasound is undertaken by an experienced nurse who has had specialist training to determine the type of ulcer involved.

CRITICAL THINKING Box 25.13

ABPI measurement

The district nurse visits Winnie at home to measure her ABPI as part of a holistic assessment of an ulcer on her right leg. Winnie's ABPI measurement is:

Right leg 135/150 = 0.9 (indicates some problems with arterial blood supply)
Left leg 150/150 = 1.0 (indicates normal arterial blood supply)

The nurse explains the result, provides information and discusses the possible use of compression therapy with Winnie.

Student activities

- Find out how the ABPI is measured and ask if you can observe a measurement.
- What is the normal range for ABPI?

Doppler ultrasound is used to determine the arterial blood flow to the lower limb. The blood pressure (BP) is measured in the arms and compared to the BP at the ankles. The comparison between the arm and the ankle pressures gives a ratio, or index – the ankle brachial pressure index (ABPI):

Ankle systolic BP/Brachial systolic BP = ABPI

For example, an ABPI of 1 means that 100% of blood is reaching the lower leg and there is unlikely to be arterial disease (unless the rest of the assessment indicates otherwise); an ABPI of 0.85 indicates that arterial disease exists and only 85% of blood is reaching the lower leg (Box 25.13). It is vitally important to exclude arterial disease before treating venous ulceration with compression therapy, which compresses both veins and arteries. If arterial disease is present, compression will further reduce tissue oxygenation, leading to serious limb damage, amputation or even death.

The equipment needed for ABPI measurement using a hand-held Doppler is shown in Figure 25.12.

Management of venous leg ulcers

The aim of management is, where possible, to restore valve function in the veins to allow ulcer healing. It is also to protect the skin from further damage and manage venous hypertension. This will include:

- Holistic assessment and determination of ulcer type (see above)
- Measures to reduce the effects of high superficial venous pressure
- Improving venous return to the heart by encouraging ankle movement/calf muscle contraction
- Ensuring concordance with treatment by partnership between nurse and patient/client (Box 25.14, p. 724)
- Preventing complications.

Compression therapy

Compression therapy is generally used for uncomplicated venous ulcers where the ABPI is ≥ 0.8. This can be

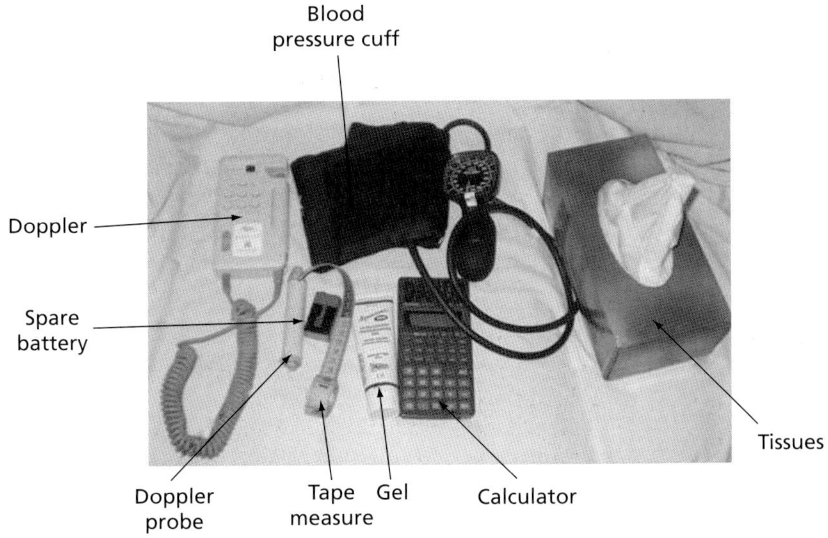

Fig. 25.12 Equipment for hand-held Doppler

applied by bandaging or compression hosiery once the ulcer is healed. A qualified nurse who has received additional training applies compression bandaging.

The veins are compressed to prevent/reduce backflow, thus reducing congestion in the leg and pressure in the superficial veins. Compression also enhances the action of the calf muscle pump, which squeezes the deep leg veins. The effects of this will be less oedema and increased comfort for the patient/client. Improvement in the circulation should allow the ulcer to heal and skin condition to improve. The precise pressures required to achieve these effects are unknown. Currently in the UK there is an approximate value of 40 mmHg; however, this will vary according to the circumference of the limb and the material used. The consensus is that some compression is better than none and it is what the patient/client will tolerate, the consistency in application and the wearing of compression bandaging/hosiery that really help healing.

EVIDENCE-BASED PRACTICE Box 25.14

Reasons for non-concordance with compression therapy

In a small study, Edwards (2003) found 'that patients did not have a clear understanding of their condition or treatment regimens. Concurrent problems associated with compression bandaging adversely affected patients' lifestyles and contributed to non-compliance.'

Student activities

Think about a patient with a leg ulcer.

- How well did they understand the cause of their leg ulcer and why compression therapy was used?
- How did compression therapy impact on their lifestyle?

[Resource: Moffatt CJ 2004 Factors that affect concordance with compression therapy. Journal of Wound Care 13(7):291–294]

Compression therapy must always include protection of the limb with a layer of padding. This helps to protect bony prominences such as the malleoli. The effectiveness of compression relies on a uniform pressure around the leg, with the pressure graduating from the ankle to the knee. The limb is not completely round so evenness can be difficult to achieve. Padding can help to distribute pressure evenly (Moffatt & Harper 1997).

The highest pressure is required at the ankle as it is furthest away from the heart with less pressure required at the knee. If the compression bandage is applied at an even pressure the shape of the limb (narrower at the ankle than the calf) ensures the pressure is graduated. If necessary, padding can be used to create a smaller ankle diameter in relation to the calf. The crucial point is that the application technique must be precise and consistent and always in accordance with manufacturer's instructions; as these vary, it must be checked before application.

Compression therapy includes:

- *Elastic systems*: These bandages apply pressure to the leg constantly and as the calf muscle changes shape the bandage resists this change to enhance the effect of the calf muscle pump. Elastic systems include long stretch, high compression bandages and multilayer systems ('4-layer')
- *Inelastic systems*: Short stretch bandages that form a rigid tube around the leg, applying low pressure when the leg is still. As the calf muscle changes shape it 'bounces' off the bandage, which redirects the force into the calf muscle. This system has a low resting pressure and a high working pressure. Some patients may find this more comfortable, particularly at night
- *Compression hosiery*: This is used after an ulcer is healed to treat venous hypertension and to reduce the risk of recurrence (Box 25.15). Sometimes it is possible to use hosiery for active ulceration if bulky dressings, which make application difficult, are not being used. Hosiery is available as below- or

HEALTH PROMOTION Box 25.15

Reducing recurrence of venous leg ulcers

Compression hosiery

- Wear hosiery as instructed
- Avoid damaging the skin when applying/removing hosiery
- Replace hosiery every 6 months.

Skin care (see Ch. 16)

- Wash legs in warm water
- Apply emollients after washing
- Pay special attention to toenails and foot care
- Visit the podiatrist as necessary.

Exercise

- Walk as much as possible and avoid standing
- Exercise toes/ankles several times an hour, even when resting
- Avoid sitting with legs crossed.

Elevation

- Position legs at heart level, e.g. lying on the bed with feet on a pillow.

Student activity

Access the article by Brooks et al (2004) and consider how the findings could be used to improve concordance with one of the aspects listed above.

[Adapted from Flanagan & Fletcher (2003)]

[Resource: Brooks J, Ersser SJ, Lloyd A, Ryan TJ 2004 Nurse-led education sets out to improve patient concordance and prevent recurrence of leg ulcers. Journal of Wound Care 13(3):111–116]

above-knee stockings and tights, but only stockings are provided on prescription in the UK. Hosiery must be properly fitted after careful measurement for the correct size. Measuring aids are available from hosiery manufacturers.

Hosiery items are classified by the pressure they deliver: Class I (14–17 mmHg), Class II (18–24 mmHg) and Class III (25–35 mmHg) (Moffatt & Harper 1997). Class III can be difficult to apply even for relatively young and able people. It can be helpful to apply two stockings of a lower class to reach the desired pressure to make application easier. There are aids available to help with application but most have to be purchased by the patient.

Summary

- While nurses have a pivotal role in the support and management of people with wounds, appropriate holistic care and management depend upon interdisciplinary working.
- Effective evidence-based care requires an understanding of wound type and aetiology.
- Knowledge of the physiology of wound healing underpins wound assessment.
- Management of the underlying condition with pressure relief, compression therapy, surgery and good nutrition are key aspects of wound management.
- Ongoing education/updating in tissue viability is both an organizational and an individual professional responsibility.

Self test

1. Give two examples of:
   a. Acute wounds
   b. Chronic wounds
2. List the stages of wound healing in chronological order.
3. What are the signs of inflammation?
4. Cold cleansing solutions can delay healing. True or false?
5. Which wound characteristics are considered during holistic assessment?
6. What criteria are used to select wound dressings?
7. Name three pressure ulcer risk assessment tools.
8. How does compression therapy help venous leg ulcers to heal?

Key words and phrases for literature searching

Dressing(s)	Pressure ulcer/sore
Healing	Tissue viability
Leg ulcer	Wound(s)

Useful websites

European Pressure Ulcer Advisory Panel	www.epuap.org Available July 2006
Leg Ulcer Forum	www.legulcerforum.org Available July 2006
Surgical Materials Testing Laboratory	www.smtl.co.uk Available July 2006
Tissue Viability Nurses Association	www.tvna.org Available July 2006
Wound Care Society	www.woundcaresociety.org Available July 2006

References

Bale S, Jones V 1997 Wound care nursing. A patient-centred approach. Baillière Tindall, London

Bergastrom N, Braden BJ, Laguzza A, Holman V 1987 The Braden scale for predicting pressure sore risk. Nursing Research 36(4):205–210

Brooker C, Nicol M (eds) Nursing adults. The practice of caring. Mosby, Edinburgh

Chaloner DM, Franks PJ 2000 Validity of the Walsall community pressure sore risk calculator. British Journal of Community Nursing 5(6):266–276

Defloor T, Schoonhoven L, Fletcher J et al 2005 Statement of the European Pressure Ulcer Advisory Panel. Pressure ulcer classification: differentiating between pressure ulcers and moisture lesions. Journal of Wound, Ostomy and Continence Nursing 32(5):302–306

Edwards LM 2003 Why patients do not comply with compression bandaging. British Journal of Nursing 12(11):S5–S16 Tissue Viability Supplement

EPUAP 1999 Pressure ulcer treatment guidelines. EPUAP, Oxford. Online: www.epuap.org/gltreatment.html Available July 2006

EPUAP 2002 Summary report on the prevalence of pressure ulcers. EPUAP Review 4(2). Online: www.epuap.org/review4_2/index.html Available July 2006

EPUAP 2003 Nutritional guidelines for pressure ulcer prevention and treatment. EPUAP, Oxford

Flanagan M 1997 Wound management. Churchill Livingstone, Edinburgh

Flanagan M, Fletcher J 2003 Tissue viability: managing chronic wounds. In: Brooker C, Nicol M (eds) Nursing adults. The practice of caring. Mosby, Edinburgh

Fletcher J 2002 Exudate theory and the clinical management of exuding wounds. Professional Nurse 17(8):475–478

Gosnell D 1982 Pressure sore risk assessment: a critique. The Gosnell scale, Part 1. Decubitus 2(3):32–38

Günnewicht B, Dunford C 2004 Fundamental aspects of tissue viability nursing. Quay Books, London

Keicolt-Glaser JK, Marucha PT, Malarkey WB et al 1995 Slowing of wound healing by psychological stress. Lancet 346(8984):1194–1196

Leaper DJ, Harding KG (eds) 1998 Wounds: biology and management. Oxford University Press, Oxford

McClemont E, Woodcock N, Oliver S et al 1992 The Lincoln experience – Part 1. Journal of Tissue Viability 2(4):114–118

Moffatt C, Harper P 1997 Leg ulcers. Churchill Livingstone, Edinburgh

Morison M, Moffatt C, Bridel-Nixon J, Bale S 1999 Nursing management of chronic wounds. 2nd edn. Mosby, London

National Institute for Clinical Excellence [now the National Institute for Health and Clinical Excellence; NICE] 2003 The use of pressure-relieving devices (beds mattresses and overlays) for the prevention of pressure ulcers in primary and secondary care. Online: www.nice.org.uk/pdf/PRD_Fullguideline.pdf Available July 2006

National Institute for Health and Clinical Excellence (NICE) 2005 Pressure ulcers: the management of pressure ulcers in primary and secondary care. Online: www.nice.org.uk/page.aspx?o=CG029 Available July 2006

Norman D 2004 The effects of age-related skin changes on wound healing rates. Journal of Wound Care 13(5):199–204

Norton D 1989 Calculating the risk. Reflections on the Norton scale. Decubitus 2(3):24–31

Reid J, Morison M 1994 Towards a consensus: classification of pressure sores. Journal of Wound Care 3(3):157–160

Singhal A, Reis ED, Kerstein MD 2001 Options for non-surgical debridement of necrotic wounds. Advances in Skin and Wound Care 14:96–103

Thomas S, Jones M, Shutler S, Jones S 1996 Using larvae in modern wound management. Journal of Wound Care 5(2):60–69

Waterlow J 2005 Pressure ulcer prevention manual. Waterlow, Taunton

Williams C, Fonseca J 1993 Evaluation of the Medley Score. Part 1: the study plan. In: Proceedings of the 3rd European Conference on Advances in Wound Management, Harrogate 19–22 October

World Union of Wound Healing Societies 2004 Principles of best practice: minimising pain at wound dressing – related procedures. MEP, London

Further reading

Bale S, Jones V 2006 Wound care nursing. A patient-centred approach. 2nd edn. Mosby, Edinburgh

Morgan DA 2004 Formulary of wound management products. 9th edn. Euromed Communications, Haslemere. Online: www.euromed.uk.com/formulary.htm Available July 2006

Morison MJ, Ovington LG, Wilke K 2004 Chronic wound care. A problem-based learning approach. Mosby, Edinburgh

Morison MJ, Moffatt C, Franks P 2006 Leg ulcers. A problem-based learning approach. Mosby, Edinburgh

NHS Quality Improvement Scotland 2005 Best practice statement: pressure ulcer prevention. Online: www.nhshealthquality.org./nhsqis/qis_display_home.jsp;jsessionid=D0C3FE2356207E2E980186B8D453C740?p_applic=CCC&p_service=Content.show&pContentID=43& Available July 2006

Answers to self tests

Appendix

Chapter 1

1. The WHO (1946) definition of health states 'health is a state of complete physical, mental and social well-being and not merely the absence of disease or infirmity.'
   Multidimensional refers to the inter-related and holistic nature of health comprising six dimensions – physical, mental, emotional, spiritual, social and societal.
2. Key determinants of health include core factors, e.g. age, sex and ethnicity; others include lifestyle, living and working conditions, community and environmental issues as well as the sociopolitical climate. The greatest determinants of health are poverty and inequality.
3. Absolute poverty is the inability to meet basic biological needs such as food, warmth and shelter. Relative poverty is usually defined in comparison with a country's average living standards.
4. Ancient health beliefs still expressed today centre on moral behaviour causing ill-health, miasma issues related to damp atmosphere and cleanliness and the increasing popularity of non-Western beliefs such as those underpinning complementary therapies.
5. Health promotion and health education approaches are similar, both using top-down and bottom-up approaches:
   a. Health promotion approaches are medical, educational, behavioural change, client-centred and societal
   b. Health education approaches are medical, educational, media/propaganda, community development and political action.

Chapter 2

1. See page 38.
2. See page 44.
3. See page 41.
4. 1919.
5. See page 48.
6. See Box 2.7.
7. See page 67.

Chapter 3

1. 1948.
2. Disease, idleness, ignorance, squalor and want.
3. See page 72.
4. See page 79.
5. See pages 87–88.
6. For example, clinical governance, ICPs, benchmarking, clinical guidelines, Healthcare Commission, National Patient Surveys, etc.

Chapter 4

1. a.
2. d.
3. d.
4. b.
5. b.
6. a.

Chapter 5

1. Possibly based on those offered in Box 5.1 (p. 124), which should make reference to: making decisions and/or solving clinical problems; searching the literature for examples of current, best available, systematic research evidence; evaluating/critically appraising the evidence; make conscientious, explicit and judicious use of the evidence as it pertains to a particular situation; and integrating the evidence with individual clinical experience.
2. Questioning practice, refining question, finding the evidence, appraising the evidence, using the evidence, and evaluating practice/audit changes.
3. RCTs, systematic reviews, qualitative research, expert opinion and guidelines.
4. AMED (Allied and Alternative Medicine), BNI (British Nursing Index), CINAHL (Cumulative Index of Nursing and Allied Health Literature), Cochrane Library and MEDLINE.
5. PICO is an acronym to help structure a search question. P = Patient or population, I = Intervention, C = Comparison, O = Outcome.
6. To facilitate an understanding of research evidence, to improve the quality of practice through use of good quality evidence, to identify the credibility and value of evidence.
7. Qualitative research seeks to explore subjective narratives to gain an insight into experiences and perceptions of phenomena; quantitative research seeks to measure phenomena and applies control to a study.
8. RCTs, qualitative, survey and systematic review.

Chapter 6

1. See pages 148–149.
2. See pages 150–151.
3. See pages 155–156.
4. Employer, professional, civil courts, criminal courts.
5. d.
6. See pages 160–161.

Chapter 7

1. The Nursing and Midwifery Council:
   - Regulates preparation for practice of nursing students
   - Stipulates criteria for registration as qualified practitioners
   - Maintains a register of practitioners
   - Supervises post-registration practice of practitioners via periodic re-registration
   - Investigates allegations against practitioners of misconduct or unfitness to practice
   - Takes appropriate action if allegations of misconduct or unfitness to practice are upheld
   - Provides advice for nurses in relation to standards of professional practice.
2. *The code of professional conduct: standards for conduct, performance and ethics* (NMC 2004).
3. *An NMC guide for students of nursing and midwifery* (NMC 2002b).
4. The purpose is to:
   - Inform the professions (nursing and midwifery) of the standard of professional conduct required of them in the exercise of their professional accountability and practice.
   - Inform the public, other professions and employers of the standard of professional conduct that they can expect of a registered practitioner.
5. a. Ethics: a formal identification of values, attitudes, beliefs and behaviours that a society or culture considers necessary for its moral functioning.
   b. Morals: behaviours considered commensurate with the ethics of a society or culture.
6. a. Non-maleficence: the ethical principle that individuals should not harm others.
   b. Beneficence: the ethical principle that individuals should do good to others.
   c. Autonomy: the ethical principle that individuals should make their own decisions about their lives.
   d. Respect for persons: the ethical principle that all individuals should be accorded respect, i.e. due regard and consideration.
   e. Justice: the ethical principle that individuals have rights, e.g. dignity, privacy, and that others have a duty to comply with these rights.

Chapter 8

1. i – c; ii – a; iii – b.
2. a.
3. Reconstituted family.
4. See Figure 8.3.
5. c.
6. All except e.
7. b.
8. Formal operational (Piaget).
9. From 6 months to about 3 years.
10. Stage 5: Identity versus role confusion.

Chapter 9

1. See page 224.
2. Environmental noise, pain, distress, etc.
3. See Table 9.1 (p. 227).
4. See page 237.
5. See page 231.
6. Preorientation, orientation, working, termination.
7. Intonation, emphasis, loudness, etc.

Chapter 10

1. True.
2. True.
3. False.
4. b.
5. See pages 264–265.
6. d.
7. b.

Chapter 11

1. See pages 277–278.
2. Affect, cognition, behaviour and physiology.
3. See Figure 11.1 (p. 279).
4. Alarm, resistance and exhaustion.
5. b.
6. Search for meaning, sense of mastery, enhanced self-esteem.
7. Hope, personal responsibility, education, self-advocacy, support.

Chapter 12

1. See pages 300–301.
2. See pages 309, 311.
3. General nurses, medical staff, district nurses, GPs, specialist palliative care nurses and doctors, physiotherapists, occupational therapists, psychologists, religious figures, etc.
4. See Box 12.2 and pages 301–303.
5. See pages 307–308.
6. See Box 12.15 (p. 316).

Chapter 13

1. b.
2. c.
3. c.

4. c.
5. b.
6. c.
7. d.
8. b.

Chapter 14

1. b.
2. c.
3. c.
4. a.
5. d.
6. b.
7. c.
8. d.

Chapter 15

1. Must wash hands: b, c, d, f, g; Not necessary: a, e.
2. b and d.
3. a.
4. All.
5. a.
6. Is at risk: a, c; Is not at risk: b, d.

Chapter 16

1. These can be found in the glossary.
2. A, B, C – meaning assess airway, breathing and circulation.
3. See pages 429–430.
4. See Box 16.11 (p. 432).
5. They were devised by the Department of Health to enhance aspects of patient care in which there was widespread room for improvement.
6. See pages 446–447.
7. See Box 16.28 (p.452).

Chapter 17

1. Coronary arteries.
2. b.
3. See page 480.
4. See page 486.
5. See page 471.
6. c.
7. Makes the secretions less viscous and easier to expectorate.
8. True (see p. 493).

Chapter 18

1. Assess the **T**ask, the **I**ndividual characteristics of the handlers, the **L**oad and the **E**nvironment (TILE).
2. Active exercises are initiated by the patient. Passive exercises involve the application of an external force, e.g. a piece of equipment or a physiotherapist, to initiate the movement.
3. Nurses, physiotherapists, occupational therapists, doctors and liaison nurses all work together to promote independence. Each profession brings its own skills to assist with such aspects of care as pain control, assistance with mobility, prevention of boredom and assistance in carrying out the activities of living.
4. Rest, ice, compression, elevation.

Chapter 19

1. See page 532.
2. See pages 538–539.
3. a. 42; b. 125 mL.
4. Carbohydrates, fats and proteins.
5. See page 557.
6. BMI 18.2; underweight.
7. See page 561.

Chapter 20

1. Filtration, reabsorption and secretion.
2. See Table 20.3 (pp. 578–579).
3. See Box 20.2 (p. 574).
4. Clean catch, midstream and specimen bags, or suprapubic aspiration.
5. See pages 582–583, 585, 587.
6. See pages 584–585 and Box 20.16 (p. 584).
7. See Table 20.4 (p. 586).
8. 23–26 cm, Ch 10–12.
9. Ensure that the catheter bag is securely attached to a catheter bag stand or the person's leg, making sure that the bag does not get dragged along or the tubing to become caught up or twisted.

Chapter 21

1. d.
2. c.
3. See Box 21.2 (p. 602).
4. See Table 21.1 (p. 605).
5. See Box 21.19 (p. 614).
6. See page 617.

Chapter 22

1. Two tablets.
2. Half a tablet
3. 10 mL.
4. 450 mg.
5. a. 0.9 mg; b. 0.9 mL.
6. a. True; b. True; c. True; d. False; e. False.
7. a. Intramuscular; b. Intramuscular; c. Subcutaneous.
8. 30 seconds.

Chapter 23

1. See pages 654–656, Figure 23.1 (p. 654).
2. See pages 656–657, Figure 23.3 (p. 656).
3. True.
4. See page 666, Figure 23.5D (p. 665).
5. Peripheral side-effects, e.g. constipation and dry mouth.
6. True, see Figure 23.9 (p. 671).
7. c. Disturbed sleep pattern reduces the ability to cope with pain and fatigue can open the 'pain gate'. Sleeplessness is frequently a problem in the hospital environment and for patients with chronic pain.

Chapter 24

1. See pages 683–684.
2. See page 685.
3. See page 690.
4. See page 692.
5. See page 692.
6. See page 698.
7. See pages 700–701.

Chapter 25

1. a. Surgical wound, burn.
   b. Pressure ulcer, leg ulcer.
2. Vascular response–inflammation–proliferation–maturation.
3. See page 705.
4. True.
5. Cause, size, location, exudate, condition of surrounding skin, tissue type, odour, pain.
6. See page 714.
7. See Table 25.3 (p. 718).
8. See pages 723–724.

Glossary

Accountability (Chs 2, 7) – responsibility for something or to someone that applies when someone is answerable for what they do.

Active exercises (Ch. 18) – movements initiated by an individual that exercise muscles and joints.

Acute pain (Ch. 23) – pain of brief duration commonly associated with tissue injury (nociceptive pain) which subsides as healing takes place.

Acute wound (Ch. 25) – one that heals in an uncomplicated way; usually a surgical incision or uncomplicated trauma.

Adaptation (Ch. 11) – alterations or adjustments in physiology, cognition and behaviour in response to changes in the environment. Adaptation implies that these changes improve the individual's condition in relation to the changed situation.

Adjuvant (Chs 12, 23) – additional treatment such as a drug that acts synergistically to increase the action of other drugs or therapy. Especially used to describe the use of drugs such as corticosteroids and anti-depressant therapies in the management of pain.

Adverse drug reaction (Ch. 22) – any unwanted effects of drugs.

Allopathic (Ch. 10) – practice of conventional medicine.

Alternative medicine (Ch. 10) – any medical system based on a theory of disease or method of treatment other than the conventional/orthodox science of Western medicine, e.g. complementary medicine.

Anaesthesia (Ch. 24) – loss of feeling or sensation.

Analgesics (Ch. 23) – drugs used to relieve pain.

Anuria (Ch. 20) – the absence of urinary output.

Apnoea (Chs 14, 17) – the absence of breathing.

Arousal (Ch. 11) – a state of heightened activity that includes cognitive, affective, physiological and behavioural changes.

Arrhythmia (Chs 14, 17) – an abnormal heart rhythm.

Aseptic technique (Ch. 15) – procedures that exclude pathogenic microorganisms from a particular environment, i.e. the use of sterile equipment and non-touch technique.

Asperger's syndrome (Ch. 4) – a form of autism.

Assessment tool (Ch. 14) – a validated method of eliciting specific information that can minimize risk to individuals and augment holistic assessment.

Audit (Ch. 3) – the systematic, critical analysis of the quality of care including the procedures used for diagnosis and treatment; the use of resources and the resulting outcome and quality of life for the patient. When these are carried out against clinical standards it is referred to as clinical audit.

Auscultation (Ch. 14) – listening to sounds within the body using a stethoscope.

Autism (Ch. 4) – a lifelong condition that impinges on how an individual communicates and relates to others.

Autonomy (Chs 2, 7) – the ethical principle that individuals should make their own decisions about their lives.

Bacteriuria (Ch. 20) – bacteria in the urine. Bacteriuria can be symptomatic or asymptomatic.

Beneficence (Ch. 7) – the ethical principle that individuals should do good to others.

Bereavement (Ch. 12) – the loss of somebody or something of value, especially through death.

Bibliographic database (Ch. 5) – an electronic and searchable collection of information about articles within a specific subject area.

Biological body clock (Ch. 10) – an inherent timing mechanism that controls physiological processes and is not dependent on external factors.

Biopsy (Ch. 24) – tissue removed for laboratory examination.

Biorhythm (Ch. 10) – the cyclical patterns of biological functions unique to each individual, e.g. sleep–wake cycles.

Blood pressure (Ch. 14) – the force of blood against the arterial walls which varies during the cardiac cycle. Two pressures are measured: systolic, which represents the greatest pressure in the main arteries following contraction of the left ventricle, and diastolic, which is the lowest pressure in the main arteries and occurs at the end of ventricular relaxation while the heart is at rest, before the next cardiac contraction.

Body language (Ch. 9) – that part of communication which is not reliant on words.

Bradycardia (Chs 14, 17) – a heart rate slower than that expected for age. Less than 60 beats per minute in an adult at rest.

Breathing (Ch. 17) – the mechanical process by which air moves in and out of the lung.

Burnout (Ch. 11) – a state caused by work stress in which a person feels unmotivated, tired, less able to cope and low in mood.

Cachexia (Ch. 12) – emaciation resulting from rapid weight loss, often seen in patients with gastrointestinal or lung cancers as a result of complex metabolic changes.

Cardiac arrest (Ch. 17) – the total cessation of effective output of blood from heart function.

Catheterization (Ch. 20) – insertion of a hollow tube into the bladder for the purpose of draining urine or instillation of medication into the bladder; catheterization can be urethral (via the urethra) or suprapubic (via the abdomen).

Chemotherapy (Ch. 12) – the use of anti-cancer (cytotoxic) drugs to destroy cancer cells.

Chronic pain (Ch. 23) – has a longer duration than acute pain – 3 months or more; it is further subdivided into malignant and non-malignant pain.

Chronic wound (Ch. 25) – one that has delayed healing for a variety of reasons, most commonly pressure ulcers, leg ulcers and diabetic foot ulcers.

Circadian rhythm (Ch. 10) – biological pattern based on a cycle approximately 24 hours in length.

Civil law (Ch. 6) – deals with the conduct and conflicts between people. A person (the claimant) who has suffered a perceived wrong can seek redress by bringing an action or claim in the civil courts. The claim may be settled with an award of financial compensation or damages, an order (injunction) banning an unlawful act or an order that requires some action.

Clinical governance (Ch. 3) – the system whereby NHS organizations are accountable for continuously improving the quality of services and safeguarding high standards of care by creating an environment in which clinical excellence will flourish.

Clinical nurse specialist (CNS) (Ch. 2) – a registered nurse who has acquired additional knowledge, skills and experience, who practises at an advanced level and who may have sole responsibility for a particular care episode or patient/client group.

Code of Conduct (Ch. 7) – the written expectations that the Nursing and Midwifery Council (NMC) has of registered nurses.

Colloid solution (Ch. 19) – a solution that contains particles (solutes) that stay in the blood because they are too large to pass through the capillary membrane (e.g. gelatin solutions). Used intravenously to increase blood volume.

Colonization (Ch. 15) – a state where pathogenic microorganisms reside on or in the body without causing any disease symptoms.

Commensal (Ch. 15) – a microorganism that lives in close association with its host (*see* Normal flora). Commensals may become pathogenic if the host is immunocompromised.

Communication (Ch. 9) – the exchange of information between at least two people.

Complementary therapy (Ch. 10) – the use of skills and practice alongside conventional treatments to enhance patient welfare.

Compliance (Ch. 22) – the extent to which a patient/client uses their medication in relation to their prescription.

Compression therapy (Ch. 25) – the application of graduated pressure to the lower limb to reverse venous hypertension. Usually applied using compression bandages or hosiery.

Concordance (Ch. 22) – an agreement between a patient/client and the healthcare professional that is negotiated in relation to the use of prescribed medication.

Confidentiality (Chs 6, 7) – information given on the understanding that it will not be divulged without the consent of the person who is giving the information, except under specified circumstances.

Consequentialist ethics (Ch. 7) – a theory in which the ethical focus is on the consequences of actions or inactions.

Constipation (Ch. 21) – an alteration in normal bowel movements, resulting in the less frequent and uncomfortable passage of hard stools.

Criminal law (Ch. 6) – deals with criminal offences relating to people and property and results in a prosecution, and, if the defendant is convicted, usually results in punishment (discharge, fine, community penalty or a custodial sentence).

Crystalloid solution (Ch. 19) – A clear solution that moves between the bloodstream and the tissue fluid, e.g. 0.9% sodium chloride. Used intravenously to maintain hydration and electrolyte balance.

Culture (Ch. 8) – the way in which a society or group lives their lives together.

Cyanosis (Ch. 17) – bluish hue to the colour of the skin and mucous membranes.

Débridement (Ch. 25) – removal of devitalized (dead) tissue that is adherent to the wound bed or the removal of foreign material embedded in the wound.

Dehiscence (Ch. 25) – breakdown and bursting open of a wound, usually due to wound infection.

Dehydration (Ch. 19) – the loss of water and usually with varying degrees of electrolyte imbalance. It occurs when fluid intake fails to replace fluid loss.

Demography (Ch. 1) – the study of populations, e.g. the age, gender and size of subgroups and their vital statistics.

Deontological ethics (Ch. 7) – a theory in which the ethical focus is upon duties.

Diarrhoea (Ch. 21) – a loose watery stool that occurs frequently.

Discharge planning (Ch. 14) – based on needs assessment, this aims to prevent readmission and provide seamless care to patients/clients and their families.

Disinfection (Ch. 15) – a process that reduces the number of viable microorganisms.

Dislocation (Ch. 18) – displacement of a body part, usually a bone, that affects joint movement.

Distress (Ch. 11) – bad stress (opposite of eustress), which occurs when there is excessive adaptive demand. Health may suffer in response to this type of stress.

Diurnal rhythm (Ch. 10) – biological pattern based on a daily cycle; also called circadian rhythm.

Duty of care (Ch. 6) – the professional obligation and responsibility that nurses have to a patient/client, while caring for that patient or client.

Dyslexia (Ch. 4) – involves a variety of abilities or problems that affect several aspects of learning, including reading, spelling, writing and numbers.

Dysphagia (Ch. 19) – difficulty in swallowing.

Dyspnoea (Ch. 17) – difficult or laboured breathing.

Dysuria (Ch. 20) – usually taken to mean pain on passing urine, but can also mean difficulty and/or pain in passing urine.

Elective surgery (Ch. 24) – planned surgical treatment.

Electrolyte (Ch. 19) – any substance, such as sodium chloride, which when dissolved in water dissociates into electrically charged particles called ions and will conduct electricity.

Emollient (Ch. 16) – an oil-based substance applied to soften dry skin that acts by reducing water loss through the skin surface.

Empathy (Ch. 9) – the ability of a person to put him/herself in the other person's position and attempting to understand the world as they see it.

Encopresis (Ch. 21) – the repeated involuntary or voluntary faecal soiling of clothing by a child over 4 years of age.

End-of-life care (Ch. 12) – also known as terminal care, this is care given at the very end of life, e.g. last few days or week.

Endoscopy (Ch. 24) – visualization of hollow structures and organs using an endoscope, e.g. the stomach (gastroscopy).

Enema (Ch. 21) – fluid introduced into the rectum or lower bowel to produce a bowel movement. Medication enemas for retention can also be given.

Enteral (Ch. 19) – within the gastrointestinal tract, such as enteral nutrition given orally or through a nasogastric or gastrostomy tube.

Epidemiology (Ch. 1) – the study of the occurrence, patterns and spread of disease in the population.

Epithelialization (Ch. 25) – epithelial cells move across the wound, once it is filled with granulation tissue, to resurface the wound.

Ethics (Ch. 7) – a formal identification of values, attitudes, beliefs and behaviours that a society or culture considers necessary for its moral functioning.

Eustress (Ch. 11) – good stress (opposite of distress) and focuses on the optimal level of stress needed to promote growth and health. Eustress is often seen in action when stressful events enhance performance and feelings of pleasure or achievement.

Evidence-based practice (Ch. 5) – to base practice on the best available evidence in order to ensure the best quality care is delivered to patients and/or populations.

Exudate (Ch. 25) – fluid produced from the wound.

Faecal incontinence (Ch. 21) – the leaking of faecal fluid from the bowel.

Family (Ch. 8) – a group of related individuals who live in close proximity and share resources.

First aid (Ch. 13) – the initial treatment given in an emergency situation, with the aim of saving life, before the arrival of an appropriately qualified healthcare professional.

Flatus (Ch. 21) – an accumulation of gas in the bowel causing discomfort due to stretching of the bowel wall.

Flexibility (Ch. 18) – range of normal movements available at a joint.

Fomite (Ch. 15) – any non-living object that can spread infection.

Fracture (Ch. 18) – break in the continuity of bone.

Free-text term (Ch. 5) – words that describe an idea. These may include alternative spellings (including Americanisms), plurals, synonyms and abbreviations.

Frequency (Ch. 20) – the need to pass urine more often than is acceptable to the person. It can be a symptom of urinary tract infection.

Gate control theory (Ch. 23) – proposes that active processing occurs at the dorsal horn of the spinal cord, where the pain sensation first enters the central nervous system (CNS). The dorsal horn gate is opened or closed depending on the combination of sensory ascending inputs from the periphery or descending signals from the brain. Thus pain will only be appreciated if the gate is open.

Glasgow Coma Scale (GCS) (Ch. 16) – a scale use to assess level of consciousness.

Granulation (Ch. 25) – the formation of new capillaries and the growth of new, healthy, moist, red tissue in the wound bed.

Grief (Ch. 12) – describes the emotional reaction to loss or death.

Haematuria (Ch. 20) – blood in the urine.

Harm reduction (Ch. 13) – any intervention that reduces the likelihood of injury or impairment occurring to an individual.

Hazards of immobility (Ch. 18) – predictable problems that arise when mobility is restricted, e.g. pressure ulcers.

Health determinant (Ch. 1) – a factor that influences or determines health, e.g. poverty.

Health education (Ch. 1) – communication activity aimed at enhancing positive health and preventing or diminishing ill-health.

Health promotion (Ch. 1) – the process of enabling people to increase control over, and to improve, their health.

Healthcare (Ch. 3) – the systems and the professionals who help maintain, attain and regain good health and prevent illness.

Healthcare-associated infection (Ch. 15) – an infection that does not show any evidence of being present, or incubating, at the time of admission to hospital but is acquired as a result of a hospital stay.

Hierarchy of evidence (Ch. 5) – a ranked structure of different types of evidence based on the ability of such evidence to predict effectiveness, remove bias and control confounders.

Holistic (Ch. 10) – a doctrine that considers the treatment of any subject as a whole integrated system; for example, in treatment of disease, the complete person – physically and psychologically – is considered.

Holistic assessment (Ch. 14) – a comprehensive collection of information from primary and secondary sources to assist in decision-making for planning appropriate and individualized care.

Hospice (Ch. 12) – a place where people with palliative care needs may receive specialist care and attention.

Humanism (Ch. 2) – a system of beliefs concerned with the interests, achievements, capabilities, values and worth of human beings.

Hypertension (Chs 14, 17) – blood pressure that is greater than that expected for age.

Hypervolaemia (Ch. 17) – a high circulating blood volume.

Hypodermoclysis (Ch. 19) – the administration of fluids by subcutaneous infusion.

Hypotension (Chs 14, 17) – low blood pressure that is insufficient to maintain tissue blood flow and oxygenation.

Hypothermia (Ch. 14) – core body temperature below 35.0°C.

Hypovolaemia (Ch. 17) – a low circulating blood volume.

Hypoxaemia (Ch. 17) – reduced oxygen in arterial blood.

Hypoxia (Ch. 17) – reduced oxygen level in the tissues.

Immobility (Ch. 18) – lack of movement in any muscle or group of muscles, caused by congenital disorders, trauma or disease. The loss of movement may be temporary or permanent.

Incontinence (Ch. 20) – involuntary or inappropriate passing of urine that has an impact on social functioning or hygiene.

Indexing term (Ch. 5) – a word assigned by a database producer to describe the content of an article. These words are arranged in a hierarchy from broad subject area to detailed specialism.

Infestation (Ch. 16) – invasion by a parasite that lives on a host, e.g. head lice.

Informed consent (Ch. 6) – information giving that is sensitive and informative over a period of time wherein the person may agree or disagree in making an informed decision.

Integrated care pathways (Ch. 3) – the multidisciplinary outline of anticipated care, placed in an appropriate timeframe, to help patients/clients with a specific condition, or set of symptoms, move progressively through a clinical experience to a positive outcome.

Integrated medicine (Ch. 10) – combining or adding parts to make a unified whole, e.g. the combination of conventional and complementary therapies.

Intermediate care (Ch. 3) – care given after traditional primary care and self-care, but before or instead of care that is available inside acute hospitals, such as pre-admission assessment units, early and supported discharge schemes, community hospitals.

Interpersonal skills (Ch. 9) – the skills and capabilities to engage people in communication acts.

Interprofessional working (Ch. 3) – a group of professionals working together to plan care for specific patients/clients and may include social care workers, healthcare workers and voluntary or private healthcare workers.

Intertrigo (Ch. 16) – irritation that develops between two moist skin surfaces, e.g. under the breasts, between the buttocks.

Jet lag (Ch. 10) – fatigue and interruption of the sleep–wake cycle caused by disturbance of normal body biorhythms as a result of travelling across different time zones.

Justice (Ch. 7) – the ethical principle that individuals have rights, e.g. dignity, privacy, and that others have a duty to comply with these rights.

Language (Ch. 9) – the agreed sounds, symbols and expressions used to express information, ideas and feelings.

Laxative (Ch. 21) – a medication used to stimulate or increase the frequency of bowel movements, or to aid formation of a softer, bulkier stool.

Learning (Ch. 4) – specific knowledge, skills and/or attitudes that someone has accomplished after participating in some form of instruction.

Learning outcomes (Ch. 4) – specific measurable results that are expected after participating in a learning experience. Outcomes may involve knowledge (cognitive), skills (behavioural) or attitudes (affective) that provide evidence that learning has occurred at the end of a specific learning experience.

Learning strategy (Ch. 4) – the way in which a person approaches a learning task.

Learning style (Ch. 4) – this reflects a person's typical way of thinking, remembering or problem-solving.

Learning theories (Ch. 4) – proposed explanations of how human beings learn.

Leg ulcer (Ch. 25) – wound of the lower leg related to a variety of underlying aetiologies (causes).

Listening (Ch. 9) – the visual, auditory and sometimes tactile process of perceiving language.

Literature review (Ch. 5) – the process of finding and appraising information, usually from a range of sources.

Maceration (Ch. 16) – softening of the skin caused by continual exposure to moisture.

Malnutrition (Ch. 19) – a disorder caused by dietary intake that is defective in either quantity or content, malabsorption or an inability to utilize nutrients.

Melaena (Ch. 21) – black tarry faeces, indicating the presence of partly digested blood from the upper gastrointestinal tract. It can also be due to disease such as cancer in the small intestine or upper colon.

Melatonin (Ch. 10) – hormone secreted by the pineal gland, thought to have a role in controlling daily biorhythms.

Milestone (Ch. 8) – competency usually attained at a given age, e.g. walking by 18 months.

Morals (Ch. 7) – behaviours considered to be ethically appropriate by a society or culture.

Morbidity (Ch. 1) – ill-health or disease.

Mortality (Ch. 1) – death, death rates and specialized mortality rates are explained in Chapter 1.

Motivation (Chs 4, 8) – what drives an individual and is closely related to their needs, emotions, beliefs, values and goals. The underlying causes of actions.

Moving and handling (Ch. 13) – the application of force to push, pull, lift, carry or support an inanimate object, or to support, roll, slide or move a person.

Multiagency team (Ch. 3) – practitioners from a range of different backgrounds or professions who work together with patients/clients to achieve results that could not be achieved by any one agency alone.

Multidisciplinary teams (Ch. 3) – groups of different healthcare professionals working together to plan and deliver care for patients/clients and may include nurses, doctors, physiotherapists, occupational therapists and social workers.

Nausea (Ch. 19) – a feeling of sickness that may be accompanied by sweating, pallor and excess amounts of watery saliva.

Necrosis (Ch. 25) – dead tissue caused by a lack of oxygen supply to the local area.

Negligence (Ch. 6) – an act with any element of carelessness or lack of regard resulting in injury, harm or loss. Any act or omission that falls short of a standard to be expected from 'the reasonable man'.

Neurological (Ch. 16) – of the nervous system.

Neuropathic pain (Ch. 23) – the experience of pain in the absence of any identifiable tissue damage due to abnormal processing of sensory input by the nervous system. Associated with chronic non-malignant pain.

Nociceptive pain (Ch. 23) – pain associated with tissue damage, which subsides as healing takes place.

Nocturia (Ch. 20) – waking up and needing to pass urine at night.

Non-maleficence (Ch. 7) – the ethical principle that individuals should not harm others.

Normal flora (Ch. 15) – microorganisms that colonize a host without causing disease.

Normalization (Ch. 8) – the process of becoming able to adopt the lifestyle usually expected of a member of society.

Nosocomial infection (Ch. 15) – *see* Healthcare-associated infection.

Nurse consultant (Ch. 2) – an expert practitioner who works with a specific group of patients or clients, influencing the quality of care through expert practice, professional leadership and consultancy, education, research and service development.

Nurse specialist (Ch. 12) – a nurse who works as part of a large multidisciplinary team, giving specialist advice, education and support to specific patients/clients and their carers, e.g. palliative care patients and carers, or patients/clients with a specific condition such as lung cancer or heart failure.

Nursing model (Ch. 14) – a framework to guide nurses, which is used with the nursing process to provide a unique perspective of nursing knowledge and practice.

Nursing process (Ch. 14) – a cyclical, problem-solving approach to providing nursing care that is based on the stages of assessment, planning, implementation and evaluation. Sometimes nursing diagnosis is made between assessment and planning.

Nutrition (Ch. 19) – the process of receiving and utilizing the materials needed for survival, growth and tissue repair. Alternatively, the science of food and its use by the body.

Oedema (Ch. 19) – an abnormal collection of tissue fluid within the tissues such as around the ankles and lower legs.

Oliguria (Ch. 20) – reduced urine output; includes very dilute/isotonic urine with a volume of less than 0.5 mL/kg/h.

Opportunistic infection (Ch. 15) – caused by a micro-organism that does not ordinarily cause disease but can become pathogenic under certain circumstances.

Orthopnoea (Ch. 17) – difficulty breathing when lying down.

Oxygen saturation (Ch. 17) – percentage of oxygenated haemoglobin present in the blood.

Pain modulation (Ch. 23) – inhibition of nociceptive impulses.

Pain threshold (Ch. 23) – the least or minimum experience of pain that an individual is able to recognize.

Pain tolerance (Ch. 23) – the intensity or duration of pain, and the maximum amount of pain that an individual is willing or capable of enduring.

Palliative care (Ch. 12) – 'palliative care improves the quality of life of patients and families who face life-threatening illness, by providing pain and symptom relief, spiritual and psychosocial support from diagnosis to the end of life and bereavement' (WHO 2004).

Parenteral (Ch. 19) – outside or apart from the gastro-intestinal (alimentary) tract such as parenteral nutrition given intravenously.

Passive exercises (Ch. 18) – movements of joints initiated by an external force, e.g. a physiotherapist, nurse or machinery to exercise muscles and joints.

Patient allocation (Ch. 2) – a system of workload allocation that enables nurses to be responsible for specific patients/clients rather than a series of tasks.

Peak expiratory flow rate (PEFR) (Ch. 17) – the greatest rate of airflow out of the lungs measured during a forced expiration.

Perioperative care (Ch. 24) – that given from arrival in the anaesthetic room, during a surgical intervention or operation and in the recovery area afterwards.

Person-centredness (Ch. 2) – respecting of the rights of each individual to make rational decisions and to determine their own ends, enabling them to reach their own decisions.

Pharmacology (Ch. 22) – the study of chemical substances, e.g. drugs, medications and other substances, that interact with the body.

Plaque (Ch. 16) – a sticky film of bacteria that continuously forms on the teeth and is removed by brushing.

Polypharmacy (Ch. 22) – the prescribing of four or more different medicines, which increases the risk of adverse drug reactions and readmissions after hospital discharge, and reduces compliance.

Polyuria (Ch. 20) – excretion of large volumes of dilute urine.

Positive regard (Ch. 9) – the ability to hold and convey feelings for other people that are not based on negative beliefs about the person.

Postoperative care (Ch. 24) – that given following surgery.

Preoperative care (Ch. 24) – that given before surgery.

Pressure ulcer (Ch. 25) – a wound caused as a direct result of pressure, friction, shear or any combination of these.

Primary care (Ch. 3) – care provided in the community by GPs, the practice team and associated health professionals.

Primary intention healing (Ch. 25) – occurs where there is little tissue loss and it is possible to draw the wound edges together.

Primary nursing (Ch. 2) – a system of workload allocation whereby patients/clients are allocated to the care of an individual registered nurse rather than a team of nurses. The focus is on individual, holistic care, where the participation of patients/clients and relatives is encouraged.

Professionalism (Ch. 2) – to guarantee and provide a consistently high standard of knowledge, skill and competence agreed between individuals, the professional body and society.

Proficient (Ch. 2) – possessing the skills and abilities required for legal, safe and effective professional practice without direct supervision.

Prophylactic (Ch. 24) – an agent or treatment that can prevent or reduce the incidence of a disease.

Prosthesis (Chs 16, 24) – an artificial part that replaces a missing or dysfunctional body part, e.g. an artificial eye.

Proteinuria (Ch. 20) – the presence of protein in the urine.

Psychology (Ch. 8) – the study of mental processes and behaviour.

Public health (Ch. 1) – the science and art of preventing disease, prolonging life and promoting health through the organized efforts of society.

Pulse (Ch. 14) – rhythmic expansion and relaxation of an artery caused by ejection of blood from the left ventricle during systole.

Pyrexia (Ch. 14) – elevation of core body temperature above 37.5°C.

Pyuria (Ch. 20) – the presence of white blood cells (WBCs) in the urine, indicating an inflammatory response of the urothelium (bladder lining) to bacterial invasion.

Qualitative research (Ch. 5) – an approach to research that explores experience, perceptions and subjective phenomena.

Quality assurance (Ch. 3) – planned system to provide service to an agreed standard within established resources and timescales.

Quantitative research (Ch. 5) – an approach to research that attempts to measure phenomena using objective, validated measures.

Radiotherapy (Ch. 12) – the use of high energy X-rays to destroy cancer cells, but which causes as little harm as possible to normal cells. May be used as curative or palliative treatment.

Reflection (Ch. 4) – a deliberate process of examining one's own and other people's behaviours, practices and effectiveness which leads to professional growth and greater understanding of oneself and others.

Relationships (Ch. 9) – the bond between people that maintains an effective connection.

Resident flora (Ch. 15) – *see* Normal flora.

Respect for persons (Ch. 7) – the ethical principle that all individuals should be accorded respect, i.e. regard and consideration.

Rest (Ch. 10) – relaxation from exertion or labour, relief from worry or something troublesome.

Retention (Ch. 20) – inability to pass urine; can be caused by urethral obstruction or the inability to contract the bladder.

Risk assessment (Ch. 13) – the first stage of risk management that helps to identify the hazards to people's health.

Risk management (Ch. 13) – the whole process of identifying potential hazards and putting systems in place to decrease the likelihood of harm occurring.

Roles (Ch. 8) – behaviour expected of people in their varying social capacities.

Search strategy (Ch. 5) – the terms used to search a bibliographic database for a particular subject area.

Secondary care (Ch. 3) – hospital-based healthcare services: inpatient, outpatient and emergency care.

Secondary intention healing (Ch. 25) – occurs where there is loss of tissue and it is not possible or desirable to draw the wound edges together. The wound fills from the base with granulation tissue.

Self-awareness (Ch. 9) – exploration of thoughts, feelings and behaviours, including an understanding of how internal and external events influence people and how they behave.

Shift work (Ch. 10) – system of employment where an individual's normal hours of work are in part outside the period accepted as the normal working day, i.e. '9 to 5'.

Skin flora (Chs 15, 16) – the community of micro-organisms that colonizes the skin.

Sleep (Ch. 10) – an altered state of consciousness occurring naturally in humans in a 24-hour biological rhythm.

Sleep disorder (Ch. 10) – change in normal sleep pattern or rhythm.

Slough (Ch. 25) – creamy yellow soft tissue comprising cellular debris, which rises to the surface of the wound.

Social care (Ch. 3) – a wide range of services provided by local authorities and the independent sector. Social care includes care at home for older people and for people with disabilities, care in day centres, residential or nursing homes as well as fostering services.

Social services (Ch. 3) – personal social services include social care and social work carried out through local authority Social Services Departments and other statutory, private and voluntary agencies.

Socialization (Ch. 8) – the process by which a culture is transmitted from one generation to another, ensuring its continuity, e.g. the survival of its language, knowledge and way of life.

Sociology (Ch. 8) – the study of societies, their component groups and individual interactions.

Sprain (Ch. 18) – damage to the supporting ligaments surrounding a joint.

Sputum (Ch. 17) – mucus and other material coughed up (expectorated) from the lower respiratory tract.

Standard precautions (Ch. 13) – set of practice guidelines for infection control and precautions used to prevent contact with body fluids, secretions, non-intact skin and mucous membranes.

Statutory bodies (Ch. 1) – agencies such as Strategic Health Authorities, duty-bound by law to undertake health work on behalf of government.

Sterilization (Ch. 15) – a process that renders an item sterile by eliminating all living microorganisms including bacterial spores.

Stoma (Ch. 21) – an artificial opening where the bowel is brought to the surface of the abdominal wall, e.g. a colostomy.

Stool (Ch. 21) – faeces which is passed from the anus.

Strain (Ch. 18) – overexertion of a muscle.

Stress (Ch. 11) – a reactive state to demands or potential demands made on the adaptive capacities of the mind and body.

Stressor (Ch. 11) – a physical or psychological event that produces stress (positive or negative).

Suppository (Ch. 21) – medication in a solid base that melts at body temperature. Inserted into the rectum to either produce a bowel movement or deliver medication, e.g. analgesics.

Symptom management (Ch. 12) – management of any physical, psychological or social occurrence or event that causes notable concern to a patient.

Tachycardia (Chs 14, 17) – a heart rate at rest that is greater than that expected for age. In the adult this is in excess of 100 beats per minute.

Task allocation (Ch. 2) – also known as functional nursing, this is a mechanistic approach to the delivery of nursing care, where completing tasks and maintaining the ward routine takes precedence over the needs of individual patients/clients.

Team nursing (Ch. 2) – a group of registered and untrained nurses working together to provide individual care to a specific group of patients.

Terminal care (Ch. 12) – *see* End-of-life care.

Tertiary care (Ch. 3) – hospital care for a patient with an unusual condition, or needing highly specialized treatments in a specialist centre such as a teaching hospital or regional centre.

Tissue viability (Ch. 25) – prevention of tissue damage and maintenance of tissue in a healthy state.

Transient flora (Ch. 15) – microorganisms that are present on a host for a short time without causing disease.

Trespass against the person (Ch. 6) – any interference with the person's bodily integrity and liberty, it includes assault and battery.

Values (Ch. 9) – those concepts that a person holds dear and are deeply important to them.

Vicarious liability (Ch. 6) – describes an employer's liability for the wrongful acts and omissions of an employee during the course of their employment.

Violence and aggression (Ch. 13) – includes verbal and physical abuse towards an individual.

Virtue ethics (Ch. 7) – a theory in which the focus is upon promotion of intellectual and moral qualities that may enable individuals and communities to flourish.

Vital force (Ch. 10) – in early biological theory, a hypothetical force independent of physical and chemical forces regarded as being the causative factor of the evolution and development of living organisms.

Vital signs (Ch. 14) – indicators of body function such as blood pressure, temperature, pulse and respirations.

Reference

World Health Organization (WHO) 2004 Palliative care. Online: www.who.int/cancer/palliative/en Available July 2006

Index